Compendium

of

Tick-Borne Disease

A Thousand Pearls

Compendium
of
Tick-Borne Disease

A Thousand Pearls

K. Spreen, DO

Pocopson, Pennsylvania
2013

Compendium of Tick-Borne Disease: A Thousand Pearls

The Lyme Disease Association, Inc. provided funding and support for this project. A portion of the profits from sales of this text will go to support Lyme advocacy programs.

Published by
Pocopson Publishing, LLC
P. O. Box 412
Pocopson, PA 19366-0412

ISBN-13: 978-0-9893806-0-7
ISBN-10: 0-9893806-0-2
Library of Congress Control Number: 2013908121

10 9 8 7 6 5 4 3 2 1

Orders can be placed at www.tickpearls.com
Books are available at a discount when purchased in quantities of 10 or more.

Printed in the United States of America

Dedication

Chris

All the patients and caregivers who have suffered from tick-borne illnesses without the understanding of their health care providers

For all those health care providers with the courage to listen and think

Acknowledgements

James Zanoni	*Larry Linford*
Albert and Joan Roose	*Anita Swayne*
Lyme Disease Association, Inc.	*Joseph Schmuckler, PhD*
Pat Smith	*Janet Shepherd*
Lymedisease.org (formerly CALDA)	*Lyme Disease Association of Southeastern PA, Inc.*
Lorraine Johnson, JD MBA	*Connie Patterson*
Jeanette Page	*Phyllis Mervine*
Doug Fearn	*Time for Lyme*

Contributors

Christopher Spreen	*Doug Fearn*
Elaina Karayannis	*Russ Sprague*
Hannon C. Fearn	*Ron Hamlen, PhD*
Emily Zimovan	*Harvey Kliman, PhD*
Keith Ryan, PhD	*Christa Vanderbilt, PhD*

Note: CALDA is referenced in the text for historical purposes. The current name is Lymedisease.org. Both LDA and LDASEPA are incorporated and Inc. is implied with every reference.

Table of Contents

Foreword

This textbook is a primer for those wanting to become better versed in the field of tick-borne disease. The target audience is the pool of health care providers who want to learn more about recognizing and managing TBDs. For the many caregivers and patients who have already educated themselves regarding these diseases, this text should provide them with additional information and strategies. This book is less rigid and more accessible than the average medical text so it can be used and understood by a variety of readers. Every effort is made to credit all original sources, but the book is built around the knowledge and practice of a number of practitioners and the reading of thousands of articles and observing what works in this complex patient population. Dr. Spreen functions as the coordinating author and narrator.

Disclaimer

The world of tick-borne disease is complex, convoluted, and controversial. This book should assist physicians and other health care providers in clinical decision-making by describing a range of generally acceptable approaches for the diagnosis and treatment of these conditions. The intention is not to replace sound clinical judgment in the delivery of health care. Recommendations for evaluation and treatment change rapidly and opinions can be controversial; therefore, physicians and other providers are encouraged to inform their patients of the various treatment options available. Each decision should be made on a case-by-case basis in the best interest of the patient. Since there is no single correct way to treat any condition, the ultimate judgment regarding a particular case must be made by the physician and the patient in light of the specific circumstances presented. The checklists and sample forms are not designed to be all-inclusive and are only as current as publishing deadlines would allow. All information provided about drug selection, doses, and lab testing represent only alternative approaches to consider. Compiled from hundreds of sources, the suggestions may or may not be pertinent to a specific case. This material is not intended to provide medical advice to patients, who should consult with their physicians for diagnosis and treatment. While this book outlines the methods and philosophies used by recognized experts in tick-borne disease, it also provides options for health care workers and educated patients and caregivers. The goal is to explore various diagnostic and treatment approaches that may help many, but not all, patients.

Caveat from K. Spreen

Although I cite nearly 700 sources, I gathered, sorted, and interpreted this material myself and any conclusions drawn are mine. My intention was to review and filter the vast amount of often confusing and contradictory material and condense it into usable form. I wanted the readers to be aware of their options and have practical guidance available when needed. With that being said, it is possible that I could have misinterpreted, miscalculated, or transposed data.

When reducing large volumes of material into a short summary paragraph, such as when I describe MRI technology or the features of petit mal seizures, accuracy might have been sacrificed to brevity. Sometimes in order to simplify ideas, the logic flow was disturbed. The goal was to present enough of a basic foundation about each topic to help readers make the best decisions possible in each situation they might be facing.

Any references to the opinions of published authors are my interpretation of their work and I do not presume to speak for them. In the cases of Jerome Groopman and many of the other fine authors that I cite, I appreciated their ideas and wanted to expose readers to their thoughts. I give them full credit for their theories and take the blame for any misrepresentation. Because I mention these writers, does not mean they agree with me. Because I mention them, does not mean I agree with them on everything either. Again, selecting only part of their work may not have captured their full intent and I apologize for any distortion or misdirection. My goal was to share the concepts that might pertain to patients and health care providers dealing with tick-borne disease.

Sections such as the history of the controversy around Lyme disease have hundreds of published articles, many in contradistinction, one with the other. Even the precise chronology of some of the events was difficult to corroborate. I had to pare down volumes in order to provide what I believe is a bare-bones outline of an important part of the foundation knowledge around illnesses carried by ticks. Every concept presented in the controversy section can be supported in the published literature. Of course, the exact opposite theory can be found with just as many supporters and enthusiastic rhetoric. I am trying to convey concepts more than precise detail.

With regard to treatment regimens and drug doses, I never want to dictate how to practice medicine. I want to introduce providers and patients to options from which they might make the best decisions, targeted toward a particular individual at a specific time. For Lyme, dozens of alternative regimens were presented in the literature. Some authors swore by a single approach, while just as many detractors proclaimed that you could permanently harm the patient if you even considered that regimen. I checked and double-checked. The treatment strategies and drug doses are gathered from a variety of practitioners who found success from a particular way of doing things. That doesn't mean one philosophy will work for the next patient or for anyone else, ever. These ideas are options to consider when deciding how to tackle a particular case. Remember the "official" doses in the label, with the exception of Ceftin, are not indicated for most tick-borne diseases. In each case, review the package insert to get yourself in the ballpark and then make the best decisions for the person you have in front of you. The information presented with regard to treatment regimens, doses, and durations are based on the experience of many tick-borne disease specialists, the literature, lectures, and personal communications. Do what makes sense for this patient, in this case, at this time. Adjust as needed.

My goal is to provide information and options to patients, providers, and caretakers. Use this knowledge judiciously, in the best interest of those who are suffering.

Permissions, Copyrights, Trademarks, and Brands

The following brand names appear in this text and are all assumed to be either a trademark ™ or registered trademark ®: 7Up, Abilify, Accutane, Actigall, Advil, Aleve, Alka-Seltzer, Alli, Ambien, Amoxil, Antabuse, Aquaphor, Aralen, Artemisinin, Atarax, Ativan, Augmentin, Bactrim, Band-Aid, Benadryl, Benefiber, Beneful, Benemid, Biaxin, Bicillin, BuSpar, Catapres, Ceclor, Cedax, Ceftin, Cialis, Cipro, Citrucel, Claforan, Cleocin, Clorox, Coartem, Coca-Cola, Coke, Colace, Compazine, Correctol, Crisco, Culturelle, Dalmane, Damminix, Diflucan, Dilantin, Doryx, Dulcolax, EES, EMLA, E-Mycin, EpiPen, ERYC, Ex-Lax, Flagyl, Florastor, Floxin, Gore-Tex, Halcion, Helioplex, Imodium, Indocin, Insect Shield, Ivory Soap, Jello, Karo syrup, Ketamine, Ketek, Kleenex, Klonopin, Lariam, Laura Ashley, Levaquin, Lexapro, Lidocaine, Lomotil, Lorabid, Luvox, Lysol, Maalox, Macrobid, Malarone, Medrol, Mefaquin, Megace, Mepron, Mercedes, Metamucil, Minipress, Minocin, Motrin, Mr. Bubble, Mycelex, Mycobutin, Mycostatin, Mylanta, Namenda, Naprosyn, Neti Pot, Neurontin, Nizoral, NoDoz, Nuprin, Omnicef, Pediazole, Pepto-Bismol, Percocet, Phenergan, Plaquenil, Pledge, Pomodoro method, Primaquine, Primaxin, Provigil, Puffs, Q-tips, Qualaquin, Questran, Relenza, Remeron, Rifabutin, Rifadin, Rifampicin, Rifampin, Rife, Rocephin, Rogaine, Rohypnol, Rynoskin, Sam-e, Scotch Tape, Senokot, Septra, Serax, Seroquel, Sevin, Shake n Bake, Skin So Soft, Sonata, Speedo, Sumycin, Suprax, Tamiflu, Theralac, Tigan, Tindamax, Trazadone, Tygacil, Tylenol, UltraFlora, Ultrathon, Valium, Vancocin, Vaseline, Viagra, Vibramycin, Vicks VapoRub, Vicodin, Vistaril, Wellbutrin, Wii, Xanax, Xenical, Zithromax, Zofran, Zoloft, Zovirax, Z-Pak

The following titles or phrases are assumed to be copyrighted: Guns, Germs and Steel, Monthly Prescribing Reference, The Price is Right, Dallas Cowboys, The Jerry Springer Show, various Kardashian shows, Washington Manual, Harriet Lane Handbook, Merck Manual, How Doctors Think, Cure Unknown, AMA Code of Medical Ethics, War and Peace, The Fever, Bull's Eye, Harry Potter, The Three Stooges, Andy Griffith, I Love Lucy, The Cosby Show, The ABCs of Lyme Disease, Top Ten Tips to Prevent Chronic Lyme Disease, Catch 22, Alice in Wonderland, Flesh and Blood, The End of Overeating, O Magazine, Dr. Oz, Recipes for Repair, The Lyme Disease Solution, Saddle Up, Danny Boy, Eat, Pray, Love, Groundhog Day, Shrek, Toy Story, Caddyshack, Looney Tunes, Sponge Bob, To Kill a Mockingbird, The Catcher in the Rye, World Wrestling Federation, WWF, Extreme Sports, Dudley Do-Right, Betty Crocker, Barney, Popeye, Snidely Whiplash, Nell, Sports Illustrated, Cliffs Notes, Patch Adams, Oprah, Criminal Minds, The Help, Walmart, Jazzercise, Facebook, Beatles, 12-Step Program, Zumba, Pilates, Hawaii, Klingon, MapQuest

Permission to use images was received from Doug Fearn, Ron Hamlin, Harvey Kliman, Keith Ryan, and Christopher Spreen. All other images are in the public domain.

If I missed listing anything referred to in the text, I apologize, but I must say, in that case, someone is reading this book way too carefully.

Guidance on Using this Text

Do not expect a traditional textbook. My goal was to allow easy access to multiple topics important to the understanding of tick-borne illnesses. Much of the information in the text will be summarized in charts on the inside book covers. These charts include concise synopses on co-infections and treatment options. This does not mean you should not read the text. You will miss many clever jokes if you do not digest each page word-for-word. Understanding the science that underscores the material in the cover charts will enable you to make better decisions. I want you to be able to locate what you need quickly and, then later, take your time in perusing the foundation material in the body of the text. My feelings will not be hurt if you do not read every word.

My name is Kathy Spreen and I am a physician, Lyme patient, and caregiver for my family members with TBIs. In the pharmaceutical industry, I was responsible for writing many peer-reviewed journal articles for specialists in a number of therapeutic areas. Most of the credited authors never wrote a word and many barely reviewed the paper when it was done. I can attest that I wrote every word in this book based on the ideas of top experts in the world of TBD. Much of the work on sample forms, interpretation of drug labels, causality assessment, and visit content is entirely based on my own experience in visiting hundreds of specialists' offices while managing clinical research and in witnessing the treatment (and mistreatment) of many TBI patients over the years. Panels of technical experts and professional editors have spent eons reviewing every sentence, page-by-page.

The beauty of being the author is that I am able to decide the flavor of the work. I write in the first person because the syntax became too weird to handle any other way. My goal is to make you feel as though I am speaking directly to you rather than you enduring yet another chapter in a textbook. Still, there are hundreds of pages of informational text and you should find what is pertinent to you or your patient and leave the rest. You might need that information another day. I try to provide insight on topics that I wish were available to me when I was struggling with TBD.

The material compiled in this text was gleaned from the top names in the field of TBIs. These specialists contributed the foundation knowledge in this therapeutic area and are responsible for a number of the innovations in the field. I gathered the information either from their written work, clinical observations, lectures, or personal discussions and put it all together in one place. I sorted through dozens of conflicting opinions and questionable "facts." Then I outlined the alternatives and explored the options and presented the ideas in such a way as to help in medical decision-making. My goal was always to advocate for TBI patients.

You will find certain ideas repeated, sometimes more than once. That is intentional. One goal of the book is to be an easy access reference. A health care provider might just want to look up first-line treatment for babesiosis. If it is only found in one location, the quest for information may take more time than she has available. So, several chapters may contain repeats of the same concepts. I would rather you read it twice than miss something important, or waste a lot of time looking.

Here are some conventions I have followed: 1) When discussing genus and species of pathogens, the genus is capitalized and the species is in lower case and italicized (Borrelia *burgdorferi*). After the first mention, the genus is abbreviated (B. *burgdorferi*). 2) The brand name of drugs is capitalized (Advil) and the generic name appears in lower case (ibuprofen). 3) Abbreviations/acronyms are generally shown in parentheses after the first mention of a term and the abbreviation/acronym is usually used thereafter. The context should help you with the meaning. Sometimes in the heat of the prose, an acronym will appear pages from its initial introduction. Sometimes, I just spring them on you. Then, the acronym list in the front of the book will come in handy.

Not all chapters are laid out in the same fashion because many do not lend themselves to identical formatting. Hopefully, the *Glossary, Index*, and *Table of Contents* (TOC) will allow quick reference when the patient is sitting in front of you. Several chapters (*Gentle Immunology* and *Understanding Medicines* come to mind) have much more detailed information than you might want or need. Nonetheless, other readers have requested additional background. I found that it was impossible to refer to some of the more complex material in later chapters without at least providing an overview of the basic scientific concepts as they pertain to TBDs. For example, you will not know when to order HLA-DR2 and DR4 testing unless you have at least a vague notion of the immunologic concept of HLA; nor would you be able to interpret the test results. Each subdivision of the *Physical Examination* chapters also includes pertinent differential diagnoses related to that body system.

I am hopelessly inconsistent in the ways that I show emphasis throughout the text. I am more concerned about getting my point across than being grammatically correct. Usually I use **bold** for headings, titles, and newly introduced terms that you are also likely to find in the *Glossary*. Clinical *PEARLS* appear throughout the book and are italicized. I use ALL CAPS, "quotes," *italics*, and <u>underlines</u> for emphasis, sometimes doing so for an entire sentence or paragraph. I wish I could say there is a reasonable pattern, but there is not. I used what my mood indicated. If I use all these modalities at once, I'm probably really "***MAD****!*"

The foundation material is based on my observations of multiple TBI practitioners. I witnessed outstanding medical practice as well as abysmal care being doled out as though one was bestowing a favor. With that being said, much supportive information was gleaned from thousands of published articles and any number of other sources including books, lectures, personal communications, legal proceedings, and websites. A number of sources that were repetitive or contradictory or obviously scientifically shaky did not make it into the *Bibliography*. The resulting chapters are compilations from many sources. Since information around TBIs is so controversial and ever-changing, my goal was to capture the basic philosophy of patient care used by the experts. If I had my way, I would have mentioned the top most valuable supportive sources and not have troubled you with the 100s that did make the *Bibliography*. The editors would not allow that indulgence.

My goal was to enable you to easily find additional reference material when needed in order to better understand diagnoses, lab testing, drug safety, and how to best use available information when selecting medications. Be patient as the text builds the vast foundation needed to care for these very sick people. A mini-TOC appears prior to those chapters where it might be useful.

I change audiences frequently, most often talking to health care providers (HCPs), but many times I speak directly to caregivers and patients. As in my personal experience, sometimes one person can fit all these roles at the same time or sequentially. On other occasions, I will be addressing school nurses, guideline authors, grandparents, government agencies, or any number of other potential readers. I hope the context makes the intended audience clear. Unless I am being snide or critical, assume that I am talking directly to you. For those times when the target is murky, keep reading. Perhaps clarity will manifest through luck, if not by writing skill.

Hyphens were the bane of my existence and I probably wasted months reconciling hyphens. Please know that of all the rules in life, those pertaining to hyphens are probably the most fluid. Many terms appear in the literature with hyphens as often as they do without (evidence-based, postoperative, on-going, antineuronal, co-infection, P450 to name a few). One helpful grammar book advised: "If you can use the articles "the" or "a" in front of the words "follow up" then there is a hyphen." This rule allows you to follow up on a follow-up plan. How did I live all these years without knowing that? In many cases I had to simply decide and move on. Although I tried to be internally consistent, I cannot guarantee that an inappropriate hyphen or two did not slip by. As soon as I finish this book I plan to ban hyphens from my life for eternity. I will live a hyphen-free existence.

Sometimes I use grammar that I know is incorrect because to use the proper form sounds too pretentious. No one knows that better than me. Although several contributors provided excellent color images to be used in this text, I elected to use black and white only in order to keep the cost of the text as reasonable as possible.

PEARLS are distributed throughout the book. For the most part, these comments are based on insight I gained from listening to the experts. Sometimes, I picked up a tidbit from other sources or I learned something myself from the school of hard knocks. For whatever reason, I thought the *PEARL* might be useful to you. Occasionally a *PEARL* is a snippet of information that I wanted to share that didn't fit well with the logic flow of the text but I couldn't bear to leave out.

You will find a quotation at the beginning of each chapter, just under the title. Sometimes the quotes relate to the subsequent material and sometimes they are simply stuff and nonsense. Rummaging through my collection of clever quotations helped maintain my sanity through the four year writing process. Please recognize that I used the most accurate source available when attributing these sayings to a particular individual. That does not mean I got it right. There is as much controversy about who said what as there is about Lyme disease. There are about a hundred versions of each of the most famous quotes by Lincoln and Churchill and Twain. In many cases these individuals would not recognize the sayings ascribed to them.

Finally, I refer to a local ER nurse with the pseudonym Lilith. She represents all I find unprofessional and disrespectful in medicine. I give background on Lilith in the *Introduction*, but if you choose not to read the *Introduction* or you forget the many reasons for my disdain, the *Glossary* gives the rationale for this name selection. A footnote appears on each page where Lilith is mentioned so that you can refer to the *Glossary* every time you want to understand how inspirational bad medical care can be.

K. Spreen, DO MS MPH

P.S. Remember, FINAL THOUGHTS, found just after Chapter 34, summarizes the entire book in one page.

Acronym and Abbreviation List

@	About, Around, At
α	Alpha
Ab	Antibody
Ab/Ag	Antibody/Antigen Complex
ABGs	Arterial Blood Gases
ACE	Angiotension-1-Converting Enzyme
Abn	Abnormal
ABS	Antigen-Binding Sites
ADA	American Dietetic Association
ADA	Americans with Disabilities Act
ADD	Attention Deficit Disorder
ADE	Adverse Drug Event
ADHD	Attention Deficit Hyperactivity Disorder
ADL	Activities of Daily Living
ADR	Adverse Drug Reaction
AE	Adverse Event
AG	Attorney General
Ag	Antigen
Ag/Ab	Antigen/Antibody Complex
AIDS	Acquired Immunodeficiency Syndrome
AKA	Also Known As
Al	Aluminum
ALP	Alkaline Phosphatase, AP
ALS	Amyotrophic Lateral Sclerosis
ALT	Alanine Transaminase
AMA	American Medical Association
ANA	Antinuclear Antibody
ANS	Autonomic Nervous System
ANSI	American National Standards Institute
AODL	Activities of Daily Living
AOL	Activities of Living
AOM	Acute Otitis Media
AP	Alkaline Phosphatase, ALP
AP	Anterior-Posterior
APA	American Psychiatric Association
APC	Antigen-Presenting Cell
API	Active Pharmaceutical Ingredient
AR	Adverse Reaction
Ar	Arsenic
ARF	Acute Renal Failure
ARDS	Adult Respiratory Distress Syndrome
AS	Ankylosing Spondylitis
ASAP	As Soon As Possible
ASD	Autism Spectrum Disorder
ASD	Atrial Septal Defect
AST	Aspartate Transaminase
ATP	Adenosine Triphosphate
AV	Atrioventricular
β	Beta

Bb	Borrelia *burgdorferi*
BBB	Blood Brain Barrier
BBB	Bundle Branch Block
BCE	Before the Common Era
BCPs	Birth Control Pills
BG	Basal Ganglion
BID	Twice a Day, 2 x/day, Latin: bis in die, bid
BLO	Bartonella-like Organisms
BM	Bowel Movement
BMR	Basal Metabolic Rate
BP	Blood Pressure
BPA	Bisphenol A
BPM	Beats per Minute
BR	Bilirubin
BS	Bowel Sound
BS	Breath Sound
BUN	Blood Urea Nitrogen
C	Centigrade
C	Complement
Ca	Calcium
CALDA	California Lyme Disease Association (now Lymedisease.org)
CAM	Complimentary & Alternative Medicine
CAP	College of American Pathologists
CAT scan	CT Scan or Computed Axial Tomography
CBC	Complete Blood Count
CBT	Cognitive Behavioral Therapy
cc	Cubic Centimeter
Cd	Cadmium
CD	Cluster of Differentiation (CD4, CD8, CD57)
C3d	Fragment of Complement C3
CDC	Centers for Disease Control
CDC-P	Centers for Disease Control & Prevention
CDD	Childhood Disintegrative Disorder
C. *diff*	Clostridium *difficile*
CE	Common Era
CEO	Chief Executive Officer
CFIDS	Chronic Fatigue and Immune Dysfunction Syndrome
CFS	Chronic Fatigue Syndrome
CHF	Congestive Heart Failure
CHO	Carbohydrate
CI	Contraindicated or Contraindication
CIDP	Chronic Inflammatory Demyelinating Polyneuropathy
Circ	Circulation
CMI	Cell-Mediated Immunity
CMR	Cell-Mediated Response
CMV	Cytomegalovirus

CN	Cranial Nerve		DVT	Deep Vein Thrombosis
CNS	Central Nervous System		DX	Diagnosis
COI	Conflict of Interest		EAP	Employee Assistance Program
COPD	Chronic Obstructive Pulmonary Disease		EBM	Evidence-Based Medicine
COX	Cyclooxygenase		EBV	Epstein-Barr Virus
CPAP	Continuous Positive Airway Pressure		E. *coli*	Escherichia *coli*
CPK	Creatinine Phosphokinase		ECP	Eosinophil Cationic Protein
CR	Continuous Release		ECP	Extracorporeal Photopheresis
CREST	Cutaneous Scleroderma		ED	Emergency Department
CRO	Clinical Research Organization		EEG	Electroencephalogram
CRP	C-Reactive Protein		ELISA	Enzyme-linked Immunosorbent Assay
C&S	Culture and Sensitivity		EFA	Essential Fatty Acid
CSD	Cat Scratch Disease		E.g.	For Example, e.g.
CSF	Cat Scratch Fever		EKG	Electrocardiogram, ECG
CSF	Cerebral Spinal Fluid		EM	Erythema Migrans
CSs	Cephalosporins		EMF	Electromagnetic Fields
CT	Computerized Tomography		EMG	Electromyography
CT	Connecticut		EMLA	Topical Anesthetic
Ct	Connective Tissue		EOM	Extraocular Eye Motions or Muscles
CTF	Colorado Tick Fever		Epi	Epinephrine
CVA	Cerebrovascular Accident		EQ	Emotional Quotient
CVA	Costovertebral Angle		ER	Emergency Room
CVD	Cardiovascular Disease		ER	Extended Release
CVS	Cardiovascular System		ESR	Erythrocyte Sedimentation Rate
CXR	Chest X-ray		et al	And others
CYP	Cytochrome P450 metabolic enzymes in liver		etc.	Et cetera, etcetera, and so forth, and other things
D	Day, d			
2-D	Two-Dimensional		F	Fahrenheit
3-D	Three-Dimensional		FA	Fatty Acid
d/c	Discontinued		FB	Foreign Body
DC	Doctor of Chiropractic		FDA	Food and Drug Administration
DD	Differential Diagnosis		Fe	Iron
DDMAC	Division of Drug Marketing, Advertising and Communications, now called OPDP		FH	Forehead
			FISH	Fluorescent In-Situ Hybridization
DES	Diethylstilbestrol		FB	Foreign Body
DHHS	Department of Health and Human Services		FM	Fine Motor
DIC	Disseminated Intravascular Coagulation		FUO	Fever of Unknown Origin
DIP	Distal Interphalangeal Joint		γ	Gamma
DJD	Degenerative Joint Disease		GABA	γ-Aminobutyric Acid
DM	Diabetes Mellitus		GAD	Generalized Anxiety Disorder
DNA	Deoxyribonucleic Acid		GB	Gallbladder
DO	Doctor of Osteopathy		GBS	Guillain-Barre Syndrome
DOB	Date of Birth		GC	Gonorrhea
DOC	Drug of Choice		GCP	Good Clinical Practices
DOC	Department of Corrections		GERD	Gastroesophageal Reflux Disease
DOE	Dyspnea on Exertion		GFR	Glomerular Filtration Rate
Doxy	Doxycycline		GG	γ-Globulin or IgG
DR	Delayed Release		GGT	Gamma Glutamyl Transpeptidase
DS	Double Strength		GHB	Depressant, Drug of Abuse
DSM	Diagnostic and Statistical Manual		GI	Gastrointestinal
DTRs	Deep Tendon Reflexes		GI	Glycemic Index

GM	Gross Motor	I	Iodine
GMP	Good Manufacturing Practices	IBD	Inflammatory Bowel Disease
GPA	Grade Point Average	IBS	Irritable Bowel Syndrome
G6PD	Glucose-6-Phosphate Dehydrogenase Deficiency	IC	Interstitial Cystitis
		ICD	International Classification of Disease
GSH	Glutathione	ICP	Intracranial Pressure
Gtt(s)	Drop(s)	ICU	Intensive Care Unit
GU	Genitourinary	ID	Infectious Disease
GvHD	Graft versus Host Disease	IDEA	Individuals with Disabilities Education Act
GYN	Gynecological, Gynecologist	IDSA	Infectious Diseases Society of America
H	Hour, hr, h, q 4 h is every 4 hours	i.e.	That is
HA	Headache	IEP	Individualized Education Program
HA	Human Anaplasmosis	IFA	Immunofluorescence Assay
HAV	Hepatitis A Virus	IFN	Interferon
Hb	Hemoglobin	Ig	Immunoglobulin (antibody)
HBO	Hyperbaric Oxygen	IgA	Immunoglobulin class A (Antibody class A)
HBOT	Hyperbaric Oxygen Therapy	IgD	Immunoglobulin class D (Antibody class D)
HBP	High Blood Pressure	IgE	Immunoglobulin class E (Antibody class E)
HBV	Hepatitis B Virus	IgG	Immunoglobulin class G (Antibody class G)
HCG	Human Chorionic Gonadotropin, hCG, Pregnancy Test	IgM	Immunoglobulin class M (Antibody class M)
		IL	Interleukin
HCP	Health Care Provider	ILADS	International Lyme & Associated Diseases Society
Hct	Hematocrit		
HCV	Hepatitis C Virus	IM	Intramuscular
HD	Hyperactivity Disorder	IMF	International Monetary Fund
HEE	Human *ewingii* Ehrlichiosis	IMIG	Intramuscular IgG
HEENT	Head, Eyes, Ears, Nose, Throat	INR	International Normalized Ratio
Herx	Herxheimer Reaction	*in utero*	Happening while in the uterus
Hg	Mercury	*in vitro*	Occurring in a non-living system
HGA	Human Granulocytic Anaplasmosis	*in vivo*	Occurring in a living system
HGE	Human Granulocytic Ehrlichiosis	IOM	Institute of Medicine
H&H	Hemoglobin & Hematocrit	I&P	Incidence and Prevalence
HHV	Human Herpes Virus	IP	Interphalangeal Joint
HIPAA	Health Insurance Portability Accountability Act	IQ	Intelligence Quotient
		IU	International Unit
HIR	Humoral Immune Response	IVF	*In Vitro* Fertilization
HIV	Human Immunodeficiency Virus	IV	Intravenous
HLA	Human Leukocytic Antigen	IVIG	Intravenous IgG, IV IgG
HME	Human Monocytic Ehrlichiosis	JAMA	Journal of the American Medical Association
H&P	History and Physical	JD	Juris Doctor
HPA	Hypothalamic-Pituitary-Adrenal Axis	JIA	Juvenile Inflammatory Arthritis
HPV	Human Papilloma Virus	JRA	Juvenile Rheumatoid Arthritis
HR	Heart Rate	K	Potassium
HR	Hour, hr, h, q 4 hr is every 4 hours	kg	Kilogram
HS	At bedtime, hs	KOL	Key Opinion Leader
HSV	Herpes Simplex Virus	KVO	Keep Vein Open
Ht	Height	L	Left
HTN	Hypertension	LBP	Low Back Pain
HX	History	lbs	Pounds
Hyper	Excess, more	LD	Lyme Disease
Hypo	Less, under, below, beneath	LDA	Lyme Disease Association

LDASEPA	Lyme Disease Association of Southeastern PA	NIAID	National Institute of Allergy and Infectious Diseases
LDH	Lactate Dehydrogenase	NIH	National Institutes of Health
LDL	Low-density Lipoprotein	NJ	New Jersey
LDN	Low Dose Naltrexone	NK	Natural Killer Cell
LE	Lower Extremity	NO	Nitric Oxide
LE	Lyme Encephalopathy	NOS	Not Otherwise Specified
LFT	Liver Function Test	NP	Nurse Practitioner
LI	Large Intestine	NP	Neuropsychiatric
LLN	Lower Limit of Normal	NS	Nervous System
LLQ	Left Lower Quadrant	NSAIDs	Nonsteroidal Anti-inflammatory Drugs
LOC	Level of Consciousness	NSF	National Sleep Foundation
LOC	Loss of Consciousness	NSR	Normal Sinus Rhythm
LP	Lumbar Puncture	NS	Nervous System
LRI	Lower Respiratory Infection	NSS	Normal Saline Solution
LMN	Lower Motor Neuron	NTK	Natural T Killer Cell
LUQ	Left Upper Quadrant	NY	New York
Lytes	Electrolytes	O_3	Ozone
MAOI	Monoamine Oxidase Inhibitor	OA	Osteoarthritis
Max	Maximum	OB	Obstetrician
MBA	Master of Business Administration	OCD	Obsessive-Compulsive Disorder
MCP	Metacarpophalangeal Joint	OCPs	Oral Contraceptive Pills
MD	Medical Doctor	ODD	Oppositional Defiant Disorder
Meds	Medicines	O/E	Observed versus Expected
METS	Metabolic Equivalent of Tasks	OM	Otitis Media
mg	Milligram	OPDP	Office of Prescription Drug Promotion, formerly DDMAC
Mg	Magnesium		
MG	Myasthenia Gravis	OS	Osgood-Schlatter Disease, OSD
MHC	Major Histocompatibility Complex Molecule	OSP	Outer Surface Protein, Osp
MI	Myocardial Infarction	OT	Occupational Therapy
ml	Milliliter	OTC	Over-the-counter
M&M	Morbidity and Mortality	P	Phosphorus
MOA	Mechanism of Action	PA	Physician's Assistant
MOM	Milk of Magnesia	PA	Pennsylvania
MPH	Master of Public Health	PAND	Pediatric Acute-Onset Neuropsychiatric Disorder
Mph	Miles per Hour		
MPR	Monthly Prescribing Reference	PANDAS	Pediatric Autoimmune Neuropsychiatric Disorders Assoc w/ Streptococcal Infection
MRE	Meal Ready to Eat		
MRI	Magnetic Resonance Imaging		
MRSA	Methicillin-Resistant Staphylococcus *aureus*	PANS	Pediatric Acute-Onset Neuropsychiatric Syndrome
MS	Master of Science		
MS	Multiple Sclerosis	PAS	Pain Amplification Syndrome
ms	Millisecond	PAT	Paroxysmal Atrial Tachycardia
MSDS	Material Safety Data Sheet	Pb	Lead
MTP	Metatarsophalangeal Joint	PCN	Penicillin
MVP	Mitral Valve Prolapse	PCP	Primary Care Physician
NA	North America	PCP	Pneumocystis *carinii* Pneumonia
NDA	New Drug Application	PCR	Polymerase Chain Reaction
NE	Norepinephrine	PD	Pharmacodynamics
NE	Not Examined or Evaluated	PDD	Pervasive Developmental Disorder
NEJM	New England Journal of Medicine	PDR	Physician's Desk Reference
NGC	National Guideline Clearinghouse	PE	Physical Examination

Per	/, 1 mg/kg/day is one milligram per kilogram per day
PERLA	Pupils Equally Reactive to Light and Accommodation
PET	Positron Emission Tomography Scan
PFT	Pulmonary Function Test
pH	Acid-Base Scale
PhD	Doctor of Philosophy
PI	Package Insert
PICC	Peripherally Inserted Central Catheter, a Central Line
PID	Pelvic Inflammatory Disease
PIP	Proximal Interphalangeal
PK	Pharmacokinetics
PMDD	Premenstrual Dysphoric Disorder
PMN	Polymorphonuclear Leukocytes
PMR	Progressive Muscle Relaxation
PMS	Premenstrual Syndrome
PND	Post Nasal Drip
PNS	Peripheral Nervous System
PPI	Proton Pump Inhibitor
PPV	Positive Predictive Value
Pre	Before or prior to
Prep	Preparation
PO	Per os, Taken by Mouth, po
Post	After
POW	Powassan Viral Encephalitis
PPI	Proton Pump Inhibitor
PPV	Positive Predictive Value
PSA	Prostate Specific Antigen
PSNS	Parasympathetic Nervous System
PT	Physical Therapy
PT	Prothrombin Time
Pts	Patients
PTSD	Post-Traumatic Stress Disorder
PTT	Partial Thromboplastin Time
PVG	Pharmacovigilance, PV
PX	Prognosis
Q	Every, q, q 4 h is every 4 hours
q	Every
QD	Once a day, Latin: quaque die, qd
QID	Four times a day, Latin: quarter in die, 4 x/day, qid
QOL	Quality of Life
QT	EKG Interval between Q and T
QTc	Corrected Interval between Q and T
R	Right
R/O	Rule out, r/o
RA	Rheumatoid Arthritis
RBC	Red Blood Cell, rbc
REMS	Risk Evaluation and Mitigation Strategy
Reps	Representatives or Repetitions
RF	Rheumatic Fever
RF	Rheumatoid Factor
RIA	Radioimmunoassay
RLQ	Right Lower Quadrant
RMSF	Rocky Mountain Spotted Fever
RNA	Ribonucleic Acid
ROM	Range of Motion
ROS	Review of Systems
RR	Interval between R waves on EKG
RR	Respiratory Rate
RSV	Respiratory Syncytial Virus
RTC	Return to Clinic
RUQ	Right Upper Quadrant, URQ
Rx	Prescription
S1, S2	Normal Heart Sounds
SBS	Sick Building Syndrome
SC	Subcutaneous, Under the Skin, sub-q, sq
SDD	Specific Developmental Disorder
SDD	Sensory Deficit Disorder
Se	Selenium
SG	Streptococcal Glomerulonephritis
S/he	She or he
SI	Sacroiliac
SI	Small Intestine
SID	Sensory Integration Disorder or Deficit
SJS	Stevens-Johnson Syndrome
SL	Sublingual, Under the Tongue
SLE	Systemic Lupus Erythematosus
SNRI	Serotonin-Norepinephrine Reuptake Inhibitor
SNS	Sympathetic Nervous System
SOB	Shortness of Breath
SOC	Standard of Care
SOP	Standard Operating Procedure
S/P	Status post, after
SPECT	Single-Photon Emission Computed Tomography Scan
SPF	Sun Protection Factor
SQ	Subcutaneous, under the skin, sub-q, SC
SSN	Social Security Number
SSRI	Selective Serotonin Reuptake Inhibitor
Staph	Staphylococcus genus of bacteria
STARI	Southern Tick-Associated Rash Illness
Stat	Immediately, Highest Priority, Latin for Statim, Urgent
STDs	Sexually Transmitted Diseases
Strep	Streptococcus genus of bacteria
Sub-Q	Subcutaneous, under the skin, sub-q, sq, SC
Sxs	Either Signs or Symptoms when it doesn't matter which
TA	Teaching Assistant

Tab	Tablet	UA	Urinalysis
T1H	T Helper Cell Type 1, TH1	UC	Ulcerative Colitis
T2H	T Helper Cell Type 2, TH2	UE	Upper Extremity
TB	Tuberculosis	UGI	Upper Gastrointestinal Tract
TBD	Tick-borne Disease	ULN	Upper Limit of Normal
TBI	Tick-borne Illness	UMN	Upper Motor Neuron
TBRF	Tick-borne Relapsing Fever	URI	Upper Respiratory Infection
TCM	Traditional Chinese Medicine	URQ	Upper Right Quadrant, RUQ
TCN	Tetracycline	US	Ultrasound
Temp	Temperature	USDA	US Department of Agriculture
TEN	Toxic Epidermal Necrolysis	UTI	Urinary Tract Infection
TENS	Transcutaneous Electric Nerve Stimulation	VA	Veteran's Administration
TF	Transfer Factor	VA	Visual Acuity
TH	Helper T Cells (Egs: T1H, T2H or TH1, TH2)	VEGF	Vascular Endothelial Growth Factor
TH1	T Helper Cell Type 1, T1H	V/Q	Ventilation/Perfusion Scan
TH2	T Helper Cell Type 2, T2H	WB	Western Blot
TIA	Transient Ischemic Attack	WB	Willy Burgdorfer
TID	Three times a day, Latin: ter in die, 3 x /day, tid	WBC	White Blood Cell, wbc
TM	Transcendental Meditation	WHO	World Health Organization
TM	Tympanic Membrane, Ear Drum	w/	With
TMJ	Temporomandibular Joint	WNL	Within Normal Limits
TNF	Tumor Necrosis Factor	w/o	Without
TOA	Tetracyclic Oxindole Alkaloids	WSJ	Wall Street Journal
TOC	Table of Contents	Wt	Weight
TOC	Treatment of Choice	w/u	Work-up
TRF	Tick Relapsing Fever	XR	Extended Release
tsp	Teaspoon	y/o	Year(s) old
TX	Treatment	Z-Pak	Branded prepackaged form of azithromycin

Introduction

MY STORY

Kathy Spreen, Author

Although I misdiagnosed my first case of Lyme in 1985 (I thought it was ringworm), the real world of tick-borne illness began for me in 2001. Since my family lives in Chester County, Pennsylvania, where both deer and ticks are ubiquitous, we all had Lyme disease at one time or another. My husband's case manifested with fatigue and shoulder pain and after weeks of complaining and me saying, "You probably have Lyme. Go get checked," he finally did. He responded to 14 days of doxycycline, and we didn't think about Lyme again until I was treated for Lyme twice about a year later. My symptoms included fatigue and pain in the right knee. We never wondered why, if I had been cured the first time, I needed to be treated again. At that point in my medical career, I was one of those doctors who were too busy to listen and think. I believed that two weeks of doxy would take care of any Lyme. I had never heard of co-infections. If I needed re-treatment that was just how things were.

On September 10, 2001, I had just arrived home from a business trip to Brazil. For about three weeks I had felt achy and tired. I had been troubled by sensitivity to odors that made me nauseous. My fellow travelers could detect a natural cedar tree smell, but they were not bothered by the scent. We traveled non-stop within the country, setting up clinical trials, and I believed my fatigue was due to overwork and my aches due to uncomfortable travel conditions. Nevertheless, by the time I arrived home my right knee was so painful that I could barely walk off the plane. Well, the next day was September 11th and the events of that week delayed any thought of seeking medical care. By the time I got my second expert opinion, I needed surgery to clean out the debris in my knee joint, and both orthopedists felt that Lyme *probably* caused my problem. At that point no one, including me, even considered that I might need further treatment for Lyme, since I had already been "cured" twice. Seven years later, I was informed that I would need a knee replacement because of the extensive damage.

In the summer of 2007, I was quickly enlightened about the true scope of tick-borne diseases. My son Chris was 20-years-old and working as an aeronautical engineering intern at Dassault Falcon in Wilmington, Delaware. We had a house full of company from Italy, and we wanted to show them a great time. We were taking them places like Washington, DC, and the Camden Aquarium. One day my son came home from work and showed me a deer tick on his flank and asked, "Does this matter?" I was quite busy with our guests so I said that he should pull out the tick, save it, wash the area with soap and water, and we would watch to see if anything happened. (Keep in mind that I am a physician with two Master's degrees - one in Public Health - and two board certifications - one in Preventive Medicine, who had surgery due to Lyme and who should have been a bit more attentive.) The next day Chris went to work, but he felt tired and had a headache. Within 12 hours he had a 6-inch by 4-inch maroon lesion with a small scab in the center where the captured tick had bitten him.

At this point, we followed all the rules of the medical system. We went to the family doctor who said that the lesion was not round enough to be Lyme (even though he had a bite mark in the middle of a classic EM rash, was symptomatic, and had the actual deer tick in the jar). By then Chris was so sick that the doctor agreed to treat him for Lyme with doxycycline 50 mg twice a day for 28 days. He took the doxy religiously and felt a little better. (By now I was back on the planet and paying attention, but no more knowledgeable than I had been the week before.) On the third day of antibiotic (6 doses), Chris took a turn for the worse and had a fever near 106° with rigors. Again, we called the family doctor who said Chris was now too sick for him to handle and recommended an infectious disease doctor at the nearby hospital. I called the specialist's office and talked to the nurse. By this time, Chris was on the floor lapsing in and out of consciousness. She conferred with the doctor. They agreed that he was too sick to wait for a routine appointment and that we should go to the emergency room where she would see him. On our arrival, the ER was to call the specialist.

By now, I was having trouble rousing Chris. His dad was rushing from work to meet us at the hospital. I got Chris to the ER. At the reception desk we got the old roll of the eyes from the RN. Let's call her Lilith[1]. Lilith said, "Why didn't you just go to the family doctor?" I relayed the story to her and said the specialist told us to bring him to the ER and to call her when he got there and she would see him. With a second eye-roll, Lilith said, "He's already on doxy, what more do you want?" When I said, "Consciousness," she said, "It's not like he's dying or anything."

---

1 See Glossary for name origin

He had to sit shaking for three hours. When we asked for a blanket, we were told that they liked to keep their cold patients cold so they didn't get a fever. (Huh?) We rejoiced when a nurse came to the waiting area and said, "Chris?" We got him back into a room, onto the gurney, and into a gown. The nurse came in and said, "How far did you fall?" He said, "I didn't fall. I'm really sick and I have a fever." She said, "You must have fallen. It says so right here on your chart." I said, "You have the wrong patient." Yes, indeed, she had the wrong patient. Instead of leaving the poor sick kid there, he had to put his clothes back on and go and sit another three hours in the waiting area—in rigors, without a blanket.

To make a long story (filled with incompetence, arrogance, and malpractice) short, he was again told that his skin lesion was not "classic." "You know if he really had Lyme, this would be rounder and not so oval." In the meantime, (Are you listening HIPAA regulators?) I could hear every word being said about the other patients in the vicinity. A 5-year-old boy had been brought in by his frantic parents. He had been diagnosed with Lyme and treated and now was barely conscious and not able to move his neck. The pediatrician thought he might have meningitis and so told the parents to take him to the ER. After the preliminary results of the spinal tap came back, I heard the eye-rolling Lilith[2] say, "He doesn't even have meningitis. They should send him home." They did.

At this point, Chris had been in the ER for nearly 8 hours. I heard every word when the ER doctor finally called the specialist, who said that it was so long since she had told us to go to the ER that now it was too late for her to come in. They should have called her at noon. Chris went home as sick as he came in. But not before we paid our co-pay.

This is where the story takes a turn for the better. While all this was on-going, Chris's father was doggedly trying to find someone who knew tick-borne illnesses so that we could get help. After searching the web, calling everyone we knew who had Lyme, (as I mentioned Southern Chester County is the tick capital of creation so we made a lot of calls), we came across the Lyme Disease Association of Southeastern Pennsylvania (LDASEPA). Doug Fearn pulled all the favors he was ever owed and found a physician to see Chris within 12 hours. He was diagnosed with Babesia and Lyme and treated appropriately. The diagnoses were *confirmed* with lab testing. (The lab tests at the local hospital were negative.) He was treated aggressively for 6 months and is now a graduate student working on his PhD in rocket science at Purdue University.

One could argue that everything might have turned out as well without the long-term aggressive treatment, but I do not ever want another child and her family to go through what we went through. If I, as a physician who supposedly knows "the system," cannot get care for my child, who can? I became an

advocate. Since I had retired the year before these incidents, I was able to study and try to learn all I could. I vowed that I would never again say, "It's only Lyme. Just put him on a little doxy, and he'll be fine in a few days."

I was shocked to learn how much I didn't know. I started to do preceptorships sponsored by Time for Lyme. I was beginning to work on setting up an indigent clinic for tick-borne illnesses, but I didn't think I knew enough at that point. Again, my friends at the Lyme Disease Association of Southeastern Pennsylvania came to the rescue. They said, "You have got to do preceptorships with some of the experts." And……

A BOOK IS BORN

I knew there were problems with the medical system but I had no idea how difficult it could be to find an HCP who had any idea of what to do with these complicated TBI cases. While I learned during my various preceptorships, I also witnessed considerable inefficient medicine. There were thousands of articles and books, but much information was conflicting and just plain wrong. I couldn't believe some of the outrageous things I was reading. Worse was finding a bit of information in one place and a week later finding another bit on the same topic in another place. The situation was mind-boggling as I tried to pull it all together. Since my son had suffered so much and because I feel that he might not be alive today without LDASEPA's intervention, I knew I had to do something to give back. I figured the book would be about 250 pages and take me about 6 months to write.

LABOR PAINS

No book is easy to write, but this one was a doozy. I soon found myself echoing the same complaints of many of the patients who had tried to educate themselves: Too much information and about 99% of it is junk. For every absolute, positive, 100% certain fact I found, I correspondingly located the exact opposite statement purported to be just as true, honest, and reliable. If I had read the phrase "evidence-based medicine" in front of just plain nonsense one more time, I would have screamed. The EBM term, while starting off with good intentions, has become an excuse for doctors not to think and to mindlessly follow algorithms without considering the patient suffering in front of them.

Old reliable resources that I had used for years without question were filled with inaccuracies about Lyme. Even the latest editions were outdated in terms of tick-borne illnesses and often contained potentially harmful suggestions on diagnosis and treatment. What other misinformation had I blindly ingested over the years?

After working as a researcher in the pharmaceutical industry for decades, there is one thing I know for sure. You can

---

2 See Glossary for name origin

make data say just about anything you want it to. I had been schooled by some of the best clinical researchers, statisticians, and technical writers. I had been grilled by regulatory bodies around the world over scientific papers and data analysis. If I knew anything, it was how to look at a published paper or data set and pick it to shreds.

There was little real science in the literature about tick-borne illnesses. While there were some retrospective compilations, there were very few prospective, controlled clinical trials that could show what was happening with these patients. Unbelievable, unscientific decisions made by government agencies and professional organizations, whose personnel should have known better, made the available resources very unreliable.

So what could I do to gather scientific, robust information without trusting the many authors who have secondary agendas? How could I identify those whose publications were based on their next payment from the insurance companies or whose desire to be right overwhelmed their oath to first do no harm? Even the state of Connecticut recognized that there were too many special interests in this fight. Both houses of their legislature unanimously passed a law recognizing that the controversy had gone too far. Health care providers were being prevented from providing the care that patients needed. Personal agendas were clouding good medicine.

I needed to rely on the experience of others. In most cases, TBI patients see a multitude of doctors before they find someone with enough expertise to help them. Just like me, most front-line practitioners have no idea what to do aside from: "give 'em a little doxy." I have observed HCPs who have seen thousands of TBI patients and they know both the frustration and satisfaction that comes from dealing with these complicated cases on a daily basis. I have learned to never give up on a patient or a book.

I am well qualified to assess a physician's bedside manner and technical competence, not because I am such a hot doc myself, but because I did just those kinds of evaluations for many years. In the military as Deputy Commander of Clinical Services at Aberdeen Proving Ground, I managed a large group of physicians in a number of therapeutic areas. I was responsible for reviewing all charts. I wrote the standard procedures for audit for a number of companies, including audits by the US Food and Drug Administration in assessing drug efficacy and safety parameters and analyzing data sets. Over the years as a researcher, I visited hundreds of research sites (including those that figure prominently in the history of Lyme) to assess their competency in performing research studies and the caliber of their principal investigators. I reviewed their credentials and ensured Good Clinical Practices. I know the difference between a law, a regulation, and a guideline.

Further, in clinical studies where I was the lead medical monitor, I visited as many of the sites as possible and saw patients with the specialists. I saw good doctors and bad. I saw those who did not deserve the name and those who should be sainted. I was able to see patients with local doctors all over the world. I saw patients lying in the streets where health care providers were doing what they could with what they had. More shocking was that I saw some of the worst medicine practiced in some of the "best" places where they should have known better – places like New Haven and New Orleans where politics and greed trumped patient care.

As a clinical researcher, I spent nearly two decades looking at data and searching for patterns and trends. As I reviewed the most recent medical journals and books for this text, I realized that at least half of what I was taught in med school is no longer held to be true.

While leeches and thalidomide are making comebacks, things like hormone replacement and the thousand "clinically-proven" diet programs are getting closer scrutiny. For example, have you ever observed a hospitalized diabetic? The amount of sugar put on the patient's hospital tray is astounding. You would have to try hard to consume that much pure sugar on your own. When I asked one hospital dietician what all that sugar was about, she mentioned that she strictly followed the food pyramid[3] for each patient. "Besides," she said, "All really high sugars are covered with insulin shots." It didn't matter that the person was getting sicker as long as no one could criticize the dietician for not adhering to the latest pyramid. There was no room for the individual patient. With the delusion of infallibility provided by the shield of the food pyramid, this dietician was doing everything right. Why did my mother's blood sugar go to 544 after macaroni and cheese, sugar filled ice cream, bread, and cake? Same reason it did the next meal with spaghetti and garlic bread, full-sugar popsicles, two sugar packets for her coffee, and salad dressing made mostly of high fructose corn syrup. This time the sugar went to 611. No fault of that dietician. She can point to all the proper places on the pyramid. Absolutely no thought was required on her part; she was practicing evidence-based medicine at its finest. If complete failure in patient management doesn't inspire health care providers like this dietician, what will?

How about this? Consider an article published in *The Wall Street Journal* on February 9, 2010, titled "Are Doctors Following the Rules?" Someone is very interested in how doctors practice medicine. The insurers mentioned in the article say they are trying to save money by making oncologists conform to specific guidelines. Clearly, insurers do not want to pay for expensive medicines or treatments if they don't have to. In the article, the insurer did not once mention concern for patients and how each individual may present cancer differently and respond uniquely to treatment. You may only have

---

3 Pyramid since revised

your cancer *their* way. I wonder what happens when an insurer's child gets cancer and has the audacity to not fit into the pre-defined pigeonholes. As you read this *Compendium* you will find parallels to tick-borne illnesses. Just be aware that there are many interests out there who want to have a say in the diagnosis and treatment you are able to give and that your children are able to receive. They are not all your friends.

Remember this text is a compilation of the knowledge and experience of a number of specialists. Please don't think, as you read along, that I am against evidence-based medicine, the goal of which is better medical decision-making. I'm all for that. By definition, evidence-based medicine uses robust scientific methods to gather evidence that will help health care providers and patients evaluate the risks and benefits of various assessments and treatments. This should allow for reasonable comparisons between different diagnostic methods and alternative therapies. Sounds good, right? Who could be against that?

What I am against is the deliberate *cherry-picking* of data in order to make a case for an opinion already held. I resent the inability of some to keep an open mind in reviewing new data. When it comes to analyzing data and drawing conclusions, an introspective statistician once told me, "If you torture a number long enough, you can get it to say anything you want." People who believe themselves to be scientists often draw conclusions from data that have been mined or skewed. Personally, I become frustrated by intractability fueled by greed, hubris, and conflict of interest rather than the desire to help patients. Please remember that just because someone is a physician does not mean that person is a scientist. Likewise, just because someone is a researcher does not make him or her a good physician. Few can claim to be good at both.

AND....while evidence-based medicine has done a great deal of good, it has a definite downside. By making each patient fit into the exact same mold, you are going to either over-diagnose or under-diagnose and you are going to force some people into treatment paradigms where they do not belong. Every patient is an individual, and that is how each patient should be treated. Target the needs of the person and not the checkboxes.

I considered providing a number of specific examples here to illustrate my point of how science can be biased, but I will spare you. Just when I think I have seen it all, someone comes up with another creative way to skew the data. My personal belief is to never fear the real data. Data just is what it is. As long as you know how your data was collected and what it can and cannot describe, wouldn't you really rather know the truth? I guess that answer for some people is NO.

Now after saying all that, I can attest that this book was hard to write. With thousands of papers and dozens of books on the subject, I had to endlessly gather information as well as review each study design. To say that this type of endeavor builds character is an understatement. I was given hundreds of articles to read by Bransfield and Johnson alone. Sometimes I would feel very sorry for myself as I started on their reference lists.

I intentionally tried to get out all my anger and frustration against the worst parts of the traditional medical system in this *Introduction.* That does not mean that I can guarantee that no bias will seep out in some places like the chapter called *Controversies around Lyme.* Once you have seen your child harmed by the rigid thinkers, it is hard to let some of that emotion go without at least some venting. People can always tell where I stand on an issue. But after my occasional rants, I promise to do my best to keep the textual parts as objective as possible.

I will now go back to the original intention of this book: To provide health care providers, patients, and caregivers with useful information that has never before been compiled in one place. Here the information is organized in a way that is easy to use, simple, and direct, with relatively quick access to what you need when the patient is sitting in front of you. I hope none of us is disappointed.

Kathy Spreen, DO MS MPH

Chapter 1

THE CHALLENGING WORLD OF →TBI
TICK-BORNE DISEASE

If I have seen further than others it is by standing upon the shoulders of giants.

Isaac Newton

Most of us enter the realm of tick-borne disease quite by accident. Few are volunteers. We were minding our own business when suddenly we became sick, our child got sick, or we misdiagnosed our first case. Sometimes we were introduced to this strange world by a tick, other times we never knew what hit us.

I am a TBI patient, caretaker, and health care provider – sometimes all at the same time. I have experienced TBD from all angles. Believe me, the hardest part was watching my child suffer and being helpless to change his course. I was willing to do anything.

As a physician, I remember my first Lyme misdiagnosis over 25 years ago. A dozen HCPs looked at the concentric circles on that toddler and agreed it was ringworm. In dealing with Lyme we're occasionally gifted with a tick in a jar and a patient with a classic rash. More often we're confronted with a perplexing set of symptoms and no idea which way to go to solve our patient's problem.

Initially, TBIs tend to manifest with general signs of inflammation. Diseases like Lyme are great imitators, confounding us at every turn. Some of these tick-associated conditions have pathognomonic indicators, most do not. The available diagnostic testing is fraught with low yields and insensitive results. Our lives become overrun with false negatives. Unfortunately, this is life in the world of TBD.

When my son got sick, I felt rudderless. I was getting conflicting stories at every turn. He did have Lyme. He didn't have Lyme. He was already being treated for the Lyme that the ER doctor said he clearly did **not** have, despite an EM rash, a tick in a jar, and corroborating symptoms. If I couldn't navigate the medical system as a physician, who could?

When I looked things up I found conflicting and contradictory information and obvious inaccuracies. One doctor's opinion was the exact opposite of the next. I wish now that I had help in navigating that tick-infested jungle. Over time, as my son started to come out of the TBI haze, I realized the best way to help others was to put this all together in a book that would

allow readers to find what they needed when they needed it, not months or years later. I wanted other families, HCPs, and patients to have one master source that they could refer to and find what was pertinent for their situation at that moment. I spent weeks trying to figure out what was going on with my son. I really would have liked the options laid out in front of me. I wanted to be able to review and weigh both sides of the debates so I could make rational decisions. I would have preferred to have the science, such as it was, to be handy so I could actually understand what was happening and not have to rely on others to form my opinions.

As you will learn repeatedly in future chapters, many times a delay in diagnosing and treating TBIs can lead to permanent adverse consequences and disability. "Wait and see" is usually a poor strategy in managing TBIs. My son still suffers on account of my dithering and the lack of knowledge and experience of his initial HCPs.

I knew something was terribly amiss with my son's lack of progress. Let's just say he was crashing despite what was supposed to be sanctioned Lyme treatment. I wish I had this *Compendium* to help me make the case for additional and possibly life-saving intervention. His earliest HCPs were wrong on every count. I was lucky that the local Lyme advocacy group was able to quickly steer me in the right direction. I do not like to think of what might have happened otherwise.

But if I, as a physician, had trouble plugging effectively into the system, how were laypeople expected to manage? Although I know a lot about different medicines and am a skilled and successful clinical researcher, I was a groveling novice around TBIs. I was begging for help as my son lay unconscious. I researched and found thousands of references but most were confusing or obviously inaccurate. Many were ranting diatribes that did not provide practical guidance. I wanted (un)common sense on all aspects of TBDs, located in one place, at my disposal.

What were these diseases? How could they be diagnosed? What were the treatment options? Is there science to support the alternative approaches? Why do these tick-disease people fight so much? How should I treat my son's fever, his rash, his pain? What should he be eating? How active should he be? What else could be going on? Are there any other things I can be doing to help him? What are the next steps I should be taking? Or the most important question at the time: Is he going to die?

With the help of the LDASEPA, I interacted with experts in all areas of TBD. From a PhD entomologist to the top clinicians in the field, I gathered information. I researched and questioned and checked and rechecked. I included all the information I needed four years ago. If I knew then what I know now, my son would have been spared considerable angst. If I knew all this 10 years ago, I would not have needed a knee replacement or suffered a fall that disabled me for three months. I want to help you avoid the same fate.

I.   WHAT SETS TICK-BORNE ILLNESS APART?

Why am I gathering expert opinion on various aspects of TBIs? What makes the diagnosis and treatment of tick-borne disease so challenging? Actually these conditions are not so different from many other diseases early in their discovery cycle. When people first confronted syphilis and AIDS and epilepsy, there were many misconceptions. Much of the clinical medicine initially used to diagnose and treat those syndromes would be considered malpractice today. While Lyme and Rocky Mountain spotted fever are probably the most familiar TBIs, others are coming on strong and may even be more frightening and intractable than those with which we are better acquainted. I think it's safe to say we hardly know most of these uninvited guests.

Although we are learning that TBIs have been around for thousands of years, in most cases we are just recognizing the responsible pathogens. Instead of a familiar disease like malaria that society has dealt with for millennia, we are working with some pathogens that have been recognized for less than a decade. On August 30, 2012, a new tick-borne virus was reported in the news media. After intense investigation a kind of Hantavirus, called phlebovirus, was diagnosed in two cases in Missouri and referred to as the Heartland virus. We certainly cannot expect to manage something we have known for a week as well as we might a condition that we have struggled with for hundreds of years. Further, microbes rarely travel solo these days. Co-infections can complicate both diagnosis and treatment. For most of the TBIs, we still do not have clear diagnostic parameters or well-defined treatment protocols. Nonetheless, many experts realize that with proper diagnosis and adequate treatment, TBI patients can and do get well.

After witnessing very little knowledge and experience (not to mention compassion) in the treatment of TBD patients, I wanted the primary target audience for this book to be HCPs. This book was developed for practitioners who want to help patients struggling with any of the perplexing tick-borne illnesses. With that being said, I also wanted to provide patients and caretakers with advice they can use in navigating this complex world. No one knows better than me that even HCPs can get confused when their child is sick and things are coming at you like a hailstorm. Even though direct-to-consumer advertising on TV wants you to ask your doctor if "Brand X" is right for you, the advertisers only say that because they are required to. Everyone knows that most doctors don't know any more about "Brand X" than you do. Yes, even doctors might need advice on fungal overgrowth and exercise tolerance and various supportive treatments in TBI patients. If all parties including HCPs, patients, and caretakers have access to the same body of information they might be better able to collaborate in making the best decisions for the individual case.

Where we stand today is in the middle of a minefield filled with ticks. We have many TBDs, known and unknown, that we are dealing with. We have overlapping signs and symptoms affecting essentially all body systems and limited access to reliable diagnostic testing. What fun!

II.   THERE IS HOPE

Despite all my personal and professional frustrations in dealing with TBDs, I come away after all these years with HOPE. I have seen patients get well with appropriate and diligent case management. This endeavor is not for the faint of heart. Surviving in the tick-borne world requires stamina and determination, no matter what your role. If you are dealing with chronic disease you will be surprised at the amount of courage, creativity, flexibility, and persistence required to come through the storm. You also need to know A LOT of medicine. I hope this text will help. As I often say in the body of this *Compendium*, take what is useful to you and leave the rest. You might need that information another day.

There is hope. I have seen too many success stories to think otherwise. The progress I witnessed was due to the combined determination of their caregivers and doctors and their own GRIT. You are now in a world where diagnostic criteria are muddled and reliable testing is hard to find. Sometimes you will discover that symptoms persist despite doing everything right. Then you will need to accept that in this arena we are far from knowing everything. You might need to rethink your strategies and try new approaches as you face your insecurities and prepare to regroup.

In my work in clinical research, I have seen patients on six continents with specialists in nearly every therapeutic area. I observed both good and bad clinical practice. I know the kind of physician I want to be and exactly who I prefer to take care of my child. There are certain characteristics that the "best" doctors display. The rest of this chapter will outline those traits and actions that I witnessed that I believe lead to the best outcomes. That doesn't mean you MUST do these things. Just consider the possibilities.

HCPs should read the following list in order to become better healers. Caregivers and patients should read these strategies to recognize what a top notch clinician can be. Both audiences should have high expectations regarding the possibility of quality patient care. These strategies may seem obvious, but you would be surprised at how many HCPs have no idea how to build a successful relationship that facilitates optimum results. Fortunately, you are no longer alone as you confront these complex and frustrating diseases.

III. HCP STRATEGIES FOR SUCCESSFUL OUTCOMES:

- Concentrate on the patient.

- Observe the person from the beginning of the contact to the end.

- Even when seemingly focused on something else, gather information about the patient and the overall family dynamics.

- Make eye contact. Talk to the patient. Allow the patient to respond. Many times she will tell you what you need to know.

- Invite anyone who cares about the individual into the office. Social interactions can provide a wealth of information. Of course, if the patient wants privacy, respect that request as well.

- Know the medicine. TBIs are way too complicated to "wing it." Maybe this book will help.

- Don't rush. Make sure your schedule gives you the cushion you need to give each patient the time he deserves.

- Believe the patient and the caregivers.

- Always have a plan B and C and D.

- Exude optimism. If you don't believe the patient can get well, why should she?

- With that being said, be realistic and do not give false hope. Balance expectations.

- Do not lose track of your case. Refer to consultants but do not abdicate your TBI responsibility. If you are the primary TBI physician, coordinate the overall effort.

- Treat every patient as you would want your child treated.

- Don't just treat and run. Follow up.

- Care.

- Learn from experience. Remember what has worked and what hasn't in certain situations.

- Remember that what doesn't work in one case, may work in another. How are the cases different?

- Learn how to say, "I don't know." This might take practice.

- "I don't know" doesn't mean "I give up."

- Review the chart BEFORE you bring the patient in.

- TBI medicine is hard. I have worked extensively in oncology and organ transplantation and any number of other complex therapeutic areas. Working with TBIs is the most difficult medicine I have ever experienced. In this field you need to be a detective and you need to think outside the conventional paradigms in many cases. TBIs can involve every body system, in varying degrees. The immune system is usually involved in either a hyper or hypo capacity. There are often co-infections. Management of TBIs is not for the faint-of-heart.

- This field is controversial. You have to be willing to use innovative and creative thinking. You don't necessarily want to be the first or the last to try something new. When you hear of a new treatment option, gather information. Try a novel approach when the case calls for it. Do not be easily swayed by slick marketing or promotion.

- Take your time. Whatever a specific patient needs is what that patient should get. Recently, I had a knee replacement and the resident came in and without ever making eye contact, he said, "How ya doin?" Before I could exhale enough breath to pass over my vocal cords, he had left the room. He had circled the bed and didn't even stop for one second. He is not a doctor that I aspire to emulate. And he never will be.

- Know what you know and what you don't know. Don't be afraid to admit that you don't understand what is happening with a particular case. But, then, instantly make a plan to find out. Consult other specialists such as psychiatrists, cardiologists, or endocrinologists as needed.

- Go for success. Try and try until you get a response.

- Enthusiasm for your work and your patients is probably more infectious than any pathogen. I have seen HCPs who were just miserable. How do you think patients feel coming out of their offices?

- Foster genuine empathy. Care about these people. And their caretakers. Most will have seen many doctors before getting to you. The highest number of previous HCPs that I heard was 26.

- Know that both the patient and caregivers might have been through hell with this disease.

- Laugh at yourself and use humor to relax the patient. Sometimes even the most reserved HCP does something ridiculous. You are not required to be stuffy.

- Do not get trapped in an evidence-based medicine box that you cannot escape. Do not limit yourself in the alternatives you might consider in treating your patients.

- Tailor the assessment and treatment to the individual case. Work your plan or construct new strategies until that particular patient responds.

- With young patients, small things matter. A dab of anesthetic gel at the site of a needle stick and some fluids to plump up a vein might be appreciated. Yes, this takes a few extra minutes but it is compassionate and it is how I want my child treated by the doctor. Actually, little things count with patients of all ages.

- Never give up. Never.

IV. LET ME INTRODUCE YOU...

Most of us are taken by surprise with our first encounter with a TBI. Do not panic, but don't under-react either. Use this text to help you orchestrate a reasonable response. If you are an HCP just entering this arena, use this book to help you cross over into the world of TBD.

No one knows everything about managing TBIs. No ONE. That is why I spent four years gathering information and checking and rechecking the innumerable controversies and contradictions. In fact, the medical community has only started to gather information on these diseases. We have a long way to go.

Don't be proud or foolish. Take all the help you can get. Whether you are a patient, caretaker, or HCP, you can likely benefit from the experience of others. Use this book for all it's worth. Take what you can use. Leave what is extraneous to your needs. If you are an HCP, you will be forced to exercise your clinical judgment and to weigh the pros and cons of alternative approaches to both diagnosis and treatment. Initially this task can be daunting. I hope this *Compendium* will provide you with guidance. Again, take what you can use. I would be very surprised if you could not find something helpful.

This text supplies information from experts that is compiled nowhere else, located in one place, and organized in a way that is easy to use, simple, and direct. The *Compendium* provides access to practical guidance that might be needed quickly as the patient presents in the office. The medical expertise included should help all who are interested in learning about these complex diseases. I will walk with you every step of the way from the underlying science, the concept of co-infections, controversies, as well as patient evaluation, diagnosis, and treatment. I will weigh the various options and provide guidance on solid decision-making. The many myths that have caused so much harm to patients over the years will be dispelled. You will no longer be alone in your quest to fight tick-borne disease.

TBIs are challenging, to say the least. Most of us come into this field having no idea what we are getting ourselves into. We are often inspired by our own illness or that of a family member. Accepting these challenging patients takes a brave individual, courageous enough to take on this complex, controversial field. Aspire to combine technical expertise with creativity, compassion, and flexibility.

Now let's get to work.

Chapter 2

THE TICK

Really good listeners are usually thinking about something else.
Unknown

Perhaps the best place to start a book about TBDs is with the tick. Ticks have been around much longer than humans. Fossil ticks have been found in amber formed more than 65 million years ago in New Jersey. The presence of ticks in hardened tree sap suggests that they were as prevalent then as they are now and that Jersey doesn't ever change much.

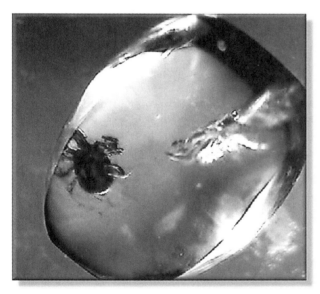

Tick in amber
Source: www.ambericawest.com/tick.
Accessed March 2013

Ticks are of the phylum Arthropod, which means they have a skeleton on the outside of their bodies. Part of the Arachnid class, adult ticks have eight segmented legs like spiders, in contrast to insects that have only six. These blood-feeding parasites can be either hard-bodied or soft and both types are important disease carriers for humans and animals all over the world. Diseases spread by ticks include those caused by bacteria, rickettsia, viruses, and protozoa.

With at least 18 different genus types and nearly 900 species, ticks represent a diverse and resilient animal group. Many kinds of ticks spread disease to humans including deer ticks or black-legged ticks, Pacific ticks, American dog ticks, Lone Star ticks, Rocky Mountain wood ticks, relapsing fever ticks,

brown dog ticks, bear ticks, woodchuck ticks, and probably many others not yet clearly identified. Some of the ticks listed here may actually be the same species, just identified in a different geographic location. We may be splitting hairs in trying to force distinctions.

There are several definitions important for understanding this topic:

Host: A host is any animal that the tick feeds upon. So humans, dogs, cats, pigs, possums, and numerous other animals can serve as hosts. A host might also be a reservoir (as in the case of the white-footed mouse), but most hosts are not reservoirs. Birds can be hosts. Some lizards can be hosts. Deer are common hosts as are raccoons, squirrels, woodchucks, pumas, coyotes, and foxes. As far as we know, most of these species are **not** capable of infecting a biting tick with Borrelia with any consistency, but ticks are happy to drink their blood.

Vector: Carrier of disease. A vector is a living organism (often an Arthropod or Insect) that transmits a pathogen from a reservoir to a host. A vector, such as a mosquito or a tick, takes the disease agent from an infected animal such as a mouse into an uninfected host, which then becomes infected. Vectors usually do not have the disease themselves. Infected does not mean diseased. For example, a tick carrying Bb is not sick with Lyme disease. The tick just happens to provide optimal living conditions for Bb and is not usually adversely affected by the presence of this pathogen.

Reservoir: In general, a reservoir can be anything that harbors a pathogen allowing it to live and multiply. A species can be a competent reservoir, which can pass the infection on to a feeding tick, or an incompetent reservoir, which cannot. A reservoir is part of the pathogen's life cycle and is not incidental. Without the reservoir, the pathogen would die out, so the pathogen needs the reservoir to survive. A species is considered a competent reservoir only if it is capable of infecting the next tick that bites it.

A reservoir can be considered a storage place or depot. Humans are not competent reservoirs, no matter how sick we are, because it is highly unlikely that we could infect a new tick that happens along and bites us. Deer are not reservoirs since they do not infect the ticks that feed on them. The only reservoir species known for the Lyme-carrying ticks in North America are white-footed mice, chipmunks, shrews, and maybe voles. Additional species may be uncovered as we learn more, but right now those are it. Reservoir animals do not get sick from the pathogen they harbor (that would be counterproductive to the pathogen), although there is speculation that the reservoir's behavior might be modified by certain microbes such as Bb in order to better serve its needs.

PEARL: Lyme infection control might then include management or elimination of the pathogen through interference with the vectors, the reservoirs, or certain hosts. A deer might be the HOST, which shelters the infected tick VECTOR, that can later expose a mouse, which then serves as the RESERVOIR for the Bb pathogen. Thereafter the mouse is competent to infect the next tick that comes along. Here control of the deer and mice populations, suppression of the pathogen with antimicrobials, and reining in of the viable ticks might all be part of an attempt to manage the Lyme epidemic. The cycle can be interrupted on many levels and the most effective management of LD might involve multiple approaches. Reduction in the deer population reduces the tick population correspondingly. Eliminate the deer and you eliminate the majority of deer ticks. Eliminate the deer tick and you should greatly reduce the incidence of Lyme disease.

PEARL: Deer are important because they amplify the tick population, but they are an incompetent transmitter of Bb. Deer are the preferred hosts for mating ticks. The gravid female ticks fall off and lay their eggs in leaf litter, where they hatch and immediately look for a mouse to feed upon. The mice are competent reservoirs for Bb, and are universally infected in some locations, so they pass the Bb infection on to the larval tick. The tick then becomes a nymph, and starts looking for a larger animal to feed on. That could be us.

A competent reservoir species is capable of passing the infection on to the feeding tick, while an incompetent one cannot pass along the disease. Since mice are a competent reservoir, essentially every time a tick feeds on a mouse, it could potentially become infected. Humans are not competent hosts. We are a dead end. We are just in the way of the bigger picture.

PEARL: One reason why humans might not be able to transmit Bb to the uninfected is that we seem to have only low levels of free-floating spirochetes in the blood stream at a given time and those only sporadically. That might be one reason why it's so hard to get a positive PCR result, as will be explained later.

Deer are best considered reproductive hosts for the ticks. Deer are essential to the life-cycle of the tick. They aren't called deer ticks for nothing. On the deer, the male and female ticks meet and mate. The female then consumes a blood meal and, now gravid, falls off the deer to lay her thousands of eggs, usually in leaf litter or foliage. The eggs hatch into larvae. The more mice in the vicinity, the more likely the larvae will find one to munch and thereby become infected.

PEARL: While deer are not a reservoir for Bb, they could very well serve as a reservoir for other pathogens. There is speculation that they may serve as such for Ehrlichia and Anaplasma.

Likewise, considerable evidence supports the contention that an increase in the number of deer amplifies the tick population. The deer are capable of hosting hundreds and even thousands of ticks at any one time. Since deer are the preferred mating site, ticks will seek them out. Deer can have 2,000 to 3,000 ticks on board that might harbor infectious spirochetes, yet the deer do not manifest symptoms (sxs) of Lyme disease. One theory is that the deer might have an immune system that clears the infecting spirochete quickly sparing them the development of systemic disease. They neither get sick from the Bb, nor are they able to pass it along. In terms of the Bb, deer would be considered an incompetent host.

The life cycle of a tick varies from species to species and even within a species depending on the environmental conditions. In general, hard ticks have distinct life stages as shown in the graphic displayed on the opposite page. This life cycle of the deer tick was compiled by Ron Hamlen, PhD, of the LDASEPA.

Larva – Deer tick larvae come out of their eggs with six legs and can be as small as the period at the end of this sentence. They take a blood meal from a host and then molt or shed their outer covering. At first the deer tick larvae are not carrying disease-causing organisms, but they can get infected with their first meal if they feed from the right infected host. Once they are infected, they can transmit the disease agent. Infected does not mean diseased. Infected ticks are not usually diseased ticks. Just as we have millions of bacteria in our guts that do not make us sick, ticks can have many organisms along for the ride that do not make them sick. If the larva does not feed from an infected host, it usually is not infected and therefore cannot transmit disease. After feeding, the larvae become inactive and later molt into nymphs.

PEARL: The bite of the Lone Star tick larva is thought to be able to transmit STARI. The infected female tick can transmit the pathogen that causes STARI to her eggs and thereby infect the larvae. The transfer of pathogen is transovarian so that these larvae are born infected. Can deer tick larvae be born infected? We don't know.

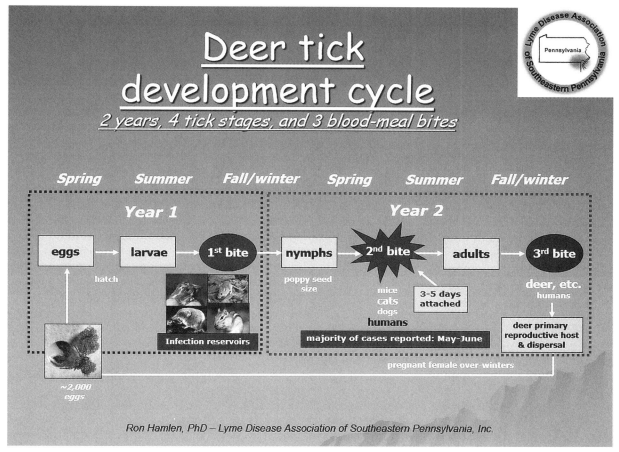

Life cycle of the deer tick
Source: LDASEPA. Ron Hamlen, PhD. Accessed October 2012

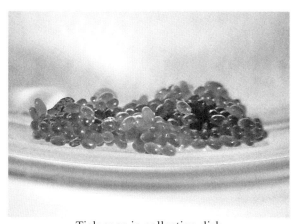

Tick eggs in collecting dish
Source: Ryan, Keith. http://www.dartmoorcam.co.uk/dartmoortick-
watch Accessed March 2013

Nymph – Deer tick larvae molt into nymphs with eight legs and are about the size of a poppy seed. Soon after the nymphs emerge, they usually become dormant for several months, usually until the next spring. As the weather warms, the nymphs become active again and look for a host, usually a small mammal. If the tick is carrying infectious agents ingested during its first feeding, it can now transmit these organisms to its next host. If it wasn't previously infected, the tick can become so now if it feeds on the right infected animal. Usually in the fall, nymphs molt into adults.

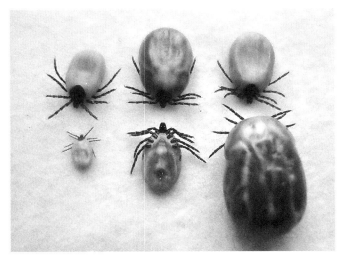

Ixodes *hexagonas*, all six taken from one hedgehog
Source: Ryan, Keith. http://www.dartmoorcam.co.uk/
dartmoortickwatch. Accessed March 2013

PEARL: Ticks generally have only three meals in their entire lifetime. The first meal prompts the metamorphosis from larva to nymph and the second from nymph to adult. The third meal prepares the female tick for laying her eggs.

Adult – The final stage of the tick life cycle, the adult, has eight legs. The females are larger than the males. If the female did not get a blood meal in the fall, she goes dormant over the winter. (The diapause state is described below.) Freezing temperatures do not kill a tick in diapause. She will look for her next meal in the spring or whenever the temperature is above freezing. When a feeding opportunity presents, the female will eat over several days and her body will swell with blood. This swelling is called engorgement. Infected females can transmit disease. The adult males may attach but they do not feed or become engorged. Since they do not mix their saliva with the blood of the host, they usually do not transmit disease. The female mates, feeds, and lays thousands of eggs. Then, she dies. The male doesn't bother to eat; he just reproduces and dies.

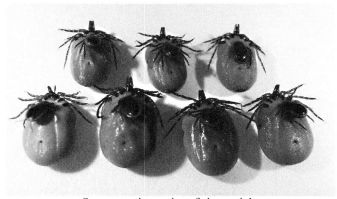

Seven mating pairs of sheep ticks
Source: Ryan, Keith. http://www.dartmoorcam.co.uk/
dartmoortickwatch. Accessed March 2013

The life cycle for the various tick species can last from a number of months to over 3 years. The cycle from egg to egg in the deer tick is typically about 2 years. The colder the climate, the longer the life cycle. In cold areas, the tick can go into diapause where its development is put on hold and metabolic activity lessens in response to adverse conditions. Once the conditions become more conducive to the tick's development, the normal cycle resumes. Diapause can last for months as the tick awaits climate changes or the availability of hosts.

The mouth parts of the tick are essential to its survival. The outside portions are two very movable palps. Inside the palps is a pair of chelicerae. The chelicerae open the host skin for insertion of the hypostome, which is a central open feeding tube illustrated in the image below. The palps move side to side while the tick eats. They do not enter the skin of the host. In contrast, the hypostome has a number of sharp protuberances along its edge and this part punctures the skin of the host. Since the projections hook backward, the hypostome anchors the tick to the host. This is why the tick can be so hard to remove and why a tiny bit of flesh often exits the host along with the tick when it is removed.

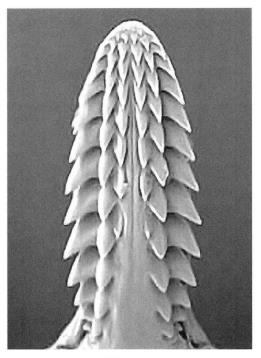

Ventral view of hypostome with barbs
Source: Ryan, Keith. http://www.dartmoorcam.co.uk/
dartmoortickwatch. Accessed March 2013

Many ticks secrete a glue-like material made in their salivary glands, which attaches the tick firmly in place. This glue dissolves after the tick is done feeding. Some hosts have shown an allergy to the saliva of ticks, and this allergy manifests in typical signs and symptoms of an allergic reaction: swelling, redness, and itch. I am unaware of any anaphylaxis reported in response to this type of allergy or any reports that the rash associated with the allergy looked like an erythema migrans rash, which is an entirely separate phenomenon. The tick saliva in some species may contain a mild anesthetic substance, which better allows the tick to remain undetected while on the host. Some researchers believe that along with pain killers, the tick also injects antihistamines and anticoagulants. This would make sense from the perspective of natural selection and survival since the antihistamine would diminish host reaction to the bite and the anticoagulant would keep the meal flowing. There is speculation that a tick can transmit nearly 100,000 pathogens in one attachment, but I do not know if this figure has ever been substantiated. Nonetheless, too often, enough of the infectious agent is transported to cause disease.

PEARL: Bb are introduced into the host skin by an infected tick. The tick saliva contains biochemicals that can numb the area, weaken coagulation so that blood flows easily, and alter the normal immune response. These actions enhance the pathogen's ability to establish itself and infect the victim.

Ticks find hosts by a process called questing. Here ticks wait in leaf litter or crawl up the stems of grass or plants, wherever they find themselves. They perch on the edge of the plant with their front legs extended. The ticks are stimulated by certain chemicals like CO_2 that are exhaled from their preferred host animals. Further, they respond to heat and movement as would be expected to emit from an animal passing nearby. Some animals, like deer and humans apparently, release pheromones that attract the tick. When a warm, exhaling, potential host brushes by, the tick grabs on and settles onto the host. The tick snags the host's fur, hair, clothing, or skin with its barbed front legs. Before I become too anthropomorphic here, the ticks are not plotting and scheming. Rather, tick behaviors have evolved in response to environmental stimuli in a way that gives them the best chance for survival.

PEARL: A pheromone is a chemical that is released by an animal into its surroundings that affects the behavior or biochemistry of other animals. Deer, humans, and possibly other animals seemingly release pheromones that attract certain tick species. Most likely the chemical developed in the eventual hosts for other purposes and the tick evolved in a way that allowed them to detect this biochemical and thereby find preferred hosts. The amount of pheromone released can be quite unique for the individual. This phenomenon has been clearly demonstrated with mosquitoes where several children can be present in the same area for the same amount of time and some of these kids will be covered with mosquito bites and others will be essentially untouched. The same process seems to occur with ticks and certain individuals.

PEARL: There may also be chemicals in deer tick saliva that aid in infectivity of the Bb and that modulate the immune

system. The saliva can carry immunosuppressive substances that enable agents to invade tissues while paralyzing the local immune response. The LD spirochete can then disseminate more rapidly and become entrenched early in the infectious process.

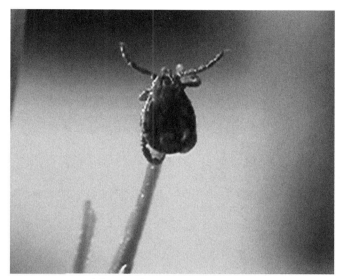

Tick questing on a blade of grass

Hard ticks can feed for days or weeks, depending on species and stage. The nymphal deer tick tends to feed for 3 to 5 days. Usually humans discover ticks and remove them as soon as possible, but many animals do not have that luxury. Once a tick latches on behind a deer's ear, it remains pretty much as long as it wants. The covering on the outside of the tick can expand to accommodate all the blood it ingests, which can be from 200 to 600 times its unfed weight. The tick will feed for varying time periods depending on its life stage, the host, and immediate needs. Some ticks have only one host in their lives, others have two or three.

PEARL: Many people never see the attached, feeding deer tick. An irritation or mild allergic reaction at the bite site may provide just enough sensation to allow the tick to be more readily detected.

How do disease-causing organisms get into and out of the tick in order to do their damage? While the tick feeds on the host blood, any organisms present in the tick are able to pass to and from the host. The tick might contain bacteria, viruses, or other organisms that can cause disease. Likewise, the host might contain bacteria, viruses, or other organisms that can cause disease. During the bite, fluids like blood and saliva are exchanged between the tick and the host. Whatever is in the host's blood and the tick's saliva is fair game. If conditions are right, the host can become infected with the disease agents. In some hosts, the infection can cause illness. Whether or not the host feels sick, the next vector who feeds on a host that happens to be a competent reservoir might pick up the infectious agent that was left behind by the original tick and transmit it again. With Bb, the tick may inoculate the host with many thousands of the spirochete along with other agents.

For many years, the idea that a tick had to be attached for 24 to 48 (or even 72) hours and become engorged before it could transmit disease was sacrosanct. However, we are now learning that symptoms have appeared in cases where the tick was not in place for more than a few hours and was not yet engorged. Since most people do not know when the tick first attached (if they did they would remove it when they first became aware), it is nearly impossible to determine exactly how long a tick was present. The point being, just because it SEEMS like a tick was not in place long enough to infect a host based on old ideas, that does not mean it wasn't. Many individuals underestimate how long the tick was attached. Therefore, always be vigilant in watching for signs of disease. The most prudent approach is to assume that every tick bite is infectious.

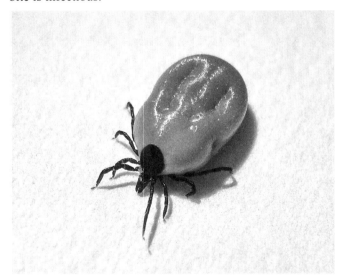

Engorged adult female Ixodes *ricinus*, 6.4 mm
Source: Ryan, Keith. http://www.dartmoorcam.co.uk/
dartmoortickwatch. Accessed March 2013

Phyllis Mervine and Ron Keith from CALDA (now Lymedisease.org) compiled information regarding length of attachment in relation to the likelihood of disease in a mouse model. The longer the tick was attached the more likely infection was transmitted. If attached for 48 hours, about half will transmit enough pathogen to cause disease. At 72 hours, transmission from infected tick to host is near 100%. While the transmission rate at 24 hours is low, it is NOT zero. This is supported by the fact that a number of Lyme cases have been reported where the tick could only have been in place for a short time and disease ensued.

PEARL: Be careful when "experts" proclaim that if a tick has not been attached for more than 24 or even 36 or 72 hours and is not engorged, there is minimal or no chance of infection. This is not true. There are a number of well-documented cases where the tick could not have been in place long before transmitting disease. One anecdote involves a toddler who just had a bath and a nap. She was with her parents when she went out to play. She had no tick on her face when she first went outside. Soon thereafter the mom found a tick near her eye. This tick would have been readily apparent had it been present earlier. Her pediatrician said not to worry because the tick had not been on long enough to transmit any organisms. The next morning the child was very ill with a high fever, painful arthritis, Bell's palsy, and an EM rash. Again the physician said there was no need to treat because these symptoms couldn't be Lyme. Apparently, an opinion once stated is an opinion that must be forever defended.[1] She was finally treated with appropriate antibiotics and responded quickly. Blood tests showed that she was loaded with spirochetes.

Organisms like the spirochete, Borrelia *burgdorferi*, are ingested by the tick when it feeds on an infected reservoir animal. Eventually the microbe reaches the midgut of the tick. Here, they find a cozy little boudoir where they multiply in a process that is much more complex than that sentence would suggest. They stay in the gut for a few weeks as they spread into the tissues of the tick including its saliva. When the tick bites and the saliva comes into contact with the host's blood, the spirochete (or any other infectious agent that happens to be present) can be transmitted to and from the host.

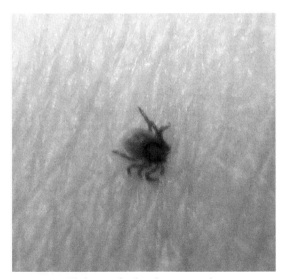

Tick attached to human wrist
Source: Ryan, Keith. http://www.dartmoorcam.co.uk/
dartmoortickwatch. Accessed March 2013

---

1 Phrase taken from work by Diane Ravitch.

The nymph midgut is the primary location for Bb multiplication. Here their density increases and that triggers a surface protein change from OspA to OspC. The pathogen then moves into the salivary glands. There is thought to be additional biochemical changes to the Bb surface proteins at attachment when feeding begins, but the trigger here is not well-defined. The altered pathogens in the salivary glands undergo the most rapid increase in their numbers from about 48 to 60 hours post-attachment, when the risk of transmission of disease is greatest. Clearly longer attachment times increase the risk of transmission both because mechanically there is a greater chance of transfer and also because the pathogen being transported has had time to be altered into a form that might be more infectious.

Still, consider any tick bites you or your family might have experienced. While you might not KNOW exactly when the tick attached, you do KNOW that it wasn't two or three days ago. Unless you are hiking the Appalachian trail, without easy ways to scrutinize some obscure body parts, you have a good idea of what is and isn't present within a 24-hour period. Any tick that I have pulled off me or my kin, or in the many patients I have ministered to in the ER, clearly was not in place for 48 to 72 hours. Still many of us became sick from these bites. The definite tick culprit in my son's most prominent TBI episode was certainly the one responsible, since it was found in the area where the EM rash soon manifested, just as he became symptomatic. This tick most definitely was NOT there 10 hours before when my son was running around the house without his shirt after showering. Even if we consider that we had missed this tick earlier, the bite site was examined less than 12 hours before, so there is really very little likelihood that this tick was present for 24 hours and probably was attached for much less time than that. This tick wasn't engorged. My point is that in the experience of many experts, despite all protestations that disease cannot be transmitted if the tick is not in place for at least a day, this is not the case and much, if not most, disease is transmitted earlier than some of the literature proclaims. Suspect that any tick bite, whatever the length of attachment, could potentially spread disease. Quibbling over whether or not the tick was in place long enough does not change the reality of the illness.

One wise sage professed that ticks are sewers. More than any other blood sucking arthropod, ticks are vectors (carriers) of multiple diseases including Lyme, babesiosis, ehrlichiosis, anaplasmosis, bartonellosis, certain types of Mycoplasma infections, Rocky Mountain spotted fever, and tularemia, among others. Ticks can carry bacteria, viruses, rickettsia, small worms like filarial nematodes, and protozoans, that we know about. A single tick may be harboring many combinations of different types of infectious agents. These days, it is nearly inconceivable that a tick would be carrying just one potential pathogen. Ticks appear to be equal opportunity transmitters.

Ticks are blood-feeding parasites that can be found in leaf litter, grasses, and low bushes where they wait to attach themselves to a passing host. Most ticks aren't especially mobile on their own, although they do climb stalks of various plants. For most of their transportation, they must hitch a ride on other animals. They are not too choosy about their transport. Migratory animals, birds, and traveling humans all help to widely disperse ticks.

Found in tall grass, near the edge of forests, in wooded areas, under leaves or shrubs, in the crevices of stone walls and woodpiles, ticks especially like areas that have been cleared next to remaining forest-land. The apparent recent increase in tick populations in suburbs may be due to wooded land being cleared for housing developments. Where lawn meets woods, the tick population seems to increase. They do not prefer lawns that are cut and maintained. Ticks are found throughout the world and are common in the grass near seashores. Since ticks can't read, they don't know where they are supposed to be and our various lists don't restrict their whereabouts. Recently a flight was delayed because a tick was found on the plane. Just because a tick isn't usually found in a certain place, doesn't mean she can't show up there.

Ticks bite dogs, wild and domestic cats, raccoons, deer, mice, voles, chipmunks, horses, squirrels, shrews, rabbits, cattle, moose, wild and domestic pigs, coyotes, opossums, bats, rodents, sheep, and numerous other mammals. One count included more than 50 types of mammals, as many varieties of birds, and at least a dozen species of lizard. They bite humans. Some of these animals subsequently get ill, but many species just harbor the pathogen.

Ticks bite and draw blood only about three times in their lives. Their first meal is usually from something small like a mouse, shrew, or chipmunk. The second and third meals are usually bigger animals like deer, dogs, or humans. Where I live in Pocopson Township in southeastern Pennsylvania we tend to blame the deer for the tick invasion and there is considerable evidence to support this contention. Usually the more deer, the more ticks are found in the same area. Deer are the preferred reproductive hosts for the ticks. In winter, the pregnant female ticks drop off the deer and overwinter near where they land.

Other sources say that the ticks are just as happy with the white-footed mice as they are with the deer. Since mice can survive in many habitats where the deer cannot, they can provide an alternative, even if it is not the first choice. While humans may be able to curtail the deer in some suburbs, mice will just move over a few feet and set up a new homestead. One theory suggests that when there are fewer deer, more mice will begin to harbor the pathogens. In fact, mice are the principal reservoir species, while deer are the preferred reproductive host. Keep in mind that overdevelopment may change the natural mix and the tick may be adapting to the new fauna distribution. Also, increasing global temperatures are allowing the spread of ticks farther north.

Once attached, the tick will gorge itself with blood and eventually drop off to wait for its next meal. The drop-off may take several days. A full tick can feed off the blood in its gut for an extended period before it needs to feed again. TBDs are not known to be transmitted from dog to cat, person to dog, or dog to the family pet pig. Although a human mother can pass along Bb and other pathogens to her offspring across the placenta, most often the microbe is transmitted by way of the tick saliva as the fluids mingle between host and tick.

> *PEARL: There are anecdotes of canine to canine transmission. These cases have been published and the circumstances were such that there was essentially no other way (such as an unrecognized tick bite) that the pathogen could have been introduced.*

The length of daylight and changes in temperature will signal a tick to seek a host. While ticks are more active in warm weather, they can attach and feed any time of the year. Apparently, they can detect heat from other animals and the carbon dioxide exhaled by their potential hosts. Populations may be denser near watering holes and close to animal trails or small mammal burrows. While ticks like warmer weather, they tend to stay out of direct sun since they can easily dehydrate. They do like high humidity, and when the humidity increases in the spring and summer months, the risk of tick bite increases. Deer ticks are quite active from May to July and the majority of cases are reported in this window.

While all the various species of tick would be fascinating to review in detail (not really!), for the purposes of this *Compendium*, the focus will be on the five ticks listed below. All are presented with their genus, then species, followed by common names.

Ixodes *scapularis* – (Deer tick, bear tick, black-legged tick, formerly Ixodes *dammini*) This tick is found primarily in the eastern and midwestern US. There remains considerable controversy about whether the northern and southern versions are the same and whether it even matters. This species is known to harbor Borrelia *burgdorferi* (Bb), Babesia, Ehrlichia, Anaplasma, Mycoplasmas, and Bartonella. Immature deer ticks cannot reproduce and tend to feed on ground-loving birds and small mammals. Both the larval and nymph stages are considered immature. A female adult deer tick needs a blood meal and will ingest a several-day supply of blood from a deer before she has enough nutrition to lay her thousands of eggs. The larva of the deer tick is as small as the period at the end of this sentence while the nymphs are slightly larger, roughly the size of a poppy seed. Tick bites are much more common than realized by the host.

The deer tick prefers the white-tailed deer as its reproductive host but will reproduce on other large mammals in the absence of deer. Therefore, the deer is an important part of the deer tick's reproductive cycle. As seen in the northeastern US, the greater the deer population the greater the population of Ixodes *scapularis*. The increase of white-tailed deer in the northeastern US corresponds with the uncontrolled spread of suburbs in this area. There is essentially an unbroken suburb tracking from Boston to Washington DC. There are now about 1.5 million white-tailed deer in Pennsylvania. More deer, and therefore more deer ticks, are being found in the southeastern US, in Virginia, the Carolinas, and throughout Florida. The humid, "Sunshine State" provides excellent tick habitat and appears to be getting an infusion of ticks from the many visitors from states that are infested with deer and deer ticks.

Deer ticks migrate by attaching to animals, birds, and people. Their habitat is expanding all over North America and they are now found in the Dakotas and well into Mexico. Deer ticks are well established along both coasts. Wherever there are large populations of white-tailed deer and white-footed mice, there is the potential for infectious deer ticks. A study conducted in the San Francisco Bay area detected antibodies to deer tick saliva in about a third of the population. Many of these people did not realize they had ever been bitten.

Mice and deer prefer the flora associated with lawns at the edge of forests. There are fewer deer in full forests than there are in recently developed areas. The only predators left in the suburbs are vehicles that leave deer on the side of the road. (Deer ticks can fall from the carcasses and the tick can continue its life cycle even though its host is gone.) Hunting is very restricted in most suburban areas. Chances of being bitten increase in spring and summer when nymphs are questing. Ticks like the shade near the edge of wooded areas where there are piles of moist leaves. They are becoming common on golf courses, and if you want to guarantee a tick bite, stop at one of the rest stops along the Pennsylvania Turnpike on a warm day and walk your dog.

Ixodes *pacificus* – (Western black-legged tick) This particular species is found in the western part of the US especially in California along the coastal range up along the coast of British Columbia into Canada. These ticks are slightly different morphologically than Ixodes *scapularis*. They also sometimes use lizards as hosts, which is somewhat unusual for ticks, since they tend to prefer mammals. I. *pacificus* is known to transmit RMSF and has been implicated in Lyme and other diseases. A west coast rat species is the suspected reservoir. Various stages of I. *pacificus* are shown in the next photograph.

PEARL: Be careful. I. scapularis *is the black-legged tick and I.* pacificus *is the WESTERN black-legged tick.*

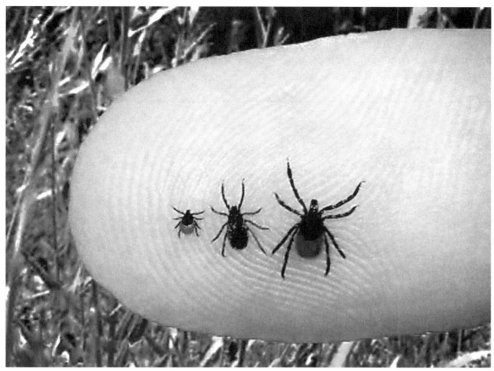

Various stages of I. *pacificus*
Source: www.doh.wa.gov.
Accessed April 2013

Amblyomma *americanum* – (Lone Star tick) This tick has a white dot or "lone star" on the back of the adult females which is occasionally seen on adult males. A. *americanum* transmits a Borrelia species, which is at least similar, if not identical, to the Bb that causes Lyme disease. The resulting disease has been called STARI or Southern Tick-Associated Rash Illness. Lone Star ticks are thought to be more mobile and aggressive than many other ticks. Some reports suggest they will actively move toward a potential host. The larvae have been suspected of biting people. Their geographic range is thought to be expanding rapidly, since they have been found as far north as Maine. John Carroll, an entomologist with the US Department of Agriculture, believes that the Lone Star tick can possibly transfer Borrelia species across the ovary so that the larvae are born infected.

PEARL: On August 30, 2012, a new tick-borne virus was reported in the news media. After intense investigation a kind of Hantavirus, called phlebovirus, was diagnosed in two cases in Missouri. This infection was thought to be transmitted by Lone Star ticks. The CDC staff mentioned that making the diagnosis was challenging because the sxs were similar to so many other infectious diseases. You will run across that concept many times in this text.

Dermacentor *variabilis* – (American dog tick) Before Lyme focused our attention on the deer tick, the dog tick was our most familiar tick nemesis, found commonly on dogs and other domestic animals. Located usually east of the Rockies in the US and Canada, this tick is also becoming more common in Mexico, the Pacific northwest, California, and in the midwest. Usually the dog tick has 3 hosts beginning with small mammals as larvae and nymphs, then moving to larger mammals as an adult. The larvae have 6 legs, while adults have 8. These ticks are usually a reddish-brown color with grey markings on their dorsal shield. A fully-fed female will be a pasty grey color. An engorged female can be 15 mm long and 10 mm wide but most top out smaller than that. The nymph can survive 6 months without a blood meal and adults can survive 2 years without feeding. Mating occurs on the host. After mating the female gorges and within a week or two drops from the host to lay her eggs and then dies. Dog ticks overwinter in the soil. Adults can be active somewhat earlier than the deer tick, springing back to life as early as April. Dermacentor ticks are the primary vector for the Rickettsia *rickettsii* that causes RMSF and are known to spread tularemia and canine tick paralysis. Their role in human tick paralysis is not clear. Bartonella have been found in dog ticks. Initially the dog tick was thought not to carry Lyme disease, but there are recent suspicions that Bb have been found in the dog tick in southeastern Pennsylvania. This has yet to be confirmed, but the thought does suggest that a high index of suspicion might be prudent if symptoms appear after any tick bite. Dermacentor *andersoni* (Rocky Mountain wood tick) may be the primary species spreading CTF and RMSF.

Ixodes *ricinis* –This tick is the principal tick vector of Bb in Europe, where animal reservoirs are suspected to be similar to those identified in the US. An engorged I. *ricinis* female is pictured earlier in the chapter.

The following figure shows areas of highest Lyme disease risk. We know that the map is slightly behind the reality since areas on the west coast and in Florida are now considered high risk.

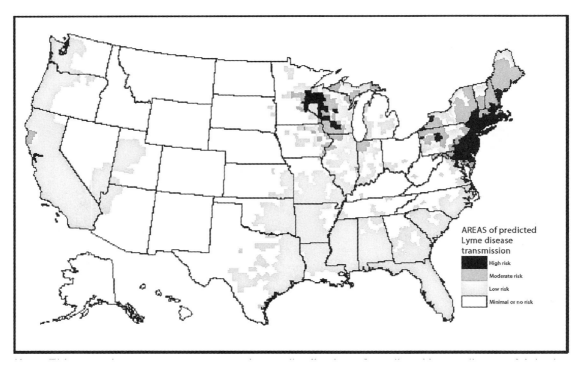

National Lyme disease risk map with four categories of risk
Source: CDC. Accessed March 2013

Initially, some researchers felt that IF the tick was NOT Ixodes *dammini* (now *scapularis*) any resulting signs or symptoms could not be Lyme. Only *dammini* could spread Lyme. While I have trouble understanding this limited focus, time has shown that a number of other species have transmitted Bb, such as I. *spinipalis* and I. *muris*. Depending on the locale, between 1% and 90% of local ticks have been shown to harbor Bb. As mentioned, there is strong suspicion that Bb have been found in the dog tick in regions just south of Philadelphia, but this has not been adequately confirmed. If it is not currently true, who knows what will prove true next week, next month, or next year?

PEARL: Ticks are a perfect vector for spirochetes like Bb. From an evolutionary perspective, the spirochete is one of the oldest bacteria, which has developed for millions of years alongside the tick. Spirochetes have evolved multiple ways to survive both independently and in symbiotic relationships with tick vectors. The December 2011 edition of National Geographic *reports that* Borrelia burgdorferi *was recovered from the body of a man frozen in the Alps for 5 thousand years. The Iceman may have been the first Lyme patient. Who says Bb are not persistent?*

To reiterate, ticks are cesspools and incubators of infection. If there is a tick bite of any kind, be vigilant. Remove the tick properly and save it. Mark on the calendar the date of the tick bite. Remember that date. Consider prophylaxis. Maybe Bb and other infectious agents have not been found in all ticks everywhere because no one has had the opportunity to look at all ticks everywhere (or even some ticks in a few places). Ticks are just being ticks and getting on with their lives. If a deer, or a chipmunk, or a pet, or a child gets in the way, the tick doesn't know and doesn't care as long as she survives. To be safe, presume all ticks are infected and all tick bites transmit disease.

PEARL: When researching images to be used to illustrate this chapter, I continued to come across photographs of exceptional quality from one source in particular: The Dartmoor Tick Watch Project. This endeavor was initiated by Keith Ryan, PhD, an electron microscopist originally from Hayle, in Cornwall, England. Trained as a botanist and zoologist, Dr. Ryan managed the electron microscopy unit at the Marine Biological Association of the UK in Plymouth for over 20 years. He had never seen a tick until the summer of 2008, when he was cutting bracken with the Dartmoor Preservation Association.

One of his teammates had a dog that came out of the vegetation with six ticks. Keith took the ticks home in a jar and examined them using a stereomicroscope. His interest culminated in the year-long Dartmoor Tick Watch project. His work has resulted in much useful information as demonstrated on these pages. Once he learned of this Compendium, *Keith became an important resource and supporter. He stresses safety first and underscores the importance of disease prevention.*

Chapter 3   GENTLE IMMUNOLOGY – Detailed chapter contents

Chapter 3

GENTLE IMMUNOLOGY

Never lose your ignorance, you can't replace it.
Andy Capp comic strip by Reg Smythe

Today we have an almost overwhelming amount of information about the immune system. Yet, we still have very little understanding. While we can describe some immune processes down to the molecular level, we have yet to appreciate the complexity of this vast, interconnected system.

While there are many theories about how the immune system may impact patients with TBIs, we simply don't know enough to say with confidence how these interactions might work. One thing is clear: some foundation in basic immunology is required to understand the pathophysiology of TBDs and to assess symptoms, interpret lab findings, diagnose, and treat these patients. When I was in medical school, we barely had T and B cells to worry about. This discipline has gotten much more complex. I had to learn everything all over again when I was working on the development of treatments for autoimmune diseases.

Despite all that you will read here about the importance of a basic understanding of immunology to your overall ability to comprehend and manage TBIs, the following chapter is INTERMINABLE. Frankly, what follows is a summary of the material I had to gather and understand before I could write this book. Unfortunately, sometimes four pages of explanation was required to underscore a one-line concept presented later in the text. Still, all these ideas are ultimately related and you will be able to understand why Lyme persists and why certain guidelines are not scientifically valid based on the immunology included in this chapter. Everything does eventually make sense.

Unfortunately, no one had put all the concepts in one place before. This must be my fate, karma, kismet. My biggest fear is that reading this chapter will dampen your enthusiasm for the rest of the book, which for the most part is much livelier. I tried separating the information into two chapters and then one chapter with an appendix and hiding the chapter in the middle of the book like an intracellular spirochete. I finally had to bite the bullet and write.

Read as much as you can tolerate straight-up. Then know where to find this foundation material when you need it to understand ideas presented later on. I had to place the immunology basics up front because so much of the other core information is built on this platform. As with the remainder of the book, use what you can and leave the rest, coming back as needed to fill in any gaps. At least page through this chapter and see what's here so you can return when you need more background.

I. INTRODUCTION

I once had a specialist tell me, "All disease is just the cry of a broken immune system." While I don't know if that statement is true, immune response to insult accounts for the majority of symptoms found in many diseases. In the case of TBIs, an understanding of basic immunologic principles is needed to comprehend the complexity of these diseases in terms of clinical course, manifestations, diagnosis, laboratory confirmation, and treatment.

Recognizing that the immune system is indeed complex helps to explain why it can be so difficult to diagnose and treat many conditions. Also, the fact that most of the pathogens transmitted by ticks affect many organ systems, concurrently or sequentially with varying severity, adds to the intricacies of patient management. Further, the possibility of the immune system having to confront multiple co-infections at once means that TBIs can be the ultimate medical challenge.

Whenever you try to simplify a complex topic you run the risk of over-generalizing, skipping logic steps, and introducing inaccuracies in order to condense the material into manageable form. In my estimation, after working with many immune-mediated conditions, science has only begun to understand this area. In two decades, many of these points may be moot. As with all the topics in this text, the literature is voluminous, contradictory, and petty in many cases. I will present only the material that is most pertinent to understanding TBIs. This means that there is much immunology that is left out. I wish I could have left out more, but I couldn't leave logic gaps since the material presented here does appear in the literature and is important for comprehending TBIs.

One of my favorite novels is Joseph Heller's *Catch-22*. While funny, this book is also painfully true and the term "Catch 22" has remained in our lexicon since the novel was first published in 1961. In the story, a military pilot wants to stop flying bombing missions. He pretends to be crazy to get out. But the truth is that to want to stop dropping bombs is quite sane. You'd have to be crazy to want to keep bombing. That is the "catch." Just another example of a frustrating cycle of absurdity. The more a plan makes sense, the more impossible it becomes. Well, I find myself in a "Catch-22" situation. To summarize immunology to the degree to which it is useful in the clinic, I have to use terms that are understandable *only* if you already know the information. Repeatedly, I had to use words not yet introduced in order to define words that you do not yet know. I eventually had to accept that this was just the nature of the immunology beast. This is especially true when discussing major histocompatibility complex molecules (MHCs), clusters of differentiation (CDs), cytokines, complement, and all the convoluted processes these concepts entail.

Nonetheless, the truth remains that if the reader does not understand some basic immunology, she could get irretrievably lost in future chapters. Many times writers assume that readers have knowledge that they do not have. Forgive redundancies, since I may be repeating myself so that you do not have to shovel through past material in order to understand a concept. Remember for every section in this chapter there are multiple books written on just that topic. Many terms are defined again in the *Glossary*.

II. BASIC IMMUNOLOGY

The immune response is designed to protect an organism from harm through many layers of defense. This system is composed of proteins and other molecules, cells, tissues, and organs. The immune response is extremely efficient and can defend against just about anything from minute RNA viruses up to huge parasitic worms. This organization communicates within a complicated network with numerous bridges and cross-links so if a foreign invader gets past one level of defense, the host has just begun to fight.

Immune defense relies on being able to tell what is *self* from what is not. Once a molecule or cell has been determined to be non-*self*, the immune response ignites and either inactivates or eliminates the foreign substance so that it no longer poses a threat.

Each day, the body is assailed with thousands of potential irritants and invaders. Pollens land in the eyes and nose, and many germs are inhaled or swallowed. The body employs defensive measures at all levels. In humans the first layer of protection includes physical barriers such as skin, eyelashes, cilia in both the nose and upper respiratory tract, and earwax. These obvious barricades block entry into the *self*.

The nose, eyes, and mouth are all potential gateways into an organism. Here saliva, mucus, and tears serve to flush away irritants. Further, they contain enzymes that lyse the cell walls of some bacteria. Mucus in the GI tract and respiratory tree not only flushes foreign material, but also traps and tangles pathogens. Once an infectious agent lands in the stomach, it is blasted by stomach acid and digestive enzymes. Mast cells also line the nose, throat, lungs, and inside layers of the skin and invaders must also get past them. These systems are quite efficient. Nonetheless, with the constant bombardment of foreign proteins, some invaders manage to get through this front line.

The next level of defense will include physiologic processes such as coughing, sneezing, or vomiting to expel the foreign agents. Urine, sweat, and stool (usually diarrhea) also transport pathogens out of the body. Vomiting and diarrhea may be the first indication that pathogens have entered the GI tract, while mucus and coughing may suggest a problem in the pulmonary tree. Mucus not only flushes, it ensnares invaders that are then expelled through coughing or spitting.

Additional physiologic defenses can be employed. The enzymes found in breast milk can bind to pathogens and damage them. Proteins called defensins can kill certain pathogens or inactivate some toxins. Vaginal secretions become acidic at menarche, and semen can contain defensins that can bind to cell membranes and cause pathogens to lose essential ions and nutrients. Gastric acid in the stomach has been shown to be effective against some pathogens, and researchers are learning that patients on long-term acid suppressors may have more respiratory infections over time. Normal flora in the gut can overwhelm pathogens and alter the local environment, making life more difficult for invaders as they attempt to cross through the gut into the circulation. Similarly, healthy vaginal flora keeps pathogens in check and reduces the likelihood that infectious organisms will reach sufficient numbers to cause disease.

A number of tissue and organ systems play critical roles in immune defense. We will start with the largest and most visible organ in the body, the skin. Skin is tough and impermeable to most bacteria and viruses. The epidermis contains cells that provide early warning that an intruder has entered. Macrophages in the skin are called Langerhans cells, and these phagocytize any trespassers they can find. Skin also has substances that inactivate some pathogens, which helps explain why you usually don't wake up moldy in the morning.

The skin often presents a nice microcosm of the immune system at work. If the skin is cut, thousands of pathogens enter through the break. The body works quickly to send in the troops to prevent infection. The cut will bleed, and the blood will flush out pathogens. (Cuts can bleed a little and the world won't come to an end. Some bleeding can be a good thing.) When the bleeding stops, the body will begin to seal off the wound. Here is where your scout leader told you to wash and flush the wound with soap and water.

A puncture wound can either be sterile or dirty. (Sterile is when I was busy talking to a patient in the ER just before I started to stitch his cut. I was so distracted that I drove the clean needle through my flesh instead of his. I replaced the contaminated materials and pretended that nothing had happened.) A puncture seals off quickly, so if there is a chance of contamination, the wound should be flushed with antiseptic and water – lots of water. A good flush does not guarantee that infection will not occur. That is why a tetanus shot is given for deep puncture wounds. A tick bite is a puncture wound, and we know how dirty those are.

Most often, a cut, or a puncture, or a splinter in the skin does not get infected, but not for lack of trying. If a cut gets infected, it is usually by the common organisms on the skin. The tissue will get inflamed, and over hours, pus (accumulated white cells and debris) will gather. A red streak from the wound going toward the heart may appear. This is called **lymphangitis.** The subsequent display of redness, swelling, heat, pus, and discomfort are all signs that the immune system is active.

Similarly, a bug bite with its red, warm, swollen, uncomfortable bump is a sign of the immune system at work. A tick will often leave a bite spot on the skin that is a red or dark dot where she was attached. The mark may be just a little scab. This is *not* the same as the EM rash that is sometimes associated with Lyme disease.

Other organs involved in immune response are not as obvious as the skin and we are less likely to consider them. Nevertheless, they are just as critical to the efficient function of the entire system. The bone marrow provides all the stem cells that eventually differentiate into any number of distinct cell types. Stem cells have the capacity for self-renewal through mitotic cell division.

The thymus is a relatively small specialized organ of the immune system. As far as we know, the only function of the thymus is to produce and train T cells for their specialized duties. The thymus is especially important in the neonate and in early childhood and is the only organ thought to get smaller with age. Galen, the ancient Greek physician, observed that the thymus noticeably shrinks as the person gets older. Over time, the active thymic cells are replaced with fat. (I can attest to that.) Nevertheless, the thymus continues to produce T cells throughout life. Loss of the thymus in childhood results in immunodeficiency and a high risk of infection.

The lymph infrastructure is also important to effective immune function. This network includes lymph fluid, lymph vessels, lymph nodes, and the spleen. Much of this system provides the foundation that allows for the movement of the cells and humors (biochemicals) of the immune response. Beyond infrastructure, the lymph system also has an active role in overall host defense. I spent a day sorting the following terms, since there is even controversy and confusion about the definition of these basic elements.

- **Blood** is about half plasma and half cells: red, white, and platelets. Lymph and blood both have liquid and cellular parts. RBCs are the most predominant cells in the blood. Blood has more protein in the plasma than does the lymph, since much protein does not readily cross the capillary walls. Blood contains clotting factors including fibrinogen.

- **Plasma** is the liquid part of both blood and lymph and is mostly water. Plasma *does* contain fibrinogen, a clotting factor. Along with H_2O, plasma contains proteins (primarily albumin), glucose, ions, hormones, CO_2, and wastes. Plasma is a primary transporter of wastes.

- **Lymph** is the plasma that diffuses from the blood in the general circulation and surrounds most tissues. Lymph is considered part of the interstitial fluid that is found around cells. Eventually the lymph returns to the lymph vessels, gradually moving through nodes and onto a re-connection with the blood circulation. Like blood, lymph has both a liquid and cellular component, but no red cells. Lymph is plasma PLUS the WBCs that float around in its fluid. Lymph often carries pathogens or other foreign proteins to the nodes where they are phagocytized. Lymph transports WBCs (especially lymphocytes), small proteins, and bacteria and other microbes. Lymph differs in composition in various parts of the body. Near the intestine, the lymph (called chyle) contains more fat than lymph from other areas.

- **Serum** is the fluid part of the blood AFTER clotting factors are removed. Fluid is called *lymph* when it is part of the interstitial fluid that is found between cells and tissues. In contrast, the fluid is called *serum* when found within blood vessels carrying circulating blood. While lymph can have WBCs present, serum has: NO cells! NO clotting factors! NO fibrinogen! But, YES, serum has all the other proteins that are NOT involved in clotting. Antibodies are present. A sample of blood from a patient is often spun in a centrifuge to remove the cells, leaving a serum sample to be used in lab testing.

On its travels back to the subclavian veins where it re-enters the bloodstream, lymph passes through at least one lymph node. Here macrophages gobble up any bacteria the lymph may contain. Unlike the circulation of blood, the lymph system is open, passive, and has no central pump. Actually it's rather sloshy and fluid can build up in dependent areas such as ankles. Lymph transport depends on the kindness of others such as valves in vessels and the contraction of nearby muscle to keep the fluid moving toward the mid-chest. A patient with swollen ankles is often told to walk so that the pressure from muscle contraction will help force the lymph centrally.

Usually lymph nodes are small round, organs connected by lymph vessels. Here awaits a small fortress guarded by many phagocytes. Normally, the nodes are barely palpable. However, nodes will swell (**lymphadenopathy**) and become tender if there is an excess of pathogens and white cells present, as occurs during an infection. Enlarged nodes are most commonly found in the neck, axilla, and groin. Unfortunately, cancer cells also spread in the lymph and lodge in the nodes. Presence of cancer in lymph nodes is used to stage the spread of the malignant cells.

I have a special attachment to the spleen, since many people believe that is the proper way to pronounce my last name. (Spreen actually is derived from the Spree River in Berlin.) In fact, the spleen is a purple-grey organ found in the left upper abdomen. This organ is almost like a giant lymph node but has more responsibility, acting like a blood filter. The spleen removes old RBCs, recycles iron, and holds in reserve a supply of blood in case of emergency. For the immune system, the spleen contains the majority of the body's monocytes, which turn into macrophages and dendritic cells. The spleen holds cells that make antibodies and removes antibody-coated bacteria. If the spleen is removed there is an increased risk of infection and a decreased response to some vaccines. In infection, the spleen will become enlarged and more easily palpable. In the humoral medicine of ancient Greece, the spleen was associated with melancholy.

III. BUILDING AN IMMUNOLOGIC FOUNDATION

Despite the best efforts of these defenders, some invaders survive and begin to cause problems. Of course, the immune system is just beginning the battle. While nonspecific assaults on the invaders continue, more targeted attacks also begin. The immunologic troops are now fighting on many levels. Here is where things get almost unbelievably complex.

Once a pathogen invades, a number of factors combine to determine if the patient actually gets sick:

- The amount of infectious agent transmitted

- Whether the individual is susceptible to disease caused by that agent

- Whether the person had been exposed to that pathogen in the past

- The overall health or robustness of the immune system at the time of the attack

- The genetic predisposition of the person in terms of auto-immune reactions

- The general health of the host including nutritional status and co-morbid conditions

Remember, all a germ wants to do is to set up a happy home. The immune system will do everything in its power to prevent that. This can get ugly. If a pathogen does wind up inside a living being where it does not belong, the host organism will initiate an *innate* immune response. We are all born with some degree of immune defense. These protective mechanisms are immediate, nonspecific, and found in nearly all forms of life from plants to snails to mammals. Innate immune response depends on the body's ability to tell it*self* from foreign material. If the body cannot tell what is *self*, it does not know what to attack. A molecule can be recognized as non-*self* if it is foreign, or, if cells inside the host are tagged as damaged, injured, or otherwise stressed. These broken cells send out distress chemicals. The distinction between *self* and non-*self* is made at the molecular level. Either way, once a protein (antigen) has been tagged as "other than *self*," phagocytosis is the process that usually eliminates the foreign entity from the body.

Innate Immunity

In most cases, newborns have no prior exposure to pathogens and are especially susceptible to infection. Fortunately, several layers of **passive** protection are provided by the mother. During pregnancy, a particular type of antibody, called IgG, is transported from mom to baby directly across the placenta. Therefore, even at birth, human babies have high levels of some antibodies with the same antigen specifications as those found in the mother. Breast milk or colostrum also contains antibodies that are transferred to the gut of the baby and protect against some infections until the newborn can synthesize its own antibodies. This is passive immunity because the fetus does not actually make any memory cells or antibodies of its own, it only borrows them. Passive immunity is usually short-term, lasting a few days to several months.

In addition to this passive immune capability, the neonate has an innate, nonspecific mechanism to ward off infection. Here, a foreign protein is identified as alien or non-*self* and a sequence of events occur to minimize the impact of the invader. The response is rapid and nonspecific.

Innate immunity does not require an earlier contact with the offending substance to become active and no memory of the encounter is recorded. Each time the same foreign irritant presents, the innate system starts from the beginning with a general and nonspecific reaction.

These inborn responses rely both on cell-mediated reactions as well as on humoral components such as complement and cytokines. Complement is one of the primary humoral components of the innate immune system, while various phagocytes provide the cell support. More detail on these complicated processes is outlined below.

> PEARL: *The* **humoral** *immune response (HIR) is comprised of all the immune defenses that do* **not** *directly involve cells.*

Acquired Immunity

With all its complex biochemistry, the innate immune system serves as a bridge to the acquired or adaptive system. With the adaptive immune response, the defense is specific for the proteins on a particular pathogen. There is a time lag while recognition occurs, and the maximal response does not occur immediately. A repeat exposure to a specific antigen recalls immunologic memory.

Memory is the key differentiation between the innate and acquired immune systems. When B cells are activated, they replicate, and some of their offspring become long-lived memory cells. Thereafter, throughout their life, the memory cells will remember each specific pathogen encountered and can mount a strong response if that pathogen is detected again. (You don't catch the exact same cold twice.) This is adaptive because it occurs during the lifetime of the individual. Here the response is specific for the proteins on a distinct pathogen. Memory prepares the immune system for future challenges and can be active or passive, short-term or long-term. This memory allows the adaptive system to respond faster and stronger each time it sees an old enemy.

Again there are both cell-mediated and humoral responses in the acquired system, but here the immune response targets the specific invader. After the intruder is gone, the host can summon up the details if that pathogen should come calling again. This is a definite advantage.

The terms innate and acquired were first described decades ago. Now as we learn more, there are so many bridges and links that the distinctions are not as clear. Both the innate and acquired immune systems have cell-mediated and humoral components. A later section describes in punishing detail both the various cells involved in immune response and the various humors.

The humoral response involves antibodies and biochemicals such as cytokines and hormones that are intricately involved in body defenses. The old term would be body humors. These nominally separate components of the immune response are so busy interacting with one another that they are often hard to distinguish. B cells make antibodies that interact with T cells that stimulate B cells, while all are awash in a humoral stew. There are innumerable bridges and cross-links between

systems. Immune responses are also said to be primary or secondary, or specific versus nonspecific.

With infection, the time course of an immune response begins with the initial encounter with the pathogen (or initial vaccination) and leads to the formation and maintenance of active immunological memory. Long-term active memory is acquired after infection through activation of B cells (and a whole bunch of other stuff, but B cell activation serves our purposes). Immunity can also be generated artificially through vaccination.

Phagocytosis

No matter how the immune system is termed, labeled, or categorized, essentially all aspects use phagocytosis in some capacity to defend the host. Once proteins are identified as non-*self*, phagocytes engulf them and destroy or otherwise remove them from the host, like mini-garbage collectors. Many cells are able to phagocytize. These cells swallow pathogens and keep normal tissue healthy by removing injured or dead cells. The name phagocyte comes from the Greek meaning to eat or devour and the cells are classified as either professional or non-professional types. Professional phagocytes include neutrophils, monocytes, macrophages, and both dendritic and mast cells. They contain a molecule on their surfaces that identifies foreign antigens. One liter of human blood contains about a billion phagocytes. The non-professional phagocytes often take out foreign organisms or injured cells but are not necessarily specific. Non-pros don't have opsonins, which are substances in serum that coat the membrane of a foreign organism and increase the rate of phagocytosis. For non-professionals, phagocytosis is not necessarily their primary function.

During an infection, chemical signals attract the phagocytes to places where the pathogen has invaded the body. These chemicals can come from the pathogen or from other immune cells already present. After a phagocyte engulfs its target, it lyses and kills. The foreign material gets trapped in an intracellular vesicle and is eventually destroyed (some would say digested) by enzymes or by cell rupture.

Neutrophils and monocytes do most of their work in the blood, while macrophages function best in the tissues. Macrophages are widely distributed cells and they lie close to the spaces where tissue and blood interface, such as in lungs, liver, joints, the lining around nerves, and kidneys. Some circulating phagocytes patrol the body looking for something to gobble, while others politely wait to be called to specific locales by cytokines or other communication chemicals.

Alas, if all was perfection, no one would ever get infected to the point of disease. Pathogens have devised many ways to avoid phagocytosis including:

- The pathogens hide in places where it is hard for the phagocytes to reach them, like on the top of unbroken skin or deep in joint spaces where there may not be ample blood flow.

- The pathogens have mechanisms by which they suppress the inflammatory response to the point that the phagocytes don't know if, or how to respond.

- Some pathogens can interfere with chemotaxis.

- Certain infectious agents can trick the immune system into thinking it's part of the *self*. The spirochete that causes syphilis hides from phagocytes by coating its surface with fibronectin. Borrelia is also a spirochete, but we do not know its capacity in this regard, although we have suspicions that Bb is a master manipulator.

- Some infectious microbes seal themselves in a protective capsule.

- Certain pathogens are able to kill or inactivate the phagocyte.

- Some pathogenic species can interrupt immune signals (e.g., decrease cytokines or alter antigenic presentations).

Despite so many clever survival techniques developed by pathogens, phagocytosis remains a critical part of both the innate and acquired immune response.

Antigens and Antibodies

While phagocytosis is important in the innate system, acquired immunity makes this process much more targeted. An antibody (Ab) is part of the acquired immune system and is used to identify and neutralize foreign substances. An antigen (Ag) is simply a protein. Proteins cover all cell surfaces and some are recognized as *self*, while others are non-*self*. These proteins can ride on the surface of a pathogen but can also come from other sources as well, so the terms pathogen and antigen are not necessarily interchangeable. All pathogens contain antigens, but not all antigens are pathogens.

PEARL: Paul Ehrlich was the first to use the word antibody. He discovered that if two substances give rise to two different antibodies, then they themselves must be different. These substances were called antigens. The name antigen comes from their role as antibody-generators. Dr. Ehrlich outlined the side-chain theory to explain antigen-antibody specificity in humoral immunity. We will see his name again when we review the commonalities between syphilis and Borrelia and when we talk about Ehrlichia, a known co-infection in TBD. Dr. Ehrlich was portrayed by Edward G. Robinson in the movie Dr. Ehrlich's Magic Bullet.

While the antigens associated with TBIs are located on the microbe's surface, other antigens can be part of a toxin, cancer cell, chemical, or pollen. These antigens do not happen to be infectious. Some of these come directly from the environment such as toxic chemicals or allergens. Of course, many antigens are infectious and are called **pathogens** and include bacteria, viruses, fungi, and various other organisms.

Some antigens are produced by the pathogen inside the host. Certain bacteria form **endotoxins** that may be responsible for some of the signs and symptoms of the bacterial disease. One example is the bacterium that causes Strep throat; it makes a toxin that inflames the throat and can also damage other organs such as heart valves, kidneys, and neurons in the brain. Some antigens are harmful in certain species, but not in others. Dogs don't get poison ivy, but they are susceptible to Lyme disease.

Antigens on the body's own cells are called **autoantigens** and should be recognized as *self*, unless the cells are old, sick, damaged, or dead. Then, chemical signals communicate that it is time for these non-functional cells to be removed as though they were foreign.

Once a B cell gets wind of a foreign antigen, it matures into a plasma cell that starts to crank out antibodies, also interchangeably called **immunoglobulins** or Igs. There is a highly specific binding site between the antigen and antibody that allows the Ab to identify and bind *ONLY* with the unique Ag in the midst of millions of other molecules in the organism. While there is some limited **cross-reactivity** that will complicate our lives somewhat in future chapters, for the most part the Ag/Ab relationship is quite specific.

PEARL: Complexity alert: B cells are lymphocytes that transform into plasma cells and thereby secrete antibodies against specific antigens. Often T cells work to activate the B cells. If T cells cause the activation, an antigen-presenting cell (APC) displays an antigen (Ag) to a helper T cell, priming it. When a B cell then processes and presents that same Ag to the primed T helper cell, the T cell releases cytokines to activate the B cell. The B cell identifies pathogens when antibodies on its surface bind to a specific foreign antigen. This Ag/Ab complex is taken in by the B cell and lysed into peptides. The B cell then displays that antigen's peptides on its surface major histocompatibility complex molecule (MHC). This combination of MHC and antigen attracts a matching helper T cell, which releases various chemicals that activate the B cell. As the activated B cell then begins to divide, its offspring (plasma cells) secrete millions of copies of the antibody that recognizes this antigen. The antibodies circulate in lymph and blood and bind to the pathogens that show the antigen and mark them for destruction by complement or for removal by phagocytes. I warned you it was complex.

Antibodies are found in blood, tissues, fluids, and in secretions, such as IgE coming out of a runny nose. Antibodies can also directly bind to some toxins and interfere with receptors on pathogens that the invaders use to infect cells. When an Ab binds to the outer coat of a virus or bacteria, it can stop their movement through cell walls. The antibodies signal to the complement system to come help remove the invader. When an antibody binds to a toxin, it is called an **antitoxin.** If that toxin is from venom, the antibody is called **antivenom** (or antivenin). This binding generally impedes the action of the toxin, as someone who was snake-bit will tell you.

The **plasma cell** is the antibody factory. All antibodies have similar globular Y-shaped structures, except that each has a section at the tips of the two branches of the Y that is unique to that antibody and allows it to bind to its specific antigen. This one-of-a-kind region on an antibody that allows it to recognize its matching antigen is called an **epitope.** There is a highly specific binding site between the epitope and antibody, which allows the Ab to identify and bind *only* with its unique Ag in the midst of millions of molecules in the organism. Humans generate billions of different antibodies, each able to bind with a distinct epitope of an antigen.

The different tip structures on the antibodies are called **antigen-binding sites.** The huge assortment of antibodies allows the immune system to identify a wide diversity of antigens. Antibodies recognize an antigen and lock onto it, thereby tagging it for attack by other parts of the immune system, usually phagocytes. These Igs can activate proteins called **complement** that assist in killing infectious invaders and help in the formation of Ag/Ab complexes.

Since antibodies exist freely in the blood stream, they are said to be part of the humoral immune system. Circulating antibodies are made by plasma B cells that specifically respond to only one antigen. These antibodies contribute to immunity in several ways: they prevent pathogens from entering or damaging cells by binding to them, they stimulate removal of pathogens by phagocytes, and they trigger destruction of pathogens by stimulating other immune responses, such as the complement pathway.

In mammals, there are at least 5 distinct classes of antibodies including IgA, IgD, IgE, IgG, and IgM. More details are presented for each of these under *Humoral Response* later in this chapter. Each Ig class differs in its biological properties and locations, and each deals with specific antigen. Since structure determines function, biochemistry dictates that each antibody deals only with its own antigen like a key fitting only its unique lock. By binding to an Ag, the Ab creates an Ag/Ab complex, which can clump and precipitate. The complexes like to float on lipid rafts which make them prime targets for phagocytes. (I have a great mental image here.)

Many of the lab tests used to support the diagnoses of TBIs rely on the highly specific binding between antigens and antibodies. When the immune system finds a protein that is foreign, or non-*self,* it constructs a MATCHING antibody that can bind with that antigen in a specific lock and key fashion. One antigen, one antibody. Because of the nature of RNA and DNA, the system cannot make any other kind of antibody. Based on this premise, a number of testing methods have been developed that recognize and measure either an antigen and its corresponding antibody, or an antibody and its matching antigen. Antibody tests are indirect in that they are the response to an antigen that must have been around at some point. Usually you can't prove that an organism is present NOW, only that it had been present. Just remember, there is NO WAY an antibody can be around today if its corresponding antigen wasn't originally there to induce its formation. "This must be distinctly understood or nothing wonderful can come from the story."[1]

ELISA, Western blot, and numerous other serological and agglutination techniques depend on the ability of an antigen to bind with its specifically-designed antibody. Most of these test methods involve the adherence of a known antigen to a surface and then washing a sample of unknown antibodies over the antigen. If the antigen and antibody can bind, they will. Then, depending on the method: dyes, radioactivity, florescence, or location on a test strip, the antigen/antibody complex is recognized and documented. Serologic tests use the smallest amount of antigen (or the largest amount of dilution) to determine if binding occurs. The presence of antibodies that could only have been manufactured after exposure to a specific antigen provides supportive evidence that the antigen had been around either now or in the past. Today, thousands of antigens corresponding to hundreds of pathogens have been isolated and are available for use in diagnostic testing.

Inflammation

Inflammation is the battle that goes on inside a body in its own defense. The first response of the immune system to assault is inflammation. The term comes from the Latin meaning to set on fire. Inflammation occurs in response to pathogens, cell damage, or irritants. For example, your thumb can be red, hot, swollen, and painful because it is infected with MRSA, was hit with a hammer, or has a nasty case of poison ivy. Inflammation is a protective mechanism that tries to remove the irritant while it stimulates healing. Without inflammatory processes, wounds would never heal.

Since ancient times, four primary signs and symptoms of inflammation have been recognized.

---

1 *Narrator in Charles Dickens' A Christmas Carol*

Calor	-	Warmth
Dolor	-	Pain
Tumor	-	Swelling
Rubor	-	Redness

These four manifestations are due to increased blood flow into the affected area and the release of cytokines and eicosanoids by injured cells. There are four types of eicosanoids, but prostaglandins and leukotrienes are most pertinent in the study of TBIs. Prostaglandins produce fever and the dilation of blood vessels that account for the warmth and redness. The blood vessels become more permeable and plasma leaks out, causing swelling. Blood vessels engorge causing redness. Blood is warm, and when the tissue gets swollen and hot, it can hurt. Consider a simple bee sting. Almost instantaneously, the area becomes red, hot, swollen, and painful. That's inflammation.

Leukotrienes, a second type of fatty eicosanoid, are also important in the inflammatory process, especially in terms of **chemotaxis**. Leukotrienes attract neutrophils and other responding cells and recruit them to the inflamed area. Chemotaxis causes these motile cells to move toward higher concentrations of a chemical.

This movement of responder cells and release of potent biochemicals is beneficial in terms of helping the immune system mount a defense, but can be bad in that some responses can result in severe symptoms for the patient. Leukotrienes are largely responsible for the common manifestations in asthma and allergies. They cause vascular permeability and constriction of the airway and are closely associated with histamine reactions. I was involved in working on the first leukotriene antagonist for treating asthma. Unfortunately, the biochemistry was not understood well enough at the time to develop the drug in the best way. Today, the role of leukotrienes in conveying messages both in the immune system and CNS is just beginning to be explored. There is some evidence that these complex chemicals may play a more significant role in cardiac and neuropsychiatric illnesses. There is a hypothesized connection between leukotriene action and the neuropsychiatric manifestations of TBDs. Leukotrienes are also important in sustaining the inflammatory response, which is great if the patient needs it, but can be catastrophic for the patient in status asthmaticus or in the throes of chronic TBI.

PEARL: What is the mechanism by which the profound fatigue found in Lyme and certain other diseases occurs? The brain of a healthy person is usually isolated from the potentially caustic effects of the immune response by the BBB. Contrarily, patients with chronic inflammation may have immune cells infiltrating their brains. These cells, in the course of trying to do their job, release a number of powerful chemicals that have been associated with fatigue, tiredness, and a listless feeling, as well as numerous other neuropsychiatric symptoms. In the case of Lyme, both the physical presence of the spirochetes and the biochemical assault from the immune humors might contribute to what the patient experiences.

When calor, dolor, tumor, or rubor are observed, then the inflammatory process is underway. These are signs that a battle has begun inside the body in its own defense. Signs of inflammation may be the first indication that there is a problem. The response will continue and adjust its intensity until the body feels that the threat is gone.

Many infectious processes cause a similar underlying pattern of signs and symptoms. When you cough, sneeze, get a sore throat, aches, fatigue, headache, and fever, you know you are "coming down with something." You just don't know what. Every layperson with a cold thinks they are dying from some terrible bacteria, while every HCP knows that it's a mild viral URI. Try *not* giving this patient antibiotics.

Almost *all* systemic infections whether bacterial, protozoal, viral, fungal, etcetera, will cause a similar pattern of basic underlying signs and symptoms. From the common cold to full-blown AIDS, there is likely to be a baseline symptom pattern of fatigue, headache, generalized aches, appetite changes, weakness, mental fog, fever, sleepiness, irritability, GI upset, etc. This is the immune system at work, and that's a big reason why there is so much misdiagnosis. There are thousands of pathogens that cause at least some of these symptoms. With TBIs, when you are likely to be dealing with multiple pathogens, you have your work cut out for you.

One problem with diagnosing TBIs is that so many of the early signs and symptoms of these diseases are the general manifestations of inflammation. While each TBI may have certain symptoms as its calling card, most present, at least initially, just like every other infectious process in the history of the universe. With most infections, the usual inflammatory symptoms of headache, fever, aches, lethargy, mental cloudiness, sleep disturbances, irritability, and GI complaints manifest. These are the universal signs of inflammation, making discriminating diagnoses difficult or delayed. This overlap of symptoms is the reason so many TBI patients are told that they "just have a little virus" and other patients swear they have influenza when they have a cold. Initially, almost all infections look similar, and they can be hard to tell apart. While inflammation is a signal that the body is fighting hard against a foreign invader, the signs and symptoms are unpleasant, and the patient usually wishes that the body would tone down the defense already.

While evidence of the immune system at work should be viewed in a positive light, the signs and symptoms that result from the powerful inflammatory chemicals can make the patient miserable. For example, prostaglandins can cause fever, pain, and swelling. We often treat these manifestations of inflammation with drugs that decrease prostaglandin activity (aspirin, NSAIDs, acetaminophen, COX-2 inhibitors, and the ultimate anti-inflammatory: steroids). However, balance is the goal. If the immune system is prevented from performing its critical function, healing may be significantly delayed.

Inflammation is considered to be either acute or chronic. Acute signs and symptoms occur after an injury or an invasion by a pathogen. Neutrophils, monocytes, and macrophages are the first responders. The chemicals involved are primarily vasoactive compounds and eicosanoids. The reaction starts immediately upon insult and continues for a few days. Either the acute reaction resolves, an abscess forms with neutrophils accounting for the majority of the pus, or the process moves into a chronic state.

In chronic inflammation, an immune response persists because 1) the pathogens are still present, 2) there is an on-going irritant or stimulus, or 3) an autoimmune component is in play. Supplementing the monocytes and macrophages, both B and T cells, as well as fibroblasts, are involved. Signs of chronic inflammation may be due to increased cytokines, which are responsible for further signs of inflammation such as fatigue, overall discomfort, GI problems, sleep disorders, and an increase in stress hormones. In addition to increased cytokine levels, chronic inflammation is associated with higher levels of γ-interferon. Chronic inflammation may continue for months or years and result in tissue destruction, fibrosis, and necrosis.

One more caveat before we move on. Unfortunately many people, including HCPs, use the terms inflammation and infection interchangeably. Infection is just one way to induce inflammation. The suffixes *-osis* and *-itis* can help here. Use *-osis* when a tissue is inflamed and *-itis* when the tissue is infected. These conventions are not used universally, but they are supposed to be. Likewise, half the people carrying around an EpiPen sincerely believe they are allergic to bee stings when, in fact, they have an inflamed area around the site. Try *not* giving them an EpiPen.

Cell-mediated Immune Response

Immune response is somewhat artificially divided into the role of the cells and the role of the biochemicals. Cell-mediated response, or CMR, is any response by the immune system that is performed by its cells and not by the numerous chemicals, hormones, or humors that are also involved. We now know that these two categories are so interrelated that it is quite difficult to separate them. Nonetheless, when we are trying to understand new or complex material, some sorting is required.

The **stem cell** is the fundamental cell of the immune system as well as many other systems. The majority of cells that have

a function in immune response start out as stem cells. These cells, which have been the subject of never-ending debate recently, can differentiate into a diverse array of specialized cells. (Before some folks get upset because I even dare mention the controversial term stem cell, the cells we discuss here are all *in vivo*, and while they have the potential to transform into a number of different cell types, if you water one like a seed it will *not* grow into a baby or a dandelion or a hedgehog, so relax.)

By definition, a stem cell must be able to renew itself through mitotic cell division (while remaining undifferentiated) *and* have the potency to evolve into many other distinct cell types. As a class, stem cells are busy. In adults, these cells act as a repair system, fixing many kinds of broken tissue. In the embryo, stem cells evolve into all manner of specialized cells capable of performing distinct functions *and* at the same time, they regenerate cells in organs such as blood, skin, and the GI tract. The more potent a stem line is, the more kinds of cells it can form.

Cell-mediated response is any response by the immune system that is performed by its cells and not by the numerous biochemicals, hormones, or humors that are also involved. Cellular immunity can begin with activated T cells that are able to cause apoptosis or death in cells that present foreign antigen. These activated agents are responsible for the stimulation of various immune cells and can even target pathogens that have survived inside other cells. One cell stimulates another, and that one activates the next, which rouses the subsequent cell, which motivates the one after that, until my thesaurus runs dry. This is the ultimate immune cascade that branches like a tree from trunk to twig with cells intimately involved throughout. Immune cells are involved in both the innate and acquired immune systems.

PEARL: A mature oak tree might have 500 million root tips and the complexity of the immune cascade makes the tree analogy seem simple.

Cells of the immune system are called white blood cells (WBCs) or **leukocytes**. They start as undifferentiated stem cells that ultimately evolve into blood cells, and then further discriminate into about a half dozen principal kinds of immune cells. By measuring the proportion of the different kinds of white cells, an HCP can gather clues about whether a bacteria, virus, parasite, or allergic process is the source of the problem. Much of the terminology is based on old staining methods from decades ago. Sometimes this nomenclature does not make sense in 2013, but it gives us a place to start. Basically there are two main categories of leukocyte: granulocytes and agranulocytes and everything cascades from there.

Leukocytes: White blood Cells

A. **Granulocytes** – These white cells contain granules in their cytoplasm and have multilobed nuclei so they are sometimes called polymorphonuclear leukocytes or PMNs. There are three types of granulocytes named after what stains them best. Overall granulocytes comprise 50% to 70% of all WBCs. Granulocytes are divided into 3 classes:

1. **Neutrophils** are also called polymorphonuclear neutrophils or PMNs as though they were the only granulocytes around. Since they do comprise the vast majority of PMNs, the term is often used synonymously to only refer to neutrophils. The bone marrow produces trillions of neutrophils every day and releases them into the blood stream. Their life span is less than 24 hours. Once in the blood, neutrophils can move through capillary walls into tissue. They are attracted to foreign material, inflammation products, and bacteria. If you get a splinter, cut, or other insult, neutrophils are attracted to the site by chemotaxis, which causes the cells to move toward higher concentrations of alarm chemicals. Once at the location of the problem, the neutrophils engulf foreign cells and release enzymes, hydrogen peroxide, and other chemicals from its granules to kill the bacteria.

   Neutrophils make up between 35% and 70% of all WBCs, depending on patient age. They are readily attracted by chemotaxis and, along with macrophages, are the primary phagocytes of the immune system. Neutrophils are often the first defenders against bacterial invasion. During an inflammatory process, neutrophils can be broken or killed and in the process, release enzymes that can damage surrounding cells. The debris results in pus, which is mostly dead neutrophils and other trash.

   In severe inflammation or an autoimmune state, neutrophils may attack normal cells and cause damage as is seen in ARDS, IBD, RA, etc. If neutrophils are low, the patient is at additional risk of systemic infection. If neutrophils are high, the patient can be assumed to be mounting an immune response. Neutrophils often increase postoperatively or after a significant burn.

   Note that a few infectious processes can actually decrease neutrophils including Gram negative sepsis, typhoid, brucellosis, and viruses such as hepatitis, mononucleosis, influenza, chickenpox, Colorado tick fever, and HIV. Logically, bone marrow depressants might decrease neutrophils as they might diminish any cell that originates in the marrow. Some conditions including SLE, RA, or other autoimmune-type conditions may cause the neutrophil count to fluctuate.

Neutrophils play a big role in the humoral immune response by releasing proteins and other mediators. These can cause a number of the signs and symptoms of inflammation. For example, if a neutrophil releases its granules in the kidney, this discharge can damage the glomerular cells. Leukotrienes that might be present can increase this damage. Likewise, in the lung, neutrophils can cause damage if granules are released. Conversely, if the neutrophil count in the lung is too low, the person is at increased risk of infection. Neutrophil counts may help determine the type and stage of infection. A guide for interpretation of a differential white cell count is presented in Chapter 19: *Scientific Basis & Interpretation of Study Results.*

PEARL: In medical school many of us learned to look at the neutrophil as a sign of bacterial infection. Today we are beginning to suspect that Lyme disease patients may not use PMNs in the way that we have come to expect. Bb may stimulate largely a monocyte response. This may account for some of the clinical manifestations that seem to be unusual or confusing to us. We are looking for the typical pattern elicited by the neutrophils and we are getting an unfamiliar presentation due to monocyte activity. This is not to say that PMNs are not involved but that their impact may be overshadowed by monocytes. Since monocytes and neutrophils are quite different physiologically, we might expect a different clinical picture. This work is just beginning and may shed future light on why TBIs are so confounding to modern medicine.

PEARL: When Alan MacDonald found evidence of spirochetes in cases of gestational Lyme, detractors said this could not be Lyme because there was not sufficient PMN evidence of inflammation. They were looking for PMNs when they probably should have been looking for monocytes or macrophages.

2. **Eosinophils** are much less common than neutrophils, and their role focuses primarily on parasites in the skin and lungs and their contribution to allergic reactions. While eosinophils are designed primarily to fight parasites, they also play a role in the defense against certain viruses through the RNAases in their granules.

   Eosinophils comprise only a small percentage (1% to 6%) of the circulating white cells. They develop in the bone marrow, and then travel in the blood for several hours before migrating into inflamed tissues where they can remain for about 8 to 12 days. In addition to congregating in infected tissue, they tend to accumulate in the thymus, lower GI tract, spleen, and lymph nodes. There are few, if any, found in healthy lung, skin, or esophageal tissue. If excessive eosinophils are present in these organs, there is pathology present.

Eosinophils respond to calls from chemokines and leukotrienes to sites of parasitic infections caused by intestinal worms called helminths. Over three billion people worldwide are infected with parasitic worms, and eosinophils diminish the ability of the worms to colonize. The helper T cells (TH2) release the activators of the eosinophils and, in turn, the eosinophils present antigens to the T cells.

Eosinophils have an extremely complex biochemistry which enables their multiple functions. Eosinophils contain granules in their cytoplasm that hold powerful chemical mediators with the potential to become involved in multiple immune reactions. We are only beginning to understand these processes. Once activated, they release chemical mediators by degranulation. These chemicals can harm their targets but also injure healthy host tissue as well. As a result, eosinophils have been called the mischief makers of the immune system.

Along with basophils and mast cells, eosinophils mediate the occurrence and severity of allergic and asthmatic reactions. They can release histamines and can stimulate mast cells to do the same. Eosinophils are involved in innumerable bioprocesses including the production of lipid mediators like eicosanoids. They facilitate formation of prostaglandins, enzymes such as elastase, growth factors, and cytokines such as ILs and TNF-α.

Eosinophil levels are high in parasitic diseases, allergic and asthmatic conditions, collagen vascular diseases, GI problems, fungal infections, and to a lesser degree after use of certain drugs like penicillin. With regard to the evaluation of TBI patients, eosinophils may help identify the type of infectious agent or if there is an underlying allergic process. A complete guide for interpretation of a differential white cell count is presented in Chapter 19: *Scientific Basis & Interpretation of Study Results.*

PEARL: Eosinophil cationic protein (ECP) is a biomolecule that is released during degranulation of eosinophils and is related to inflammation, asthma, and parasitic infections. ECP testing is sometimes used to assess level of inflammation, disease progression, and response to treatment. ECP is toxic to neurons so in patients with neuropsychiatric symptoms, measurement of this protein could provide additional information.

3. **Basophils** are the least common granulocyte in the circulation, comprising only 0.01% to 0.3% of the total population. Their name originated because they stain best with basic dyes. Basophils are essential to the nonspecific immune response (innate). These cells have such large granules that their nuclei can barely be seen under the microscope. Basophils carry histamine and, along with mast cells, are important in causing inflammation. Recall that from the immune system's viewpoint, inflammation is a good thing, bringing in more blood and dilating capillary walls so that more immune cells can get to the problem site.

Basophils are similar (perhaps identical) to the mast cells found primarily in tissues. Both store histamine and therefore induce symptoms of allergies. Basophils can also be recruited out of the blood into the tissue when their services are needed. They are involved in many inflammatory reactions. Not only do their granules hold histamine, they also contain heparin which is an anticoagulant. Since histamine is a vasodilator, it increases blood going to the tissues.

When a basophilic granule disintegrates, many other chemicals are released including chondroitin, enzymes such as elastase and lipase, and lipid mediators like leukotrienes and cytokines, many of which contribute to inflammation. Despite all the advertisements touting processed chondroitin as a treatment for osteoarthritis, it is actually a natural molecule. Chondroitin is a major part of the cartilage which helps cushion joints. Chondroitin blocks enzymes that break down the connective tissue and helps make new cartilage while keeping it healthy by drawing fluid into the joint.

Basophils are needed to release IL-4, one of the cytokines in the development of allergies which can influence IgE antibodies. Basophils also help regulate T cells and mediate the magnitude of the secondary immune response. In laboratory testing, basopenia is usually only found in autoimmune urticaria, while basophilia is uncommon and appears occasionally in leukemia or lymphoma. In terms of TBI patients, a high basophil count may suggest allergy, parasites, or response to pollens. With Lyme so often impacting multiple systems, basophil counts may provide clues to what is happening with the patient, or at least lead to better questions.

B. **Agranulocytes** - In contrast to their granular cousins, these WBCs have one-lobed nuclei and few or no granules in their cytoplasm. This does not mean they are not biochemically complex. A sample of the gordian nature of these cells is outlined in a box at the end of this chapter entitled *Immune Markers Applicable to TBIs.* As I refer to CDs, MHCs, and HLAs, look to the box for a more detailed explanation of these concepts. There are primarily two types, with a number of subsets under each group.

1. **Lymphocytes** - As with almost all blood cells, the lymphocytes originate as stem cells. Lymphocytes are present in both blood and lymphatic tissue and account for between 20% and 40% of the total circulating WBCs. They travel from the blood to the lymph and then into the nodes and eventually back into the circulation. In general, lymphocytes recognize foreign antigens, produce antibodies, and help modulate the overall immune response to prevent excessive tissue damage. Distinct lymphocytes have both overlapping and unique functions. B and T cells interact with each other in a mind-boggling fashion: activating, suppressing, and communicating in ways still largely undiscovered. Lymphocytes start out in the bone marrow and either stay there and mature into B cells or leave for the thymus gland where they mature into T cells. (Get it? B for bone marrow and T for thymus.)

   a. **B cells** - Humoral immunity is the immunity that comes largely from antibodies, and antibodies come from B cells. They are formed in the pluripotent stem cells in the bone marrow, and thereafter, they go to the spleen, nodes, and other lymphoid tissue where they are activated by the presence of antigens. B cells get their name from the B in bone marrow. (Not deep, but at least it makes more sense than many of these other names.)

      After a B cell comes into contact with an antigen, the cell begins to mature and is able to independently identify foreign antigens. All B cells are antigen-specific and respond to only one foreign protein. B cells carry receptor molecules that recognize these specific targets. Think of them as military intelligence, seeking out targets and sending out spies to lock onto them. A specific B cell is tuned into a specific pathogen. When the specific pathogen presents again in the body, the B cell clones itself and produces millions of antibodies designed to eliminate the germ. A typical B cell has 50,000 to 100,000 antibodies bound to its surface.

      The B cell antigen-specific receptor is an antibody molecule on the B cell surface that recognizes whole pathogens without the need for antigen processing. Each line of B cell expresses a different antibody so the complete set of B cell antigen receptors represent all the antibodies that the body can make.

      The spleen contains many immature B cells that, because of the large amount of blood passing through the spleen, become exposed to new antigens. Each mature B can be stimulated by a specific antigen.

Activated B cells differentiate into either antibody-producing plasma cells that secrete soluble immunoglobulins *or* memory cells that survive in the body for years. Immunologic memory allows the immune system to remember the antigen and respond faster upon future exposure.

   i. **Plasma cells:** Also called plasmacytes, these offspring of the B cells secrete antibodies, also called immunoglobulins or Igs. Once aware of the presence of foreign antigen, some immature B cells evolve into plasma cells that manufacture antibodies. These plasma cells are the only manufacturer of the Igs. After the plasma cell becomes sensitized to a foreign antigen, the resulting antibodies are able to identify the foreign invader. Each Ig class differs in its biological properties and deals with different antigens. There are five primary types (or isotopes) of Igs with different structures and thereby different functions. In mammals, these include IgA, IgD, IgE, IgG, and IgM. Details on these antibody classes are provided in the *Humoral Response* section that follows.

PEARL: Antibodies are specifically made in response to the protein of a particular antigen. The antigen and antibody fit together like a lock and key and, forsaking all others, the mass-produced antibodies go forth to recognize antigen by forming Ag/Ab complexes that target a certain antigen for destruction. Formation of these Ag/Ab complexes usually consumes complement.

   ii. **Memory cells:** In addition to evolution into plasma cells, B cells can also differentiate into memory cells that recall previously identified Ags and allow for faster response upon future exposure to that Ag. The job of memory cells is to hold a grudge. Progeny of the B cell, memory cells come into play if the same antigen returns in the future. Memory cells enable the body to produce antibodies quickly when confronted by an antigen it knew in the past. Some memory cells can be classed as either CD4+ or CD8+, but for most of the TBIs, immunologic memory is poorly understood. For Lyme, it seems that there is little immunity after initial exposure, and the patient can become infected over and over again. With most other TBIs, too little is known to say whether immunity occurs after first infection. As we gain knowledge in this area, we may better understand the difficulty in developing vaccines to these pathogens.

   b. **T cells** - These cells start as hematopoietic stem cells in the bone marrow and then migrate to the thymus where they begin to mature. They get their name from the T in thymus. T cells in many forms can be found in the circulation and are essential for the specific immune response. Overall, T cells straddle the border between innate and adaptive immune response in ways that are not yet well understood.

Numerous subpopulations of T cells perform specific functions. Ts carry receptor molecules that distinguish between specific proteins. T cells recognize a non-*self* target, such as a pathogen, *only* after an antigen has been processed and presented in combination with a *self* receptor called a major histocompatibility complex (MHC) molecule. One analogy is that the T cells are sent on a mission to destroy the invaders that the military intelligence forces have identified. These are the soldiers, the ground troops, that actually bump up against cells and kill them.

A number of distinct, as well as overlapping, categories and subpopulations of T cells include the following:

i.   **Helper T cells**: Many T cells are vicious creatures that live to gobble up others. Not the helper cells. T helper cells are unusual in that they have no cytotoxic or phagocytic activity themselves. Instead, they activate and direct other cells and are essential in multiple immune functions. They stimulate growth of many cells and influence the efficient activity of phagocytes.

Helpers become activated when presented with peptide antigens that are expressed on the surface of the antigen-presenting cells (APCs). Once primed, they divide fast and secrete small proteins called cytokines that regulate or assist in the active immune response. Helper Ts are needed to help produce Ab for a specific Ag. These cells are involved with B cell maturation into plasma cells and the activation of cytotoxic Ts and macrophages.

A burst of helper Ts will cause stimulation of both B cells and macrophages. Cytokine signals from the helper T cells increase the -cidal action of macrophages and the action of killer Ts. T cell activation also causes upregulation of molecules expressed on the T cell's surface, such as specific CDs, which provide extra stimulation signals needed to activate B cells to make antibodies.

PEARL: Clusters of differentiation or CDs are a group of protein markers on the surface of white blood cells. They are used to classify immune cell types and establish international nomenclature standards. Each marker identifies a specific function within the system like passing along biochemical signals. CD levels are measured as a percent of total lymphocytes. T cells are mostly labeled CD1 through CD8, while B cells are categorized generally from CD19 to CD24. Additional information on CDs is provided in the box at the end of the chapter.

Mature T helper cells probably always display the surface protein CD4 and are then said to be CD4+. They usually have a defined role as helpers in the system and are expressed through various subtypes including T1H, T2H, T3H, etcetera, which produce different types of cytokines to facilitate specific types of immune responses.

- **T1H:** These helpers aid in regulating the immune system and are integral to both the innate and adaptive immune responses. T1Hs help determine which types of immune responses the body will make to a particular pathogen. They have no cytotoxic activity and do not kill directly. They help control the immune response by directing other cells to perform these tasks. T1H is hypothesized to be dominant in certain kinds of autism and autoimmune conditions.

- **T2H**: These cells help modulate the immune system. They send antibodies to go after invaders like bacteria. T2H is thought to be dominant in allergies, frequent infections, and cancer.

PEARL: Both T1H and T2H make cytokines, which cause inflammation. Some cytokines can adversely affect certain organs or systems. Cytokines can significantly impact the brain and nervous system resulting in increased depression, anxiety, or behavior changes, and interfere with sleep. They may be significantly involved in the Lyme symptom called "brain fog." In addition to affecting the nervous system, this inflammation can affect joints, the GI tract, and other areas.

Apparently, the body adjusts the amounts of both T1H and T2H as needed. Many confounders impact this delicate and vigorous system and the key to good immune health is balance. Once T1H and T2H ratios become skewed, the entire system can experience disequilibrium.

ii.   **Natural Killer T cells:** A subset of T cells, NKs are a heterogeneous group that share the properties of other types of T cells. NKs, therefore, can perform the functions of other T cell lines as well as production of cytokines and instigation of cell destruction. Serving as a bridge between the innate and adaptive immune responses, NKs are large lymphocytes that bond to cells and lyse them by releasing cytotoxins effective against viruses and some tumor cells. They detect cells in the body that are harboring viruses and then kill them. NKs identify Ag presented by CD1d. They are proliferated by γ-interferon, IL-2, antibodies, retinoic acid, and prostaglandin E.

iii.   **Regulatory Ts**: These T lymphocytes used to be called suppressor T cells. (Suppressor sounds so tyrannical, while regulatory sounds like a government bureaucracy.) There remains controversy today about whether suppressor cells are a distinct category or simply a regulatory cell by another name. Regulatory cells come out near the end of T cell-mediated immune response to suppress the processes so there isn't an overreaction. Note that a malfunction of regulatory (or suppressor) T cells is hypothesized to be involved in some autoimmune reactions. In these cases, the T cells continuously stimulate the B cells and keep the immune response going long after it has performed its initial duty. Relentless stimulation results in over-response, including attack of the body's own *self* proteins, that results in symptoms of inflammation.

iv.   **Cytotoxic Ts**: Cytotoxic T cells are part of the innate immune system, and they do what their name implies. They are toxic to their targets, focusing on cells infected with viruses or other pathogens as well as cells that are damaged or impaired. They distinguish *self* from non-*self* and kill their quarry.

The cytotoxic cells travel through the body in search of cells where the MHC I receptors contain a specific antigen. When an activated T contacts such cells, it releases cytotoxins that disrupt the target cell's plasma membrane allowing water, ions, and toxins to enter, which causes the target cell to undergo apoptosis. The killing of these cells is important in preventing the replication of viruses. T cell activation is extremely well controlled and requires a strong MHC:antigen activation signal or additional stimulus provided by helper T cells.

These cytotoxic Ts not only are able to defend against viruses and attack tumors, but also are probably involved with transplant rejection as well. Some cytotoxic T cells are also called killer cells, but the distinction between them and the NK cells listed above is not worth making for our

purposes. (Scientists even argue over whether the distinction is real.)

2.   **Monocytes** – Originating from myeloid stem cells, monocytes circulate in the blood for about 24 hours before they move into the tissues. There they mature into **macrophages,** which are Grade A super-phagocytes.

The macrophages devour pathogens and damaged cells, especially in tissue fluid. Monocytes account for about 3% to 8% of the total WBCs. Monocytes and macrophages are a first-line of defense in the inflammatory process. A macrophage is a monocyte that has left the circulation and moved into tissue, where it may enjoy a relatively long life. **Histiocyte** is a general term for any monocyte that has become a resident in tissue. Macrophages often take their mature names from the tissue in which they reside, for example:

- Macrophages in the liver are called Kupffer cells.

- Macrophages in the brain are called microglia.

- Macrophages in the skin are called Langerhans cells.

Each of these histiocytes has even more alternative names, and there are macrophages present in most other tissues as well.

Along with neutrophils, macrophages are the primary phagocytic cells of the immune system. They have the ability to recognize and ingest foreign Ags through receptors on the surface of their cell membranes. These antigens are then destroyed by lysosomes. Macrophages in organs and peripheral lymphoid tissues serve as primary scavengers. They clear the blood of abnormal or old cells and debris as well as pathogens. Macrophages also serve a vital role in processing Ags and presenting them to T cells, thereby helping to activate the specific immune response. They release many chemical mediators that are involved in the body's defenses including IL-1 and complement.

PEARL: Lyme disease patients appear to mount a largely monocyte response against the Bb pathogen. In many other cases of infectious disease the presence of neutrophils signifies inflammation. While some PMNs may be present, they are likely to be overshadowed by monocytes. Since monocytes are resident as macrophages in most tissues, this predominantly monocytic immune response may also help explain Lyme's propensity to affect so many organ systems so profoundly. Whereas PMNs are largely present in the blood and lymph, macrophages remain localized in tissue. Whether the monocytes or the microbe settle in the tissue first, I have no idea. Maybe the pathogen has an affinity to certain tissue and its presence attracts more monocytes into the organ. This is all pure speculation on my part but it gives us something to consider. Monocytes are amazingly complex from a biochemical standpoint. We are just beginning to learn about them in general and how they contribute to the illnesses caused by specific pathogens. I suspect we haven't heard the last of the role of monocytes in the immune defense against Bb.

3. **Other agranulocytes:** There are other immune cell types that are somewhat harder to classify but may be important to TBI patients. Since they don't seem to fall under the granulocyte heading, they have the distinction of being labeled "other."

    a. **Dendritic cells -** Specialized phagocytic antigen-recognizing cells, dendritic cells have long outgrowths called dendrites that help to engulf microbes. Dendritic cells are in contact with the external environment (primarily skin, and the lining of the nose, lungs, stomach, and intestines). Once activated, they mature and migrate to the lymph tissues and interact with T and B cells to activate the adaptive immune response. Mature dendritic cells stimulate T helper cells and cytotoxic T cells and interact with macrophages and B cells to activate them as well. They can influence the type of immune response produced. There are two recognized forms of dendritic cells: sessile and migratory. When dendritic cells travel to the lymphoid areas where T cells are held, they activate the T cells which can then differentiate into cytotoxic T cells or T helper cells.

PEARL: Dendritic cells that stimulate the T helper cells may arise from monocytes, which may prove to be the body's primary defender against Lyme.

    b. **Mast cells -** Found in the connective tissue of vertebrates, mast cells contain heparin and histamine and function like gate keepers. They are very similar, and may be identical, to circulating basophils. Masts interact with dendritic cells as well as with B and T cells to help mediate adaptive immune responses. Mast cells express MHC class II molecules and consume Gram negative bacteria like salmonella. They specialize in processing the fimbrial proteins on the surface of bacteria, which are involved in adhesion to tissues. This is an important part of the destruction of microbes, because released cytokines attract more phagocytes to the site of infection. In fact, mast cells produce cytokines that promote the overall inflammatory response. They appear to be an important inducer of hyperreactivity to allergens (antigens) and are prominent in late phase inflammation. Since mast cells contain extremely irritating chemicals such as histamine, they contribute to itching, swelling, and fluid leaking from cells.

The location where the allergen contacts the host will determine the allergic manifestations prompted by the powerful biochemistry of the mast cells. If the allergen contacts the eye, there will be itching and prolific watering. If skin is the first contact, then irritation, swelling, and itch will predominate. Airway exposure can cause an irritated throat, wheezing, tightness, cough, shortness of breath, and constriction.

While the immune system's work is divided into the cell-mediated response and the humoral response, this division is somewhat artificial since their activities are interconnected, overlapping, and quite dependent on each other for optimum function. One does not perform without the other. How can you separate a B cell from the immunoglobulin antibody that it makes? But when dealing with such a complex and voluminous process, some sorting and categorizing must be done to be able to understand the system at all.

Humoral Immune Response

The humoral immune response (HIR) is comprised of all the immune defenses that do **not** directly involve cells. Effective immune response requires numerous substances found throughout the fluids of the body. These biochemicals include secreted antibodies and the various molecules that are needed to stimulate their production. In addition to antibodies, the HIR includes all the essential immune compounds such as interferons, ILs, tumor necrosis factors, chemokines, and selected hormones. While considering the humoral response, never forget that all the cells and humors are part of the same immune system with cross-links, bridges, and awe-inspiring cascades. No part of the system stands alone. Cells need humors to activate and differentiate, and humors are manufactured and released by essentially all immune cells. The HIR then involves all the processes needed for antibody and cytokine production, without focusing on the cells that are integral to their formation.

Components of the humoral response:

A. **Immunoglobulins (Antibodies)** Some authors say that antibodies are the most important part of the humoral immune system, but I never know why humans have to make everything competitive. All the parts are equally important. (I don't want any component to feel disenfranchised.) Igs are made by the mature B cells, called plasma cells. Each antibody class has specific roles and responsibilities, but that doesn't stop them from minding their neighbor's business plenty.

1. **IgA**: This immunoglobulin is found primarily in the mucosal areas of the respiratory tree, GI tract, and GU system where it prevents colonization by pathogens. Mucin secretions in saliva and tears contain high concentrations of IgA. The exocrine secretions in breast milk, which can be pertinent to TBI patients, contain high amounts of IgA. In colostrum, IgA helps protect breast-fed newborns from infection. Low IgA is the most commonly recognized deficiency of antibodies but the significance of this finding in TBI patients is not clear.

2. **IgD**: IgD is a receptor found on cells that have not yet been exposed to antigens. The function of IgD is less defined than that of the other isotypes. When a B cell begins to express IgM as well as IgD, it is considered mature, so IgD may help develop its parent B cell.

3. **IgE**: The IgE antibodies have several extremely important roles. IgE is involved in allergic reactions through binding to allergens and triggering histamine release. Anaphylactic reactions are also thought to be a result of IgE. This Ig is found primarily in mucus where it binds to allergens and attaches to mast cells in the respiratory tract and causes these cells to release additional histamine. More than half of the patients with allergies have high IgE levels, which also play a role in atopic hypersensitivity. Also, IgE protects against parasites, especially helminth worms. When you observe high IgE levels, think allergy or parasites.

4. **IgG**: IgG is the principal Ig in human serum and provides most of the antibody-based immunity against invading pathogens. In general, IgG levels increase as IgM starts to decline and they can linger after the infection is gone. IgG can remain high weeks or months after the active infection has dissipated. IgG is the key antibody after re-exposure to a pathogen due to the memory response. IgG crosses the placenta to give passive immunity to the fetus before birth. This antibody class protects against bacteria, viruses, and toxins. IgG activates complement and serves in the role of **opsonin**. Measurement of IgG is thought to provide information about active, on-going, chronic, or past exposure. Usually, IgG is said to come on *late* in an infectious process. As injectable γ-globulin, IgG is given to provide temporary resistance against hepatitis and other viral conditions and to compensate for immune deficiencies. A new role for IgG may be in treating patients found to have high antineuronal antibodies who are exhibiting neuropsychiatric symptoms secondary to Strep infections or possibly TBIs. IgG seems to be prominent when there is an autoimmune component to the immune response.

Most of the Ab-based immunity is due to IgG fighting against invading pathogens. IgG is more likely to be detected as IgM dissipates.

PEARL: New theories regarding the function of IgG and IgM suggest their roles may be somewhat reversed in Lyme patients, with IgM persisting far longer in the clinical course than previously expected. Again, this difference from what we traditionally expect would help explain why we remain so confused about this disease. Stay tuned.

5. **IgM**: IgM is the first Ig to appear in measurable levels in response to infection especially viral parasitic pathogens. IgM is thought to be the first antibody formed after exposure to a new antigen. This antibody is found on the surface of B cells and eliminates pathogens *early* on in B cell-mediated immunity *before* there is enough IgG made to fight the invasion. This fact may be important in interpreting lab results in TBI patients, although Bb may not follow the early/late rule as rigidly as other pathogens. IgM is involved in almost all immune reactions including autoimmunity. IgM provides the blood group (A B O) antibody reactions and is the best Ig at stimulating complement. Some say IgG is the only antibody to cross the placenta, but IgM might do so as well.

PEARL: In terms of Ab/Ag testing for Lyme, IgM 31 may take the better part of a year to appear.

B. **Cytokines** Since cytokines are biochemicals in the blood, they are considered part of the humoral immune response. Made primarily by WBCs, cytokines provide the biochemical signals that regulate immunologic processes, especially the magnitude of the response.

Cytokines are non-immunoglobulin peptides that are secreted chiefly by T cells and monocytes. Each cytokine is manufactured by a specific cell in response to a particular signal. They influence events both near and far by interacting with specific cell surface receptors. By binding to receptors on the cell surfaces, cytokines regulate the behavior of their target cells and are largely responsible for the communication between WBCs. This binding triggers a variety of responses depending on the target and the type of cytokine. Cytokine signals have numerous effects on cells, tissues, and organs.

These messengers also mobilize other components of the immune system and can be considered modulators of the immune response, increasing or decreasing inflammation. Often they are released by injured or infected cells and *recruit* immune cells to the site of insult. Some cytokines promote healing of damaged tissue after removal of pathogens by phagocytes.

Cytokines are thought to be responsible for a number of the symptoms observed in TBI patients. In addition to their influence on inflammation, cytokines can significantly impact the brain and nervous system. These effects can increase depression, anxiety, behavior changes, and interfere with sleep. They are theorized to be significantly involved in the common symptom called "**brain fog**." Further, the inflammation enhanced by cytokines can affect joints, the GI tract, and other body systems.

Cytokines are secreted primarily by monocytes and lymphocytes in response to awareness of antigens including pathogens, endotoxins, poisons, or even other cytokines. Cytokine activity itself is **NOT** antigen-specific so cytokines bridge between the nonspecific and specific immune responses (innate and adaptive).

PEARL: Cytokines are thought to increase quinolinic acid which is a neurotoxin that potentially contributes to the many neuropsychiatric symptoms associated with Lyme disease, especially those involving the hippocampus.

In summary, cytokines are simply biochemicals that activate, recruit, arouse, draft, stifle, motivate, dampen, invigorate, restrain, smother, control, repress, promote, accelerate, excite, inspire, encourage, beckon, stimulate, suppress, incite, riot, and hire assassins. And this is just when they're being nice. More than a hundred types of cytokines have been identified so far. Those most commonly cited in TBI literature include:

1. **Interferons** (IFNs) – Just when you think none of this makes sense, interferons get their name because they *interfere* with the ability of viruses to colonize a host. What could be more logical than that? IFNs are made by most cells in the body so the majority of cells have some capacity to fight viral pathogens. They perform their antiviral effects by diminishing the ability of the virus to synthesize protein. When a cell detects interferon, it begins to produce proteins that prevent viral reproduction in the vicinity. IFNs, which include α, β, and γ forms, have a number of roles, such as serving to signal other parts of the immune system.

   - α-**IFN** inhibits viral replication and tumor growth. This interferon class enables host cells to produce MHC class I surface antigens so that the invader is more easily recognized and destroyed. IFN-α also increases MHC class II and NK activity and modulates antibody responses.

   - β-**IFN** is found in fibroblasts.

   - γ-**IFN** has been observed in T cells and NK cells and appears to have numerous functions. These

glycoproteins have antiviral and other immunologic properties. They inhibit viral reproduction. Sometimes γ-interferon is used in the treatment of certain viral infections such as hepatitis. As with all extremely active molecules, while they may have positive treatment effects they also have the potential to cause adverse reactions.

2. **Tumor Necrosis Factor** (TNF) – This family of protein mediators has many powerful and sometimes conflicting actions that are only beginning to be explored. TNF cytokines are released primarily by macrophages and T lymphocytes and help regulate the immune response including the death of targeted cells through apoptosis. TNF presents another "Catch-22" to the body. Sometimes the more it helps, the more it hurts. Actions attributed to TNF include: fever, sepsis, inflammation, cell death signaling, direct cell death, cachexia or wasting, tumor inhibition, restriction of viral replication, and vascular changes that can lead to constriction in some cases and dilation in others. Shock occurs when TNF is released into vital organs causing vasodilation and subsequent pooling, which decreases the volume of blood in the circulation. Dysregulation of TNF has been associated with Alzheimer's, cancer, depression, and IBD. Whether there is a causal relationship has not been solidly established. While a number of cells can discharge TNF, the most common source is the monocytes in the circulation and the macrophages in the tissues. Since monocytes may be the predominant cell responder to Bb, this could be the TBI connection. We do not yet clearly understand the role, if any, of TNF in Lyme or other TBIs. Still, TNF is occasionally measured as part of an initial TBI work-up.

   - TNF-α: Generally when TNF is referred to nonspecifically, TNF-α is what is meant. Tumor necrosis factor-α is a cytokine that is sometimes measured to assess the degree of chronic inflammation. This molecule is a growth factor for both immune cells and the osteoclasts that break down bone. TNF-α affects the hypothalamic-pituitary-adrenal axis, suppressing appetite, increasing insulin resistance, and elevating CRP. This cytokine is known to attract neutrophils and enhance phagocytosis and so can be assumed to have some responsibility in fighting infection. Sometimes TNF is measured as part of a broader cytokine panel. High levels have been associated with shock. Since TBIs can be associated with significant chronic inflammation and on-going infections, elevated TNF-α could be measured in these patients, although the definition of a normal level remains unclear. As always, know what you will do with a test result before you order the test.

3. **Interleukins (ILs)** – This type of cytokine facilitates communication between white cells and other mediators of the immune system. The primary sources of ILs are the monocytes, macrophages, T cells, and mast cells. ILs promote additional mediators and not just as part of the immune response. These cytokines are biomolecules that help regulate the immune system, inflammation, and the formation of blood cells. Various IL families are made by different cells and have unique roles. ILs appear critical to normal function of the CNS in ways not clearly understood but seem to impact the hippocampus and its role in memory, learning, and nerve signal potentiation. Reading the last sentence would suggest that ILs could have a role in the neuropsychiatric manifestations of Lyme and other TBIs.

ILs also facilitate the manufacture of colony-stimulating factors, transforming growth factors, and numerous modulators in many organs. When ILs circulate, they can cause fever, sleepiness, anorexia, and inflammation. Of course, these are symptoms found in many infectious processes. ILs activate both B and T cells and influence their growth. ILs are also somehow involved with mast cells.

Specific ILs have specific roles. IL-1 is the cytokine involved in fever production and other signs and symptoms of inflammation. The raised temperature of a fever is known to kill certain bacteria. IL-1 is manufactured by macrophages after they devour a foreign cell. This interleukin also seems to cause fatigue when it reaches the hypothalamus. IL-2 is activated primarily by CD4+ helper T cells and has many functions and may be involved in the complex differentiation between *self* and non-*self*. IL-3 promotes production of bone marrow stem cells and is involved with mast cell physiology. IL-6 is occasionally ordered as an assessment of the immune function of TBI patients. IL-8 is a chemokine and induces chemotaxis of neutrophils and T cells. There are a number of others.

ILs currently play a role in assessment and treatment of certain cancers such as melanoma and kidney carcinoma. ILs have been measured in conjunction with TBIs, but the specifics of their possible role has yet to be clearly defined. Some researchers and HCPs use measures of ILs such as IL-6 and IL-1B in TBI patients to get clues about immune response and inflammation. Future work may reveal a less ambiguous function for these molecules.

PEARL: The terms leukotriene (which refers to hormones involved in inflammation, chemotaxis, allergy, and asthma) and interleukin are easily confused.

4. **Chemokines** – Sources of chemokines are variable but include CD8, NK, and mast cells. Chemokines induce chemotaxis of T cells and NK cells and call neutrophils and monocytes to come help defend a site from invasion.

5. **Others** – By definition, a hormone is a compound produced by one tissue and then transported through the circulation to the cells of another tissue where it has an effect. One hormone that is referred to as a cytokine is erythropoietin, the substance that controls the production of red blood cells (RBCs). Practically, interferons and ILs could be thought of as hormones made by the immune system. Other cytokines include lymphokines made in parts of the immune system.

This "Other" category is included to illustrate that we are just beginning to uncover all the chemicals involved with immune communication. As with many of the classification schemes I have had to employ, this one is artificial and used to make sure that you are aware that multiple cytokines might yet be defined. To complicate our understanding, some of these "other" hormones, like endogenous steroids, suppress the immune system. In contrast, tymosin, a compound produced by the thymus, enhances lymphocyte production. Vitamin D is a hormone produced by the body in response to sun energy, but often not in sufficient amounts. Because supplements are needed in many cases, this hormone is referred to as a vitamin. Don't let the complexity overwhelm you. Just be aware of what the TBI patient is up against.

C. **Complement** – Complement is another intricate immune process, the complexity of which is astounding. Nonetheless, we must know a few basic concepts since complement is an integral part of the body's defenses and the term appears in the TBI literature. Complement is a group of proteins that play an important role in immune response through a complex cascade of reactions. Considered part of the humoral immune response, complement protein does not involve cells. Instead, these molecules tend to lie inactive in the blood until called upon to perform. With complement, the phrase "immune cascade" is especially relevant. One reaction begets another and that one sparks a third, etcetera, in a sequential activation of this intricate system. Antibodies can't do all the work themselves. They need their action to be *complemented* by this additional immune component. Complement impacts both innate and acquired immunity.

Complement is comprised of proteins in the serum that act to destroy foreign invaders. For example in the **classical** complement pathway, antibody-binding initiates the immune cascade calling in other immune molecules to help. An **alternative** complement pathway works without needing antibodies to start the process. Repeated activation of the complement process uses up the available complement proteins. When complement levels are low, complement is probably being used in the formation of antigen/antibody complexes. This result can be deemed good in that the complement is being consumed in mounting a defense. But complement consumption can go too far and when too much is consumed before it can be replenished, there is not enough complement around to help form the Ag/Ab complexes.

Once complement is activated it will begin to work with or without the antibodies to punch holes in the cells of the pathogen eventually destroying the invaders. Complement is a series of plasma proteins that work together. There are millions of different antibodies in the blood but only a small number of proteins in the complement system, which float freely in the blood. Once the complement chemicals are triggered to respond, a rapid killing spree is initiated, essentially a catalytic cascade of reactions. First, the binding of the antibody and the complement molecule tags the microbe for ingestion by phagocytes in a process called **opsonization**. Simply put, opsonization is the coating of a microorganism with antibody and/or complement making them easier to identify. Complement may act directly by killing through lysis of the pathogen's plasma membrane.

Complement increases inflammation, chemotaxis, and B cell response. After complement proteins bind to the pathogen, they activate their protease enzymes, which set off other complement proteases, which produce a cascade that magnifies the initial signal through controlled feedback. This intricate cascade also attracts other immune cells and increases vascular permeability. (You can see where this might get a little complicated.)

Complement does its job through signal amplification, sequential activation of reactions, and transmission of biochemical messages that tell the clean-up crews to come remove the mess. The activation of the complement pathway is multifaceted. Some of the activation pathways require antibodies to begin. Antibodies that bind to surface antigens attract the first components of the complement cascade called the "classical" pathway. This results in the killing of bacteria in two ways. First, the binding of the Ab and the complement molecules marks the microbe for ingestion. Phagocytes are then attracted by certain complement molecules generated throughout the cascade. Second, some complement components form a membrane-attack complex to assist antibodies in killing the bacterium directly. "Alternative" complement pathways are nonspecific and do not need antibodies to get started.

Different complement proteins are labeled C1 through C9. Contemporary scientists know most about C3 and C5. Details of the specific roles for the various complements are not yet well-defined. We do understand that lack of C3 increases the risk of bacterial infection. Deficiencies of C5 through C9 are often associated with autoimmune disorders especially SLE and glomerulonephritis.

Individual complement levels have been measured in the management of TBI patients. The measurement of complement is starting to be used in the search for understanding and ultimately in diagnosing inflammatory, autoimmune, rheumatologic, and infectious diseases. Their role in TBIs is just beginning to be explored. Levels of circulating immune complexes can be measured serially to determine the effect of treatment or help assess clinical status. Tissue from biopsies can be used to look for Ag/Ab/complement complexes.

PEARL: In summary, complement is a group of proteins that play an important role in immune response through a complex cascade of reactions. Antibodies can't do all the work themselves. They need their action to be complemented by this additional immune component. Complement is known to be consumed when antigen/antibody complexes are formed. These proteins then allow for lysis of foreign microbes. Complement impacts both innate and acquired immunity.

Why would readers interested in TBIs need to know anything about complement? Measurement of complement can provide information on the status of the immune response to infection. Complement is the stuff that allows for the formation of the critical Ag/Ab complexes. The more complexes that are formed, the more complement is consumed. By measuring the amount of complement remaining after a reaction, the HCP can get information on how well a specific antigen binds with an antibody in a test sample.

PEARL: Complement fixation techniques are blood assays used to determine if Ag/Ab reactions have occurred. After complement combines with antigen and antibody to form a complex, it is no longer available to lyse RBCs in vitro. The degree of complement fixation can then be determined by the number of RBCs destroyed, which indicates the amount of free complement not bound. Complement fixation can suggest the severity of an infection because it helps indicate the extent and effectiveness of the Ag/Ab reactions occurring in the system.

In the initial work-up of a TBI patient, some HCPs order measures of a number of these humoral chemicals to get a handle on the patient's immune status. These tests might include: Complement affixed to subclasses IgA,

IgM, IgG and IgE, as well as other specific complement molecules.

1. **Complement C1Q** can be measured with an assay of binding sites on immune complexes. Ag/Ab complexes attach to the complement fixation sites and the C1Q levels should reflect the amount of these immune complexes in the circulation. Consider ordering C1Q complex levels in puzzling cases. If levels are low, the result could suggest an autoimmune mechanism in play. If high, a persistent, on-going infection is likely. C1Q inhibits immune complex-induced interferon production and is linked to SLE and other immune diseases. Lack of C1Q is the biggest indicator for SLE. Almost everyone with a deficiency of C1Q gets lupus, and especially low levels will correspond with a flare. C1Q has a role in the overall cytokine production processes such as the regulation of production of IFN-α and influencing other complement activities.

2. **Complement C3** is the type of complement found in the highest concentrations in plasma and is elevated in a number of inflammatory conditions. C3 is low in lupus, bacterial endocarditis, some kidney diseases, bacterial septicemia, end-stage liver disease, as well as some fungal infections, possibly because the complement is being used in the formation of Ab/Ag complexes. When antibodies bind to a foreign protein, C3 attaches to the complex and calls for help from other parts of the immune cascade. Measurement of C3 levels is used in the diagnosis and management of diseases such as kidney problems and lupus and in many inflammatory conditions. **C3d** is a fragment of C3 that serves as a signal to certain B cells. These molecules are thought to reflect the prevalence of toxins and infectious agents and may prove to be a good monitor of overall pathogen burden and indicator of an on-going inflammatory process. A result > 40 is an index of persistent inflammation. If the person seems to be improving, but C3d levels are still at 40 or above, something pathological is probably still going on inside this patient, either a simmering infection or an autoimmune process. C3d may suggest that a persistent infection is driving an autoimmune clinical presentation. Low levels probably means C3 is doing its job. (You didn't think this would be comprehensible, did you?)

3. **Complement CH50** levels can be used to monitor complement deficiencies and to watch disease progression in patients with lupus, nephritis, or a variety of infections. One source lists the normal reference range in serum as 35 to 55 CH50 units/ml. CH50 is a measure of the overall health of the complement system and indicates how much complement is available to mount an attack. CH50 can be used to follow auto-immune conditions.

4. **Complement individual immunoglobulin profiles:** Quantitative measures can be done for each of the distinct complement/antibody complexes such as IgA, IgD, IgE, IgG, and IgM. In many specialized diagnostic tests, both IgM and IgG should be ordered to help establish the chronology in each individual's case and to avoid missing the presence of antibodies due to fluctuating levels in the blood. Each result could have potential clinical significance.

PEARL: No one knows everything. If you can't decide whether a measurement of complement in a particular patient will be beneficial, talk to a trusted lab before you order the test to make sure you are requesting exactly what you want and that you will understand how to interpret the results when they come back.

PEARL: Do not get complement (C), a group of proteins that help Ab and Ag bind in complexes, mixed up with clusters of differentiation (CD,) which is a system of naming certain white cells according to their immune function.

IV. WHEN GOOD IMMUNOLOGY GOES BAD

The immune system is usually well regulated and balanced by internal controls. Many of the signs and symptoms of disease are simply the immune system doing what it is designed to do. For example, during infection, the headache, fever, and aches are likely a result of the inflammatory process. Recognition of the functioning immune system has been around at least since the plague of 430 BCE when Thucydides noted that those who had the plague and recovered could now nurse the sick without getting sick again themselves. Thucydides recognized that something was happening, but he didn't know what. We also recognize that something is happening and we still don't know exactly what that might be.

From an immune perspective, we all seem to fall on a spectrum where our immune system is normal most of the time, but at other times, it can be hypoactive or hyperactive. Many individuals are exposed to the same infectious agents over time. Some get sick and some don't. Some respond to treatment and some don't. Some go into remission, while others relapse. Some are cured with minimal or no intervention. We don't even know if the terms relapse and recur are the same or different. We are just beginning to understand how many confounding factors impact an individual's immune response.

Despite Thucydides' insight 2400 years ago and definite advances in some areas today, we still are largely at the mercy of our ignorance. We do know enough to recognize that while the immune response is amazing, and at times miraculous, problems do occur. The system can be hypoactive, hyperactive, or broken.

A. Too Little Immune Function

In the case of immunodeficiency, parts of the process are either hypoactive or inactive. Here, the immune system does not respond to pathogens normally or is weak or non-existent in its response. Many conditions can impact the full function of the immune system including stress, obesity, poor nutrition, alcohol, drugs, etc. Malnutrition is the most common cause of immunodeficiency in developing countries. Diets that lack adequate protein present numerous problems with regard to mounting an effective immune response. Further, deficiencies of certain nutrients such as zinc, iron, copper, selenium, and Vitamins A, C, B6, E, and folic acid can reduce immune efficiency. The loss of thymic function at an early age causes severe immunodeficiency and makes the individual quite susceptible to infection. AIDS, splenectomy, and certain cancers are also responsible for some of these secondary immunodeficiencies. In contrast, primary immunodeficiency is the term used for a group of diseases that are inherited through errors in the genes that code for parts of the immune system. These conditions can be mild or severe. These patients lack one or more of the proteins, cells, or tissues needed for optimum immune function. There are more than 150 documented different manifestations of primary immunodeficiency. In general, immunodeficient individuals get more infections and are slower to recover even with appropriate antibiotics. Although the metastasis of cancer is multifactorial, one cause of spread may be that the immune system becomes overwhelmed by the proliferation of the abnormal cells, rendering it ineffective against the assault.

PEARL: When the immune system is overwhelmed, usually by a massive quantity of pathogen or multiple infectious agents invading at once, the system can shut down completely in an event termed **immune paralysis**. *If a large amount of Ag influxes at any one time, the immune system might be temporarily incapacitated. In the case of a large transmission of Bb, by the time the immune system regroups and resumes function, the pathogen has gone intracellular. As far as we know, paralysis can last several days. As immune activity returns, there is no recollection of having been infected, almost like post-traumatic stress disorder at a cellular level. There are no memory cells in evidence. The immune response has to start from the beginning. Initially, the patient tests sero-negative, even with known infection. As the patient begins treatment, the pathogens gradually re-emerge and antibodies begin to appear. This revitalization of the system can take weeks, months, or years. Immune paralysis might also occur in some cases when multiple vaccinations cause antigen overload.*

B. Too Much Immune Function

If you've ever had poison ivy, you know what happens when the immune system gets overzealous. Frightful. Miserable. Uncomfortable allergy symptoms are the result of overly aggressive immune response, or hyperactive immunity. Some people have severe and even fatal reactions to peanuts, while others never react no matter how many times they are exposed. In hyperactive immunity, the system reacts to an allergen (antigen) that should generally be ignored: such as some foods, pollens, drugs, animal danders, etc. A person allergic to pollen will likely get a runny nose, watery and itchy eyes, and sneeze repeatedly. This reaction is caused by mast cells in the nasal passages. In response to the pollen, the mast cells release histamine which causes inflammation. Fluid then seeps from blood vessels causing a runny nose. Histamine is responsible for the itchy, irritated eyes. Antihistamines are often used to relieve these symptoms.

Hypersensitivity Reactions

Hypersensitivity reactions are immune responses that damage the body's own tissues. These types of immunologic reactions depend on previous exposure to the antigen. You can't be allergic to something you have never experienced. There are four types of hypersensitivity reactions that depend on the time course and on the mechanisms involved in that particular reaction:

- **Type I**: **Immediate** or **anaphylactic** reactions are often associated with allergies. Here symptoms range from mild discomfort to death. These reactions are mediated by IgE, which causes degranulation of mast cells and basophils when cross-linked by antigen. Atopy is a predisposition to develop Type I hypersensitivity reactions and may be a genetic susceptibility. Atopy can refer to any IgE-mediated reaction or only to those that are excessive.

- **Type II**: In Type II hypersensitivity, antibodies bind to antigens on the patient's own cells marking them for destruction. This is also called **antibody-dependent** (or cytotoxic) hypersensitivity and is mediated by IgG and IgM antibodies.

- **Type III**: **Immune complexes** (aggregates of antigens, complement, and IgG and IgM antibodies) deposit in tissues and trigger Type III hypersensitivity.

- **Type IV**: **Cell-mediated** or **delayed** hypersensitivity takes about 2 to 3 days to develop. This Type

IV reaction is involved in many autoimmune and infectious diseases and in contact dermatitis such as poison ivy. Just when you think you are out of the woods unscathed, two days later a reaction.

Transplant rejection, while it is not a desired outcome for the patient, is the immune system doing its job extremely well. Getting a donor that matches as closely as possible helps decrease the problem of rejection. Often with transplant rejection, immunosuppressants are used to help the patient tolerate the new organ. While this suppression often helps, or at least buys some time, muting the immune response opens the patient to all sorts of opportunistic infections and other adverse events.

C. Immune System Mistakes

Overall, mistakes made during an immune response are few, considering the complexity of the system. Autoimmunity occurs when the immune system attacks its own body in the same way that it would attack a germ. This results in cell and tissue damage and occasional organ failure. Certain common diseases are thought to be the result of autoimmune action. Juvenile onset diabetes causes the immune cells to attack the pancreas thereby interfering with the production of insulin. Rheumatoid arthritis (RA) is the immune system attacking tissues inside the joints.

PEARL: Autoimmune diseases are conditions that result when the body cannot distinguish self *from non-*self. *The body attacks it*self *and the overall inflammation can grow out-of-control. Everyone has some degree of autoimmunity but usually the body keeps the response under control. Some components are genetic. The degree of autoimmune response may depend on the condition of the immune system when it confronts yet another insult. Autoimmunity can damage joints, skin, blood vessels, lungs, kidneys, heart, and brain. The condition can be chronic with flares and remissions. The body produces antibodies against its own tissues. Abs bind to self-antigens activating complement and other biochemicals causing damage to organs, blood vessels, and other tissues.*

In autoimmunity, the immune system seems no longer able to distinguish between *self* and non-*self* so healthy tissue could be inadvertently damaged. Under normal conditions, special cells in the thymus and bone marrow "educate" young lymphocytes and eliminate those that attack *self*-antigens in an attempt to prevent autoimmunity.

PEARL: In addition to the well-known autoimmune conditions such as diabetes mellitus (DM) type I, RA, and SLE, there are many lesser known diseases that are thought to have an autoimmune component including: pemphigus, amyotrophic lateral sclerosis (ALS), Addison's disease, hepatitis, aplastic anemia, atopic dermatitis, asthma, celiac disease, cardiomyopathy, Cogan's syndrome, Cushing's disease, glomerulonephritis, Crohn's disease, autism, CREST, arteritis, Dressler's syndrome, Evans syndrome, Hughes disease, eczema, infertility, encephalitis, purpura, meningitis, adrenal problems, Kawasaki's disease, Meniere's disease, connective tissue diseases, multiple myeloma, multiple sclerosis, myasthenia gravis (thymus disorder), myositis, Hashimotos's thyroiditis and other types of thyroid inflammation, ulcerative colitis, uveitis, vitiligo, Wegener's granulomatosis, Alzheimer's, polymyalgia rheumatica, polymyositis, Goodpasture's disease, cirrhosis, Wilson's syndrome, psoriasis, Raynaud's, Reiter's syndrome, sarcoid, scleroderma, Still's disease, Sjogren's syndrome, vasculitis, pediatric autoimmune neuropsychiatric disorders (PANDAS), Behcet's disease, chronic fatigue, antiphospholysis, some seizures, some blood disorders, Guillain-Barré, irritable bowel, autoimmune inner ear disease, chronic otitis media, and probably dozens of others. Autoimmune reactions may be one reason why some kids get rheumatic fever after Strep throat, while most do not. Autism may be linked to the mom's autoimmune status. Repeated miscarriages are also thought to have an autoimmune component, but more research is needed to confirm this theory.

When the body attacks it*self* the signs and symptoms can range from mild to fatal and appear general or specific. Overall, inflammation can seem out-of-control. Everyone probably has a degree of autoimmunity at some point. No one knows definitively how much autoimmunity is genetic and how much is sparked by environmental influences. Maybe repeated insults to the immune mechanisms result in significant dysfunction manifesting as autoimmunity.

Consider what happens to a patient who has an autoimmune component to his pathology. Often these patients are misdiagnosed for years and many are told that their problems are all in their head. Here is a good place to consider the multiple cascades of the immune system and how they are similar to a multi-branching tree. My friend Debbie has multiple autoimmune diagnoses including: RA, SLE, diabetes, Sjogren's, kidney problems, anxiety, depression, hypersensitivity reactions, etc. Debbie has a half-dozen doctors, all of whom only handle their one thing: the arthritis and lupus doctor, the endocrine doctor, the psychiatrist, the nephrologist, the internist, etc. None of them will look beyond their twigs to the trunk of the tree. What if all these autoimmune symptoms that are causing Debbie so much suffering are due to a break in the system higher up and closer to the trunk of the tree? What if there is damage or malfunction high in the cascade that then affects many other processes that result in joint problems, endocrine problems, neuropsychiatric problems, kidney problems, etc. Debbie has never been tested for Lyme or TBIs. Debbie's son, 23, is now experiencing many of the symptoms that Debbie has encountered over the years. Here's hoping that someone will take the time to look at the trunk of the tree in trying to help this kid.

PEARL: An antineuronal antibody is an antibody that attacks the nerve cell of the individual. The human genome is about 90% identical to that of bacteria. Because of this molecular mimicry, when the immune system is assaulted and is in combat mode, it is understandable that some of the less specific components may mistake self-antigens for bacterial antigens. An autoimmune reaction may result where neurons in the nervous system are mistakenly targeted for elimination. This phenomenon has been well-described in some children with Strep infections. Termed pediatric autoimmune neuropsychiatric disorders associated with Streptococcal infections (PANDAS), these conditions present with sudden onset or change in intensity of OCD, tics, anxiety, panic, aggression, and other intense neuropsychiatric problems.

The role of antineuronal antibodies is just beginning to be explored primarily as they relate to the symptoms of PANDAS. Initially, these disorders were only thought to follow the body's mismanagement of a Strep infection. Now the possibility that some TBI pathogens may also cause the body to make antibodies against its own neurons is appearing more likely.

Madeline Cunningham, at the University of Oklahoma, is investigating how and why the body might be making these antineuronal antibodies against its own nervous system. This research is part of a larger PANDAS study that might help explain a few important loose ends around TBIs. Several TBIs, such as Lyme, bartonellosis, and M. fermentans, manifest with significant neuropsychiatric symptoms. The possibility that antibodies made to fight these organisms might also be damaging self-nerve tissue would account for the virulent autoimmune presentation seen in some patients. This mechanism might help us understand why so many infectious processes manifest with similar neuropsychiatric symptoms.

Bb loves central nervous system (CNS) tissue and is sometimes present in high concentrations around the brain and other nerve cells. If the immune system is mounting an aggressive defense, sometimes the program seems to get stuck on "GO" where the T cells relentlessly stimulate the B cells and an autoimmune presentation occurs. In addition to destroying pathogen, self-tissue is also damaged. This mechanism appears to offer a solid scientific rationale for the Strep-induced PANDAS syndrome and now may also be valid in explaining some neuropsychiatric symptoms in

TBIs. One estimate is that between 40% and 60% of PANDAS patients are positive for Bb.

The molecular mimicry that results in this tendency toward an autoimmune presentation might cause similar signs and symptoms in response to a number of infectious agents. Of course, this complicates the differential diagnosis but overall may help us understand the confusion and delays in making many of these fine distinctions.

Currently, the testing for antineuronal antibodies conducted by Dr. Cunningham is not yet commercially available. However, Quest will conduct somewhat less specific tests called the anti-ganglioside antibody panel 3. These studies measure anti-lyso-ganglioside, anti-tubulin, and anti-dopamine 1 and anti-dopamine 2. If even one of these parameters is found to be present, there can be interference with nerve transmission in the patient. Some insurance plans cover this testing.

Dr. Cunningham is exploring the possibility of treating these patients with IV γ-globulin and targeted antibiotics. After treatment, plasmapheresis is used to clean up the immunologic debris.

There are a number of well-documented cases of TBI patients with life-altering neuropsychiatric symptoms. The possibility for this research to change the life of a patient is encouraging.

D. Regulating a Broken Immune System

If we're lucky we recognize those occasions when the immune system is either underperforming or overperforming, or that there is some other break in the works. Recognition is half the battle. Then we can endeavor to boost, suppress, or mend the system in an attempt to normalize function.

HCPs have tried to regulate the immune system for millennia. **Suppression** of intense immune responses has been tried with herbs, food, baths, ointments, and many other potential remedies. Likewise, many methods have been tried to **boost** immune response. When you read about patients going to Mexico for alternative cancer treatments, many of the modalities they seek are efforts to enhance the immune response.

To date, there is some evidence that the immune system will respond to a number of healthy behaviors, such as maintenance of good nutrition, reasonable body weight, consistent exercise, high quality sleep, and adequate rest. Minimizing stressors is also helpful. We know, for example, that cardiac workouts boost immune responses. Researchers at McMaster University in Canada examined the impact of exercise on the efficacy of the immune response. They found that regular aerobic activity boosts the immune system and helps reduce chronic inflammation.

Optimal function of the immune system requires adequate nutrition. Malnutrition clearly leads to immuno-compromise. You can't build defenses from protein if you do not have the building blocks available. Similarly, too much nutrition leads to obesity and diabetes, which are well-known to impede immune efficiency.

Further, scientists have documented that biotoxins bind preferentially to adipose tissue (i.e., fat cells). The more fat, the more toxin might be stored for indefinite periods. Biotoxins bound to cell receptors increase cytokines, which cause inflammation. Immunity seems to work best when the patient is in the normal weight range.

The immune system is greatly impacted by sleep and rest. Immune function is reduced by sleep deprivation. Complex feedback loops involving cytokines such as IL-1, produced in response to infection, also appear to play a role in sleep. Therefore, the immune response may result in changes in sleep patterns and account for some of the symptoms associated with many infections and other diseases. Likewise, poor sleep can impact the ability of the immune system to mount a full response.

The problem with all these methods to boost immune function is twofold. First, to reap the benefits from these healthy behaviors requires considerable time. Second, most people convert to the righteous path for a few days and then skip the next 6 months. Unfortunately, this laxity is true for most of us no matter how motivated we are toward compliance. A study of people dying from the effects of graft versus host disease after organ transplantation proved that even though they understood how important taking their medication was to saving their lives, many were not compliant. Rather than admit to their HCPs that they missed multiple doses, patients were filmed as they secretly threw their extra pills into the base of a large planter outside the medical building. Even the real possibility of dying could not keep these patients compliant. Especially when eating right and exercising take so long to show their positive results, the average person just doesn't have the patience. While some medicines are under development to stimulate the immune system, there is currently no fast-acting, effective, and safe drug to enhance immune response.

In contrast, there are a number of medications that are quite effective in muting or suppressing immune reactions. These drugs are in great demand, because the signs and symptoms that result from an over-eager immune system can be quite uncomfortable. Think of a patient with a severe asthma attack or a kid covered in poison ivy. The classic hallmarks of infection including fever, aches, fatigue, and GI upset, usually scream for relief. The drugs used to address these problems are called anti-inflammatories and include aspirin and all those drugs promoted endlessly on TV: Advil, Motrin, Celebrex, Nuprin, Indocin, Aleve, Naprosyn, etc. As a drug class they are referred to as NSAIDs or nonsteroidal anti-inflammatories. These drugs are quite effective, but they are not without their problems. GI upset, bleeding, and liver problems are at the top of the list.

PEARL: Be aware of the ads touting agents for arthritis and psoriasis that warn against recurrence of TB or susceptibility to certain fungal infections. Warnings are necessary because the treatments suppress the immune system to such a degree that the host can no longer put up a decent defense against these infections.

Perhaps the most effective modulators of excessive immune response are steroids. Nothing beats down an aggressive immune system better than a good steroid. As might be expected, no one knows exactly how steroids mute the immune response. Their effects can be paradoxical, where they diminish overactive cytokines in one case and stimulate underactive cytokines in another. Unfortunately, steroids can have many untoward side effects including bone loss, high blood sugars, fluid imbalance, growth disturbances, and obesity. Steroid use is discouraged in TBI patients since it is hypothesized that the spirochete may burrow deeper into the tissue if the inflammatory response is dampened. This might not be all bad since then the pathogen can be hit hard with appropriate antibiotic when it resurfaces.

PEARL: An alternative hypothesis as to why steroids might not be a good idea in Lyme patients explores the possibility of steroids allowing a subtle, on-going, low-grade infection to simmer that is hard to manage.

Extracorporeal photopheresis (ECP) also modulates excessive T cell activity primarily in cutaneous T cell lymphoma and possibly in other T cell-mediated disorders. Here ultraviolet radiation causes apoptosis of certain T cells, perhaps focusing most on the abnormal Ts. ECP may also cause monocytes to differentiate into dendritic cells that then clean up the Ts that were broken in the apoptosis induced by the ECP. ECP functions to suppress excess immune response just as steroids do. If the mechanism of action of steroid immunosuppression is poorly understood, then ECP is even less well comprehended. ECP is mentioned here as another option for HCPs who feel they are out of alternatives for the patient with an out-of-control immune response. ECP seems to have fewer side effects than long-term steroid use but, then again, it may be less effective.

Other drugs can dampen the immune response as part of their MOA. These are not used to purposely decrease inflammation but they secondarily harm the immune system as a side effect of their action. Some cytotoxic drugs actually kill certain immune cells such as activated T cells. Others can prevent T cells from responding to signals and thereby neutralize immune response.

V. ANTIBIOTICS AND THE IMMUNE SYSTEM

Sometimes the immune system is not able to activate itself fast enough to curtail the reproduction of a pathogen. In other cases, bacteria are making toxins so fast that permanent damage or death could occur before the immune system can get the upper hand. This is where antibiotics come in. Antibiotics help tip the recovery balance in favor of the host.

Antibiotics help the immune system do its work. If effective, this assistance usually allows the patient to feel better sooner compared to the immune system working alone. Antibiotics kill or cripple the pathogens directly. They work on bacteria and certain other pathogens but _not_ viruses. Usually, the antibiotics damage the bacterial cells but not the host cells.

Antibiotics hurt bacteria through a number of mechanisms such as cell wall inhibition. Different antibiotics work in different ways, so some will be effective against certain bacteria but not at all useful against others. Some antibiotics work just by decreasing the bacterial numbers by not allowing the bacteria to divide and increase their populations. Still, the antibiotic cannot function alone and needs the infrastructure of the immune system to complete the task.

Usually patients start to feel better after a few doses of the antibiotic (if they are lucky enough to have an HCP who selected the correct medicine at the right dose). In general, an antibiotic takes about 7 to 10 days to reach maximum effect. In most cases, the patient will feel better before the antibiotic has done all it could. That is why patients are often told to take all the prescription even if they feel better. (Now be honest… how many bottles of half-used antibiotics are in your medicine cabinet? That's okay; you probably had a virus anyway.)

To be effective, an antibiotic needs reasonable access to the pathogen. The survival of a pathogen depends on how well it can evade the host's defenses at every step. If the skin or cilia keep it out, then that particular pathogen doesn't need to worry if there are antibodies or antibiotics waiting for it down the line. But, of course, pathogens have evolved many ways to escape and ultimately infect the host. Some bacteria can secrete enzymes that digest barriers. Still others can manufacture chemicals that can shut down specific parts of the host's defenses. Some pathogens can avoid the innate immune responses by hiding inside host cells (intracellular pathogenesis).

In intracellular pathogenesis, the invader spends most of its life cycle inside the cells of the host. There it is shielded from immune cells, antibodies, antibiotics, and complement. Examples of intracellular pathogens include viruses, Salmonella, malaria parasites, Babesia, and Borrelia. Other bacteria such as Mycobacteria and Bb can live inside protective capsules that prevent lysis by complement. To be effective in these cases, the antibiotic needs to be able to penetrate the capsule. Some pathogens secrete compounds that lead the host's immune responders on a wild goose chase. Other microbes form biofilms that protect them from many of the defenses of the immune system. Biofilms have made a number of pathogens very effective infectious agents since the biofilm might shield the pathogen from antibiotics as well. A few bacteria can generate surface proteins that bind to antibodies making them ineffective. Others take a different tack and damage or destroy the immune cells themselves. Unfortunately the TBIs, especially Bb, seem to have mastered many of these techniques in order to survive.

Invaders can also elude the adaptive immune system. One way is by mutation. Some pathogens can quickly change epitopes on their surface. The infectious agent changes non-essential epitopes, while hiding essential ones. This is termed **antigenic variation**. A good example is HIV. The proteins on its viral envelope are always changing – one reason that development of a vaccine for HIV has been so elusive. Some parasites use similar strategies, always switching one kind of surface protein for another so it is always one step ahead of the host antibodies. Other pathogens avoid detection by masking their antigens with host molecules. While this is all just biochemistry, it's hard not to anthropomorphize.

To make a complex story short, the immune system is always trying its best to respond to any foreign invader. Sometimes, its best just isn't good enough. The system can be overwhelmed. Whether it can pull off an upset over time is unknown, at least unknown at the point when we first recognize a problem. Antibiotics are simply another weapon in the arsenal, another tool in the chest, another utensil on the table. Many patients will get better without any antibiotics. But some die without help, and even more just feel terrible or sustain long-term damage if antibiotics are not introduced.

The concept of resistance and the pros and cons around antibiotic use will be discussed in Chapter 23: *Understanding Medicines*.

VI. VACCINES AND THE IMMUNE SYSTEM

I don't know how many lives vaccines have saved, but let's just say it's been a bunch. There would be no vaccines without some understanding of immunology. The principle behind vaccination (also called immunization) is to introduce an antigen from a particular pathogen into the host, in a controlled fashion, in order to stimulate antibody production. Once the B cells evolve into plasma cells and memory cells, then very specific immunity against that particular pathogen can be established without causing the disease usually associated with that organism.

Active immunity can be generated naturally from surviving an infection or artificially through vaccination. Deliberate induction of an immune response through vaccination is successful because it exploits the natural specificity of the immune system as well as its inducibility. Vaccination is the most effective manipulation of the immune system ever developed.

The miracle is that this process was introduced by scientists like Pasteur when the basics were barely recognized. Pasteur had to endure considerable ridicule for daring to say that germs might cause infection. But there had been hints for a long time. Remember that Thucydides had an inkling back in 430 BCE that those who survived the plague could nurse new plague victims without getting sick again themselves.

Actually, there are many diseases, like measles, that you do not get a second time. The measles pathogen makes its way into the body and starts to reproduce. The immune system recognizes this intrusion and gears up to fight back. There are already B cells in the body and once they get the message, these B cells turn into plasma cells, start cloning themselves, and pump out antibodies specific for measles. This process takes time, but the symptoms of the disease are eventually eliminated from this host. In the meantime, the disease runs its course. While many of the B cells are occupied in making antibodies, other memory B cells specific for the measles virus remain in the body for years. If the same measles strain reappears, the body is able to handle it almost immediately before it has a chance to cause disease.

A vaccine is a weakened or dead form of the disease pathogen. Once vaccinated, the immune system reacts as though it is infected. The immunized person gets few or no symptoms of the disease but the immune system gears up, complete with the B cells that remember the pathogen from the vaccination. Later when the real disease presents itself to the immunized person, the body can react quickly before the pathogen can take hold.

There are vaccines now against many pathogens. Some pathogens such as the viruses that cause the common cold and other URIs either mutate so fast or have so many slightly different strains in the wild that no practical vaccine is available to date. Each time you get a flu shot, you get a somewhat different strain of the pathogen. Some infectious pathogens like HIV (and perhaps Bb) change so rapidly that a vaccine has so far not been possible.

VII. CANCER AND THE IMMUNE SYSTEM

In my role as clinical researcher, I was once called by an academic who told me that he had cured cancer. This was based on apoptosis of some white cells in 12 patients that he was treating for other conditions. He, like most of the rest of us, did not understand the immune system very well, especially when it comes to cancer or TBIs. Know what you don't know before you call your grant sponsor to come to New Haven only to be disappointed.

The immune system is designed to identify and eliminate tumors. The altered cells found in tumors present antigens not found in normal cells. To the immune system, these antigens should appear foreign. Immune cells should attack and eradicate them. Inducers of cancer include viruses, UV light, toxins, *self*-proteins that have been altered, and proteins involved in regulating cell growth and survival. Any of these can mutate into cancer-causing molecules called **oncogenes**. Once a cell takes on the characteristics of cancer, the host should recognize that cell as abnormal and eliminate it.

Killer T cells are one modality used by the immune system to identify and destroy these abnormal cells, with assistance from helper Ts. In some cases, antibodies are generated against cancer cells allowing their destruction by complement. TNF also seems to be involved in reducing the cancer load. Nonetheless, some cancer cells either escape or overwhelm the immune system and become pathologic.

Cancer cells are able to multiply and spread because they *either* 1) evade detection, 2) release substances that inhibit the immune response, 3) suppress phagocytes, *or* 4) the host develops tolerance for the tumor antigens. Any of these methods, and probably many that we have not yet identified, cause the immune system to no longer adequately attack cancer cells. Some parts of the immune system may actually promote tumor growth. Cytokines can attract macrophages, which make more cytokines and various growth factors that nurture tumor development. Other cytokines, also made by macrophages, seem to facilitate metastasis (spread of cancer). So is cancer an immunologic disease? (Is Lyme an immunologic disease?)

Some researchers theorize that we all have cancer cells in our bodies all the time. Under normal circumstances, our immune systems are extremely efficient in removing these abnormal cells. But for the millions who receive a cancer diagnosis each year, some combination of conditions allowed the cancer to take hold and cause disease. While every disease seems to be multifactorial to some degree, cancer seems to depend on a deficient immune system in order to thrive.

PEARL: The Bb organisms tend to gravitate to areas that are injured or that are affected by tumefaction (swelling either from excess fluid or the formation of new tissues).

Therefore, it is not uncommon to find Bb in gliomas as well as other brain tumors. Borrelia have also been identified in skin tumors and lipomas. Here the organisms are not causal agents of the cancer, but rather opportunistic pathogens.

PEARL: At the June 2012 American Society of Clinical Oncology meeting in Chicago, the focus was on targeted treatments for cancer. The immune system was proposed as a cancer fighting tool – a concept that TBI experts have been suggesting for years.

In 2013, we have barely touched the surface of cancer immunology. What makes some people think they might have a better understanding of the relationship between TBIs and immunology?

VIII.   TBIs AND THE IMMUNE SYSTEM

Is long-term Lyme an infectious disease, or does it result from a defect in the immune system? Many TBI experts feel strongly that recurrent manifestations of Lyme disease are due to live spirochetes reasserting themselves. Much of the controversy around Lyme involves debate over chronic Lyme and the role of the immune system. While I will not be able to resolve this disagreement within this text, some discussion around the role of the immune system in TBIs may prove helpful.

All infectious diseases depend in some way on the host's immune system. We all get "infected" many times, after which we never manifest any signs of disease. I read yesterday that 50% of all shopping carts have E *coli* on their handles. Then why aren't we all constantly running to the bathroom? We are exposed, why aren't we sick?

Whether or not we get sick may depend on the robustness (or the lack thereof) of the individual immune system. We are all familiar with college students who hold it together until after finals and then get a "terrible" cold that flattens them for days. Run-down and depleted individuals and those with known immune compromise (AIDS, splenectomy, etc.) are more susceptible, of course. Bb seem to hit hardest in those who are somehow immune deficient and in these cases can be considered an opportunistic disease.

While more discussion around the individual TBIs and their relationship to the host immune system is presented in their specific chapters, some general comments are appropriate here. Why did my son, who was healthy as an ox, get so sick with babesiosis? Did his chronic otitis media as a baby portend his proclivity to poor immune response? Is there something wrong with his immune system? What is it? Who are the people who get the Lyme rash? Are they immunologically different from those who do not? Does the rash predict a more severe clinical course? Is it a sign of a defective immune system? Did the fact that Chris had a number of co-infections contribute to the severity of his illness?

Why do some people with a tick bite get sick while others, with all other factors the same, don't get any signs of disease? Some get far sicker than others. Some Lyme patients recover with a short-course of antibiotic and some recover with no treatment at all. If you are reading this book, you might know someone who has had recurrent or persistent symptoms, or who has actually been disabled by a TBI. Who are these people immunologically?

We can safely say that in terms of TBIs, the immune system impacts the disease and the disease impacts the immune system. Where are the sickest patients on the immune spectrum? Do they get so ill because of the circumstances of their infection (amount of exposure, strain of pathogen, co-infections, etc.) or the condition of their immune system when the infestation occurred? Can the severity of illness be attributable to all these factors? Why would this pathology be restricted to one mechanism or the other?

We are far from answering any of these questions but, little by little, data are accumulating that may shed some light. Studies were done by Janis Weis at the University of Utah on hundreds of mice exposed to Bb, comparing those who could not mount *any* immune response to those who could only grossly *over-react.* Although an over-reactive response was found to be bad, no immune response was worse. With no response, the infection was quickly out-of-control and these mice were the sickest. Weis found the receptor that Bb needs to lock onto in order to cause an immune reaction. The mice that could not mount an adequate response quickly became overwhelmed with the infection.

Bb are thought to invade immune cells and harm them. Some cells are destroyed and others significantly inhibited. The longer a patient harbors Bb, the bigger the impact on the immune response. Further, the larger the spirochete load, the greater the potential effect on the host immune system. Clearly, in terms of Lyme, the status of the host immune system does impact the presentation and clinical course of the disease. Weis thinks that these findings might explain why there is so much individual variation in response to Bb infection. Some immune system alterations that have been associated with on-going Lyme disease include: likely presence of antineuronal antibodies, higher levels of nonspecific immune activity, higher levels of IL-2 and IL-10, elevated nerve growth factor, as well as immune hyperactivity and dysregulation. This malfunctioning of the immune system in relation to Bb infection can also leave the host susceptible to the activation of previously dormant infections. Think cold sores and shingles. The Lyme itself may flare or wax and wane. Some Lyme patients experience an exacerbation after receiving certain vaccines which may suggest an immune overload.

PEARL: Some think that the immune dysfunction that results from Lyme infection is irreversible. While in some cases this may be true, there are a number of reports where these problems reverse with adequate treatment.

With regard to TBIs, certainly some signs and symptoms are due to the specific pathogen. For example, Bb loves collagen, so many of the disease manifestations seen in Lyme would be expected to affect the tissues with the most collagen. Collagen is a primary component of connective tissue and is found in high concentrations in skin, valves in blood vessels and the heart, tendons and ligaments in the joints, bone, and the GI tract.

But a number of other Lyme symptoms are due to the response of the immune system. For example the fever, aches, headache, fatigue, and GI upset are familiar manifestations of the immune response to almost any pathogen. The majority of infections present with these common complaints. That might be a good reason why HCPs have so much trouble diagnosing. Frankly, it's often hard to differentiate between a virus and a bacterium. Even harder is the parsing of what symptoms are coming from one TBI versus another. In the previous pages, I listed how parts of the inflammatory process contribute to fever, aches, and nausea, etcetera, and how cytokines adversely impact the brain and nervous system causing depression, anxiety, behavior changes, and sleep problems. As mentioned earlier, whenever a patient complains about brain fog, think about unbridled cytokines. There is a lot of malicious biochemistry going on in these very sick people. The reaction of the immune system is at least partially responsible.

The brain is usually rather isolated from the general immune response. Cells need to pass the blood brain barrier (BBB) before they can enter the inner sanctum. Why, then, do some infections such as the TBIs make patients so tired? Some of the fatigue associated with TBIs is quite debilitating, with patients confined to bed for days, weeks, or months. There are a number of theories concerning the mechanism by which inflammation contributes to fatigue and listlessness. Seemingly, some cells such as Bb, are able to pass the BBB. How? Probably some of the cytokine messengers open a pathway through mechanisms not yet understood. Something must open the gates. That something just might be our immunologic humors.

Chronic inflammation appears to allow additional breach of the BBB, thereby resulting in more neurologic symptoms such as incapacitating fatigue, behavioral changes, and apathy. More immune cells can release more chemical messengers. Eicosanoids, such as prostaglandins and leukotrienes, are also important messengers in the CNS. Their pathways are some of the least understood and most perplexing in the body. Nonetheless, they seem to have a relationship to the symptoms so often experienced by TBI patients. Their multiple

functions may explain why so many serious CNS manifestations have been associated with TBIs. Of course, spirochetes do find their way into brain tissue as demonstrated repeatedly by Alan MacDonald and others. Is it the spirochete, the modulator, or both causing the symptoms?

Finally, to relate all this immunology to TBIs, let's just say that the immune system usually dances for a reason. In terms of those Lyme patients with intermittent, on-going, low-level, or rip-roaring episodic symptoms, something must have inspired the recurrence. There must be some explanation for the reappearance of so many inflammatory-type signs and symptoms (assuming there is not a new infection).

Many TBI specialists believe the explanation is on-going infection. We can easily understand the early inflammatory signs that are observed due to initial invasion and establishment of a Bb infection. Then why would Lyme symptoms reappear after the patient was told they were cured by a course of antibiotics? Because the Bb, whether it was lurking, hiding, active, dormant, encapsulated, etcetera, resurfaces for a number of reasons. When the Bb reappears, so do the signs and symptoms of the inflammatory response. Now whether that response is the same in that individual the second time around or somehow different, who knows?

For the individual patient, sometimes the response to recurrence of active Bb are the same as it was in the past and sometimes it is not recognizable. The patient's reaction may be similar to the secondary reaction of others or quite different. Is the individual's response maladjusted? Is her immune system over or under-reacting? Will her defenses become overwhelmed or overaggressive? Whatever the response, something must have started this ball rolling again. The reason the music restarts is that the pathogen again strikes up the band. The infection is calling the shots and befuddling us over and over again.

I am not convinced that we will answer these questions in my lifetime. All we know is that we have a sick patient in front of us and someone has to do something. Additional detail about how the individual co-infections affect (or are affected by) the immune system is presented in the separate pathogen chapters.

IX. PRACTICAL USES OF IMMUNOLOGY IN ADDRESSING TBIs

You have suffered enough. I promised practical application around diagnosis and treatment for TBIs and here it is. The basics of immunology give us some clues in understanding the signs, symptoms, and clinical course of TBIs. Further, measurement of specific cells and modulators of the immune system can provide helpful information regarding diagnosis and treatment effect.

When a patient visits an HCP complaining of a fever or other indicators of infection, one option is to order a WBC with differential. This test counts all white cells in the blood and either manually or mechanically tallies the various kinds of cells present. A simple high white count usually says infection, but by enumerating the various types of cell that are responding to the invasion, we can learn much more. We would then know how many neutrophils, eosinophils, etcetera, are on hand. By knowing the USUAL number of these cells found in a healthy person at a specific age, we can tell if our patient has more or less than expected. By comparing these results to those of known pathology, we can get hints regarding whether there is an infection. Further, the results might suggest whether that infection could be viral, bacterial, or parasitic, or if the inflammatory reaction is more likely due to allergy than infection. Of course, the results can get quite muddy when co-infections are involved, but we will take all the help we can get.

Trust me, as an old ER doc, this information can provide HINTS, but never 100% guaranteed diagnostic truth. Nonetheless this data can be used, in conjunction with the other information gathered from the history and physical etcetera, in assisting the HCP in drawing conclusions.

In assessing TBIs, considerable information can be gathered from measuring antibodies. Detection of particular antibodies is a common form of medical diagnostics. Serology is the study of the blood serum, along with other body fluids, used most often in trying to identify specific immunoglobulins in the serum. For example, testing can be done looking for antibody against an infectious agent, foreign protein, toxin, etc. Familiar examples are the identification of foreign proteins in a mismatched blood transfusion or one's own proteins in cases of autoimmune disease. Antibodies against hCG antigen are used in pregnancy tests.

An antibody profile, where the levels of the different Ig classes are measured, can be done in Lyme patients. Assessments can be made regarding acute versus chronic status. Of course, useful information can only be gathered if the appropriate test is ordered, the test is sensitive and specific enough, and the results are interpreted by someone who knows what they are doing. For example, a test sample looking for antibody titer directed against Epstein-Barr virus, Lyme disease, or ehrlichiosis could be examined. If there are no antibodies, then 1) the person is not infected, 2) the wrong antigen was used to bind with the antibodies in the test, or 3) the infection was so long ago that the memory B cells have naturally decayed.

A blood test measuring HLA-DR2 and HLA-DR4 might be considered in essentially all Lyme patients to determine if they will tend toward an autoimmune-type response to Bb infection. If positive, these patients might benefit from an alternative treatment approach including hydroxychloroquine (Plaquenil).

Another test of the immune system that might prove helpful is measurement of specific clusters of differentiation (CDs). CDs are protein markers on the surface of cells that assist in the immune response primarily against viruses. Probably the most commonly used CD measurement is CD4 levels in the estimation of the severity of HIV infection. CD4 levels lower than 200 are a prerequisite for the diagnosis of AIDS. The lower the CD4, the more severe the illness, so CD4 is used as a marker of clinical status. For TBI patients, some practitioners use CD57 as a marker to determine when treatment can be discontinued. In children, CD57 measures might not be as consistent as they can be in adults. Before making a determination about how the patient is doing based on the CD57 level, consider the patient's or caregiver's assessment of the clinical status. Tests of immunoglobulins, complement, and HLA subsets can provide information and are included in Chapter 18: *Ordering Appropriate Tests*.

Let's look at just one case where the immunology can be used in practical application in Lyme disease. This will be a brief diversion to illustrate the complexity of the overall system. This same material is reviewed again in Chapter 10: *Borreliosis,* but inclusion here underscores the importance of understanding the immune system in order to better comprehend TBIs. This is a practical application of the new knowledge you gained by making your way through this chapter.

Outer surface proteins (OSPs) are proteins located on the outside of the Bb cell. Genes that code for seven distinct OSPs on Bb have been recognized. These are all antigens that can inspire the production of specific antibodies. OspA and OspB are likely the most common, but OspC may be the most clinically significant. OSPs seem to be correlated with virulence.

Bb are able to shift their OSPs making them unrecognizable to the host's immune system. This genetically-engineered shift allows for a new generation of spirochetes that aren't susceptible to identification by the antibodies that were made against the original OSPs. The antibodies were produced based on the information they discerned from the original proteins on the Bb.

When first available those antibodies attacked the original Bb and the host felt the symptoms produced by that inflammatory response. When the antibodies and the rest of the immune system were effective in defending the host, the person responded by feeling better. The fever and other signs of inflammation abated until a new batch of modified Bb appeared causing another immune response and another set of corresponding sxs. This would be perceived as a relapse. This shift in OSP composition is a defensive strategy used by Bb to avoid detection and destruction.

Bb are quite adept at changing their protein coats constantly, thus eluding the antibodies that destroy most other germs. As the individual makes antibodies against one set of Lyme proteins, the spirochete cloaks its outer surface with an entirely new set of proteins, making it unrecognizable to the immune cells targeting it. So Bb turn into moving targets that can elude the immune system for months or years.

In the journal *Cell*, Norris describes the special segment of DNA in Bb that constantly churns out new gene sequences. These novel genes then direct the production of new proteins. As the proteins (antigens) change, the outer coat of the spirochetes change, rendering the immune molecules that might once have killed them impotent. Norris comments on "promiscuous recombination" that constructs a vast array of proteins at a rapid pace potentially producing millions of antigenic variants in the host. If in serology testing, the antibody from the patient is matched against test antigen that has significantly changed OSP, the odds of getting a positive test could be diminished. Immunology matters in TBIs.

X. RELATIONSHIP BETWEEN THE IMMUNE SYSTEM AND OTHER BODY SYSTEMS

I know I sound very Zen here but, in truth, the immune system cannot be distinguished from the other systems of the body. Immune response is intimately involved with essentially every other organ system. To say that the immune system is a separate entity from the GI tract, the skin, the liver, or the endocrine system would be false and artificial. Can we really separate the bone from its stem cells and their products? How can we deny that modulators from both the immune system and the endocrine system affect the brain and nervous system accounting for much of the neuropsychiatric symptomatology found in disease?

One example is the ability of hormones to act as immunomodulators that change the sensitivity of the immune system. This activity could impact the immune system's ability to communicate and the capacity of the infected organism to heal over time. Female sex hormones are known immunostimulators. Male sex hormones appear to be immunosuppressants. Some diseases seem to be affected by puberty and, later, the progressive decline of hormones may account for weakened immune response in the elderly. Thyroid hormone seems to be especially impacted by the immune system. Vitamin D is a hormone. Before your head starts spinning, do you see the interconnections here that might affect TBI patients? Does it really matter if we call one set of functions the immune system and another group the endocrine system or the nervous system?

As scientific knowledge accumulated over decades, we became desperate to organize the material to make it manageable. When we find similarities between things, we can declare that they belong together. When we find differences, we can say that an entity does not belong. Once we label something, we no longer need to think about it as hard. Keep it with its group and never stray. A place for everything and everything in its place. We become restricted by our own organizational scheme. Nonetheless, we have learned a lot since 9th grade biology class when everything could be contained in its own little book chapter. Now the interrelationships between systems are so overlapping and intricate that we should stop trying to force every new idea into the old framework. We need ways to simplify this enormous amount of material, but we do not need to be limited by our own logic. The more we learn, the more flexible we need to become in order make good use of our progress. We need to keep gathering and organizing information. But we also need to LOOSEN UP!

Personal note: According to Christopher Hitchens, several things in life are grossly over-rated including champagne, lobster, and picnics. To that I would add natural childbirth, owning your own business, and writing a chapter on Gentle Immunology *and TBIs.*

IMMUNE MARKERS APPLICABLE TO TBIs

Immune markers: Many immune cells, with their protein coats, have characteristic markers that can be used for identification and classification. There are entire encyclopedias written on each of these marker designations as well as on-line catalogs identifying the various molecules, categories, and groupings. The complexity here can be mind-boggling. Not being a masochist, I was desperate to skip this section. Unfortunately, I do not have that luxury since these markers have been shown to be important in the understanding and management of Lyme. I am providing the minimum information needed to understand just enough to use these concepts to help TBI patients.

Major Histocompatibility Complex (Human Leukocyte Antigens): The Major Histocompatibility Complex (**MHC**) proteins are antigens present on the surface of many kinds of cells. In humans, the MHCs that mark white cells are referred to as human leukocyte antigens or **HLA**s and these molecules help mediate the action of leukocytes. Cells present their antigens to the immune system by way of these MHC molecules. Depending on the antigen presented and the type of histocompatibility molecule, several types of immune cells can then become activated.

The importance of the MHCs comes back to being able to tell the difference between *self* and non-*self*. How does the immune system determine what belongs and what doesn't? How do WBCs and other parts of the immune response know what to attack and what to leave alone? Every cell in the body has a built-in system to answer that question. There are thousands of antigens on cell surfaces serving as identifiers so that we don't eat ourselves up. MHC marks a cell as *self*. Anything that doesn't have the correct *self* mark then becomes non-*self* and is tagged to be eliminated. Simply, MHC tells the system what should stay and what should go.

Each MHC molecule displays a fraction of protein called an **epitope** outside the cell, like a hot dog that is too long for its bun. (The hot dog being the epitope and the bun being the MHC molecule.) Many white cells display these HLAs on their surfaces. These markers serve as the identification card or fingerprint for a cell. Antigens on the body's own cells are called **autoantigens** and should be recognized as *self*.

MHC molecules are important to the immune response. They allow cells that have been invaded by an infectious agent to be recognized as non-*self* and thereafter be targeted by T cells. Depending on the antigen presented and the type of histocompatibility molecule, several types of immune cells can become activated. When the MHC protein is displayed on the surface of the cell, it's detected by a nearby immune cell (often a NK cell or other cell in the T cell lines). If these nearby defenders recognize the protein as non-*self,* it will kill the infected cell and any other cells displaying that non-*self* MHC protein.

HLA antigens were first explored as a way to find compatible donors for transplants. Tissue donors with a similar HLA profile to the recipient would be more likely to donate organs that would not be rejected. More recently, HLA markers are used to identify potential for autoimmune reactions, vaccine efficacy, and response to various drugs. For example, most Caucasians with Grave's disease display HLA-B8 but not HLA-B7. Further, patients with HLA-B1502 using carbamazepine may have a higher risk for developing Stevens-Johnson syndrome.

Everyone has their own unique HLA fingerprint. HLA markers are divided into two distinct types of molecules that verge on the incomprehensible, but come in handy in assessing TBI patients:

HLA Class I: HLA-A, HLA-B, and HLA-C

Class I: HLA-A, HLA-B, and HLA-C are present on most nucleated cells and platelets and they function to present those peptides made in-house to the CD8 T cells. Class I HLA molecules indicate the **internal** contents of the cell and display this identification on the cell surface. When the internal contents change, the HLA molecule should change. This change might signal that something is amiss thereby sounding the alarm. This HLA presentation is critical to the distinction between *self* and non-*self*. This class presents antigen to cytotoxic T lymphocytes by using the CD receptor on the cytotoxic T cells. They also bind inhibitory receptors on NK cells, perhaps via CD8. HLA class I thereby mediates the destruction of a specific antigen. Each of the HLA I classes can express six different types of molecule. (This is due to complicated genetics, which we do not need to know here.)

HLA Class II: HLA-DR, HLA-DQ, and HLA-DP.

Class II: HLA-DR, HLA-DQ, and HLA-DP are found on antigen-presenting-cells (like those on macrophages and B cells) and exhibit the foreign peptides that were made **external** to the *self* to CD4 T cells allowing for specific immune action. In transplants, the degree to which the donor and recipient match in terms of HLA or "tissue type" will help determine success. Fragments are presented to helper T cells, which then stimulate an immune reaction from other cells. MHC Class II markers present their antigen fragments by binding to the CD4 receptor on the T helper cells. Class II HLAs sound the alarm when foreign antigen is present recruiting additional components of the immune cascade to help defend the host.

HLA markers become important in the management of Lyme disease. About 15% of the general population has specific HLA markers that identify them as a subpopulation that will not react predictably to the Borrelia *burgdorferi* infection. HLA-DR2 and HLA-DR4 are just two of the thousands of antigen markers present in humans. Recently scientists have learned that individuals with these two specific markers are at an increased risk of developing an autoimmune-type reaction when infected with Bb. About 15% of the populace has HLA-DR2 markers and about 15% have HLA-DR4. Some have both. This autoimmune presentation of Lyme might include increased joint involvement and muscle pain along with a more aggressive inflammatory response (since, in addition to attacking the foreign Bb, they are also assaulting the *self)*. The genetics of these patients predispose them to a more difficult clinical course and they do not seem to respond to traditional therapies very well. Addition of Plaquenil (hydroxychloroquine) appears to help alleviate these symptoms and may lessen the autoimmune reaction.

If HLA testing can recognize those at risk for this atypical presentation, they might be helped sooner and more efficiently. Consider testing for the presence of HLA-DR2 and HLA-DR4 in Lyme patients as early in the work-up as possible. These studies potentially identify those who might have an increased risk of an autoimmune tendency, especially those who present with intractable, intense, or atypical presentations of Lyme. The presence of these markers can significantly impact treatment decisions. An individual's HLA markers should not change over time so, once ordered, there is no need to repeat, unless you feel the test was not valid when first run.

Of course, nothing about this could be simple. Not all individuals with HLA-DR2 and HLA-DR4 markers trigger this type of immune reaction. For those who do react with autoimmune manifestations, there appears to be a correlation with the antibody bands 31 or 34 on Western blot that makes them more inclined to present in this way. Antibodies 31 and 34 may take a year to evolve after initial tick exposure. Knowing the patients' proclivities could help in their case management. They can be treated, just not in the traditional way.

PEARL: MHC is a gene region that codes for protein, including both self-proteins and non-self-proteins. An MHC molecule can take a bit of any of this protein and display it on the cell surface. In humans, MHC molecules are encoded by genes clustered on the short arm of chromosome 6. Each of these genes has a number of different alleles (alternate forms of the gene). So it is VERY rare for two people to have the same set of MHC molecules, which collectively are called a tissue type. This knowledge may be useful in interpreting lab results. Think of the HLA markers as a fingerprint or identification card, and the immune system as the bouncer who will 'card' you at the door. We are most familiar with the use of HLA markers in finding the best matches for organ transplant patients, in blood compatibility, and in paternity testing.

PEARL: Because the MHCs must defend against large varieties of foreign proteins, they must be diverse. MHC genes vary greatly from individual to individual and may account for the range of responses that can be observed in an infected population. This diversity of MHC alleles makes sure that somewhere in the population there is that special someone with the correct genotype to recognize a specific microbe and deal with it. This individual would have a chance to survive an epidemic and then find the other person that survived and mate. This might be especially pertinent in understanding the vast differences in individual patient response to TBIs. But, who knows?

PEARL: Humans have great diversity in the genetic codes that make MHC molecules. Why is diversity important? In 2007, low MHC diversity was associated with the increased susceptibility to tumors in Tasmanian devils on the isolated island of Madagascar. Because of in-breeding there was little diversity in the MHC molecules making it more difficult for the immune system to distinguish self from non-self and nearly wiping out the species.

Another HLA has been used in paring down the differential diagnosis of TBIs. The presence of marker HLA-B27 can be useful in sorting through the differential diagnosis in TBI cases. HLA-B27 is more often found in individuals with ankylosing spondylitis, irritable bowel syndrome, and an increased tendency to experience generalized achiness. JRA might be hard to distinguish from Lyme disease and the presence of HLA-B27 may point more in the direction of JIA than Bb.

PEARL: HLA-B27 is one of thousands of identifying markers found on cells. This particular antigen on the cell surface is associated with ankylosing spondylitis. About 6% of the Caucasian population has the HLA-B27 marker which is associated with back pain including ankylosing spondylitis and IBS. These people tend to have more general aches and arthralgias. Not everyone with HLA-B27 has ankylosing spondylitis but essentially everyone with AS has the B27 marker.

Clusters of differentiation (CD): In 1982, a group of immunologists met in Paris for the First International Workshop and Conference on Human Leukocyte Differentiation Antigens. (What a waste of Paris!) At that time, considerable work was being done on monoclonal antibodies and scientists needed a way to standardize communication between labs.

Toward that goal, the scientists decided to use the distinct protein markers displayed on the cell surface membranes as a means to identify and class the different molecules. These **clusters of differentiation** could be used to sort and classify cell types and establish international nomenclature standards. A cluster of differentiation is a group of proteins on the surface of many cells, although in Paris the focus was leukocytes. For our purposes, the term CD refers to the identifying clusters on B and T lymphocytes. Each cluster is unique. Today over 300 distinct clusters have been identified and cataloged.

Cell populations are usually defined as being either + or − for a particular CD depending on whether or not they display a specific molecular cluster. For example, **all** leukocytes are CD45+. Granulocytes are also CD15+ and monocytes are CD14+. Helper T cells express CD4+, while CD8+ identifies cytotoxic T cells. So, while all leukocytes might have the last name "Smith" they would have various first and middle names further distinguishing them from others in the Smith clan.

Although recognition of the unique CDs is useful to scientists for classification purposes, the different cluster groups appear to have distinct roles and functions beyond simple cataloging including: Ag recognition, biochemical communication, and stimulation of certain immune activities. Each CD marker has a specific function in the cell such as passing a signal from the T cell receptor to the cytoplasm. A CD receptor is a receptor specific to one type of cell such as mature T lymphocytes. These T cells, along with the major histocompatibility complex (MHC), help in the recognition of antigens. Receptor molecules CD2, CD3, CD4, among hundreds of others, have been identified.

There are many CDs, and most cells express more than one. The differences lie with the antibody onto which they eventually bind. An antibody recognizes a specific cluster of differentiation on a cell surface and can then bind to that unique area. CDs have traditionally been numbered sequentially. CD1 was the first identified and is most often associated with immature T cells. CD4 is found on all mature T helper cells and they are said to be CD4+. Measures of CD4+ are common in the clinic. When levels of T cells marked with CD4 decrease, HIV activity may be increasing in AIDS patients.

CD levels are measured as a percent of total lymphocytes. T cells are mostly labeled CD1 through CD8, while B cells are generally categorized from CD19 to CD24. Of course, there are exceptions. CD subsets that are often mentioned in the literature and that may be important for the TBI patient include:

CD2 markers are found on some T and B cells and macrophages.

CD4 is a unique cluster of proteins on the surface of cells that appears to have a significant role in the immune response to infections. This grouping is found on essentially all T helper cells and some macrophages (monocytes) and even a few B cells which are then labeled CD4+. The CD4 proteins are expressed on the surface of T helper cells, regulatory T cells, monocytes, macrophages, and dendritic phagocytes. The CD4 cluster involves the MHC class II molecules on the surface of the antigen-presenting cell. CD4 is responsible for sending signals from the T cell receptors and functioning as a co-receptor. Somehow, CD4 clusters amplify the signal using an enzyme that is also necessary for activating many other molecules in the immune cascade. The CD4 receptors on T lymphocytes are the sites where HIV binds. HIV attaches itself to this protein and from there causes the CD4+ WBCs to be attacked, eventually causing a failure of the host defenses. Near the end-stages of HIV infection, the functional number of CD4+ cells decreases, limiting immune response, which leads to the symptoms associated with AIDS. CD4 levels less than 200 are considered a prerequisite for the diagnosis of AIDS. The lower the CD4, the more severe the illness, so CD4 is used as a marker of clinical status. By measuring CD4+ levels, HCPs can gauge where the AIDS patient is clinically and where that patient might be going. CD4 levels are sometimes ordered as part of an immune evaluation in TBI patients.

> *PEARL: Since monocytes MIGHT be more involved in the immune response to Lyme than previously recognized, eventually measurement of the CDs more specifically associated with monocytes could become more useful for the monitoring of Lyme disease. Wouldn't that be nice?*

CD8 is found on T suppressor and T cytotoxic cells which are important in the defense against viruses. Markers for CD8 are measured to identify cytotoxic T cells. Like CD4, CD8 is a unique protein cluster that serves as a co-receptor for the T cell. CD8 binds to MHC Class I and interacts with a specific alpha part of the MHC Class I molecule. Cytotoxic T cells with CD8 surface protein are said to be CD8+ T cells.

CD57 marks a subpopulation of NK (natural killer) lymphocytes. These are thought to be suppressed **ONLY** in Lyme disease. In theory, the lower the CD57, the more suppression of these Lyme-specific NK cells and the more active the Lyme disease. So, the lower the count, the sicker the patient. Some practitioners use measurement of CD57 to help determine how active a Lyme infection is, how well treatment is working, and whether treatment can be reasonably discontinued. Further, after treatment ends, CD57 might provide clues as to whether a relapse is likely to occur. Suggestions on interpretation of CD57 levels are outlined in Chapter 19. Note that kids and teens do not make NK cells in the same amount as adults, so measurement of CD57 may not be as useful in the pediatric population. Further, this subpopulation of NK cells may also be low in some autism cases. As always, treat the patient and not the lab report.

Chapter 4

HISTORY OF TICK-BORNE DISEASES

If you can't get rid of the family skeleton, you might as well make it dance.
George Bernard Shaw

Pam Weintraub has outlined the history of TBIs clearly and comprehensively in her book, *Cure Unknown: Inside the Lyme Epidemic,* which is referenced often in this text. She captures the politics that have shaped this history in ways that were often detrimental to patients. Thanks to advocacy groups like the LDA, the tide is slowly turning in terms of recognition of these diseases and the loosening of restrictions on the diagnosis and treatment of TBI patients in states like Connecticut. There, physicians are now allowed to treat the patient as they see fit, instead of checking off boxes on guidelines that were written by persons with clear secondary agendas – at least according to the state Attorney General.

We know that TBD has plagued humans and animals for millennia. Since we still don't recognize and understand most of the TBIs, we can't possibly expect an accurate chronology. The history of each co-infection is captured in the individual chapters, at least as much as I could glean out of the literature. Strange that the "history" of many of these diseases is very recent. Either we had no idea what we were seeing, as people died all around us, OR we were calling TBIs by any one of a number of inaccurate names like apoplexy and grippe. Have some of these pathogen strains just appeared in the last few decades? If so, where did they come from? If not, we must have been missing something.

As with so many diseases, the history of TBIs is fraught with a "blame the patient" mentality that causes much suffering until more rational minds eventually prevail. Usually, several generations must endure controversy before the traditional medical community catches up. Remember that Joan of Arc was seen as a saint by one side of the battle and was burned at the stake by the other. (Actually the same side that burned her later sainted her after they saw the error of their ways. By the way, Joan was probably schizophrenic.) As with epilepsy, depression, ADHD, autism, CFS, fibromyalgia, leprosy, schizophrenia, AIDS, and innumerable other conditions, once the flogging and eye-rolling stop, we can all get down to work and focus on helping patients.

Lyme disease is named after the town of Lyme, Connecticut, where the first cases were recognized in the 1970s. While the connection to ticks was made early on, the pathogen was not identified until 1981 through the intense work of Willy Burgdorfer. The species now appropriately bears his name. A disorder similar to what we now call Lyme was described in Europe earlier in the 20th century. Fortunately, Dr. Burgdorfer kept up with the scientific literature and was able to make the connection.

In fact, ticks were causing human disease long before any modern discoveries were made. Otzi, a 5300-year-old mummy found in the Tyrolean Alps (near where my grandfather was born), was found to have DNA from Bb co-mingled with his DNA. Otzi is now considered the first case of Lyme disease. Unlike many others, Otzi did not die from his LD. He was about 45-years-old when a flint arrowhead shot into his left shoulder likely finished him off. Otzi also had arthritis and heart problems. Not only was he the first case of Lyme, I submit he was the first case of chronic Lyme.

In the 1960s, Polly Murray and her family in CT began to experience mysterious symptoms that no doctor was able or willing to explain. By 1965, eight neighborhood kids were diagnosed with JRA. Several of the kids on the same street recalled being bitten by a tick. They complained of severe malaise, fever, and headache. Doctors soon recognized that antibiotics helped in these cases.

A few HCPs in Connecticut in the 60s started to notice a pattern like JRA in a number of patients. But UNLIKE juvenile rheumatoid arthritis cases, these kids had headaches, debilitating fatigue, and none of the markers usually associated with JRA. Treatment with antibiotics made the arthritis go away. Some of these kids also had Strep and the majority of these cases responded if treated early enough. Sometimes the patients had a strange expansive skin lesion. As time went on, several HCPs recognized that this syndrome was a multisystem disease and that there was often arthritis, fever, headache, and overwhelming fatigue but not always a rash. Other body systems like GI, GU, cardiac, endocrine, immune, and especially the neuropsychiatric organs might be involved. There could be fasciculations, paresthesias, and hyperactive senses. The earlier the condition was treated with appropriate antibiotics, the less likelihood of a persistent Lyme-syndrome occurring, which could become progressively harder to treat as time went on.

Early in the modern history of TBIs, the fighting began between rheumatologists and dermatologists competing over who owned Lyme disease. Stupendously bad decisions were made that continue to impact patients today. (Think steroid blasts, mandated ELISA testing, incomprehensible WB bands, and rigid short-term antibiotic regimens that continue to be promoted despite evidence of on-going infection in incapacitated patients begging for help.) These sad, indefensible bungles are all subjects of additional discussion later in this text.

Until very recently, HCPs did not realize that TBIs were caused by some of the most complex and confounding pathogens on the planet. We are only beginning to scratch the surface of what we will need to know in order to deal with this tick-borne epidemic. Finally we are recognizing that Bb sometimes have traveling companions that greatly complicate diagnosis and treatment. Further, all of these microbes might impact the host's immune system in ways that we had not previously considered.

The story of TBIs is dynamic and on-going. History is constantly in the making. We have reached the point where traditional medicine is beginning to accept the concepts of co-infection and chronicity with respect to these conditions. Considerable strides are being made in areas of immune response to Lyme and other TBIs, as well as autoimmunity, which should enable a more comprehensive and compassionate approach to these diseases. Keep an open mind and watch as the history of TBIs takes an optimistic turn.

Chapter 5

THE CONCEPT OF CO-INFECTION

You did then what you knew how to do, and when you knew better, you did better.

Maya Angelou

A solitary tick can carry dozens of different potential pathogens. The lowly tick might pick up many possible infectious agents in its two or three-bite life. The idea that a tick would transmit only a single prospective infectious organism to its victim seems rather naïve in 2013, yet every day HCPs fail to consider the likelihood of co-infections. Instead, the term "Lyme" is often used to describe what is really a polymicrobial condition. While Bb are often part of the mix, they are rarely the only pathogens present in a TBI patient these days. One estimate suggests that at least 40% of TBI patients have co-infections rather than a single pathogen causing disease.

When I was in medical training in the 80s, we certainly understood that more than one pathogen could be active in a host at a given time. However, we rarely thought that two or more infectious agents might arrive through the same vector. In the last two decades however, the concept of co-infection has become more familiar because of the AIDS pandemic and with the increased prevalence of TBIs.

With HIV we now recognize a number of common co-infections such as hepatitis, sexually transmitted diseases, and the many opportunistic infections that take hold as the immune system deteriorates. Since I was just coming into medicine when HIV/AIDS was first uncovered, I know that we were often quite surprised to find multiple infections either along-for-the-ride or taking advantage of a bad situation. We had a lot to learn then and we still do.

Pathogens can affect the host through multiple mechanisms. More than one pathologic process can be occurring at the same time including: 1) microbes invading the tissues and cells thereby causing direct physical damage, 2) genetic material from the pathogen incorporating into the genetic material of the host, 3) release of toxins by the infecting organisms, 4) discharge of harmful biochemicals from the host's immune response, and 5) changes in overall immune processes. Co-infections can act synergistically or independently and this may be one reason that the clinical presentation of TBIs can be so variable and confounding.

While there may be more recognition and reporting of co-infections in recent years, there actually may be more disease to recognize and report. In the coming decades, there will continue to be increased opportunity for ticks and humans to mingle. As we change our environment from pure urban-dwelling and untainted farmland to glorious, woody suburbs, we are encountering more of our blood-thirsty friends. The ticks are loving the backyard resorts we have established for them. Many humans dream of raising their families in the quiet suburbs. So do many ticks.

A few definitions might be helpful here. These terms are often used interchangeably, but there are fine distinctions.

Concomitant – Occurring along with something else. In drug development, we used this term to refer to all the medicines a patient was taking at the same time.

Concurrent – Happening together. The term concurrent is often used to refer to diseases that are simultaneously affecting a patient such as diabetes, obesity, and heart disease. They may or may not have the same etiology. For example, the patient with diabetes and heart disease could also have bunions. All these conditions would be considered concurrent, while not all might have the same root cause.

Co-infection – The simultaneous infection of a host by two or more different pathogens. When considering TBIs, we usually consider that these infections arrived TOGETHER, riding on the same vector. So while a TBI patient may also have a viral respiratory infection and a fungal skin disease, these would be considered concurrent illnesses, while her Lyme and babesiosis would be called co-infections.

A deer tick is thought to infect its victim with thousands of Lyme spirochetes in one feeding. Any other microbes in the vicinity at the time of the bite will likely flow along. Some of these infectious agents may or may not be pathogenic to the host. The following list outlines the most commonly transmitted tick infections in the US in mid-2012. Remember that we might have identified only the tip of the iceberg. Over 3 dozen additional viruses have been hypothesized to co-transmit along with Bb during a tick bite. We are very early in the information gathering and understanding of co-infections.

The "knowledge" presented below is based on sparse documentation of "facts" from sources that may not be entirely reliable. Much of the literature is contradictory or confusing and often it is hard to determine whether some or all these conditions are separate diseases or not. Each TBI marked below with an asterisk* has its own chapter in this text since these are the diseases most likely to present in clinical practice. All others are described in Chapter 12: *Other Recognized TBIs*. Use this list as a way to make sure you are considering diagnostic alternatives in assessing your TBI patient.

Most Commonly Transmitted Tick Infections in the United States

- **Lyme Disease***: The best known TBI, Lyme is transmitted primarily by the deer tick but also by the western black-legged tick and possibly the Lone Star tick and various dog tick species. The pathogen causing Lyme is usually Borrelia *burgdorferi* but some researchers also include B. *lonestari* as a causative organism as well. Lyme is found primarily in the northeast, west coast, and the upper midwest US, but its range is expanding rapidly. Most commonly, patients experience aches especially in joints and head, flu-like symptoms, fevers, and neurologic signs and symptoms such as paresthesias and cognitive deficits especially brain fog. Bell's palsy may be present in as many as 10% of Lyme patients. Estimates of those presenting with an EM rash range from about 7% to nearly half. Symptoms may wax and wane. Really severe Lyme disease is a red flag for co-infection.

  PEARL: Despite all my research and much discussion and debate, I still do not know whether STARI is the same as Lyme or not. Despite a zealous letter from a DHHS worker to Pat Smith, (President of the LDA) suggesting that the two conditions were NOT the same, in my opinion, this knowledge base is too new and unexplored to draw definitive conclusions. With the multiple and diverse presentations of Lyme, how can anyone be certain that STARI is not simply another manifestation of Lyme? STARI is currently treated the same way as infection caused by Bb, and the most important consideration is that borreliosis be recognized and managed. As more data is collected, hopefully the significance of any distinction will become clear.

- **Babesiosis***: This TBI is probably the most common after Lyme and is the most frequently identified co-infection. Unfortunately, incidence and prevalence data are sparse since few practitioners test for Babesia and it is grossly under-diagnosed. Babesia microbes probably share the same tick vectors as Bb. In the northeast, incidence of babesiosis may soon exceed that of Lyme. These protozoal pathogens include Babesia *microti* and *duncani* (also known as WA-1). Symptoms include a malaria-like fever that is usually more significant than the fever experienced with Lyme alone and may include night sweats and severe chills. Because Babesia damages RBCs, significant hemolytic anemia can occur, and the urine can become bloody and the skin jaundiced. There are more respiratory issues such as cough, air hunger, and shortness of breath than seen with only Lyme. Many patients also experience fatigue, weakness, nausea, abdominal pain, diarrhea, unrelenting headache, along with neck and back pain. Babesiosis can be fatal, so a high index of suspicion is recommended.

  PEARL: The severity of the arthritis documented in mice is greater when the mice are co-infected with both Bb and Babesia than with either pathogen alone. These two organisms appear to be much more disabling together than when present by themselves. Since Babesia does not respond to the same antimicrobials as Bb, the symptoms of one co-infection may flare if only the other condition is being treated. In untreated co-infection cases, symptoms can persist despite adequate Lyme treatment. With Babesia co-infection, Krause et al detected circulating spirochetal DNA three times more often when Babesia was present than when Bb was alone. I don't know what happens when there is a third or fourth pathogen.

- **Ehrlichiosis/Anaplasmosis***: The pathogens here include Ehrlichia *chaffeenis* and Anaplasma *phagocytophilum*. The deer tick is again the most commonly implicated vector but others include the Pacific tick, American dog tick, and the Lone Star tick. These diseases are most commonly found in the upper midwest and northeast. Ehrlichiosis can be fatal and symptoms include fever, chills, headache, muscle pain, rigors, GI complaints, anorexia, and fatigue. The headache and muscle pain can be intense. Ehrlichiosis has the questionable distinction of being the first recognized co-infection.

- **Bartonellosis***: This pathogen is transmitted by ticks, fleas, and cats. The infectious bacterium is most often Bartonella *henselea*, but B. *quintana* has also been implicated and there is much taxonomic confusion. The infection transmitted by ticks may be due to Bartonella-like organisms (BLOs) and not the traditionally implicated B. *henslea*. Diseases due to Bartonella species are found worldwide and symptoms include fever, chills, headache, gastritis, weight loss, neurologic problems, cold extremities, sore throat, lymphadenitis, and red, papular skin lesions. Distinctive features of tick-borne bartonellosis include severe pain in the tibia and sole, disproportionate neuropsychiatric symptoms, violaceous striae, and subcutaneous nodules. In the northeastern US, Bartonella may be more common than Bb.

  PEARL: If a patient is not responding to the treatment plan that you believe should be hitting the organism responsible, think co-infection. In these cases, symptoms persist despite on-going treatment for other TBIs. When the fatigue or headache is intractable, the arthritis is especially resistant, there is a new onset of seizures, the lymphadenopathy is pronounced, the encephalopathy persists especially with cognitive defects, or visual problems are prominent such as loss of acuity or retinitis, make sure you have considered that Bartonella might be confounding the clinical picture.

- **Mycoplasma** *fermentans**: This pathogen may not cause a specific illness itself but rather contributes to the pathology caused by other TBIs. Smaller than bacteria, these organisms lack cell walls and are able to invade human tissue and disrupt the immune system. Symptoms include fatigue, headache, GI symptoms, joint and lymph node discomfort, breathing difficulty, and muscle soreness. M. *fermentans* can cause significant cognitive problems, behavior changes, and depression. These neuropsychiatric problems might be the most distinguishing feature of M. *fermentans*. Mycoplasma are notoriously slow growing and so are not readily susceptible to antimicrobials. M. *fermentans* may be the biggest treatment challenge in TBIs. Other species of Mycoplasma may be involved in the pathology of TBIs, but little is known about their status as co-infections.

- **Colorado Tick Fever**: This TBI is also called American tick fever and is thought to be transmitted mostly by the Rocky Mountain wood tick. The infection is due to a virus creatively called the Colorado tick fever virus, which was first isolated in humans in the 1940s. Found primarily in the western US, the pathogen lodges inside blood cells. Usually there is a bout of fever that resolves, only to recur again. Many patients complain of high fever, severe headache, chills, fatigue, muscle pain, back pain, pain behind the eyes, light sensitivities, nausea, vomiting, and diarrhea. Because the RBCs are affected, the disease is also thought to be transmissible through blood transfusion.

- **Powassan Viral Encephalitis**: The woodchuck tick is the usual vector for this flavivirus. Found in the eastern and western US, this TBI presents with fever, headache, pain behind the eyes, light sensitivity, lethargy, and muscle weakness. Since the virus invades the brain, symptoms can progress to brain inflammation with seizures, paralysis, disorientation, and meningoencephalitis leading to coma. Also called tick-borne encephalitis, Powassan fever has a 10% fatality rate and 50% of patients have neurologic sequelae that can be permanent. Note that West Nile virus and the agent that causes yellow fever are also flaviviruses.

- **Q Fever**: The brown dog tick, Rocky Mountain wood tick, and Lone Star tick are all known vectors for Coxiella *burnetii*. Found throughout the US, this pathogen causes acute fever, chills, sweats, and other symptoms. Suspect Q fever in TBI patients with pneumonia and abnormal liver function. These bacteria are thought to be carried by cattle, sheep, and goats, but this is not definitive.

PEARL: If the Lone Star tick has been implicated in transmitting Coxiella, why is one government staffer, described later in the text, absolutely positive that it cannot transmit Bb?

- **Rocky Mountain Spotted Fever**: (RMSF) The American dog tick and the Rocky Mountain wood tick spread Rickettsia throughout the US, and not just in the Rocky Mountain area. The disease is especially prevalent in the southeastern US. This pathogen invades the cells lining the heart and blood vessels causing sudden, high fever and a maculopapular rash beginning on the soles of the feet and palms of the hands that spreads over the entire body. Patients also complain of severe headache especially behind the eyes and bleeding problems. This bacterium, called Rickettsia *rickettsii*, has a 30% mortality if left untreated and a 3% to 5% mortality rate even if treated with an appropriate antibiotic regimen.

- **Tick paralysis**: A neurotoxin excreted from the salivary glands of the American dog tick, the Rocky Mountain wood tick, and the Lone Star tick is thought to cause tick paralysis. Ixodes *holocyclus*, called the paralysis tick of Australia, has also been implicated. Found throughout the US, symptoms begin with fatigue, followed by flaccid paralysis, loss of function of the tongue and facial muscles, progressive paralysis beginning in legs and moving over the body within hours, convulsions, and death. The paralysis is a toxic reaction to the saliva of certain female ticks, which seems to reverse fairly quickly after the tick is removed.

- **Tick Relapsing Fever**: The relapsing fever tick transmits the spirochete Borrelia *hermsii* causing disease in some hosts. Found most often in the western US, this TBI presents with cycles of high fever, sudden chills, eye inflammation, cough, jaundice, and petechial rash.

PEARL: Technically tick relapsing fever would be considered a borreliosis and should appear as such in Chapter 10: Borreliosis. *While it is included as a borreliosis in that context, Chapter 10 must focus on Lyme primarily (and to a lesser degree the confounding STARI), so that we don't all stress out over splitting these hairs. Information overload can keep us from managing the material productively. In fact, Lyme clearly qualifies as a relapsing fever and maybe it should be listed here instead of boasting its own chapter. We must strive to keep the artificial nomenclature from driving the logic.*

• **Tularemia**: Also called rabbit fever, this TBI is carried by the American dog tick, Rocky Mountain wood tick, and Lone Star tick. Identified throughout the US, Francisella *tularensis* are bacteria that cause skin ulcers, swollen and painful lymph nodes, inflamed eyes, fever, chills, fatigue, sore throat, mouth sores, diarrhea, and vomiting. The ulcers and mouth sores can be slow healing. Symptoms can progress to pneumonia and death can occur.

> *PEARL: If the Lone Star tick has been implicated in transmitting Francisella, why is one government staffer absolutely positive that it cannot transmit Bb? But I repeat myself.*

In TBI management, the existence of co-infections complicates everything: presentation, clinical course, diagnosis, and treatment. Unfortunately, most TBIs *initially* present with the nonspecific signs and symptoms found in most infections. These include the classic inflammatory responses such as generalized aches, fever, fatigue, and anorexia. These manifestations are common to many, if not most, infectious processes. These broad reactions may be predominant for days before more specific and distinguishing signs of the individual pathogens become apparent (if they ever do). Since the majority of TBI patients do not recall a tick bite, many patients get misdiagnosed with routine viral infections or flu.

> *PEARL: Co-infections can contribute to a confusing clinical picture. Symptoms may overlap or intensify depending on the pathogens involved. With diagnostic testing so unreliable in most cases, the clinician will have to use good medical judgment including weighing the patient's response to various treatment approaches. When multiple microbes infect concurrently, they can change the immune response and they themselves can be altered in the process. Therefore, co-infections may not present together as they would separately. Further, the HCP might have a hard time parsing out which manifestations are due to co-infections and which might be the multifaceted nature of some of these pathogens.*

Those patients with multiple TBIs seem to get sicker and stay sick longer than those with a single active pathogen. Recovery time could be compromised and there can be permanent sequelae that might have been avoided if only one pathogen was operating. This increase in severity could be due to the impact of multiple TBIs on the immune system, OR due to a delay in appropriate diagnosis and treatment, OR a combination of these factors. Most HCPs agree that a delay in proper treatment exacerbates the clinical course and makes a full recovery less likely.

> *PEARL: The sickest kids and those hardest to treat probably either have an immune vulnerability to TBDs or they have more than one co-infection. If they have both, case management will be a challenge.*

We used to think that Lyme was "the" TBI and everything else was just a tag-a-long. Many uninformed HCPs felt that all TBIs should get better with 2 weeks of low-dose doxy. If patients didn't improve as expected, then there was something wrong with the patient not the diagnosis and treatment. While most TBI patients DO have Lyme, many have other pathology as well. In fact, the existence of multiple co-infections was first uncovered when some Lyme patients were not getting better as expected with their low-dose doxy for 2 weeks. After my son was much worse after 3 days of doxy, lying unresponsive with savage rigors, the ER nurse Lilith[1] asked, "He's already on doxy what more do you want?" How about an antibiotic that hits what he actually has? While he did have Lyme, which made him seem to be improving after the first few doses of antibiotic, the doxy was not up to handling the Babesia, which flared spectacularly causing him to crash. Lilith assumed that since Chris was being treated for Lyme, he was being adequately treated. This proved to be a dangerous misconception. Clearly, co-infections can alter and complicate the course of LD and will likely make the infected person more difficult to treat.

Because Lyme is thought to be more common that the other TBIs, many HCPs will stop at Lyme and never consider the more recently recognized TBIs. In fact, other TBIs such as babesiosis and bartonellosis might be more common, just less identified. Some HCPs agree to humor the caregiver and treat the person for Lyme. Then they think their responsibility is over. They figure that 2 to 4 weeks of doxy won't hurt and they can have the patient in and out of the office in less than 4 minutes. This is great for those patients who are at the point in their disease where the doxy might be all they need, but what about those who aren't? What about those cases where the solo agent just serves to force the pathogen into cells or cysts where it can resurface at a later date?

Some authors believe that unrecognized co-infections are the cause of what is called chronic Lyme (or Category 4 Lyme or persistent Lyme). While this is probably true in some cases, chronic Lyme is also a distinct entity, separate from other infections. Clearly, Lyme affects the course of co-infections just as they impact the course of Lyme. In most cases, co-infections are thought to delay appropriate treatment and thereby prolong recovery time. Sequelae may be permanent. The patient suffers more.

If the person is not responding to treatment, ask:

1. Have all possible co-infections been considered? What else could this be?

2. Have I noted any distinctive signs or symptoms to see if clues are pointing to a specific pathogen?

---

1 See Glossary or Introduction for name origin

3. Would additional diagnostic testing help?

4. Am I just doing the minimum because I have 12 more patients waiting outside?

5. Have I done all I could to address what is happening with this individual?

6. What am I missing?

Today, co-infections are thought to be the rule rather than the exception. In one regional sample, 80% of mice that carried deer ticks were infected with either Borrelia, Babesia, or Ehrlichia, and 40% had two of the three. In one TBI practice, the typical child has two to five co-infections with an average of three. That we know of…

One theory of the pathophysiology of co-infections suggests a cyclic pattern:

1. One infection impacts the organs and the immune system, which…

2. Causes the patient to feel ill, which…

3. Allows other pathogens that may have arrived on the same tick, or found their way into the host by other means, to establish a presence and…

4. Their reproduction and proliferation may be enough to cause additional symptomatology in the person. …

5. These pathogens, which may or may not have manifested signs of disease if infecting as a solitary agent, now have the "opportunity" to multiply and cause their own set of signs and symptoms. …

6. This may alter the clinical presentation of both pathogens and the patients feel sicker than they would have if only one microbe was the underlying cause of the problem. …

7. There is additional organ damage and…

8. The immune system may be more compromised. …

9. The patient feels worse and may display additional or more intense symptoms. …

10. The active pathogens continue to impact the organs and immune system and the cycle starts over.

The presence of co-infections may also account for the various presentations thought to be due solely to Lyme. One reason that Lyme may present with so many faces might be that it's not just Lyme. The presence of multiple pathogens may account for the discrepant responses to treatment.

HCPs, remember that your lack of awareness of co-infections can be disabling or even fatal for the patient. Some of the co-infection literature recommends going to the doctor immediately after finding any tick bite or as soon as any symptoms appear. The premise is that proper diagnosis and prompt, appropriate treatment can be critical to ameliorating the severity of the disease. While this may be prudent advice, just try to tell your concerns to a busy HCP. Even with the deer tick in a jar and an EM rash, my symptomatic son was told he couldn't possibly have Lyme, since the skin lesion was too oval. Even when he was unresponsive, some of the local HCPs didn't want to hear that he might need more than doxy. The nature of the medical system today mandates that there will always be some kind of delay in getting care. Therefore, if you have concerns, err on the side of the conservative and make an appointment asap. But be prepared for your local Lilith[2] to roll her eyes and say, "It's not like he's dying or anything."

Some practitioners think that each co-infection should be managed sequentially and they prefer to handle one before they tackle another. I happen to disagree with this. I have a hard time understanding how you can know that a pathogen is at work in your body and not want to be addressing the situation. What if the first co-infection you pick to treat does not respond to treatment or your regimen does not lead to a cure? Would you still continue to wait while you beat on the first infection before you address the second? Since we often do not even recognize all the co-infections to start with, why would we allow some to run rampant while we addressed only part of the problem? Ultimately, my son did not have that option. Only one of his TBIs was being addressed (and even that one inadequately) and a co-infection flared and nearly killed him. I think if you recognize an infection you should address the conditions as effectively as possible. Of course, try to select antimicrobials that hit both (or all known) infections concomitantly. Of course, try not to add medicines that are redundant or unnecessary. Chapter 24: *Antimicrobials* has charts listing therapy options for the various co-infection combinations.

As always, I ask the HCPs to listen to the patients and to the caregivers. When a caregiver tells you that the person is not getting better on current treatment, consider that you might not be treating the right thing (or not all of it, anyway). And for goodness sakes, NEVER roll your eyes. Someday it might be your child sitting in that chair.

In the following chapters, we will always be aware that *in every case* we might be dealing with more than one pathogen. Borrelia will get the most attention because that is where most of the information has been gathered and where most of the

---

2 See Glossary or Introduction for name origin

controversy has settled. Separate chapters are presented for the most common co-infections seen in TBI-focused practice.

PEARL: As I often claim, the veterinary community appears further ahead of the human medical establishment in understanding TBIs including the concept of co-infection. Further, vets don't get too excited about what kind of tick was the culprit. They consider that multiple pathogens could possibly be transmitted by a variety of ticks. For example, dogs bitten by either deer or dog ticks can experience the following co-infections:

Lyme disease: Presents with lameness, fever, swollen joints, kidney failure, anorexia, and the dog not acting normally. Neurologic and behavior problems may be prominent. Lyme can cause permanent joint damage and fatal kidney disease.

Anaplasmosis/Ehrlichiosis: Presentation in dogs can be mild to severe with loss of appetite, lack of energy, depression, high fever, very painful or swollen joints, chronic joint problems, bleeding complications such as bloody nose and pale gums, vomiting, diarrhea, very low platelet and WBC counts, and neurological signs. These conditions can result in permanent blindness, autoimmune presentations, and death.

Babesiosis: Usually due to B. canis *or B.* gibsoni, *about 13% of shelter dogs in California are positive for Babesia. These dogs might develop what could be termed a form of red water fever with red urine, anemia, jaundice, lymphadenopathy, inflammation of the liver or kidney, and an enlarged spleen. Treatment includes antiprotozoals and blood transfusions.*

RMSF: While canines with RMSF may present with a rash this finding is inconsistent in dogs (as with humans). Fever, petechiae, ecchymosis, vasculitis of the mucosa in the mouth, edema in the extremities or in low hanging ears, myalgia, and neurologic abnormalities including ataxia and eye problems have all been associated with RMSF in dogs.

These afflictions can all present as "silent infections" as well. If left untreated any of these co-infections can progress. Treat all but babesiosis with doxy or TCN. This information was obtained through personal communication with vets I trust plus additional research. Thank you Dr. Coats, Dr. Svonavec, and Dr. Spancake.

Chapter 6

BABESIOSIS

And the LORD spake unto Moses, Say unto Aaron, Take thy rod, and stretch out thine hand upon the waters of Egypt, upon their streams, upon their rivers, and upon their ponds, and upon their pools of water, that they may become blood; and that there may be blood through all the land of Egypt.

Exodus 7:19

Background: Just for the sake of argument and a little excitement, let's consider a theory that a number of biblical scholars have suggested. Let's say that God used Babesia to smite Pharaoh. Those of us from the western religious traditions have all heard of the ten plagues of Egypt. Each time Pharaoh refused Moses' request to free the Hebrews, another plague hit the land. If you add the red rivers to the swarms of arthropods and the death of all the Egyptian livestock, skin lesions, and the demise of the firstborn, God could not have picked a better agent for getting Pharaoh's attention. Forget that the Bible says lice. If we can't properly classify ticks in the 21st century, the ancient entomologists shouldn't be expected to do better. As a mother who saw her firstborn nearly succumb to Babesia, I certainly believe this organism can wreak havoc of biblical proportions.

Let me take the analogy a bit further. Why would the waters run red? As we have learned over the last two centuries, Babesia in cattle has made the water run red in many locales. In fact, in recent history when Babesia caused disease in cattle in Texas and Mexico, it was called red water fever. As I review the pathophysiology below, you will see how invasion and disintegration of red blood cells causes the infected animal to develop an anemia so severe that the damaged cells are poured out in crimson urine in such large quantities that the rivers literally run red.

Even the biblical timeline would be compatible with Babesia infestation. The water running red would be the early stage of disease, then people would start noticing the arthropod vectors, and soon they would see that the livestock were dying off in huge numbers. Skin lesions on all forms of mammals would develop (from co-infections, of course) and finally death of the firstborn of all creatures. I can't account for the frogs in the ovens, or the hail, or why the Hebrews weren't affected. I guess that's where God comes in, but this speculation was certainly fun for me. Of course, there are a hundred other hypotheses used to explain the ten plagues, but none of the others fit a textbook on TBIs.

Forgive me if I spend more time on Babesia than the other co-infections. I have a personal vendetta that drives me. Besides, I was able to find more information on this disease than many of the other TBIs. This wealth of knowledge may be due to the economic impact of Babesia on the global cattle industry over the years. Dozens of articles can be found discussing the infection in donkeys and llamas. In contrast, many papers outlining the human condition are superficial, dismissive, and without scientific merit. While some Babesia infections in humans can be mild or even asymptomatic, others are fatal. Until an HCP has witnessed the suffering that accompanies a severe, acute episode of babesiosis, a dismissive attitude is not warranted.

Aliases: Babesiosis, Nantucket fever, American malaria, Northeastern malaria, formerly called piroplasmosis, continues to be called equine piroplasmosis in horses and red water fever in cattle. Some sources now refer to animal babesiosis due to B. *microti* as theileriosis.

Pathogen: The genus Babesia comprises more than 100 species of tick-borne protozoal pathogens formerly known as Piroplasms. When I started to research Babesia, I didn't immediately realize there had been a name change from Piroplasm. This caused considerable angst. As I got up to date, I could translate the articles that had been written prior to the name change. The hard part was trying to figure out what was happening in the current literature. Some authors refused to make any changes. Were these writers obstinate or just ignorant of the new conventions? Others made no reference to the Piroplasms at all, as though the old name had never existed. My favorite, though, were those authors who used both names in the same article, and not because they were attempting to dissipate the current confusion, but because they were still plenty confused themselves. Just be careful if you should ever try to read this literature. For the first month, I was dumb as a bag of hair and much time was wasted.

PEARL: Some recent literature calls B. microti by a new name, Theileria microti, apparently because RNA comparison found this microbe to be more like the Theileria genus than the Babesia. Perhaps that explains why the distinct Babesia species respond to different treatment regimens. Since almost none of the TBI literature uses this new terminology as yet, this text will retain the Babesia nomenclature. Be aware. I was just getting over the change from Piroplasm.

Formerly called Piroplasma, Babesia are tick-borne protozoans that used to be in the kingdom of protists. Even though protists no longer have a separate kingdom, they are now defined as a group of eukaryotes, which are organisms that have cell membranes and complex internal structures like nuclei. They include such disease-producers as Amoebas, which can cause severe dysentery, and Plasmodia that initiate malaria. The Babesia that cause disease are different from many other protists in that they have no cilia or flagella to help them move. Instead they get around through vectors and the pumping of blood.

Currently, we recognize several Babesia species to be human pathogens. At least a dozen have been identified in ticks and most of these have been implicated as causing disease in people. More are being associated with human disease all the time. Some are little more than a name in the literature. As of January 2013, here is a modest list.

Babesia *microti*	Likely the primary organism causing babesiosis in the US. Some recent sources now list new nomenclature for this organism as Theileria *microti*.
Babesia *divergens*	Primary organism causing babesiosis in Europe
Babesia *duncani*	In addition to B. *microti,* B. *duncani* causes babesiosis in the US on both coasts. Currently, most authorities consider the organism that used to be called WA-1 to be the same as B. *duncani.* In the future, we may learn that B. *duncani* is actually more prevalent than B. *microti* in the US, but that has yet to be confirmed.
Babesia *WA-1*	Today, most sources believe that WA-1 is the same as B. *duncani.* I list them separately here because some of the literature makes this distinction. Found primarily in northern California and Washington state (hence the WA) this strain may be more difficult to treat than other strains. Serologic surveys in northern California show an especially high seroprevalence for WA-1 antigens, which appear most closely associated with bovine disease.
Babesia *canis*	In Mexico, human disease has been found to be caused by this species that more often afflicts dogs.
Babesia *MO-1*	Named after Missouri where first identified

Read quickly. They are probably changing the taxonomy as you turn the page. There are likely many species yet to be uncovered. These distinctions are important since some organisms respond differently to treatment. As a pathogen, Babesia can work alone or as one of a number of co-infections transmitted by the same vector.

Vector: Round up the usual suspects. Babesia shares the same tick vectors known to transmit Lyme, primarily deer ticks and Pacific black-legged ticks. Transmission of Babesia *microti* from a reservoir to a host generally takes place through direct tick contact. In the northeastern US, the cycle is maintained principally by the interactions between immature black-legged (deer) ticks and white-footed mice. Larval ticks of genus Ixodes acquire the infection when feeding on B. *microti*-infected mammals. The larvae change into nymphs, which are most often responsible for spreading the disease during their next feed.

In the US, the black-legged deer tick, Ixodes *scapularis* (formerly known as Ixodes *dammini*) is the primary vector for the parasite; while in Europe Ixodes *ricinis* appears to be the primary tick vector. In both locations, the Ixodes tick carrier for Babesia is the same that locally transmits Borrelia *burgdorferi,* the agent implicated in Lyme disease. The primary US animal reservoir is the white-footed mouse, Peromyscus *leucopus*. White-tailed deer serve as transport and reproductive hosts for the adult tick vector, I. *scapularis*. In Europe, an important animal host is cattle.

Known mammalian hosts include wild and domestic mammals, opossums, deer, rodents, bats, cattle, sheep, voles, and dogs. In the suburbs there has been a complete removal of deer predators. Most sources report that as the deer populations grow, deer tick populations swell, resulting in a corresponding increased incidence of babesiosis.

Distribution: From Egypt to Milwaukee to the Pacific Northwest, Babesia abound. These protozoans are one of the most common infectors of animals worldwide and are prevalent in rodents, carnivores, and cattle. Infections in humans are only beginning to be recognized in endemic areas.

Most cases of babesiosis in the US are reported in the northeast and on the west coast. Babesiosis used to be rare except off the coast of Massachusetts, where the name Nantucket fever originated. Incidence is increasing with new cases being reported as far apart as Oregon and Tennessee. In 2001, there were five cases reported in the Hudson Valley, 10 years later there were 120 cases from that same geographic region. With the revitalization of the suburban deer populations, decreased hunting, and an increase in outdoor activities, a swell in the incidence and prevalence can be expected.

In the Mid-Atlantic States and other endemic areas, babesiosis should always be considered as one cause of infection in symptomatic tick bite patients. No one knows how often Babesia rides alone, but pairing with the Borrelia that causes Lyme seems to be widespread. In some locations, more than 60% of Lyme cases also include Babesia. Subclinical infections are often undetected, at least initially, because the symptoms are said to be "just Lyme." The full extent of the co-infection may not manifest until the Borrelia symptoms begin to subside. My son, who had both Lyme and babesiosis, got better in the first 36 hours of Lyme treatment and then crashed as the Babesia infection became prominent. Other co-infections and co-morbidities may further complicate the picture.

Most cases of babesiosis are reported from May through September. The ratio of males to females is approximately 1:1. All ages can be affected, but most reported cases are from people in middle age.

Just as with its cousin malaria, babesiosis can be transmitted in ways not involving an arthropod vector. Transplacental transmission is possible. Babies born of mothers with babesiosis can be extremely ill. They can present with severe anemia, heart failure, pulmonary edema, and varying degrees of respiratory distress. They will likely need hospitalization for respiratory support and stabilization. Anecdotally, a number of cases of children born with babesiosis have been recognized. In those not stillborn, many are in dire straits at birth. Often Babesia were identified on their blood smears. Several have responded to treatment including Mepron (atovaquone) in combination with Zithromax (azithromycin) and blood transfusions. Currently, perinatal babesiosis is rare with only a handful of cases annually in the US. Nonetheless, a case was identified in July of 2012.

Protozoal disease can also be spread via blood transfusions. Over the past decade about 100 people in the US acquired babesiosis through tainted blood. At least eleven died. All the donors in these cases had lived or traveled through endemic areas. While incidence and prevalence data are sketchy and may not be entirely accurate, regulators believe that about 5% of stored blood is infected with B. *microti*. Blood banks are trying to protect the blood supply but many who are infected with Babesia do not know they could be transmitting a pathogen. Even though potential donors are asked if they ever had babesiosis, about one out of a hundred who pass the screening actually harbor the organism.

Right now screening all donor blood for Babesia is considered too labor intensive and costly and too slow to be used on the millions of pints collected each year. Unfortunately, patients who contract babesiosis from blood transfusions require treatment that is labor intensive and costly as well. A high percentage of these patients get severely ill and recovery is slow. Rhode Island is trying to start a program where clean units are set aside to be used only in the most vulnerable patients.

Because many HCPs, like me, have not kept up with Babesia until we are forced to do so, infection has been overlooked and undertreated. Accurate incidence and prevalence data will take years to compile, especially if HCPs, like those in one tick-infested county in southeastern Pennsylvania, continue to deny its existence even as patients lie unconscious in rigors before them. Are you listening, Lilith[1]?

PEARL: The medical staff at the local hospital did not even consider babesiosis in my son's case despite my continuing to plead that his presentation didn't look like garden-variety Lyme to me. Their failure to recognize a classic case placed him and his future blood recipients at risk. Had another HCP not made the diagnosis, Chris would have continued to donate blood (had he recovered enough to do so). Sadly, HCPs in this endemic area were not even aware of the possibility. The ER doc argued both that he had Lyme and no further treatment was needed – AND that he didn't have Lyme because his EM rash was oval instead of round. She didn't even entertain the idea of babesiosis or co-infection. Is it any surprise that three years later we are reading that Babesia in the blood supply is becoming widespread and impacting the amount of usable blood available for transfusion? I wonder how many other cases were missed by that doctor in that ER. After I learned the diagnosis, I tried to call the hospital to tell them. I couldn't even leave a message because the voice mailbox was full. Do these people feel any responsibility for public health?

History: In the 1880s, a devastating red water fever decimated the cattle herds in Texas and Mexico. Theobald Smith and F. L. Kilborne discovered that ticks carried the disease and red water fever became the first vector-borne illness described in the scientific literature. At about the same time, Victor Babes found that this tick parasite was a protozoan, which was named Babesia after him. In 1885, he published the first known treatise of bacteriology after working in the Pasteur Laboratory in Paris. Recall that these discoveries were barely 20 years after Pasteur provided evidence that germs caused infectious diseases and there were many skeptics, then as now.

Other cattle infestations at the turn of the century killed millions of cattle in Australia within a week and again cut the herds in Texas by half. From this devastation came tick control methods like dipping cattle, pesticides to control the tick population, inoculating calves with a mild form of the disease, and limiting the movement of herds so they could not go into infested areas. New medicines allowed some cattle to recover after infection. These efforts met with considerable success since babesiosis in cattle has largely been eradicated from the US. As is often the case, the veterinary community was more progressive in its thinking than traditional human medicine has been. Unfortunately, red water fever remains a problem in Mexico and Central America.

---

1 See Glossary or Introduction for name origin

In the recent past (like when I was in medical school), Babesia were called Piroplasma, so when my son was diagnosed with acute disease, I had to go home and look it up. I had never heard of Babesia. We didn't even know how to pronounce it (Bab-EEE-See-ah). Chris and I would practice saying Bab-EEE-See-O-sis on the way to the doctor's office so we wouldn't look like uneducated fools when we got there. Chris would say, "What do I have again?" Bab-EEE-See-O-sis.

The first *suspected* human infection was in 1908 and the first clear case was found in an asplenic Yugoslavian farmer in 1957. In the US, the earliest case was described in Nantucket in the late 1960s. This "fact" illustrates one of the frustrations in writing this book. I found four different years listed in the literature as the "exact" year the first US case was reported on Nantucket Island. Since the precise year is not critical to how well you take care of your patients, I did not bother to call the Nantucket Health Department to check. Would I have trusted the local health department to get this right? Is there a Nantucket Health Department?

While babesiosis can be severe and even fatal, many cases are subclinical. Even in recognized cases, the symptoms can fade over time, so knowing who was infected and when, is impossible to say. Infections with B. *microti* and B. *divergens* are the most common in humans with the European variety having a much higher mortality. Infections by other strains have either been poorly documented or limited to a few isolated cases.

Pathophysiology: Some articles on the life cycle of Babesia are so complicated as to be unreadable. After days of trying to decipher this jumble, I accepted that HCPs need to know very little about the details of the Babesia life cycle in order to help their patients.

Babesia belong to the phylum Apicomplexa that are almost entirely parasitic (none free-living). The Apicomplexa have a group of organelles at the apical end of the organism called the *apical complex* (Get it? Apicomplexa.) This organelle plays a role in the parasite-host interaction and enables the parasite ultimately to invade the host. As part of their life cycle, the Babesia have various stages, rounds, cycles, and processes, which have repeatedly been resorted, renamed, redefined, and debated. Much has yet to be discovered.

In the case of babesiosis, an infected reservoir mammal is bitten by a vector tick. The tick ingests contaminated blood from the host. The next time the tick goes for a meal of mammal blood, it infects that new host. In short, a tick bites a mouse that is infected with Babesia. Now the tick is infected. When the tick then bites again, the Babesia is transmitted to the new host, which just might be you, or your dog, or a chipmunk, or Grandma. Tick spit is needed to facilitate the transfer of the organism into the host and back out into the tick. So not only can the process cause severe illness, it is disgusting as well.

Note that infected does NOT mean diseased, it just means that the organism is present.

As the infected tick sucks blood from the host, its saliva mixes with the blood of that host. In the salivary gland of the tick is a sporozoite, which is the infective stage of the Babesia parasite. Actually there are thousands of Babesia sporozoites. The next time the tick bites a mammal, the sporozoites get into the blood of that animal. The tick is trying to gorge itself with blood, so the contaminated saliva has plenty of time to get into the host. Once the Babesia contact blood, they quickly invade the RBCs. The host has now been infected. In the RBC, the Babesia matures to its next stage, which reproduces. They reproduce so well that some of the RBCs explode from the volume of the parasite.

These bursting RBCs can result in symptoms manifested by the host (anemia, weakness, air hunger, and signs of infection and inflammation). The RBCs that do not break contain the Babesia parasite and are pumped around the mammal's blood stream. When the next tick comes along, if she wasn't already infected, she can become so when she mixes her saliva with the blood of her new target. So the life cycle of the Babesia continues. To be infectious to the next animal, however, the Babesia must leave the intestine of the tick where they were drawn and migrate to other cells, like the tick ovary, where they undergo other aspects of their life cycles. These Babesia then travel all around the tick including the salivary glands, which can become swollen. Imagine a tick with mumps. At this point, the cycle has come full circle.

PEARL: One theory is that the infected RBCs can become deformed and get wedged in small tissue capillaries and cause a number of the presenting signs and symptoms.

Since many protozoans have both an active phase as well as a dormant, cystic phase, the clinical picture can be complicated and is just beginning to be understood. Some cysts can survive in the harshest conditions for long periods, resurrecting at later dates when the initial Babesia infection may be forgotten and no longer suspected.

The signs and symptoms experienced by diseased animals and humans are directly due to the pathophysiology of the Babesia. Because RBCs are bursting, there may be breakdown products in the serum including pigments causing a yellow or orange discoloration of the eyes (icterus), skin (jaundice), as well as the urine (hemoglobinuria). Anemia can be severe and MIGHT be correlated with the amount of parasite load. In contrast, some patients have no signs of anemia and this may be strain related. If parasites are present in more than 25% of RBCs, anemia can be severe. Not only are RBCs bursting, they are also maimed and deformed enabling them to get stuck in tiny organ capillaries and potentially causing debilitating problems. Broken RBCs may contribute to respiratory distress in the sickest patients.

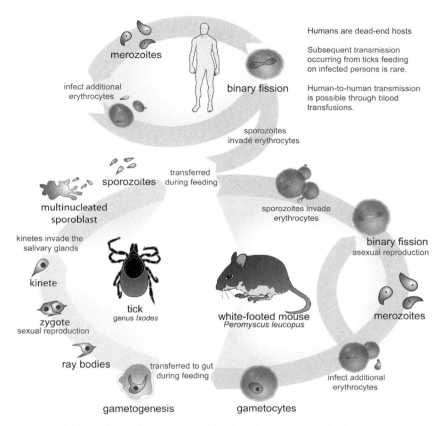

Life cycle of the parasite Babesia, (B. *microti* or B. *divergens*)
Source:http: //commons.wikimedia.org/wiki/File:Babesia_life_cycle_human_en.svg
Accessed March 2013

PEARL: B. duncani *seems to affect the lung with more breathing difficulties than B.* microti. *In contrast, B.* microti *appears to have more of an effect on the RBCs which eventually could manifest as anemia. The anemia may then indirectly affect the host's oxygenation also causing air hunger.*

Symptoms are most severe in the immunocompromised such as those who have had their spleen removed or those who are just born. In theory, Babesia is believed to significantly impact the immune system of the host. Defenses are compromised and signs and symptoms of co-infection may be substantially enhanced. Target organs can be hit harder with permanent damage resulting. Response to treatment can be impacted and recovery greatly prolonged.

If acute symptoms develop, they usually do so after about a week's incubation period. However, months or years may pass before symptoms appear. Some infected individuals never show signs of disease. Different species may have slightly different modus operandi: B. *microti* cause RBC explosions, whereas B. *duncani* cause fluid imbalances that lead to the lung becoming edematous. We do not know enough yet to go beyond speculation.

One of the first signs of acute babesiosis can be paroxysms of rigors. When I told Lilith[2] of the rolling eyes in the local ER that Chris had rigors she had never heard that term. Spreen Corollary: Just because you haven't heard of something doesn't mean it's not real; just means you need to hit the books.

Here is the official definition of rigors, Lilith: alternating severe paroxysms of fever and chills. The <u>cold</u> stage involves a sudden high temperature with a feeling of chills, followed by a <u>hot</u> stage, which is a sense of heat and profuse sweating. The rigors correspond to the release of the parasite from broken RBCs. The paroxysm can cycle from daily to every 48 to 72 hours, depending on the strain of pathogen and the individual's response.

---

2 See Glossary or Introduction for name origin

The clinical course of Babesia is built around these parox-ysmal cycles and based on the pathophysiology. The natural history of this organism also impacts diagnostic testing. Apparently, since Babesia breed like bunnies, very little initial inoculum is needed to eventually cause disease. This means that diagnostic lab tests such as antibody testing, FISH, and PCR can remain negative even after the patient is quite sick. Negative tests do not mean not infected, just not detected. Further, the Maltese crosses, which are clusters of pathogen inside the red cells, might only be apparent at certain times during the course of the infection.

PEARL: Levels of parasitemia may correlate with sever-ity of illness. Patients who are mildly ill may have less than 1% parasitemia, and patients who are very sick may have greater than 85% involvement. Parasite lev-els seem to be especially high in those patients with no spleen. In line with the pathophysiology, haptoglobin levels may be decreased and urine may show hemoglo-binuria, proteinuria, and a dark color from bilirubin.

Malaria: Lessons from a Similar Pathogen

Both babesiosis and malaria are caused by protozoa. Both are transmitted by arthropod vectors: Babesia by ticks and Plasmodium by mosquitoes. Both affect the red blood cells of the victims and have similar patterns of signs, symptoms, and a cyclic clinical course. Hopefully we can gain some insight about how to manage patients with babesiosis by learning from the mistakes made over the years in handling malaria.

For many years the organism that causes malaria was dis-counted as insignificant. Not quite a bacterium, this microbe was thought to be inconsequential. Since this pathogen ap-peared different from any previously acknowledged infec-tious agent, the medical establishment preferred to pretend it didn't exist. How dare it not fit easily into what was already known? But as the horrendous consequences of malaria piled up, the toll on human health had to be addressed. Malaria flat-tened a number of US presidents, (James Monroe, Teddy Roo-sevelt, James Garfield), turned back Alexander the Great from India, decimated Attila and his Huns, relocated the Vatican, killed King Tut and four popes, slayed Dante, contributed to the US defeat in Vietnam, sickened Osama bin Laden before the Navy Seals got him, and helped in the fall of the Roman Empire. Not bad for a little microbe that was not considered worthy to be called a bacteria.

PEARL: To paraphrase Sonia Shah in her book, The Fe-ver, *the Plasmodium malaria pathogen is a supervillain: a complex, brilliant, and mysterious foe that resists all at-tempts to control it. Currently 1 out of 14 humans carries genetic mutations that evolved solely to fight malaria. Still*

the Plasmodium is winning. This pathogen should never be underestimated. The same can be said of Babesia.

In 2008, malaria infected 244 million people worldwide, kill-ing almost a million. A child dies of malaria every 30 seconds. A new epidemiologic report issued early in 2012 suggests that malaria is actually killing twice as many people than had previously been recognized. The idea that Babesia operates in much the same way as the agent that causes malaria should set off alarm bells in all rational HCPs. Both pathogens can cause asymptomatic infection, as well as forms that are dor-mant, acute, fulminant, and fatal. Neither seem to confer suf-ficient immunity to prevent reinfection and both can contami-nate the blood supply.

Malaria and babesiosis are both characterized by paroxysms of chills called rigors which coincide with the release of the pathogen from ruptured red blood cells. Fever can be very high – up to 106° with profuse soaking sweats. Malaria is known to cause cerebral sxs and babesiosis may do so as well. In both conditions, some of the microbes can occasion-ally be seen within the cells on blood smears. Malaria has more extracellular parasites than Babesia and so is thought to be capable of causing more liver damage. If the Maltese cross is seen on the blood smear, the diagnosis is likely Babesia. If the smear has parasites visible extracellularly, then the diag-nosis is more often malaria. Untreated infection during preg-nancy can cause problems for the neonate. Both pathogens are treated with similar antiprotozoal agents.

With considerable effort, some progress has been made in controlling the malaria pathogens and the vectors. Nonethe-less, malaria still kills nearly a million people annually, and babesiosis is spreading as a human disease. Both of these types of protozoans have extremely complex life cycles with schizogonic (active) phases from invasion of the host cell up to cell rupture. The pathophysiology correlates closely to the clinical presentation in both cases. Looking for ways to inter-rupt these cycles may help control these rampant diseases in the future.

Despite being an epidemic, malaria is often missed on blood smears, as is babesiosis. In both cases, an experienced reader is more accurate and can mean the difference between a "true positive" and a "false negative" test result.

While clearly malaria has a more direct effect on human health in the early 21st century, babesiosis has as much im-pact on human well-being with its devastation of cattle herds and other domestic food sources. With the spread of babe-siosis globally, public health advocates must be vigilant that Babesia does not eventually contribute the same degree of human misery as does malaria. Authorities are attempting to control the arthropod vectors in order to lessen the spread of disease.

An initial public health step may be found in the parallels between Babesia and Plasmodium in the human blood supply. Both are readily transmitted by infected RBCs during blood transfusions. In both scenarios, many donors do not realize they have the infection in their blood. Malaria organisms can remain dormant and transmissible for 10 to 15 years. While blood collection programs are doing a fairly good job in identifying donors who could potentially transmit malaria, work is just beginning with babesiosis. Yes, the donor questionnaire in Chester County, Pennsylvania, asks if the donor ever had babesiosis. But if the doctor in the local ER had never heard of it, and the family practitioner had never heard of it, and the infectious disease specialist was too self-important to be bothered with it, how can the average person sitting at the Red Cross table be expected to know if the donor could be passing along a fatal disease? Awareness and education must continue. We are ethically obligated to learn from malaria.

––––––––––––––

Clinical course: Having seen a dozen cases of malaria at Walter Reed as a medical student, my first thought when I saw my unconscious son with savage rigors was, "He has malaria." At that point, I had no idea that babesiosis was also called American malaria or Northeastern malaria.

Babesiosis is often a cyclic disease with signs and symptoms presenting themselves at intervals ranging from 24 to 72 hours. Some sources say the cycle is closer to 4 to 6 days. Episode length will vary depending on the strain of pathogen, microbe load, and the individual's response. Other co-infections have periodic manifestations as well. Some HCPs believe these cyclic patterns are so distinctive as to help identify the infectious agent. A sign and symptom calendar is sometimes used to track possible patterns. Not only do acute symptoms cycle, but the entire course of these diseases can demonstrate intervals. For example, Babesia symptoms are thought to cycle about every 2 to 3 weeks while Borrelia can have a longer 3 to 4 week cycle. Of course, to complicate matters, some patients never show any episodic patterns.

As many as 25% of infected patients have no inkling they were ever contaminated with Babesia. A silent Babesia infection may persist for years, but the status can change into active presentation at any time. Others develop a "barely there" syndrome that they may never associate with a TBI. When symptoms occur, the most common include fever, chills, headache, fatigue, sweats, and muscle aches. With some Babesia strains anemia is common and with others air hunger is more prominent.

With co-infections, all bets are off. The clinical course seen with multiple co-infections may not resemble any pattern that might be expected for the individual diseases. In these cases, intensity of all signs and symptoms can increase significantly.

Treatment may need to go on for months. If relapse or reinfection occur, then the patient will need to resume therapy. A high index of suspicion is recommended. Lilith[3], you must acknowledge that something can possibly exist before you can deny its existence. Recognizing the presence of Babesia as a co-infection may help explain many of the conundrums currently around TBIs.

Babies born infected with Babesia can be near death, with jaundice, severe anemia, and high fevers. Those not stillborn can have heart, liver, and kidney failure. Since they are so infested with pathogen, the Maltese cross can more often be seen in their blood smear. They must be aggressively treated or they can die quickly. Antiprotozoals and multiple blood transfusions will likely be required as well as intensive respiratory support.

> *PEARL: Look for the rooting reflex in neonates born with Babesia. Without this reflex, nursing might be adversely impacted. With appropriate treatment, the reflex returns.*

Babesia infections can be totally asymptomatic. If the patient becomes symptomatic soon after the tick bite, it is usually after an incubation period of between 1 and 4 weeks. Some believe that the more compromised the immune system, the sooner the symptoms will appear and the more severe they may be. Others think that the immune system does not play as much of a role as the parasite load at the time of infection. These mechanisms are not mutually exclusive and both may be in play. Splenectomy may cause an asymptomatic patient to develop symptoms. The disease is thought to be more serious in the immunocompromised and in those over 50.

Seeing an acute presentation of babesiosis is relatively rare. At least, seeing an acute presentation that is recognized as such is rare. More often, a patient presents after having previously undiagnosed episodes of cyclic or recurrent symptoms that suggest that Babesia may be the etiologic agent.

An on-going record of temperatures might show a clear cyclic pattern. These cycles may occur once or twice a day or over 2 to 3 day intervals. In contrast, temperatures may rise quickly and then stay elevated for days. The extreme temperatures may result in delirium and changes in consciousness. The patient may be hard to rouse. A record of temperatures showing cycles of fever spikes may help the HCP make a diagnosis. Patients may refer to periods of intense symptoms as flares.

Signs & symptoms: Babesia infections can range from asymptomatic to life-threatening, malaria-like diseases. Every patient with babesiosis is unique and presents in his own way. The most common symptoms include fever, chills, headache, fatigue, sweats, and muscle aches. Acute symptoms may come

––––––––––––––

3 See Glossary or Introduction for name origin

on suddenly and be extremely intense. Heart palpitations can occur and the neck pain and stiffness can be incapacitating. As the disease progresses, or in gestational babesiosis, anemia can be a prominent feature.

Signs and symptoms that should make HCPs think about babesiosis are rigors, night sweats, and intractable headaches. Rigors are alternating paroxysms of fever and chills. There will be a sudden high temperature with a feeling of being very cold with intense, shaking chills followed by a profound sense of heat with drenching sweats. These sweats mostly occur at night but can occur at any time of the day. Teeth may chatter audibly. Night sweats can be very uncomfortable, requiring numerous bedding changes. The savage shaking with these chills can exhaust the patient. They may appear to be seizing. Although fevers can be quite high with several of the TBIs, Babesia tends to cause higher fevers than most, with readings of 105° or 106° F not uncommon. Patients can be so fatigued and weak that they cannot stand and walk even a few steps to the bathroom by themselves. Fatigue becomes prominent. It does not clear with rest and becomes worse with exercise. These patients are *tired*.

While air hunger is not necessarily common with Babesia infection, when it occurs, Babesia should be included in the differential diagnosis. Air hunger can be subtle or intense. If you do not have enough circulating RBCs you might feel somewhat oxygen deprived. Likewise, if the pathogen causes excessive fluid to build up in the lungs that can also cause the perceived need for more oxygen. Air hunger can range from excessive sighing and yawning to the inability to take a satisfactory deep breath. Eventually frank shortness of breath and respiratory distress could ensue. Shortness of breath can become serious quickly, and the patient may need hospitalization for respiratory support. B. *duncani* might affect the lungs more than B. *microti*.

> PEARL: *Initially academics thought that Babesia-induced air hunger was due to the anemia and that certainly can contribute to the problem. More likely, B.* duncani *seems to cause lung tissue edema that impedes adequate oxygenation.*

Anxiety can be one of the presenting symptoms of babesiosis. Some children develop an autism-like syndrome. (Again, it's hard to tell if some of these things are due to the Babesia or to various co-infections.) Other symptoms such as paresthesias, chest wall pain, along with severe bone and muscle pain can suggest the presence of Babesia. Not every patient will have all the listed symptoms and some may have only a few.

The babesiosis headache has been described many ways: severe, dull, unrelenting, global, involving the whole head, or restricted to the top of the head only. Some complain that they cannot move their head because the pain is so severe. Others become extremely sensitive to light. The onset of the headache can be rapid and surprisingly severe. One person described the headache as a football helmet of pain. Another claimed his head was in a vise. Neither sounds pleasant. Neck pain can be severe and stiffness can be incapacitating.

A number of other nonspecific signs and symptoms have been noted including: fatigue, conjunctivitis, eye pain, blurred vision, night blindness, sole pain (plantar fasciitis), listlessness, dullness, changes in appetite, nausea, vomiting, dry heaves, neck cracking, dark circles under the eyes, blue knuckles, vibrating sensations, back pain, migrating joint pain, myalgias, bone pain, shooting pain, burning sensations, feelings like electric shocks, tingling, numbness, heart palpitations, anxiety, panic, sleep problems, light sensitivity, mental dullness, neuropsychiatric symptoms, dry cough, lymphadenopathy, disorganized thinking, light sensitivity, itching, disrupted senses, and changes in consciousness. Whether these sxs are due to Babesia or co-infections is anyone's guess. While some say their appetite decreases, others say that the desire for food is the one parameter that stays normal throughout the course of the disease. A few gain weight. Most of the TBIs can present with some of these clinical manifestations and diagnostic distinction can be difficult in the presence of co-infections. Be careful blaming a symptom set on just one pathogen, especially if the patient is not improving as expected.

There may be RBC breakdown products causing icterus, jaundice, and hemoglobinuria. Internal organs can be affected especially through enlargement (organomegaly, primarily of the liver and spleen) or suboptimal function (lung and heart). Central nervous system signs may be due to low oxygen levels or to damaged or abnormally shaped RBCs clogging the small vessels in and around the brain. Early on, the patient may feel unstable or dizzy. Mental dullness and slower reactions and responses are common. The patient may lapse in and out of consciousness, experience delirium, or go into a coma.

As the patient gets sicker, complications of babesiosis include poor oxygen exchange, low blood pressure, cardiac compromise, and kidney dysfunction. SOB can get serious quickly. These problems can progress to respiratory distress, heart failure, shock, disseminated intravascular coagulation (DIC), and kidney failure. At this point, the condition is life-threatening and, if not aggressively managed, can lead to death. Hospitalize sooner rather than later.

Lab testing to follow the clinical course of babesiosis includes: CBCs to monitor for anemia, peripheral smears early in the disease process, LFTs to watch both liver function associated with the disease and to assess any problems from medication use, and clotting studies since hypercoagulability is common with Babesia. Evaluation of kidney function is critical. If the patient is essentially peeing blood and red cell debris, there is likely to be some impact on the kidney. The muscle component of CPK can be high, perhaps from the intense muscle action associated with rigors. In some cases, there is significant involvement of the skeletal muscles, with an almost muscular dystrophy-like presentation. Haptoglobin levels can be low with hemolytic anemia. Measured serially, haptoglobin can be used to monitor the degree of anemia. If signs of anemia or liver involvement appear to be getting worse, the patient could be getting into trouble.

In my research, both when my son was sick and for this text, I realized that many people writing about TBIs have never actually seen a case. Or, worse, they don't recognize it when they do see it. I realize now that Lilith's[4] ignorance could lead to sad repercussions for the innocent patient.

Diagnosis: Babesiosis, like most TBIs, is a diagnosis based on clinical judgment. HCPs must take clues from the history and physical exam, combined with any supporting evidence from diagnostic tests, and formulate a diagnosis. They must consider the full differential diagnosis and come out with a conclusion that best matches the clinical presentation. In all cases, a high index of suspicion is needed to make the right call. You can't diagnose something unless you recognize its existence.

- **To diagnose babesiosis based on clinical judgment, consider:**

  1. History of tick bite or diagnoses of other TBIs

  2. Description of cyclical symptoms especially fevers and chills

  3. Abrupt onset of acute symptoms including headache, high fever, chills, rigors, drenching sweats, red or discolored urine, and incapacitating fatigue. Air hunger and bone pain also suggest Babesia.

  4. Physical exam results can be indicative of babesiosis. A drenched patient in rigors should tell you something. Signs of anemia, such as pale conjunctiva and mucus membranes, along with weakness are suggestive. Air hunger is prominent in some cases.

  5. Incorporation of diagnostic test results that can help support the diagnosis

- **To use test results in support of a diagnosis, review:**

  1. **Routine lab work:** Listed here are tests to support diagnosis. To follow the progress of the disease or

to assess for adverse drug effects, other tests may be needed and should be based on the individual presentation.

a. **CBC** may show a moderate to severe anemia. Note that depending on the infecting strain, some patients show little or no evidence of anemia. Absence of anemia does not rule out babesiosis. In cases of hemolytic anemia, haptoglobin levels may be low.

b. **Urinalysis** may show blood or bilirubin in the urine. Not all strains of Babesia cause bloody urine. Presence of blood can be suggestive of Babesia, but absence is meaningless. Some HCPs recommend using home dipsticks to see if blood becomes apparent during the course of the disease. Home dipsticks may not be sensitive enough to pick up low levels of blood.

c. **Abnormal clotting panels** may indicate hypercoagulability, a common finding in babesiosis.

d. **A peripheral blood smear** looking for the characteristic Maltese cross formation can be useful. Blood smears are relatively inexpensive tests that can provide rapid results. Since Babesia reproduce in the RBCs, they often form a cross-shaped body composed of a tetrad that forms the shape of a cross. I regret to inform you that when you see a Maltese cross, you are actually witnessing Babesia sex. The arms of the cross are the asexual buds of B. *microti*. Under the microscope, crosses can be seen inside the RBCs, often with a pale center. One RBC can hold about 8 parasites.

Use of the Maltese cross smears is reliable for only about the first 2 weeks of the infection. A Giemsa stained blood smear is placed under a high-powered microscope and the search for the Maltese crosses begins. Machine readings are notoriously insensitive. They can't easily see the pathogenic crosses inside the RBCs. Write "manual read please" on the lab order slip. This test must be done by an experienced lab technician; otherwise the cluster formations can be missed.

---

4 See Glossary or Introduction for name origin

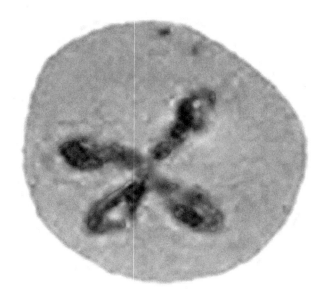

Maltese cross
Source: CDC. Accessed March 2013

When 80% of the RBCs contain Maltese crosses, interpretation is easy. The problem comes with those specimens where only 1% or 2% of the cells are involved. These are the cases that will be missed if the examiner is not careful. Often these tedious tasks are delegated to the technician with the least seniority rather than the person who has actually seen a Maltese cross before. If the tech is in a hurry or rushed, there is more chance for a false negative. How long will the tech look if Maltese crosses are not as ubiquitous as Kardashians?

PEARL: Half of the highly educated, otherwise-worldly editors reviewing this book have never heard of the Kardashians. They worry that the audience will not know who these reality TV personalities are in a few years. I worry that they will.

I have had good luck in establishing close collaborations with the staff in the local labs. Just like my trusted local pharmacists, these guys know everything. They often appreciate the opportunity to "connect" with a real patient once in a while. When you explain to them the importance of the blood smear for a very sick child, they will understand the significance of determining if there is actually pathogen present. I have always found that they were as interested in these special cases as I was. (Thank you, Larry Bowman at Riverside Hospital in Wilmington, Delaware.)

There are techniques that help to enhance the sensitivity of the peripheral smear reading. Enhanced smears use buffy coat technology, longer scan times of several hours, digital photography, and customized microscopes to increase sensitivity. Nonetheless, positive results will sometimes be missed, but at least not as often. These enhanced techniques may improve recognition of more species but still might not be useful in detecting infection later in the clinical course or when the germ load is too light to be observed.

PEARL: Some strains of Babesia show more parasites in the blood smear than others, even though both can be equally symptomatic.

2. **Specialized diagnostic tests**: With varying degrees of utility, a number of laboratory tests are available to help identify an etiologic agent. Currently, PCR looking for DNA, FISH looking for RNA, and IFA are all performed looking for evidence of Babesia. Chapters 18 and 19 contain the science underlying these test modalities.

   a. **Serology** – Titers can be used to measure the presence of antigen or antibody. Persistently positive titers or WBs suggest on-going infection which is not surprising since endurance appears to be a characteristic of Babesia in the same way that it is for malaria.

   b. **PCR** – The polymerase chain reaction looks for DNA. The DNA sample of interest is concentrated and amplified using primers. These primers contain Babesia-exclusive nucleotide sequences that bind specifically to the organism of interest. Here they do not bind to anything other than the Babesia. Then the PCR-amplified Babesia DNA fragment is identified using electrophoresis. The amplified DNA bits that are the right size will show up as a band on the electrophoresis gel. This band is specific for Babesia. The PCR method can be quite sensitive and specific for B. *microti*. For B. *duncani* (formerly WA-1) and the myriad other strains, methods are still under refinement.

   A positive PCR result for Babesia means that the actual DNA of the organism was found. A negative result means *only* that no Babesia DNA was found in this sample, *not* that there was no Babesia in this patient now or ever. As always, a negative test does not exclude the diagnosis.

   PCR testing is more sensitive than smears but currently good only for B. *microti*. Note that compiled PCR results showed that Lyme DNA was detected more often, and remained in the blood longer when a patient was also infected with Babesia than with Lyme alone. I don't know why.

In the case of a new baby with an infected mom, consider DNA PCR at birth for babesiosis, bartonellosis, and Borrelia *burgdorferi*. Take samples from the placenta, cord, cord blood, and the foreskin remnant. Send the specimens to a lab that knows what to do with them. Call the lab first to make sure you are sending them exactly what they need to give you the results you are looking for. Do not be responsible for wasting such a precious sample.

c. **FISH** – In contrast to PCR, the fluorescent in-situ hybridization assay looks for RNA. FISH uses thin blood smears and looks for ribosomal RNA from Babesia and can indicate an active infection. If the result is positive, FISH provides very strong supportive evidence for the presence of Babesia. This technique may eventually be able to detect other species of Babesia besides *microti*. Since blood smears have little value after the first few weeks of the infection, a FISH test might provide more useful information. FISH testing may be 100 times more sensitive than standard smears for B. *microti*. Instead of standard stains, FISH uses a fluorescent RNA probe and UV light which is easier to see when scanned. Currently only B. *microti* can be scanned in most labs performing this test. Since we know this species is not the only bagpiper on the hill, FISH has limitations.

d. **IFA** – In general, the cutoff for positive Babesia titers using indirect immunofluorescent assays are 1:160 or higher. Early on in the infection, the titer may be as high as 1:1280. The titers should fall as the treated disease proceeds along its course. If samples are tested again after about a month, titers should be lower if treatment is adequate. Positive results can vary between labs. A positive result must be statistically different from a negative one and has meaning only if correlated with the clinical picture. Further, a negative result simply means "not detected." The patient could still have been infected.

Repeating the test in 4 to 6 weeks may increase the chance of confirming the diagnosis. Unlike results found with Borrelia *burgdorferi*, which causes Lyme, Babesia titers can suggest infection status. Persistently positive titers or Western blot suggest on-going infection.

IFA testing may not always be reliable for several reasons. With babesiosis, a patient with fever may not have an established antibody presence until the fever abates. Further, antibodies to the original Babesia antigens can linger long after symptoms are gone. Using polyclonal antibodies in the testing may decrease specificity.

In all cases of laboratory tests used to support diagnosis, if you or your staff are not *very* familiar with how to order, collect, pack, and ship the sample, call the lab you intend to use and *ask* for instructions. These tests can be extremely expensive and insurance does not always cover them. You do not want to be the reason a specimen is useless. The cost of the test should not be a surprise to the person responsible for paying for it. Stories have been told of panicked parents pawning wedding rings and taking out second mortgages to pay for these studies.

PEARL: Do not assume that your local lab knows these specialty techniques. Call.

While blood and serum can be used for a number of these tests, tissue samples are usually more reliable. One group of patients tested negative for Babesia using blood samples. When tissue from biopsies taken during endoscopy and gall bladder surgery were used instead, the same patients all tested positive. Except in extreme circumstances, resist invasive tissue samples for the sole purpose of diagnosis. However, if tissue becomes available during a procedure, take advantage of the opportunity to obtain more sensitive test results. If you are aware of a procedure your patient will be undergoing, don't let tissue be discarded without considering if useful information could be gathered.

IGeneX performs IFA, FISH, and PCR. Medical Diagnostic Laboratory (MDL) does ELISA and PCR. Specific contact information for these labs is found in Chapter 18: *Ordering Appropriate Tests.*

- **Diagnosis in special populations**

  Transfusions: In transmission of Babesia through blood transfusions, a high index of suspicion is the patient's only hope. Otherwise, you will be wasting time thinking of blood group incompatibility and serum sickness when you should be hanging antimicrobials and preparing for a clean transfusion. In some cases, essentially all blood has to be replaced. Have an experienced pathologist look at a peripheral smear.

  Neonates: The diagnosis of babesiosis in the newborn should be based on the pregnant mother's history. The attending HCP should be aware and prepared for neonatal intensive care before the delivery. At birth, do a DNA PCR for Babesia as well as for Bb and Bartonella. Take samples from the placenta, cord section, cord blood, and foreskin remnant. Send the specimens to a lab that knows what it's doing, like Clongen. Call the lab first to make sure you know what **you** are doing and to be sure you are giving them exactly what they need. Note that with sick neonates, a peripheral blood smear might be especially useful. These tests can be done locally, quickly, and cheaply. Stress to the lab personnel the importance of an accurate reading – literally, life or death.

PEARL: News flash from July 2012: Baby born with babesiosis. This is not news to the TBI community.

- **Diagnosis in the presence of co-infections**

What else could this be? Why is this patient still so sick, after being treated for Lyme? Is the illness more severe than would be expected with a single etiology? Is this the worst Lyme you have ever seen? Maybe it's not just Lyme. Do the symptoms go on and on despite seemingly appropriate Lyme treatment? Are the clinical course and presentation confusing and confounding? With the high incidence and prevalence numbers for co-infections, an HCP should never think of one TBI without at least considering that there might be more than one. If you see hypercoagulability, think Babesia and Bartonella. If you see muscle pain, put both Babesia and Ehrlichia on the list.

PEARL: Hints that should make you think babesiosis: rigors, sweats, more severe Lyme than usually seen, patient gets worse when only treated for Lyme, or a cyclic pattern to the symptoms. In the northeastern US, whenever Lyme crosses your mind, Babesia should be right there along with it.

Consider Babesia whenever a person presents with a fever of unknown origin (FUO) with even a possibility of exposure. The actual exposure can be well hidden. There is rarely a smoking tick. A tick could have come and gone and never been seen, or it could have been mistaken for something else, or forgotten. Don't discount babesiosis as a possible diagnosis just because the tick is not handed to you.

PEARL: IDSA guidelines for babesiosis are interesting, relying heavily on the visualization of the parasites on blood smears. If the protozoa are seen, that's wonderful. BUT if they are NOT observed that proves nothing. IDSA says if no Babesia is seen on the smear or by PCR, don't treat. There are a number of reasons why the Babesia pathogen might be missed: machine analysis, tech inexperience or impatience, or the time in the disease cycle when the sample was drawn. PCR has limited specificity for most pathogens. No test is 100%. Treat the patient, not the test.

In a somewhat uncharacteristic recommendation, IDSA recommends daily or every other day smears and Hcts until the patient is well. First of all, in the county where I live, where there is thought to be one of the highest incidence rates of babesiosis in the US, it is almost impossible

to get these patients seen and diagnosed initially, let alone drawing daily labs.

IDSA says patients with Babesia should be re-treated if Babesia is seen on smears or by PCR three months after initial treatment even if the patient is asymptomatic. (That's great but a tad unrealistic. I had trouble getting a test run on an unconscious, hypoxic patient in rigors with the tick in a jar.)

Differential diagnosis: As with all TBIs, parsing out which signs belong to which pathogen can be daunting. If you are waiting for the one indicator that screams your diagnosis, that probably isn't going to happen. Buddha said something like, "Expectations lead to disappointments," and he wasn't even dealing with TBIs.

In considering the differential diagnosis of babesiosis, you are asking the question, "What else could this be?" First, start with all the other pathogens that could be traveling along with the Babesia on that Ixodes tick. Look at Chapter 18: *Ordering Appropriate Tests* for a comprehensive list of possibilities.

Clinically, the condition that babesiosis most resembles is malaria. This being said, most people do not frequent overlapping endemic areas. If the Maltese cross is seen on the blood smear, the diagnosis is likely Babesia. If the smear has parasites visible both in the RBCs as well as extracellularly, then the diagnosis is more often malaria. I do not know what happens if the patient has both malaria and babesiosis at the same time, but at least they would be treated using similar antimicrobials.

In ERs and HCP offices, babesiosis has been mistaken for URIs, acute asthma attacks, "just a virus," FUO, anemia, psychiatric conditions, flu, Lyme, fibromyalgia, CFS, or a sleep disorder. In the northeastern US, babesiosis is not often mistaken for malaria because HCPs rarely see malaria. Unfortunately, these two conditions do not easily come to mind no matter how clear the indicators.

Most general docs forget they ever heard of Babesia, Ehrlichia, Bartonella, etc. It's hard to diagnose something you haven't heard of in 10 years, if ever. The last time they may have seen these names was when they were studying for boards and there was a list of pathogens to memorize. Most had very different names back then (Piroplasms anyone?) or the species hadn't even been discovered yet. Most doctors in areas with endemic TBIs have never seen a case of malaria. The doctor who initially saw my son, said he just had Lyme and would be better in a few days on the doxy. Except a few days had already passed and he was worse and he was presenting like he had malaria, not Lyme.

PEARL: Some HCPs think if there is no anemia there is no babesiosis. That's not true. In fact, B. duncani does not appear to cause anemia as often as microti *and some patients show little, if any, signs of anemia.*

Treatment: Assuming Babesia is recognized, the battle is just beginning. Few of the antimicrobials used for the other co-infections hit Babesia. Further, different species of Babesia respond to different treatments. In general, babesiosis is treated like malaria with all the same frustrations. Here, I prefer to use the term *antiprotozoals*, instead of *antimalarials*. In this chapter, I outline one treatment approach for babesiosis. Detailed information about each of the listed agents and other potentially useful medications is included in Chapter 24: *Antimicrobials*.

The two species of Babesia causing the most disease in the US do NOT respond to the same antimicrobials. Even if laboratory evidence for one of these species exists, that confirmation does not rule out any of the other potential pathogens, many of which have no reliable means of detection to date. The most prudent approach is to treat *simultaneously* with both regimens if babesiosis is diagnosed.

Duration of treatment depends on how sick the patient becomes, how long she was sick prior to diagnosis, general health, immune status, and potential for co-infections. While acute symptoms usually diminish in about 3 to 4 weeks, the natural history of this pathogen suggests a minimum of 4 months of treatment, and 6 months is probably prudent. Still relapses can occur.

Treatment of B. *microti*:

1st option: Atovaquone (Mepron) PLUS azithromycin (Zithromax)

2nd option: Replace Mepron with Malarone (combination of atovaquone and proguanil)

3rd option: Replace azithromycin with a different macrolide or ketolide, such as clarithromycin (Biaxin) or telithromycin (Ketek)

4th option: Increase doses

5th option: Consider a role for Septra (Bactrim), Cleocin (clindamycin), Biaxin (clarithromycin), Lariam (mefloquine), Flagyl (metronidazole), Plaquenil, or even quinine. For example, a combination of Biaxin and Flagyl has been documented as effective, and will have the benefit of hitting borreliosis and babesiosis at the same time. Unfortunately, not everyone can tolerate Flagyl.

6th option: At this point, you better make sure you have artemesia on board just in case you're dealing with B. *duncani* as well as B. *microti*. In general, always treat as though both Babesia species are present.

Older regimens such as those combining clindamycin and quinine were only partially effective and many patients could not tolerate the disabling side effects. Even in those who could put up with the untoward events, only about half of these responded to the therapy. Chloroquine appears to relieve the sxs of B. *microti*, but doesn't seem to diminish the overall parasite load. More recent formulations and regimens have been better received in terms of both efficacy and tolerability. In finding an effective treatment, HCPs will be challenged with patient allergies, intolerance, and ineffectiveness. You will have to experiment appropriately until you find what helps your patient.

PEARL: Atovaquone (Mepron) is a bright yellow suspension with a strange (not to say bad) taste and a weird texture. One child said it was like drinking a daffodil. Mepron must be taken with fatty food to increase absorption, which is pretty dismal otherwise. For kids over 13-years-old give 750 mg (which is 1 teaspoon or 5 ml) twice a day with food or 1500 mg (2 teaspoons or 10 ml) once daily with food. In small kids, use ½ tsp bid. Measure accurately. Kitchen teaspoons can vary considerably. In cases where neuropsychiatric manifestations might be due to Babesia, remember that Mepron does not easily pass the BBB. Here the patient may benefit from a switch to Lariam since that passes into the brain and CNS more readily. Treatment with Mepron is usually recommended for at least 6 months and up to 2 years. Mepron is expensive. Prices vary widely but the average is over $800 a bottle for about 3 week's therapy. Check around.

Keep in mind when dealing with TBIs, the more effective the treatment, the more intense the resulting Herxheimer reaction might be. Be prepared and prepare your patients – and their caregivers. Patients have described something called a "brain Herx" if the demise of the pathogens is too rapid or intense. For B. *microti*, treatment is recommended for about 6 months, but longer, up to 2 or more years may be needed. Shorter courses do not seem effective, especially since relapses seem more likely if therapy is of insufficient duration.

When using a combination of such big guns, follow the patient closely, both for adverse events due to the drug regimen and to assess treatment efficacy. Always consider probiotics. Be ready to regroup and reconsider your treatment plan. Monitor blood counts, LFTs, and kidney function. For more details on these medicines see Chapter 24: *Antimicrobials*.

PEARL: IDSA provides the following dosing recommendations for the treatment of babesiosis:

Clindamycin:	Use in severe cases requiring IV Adults: 300 to 600 mg q 6 IV or 600 q 8 orally Kids: 7 to 10 mg/kg IV or orally q 6 to 8, max of 600 mg/dose
Quinine:	Adults: 650 mg q 6 to 8 Kids: 8 mg/kg po q 8 maximum 600 mg/dose
Mepron:	Adults: 750 mg q 12 Kids: 20 mg/kg q 12 max 750 mg/dose
Azithromycin:	Adults: 500 to 1000 mg on day 1 and 250 mg daily thereafter Kids: 10 mg/kg on day 1 up to 500 mg/dose and then 5 mg/kg daily up to 250 mg/dose

Higher doses may be needed in the immunocompromised.

IDSA says to use exchange transfusion if indicated: if greater than 10% parasitemia, significant hemolysis, or renal, hepatic, or pulmonary compromise.

IDSA Guidelines for dosing are often inconsistent with the dosing recommendations in the product package insert and not for approved indications.

Treatment of B. *duncani*:

Since few labs test for B. *duncani*, you never know when it is contributing to the signs and symptoms of babesiosis. Consider adding artemesia when treating any potential Babesia cases. So, *in addition* to one of the options listed above, artemesia *should* be on board to make sure both kinds of Babesia are covered. Full details on the mechanism of action and use of artemesia are found in the *Antimicrobials* chapter.

To add to the confusion, artemesia is a WHO-recommended antiprotozoal that is not available by prescription in the US. There are many formulations and dosing regimens. This treatment MUST be *pulsed*, otherwise an enzyme build-up in the liver will increase metabolism of the product, rendering it ineffective. After a few days of administration, blood levels will be so low as to decrease efficacy. In children, 250 mg tid is a recognized regimen. Pulse the artemesia, dosing 4 days on and 3 days off. (Some HCPs use 3 weeks on and 1 week off, while others prefer a schedule of 12 days on and 2 days off. But the plan of 4 days on and 3 days off seems more consistent with the pharmacokinetics of the medicine.) Consider antiprotozoal treatment for a minimum of 3 months. Shorter courses have been known to make some patients worse overall.

PEARL: Artemesia MUST be pulsed to remain effective.

Artemesia seems to have less potential for Herx reactions than other treatments for Babesia, but that might mean it is less effective than other agents. It is also cheaper than Mepron and Malarone.

PEARL: From my background, I know many drugs intimately. Nonetheless, after careful consideration, I must admit that artemesia is my least favorite. Not because it doesn't work, but because it is so hard to figure out. For the last year, I have taped to my monitor some of the different spelling and formulations for this product. Right now I have over two dozen. One formulation, Artemisinin, has 250 or 500 mg capsules given 2 or 3 times a day. Some say that Artemisinin is more effective than artemesia. Just as passionate are the artemesia proponents who declare their formulation superior. My best advice is to find one that is readily available on the Internet, from a company that is fairly reputable, and stick with it. Sometimes I am able to find Dr. Zhang's Artemisinin at hepapro.com, but sometimes I can't. Unfortunately, we need this agent in our anti-Babesia arsenal, so we don't have the luxury of ignoring it.

PEARL: Recently another antiparasitic herbal called enula has been used anecdotally in treating babesiosis. Enula may eventually be found to be as effective as artemesia. Chapter 24 has more information on this herbal. Mora has also been tried with anecdotal success.

Other treatments for babesiosis: For those with significant anemia, a high pathogen load in the RBCs, or who are severely ill, consider blood transfusion. A full exchange is preferable since the pathogen in remaining cells can infect the new cells coming in. Use blood that does not contain Babesia, otherwise you might have more strains than you already had to deal with. Continue antimicrobials throughout the transfusion process. Follow the patient's progress so you can see what more may be needed.

Ancillary treatment can be helpful in making these people feel better. Unlike Lilith[5] in the local ER who would not give my son a blanket because she didn't want her patients with chills to get a fever, I prefer to attempt to keep people comfortable. First, consider probiotics for all patients who are on such a broad antimicrobial regimen. This may spare the gut some anguish. Second, provide all reasonable supportive care. Some of these people are very SICK. For Chris, we were able to modulate temperatures somewhat by administering antipyretics (alternating ibuprofen and acetaminophen). This helped keep him from exhausting himself with the rigors and diminished the delusions and lapsing consciousness that came with the near 106° fevers. At that point, my husband and I would do anything to keep him more comfortable and able to rest. To keep him warm we used warm baths, hot water bottles, microwave packs, and electric blankets. To cool off,

---

5 See Glossary or Introduction for name origin

he liked tepid baths, popsicles, and cold packs in his groin and under his arms. We changed bedding four times in 12 hours. We switched beds when he soaked through onto the mattress. We gave him whatever he felt he could eat. For the two of us it was 24/7, until the Mepron kicked in.

Duration of treatment depends on 1) how sick the individual is; 2) the length of the illness before diagnosis; 3) general health and immune status; and 4) the presence of co-infections or concurrent conditions. Usually it will be 3 weeks in acute cases before the symptoms subside. The more morbidity, the longer the treatment. Follow the patient's clinical course carefully. Even with 4 to 6 months of treatment, relapses can occur. Re-treat as needed.

In summary, if you are treating a patient for her first bout of babesiosis, a reasonable starting point might be Mepron, Zithromax, and artemesia. If this regimen is not successful, consider increasing the doses. If still not effective, start substitutions such as one macrolide for another or Malarone instead of Mepron. Go to options 3 or 4 above. Consider that the diagnosis is wrong or that additional co-infections may be confounding the recovery. Do not give up. Successful resolution of babesiosis can be a long process taking more than a year or two. Even Peter Krause in the Babesia section of the IDSA 2006 Guidelines said that Babesia could be chronic and treatment in severe cases should be open-ended until signs of the disease are gone.

Prognosis: Morbidity and mortality are highest in the newborn, elderly, and immunocompromised, especially those who have had a splenectomy. Everything is worse if there are co-infections. These patients can never donate blood and the scariest part of that restriction is that many don't know that they can't donate, which leaves the blood supply vulnerable.

Morbidity and mortality rates are difficult to estimate since it is hard to tell what problems might be caused by Babesia and what are due to co-infections or concurrent diseases. There is seemingly a higher rate of death from babesiosis in Europe. Whether this is due to more careful recognition and reporting or because of a more virulent protozoal strain than found in the US, is not known. The infected population in Europe may be different, with more immunocompromised patients getting exposed to Ixodes ticks. Maybe patients are dying of Babesia and we just don't recognize the real cause. Their death certificates say "cardiopulmonary arrest" and we never know the difference. The critical point for HCPs is that Babesia infection can cause severe illness and end in death.

B. *microti* is thought to have about a 5% to 10% mortality rate while B. *divergens* has a much higher death rate closer to 50%. While there are many theories that try to account for the discrepancy in mortality rates, no one knows for sure. In

Europe, babesiosis is considered life-threatening with over half of the infected becoming comatose and dying. Over 80% of these deaths are thought to be in asplenic patients.

Few cases are reported. Dr. Virginia Sherr relates being told by the state health department in Pennsylvania not to bother reporting since Babesia was not really a problem, just a "trendy" diagnosis. (Lilith[6], are you moonlighting?) Now that the state is in a panic over Babesia in the blood supply, I wonder if they feel the same way.

Those who were infected through blood donation had significant mortality and the survivors had long recovery periods. The American Red Cross will not permit donations from people who have *ever* been infected with Babesia. Apparently the Red Cross believes that infection is permanent even if symptoms have not been noted for many years. Due to increasing international travel, this is becoming a bigger problem worldwide. In addition to donor transmission, transplacental transmissions have been reported. In cases of live births, the neonates were in grave condition and heroic measures were needed to save them.

There is considerable debate regarding whether an initial infection with Babesia provides immunity. In my opinion, we just don't know for sure and the most prudent course is to avoid reinfection. Babesia may impair human defenses, which can then allow co-infections to be more aggressive in causing symptoms and may weaken the body's ability to fight other diseases (tick-borne or otherwise). Untreated Babesia can persist for years. If the parasite load continues to increase, by the time symptoms present, the result can be catastrophic.

Still about 25% of infected adults and 50% of infected kids are asymptomatic. What causes some to develop symptoms and others to remain symptom-free remains a matter of conjecture. For those who do get sick, treatment may need to continue for months or years. If relapse or reinfection occurs the patient will need to resume therapy.

As environmental changes make life easier for the tick, the mouse, and the deer, we should expect to see more babesiosis not less. More international travel is causing first case reports in places where Babesia has never been seen before like the Czech Republic and B. *microti* has now been isolated in Europe. For HCPs to simply recognize that Babesia can cause a TBD will be progress.

---

6 See Glossary or Introduction for name origin

Chapter 7

EHRLICHIOSIS/ANAPLASMOSIS

The only way to guarantee failure is to try to please everyone.

Bill Cosby

Background: Sometimes life is hard and confusing and complicated. Then there is Ehrlichia. In the course of my research for this book, I have found the mother lode of misinformation, bias, unscientific babbling, and opinions stated as fact. The literature on Ehrlichia was especially confusing. The scientists seem to have given up halfway through and, I guess, went off to lunch. To add to the confusion, I found the word Ehrlichia spelled three different ways (in one paragraph by the same peer-reviewed author). As I dug and dug, I learned that there were very recent changes in how these organisms are classified. As if taxonomy were not bizarre enough on a good day, now I was trying to figure out organisms that yesterday were the same, but today are different. That makes looking back into the literature (unscientific as much of it is) and trying to sort out what was going on, a rather hapless endeavor. Please read this chapter quickly before everything changes again.

The Family Anaplasmataceae now has four (or six, depending on the source) genuses including Ehrlichia and Anaplasma. Some Ehrlichia species have become Anaplasma and some have fallen into other genuses and even other categories entirely. (For example, some Ehrlichia have become Neorickettsia. Introducing the term "new" rickettsia is yet another confusing factor, since the "old" rickettsia are still around. Further, some Heamobartonella became Mycoplasma.) Other distinguishable organisms have yet to be classified according to the rules of the International Code of Nomenclature of Bacteria.

After suffering with this for days, I came to accept that some of this doesn't matter to practicing HCPs. The point is: If disease from one of these organisms is suspected, it does not necessarily matter what you call it, as long as you recognize that additional work-up and treatment may be indicated. So I stopped splitting hairs and got on with my life.

Aliases: Rocky Mountain *Spotless* Fever, human monocytic ehrlichiosis (HME), human granulocytic ehrlichiosis (HGE), human anaplasmosis (HA), human granulocytic anaplasmosis (HGA), canine ehrlichiosis, canine granulocytic ehrlichiosis, human *ewingii* ehrlichiosis (HEE), tick-borne fever, pasture fever. The *Pathogen* section below should help clear up the confusion. Or then again, you may remain confused. But in the end it doesn't really matter, as long as you help the patient. You say Ehrlichia, I say Anaplasma. We're still friends.

History: Paul Ehrlich, for whom Ehrlichia was named, was an interesting guy. His life is presented in much more detail in the *Gentle Immunology* chapter where I discuss his contributions to the understanding of antigens, antibodies, serum sickness, and the blood brain barrier. (I also reveal the actor who played him in the movie.) In 1910, Ehrlich discovered Salvarsan, a treatment for syphilis, which became the most widely prescribed medicine in the world. Salvarsan was also called 606 because it was the 606th compound Ehrlich tested. Obviously a persistent and patient person, he had two daughters, Stephanie and Marianne. I wonder how he would feel today knowing that half of his eponymous Ehrlichia are now Anaplasma. Ehrlichia were first recognized in the US as a human pathogen in the late 1980s.

Pathogen: Whatever the name, these pathogens are parasites that invade specific parts of the host's cells. Mostly they locate in the cell vacuoles where nutrients are stored and waste released. In much of the old literature, the terms ehrlichiosis and anaplasmosis have been used interchangeably. Here they will be separated for clarity since this seems to be the way of the future. Note that the clinical presentation of these conditions is similar. Under the time and resource constraints of the clinic, it may not be possible to distinguish them before treatment needs to begin.

Early on, the Ehrlichia were classified by the type of blood cell they most commonly invaded. This turned out to be premature and misleading since the Ehrlichia species have been found in other cells beside their primary target cells. Further, more than one species may cause a certain disease. The blood cells used to sort the diseases include granulocytes, monocytes, platelets, and lymphocytes. For example, you have the term human granulocytic ehrlichiosis (HGE), which some are now calling human granulocytic anaplasmosis, or HGA. Ehrlichia AND Anaplasma are round Gram negative bacteria, that some do not believe even merit the title of bacteria. Some taxonomists think they are closer to Rickettsia, and a few species have been moved into those groups. At this point, the ones who act more like bacteria than their renegade cousins remain bacteria. But, alas! The day is young.

Now comes the part where all becomes clear.

Ehrlichia *chaffeensis*

Disease caused: Human Monocytic Ehrlichiosis (HME) Note that there is controversy around whether E. *chaffeensis* is the actual causative agent.

Hosts: Humans, deer, dogs

Primary cell affected: Monocyte

Vectors: Lone Star tick as well as deer tick (black-legged tick), Pacific tick (Western black-legged tick), and the American dog tick

Range: US from the Mid-Atlantic and into the southeast and south central parts of the country. Found in Utah and Montana. Also in Africa, Europe, Central America, and South America

Clinical course: If symptoms appear, they most likely occur 1 to 2 weeks after the tick bite. Many cases are uneventful but some can be dangerous. About half of symptomatic patients require hospitalization. The immunocompromised appear to be at greater risk of poor outcomes. Fatal outcomes are estimated at 2% to 3%. There is suspicion that E. *chaffeensis* can also be transmitted through blood transfusions.

Signs & symptoms: More than half the patients will have a sudden onset of chills, fever, sweats, bad headache, and muscle aches. Few have a maculopapular rash. Some also have confusion, prostration, nausea, vomiting, malaise, and other vague confounding symptoms.

Lab findings: Morulae seen in monocytes, PCR, culture, IFA

Treatment: Doxycycline is used for both adults and children: 100 mg q 12 hours for 14 days, adjusted to patient weight and condition. Consider treatment for at least 7 days after fever is gone. If TCNs are contraindicated or not tolerated, try rifampin in combination with other antimicrobials. Doxycycline is not usually recommended in children under 8-years-old. However, this is a judgment call and sometimes doxycycline will be needed on a shotgun basis. A number of HCPs feel that short-courses of doxy in kids under 8 are indicated in some cases and the brief treatment period usually required for HME poses little risk. Always do a risk/benefit analysis and discuss options with the patient or guardian. Chapter 24: *Antimicrobials* has additional information.

Anaplasma *phagocytophilum* (Formerly Ehrlichia *phagocytophilum* or a related organism)

Disease caused: Human Granulocytic Anaplasmosis or HGA, or Human Anaplasmosis or HA, formerly called Human Granulocytic Ehrlichiosis (HGE), also called: equine ehrlichiosis, tick-borne fever, pasture fever

History: The first known case of HGA was a Wisconsin patient who experienced a high fever and malaise after a tick bite. He died within 2 weeks. Ehrlichia was suspected but cultures for E. *chaffeensis* were negative. Yet, morulae were seen inside the person's neutrophils. The clinical course suggested Ehrlichia and similar cases were identified in the midwest region at the time. Despite uncertainty the patient was diagnosed initially with human granulocytic ehrlichiosis. By 1994, DNA samples showed that this species was different from E. *chaffeensis*. Eventually a new species was named, Anaplasma *phagocytophilum*. With the name change the disease formerly known as HGE is now known as HGA, or human granulocytic anaplasmosis. This makes my head hurt.

Hosts: Humans, deer, rodents, elk, horses, llamas, sheep, cattle, bison. The primary mammalian reservoir is the white-footed mouse.

Primary cell affected: Granulocyte

Vectors: Ixodes *scapularis*, Ixodes *pacificus*, Ixodes *ricinis*, Ixodes *persulcatus*

Range: Europe, Great Britain, US, Asia

Signs & symptoms: Similar to E. *chaffeensis* with fever greater than 102° but may have more joint pain than that caused by Ehrlichia and more mental status changes, but this is speculation.

Treatment: Treatment specifics are provided in the general *Treatment* section below.

Ehrlichia *ewingii*

Disease caused: Canine Granulocytic Ehrlichiosis, Human Granulocytic Ehrlichiosis (HGE), Human *ewingii* Ehrlichiosis (HEE)

Hosts: Humans, dogs

Primary cell affected: Granulocyte (neutrophils)

Vectors: Deer tick (black-legged tick), Pacific tick (Western black-legged tick), American dog tick, and Lone Star tick are all suspect.

Range: US

Clinical course: In humans this disease is thought to be similar to HME but no deaths are known.

Signs & symptoms: Fever, chills, headache, body aches, and malaise

Treatment: Treatment specifics are provided in the general *Treatment* section below.

Ehrlichia *canis*

Disease caused: Canine ehrlichiosis. Currently E. *canis* has not been confirmed as an agent in human disease, but it is suspected as another cause of human monocytic ehrlichiosis.

Hosts: Dogs, other canines, only recently thought to infect humans

Primary cell affected: Monocyte

Vectors: Rhipicephalus ticks, such as the brown dog tick. Note that this tick species can complete its entire life cycle indoors so it may be able to initiate disease in colder climates than many other ticks.

Range: Global

Treatment: Treatment specifics are provided in the general *Treatment* section below.

Vector: Apparently, many different ticks are responsible for transmitting various Ehrlichia-like parasites, most of which have yet to be clearly differentiated. The usual suspects include: Lone Star tick, deer tick (black-legged tick), Pacific tick (Western black-legged tick), and the American dog tick.

Distribution: These bacteria have been found in more than a quarter of the ticks tested in the northeastern US. Ehrlichiosis has been recognized as a pathogen of animals for a long time. The first case in humans was reported in about 1990. (Even "facts" like the year of the first human report, which should be indisputable, are the subject of intense controversy in the literature. For crying out loud, was it 1989 or 1990? The harder I tried to answer this question, the more dates I found. The date doesn't matter. Treat the poor patient.) Case reports are about 1000 per year. The true incidence is thought to be much higher. According to the CDC, cases of ehrlichiosis grew from 200 to 957 (a 378% increase) between 2000 and 2008. Anaplasmosis tripled in the same period, but since the nomenclature changes occurred after these statistics were compiled, who knows what these numbers actually mean?

Ehrlichiosis has been documented now in at least 30 states. In endemic areas, a 12% to 35% seropositive rate has been documented in tested humans, but there is not a corresponding amount of reported disease. This means that these infections are either so mild as to be unrecognized, the symptoms are attributed to something else, or the illness is buried as a co-infection under more familiar diagnoses. I did not know until I researched this book that ehrlichiosis was nationally reportable. The incidence of ehrlichiosis appears to wax and wane. There may be few reports one year and then a resurgence occurs.

Ehrlichia tends to infect mostly in the spring and summer but reports continue into the fall. These bacteria more often affect the elderly, perhaps due to less immune defense. However, severe cases have occurred at all ages including children. The age of these patients ranges from the very young to the very old (4 to 92 in 2007 in Minnesota) with the median age thought to be about 50. The numbers may be increasing both owing to more actual cases (because of the wider tick range) and to the possible increase in awareness by HCPs and the public. One author lamented that the tick that carries Ehrlichia is moving from Long Island to New York City and to the rest of the state. I do not know what evidence he had to make these claims, but I don't dispute them.

Before the first human case was suspected in about 1990, the pathogen responsible for HGE (now anaplasmosis) was known to infect horses, dogs, and cattle. As is often the case, veterinary medicine is one step ahead.

Pathophysiology: Now that we have established that we don't know what to call these pathogens, let's see if we can hypothesize about how they might cause symptoms in humans.

Anaplasma and Ehrlichia are parasites that invade specific parts of the host's cells. They prefer the cell vacuoles where plenty of nutrients are stored. The clinical presentation of these different species (and now genuses) is so similar as to be indistinguishable. Under the time and resource constraints of the clinic it may not be possible to distinguish them before treatment needs to begin. Fortunately, they respond to the same treatment regimen. Maybe next month they will change the names back.

Ehrlichia/Anaplasma are round Gram negative bacteria that prefer to localize in the vacuoles floating in the cell's cytoplasm. Ehrlichia target the mononuclear phagocytes such as monocytes and macrophages and occasionally neutrophils. Anaplasma go after the granulocytes, especially neutrophils. We now know that both of these pathogens have been found in the immune cells preferred by the other genus. Kind of like your sister going after your boyfriend.

Both types of pathogen are small, obligate intracellular microbes that like to hang out at the buffet, which is the cell vacuole. Here they form clusters called **morulae** which are mulberry-shaped clumps of bacteria. Since the vacuole floats in the cell's cytoplasm, these morulae clusters can sometimes be seen in blood smears under a microscope. Therefore, visualization of morulae can be helpful in diagnosing ehrlichiosis and anaplasmosis.

The organism seems to affect the host through inflammation, but the mechanism of action has not been well-defined. The Ehrlichia/Anaplasma organisms cycle between ticks and small mammals. Since they share vectors and hosts with other TBIs, co-infection can occur. Anaplasma present and respond much like Ehrlichia (since many were Ehrlichia last month).

Clinical course: The clinical course of these pathogens can be difficult to define. Obviously, many people are infected that do not manifest signs of disease. In others, there is a rapid onset of initial illness. Severity ranges from asymptomatic, to mild, to severe, to fatal if untreated. As the disease progresses, more lab results become abnormal. Patients can develop kidney failure and respiratory insufficiency which can lead to death.

One source declared that symptoms occurred 12 days after a tick bite (not 11 days, not 13 days, always 12). These organisms and their clinical manifestations are not yet well understood, so any rigid pronouncements should be taken with a grain of salt. Note that the clinical presentations of these conditions from the various Ehrlichia/Anaplasma species are essentially indistinguishable and they respond to similar treatment protocols.

On-going low grade infection can occur especially in the presence of other TBIs. Elderly and immunocompromised patients fare worse. Many of these patients will require hospitalization. Significant complications have been documented including respiratory distress, persistent fever, shock, abnormal coagulation, kidney failure, hemorrhages, and central nervous system problems such as meningitis, encephalitis, coma, and seizures. Peripheral neuropathies and cranial neuritis have been described.

However, in many of these severe cases, it was not known if the patient had a pure infection from Ehrlichia or if other agents may have been contributing as well. Too little is known about these diseases in humans to state unequivocally that A caused B and *only* A caused B. Many confounding variables are at play. If treatment is delayed, serious consequences can result. Ehrlichiosis can be fatal, so do not dismiss this diagnosis.

Signs & symptoms: The symptom patterns for both anaplasmosis and ehrlichiosis are similar, if not identical. Further, the signs and symptoms seen here are quite close to those observed with other TBIs such as Lyme and RMSF.

Common symptoms associated with Ehrlichia/Anaplasma include: headaches (sharp, stabbing, shooting, or knife-like), significant muscle pain but *not* joint pain, prostration, fatigue, fever, nausea, confusion, flu-like symptoms, GI complaints, anorexia, chills, shaking, and vomiting. Fevers can be high. The headache associated with Ehrlichia/Anaplasma can be especially severe and is often localized behind the eyes. Fatigue may persist.

The onset of symptoms can occur rapidly about 2 weeks after the causal tick bite. Initial symptoms usually include fever, chills, headache, myalgias, and malaise. Of course, this pattern is common to just about every known TBI and most other infectious diseases.

HGA may have less CNS involvement than HME. Peripheral nerve problems can last months. Patients have experienced facial palsy, neuropathy, and brachial plexus problems. Respiratory distress and septic shock have been noted. Death rates may be less with HGA than with HME. Most deaths occur in immunocompromised patients with opportunistic infections such as herpes or fungus.

PEARL: Untreated ehrlichiosis has been associated with a rare but dangerous condition called hemophagocytic lymphohistiocytosis. In a case study presented at the 2011 Lyme Disease Association/Columbia University conference, Andrew Walter from A.I. Dupont Children's Hospital in Wilmington, Delaware, discussed the pathogen's invasion of the WBCs that subsequently required bone marrow transplantation and doxycycline therapy.

Rarely is there a rash seen with these pathogens. That is why the facetious moniker Rocky Mountain *Spotless* Fever has been used to refer to these syndromes. If a rash does occur, it can be diffuse, vasculitic, and involve the palms and soles. Rash is thought to occur in less than 10% of patients. This rare rash has also been described as maculopapular or petechial, involving the trunk and extremities.

As the patients get sicker without treatment, they can experience lung infections, confusion, ataxia, cranial nerve palsy, respiratory distress, on-going fever, shock, coma, kidney failure, abnormal coagulation, DIC, and hemorrhages. Central nervous system problems including meningitis, encephalitis, coma, and seizures have been recorded. Peripheral neuropathies and cranial neuritis have also been described. However in many of these cases, it was not known if the patient had a pure infection from Ehrlichia, or if other agents contributed as well. Be very careful in TBIs. Do not think that making one diagnosis ensures that there are not additional diagnoses.

Results from routine lab tests may have more significance with Ehrlichia/Anaplasma than with most of the other TBIs. These pathogens are said to have a TRIAD of lab findings that suggest their presence: low WBC, elevated LFTs, and low platelets. However, the presence of this triad is far from diagnostic and can be quite variable depending on where the patient is in the clinical course.

Probably more useful is the observation of the *morulae* as inclusion bodies in the vacuoles of WBCs. When ordering a WBC, request a peripheral blood smear. Presence of morulae should be pathognomonic. Instructions for collection and interpretation of results are provided in Chapter 19.

Recall that any TBI co-infection may cause symptoms to be worse, complicate the clinical course, make diagnosis more difficult, and postpone recovery. Whenever things aren't going like you expect, regroup.

Diagnosis: As with all TBIs, diagnosis of ehrlichiosis/anaplasmosis is based on clinical judgment. You may need to act quickly if the patient is deteriorating. Even the best supportive diagnostic tests are usually negative early in the course of the diseases since IgM and IgG are not yet at discernible levels. So while diagnostic testing for ehrlichiosis is possible, it is usually not practical in real clinical medicine.

Diagnosis of tick-borne infection by Ehrlichia/Anaplasma can be challenging for a number of reasons:

1. The symptoms are so similar to other TBIs, that these etiologic agents are over-shadowed by more familiar pathogens.

2. While under certain circumstances these diseases can be fatal, they are rarely the meanest dog in the fight. HCPs are usually busy trying to uncover other agents that they believe might be causing more harm.

3. Because Ehrlichia/Anaplasma respond so well to some of the antimicrobials used for Lyme and the more common co-infections, it can be gone before anyone knew it was there.

4. The presence of the distinguishing morulae inside certain leukocytes will not be found unless the HCP thinks to order a peripheral blood smear and then that smear is examined by an experienced technician. While this study is quick, it is also only about 25% sensitive under the best of conditions, meaning that only 25% of the time does the test capture a positive when indeed the patient is positive for the disease. Antibiotic treatment prior to testing could alter the results. Morulae may be seen slightly more often with Anaplasma smears than with Ehrlichia, but smears are still largely insensitive to the true positives.

So, should we just allow Ehrlichia/Anaplasma to plunder and pillage without any repercussions? Well, we often do just that because we don't know any better. Nonetheless, the presence

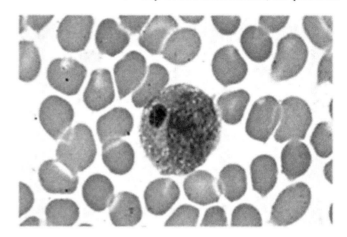

Morulae in white cells
Source: CDC. Accessed March 2013

of a surreptitious infection can complicate both the diagnosis and treatment of a TBI patient and significantly delay recovery.

If you recognize the lab triad, if the patient has exceptionally sharp headaches, if significant myalgia occurs with NO joint pain, and certainly if morulae are seen, think about Ehrlichia and Anaplasma. The best outcomes will be achieved only if we try to uncover the full clinical picture.

As previously noted, the triad of laboratory results that manifests in some Ehrlichia/Anaplasma patients is actually quite nonspecific and can occur in other infectious diseases. Nonetheless, we will take all the help we can get. The triad includes *low* white blood cell count, *low* platelets, and *elevated* liver enzymes. Many infectious diseases do present with elevated white counts (bacterial more so than viral). Since the organisms involved with HME and HGA invade the white cells and damage them, fewer white cells would be left circulating during an acute infection. Therefore if white cell counts remain low in a TBI patient, the leukopenia may be a useful clue to the presence of HME or HGA. If WBC levels go too low, the patient may become susceptible to opportunistic infections. The triad is more common in acute disease and becomes less clear if the infection is on-going.

This leukopenia usually has WBCs less than 4,500/mm^3 and thrombocytopenia with platelets less than 150,000/mm^3. The abnormal LFTs include high aminotransferases and perhaps a high bilirubin. The liver enzymes AST and ALT will often be over 100 units/L. However, a similar triad can also be seen in RMSF. Here, if a rash is present, it can help distinguish between the two since the rare maculopapular rash of ehrlichiosis is usually quite different from the common petechial rash of RMSF. Remember, the presence of other infections could easily obliterate any subtle triad.

While diagnostic testing specific for Ehrlichiae is possible, it is of limited value in real clinical medicine. Blood smears can be examined for morulae, the large mulberry-shaped clusters found in infected white cells. Positive Wright-stained smears of monocytes are diagnostic for E. *chaffeensis*. This test is quick but has only limited sensitivity (finding a positive when it is actually positive). A negative result does not rule out disease. Under the best circumstances morulae can be hard to see with standard stains. Even enhanced smears using buffy coats only raise positive yield slightly. Any antibiotic treatment prior to testing will decrease the sensitivity further. An experienced technician should be reading these smears.

Detection of antibody titers for HME and HGA are possible and Specialty Labs can turn around the results in about 48 hours. Specialty Labs will test for both IgM and IgG. Other labs may also do this testing, which can be expensive. In general, the labs can only test two species even though many more might be involved. Remember, these pathogens just got new names recently, so we might not have a good handle on what we are dealing with here.

Ehrlichia titers over 1:80 on IgG and 1:40 on IgM are considered positive. Interpretation becomes more of a problem when the titers are borderline. If only IgG is positive, this could mean past infection and not active disease. Continue to treat these cases as clinically appropriate. There may not be detectable IgG or IgM early in the clinical course. In these cases, IgM turns out to be not particularly specific and may persist long after active disease is gone and so is not useful in making the diagnosis. That is why the state of Missouri recommends making a clinical diagnosis. IgG antibodies to Ehrlichia can be high for years after acute infection.

When the patient is recovering, changes in antibody titers can be assessed using indirect immunofluorescent assays (IFA), but this is not helpful in acute illness where decisions need to be made before waiting for results. Some sources recommend taking a sample for IFA testing in the first week of the illness and then 2 to 4 weeks later. IFA of both IgM and IgG anti-Anaplasma *phagocytophilum* antibodies can be done, but turn-around may be too slow to help with any clinical decisions. Check with the lab regarding turn-around times.

Polymerase chain reactions (PCRs) can help establish the diagnosis early. The PCR is thought to have a sensitivity of 60% to 80% in E. *chaffeensis*. The sensitivity for E. *ewingii* is unknown. Again, previous antibiotic therapy will decrease sensitivity. In general, there is a poor recovery using fluids for PCR testing. Better to submit a tissue sample from biopsy or surgical procedure, if possible. If such samples are not likely to become available, try blood or other fluids and you may get lucky and get a supportive result. Again, DNA is thought to persist for a time after the causative organism is gone.

Some literature reports discuss immunohistochemical staining using samples from skin punch biopsies taken at the site of the rash. These biopsies have occasionally been shown to contain organisms because of their location within the endothelial cells of the blood vessels near the rash. Unfortunately, the rash is rare and so this method cannot be relied upon for diagnostic support. But if there is a rash you might want to take advantage of the opportunity.

E. *ewingii* has not been reliably cultured. Culture of E. *chaffeensis* has been done from blood and spinal fluid but results may take several weeks. These cultures could only be used to support a tentative diagnosis. In general, there is not much culturing in human clinical practice. In contrast, veterinary medicine makes more use of cultures to detect ehrlichiosis and anaplasmosis.

PEARL: Comparisons between human and veterinary disease maps are interesting. A few isolated disease blips will appear on human maps in areas thought to be endemic and where HCPs know enough to report incidence. Maps illustrating animal disease resulting from the same pathogens show much more widespread disease prevalence. Maps used by entomologists showing the detection of the actual pathogen-vectors are covered with ink. This discrepancy illustrates likely underreporting that may be occurring in the human population for many of the TBIs. Maybe vets do not need to practice in such a political environment and entomologists seem to be free to report whatever they find.

As always, a high index of suspicion must be maintained. Diagnosis will need to be based largely on clinical judgment. Use history, symptoms, physical examination, clinical course, laboratory clues, and the elimination of other reasonable causality. Consider ehrlichiosis/anaplasmosis in TBI patients who are not doing well. Remember that RMSF and Ehrlichiae-diseases have often been confused in the past, especially early in their clinical course.

Consider empiric therapy for patients from endemic areas who are symptomatic, especially if they remember a tick bite or had any other potential exposure. Empiric medical decisions are based on experience and observation rather than theory. Do not abandon a sick patient because you do not have 100% evidence that the diagnosis can only be ehrlichiosis. If co-infections are possible, make sure ehrlichiosis and anaplasmosis are considered.

Treatment: Anaplasma present and respond much like Ehrlichia. Here we presume that treatment is the same for both etiologies. Despite all my research, I have not been entirely convinced that these pathogens need to be considered separately in the clinic. Both respond rapidly to appropriate antibiotics. J. Stephen Dumler from Johns Hopkins wrote the ehrlichiosis section for the IDSA Guidelines in 2006. His recommendation is to treat on the basis of clinical suspicion without waiting for supportive test results.

1st choice: Doxycycline is the drug of choice for ehrlichiosis/anaplasmosis. In adults, consider 100 mg bid. For children, 4 mg/kg/day in two divided doses has been successful. Doxycycline can be given IV or po. Treatment should continue for 2 to 4 weeks or for at least 7 days after fever is gone. If doxycycline cannot be used, then other tetracyclines have been substituted. Recommendations include TCN 500 mg qid in adults or Minocin 100 bid. Doses and regimens should be adjusted for age and weight and the duration of therapy modified on a case-by-case basis. Higher doses, IV administration, and longer treatment runs have been needed for some patients. See Chapter 24: *Antimicrobials* for guidance on pediatric use of doxy.

2nd choice: Rifampin 600 mg daily. Consider adding rifamycin 1) if doxycycline cannot be used, 2) if IV or higher dose doxycycline does not work, 3) if doxycycline or other TCNs are contraindicated or not tolerated. Rifamycin is a poor solo agent. If it is used alone, resistance can mount within hours or days. Always use rifamycin as part of a combination regimen with other antimicrobials.

Azithromycin has been used in combination with the TCNs or rifamycin in these patients.

If you suspect ehrlichiosis or anaplasmosis start treatment BEFORE you get laboratory confirmation, because you might never have that. The earlier treatment begins, the better the response. Duration of therapy should continue for at least a week beyond the fever. Because of the mechanism by which these pathogens cause disease, the patient could be susceptible to permanent sequelae if therapy is delayed.

Treatment should be extended if co-infections are likely and the duration should go beyond the time of the patient's fever. Anaplasma usually respond quickly to treatment. If fever does not resolve soon after the antibiotic is started, regroup. Your diagnosis could be wrong or incomplete.

PEARL: Minocycline can be the first choice for ehrlichiosis. Doxycycline can be hard on the stomach. When doxy is the choice, often the Doryx formulation is preferred since more of the drug is absorbed in the SI. Usually the doxycyclines are not recommended for kids under 8-years-old. Yet in cases with no other reasonable options, sometimes these drugs are used in younger children. Most practitioners have not observed significant untoward effects because in these younger kids the doxy is used only short-term (one or two weeks) until an alternative regimen can be substituted. Doxycycline does have a liquid formulation. Doxy is CI in pregnancy and in those who are allergic, so rifamycin then becomes the DOC.

Prognosis: In 1999, a 22-year-old soldier in Kentucky died of HME. Since recognition of human disease is fairly recent, we do not know enough about these pathogens to make predictions about their behavior. Many of these organisms can be hidden from the body's defenses inside blood cells. For this reason, the infection may not completely clear. Symptoms can wax and wane. As the immune response recedes, the infectious organism can regroup and the host can relapse. No one knows what kind of immunity an individual has after initial infection with Ehrlichia/Anaplasma. There may be some immunity against reinfection but some patients seemingly have been acutely reinfected. Of course, they may not have had Ehrlichia/Anaplasma in the first place. We just don't understand these organisms well enough to make definitive statements about how they will act. Keep vigilant for the unexpected and remember that these conditions can be fatal.

References

I am deeply grateful to Ohio State University for their clarity on the murky topic of taxonomy around Ehrlichia/Anaplasma. I wish I had found their website sooner. Nonetheless, I feel I must mention that Purdue beat Ohio State in football in both 2009 and 2011. OSU's consolation is that they certainly have everybody beat when it comes to the taxonomy of Anaplasma.

Chapter 8

BARTONELLOSIS

The wallpaper or me, one of us has to go.
Last words of Oscar Wilde

Background: Napoleon's Grand Army had to make a hasty retreat from Russia in 1812. While the combat was savage, more soldiers died from Bartonella in this campaign than from war wounds. The men were infested with lice in the trenches. By excavating mass graves in modern-day Lithuania, researchers discovered that one third of the Grande Armee was infected with Bartonella. They suffered a form of trench fever that changed the course of history and inspired Tolstoy's *War and Peace* and Tchaikovsky's *1812 Overture*.

In 1999, Bartonella pathogens were identified in ticks, and by 2001, Lyme doctors were finding that their patients could be co-infected with Bartonella. To me, that seems shockingly recent. As with most of the organisms under discussion in this book, Bartonella was previously known by several other names. The nomenclature changes are so confusing that I decided I would continue to refer to these pathogens as Bartonella even though this might not be entirely accurate today. While both cat scratch fever and tick-borne bartonellosis are considered to be caused by Bartonella *henselea*, we know that the organisms that cause these diseases are not identified by reaction against the same antibodies and do not respond to the same antibiotics.

Joe Burrascano calls the organisms that cause the TBI Bartonella-like organisms or BLOs. Unfortunately, his recognition of the distinction between the two obviously different strains has not yet had time to be adopted into the medical literature. We are therefore stuck in nomenclature limbo. This confusion is painful and will leave your head spinning and you crying for an exorcist. But as Shakespeare would have wisely mused, "Bartonella by any other name would make you just as sick." I will attempt to rectify any confusion to the best of my ability in the remainder of this chapter.

Bartonella is a common tick-borne co-infection in TBD practices in endemic areas. In fact, Bartonella may be more common than Borrelia in some places. Since we have known Lyme longer, we usually consider it to be tick-borne royalty, with everything else just along for the ride. In reality, both babesiosis and bartonellosis may be more common, and Borrelia may be the interloper. We just don't know the incidence and prevalence numbers well enough to draw any conclusions

as yet. Nonetheless, Bartonella *henselea* is now recognized as an important human tick-borne infection. First reported in the 1990s as a pathogen, and soon after recognized as a new species, the microbe is mainly carried by cats and ticks and causes cat scratch fever, endocarditis, and a TBI.

Aliases: Many species of Bartonella cause a variety of diseases:

Cat scratch disease (CSD) or cat scratch fever (CSF): Here Bartonella *henselea* is transmitted by cat bites or scratches. Interestingly, a number of patients diagnosed with cat scratch fever have not had any contact with felines. (What else is going on?) Overall, these kinds of Bartonella infections are rather common with estimates of more than 40,000 cases of cat scratch disease each year.

Tick-borne bartonellosis: While this illness is also said to be caused by Bartonella *henselea,* clearly the pathogen is different from that which causes cat scratch fever. The two microbes do NOT react to the same antibodies or respond to the same antibiotics. Paul Ehrlich said that if different antibodies result, then different antigens inspired them. The vector for this pathogen is the tick, probably most commonly the Ixodes genus, but Bartonella is likely transmitted by any of the ticks that transmit other common TBIs. This is the microbe Burrascano calls the Bartonella-like organism or the BLO and is the pathogen that is a potential co-infection with Lyme and the other recognized TBIs.

Trench fever or louse fever: B. *quintana* is transmitted by lice and was likely responsible for Napoleon's retreat from Moscow.

Carrion disease: B. *baccilliformis* is transmitted by sand flies.

Pathogen: The genus Bartonella is a weakly staining Gram negative bacteria with more than 32 species identified. At least 8 species of Bartonella are known to cause human disease including B. *henselea*, B. *quintana*, and B. *baccilliformis*. An intracellular parasite, Bartonella can infect humans and other mammals. Yet, most species do not cause human disease. As pathogens, they are mostly opportunistic.

Vector: Bartonella is transmitted by ticks, fleas, lice, mites, and sand flies. Both Ixodes (deer and Western black-legged) and Dermacentor (dog and wood) ticks have been associated with Bartonella. In California more than 20% of Ixodes *pacificus* ticks are positive for Bartonella, which may be a higher prevalence than those that carry Lyme. The vectors are blood-feeding arthropods and the hosts are mammals such as cats (wild or domestic), rats, squirrels, mice, dogs, and humans. What's the reservoir species? Not sure. The reservoir may be the white-footed mouse. Coyotes may also be a reservoir for a human Bartonella species (even though 22% of bacteremic coyotes are seronegative). To complicate matters, infections by Bartonella have now also been associated with dog bites, crab claws, cactus spines, porcupine quills, goats, and barbed wire.

Bartonella prefers to settle in endothelial cells in the blood vessels, where they periodically are released into the blood stream. When a blood-sucking arthropod comes along, they are drawn out and carried away. When the arthropod bites another host, the bacteria can be transferred. Bartonella can move across the placenta and the disease transmitted gestationally.

Distribution: Diseases due to Bartonella species are found worldwide. Sand flies transmit the pathogens in the Andes Mountains of Peru, Columbia, and Ecuador. BLOs are found worldwide in body lice. The European sheep tick has been shown to harbor at least five pathogenic Bartonella species. More Ixodes *pacificus* ticks in California harbor pathogenic Bartonella species than Borrelia.

Bartonellosis may be a more common TBI than Borrelia infection, especially in the northeastern US. In this *Compendium*, we are trying to focus on the TBDs, but statistics on the incidence and prevalence of this pathogen in terms of co-infections in the US are either non-existent or so far-fetched as to be meaningless. As always, when considering co-infections, recognize that a certain pathogen exists in relation to other TBIs. Put Bartonella in the differential diagnosis when a patient is not doing well. While Bartonella may be a lone agent in certain conditions such as trench fever and cat scratch disease, when the vector is a tick, at least consider that more than one etiologic agent is at work.

PEARL: Work by Mordecai, Adelson, et al suggests that ticks in some parts of New Jersey may have as many Bartonella as Borrelia on board. In some cases, Bartonella may be more prevalent.

History: Napoleon's encounter with Bartonella notwithstanding, this pathogen has been plaguing humans a lot longer than

that. The organism was found in a 4,000-year-old infected tooth. While humans, both in 2000 BCE and 1812 CE, understood that they were sick for some reason, it has only been 20 years since we first isolated Bartonella in humans and began to sort through its taxonomy and pathology. Obviously, since we still have only one name for B. *henselea,* when we are likely dealing with two (or more) distinct pathogens, we have a long way to go in defining the impact of these infectious agents on human health.

PEARL: The work of Edward Breitschwerdt, an infectious disease veterinarian from North Carolina State University, has advanced the understanding of this disease in both animals and humans.

Pathophysiology: Whatever you call it, how does Bartonella do its damage? These pathogens can cause a wide array of problems of varying severities. Just as with Bb, Bartonella appear highly adapted for intracellular persistence which complicates their clinical presentation.

Whether introduced into the host by a cranky cat or by an oblivious tick, once it is inside the host, the resulting symptoms seem to depend on pathogen load and the entry site. Presumably a bite in a place where bacteria could easily enter the blood stream might be more significant that a scratch over thickened skin on the palm. The resulting disease can subsequently range from mild to serious depending on these and other factors. Immunocompromised patients appear to be at significantly more risk from a Bartonella infection than those with a fully-functional immune response.

PEARL: Bartonella has been identified in some AIDS patients for a number of years. How did it get there?

Once inside the host, the Bartonella prefer endothelial cells, which are the flat cells that line blood and lymph vessels. The theory is that cyclically, every few days, some of the Bartonella and some of the endothelial cells are released into the blood stream. They then invade red blood cells (erythrocytes or RBCs). Here the Bartonella replicate while separated by a membrane from the rest of the RBC. The bacteria replicate until they reach a critical mass. Then they wait. When a blood-sucking arthropod comes along they are drawn out and carried away. When the arthropod bites another host, the bacteria can be transferred.

In the host, the Bartonella lives mostly inside the host's cells, but also floats in the blood. The signs and symptoms eventually displayed by this pathogen are directly related to its pathophysiology. Since Bartonella reproduce intracellularly, they are largely protected from antibiotics. The following systems appear to be prime targets of Bartonella.

- **Immune System** - Bartonella seems to be able to mute the host's immune response by decreasing antibody production and by somehow diminishing the efficiency of the antibodies that do form against its antigens. Practically, this means that Bartonella should be considered as early as possible in the differential diagnosis so that antibiotics can help the immune system fight the infection before the immune response is further compromised. Several sources used the word *stealth* to refer to Bartonella's impact on the immune system. While this is a bit more anthropomorphic than I'd like, it certainly seems that Bartonella has a significant amount of control over the host's immune function, once it takes hold.[1] Note that most of the inflammatory responses to Bartonella are muted compared to those of other TBIs. There is no raging fever or wracking chills. Fevers are often low grade around 99° in the mornings with light sweats. While there may be lymphadenopathy, the enlargement is mild or moderate instead of huge and painful. One hypothesis suggests that Bartonella mutes the fevers that accompany other TBIs, making diagnosis and management of co-infections more difficult. By taking charge of much of the host's immune response, Bartonella can float freely in the blood or settle into the cells of many organ systems, contributing to the various other signs and symptoms that may accompany its presence.

- **Gastrointestinal Tract** - Bartonella can present with more GI symptomatology than any of the other TBIs. This is probably due to the highly vascular nature of the gut and the subsequent penetration of the pathogen into the cells of the digestive tract. In addition, some of the GI symptoms may be due to pathogen effect on the nerves that control the GI tract. For example, vagal nerve impairment by Bartonella has been hypothesized to cause a partial paralysis of the gut. Vascular changes will result in the observation on endoscopy of the purple-red striae similar to those seen on the skin or angiomas. Other GI manifestations associated with Bartonella include: gastritis, abdominal discomfort, mesenteric adenitis, GERD, IBD-like symptoms, cholecystitis, diarrhea, and weight loss. GI problems are common to all TBIs, so unless you observe the striae in the GI tract, you could be dealing with any of these various pathogens.

PEARL: Sometimes the only positive test for a TBI will come from a biopsy of the gut. So, if your TBI patient is having an endoscopy, make sure a sample is taken for diagnostic evaluation. So as not to waste this golden oppor-

tunity, make sure you call your trusted lab so that you can ensure that the sample is gathered and preserved properly and that you order the tests that you actually need to have run. Patients do not have endoscopies every day, especially kids, so you want to make the most of this rare opportunity.

PEARL: Virginia Sherr's article "Bell's Palsy of the Gut" discusses the possibility of Bartonella, Bb, and M. fermentans, alone or in combination, being responsible for many of the GI manifestations seen with TBIs. Martin Fried and others talk about how the presence of multiple infections in the GI tract can confound the clinical presentation. He looked at kids with abdominal pain, reflux with heartburn, and blood in the stool to uncover which microbes might be contributing to the clinical picture. Bartonella was the most common pathogen found in kids reporting abdominal sxs. Biopsy of the GI tract showed chronic inflammation and the presence of ILs 2, 6, and 10. IL-6 may be associated with the neovascularization often seen in bartonellosis. GI sxs are often found in association with Bb, M. fermentans, and H. pylori. With co-infections, sxs can overlap making it hard to tell who caused what and complicating treatment decisions. I worked in the GI therapeutic area for years and wrote a primer on pediatric GERD. I had no idea there could be an underlying infectious contribution. Looking back, this idea explains a lot.

- **Skin and Subcutaneous Tissue** - Bartonella *henselea* creates new vasculature where new blood vessels form in tissue where the pathogen is lurking. These purple streaks are referred to as violaceous striae. Once you see them, you will not soon forget. While they resemble the white stretch marks that appear during pregnancy and after significant weight loss, these are definitely violet in appearance and may not follow the skin planes like mechanical stretch marks tend to do. Usually the striae appear as violet snakes on the flanks, thighs, and sometimes under and over the breasts. Some may look more like a bruise or purple patch. Interestingly, what happens on the surface happens behind the scenes as well. On endoscopy, patients with visible striae on the skin will often manifest purple-red steaks in the gut. I know of no other condition that presents with violaceous striae, so in assessing TBI patients, these striae should be considered pathognomonic for Bartonella. Angiomas or microangiomas might be seen on the skin or on endoscopy. Spider veins or red papules are sometimes seen.

- **Coagulation and Circulation** - Bartonella floats in blood intermittently and also enters blood vessel walls. Through the circulation, Bartonella makes its way to the various organ systems. Of all known TBIs, Bartonella causes the most increase in coagulation. While a number of TBIs cause abnormal coagulation, Bartonella causes hypercoagulation. Since Bartonella has an affinity for

---

1 While I rail against anthropomorphizing, swearing that all these microbial behaviors are triggered biochemically, I can't shake the image of Snidely Whiplash from the Dudley Do-Right cartoons, tying poor Nell to the railroad tracks as his mustache blows in the wind. I see the pathogen lurking on the sidelines waiting to pounce. Only in these cases, Dudley doesn't always show up in time to make the rescue.

vascular tissue, its presence in addition to sluggish blood flow may impede circulation especially to the extremities. Patients will complain of cold hands and feet and the exam might reveal poor peripheral circulation. When tissues are oxygen-deprived, organisms like Bartonella can congregate, making the situation worse. Poor circulation can also keep antibiotics from penetrating deep into infected tissue.

Because of the enhanced vascularization promoted by Bartonella, vascular endothelial growth factor (VEGF) levels might be elevated in some patients. Additional vasculature may be the mechanism by which Bartonella gains entry into many tissues and organs. While this is a nonspecific finding, the degree of elevation could correlate with the activity of the infection and may have the potential to be used to monitor the effect of treatment and clinical course. Potentially, when VEGF returns to normal that might mean treatment has been effective. But be careful not to rely too heavily on equivocal findings that may have other underlying causes.

- **Central Nervous System** – Of all the TBIs, Bartonella and Mycoplasma *fermentans* are the most damaging to the nervous system and thereby cause the most intense neuropsychiatric manifestations. If CNS signs and symptoms are out of proportion to any other problems, think Bartonella. Presumably the pathogen uses its frequent floater miles to travel to the brain and various nerves within the body and infiltrate in a way that causes impairment. The signs and symptoms that result may be due to irritation and induced excitability of the CNS. The patient may present with signs of encephalopathy. Encephalopathy is a deterioration of brain function through some acquired mechanism such as organ failure, metabolic disease, inflammation, or infection. Characterized by a change in mental status, encephalopathy can include loss of cognitive abilities, personality changes, inability to concentrate, lethargy, irritability, combative behavior, oppositional defiant disorder (ODD), agitation, decreased consciousness, sleep problems, depression, restlessness, twitching, tremors, changes in muscle tone, nystagmus, neuropathy, and seizures.

New onset of seizures is especially suggestive of Bartonella. Other neurologic manifestations include headaches described as having an ice pick to the brain, bad photophobia, loss of vision, retinitis, decreased visual acuity, hemorrhages, exudates, papilledema, and burning pain. While most, if not all, of the TBIs might predispose a patient to many of these neuropsychiatric manifestations, Bartonella can really make the person miserable with its effects on the nervous system. NP sxs may be associated with species type.

In children, most of the presentation of Bartonella is psychiatric. Take the above list and magnify the intensity and add extreme agitation, severe anxiety, broad-range mood swings, atypical presentations of autism, outbursts, aggression, and antisocial behavior that may become violent. The child may not be able to function in age-appropriate circumstances. Clearly, Bartonella causes behavior problems in kids. Thinking can be foggy and the child may have poor insight and bad judgment. Sometimes the child will become more isolated and combative. If you see rage, think Bartonella.

Significant neuropsychiatric signs are probably the most important indication that Bartonella may be involved. Caretakers will report tantrums. "He's not the same kid." Beware of a sudden onset of new anxiety, panic attacks, new psychiatric issues, (some even become psychotic), and significant behavior problems. The school will say the child is "suddenly acting out." A number of children with Bartonella-induced ODD have been identified. Here the children have frequent tantrums and argue and oppose all direction. They are angry and disruptive. They resent any authority figure. Often there will be calls from the school. There may be new onset OCD (obsessive-compulsive disorder) and significant mood swings. Occasionally parents are confused when some of these behavioral changes coincide with puberty. Is this how teens behave? If they are sick, yes.

PEARL: If you observe neuropsychiatric symptoms way out of proportion to what you might usually expect with a TBI, think Bartonella. Especially if a patient is thought to have neuroborreliosis that is not resolving despite the best treatment efforts, consider Bartonella.

PEARL: There is strong suspicion that Bartonella may also induce antineuronal antibody activity similar to that observed with PANDAS.

- **Musculoskeletal** - Bartonella can cause plantar fasciitis (also found in babesiosis and with Bb), foot pain, and joint discomfort. Individual joints can be swollen. The sole pain can be remarkable, especially in the morning, like walking on glass. Another distinguishing finding in Bartonella, although it may not be pathognomonic, is tender subcutaneous nodules along the extremities, especially the outer thighs, shins, and occasionally along the triceps. These may be another manifestation of neovascularization or the mechanism could be entirely separate. One more distinctive feature of Bartonella may be severe pain in the tibia. Bones have become inflamed and softened, and arthritis is not uncommon. Myelitis (here referring to inflammation of bone marrow), myositis (inflammation of muscle tissue), and polyneuropathy have all been mentioned in the literature as associated with Bartonella.

PEARL: A mid-chapter review: Various manifestations, while not necessarily pathognomonic, do strongly suggest bartonellosis including plantar fasciitis, sole or shin pain, subcutaneous nodules, violaceous striae, cold extremities, and excessive neuropsychiatric symptoms, especially rage.

- **Biofilm Formation** - The science of biofilm formation is fairly new in clinical medicine. Bartonella may be the best biofilm maker of the common TBIs. This is a frightening prospect once you understand more about biofilms. A biofilm is an aggregate of microorganisms in which cells adhere to one another and sometimes to a host surface. The underlying foundation is made of mucopolysaccharides. Organisms attach forming a bladder-like structure that may be protective of pathogens and allow nutrients and communication signals to pass. This shields the organisms from antibiotics and host immune response. Environmental triggers such as microbial crowding, nutrient depletion, and the introduction of antibiotics might promote biofilm formation.

Like a small pathogen community, the biofilm separates the organism from the environment of the host. The pathogen uses the host's resources to build a structure or enclosure around its group. The biofilm provides protection and may even allow for communication between individuals. The organization is complex and the pathogen takes full advantage of the resources available inside the host. We are just beginning to recognize the role of biofilms in pathology. With Bartonella, the formation of biofilms could potentially impact the clinical course of the disease and the ability to provide adequate samples for diagnostic testing. Antibiotic regimens may need to be adjusted with higher spikes to be able to penetrate through the protective film. We simply don't understand enough about Bartonella's ability to form biofilms to know just how scared we should be.

PEARL: The concept of quorum sensing is associated with the formation of biofilms. Even the term is anthropomorphic with a human quorum referring to cases where there are enough individuals present to take a vote. Quorum sensing refers to a system of stimuli and responses that is correlated to local population density. Depending on the numbers present, some bacterial species can use peptide signals (pheromones) to coordinate behavior through gene expression. The idea is somewhat unnerving in that quorum sensing is analogous to our communication networks and seems to be almost a conscious, decision-making process. These networks involve feedback loops where more signal causes more effect on behavior.

PEARL: NIH speculates that 80% of chronic infections could be due to biofilm formation. Currently modern medicine does not have a good grasp of how to manage biofilms.

Dentists scrape them away and naturopaths propose natural products to breakdown the fibrin that may be involved. Lumbrokinase is postulated to dissolve the biofilms so that the antibiotics might then have a better chance to work.

PEARL: Work by Eva Sapi suggests that the herbal banderol might impede biofilm formation.

Clinical course: Bartonella species can cause a diverse array of symptoms of varying severities. Most infections resolve spontaneously but some cases evoke serious consequences and substantial morbidity. Bartonella can produce chronic infections in humans.

Most patients have a gradual onset of symptoms with the initial illness. CNS symptoms tend to be disproportionate to all other manifestations. As with other co-infections, the HCP may have considerable difficulty teasing out which manifestations are coming from which co-infection. Bartonella does have a few characteristics that can distinguish it from the other TBIs. For example, the violaceous striae on both the skin and the gut, the subcutaneous nodules along tendon lines, plantar fasciitis, shin pain, cold extremities, and the extreme intensity of the psychiatric symptoms, especially in children.

If untreated, symptoms can become chronic. Presence of co-infections may alter the way each of the TBI pathogens present. When part of a group of TBI co-infections, Bartonella can change the course of both its own clinical presentation as well as that of its co-pathogens by manipulation of the host's immune system. If the sole pathogen, Bartonella can be a mild condition, but serious cases can affect the entire body with a syndrome that is both difficult to diagnose and treat. As always, if you have a TBI patient who is not getting well, pull out the list of co-infections and see what might be complicating the situation.

If the Bartonella infection persists, complications might arise including berry-like lesions called bacillary angiomatosis, various other rashes, extended fevers, and bacteremia. End-stage disease can include osteomyelitis, hepatitis, brain abscesses, cardiomegaly, and endocarditis.

Signs & symptoms: Over half the patients experience fever or malaise. Also common are poor appetite, nausea, vomiting, sore throat, enlarged spleen, lymphadenopathy, fatigue, cold extremities, and headache. Immunocompromised hosts may present with more severe illness. Since the endothelial cells are part of blood and lymph vessels and therefore are found in all tissues, Bartonella can affect any organ system. There have been reports of a skin lesion at the site where the tick bite occurred. This can mimic a Lyme lesion (or can be the Lyme rash if Borrelia is a co-infection). Other skin manifestations may include papules or splotches, especially on the upper limbs, head, and neck. Lesions may appear on mucous membranes. Subcutaneous nodules have been described as hyperpigmentation. Gastritis may be marked in these patients.

There are several signs that are fairly unique to Bartonella. Be vigilant for cold extremities. If you see violaceous striae, subcutaneous nodules, or pain in the tibia, shins, or plantar fascia, think Bartonella. Rage and neuropsychiatric manifestations point to Bartonella. Symptoms that may persist despite the best-intended treatment include: fatigue, headache, resistant arthritis, intractable encephalopathy, cognitive difficulties, new onset of a seizure disorder, persistent lymphadenopathy, GI complaints, and eye problems such as visual loss and retinitis. A number of these signs and symptoms are similar to those found in other infections and deciding what might be Bartonella versus another infectious agent can be difficult. Further, deciding if the persistent complaints are due to co-infections or inadequately treated Bartonella is also difficult.

PEARL: B. henselea *appears to cause new vasculation. Blood vessels form in areas of injury causing violaceous striae to manifest in some patients. On endoscopy, these violet streaks can also be observed in the gut.*

PEARL: Babies born with gestational bartonellosis can present similarly to those with congenital Lyme with irritability and hypersensitivity and multiple other problems. Later they may be found to have sensory integration disorder and various cognitive and NP issues. These neonates may also present with multiple microangiomas.

For a detailed listing of the signs and symptoms associated with Bartonella, see the *Pathophysiology* section above, where I got carried away making the connection between the pathology and the clinical presentation.

Diagnosis: As with all co-infections, it is important to have a high index of suspicion. With violaceous striae, tibia pain, subcutaneous nodules, and disproportionate cognitive and behavior changes, consider that Bartonella might be complicating the clinical course. If any of these manifestations are present, you are on your way to making a diagnosis. Note, however, that the absence of any or all these signs does not rule out Bartonella. Unfortunately, when part of a broader co-infection, Bartonella might mute the signs and symptoms of other TBIs, confounding the diagnostic picture further.

Again, there is no diagnostic lab test that says, "This is Bartonella." In fact, testing for the Bartonella *henselea* that causes cat scratch fever is one way to get a negative result. The pathogen that causes the tick-borne bartonellosis, although referred to in the literature as Bartonella *henselea*, does not usually react to the same antibodies or respond to the same antibiotics as the pathogen that causes cat scratch disease.

In fact, some labs test for only one or two strains of Bartonella and often set the cut-off titers prohibitively high. Even if the history and physical are screaming Bartonella, the chances are quite small that you will get a positive result on a diagnostic lab test looking for the tick-borne pathogen. If you are looking for the etiology of cat scratch fever, you have a chance. Remember, we are concerned with the tick-borne pathogen here. You cannot find what you are not looking for.

So we return to one of the fundamental principles: Diagnosis of TBD is based on clinical judgment. While diagnostic testing can be supportive of a clinical decision, negative test results do not rule out a certain pathogen.

Bartonella has been grown in blood cultures. Since this organism only circulates in the blood intermittently, a number of consecutive specimens might need to be collected. A positive culture can be considered positive for infection, since there are not many ways for the specimen to get contaminated by Bartonella unless it came from the patient. However, a negative culture could mean that the specimen was collected at a time when insufficient organisms were circulating to be captured.

As with many infectious agents, we can look for evidence of Ag/Ab complexes. Unfortunately, we have the issue of B. *henselea* versus BLOs. Here we might not be testing for the same thing we are looking for in the TBD. Again, a positive result would be suggestive of some past exposure to a kind of Bartonella, while a negative result could be negative for many reasons that have nothing to do with the patient. For most diseases where antibody levels are used to help make the diagnosis, a minimum "titer" or amount of antibody is needed to say that the antigen from the pathogen was present at some point. Up to 11% of cats with Bartonella in their blood do not make antibodies against the pathogen, and so will test negative on antibody detection tests. The immunofluorescence assay (IFA) from Specialty Laboratories has been mentioned as more sensitive than some alternatives. Nonetheless, do not let a negative lab result rule out disease.

PCR testing can look for the presence of Bartonella DNA. Again, since the organism only cyclically enters the blood stream, there is not much advantage over blood culture except that the results might be obtained faster. Again, a positive can be considered positive, but a negative result could just be bad timing. If tissue can be obtained, the organism might be more likely to be captured. Except in extreme cases, resist invasive biopsies of tissue solely for the purpose of a culture or PCR test. However, if tissue is being excised for any other reason, take the opportunity to order appropriate testing. This tissue can be from surgery, biopsy, circumcision, placenta, endoscopy, aspiration, etc. Call the lab first before sending tissue to ensure that all specimens are prepared and maintained properly. Because of the intermittent cycling of Bartonella in the blood, techniques like PCR have limited usefulness unless you "catch" the specimen at a "peak." If you miss a high point, there might not be enough DNA for detection.

In an infected mom with a new baby, consider DNA PCR for babesiosis, bartonellosis, and Borrelia *burgdorferi*. At delivery, take samples from the placenta, cord, cord blood, and the foreskin remnant. Send the specimens to a lab that knows what to do with it. Call the lab first to make sure you are sending them exactly what they need to give you the results you are looking for. Do not be responsible for wasting such a precious sample.

With FISH tests looking for Bartonella RNA, positive results might be low. We don't know the sensitivity on the low percentage of positives. Are there many false negatives or was the test finding only those who were actually infected with Bartonella? When the test comes back positive, it provides strong supportive data. If negative, the test does not rule out Bartonella.

Since Bartonella stimulates vascular development, the measurement of vascular endothelial growth factor (VEGF) can suggest the presence of this pathogen. Elevated levels *might* mean that the person has been exposed to Bartonella. Changes in levels of VEGF could allow monitoring of an individual's progress. If VEGF levels decline or return to normal, then the antibiotics may be doing their job. These results could help with decisions regarding length of therapy. VEGF is performed at many commercial laboratories and cancer hospitals. Note that Bartonella is not the only reason VEGF can be elevated.

In all cases of laboratory tests used to support diagnosis, if you or your staff are not *very* familiar with how to order, collect, pack, and ship the sample, call the lab you intend to use and *ask*. These tests can be extremely expensive and insurance doesn't always cover them. Don't you be the reason a specimen is not useable. The cost of the test shouldn't be a surprise to the person responsible for paying for it.

IGeneX performs IFA, FISH, and PCR. Medical Diagnostic Laboratory (MDL) does ELISA and PCR. Specialty Laboratories is now owned by Quest but still remains a separate division for dedicated work. The blood sample can be drawn at any Quest location and shipped properly to Specialty Labs. Specific contact information for these labs is found in Chapter 18: *Ordering Appropriate Tests*.

Differential Diagnosis: When a patient presents with a tick bite and a clinical picture of fatigue, headache, and some degree of cognitive or behavioral problems, Bartonella should be considered. However, not every patient who was bitten by a tick recalls such a bite, so keep an open mind in those patients as well. If there is a fever of unknown origin in an endemic area, keep Bartonella on the list. While the neuropsychiatric symptoms in M. *fermentans* may be the most severe of all the TBIs, who can distinguish the degree of severity when all hell has broken loose in a patient? Consider Bartonella in these cases. If the TBI patient isn't getting better on what you thought was a reasonable treatment plan, your original diagnosis might be wrong, you might be using the wrong treatment approach, or co-infections could be confounding the diagnostic process. Always be willing to rethink.

PEARL: If a patient is not responding to the treatment plan that you think should be hitting the organism responsible, think co-infection. In these cases, symptoms persist despite on-going treatment for other TBIs. When the fatigue or headache is intractable, the arthritis is especially resistant, there is a new onset of seizures, the lymphadenopathy continues, the encephalopathy persists especially with cognitive defects, or visual loss is prominent including neurologic retinitis, make sure you have considered that Bartonella might be confounding the clinical picture.

Treatment: Tick-borne Bartonella can be difficult to treat, but it will respond to an appropriate course of antibiotics given for an adequate length of time. If you treat for cat scratch fever, you may not be treating for the pathogen that causes the tick-borne version of the disease. Treatment of bartonellosis in humans is often refractory to standard antibiotics possibly because of inaccessibility to the intraerythrocytic bacteria. Bartonellosis is difficult to cure with antibiotics and relapses are common when treatment is discontinued. Two months of antibiotic treatment is the minimum for immunocompromised patients, but anyone can relapse when antibiotics are withdrawn.

Consider the following medications IN COMBINATION:

1. The foundation antibiotic is a macrolide, such as azithromycin (Zithromax) or clarithromycin (Biaxin). Kids tend to tolerate Zithromax pretty well.

2. Trimethoprim-sulfamethoxazole (Bactrim, Septra) bid. This agent may be especially helpful if visual problems are part of the clinical presentation.

3. Rifamycin (Rifampin) generally dosed at 300 mg bid. Never use rifamycin as a sole agent since resistance can develop within hours. Always use in combination with other antimicrobials. Rifampin is a good choice if the patient is co-infected with both Bb and Bartonella or needs CNS penetration.

4. The fluoroquinolone ciprofloxacin (Cipro), po, in tablets or suspension, or IV. Cipro is indicated in kids only when there are limited alternatives or when the severity of the disease suggests its use. There is potential for tendon

damage. The dose ranges between 250 and 750 mg q 12 hours. An alternative fluoroquinolone might be Levaquin but this drug is not recommended in children under 18. Generally, consider Rifampin before Levaquin because of potential tendon problems with the fluoroquinolones.

5. Tetracycline such as doxycycline (Doryx) or minocycline (Minocin). With minocycline start with 50 mg bid; if there is no headache, increase to 100 mg bid after one week.

For Bartonella alone, consider a combination made up of drugs from the first 3 options above. If there are co-infections, say with Bb or Ehrlichia, consider adding a TCN. Cipro can also be added to cover additional co-infections as well as to hit the Bartonella. There is no one best drug for Bartonella. As far as I know, no drug company is working on such a magic bullet either. Note that gastritis may occur from both the pathogen and the treatment, which can sometimes be mitigated by adding a PPI to the mix. Hypothetically, PPIs may make Levaquin more effective.

> *PEARL: Anecdotal reports in kids have shown successful combinations of rifamycin and Bactrim for 1 to 12 weeks; rifamycin and azithromycin; and Bactrim and azithromycin. Sometimes you may have to explore several options to get results.*

> *PEARL: Reports of treatment for Bartonella in adults suggest that rifamycin as part of the combination therapy may be the key to therapeutic success.*

> *PEARL: In pregnant women with B. henselea consider azithromycin with Bactrim BUT Bactrim is a category C drug and may not be appropriate for use in these women. Here you would want to do a careful risk/benefit analysis.*

Treatment of tick-borne Bartonella is a balancing act. The better the response to the treatment regimen, the more likely a severe Herxheimer reaction is to occur. More information on the antibiotics listed above is contained in Chapter 24: *Antimicrobials.* Chapter 28 is called *Understanding the Herxheimer Reaction.*

Bartonella responds quickly to appropriate treatment changes. Symptoms can improve within days after antibiotics are started. But these same symptoms can recur just as quickly if medicines are withdrawn too soon. Consider treating for 3 to 6 months. Stopping prematurely may lead to relapse. Antibiotics can be administered po or IV. If the patient does not improve on the initial regimen, adjust until you find a course of therapy that works.

In immunocompromised patients, erythromycin may need to be added to the regimen. Efficacy of antibiotic therapy in immunocompromised patients is variable but these patients should be treated vigorously since they are prone to more severe systemic infections and sepsis.

Treatment for pregnant women with tick-borne BLO is extremely difficult. The first consideration would be a combination regimen that includes azithromycin. Then you need to consider what other antimicrobials might be appropriate on a case-by-case basis. Bactrim is a category C, as are several of the other options. In these cases the risk/benefit will need to be weighed in order to make a decision. In infected newborns, again contemplate azithromycin with Bactrim. Rifampin may also be tried, although it is less recommended in newborns. Taking into account the potential severity of the disease and that choices are quite limited, less attractive options might need to be placed on the table. Rifampin has been used in newborns infected through their mothers with the tick-borne version of Bartonella with considerable success and no known adverse sequelae. Nonetheless, you are between a rock and a hard place (and ticks are hiding nearby).

Since Bartonella has so many ways to defy the host's defenses, some HCPs recommend the herbal remedy cumanda. This adjunct treatment is thought to decrease the pathogen load. Consider cumanda if the original therapeutic regimen seems to be ineffective and reassess both the diagnosis and the treatment plan.

Treatment success: Look for improvement in psychiatric symptoms and focus on the response in this area. If the neuropsychiatric symptoms are caused by TBIs, they are likely to respond better to antibiotics than to psychotropic drugs alone. That being said, behavioral therapy as an ancillary treatment may be beneficial. This type of treatment is best provided by psychiatric professionals who are aware of the TBI etiology and will work with you in helping the patient.

Chapter 9

MYCOPLASMA *FERMENTANS*

Lions don't need to roar.

African saying

Background: Mycoplasma *fermentans* is unique among the TBIs. First of all, it doesn't seem to have its own disease. There is no mycoplasmosis or fermentanitis. This pathogen always seems to be a tag-along to other conditions. But what a tag-along it turns out to be! This nasty little creature can cause major diagnostic and treatment problems. As a co-infection with other TBIs, M. *fermentans* complicates the process every step of the way. If you have a TBI patient who is not doing well despite your best efforts, think about Mycoplasma.

What is real about Mycoplasma *fermentans*? Is it a common co-infection with TBIs? Is Mycoplasma the sole cause of chronic fatigue? Is it a germ warfare agent used against the US in the Middle East and a contributor to Gulf War Syndrome? Have vaccine supplies been contaminated with this pathogen? Is *fermentans* a prime factor in fibromyalgia? Was it considered before my friend's son committed suicide after writing that he could not take his depression, joint pain, and fatigue anymore? I wish I knew.

I will try to sort through all the angry blogs and the half-scientific literature to provide some useable information. There are many different species of Mycoplasma and the entire field is confusing and contentious. Whenever you have politics encroaching on medicine, consider who has reason to hide information. In a case where veterans are in conflict with government over germ warfare and contaminated vaccines, you can expect some heated exchanges.

There are a few facts that are hard to dispute about Mycoplasma *fermentans*. There are many strains of Mycoplasma and they can wreak havoc given the right conditions and a susceptible host. Most of us have been exposed to these organisms. Despite our awareness of them for years, we know far less than we should.

Mycoplasmas are never good news. While they are probably one of the most important co-infections, they remain the most elusive. They are hard to diagnose, confirm, and treat. Unfortunately, as with all the co-infections, we can't hope they will go away on their own. A high index of suspicion must be maintained since this genus can cause severe and protracted illness.

PEARL: Thomas McPherson Brown was the first to associate Mycoplasma with patients with arthritic symptoms. He made this connection before Lyme and TBIs had been identified. He treated his patients with long-term antibiotics, primarily minocycline, and the majority of patients seemed to greatly improve. His patients loved him and his detractors thought he was a trouble-maker. His biographer, Henry Scammell notes, "Nothing is likely to ruin a good reputation in medicine faster than being the first to come up with the right answer while the rest of the institution is comfortably bedded down with familiar folly." Dr. Brown was likely hitting both Mycoplasma and other susceptible infectious agents such as Bb with his regimen. His critics whined about resistance and dormant pathogens. His theories are now proving to be supported by experience over time.

Pathogen: Smaller than bacteria, Mycoplasma lack cell walls and are able to invade human cells and disrupt the immune system. M. *fermentans* may be the biggest management challenge of all the TBIs. Other species of Mycoplasma besides *fermentans* may be involved in the pathology of TBIs, but little is known about these other forms in relation to tick-borne pathology.

With no cell wall, Mycoplasma are not susceptible to many antibiotics, like penicillins, that work by impeding cell wall synthesis. They can be either parasitic or saprotrophic (feeding off dead matter). A number of Mycoplasmas are pathologic in humans including those that cause atypical pneumonias and pelvic inflammatory disease (PID).

The species of most interest in terms of TBIs is M. *fermentans*, which is thought to be an elusive and difficult tick-borne co-infection. In my research, I found at least eight names for what seems to be the *fermentans* species without counting the variations that occur when strains like *incognitus* are added to the mix. Several authors also mentioned the high frequency of rapid antigenic variation with the Mycoplasma that would cause our target to repeatedly shift as we continuously aim.

Mycoplasma are unusual bacteria in that they require sterols to make their cell membranes, and this usually is cholesterol obtained from the host. They also have relatively small genomes. Several Mycoplasma species have some of the smallest genomes of any free-living organisms sequenced to date. This means they cannot synthesize all they need on their own and are more dependent on their hosts. Nonetheless, their small genome could prove useful in the future for studying these minimal cells and their total protein content.

When first discovered, Mycoplasma were thought to be closely related to fungi. Culturing has always been difficult because of their complicated growth requirements. In the past, an organism was required to have a vertebrate host to be classified in the genus Mycoplasma, but that thinking is loosening. There remain many discrepancies involving this genus. Taxonomists appear reluctant to make any additional modifications in the near future since the medical and agricultural communities have not yet recovered from the last changes. Use caution when you read about these bacteria to ensure you are comparing apples to apples.

M. *fermentans* is a very small bacterium, more like DNA in a baggy without a lot of its own plumbing. The Mycoplasma get into the host cell and take over. These affected cells can be blood cells or just about any other tissue cells. M. *fermentans* is known to cross the blood brain barrier and the placenta. Once inside the cells, the M. *fermentans* takes the cell's nutrients, including sterols, and uses the cell's organelles to replicate itself. Since many cell types can be involved, M. *fermentans* can cause a systemic infection, involving numerous organ systems. Essentially, it can travel anywhere a WBC can go.

Vector: No one knows how contagious M. *fermentans* might be or all the ways it might be transmitted. Here we are concerned primarily with tick transmission but cannot ignore that many people who are sick with this organism have family members who are also sick. Were they also bitten by an infected tick or did they get their illness some other way? In those with Gulf War Syndrome, possibly caused by M. *fermentans,* half their spouses became ill and 100% of their children were sick. No tick seems to have been involved in these subsequent cases.

Otherwise, M. *fermentans* seems to be able to hitch a ride on any tick species that carries other TBIs. Unfortunately, Mycoplasma do not seem to be as choosy as some pathogens, and they appear to take any taxi passing by.

Distribution: No one has a glimmer of insight regarding how widespread *M. fermentans* might be. There are many confounders in assessing the distribution and epidemiology of this pathogen. Vaccines, especially those given to members of the military, may have been tainted with Mycoplasma *fermentans.* Anthrax strains may have been contaminated with M. *fermentans*, although in this case, I would be hard pressed to decide which agent was the contaminant. We likely have just touched the tip of the iceberg.

History: When did this organism begin to cause health problems in humans? Who knows? We are only beginning to recognize it as a source of significant, widespread pathology. Recently M. *fermentans* has been implicated in fibromyalgia, chronic fatigue, vaccine-associated conditions, Gulf War Syndrome, and a number of other disorders. While it may have gotten a bad rap in some of these cases, there are probably many other situations where we have not yet made the connection. In terms of TBIs, we are just starting to explore the damage this microbe may inflict. Many TBI patients who have not improved despite aggressive drug therapy may have cases complicated by this agent.

M. *fermentans* was first identified in the lower genital tract of humans in the 1950s, although any relationship to disease in the genital region was not then established. Since that time, the organism has been disproportionately found in patients with rheumatoid arthritis, leukemia, Gulf War Syndrome, chronic fatigue, and fibromyalgia. Drs. Garth and Nancy Nicolson have done a great deal of investigation into the role of M. *fermentans* in Gulf War Syndrome after their daughter returned home sick from Operation Desert Storm. Of course, there is considerable controversy around whether M. *fermentans* is the actual etiologic agent of any of these conditions or just along for the ride. My contention is that if you have a sick patient in front of you who just can't seem to get well, and you find reason to suspect M. *fermentans,* you might want to do what you can to eradicate it.

Pathophysiology: Mycoplasma get into the cells and take over. The affected cells can be blood cells or just about any other tissue cells. M. *fermentans* is known to cross the blood brain barrier and the placenta. Since many cell types can be involved, numerous organ systems can be affected, and symptoms will depend on where the pathogen has settled. Access to the CNS can result in inflammation of the brain, called encephalitis. Signs that the peripheral nervous system is involved include problems with motor or sensory conduction to the limbs or internal organs.

Mycoplasma seem to have a significant adverse impact on the host's immune system. One theory is that when the M. *fermentans* breaks down the host cell, part of the host cell membrane is released along with the Mycoplasma. As the body's immune system gears up to attack the invader, it also sees the protein from the broken cell and cleans that up too, essentially destroying its own proteins. Since the body is attacking it*self* here, that would be an autoimmune process. This would make sense since the kind of symptoms that are found with M. *fermentans* are similar to those seen in other types of autoimmune conditions such as arthritis, thyroid or other endocrine problems, myalgia, or myositis.

Further, M. *fermentans* likely affects B and T cells in the immune cascade. Interaction with B cells results in the activation of autoimmune responses and may enhance rheumatoid conditions. Further, M. *fermentans* activates the hypothalamic-pituitary-adrenal axis, which can trigger a number of limbic symptoms. In looking at the limbic system and comparing its functions to the symptoms associated with M. *fermentans* infection, important parallels can be seen. The limbic system governs emotion and behavior, memory, happiness, pleasure, decision-making, reward patterns associated with addiction, sexual drive, and the sense of well-being. Also, the sense of smell and the overall balance of the endocrine system are influenced by the limbic system. If you break it, guess what kind of symptoms might be associated with its malfunction.

There is continued investigation into whether M. *fermentans* can trigger inflammatory cytokine over-production and an increased manufacture of various ILs and TNF-α. Elevated cytokines have been suggested as the cause of many symptoms including neuropsychiatric problems. Increased ILs 1, 2, and 6 have been found in the joints of patients with rheumatoid arthritis and some theorize a role of Mycoplasma in spawning these higher levels. This effect on immune modulators may also increase the susceptibility of the host to other infections.

> *PEARL: Do not underestimate the power of M. fermentans to cause neuropsychiatric problems. M. fermentans may significantly impact the limbic system and is thought to increase microfibers, decrease NK cells, and increase inflammation and autoimmunity. M. fermentans may increase IL-1, IL-6, TNF-α and some of the neuropsychiatric manifestations may be due to the damage done by these biochemicals.*

While M. *fermentans* can activate the immune system in some ways, it then seems able to hide itself successfully within the host immune cells. The Mycoplasma appear to invade the natural killer (NK) cells. These lymphocytes are then weakened and their numbers decrease making the host more susceptible to opportunistic infections. This leaves the host with a highly dysregulated immune response resulting in severe immune suppression and a vulnerable situation for the host.

Mycoplasma are notoriously slow growing and so are not readily susceptible to antimicrobials. Since they have no cell wall, they cannot be harmed by agents that only inhibit cell wall synthesis. This organism also seems to be able to use a number of mechanisms to become drug resistant, so keep this in mind as therapy continues.

Clinical course: In essentially every TBI case in the literature, the course of action of M. *fermentans* is dependent on the course of at least one other co-infection and usually more than one. There is so much intermingling of pathology it is difficult to tease out what belongs with what. Nonetheless, there are such obvious parallels to the symptom patterns found in chronic fatigue, fibromyalgia, rheumatoid arthritis,

TBI co-infection, and Gulf War Syndrome, that whether the Mycoplasma is the *sole* source of the problem or a mere contributor, it is a force to be recognized. Don't dismiss its role just because you don't understand it.

> *PEARL: A high percentage of autism spectrum disorder (ASD) patients are infected with Mycoplasma. One estimate is that >20% are infected with M. fermentans and > 45% with M. pneumoniae.*

Signs & symptoms: Most signs and symptoms of Mycoplasma follow from the mechanism by which the organism causes disease. These findings overlap with the symptoms of several other TBIs and defining which sxs belong to which pathogen can be daunting. The red flags for diagnosis are the persistent chronic fatigue, somnolence, and neuropsychiatric manifestations. M. *fermentans* presents much the same way as Bartonella, but here the psychiatric manifestations are much worse. While psychiatric problems are responsive to antibiotics in the correct combinations, they do not usually respond very well to psychotropics alone.

Symptoms that have been associated with Mycoplasma *fermentans* include fatigue, headache, GI symptoms, joint and lymph node discomfort, breathing difficulty, and muscle soreness. M. *fermentans* can cause significant cognitive problems, behavior changes, and depression. Neuropsychiatric problems might be the most distinguishing feature of M. *fermentans*.

GI manifestations include GERD, vomiting, irritable bowel-like symptoms such as diarrhea, cholecystitis, and pain. Vagus nerve involvement may account for many of the GI symptoms.

There may be persistent arthritis and joint pain, severe chronic fatigue, prostration, persistent headaches, inability to concentrate, trouble thinking clearly, difficulty falling asleep or staying asleep, lymphadenopathy, numbness, tingling, night sweats, arthritis, cognitive impairment, memory problems, and rash. The patient can experience strange sensations in extremities, a feeling of skin burning or freezing, bone pain, muscle pain, cramps in muscles, or knife-like shooting pains.

Symptoms of M. *fermentans* might be mostly psychological. Psychiatric manifestations might include personality changes, mood swings, violence, depression that can be severe, preference for a dark room, uncontrolled anger, increased use of alcohol or drugs (presumably to self-medicate), denial, inability to concentrate at work or school, and suicidal ideation and attempts. Mycoplasma have been associated with mood disorders, Tourette's syndrome, anxiety, and depression. This may be the saddest symptom set of any of the TBIs because the psychiatric problems can go on so long without explanation. Since M. *fermentans* alters the limbic system which governs emotion and behavior, the pathogen can significantly impact memory, happiness, pleasure, decision-making, reward patterns associated with addiction, sexual drive, and overall sense of well-being. Patients complain of feeling out of balance emotionally and unable to feel happy.

M. *fermentans* seems to have the potential to devastate the immune system, leaving the host susceptible to other infections including those opportunistic types that may not ordinarily be pathogenic. In many cases, it is hard to tell which symptoms are due to M. *fermentans* and which might be secondary to other infectious agents.

Of those who have been tested, half of all members of the military who participated in Operation Desert Storm were positive for the *incognitus* strain of Mycoplasma. Whether this strain is responsible for the symptoms found in Gulf War Syndrome is still under heated debate. Gulf War syndrome presents with extreme fatigue, night sweats, intermittent fevers, irritability, memory problems, muscle pain, headaches, rashes, diarrhea, depression, bronchitis, and bloating.

Diagnosis: I know of no TBI specialist who thinks of Mycoplasma *fermentans* first when assessing a patient. Maybe we should, but the organism is just too vague and murky. I would be happy if this text makes people think of Mycoplasma when all else has failed and the patient still desperately needs help. With luck, some might think of Mycoplasma a little sooner than that.

Because M. *fermentans* is intracellular, diagnostic testing can be difficult. If possible, get a biopsy sample (the gut is the best source) and send this to a lab that knows how to test for this pathogen. Even with the best tissue sample, M. *fermentans* is very difficult to measure.

Serology has limited usefulness with M. *fermentans* although IFA is sometimes attempted. DNA PCR is the most used testing method. PCR may identify active cases but cannot be relied upon to exclude the diagnosis if negative. If the patient has been on antibiotics before the sample was taken, a false negative can occur. Even if the samples are as fresh as possible and from tissue instead of blood, it is very difficult to get a positive result. Few labs can handle this type of testing. As of March, 2010, Clongen Laboratories in Germantown, Maryland, was still performing PCR testing on solid tissues for M. *fermentans*. My recommendation if you are an initial user is to pull up the website and call any lab before you send samples for testing. See the lab information provided in Chapter18: *Ordering Appropriate Tests*.

Diagnoses of most TBIs are clinical judgments and this holds especially true for M. *fermentans*. With M. *fermentans*, keep a high index of suspicion. If you have a TBI patient who doesn't seem to be getting better with appropriate treatment, especially if they have incapacitating fatigue and cognitive or behavioral problems, consider M. *fermentans*.

Differential Diagnosis: When a patient presents with a tick bite and a clinical picture of fatigue, headache, and some degree of cognitive or behavioral problems, M. *fermentans* should be on the short list. However, not every patient who was bitten by a tick recalls such a bite, so keep an open mind in those patients as well. Also, consider Bartonella when you have considerable neuropsychiatric involvement. Before you too quickly diagnose CFS, or fibromyalgia, or an autoimmune condition of unknown etiology, consider M. *fermentans*. If the patient isn't getting better on what you thought was a reasonable treatment plan, your original diagnosis might be wrong or you might be using the wrong treatment approach. Co-infections could be in play. In these cases, it is hard to tell what signs and symptoms are due to M. *fermentans* and what might be secondary to other infectious agents. Note that professional psychological testing may help in the long-run with differential diagnosis and monitoring treatment.

Treatment: M. *fermentans* may be the biggest treatment challenge in TBIs. However, you must think of a pathogen before you attempt to treat it. Always remember that Mycoplasma is rarely the only duck in the pond. Most likely, it is only one of two or more co-infections, or other contributing factors such as contaminated vaccines. Do your best to select a treatment regimen that hits the most probable candidates.

M. *fermentans* will respond to antibiotics but it might be hell finding the right combination. Treatment can last 6 months or more. If the patient you are treating is not getting better, consider changing antibiotics. While on antibiotics, the person seems pretty well protected from reinfection, but if rebitten she could get a resistant strain. M. *fermentans* is responsive only if the right antibiotics are selected.

PEARL: Since M. fermentans *are SLOW growing they might be less susceptible to any antibiotic that works through the various cell metabolic pathways. They can certainly be a treatment challenge.*

Treatment with long courses of high dose antibiotics may be needed. Doxycycline is a bacteriostatic tetracycline. This means it slows the organism down but it does not kill it. Therefore, the patient may need to be treated over a number of life cycles of the M. *fermentans* before it is functionally eradicated. Since this strain of Mycoplasma can be slow-growing and intracellular, treatment could take 6 months or longer. With longer treatment, the host's natural immunity would have time to respond and help in the healing process. Remember M. *fermentans* uses a number of mechanisms to become drug resistant, so keep this in mind as therapy continues.

M. *fermentans* can be treated much the same way as Bartonella. Here however, the TCNs, especially doxycycline, would likely be the foundation antibiotic with all the others added to the regimen as appropriate. Macrolides might be an important part of the initial combination. Fluoroquinolones could have a prominent role. Both Rifampin and hydroxychloroquine (Plaquenil) have been used successfully in treating M. *fermentans*.

The foundation regimen begins with a tetracycline such as doxycycline (Doryx is an enteric-coated, time-release formulation that might be better tolerated) or minocycline (Minocin), *together* with a macrolide, such as azithromycin (Zithromax) or clarithromycin (Biaxin). With minocycline consider starting with 50 mg bid and then after 1 week, if there is no headache, increase to 100 mg bid.

Other agents are added as needed:

- Trimethoprim-sulfamethoxazole (Bactrim, Septra) bid

- Rifamycin (Rifampin) generally dosed at 300 mg bid. Never use rifamycin as a sole agent since resistance can develop within hours. Always use in combination with other antimicrobials. Rifampin might be a good choice if the patient is co-infected with both Bb and Bartonella.

- The fluoroquinolone ciprofloxacin (Cipro), po in tablets or suspension, or IV. Cipro is indicated in kids only when there are limited alternatives or when the severity of the disease suggests its use. There is potential for tendon damage. The dose ranges between 250 and 750 mg q 12 hours. Floxin or Levaquin have also been used.

- Hydroxychloroquine (Plaquenil): See Chapter 24 for dosing guidance.

- Chloramphenicol has been used against M. *fermentans*.

  PEARL: Individual case reports mention the combination of rifamycin and azithromycin OR Bactrim and azithromycin.

Long-term treatment is usually needed. Multiple cycles of antibiotics may be needed because of the intracellular location, slow-growing nature, and inherent insensitivity to most antibiotics. One source treats in 6 week cycles. Treat, check, and if there are still residual problems, consider treating for another 6 weeks. Then check again and treat again. Six months of treatment is often considered the minimum needed to eradicate the symptoms associated with M. *fermentans*. Remember this organism uses a number of mechanisms to resist antibiotics and the immune response, so recognize that you may be in for a long and aggressive battle.

Dosing ranges for patients over 8-years-old or over 100 pounds as part of the listed treatment options include:

Doxycycline 200 to 300 mg per day

Ciprofloxin (Cipro) 1500 mg per day

Azithromycin (Zithromax) 500 mg per day

Clarithromycin (Biaxin) 750 to 1000 mg per day

Rifampin 300 mg bid

Hydroxychloroquine (Plaquenil): Children's doses have not been established but look in Chapter 24 for dosing recommendations in other conditions.

Measure treatment success by resolution of psychiatric symptoms. Cognition and behavior should improve. With other TBIs, you might be assessing different areas of improvement such as musculoskeletal pain and function. If treatment for M. *fermentans* is discontinued too soon, relapse is possible. Do what you would do if it were your child who wasn't improving.

Prognosis: Successful outcomes in these cases can occur if you remember that M. *fermentans* could be the reason a TBI patient is not improving. With this pathogen, maybe more than any other, a number of therapeutic regimens may need to be tried before achieving success. These patients can get well. You just need to be persistent. Never give up.

Chapter 10   BORRELIOSIS (LYME) – Detailed chapter contents

Chapter 10

BORRELIOSIS

Ready! Fire! Aim!
Unofficial motto for one large pharmaceutical company

Background: Lyme disease, or borreliosis, is a complicated, multisystem disease caused by bacteria in the genus Borrelia. We are only beginning to understand its complex pathophysiology, varied manifestations, and divergent clinical paths. With this disease, apparently, numerous factors combine to determine who will get sick, how sick they will become, and whether they will respond to treatment. The Lyme syndrome is both frustrating and perplexing in many ways. Dr. Robert Bransfield talks about Lyme as a *common* human disease that presents under certain environmental *conditions* in patients with *susceptible* genes. Some individuals barely notice a Bb infection and others respond quickly to a short-course of antibiotics. Still, there remains the significant subpopulation that gets chronically ill. Sadly, Lyme can be fatal in probably more cases than are recognized.

In this chapter, borreliosis caused by Borrelia *burgdorferi* (Lyme) will be the primary focus. Other forms of borreliosis will be introduced when appropriate, but these variations are not nearly as clear-cut as you might think. The good news is that, so far, all identified Borrelia infections respond to the same treatment regimens, as far as that goes. I purposely did not feature Lyme as the initial chapter of the co-infections since infections from Babesia, Bartonella, and M. *fermentans* are probably as common, even though currently less identified. Other TBIs also have significant M&M, not just Lyme. Further, Lyme manifesting in the presence of any of these co-infections can present almost as a different beast compared to when the pathogen presents alone. Lyme is only one of many serious, confounding tick-borne diseases.

Where do I begin? I wrote this chapter last. After nearly four years of study and research, I had to finally stop searching and start writing. As I have mentioned repeatedly, much of the published material regarding Lyme is simply wrong. Entire books have been written based on flawed premises. This misinformation, even when inspired by good intent, has hurt numerous people, many of them children. Some of the material included below may be imprecise because we are just beginning to understand the pathophysiology that underscores Lyme. My primary intent in this chapter is to provide all types of readers with material to review and options to consider. Some sections had dozens of theories presented in the literature and many ideas were stated as fact with no supporting evidence whatsoever.

PEARL: A 2004 study in the Pediatric Infectious Disease Journal stated that 9 out of 19 Internet websites contained major inaccuracies. I think they are being very generous. My four years of intensive research suggests that the number of sources with significant inaccuracies and frank distortions is far greater, especially with reference to Lyme. Be very careful.

This chapter reviews a number of alternative approaches for treating Lyme. Each of the experts has their own way of doing things. As the treating HCP, you have to find what works best in each individual case. Look at the rationale provided alongside the various options listed in the *Treatment* section below. As long as the HCP is working toward the re-establishment of wellness in the patient, I am not going to quibble about small differences. The following information is compiled from the experience of TBI specialists as well as extensive examination of the literature. The reader should be able to review the various approaches and options in order to target the best strategy for the individual patient.

Lyme is not cookie-cutter medicine. The field is too amorphous and complex. If you are an HCP who only wants to follow algorithms, Lyme medicine is not a good place for you. Unlike Dante who warns to "...abandon all hope...all ye who enter here...," there is hope for the Lyme patient. But for optimism to prevail, there needs to be commitment and cooperation between the HCPs, patient, caregivers, family, and society.

Lyme disease is a *multisystem* disorder caused by a Borrelia spirochete. This pathogen affects many body structures but has an apparent affinity for those tissues with considerable collagen and connective tissue like valves in the cardiovascular system, joints, and the nervous system with its supporting structures. Bb infection can cause both acute and chronic disease, can go dormant for varying periods, can wax and wane, relapse, and become chronic. Lyme affects all ages, ethnic groups, and genders, and is almost always tick-borne. The only thing Lyme is NOT is boring.

Some people have made a career denying everything about Lyme: how to diagnose, the clinical course, treatment options, the possibility of on-going infection, and the persistence of sequelae. The local ER doctor alternatively told me that my son did and didn't have Lyme. Yes, he had a tick in a jar, an EM rash, and a history, physical, and ROS compatible with the diagnosis of Lyme. But the EM lesion was not round enough she said. I was told that the low-dose doxy he was receiving should be enough to hit the Lyme he didn't have. For a condition with such a significant M&M, many HCPs are woefully misinformed and as a result Lyme patients are often not receiving the care they need.

In *Cure Unknown*, Lorraine Johnson is quoted by Weintraub as calling Lyme "both a masquerader and a changeling, not unlike another spirochete-induced disease, syphilis," in which overt neurological and other symptoms emerged over time in a way that were not always understood to be related to the original infection. Bb causes so many various manifestations of disease we are lucky to pin it down as often as we do, which is not as often as we should.

In 2013, there are thousands of articles, lectures, books, and videos with arguments, contradictions, misinformation, and just flat-out bad science in all directions regarding Lyme. That is the world of this difficult disease. While many contributors have good intentions to help educate and understand, a few do not. While the information is evolving, HCPs are finally beginning to understand how Lyme can be complicated by co-infections as well as its own complex and confounding physiology.

To summarize my current basic understanding of Lyme in one sentence: Lyme is a multisystem disease, diagnosed using reasonable medical judgment, with the duration of treatment based on clinical response, which can be cured with enough determination, patience, knowledge, and chutzpah.

Someday we will understand so much more about Lyme and all the pieces of the complex puzzle will fit together neatly. We will know why some patients get sicker than others and why some stay sick while many quickly respond. The bottom line is that Lyme can be cured, even in those who have been chronically ill for a long time.

Essentially all chapters in this book are ultimately about Lyme. Chapter 10: *Borreliosis* will largely summarize the conclusions from the other 33 chapters. Most HCPs have too much information and not enough perspective to manage it all. Hopefully, this book will help organize all the disjointed facts and provide perspective in managing these complex, multifaceted patients. In another decade we should have things more clearly sorted. We have the genome for Bb. If only we had the sense God gave a walnut, we'd be able to figure out what to do with this tangle of facts and theories.

Let's see if we can eventually come out of this morass with some insight into how to help Lyme patients.

As a pathogen, Bb must be respected. As a disease, Lyme should never be underestimated. For whatever reason some people get sick and stay sick until the appropriate intervention can be targeted to their individual case. Our goal should be to relieve their suffering and give them back a full, productive, satisfying life.

I. ALIASES

Lyme disease, LD, LYD, Lyme borreliosis, LB, BI, relapsing fever, great imitator, new syphilis, imposter, the mimic, meningopolyneuritis, Garin-Bujadoux syndrome, Bannworth disease, Afzelius disease, Montauk knee, sheep tick fever, stealth bug, human borreliosis, modern pox

NOTE: STARI is a borreliosis which may or may not be the same as Lyme. STARI is also called Master's disease, Missouri Lyme, or Lyme-like disease.

II. PATHOGEN

Lyme disease, or borreliosis, is a **spirochetal** disease caused by bacteria in the genus Borrelia. In the US, Borrelia *burgdorferi* is the etiologic pathogen of Lyme. In Europe, B. *afzelii* and B. *garinii* are thought to be the most prevalent infectious species. From an evolutionary perspective, the spirochete is one of the oldest known bacteria and it has developed multiple ways to survive both independently and in symbiotic relationships with tick vectors.

Spirochetes are a group of genetically distinct bacteria that use axial filaments as endoflagella for motility. When the filaments of the endoflagella rotate, the spirochetes move like a cork-screw. This method of movement is thought to be an adaptation to **viscous** environments such as blood, biofilms, mucosa, intestines, vitreous of the eye, or joint spaces. As a pathogen, the spirochete is thought to be able to hide its flagella, which is antigenic, from the host's immune defenses. Spirochetes are longer than they are wide and sometimes their width is below the resolving power of many light microscopes. This feature has caused problems when labs have said no spirochetes were visible in a test sample when using technology that could not possibly have allowed them to be seen. Dark-field microscopy is best for seeing the spirochetes. This methodology uses a condenser which directs the light toward an object at an angle so the image is seen as a light object against a dark background.

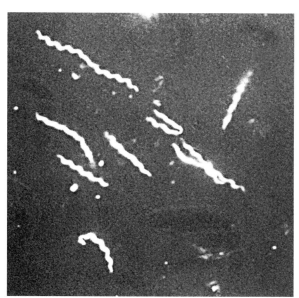

Borrelia *burgdorferi*, the spirochete that causes
Lyme disease
Source: CDC. Accessed March 2013

Remember, this chapter reviews a number of **borreliosis**, not just Lyme. In the US, Borrelia *hermsii* is tick-borne and *Borrelia recurrentis* is transmitted by a louse. Both are thought to cause variations of relapsing fevers. A number of other *Borrelia* species are likely pathogens as well, including *B. parkeri*, and *B. duttoni*, responsible for a number of African relapsing fevers that are reminiscent of the clinical syndrome called Lyme in the US. Several Borrelia species that cause relapsing fevers use rodents as reservoirs via tick vectors. Additional species such as B. *bissettii* and B. *valaisiana* may also cause human disease.

In Chapter 12: *Other Recognized TBIs*, the tick relapsing fever caused by Borrelia *hermsii* is given separate billing. Clearly this is a borreliosis. Here the tick transmits the spirochete that is responsible for disease in some hosts. Found most often in the western US, this TBI presents with cycles of high fever, sudden chills, eye inflammation, cough, jaundice, and sometimes a petechial rash. Should this TBI be listed as a separate co-infection or simply cataloged here as another borreliosis? Is it a separate disease? Does it matter? I don't know. Just be aware of both when you read the literature and as you evaluate patients with TBIs.

Currently, there is not enough reliable information to know exactly how these different Borrelia strains cause disease and how the diseases may be different or the same. Lyme has been referred to in some venues as relapsing fever. Keep a high index of suspicion and treat the patient, not the label.

PEARL: On January 17, 2013, Reuters released the headline, "U.S. researchers find new disease carried by deer

ticks." The un-labeled disease is likely due to a type of Borrelia miyamotoi *that has been identified in Japan, New England, and Russia. If untreated, the pathogen can cause recurring episodes of fever. Symptoms are similar to Lyme disease and some patients have developed a rash. However, the authors felt this illness was distinct from Lyme in that there were often relapsing fevers in these cases. There is clear evidence that at least B.* burgdorferi *and B.* hermsii *can cause relapsing fevers. Be careful. This condition is too new to proclaim that only deer ticks are infected, and too new to know if there were co-infections in these few patients, and too new to say if the clinical course is different from the various borrelioses that we already know (if imperfectly). Perhaps we need to step away from a rigid definition of Lyme and speak more often of Borrelia-induced disease. For our new nemesis, B.* miyamotoi, *it is way too early to etch any conclusions in granite. Let's all try to not repeat the same mistakes made with Lyme.*

Borrelia has at least 3 dozen recognized species and about a dozen cause Lyme-like infections. We used to think only 3 species caused Lyme: B. *burgdorferi* in NA (and recently found in Europe) and B. *afzelii* and B. *garinii* both in Eurasia. As we learn more, we realize we need to keep an open-mind as to what might actually be transpiring in the world of spirochetes.

These Borrelia that cause LD have been divided into several genospecies where the differences depend on restriction fragment length polymorphism, multi-locus enzyme electrophoresis, and ssRNA sequences and these are labeled: 1. Borrelia *burgdorferi* **sensu stricto** 2. Borrelia *garinii* and 3. Borrelia *afzelii*. The collective term referring to all 3 is Borrelia *burgdorferi* **sensu lato**. All US isolates are Borrelia *burgdorferi* *sensu stricto*. I know this paragraph seems pretentious and confusing. I just want you to be aware of terms that you might run into in the literature. I really MUST hurry and finish this book before any other nomenclature changes. Speaking of confusing and evolving,

STARI: Southern Tick-Associated Rash Illness is thought to be transmitted by the Lone Star tick with the pathogen assumed to be B. *lonestari*. A letter to Pat Smith, the president of the Lyme Disease Association, from a government staff member dated August 24, 2007, indicates that he believes that STARI is clearly a different disease from Lyme caused by a unique pathogen. Those of us who are up to our elbows in Lyme every day aren't so sure. While the Lone Star tick is demonstrably a distinct species and B. *lonestari* probably has defining features that separate it from Bb, the clinical syndrome is so close as to be indistinguishable from Lyme. While both can cause EM lesions, Lyme is thought to do so less frequently and we have no idea how often STARI does or does not cause an EM rash. Some commentators say that while the EM rash in Lyme RARELY has central clearing, the STARI EM rash NEVER has central clearing. How could anyone be sure of that? Others say the rashes are different in terms of color, degree of homogeneity, and sharpness of borders, that the STARI lesions are smaller. I had enough trouble getting several doctors to recognize my son's classic Lyme rash let alone split hairs so finely. How could anyone know these lesions so well as to make such definitive, general statements? We have recently learned that Lone Star ticks can be infected with Bb as well as B. *lonestari*. Certainly, if both pathogens are present in the tick saliva, then both pathogens could be transmitted during the same bite, just as any other co-infection. I believe it is more important to work on ways to relieve the suffering and potential long-term sequelae of these diseases rather than quibble over uncertainties. We are very early in the information-gathering phase of this recently described disease. If flawed surveillance criteria were used to identify Lyme in STARI patients we can have no confidence in a negative report. So, we simply don't know if B. *lonestari* was solely responsible for the clinical presentation seen or if Bb was along for the ride. Is B. *lonestari* a separate species, a subspecies, or a strain of Bb? I am open to modifying my perspective on STARI as more information becomes available. Hopefully, others will be as flexible when reviewing new data.

Now to save our mental health, let's focus on Bb. ...

Borrelia *burgdorferi* is responsible for most of the illness we call Lyme disease. The Bb microbe is very complicated. Porcella and Schwan suggest that the genetic structure of Bb is the most complex ever identified in a prokaryote. Also, Bb have greater strain diversity than previously imagined. These strain differences may partially explain the multifaceted clinical presentations seen in Lyme disease.

Bb are microaerophilic, which means that the organisms require oxygen for survival BUT the levels need to be at a lower concentration than that found in the atmosphere. They PREFER lower levels of oxygen, not NO oxygen. This concept has caused considerable discord in the literature where some authors argue that they are aerobic and others insist they are anaerobic. This argument has caused some sources to say that no aerobic exercise should be done by Lyme patients since the extra oxygen in the tissues would make the pathogens too happy. In contrast, you could argue that less oxygen in the tissue as might be found in anaerobic activities would make them just as jolly. (I believe that most types of moderate exercise are likely beneficial as long as not overdone and the patient tolerates the activity.)

Bb are slower growing than many other pathogens, but not as slow as microbes like M. *fermentans*. This unhurried

development may help explain some of the delays in the clinical presentation, diagnosis, and response to treatment.

When compared to the fast-replicating bacteria, Bb may require a longer course of antibiotic treatment to reach the same endpoint. Bb replicates in about 24 hours whereas organisms such as E. *coli* and Strep replicate in a few minutes. Antibiotics usually work best during replication. Therefore, for a rapid reproducer, a 7 to 10 day regimen of antibiotics provides thousands of chances to kill the bacteria. But with Bb the same number of replication cycles can take 10 to 50 times longer. If caught and treated early enough in the clinical course, most patients are symptom-free after a 6 to 8 week course of appropriate antimicrobials. If treated for less time, the symptoms may resolve, but the infection can still be present. So, instead of using rapid replicators like Strep or Salmonella as models, think more in line with pathogens like those that cause syphilis or tuberculosis.

Of course, with Bb, even something as straightforward as Gram staining would be controversial. These spirochetes are neither Gram positive nor Gram negative and are best termed Gram neutral. Actually, when stained they are weakly Gram negative by default since the last stain used leaves some residue. Bb do have outer membranes and inner membranes that more closely resemble the Gram negative type cell wall than the Gram positive. This fact will not alter the way you approach LD patients, but it sure caused some big fights in the literature.

Bb can be cultivated *in vitro* but they are very meticulous, fastidious, and difficult organisms that require complex growth medium. Bb grows best in BSK medium containing over 13 ingredients in a rabbit serum base. Optimal temperature for growth is 32°C or about 90°F. In cultures, these organisms will survive best in a microaerophilic environment. A technician with patience will also be needed since the generation time is at least 12 to 24 hours. Now you can understand why merely smearing a routine culture plate with a patient sample is not likely to yield a lot of baby spirochetes.

Again the optimal culture temperature has caused bitter disputes in the literature where various factions argue whether Bb loves or loathes heat or cold. Logically, it seems to me that a temperature above or below the 90° mark would not be as Bb-friendly as the 90° mark would be. So you will make this microbe miserable at either extreme. There doesn't seem any reason to either bake or freeze the poor patient. Still many alternative treatments advocate one or the other extreme. Obviously Bb survive in ticks over freezing winters and throughout the long, hot summers. So I'm not sure we need to torture a patient in order to attempt to inconvenience the Bb through extreme temperature variations.

For the purposes of this section, borreliosis will be assumed to be Bb-induced. The **genome** of Bb strain 31 is known, and work is underway on other strains. NIH has funded a project that has sequenced 17 strains of modern Borrelia *burgdorferi* and have published information on about a dozen. A number of other variants are beginning to be identified in places like Greece, Japan, and China. So before you become too entrenched in one intractable perspective or another, remember we have only just begun to understand this complex organism.

> *PEARL: I do not have great confidence in some of the fine distinctions made between these Borrelia species. I DO trust the work of Willy Burgdorfer that identified the* burgdorferi *species and Ed Masters who first recognized the STARI phenomenon. However, a few other authors seem to be trying too hard to establish differences that may or may not be present. The important point is that, so far, all disease caused by the genus Borrelia seems to respond to similar treatment protocols, to the degree possible.*

B31 is quite hardy and virulent. This strain is thought to have arrived in the US about 40 years ago where it was soon responsible for disease that was more infectious, with a more aggressive course, than previously experienced in North America. B31 seems to cause the worst disease and only gives the protein pattern for B31 on testing. Bb genospecies are believed to exhibit strain-dependent organotropism, where the pathogens show a predilection for certain tissue. For example, the European species B. *afzelii* seems to prefer skin while B. *garinii* favors tissue in the nervous system. Therefore different strains might manifest with dissimilar clinical presentations – the many faces of Lyme.

These multiple strain differences may be why there are so many different clinical presentations of Lyme and such divergent clinical courses. The strains may have varying virulence and pathogenicity. In Danbury, CT, the Bb cause a disease that is primarily a mix of GI, urinary, and cognitive deficits. In contrast, the clinical manifestations in Pocopson, PA, are more often rheumatic, cardiac, and especially neuropsychiatric. Both clearly Lyme, but quite different in appearance. Of course, other factors may contribute to these variations, but alternate strains are certainly something to consider. Why do certain antibiotics work in some patients but not in others? An Omnicef combination regimen might work in southern Jersey and PA, but not in northern NJ. Strain variation is probably partially responsible for this discrepancy. The best example is the apparent difference in the M&M in the Borrelia strains that cause borreliosis in North America compared to Europe.

We do know that Lyme manifestations can differ from person to person and even within a person at various times. Similar, but not identical, strains might be responsible for these variations. In each region there appears to be a mix of strains. Mul-

tiple strains also help explain why so many Ab/Ag serological tests are negative. The patient was infected with one strain, but tested against another.

Bb are thought to have at least 3 forms which appear to enable the pathogen to maneuver through life dodging antibiotics and evading the best efforts of some immune systems. The known forms include:

A. **Spirochete** with cell wall: Also called free-form, extracellular, free-floating, helical, spiral, or spirochetal form. These spirochetes can be floating free in the blood and other fluids. This is the most active version of Bb and the most susceptible to antibiotics. Since they have a cell wall they would be at risk from cell wall antibiotics like amoxicillin. In some cases, treatment of the spirochetal form may cause these pathogens to convert to the other two types of Bb, which may not be as vulnerable to the host's defenses or to antibiotics as is this spirochetal adaptation.

B. **Spirochete without cell wall**: Also called the **L-form** or spheroplast. You can't be hurt by destruction of your cell wall if you don't have one. These entities will require an advanced macrolide or other intracellular agent. Therefore, the L-forms of Bb are resistant to cell wall antibiotics such as the PCNs and CSs. Note that to earn the right to be called an L-form you must have a cell wall during one of your life phases. For example, Mycoplasma never have cell walls so they are never referred to as L-forms. The Bb that lack a cell wall and morph into the L-form appear to be critical in setting up chronic infections and treatment failures. Antimicrobials may need to be cycled or a different combination tried.

C. **Cystic** form: Encysted Bb are the most resistant of the manifestations of the Bb pathogen. To penetrate the cyst requires specific cyst-busting antimicrobials such as Flagyl (metronidazole) or Tindamax (tinidazole). When in a hostile environment (low nutrients, unfavorable O_2, extreme temperatures, or the presence of antibiotics), Bb can change from spirochete to cyst. The cyst can stay dormant until conditions are favorable again. Generally, antibiotics used against the spirochetal form are not effective against Bb's cystic manifestation. In the chronically infected, who seem to be resistant to drug therapy, try cyst-busters.

III. VECTOR

How is the Bb that results in Lyme disease spread? By deer ticks, of course. Everyone knows that. Well, this being the fantastic world of TBIs, nothing is that simple. Until very recently, patients were told that if it wasn't a deer tick, their symptoms could not possibly be Lyme. Time and money were spent on testing ticks and seeing if they were engorged "enough" to have transmitted the disease. Many people were told, "You do NOT have Lyme!" when in fact they most certainly did.

While the Ixodes genus is the primary purveyor of LD through the deer tick (black-legged tick or I. *scapularis*), there are strong suspicions that dog ticks (Dermacentor *variabilis*) and other Ixodes species like the Western black-legged tick (I. *pacificus*) are infected with Bb as well. This information is documented from analysis of the pathogens present in the ticks collected during **tick drags**.

If the ticks are infected, I cannot think of a single reason why the pathogen cannot move into a host through dog tick saliva as easily as it does by way of the saliva of deer ticks. This is the whole premise behind the co-infection epidemic that is currently underway. We now suspect that the Lone Star tick (Amblyomma *americanum)* that moves B. *lonestari* can also transmit B. *burgdorferi*. Don't be surprised if additional genuses and species appear in the literature. And never rule out a diagnosis because someone was bitten by the "wrong" kind of tick. Chapter 2: *The Tick* details the vectors associated with Lyme and other borreliosis, at least as much as we currently know. Even though estimates vary greatly, in the overall TBI patient population probably less than half the patients or parents recall the actual tick bite. So no need to split hairs. Stop looking for reasons for the clinical presentation to not be Lyme and address the needs of the sick person.

While LD is almost always tick-borne, gestational transmission occurs when the Bb spirochete infecting the mother gets into the tissues of the fetus. When the child is born with Lyme, the disease is said to be **congenital**. Bb have been found in semen and breast milk but evidence of transmission through these fluids is less clear. Bb DNA has been isolated from semen using PCR techniques. While sexual transmission and disease secondary to passage through breast milk are anecdotal, cases of gestational Lyme where active spirochete is passed from mother to child is well documented. Chapter 30: *Special Populations* details gestational Lyme.

The literature also cites cases where the Bb are thought to have been transmitted through blood transfusions, sexual contact, other intimate human contact, fleas, mosquitoes, and mites. Anything is possible, but a missed tick bite could also be the culprit. Research out of the University of Wisconsin suggests that dairy cattle and perhaps other food animals can be infected with Bb. While they do not manifest LD, raw food obtained from these animals may be contaminated with Bb. Whether this route could spread disease is debatable. Be aware of the possibilities.

In the patients that do remember being bitten, consider that the tick they see may not be the tick that caused the disease. The tick you see may not have attached, while the tick you missed may have had a great big bite of you. Something happened to transmit disease.

PEARL: The deer ticks are thought to release pheromones that attract other ticks and this increases the chance of re-bite along with reinfection. Although I did not include these pictures in the book because they were too gruesome, several websites show pictures of deer and other animals just covered in ticks. I guess when one tick finds a bounty, it's best for the survival of the species if other ticks are informed of the location of the buffet.

Chapter 32: *Prevention* clears up the misconception that the tick has to be attached for a minimum number of hours before disease is transmitted. While the longer the attachment persists, the greater the likelihood of transmission, the risk does not go to zero even if the tick has only been present a short time. In these cases infection will depend on the parasite load in the tick, skin thickness at the bite site, and how deep the tick inserted itself. While the degree of engorgement can relate to the length of attachment, the tick does not need to be engorged to transmit disease. Stop looking for reasons why this couldn't possibly be Lyme and accept what you see in front of you. I still find myself rationalizing why a certain symptom pattern couldn't possibly be Lyme.

IV. DISTRIBUTION/EPIDEMIOLOGY

Until recently, Lyme was thought to be the most common TBI in North America. However, the surge in cases of Babesia, Bartonella, and several other co-infections may alter that presumption in the future. Right now, all TBIs are grossly underdiagnosed so the actual I&P numbers are mostly guesses.

I hesitate to give any numbers provided from CDC sources since I believe these numbers are grossly understated. In 2002, the number of LD cases reported to CDC increased by 40% to 23,763. In 2012, there will likely be more than 35,000 "official" cases. (Remember these are only those cases that meet the surveillance criteria.) Since only 10% to 15% of LD cases are actually reported, the true number of cases throughout the US may exceed 300,000 annually. The highest reported incidence of LD occurs in kids under 15 with at least a quarter of the cases. According to Adler, even the CDC admits that as many as 90% of the cases go unreported. Some sources estimate that only 1 in 40 cases is reported. That's less that 3%.

PEARL: Chester County, Pennsylvania, will only report a Lyme case if they speak directly to the doctor on the phone. They will try to return a doctor's call twice and then abandon the pursuit. The LDASEPA intern could not get in touch with anyone in the appropriate office to clarify reporting standards. She made multiple attempts. How many times do you think a busy HCP will try?

Lyme is to be reported in all 50 states. I know my son's case was not initially reported, since the family doctor didn't really think the signs pointed to Lyme, despite the EM rash at the bite site, compatible symptoms, and the deer tick in the jar. The ER doctor did not report his Lyme because his labs were drawn too early in the clinical course and processed at the local lab that prides itself in the number of negative results it reports. My husband's Lyme was never reported. My Lyme was never reported. Not the first time I had it, or the second, or the third. …

> PEARL: *Numbers are all over the place. There were 27,444 Lyme cases in 2007 according to the CDC. One source says that number should be 10 times higher i.e., 274,440. Another source believes the estimate should be 100 times that number or over 2 million cases. One author thinks that a quarter of the US population may be infected. Still another believes that Lyme might contribute to half of all chronic illnesses including conditions like Alzheimer's and Parkinson's. I don't know if I can accept that as fact. I do not know how the author came to this conclusion. The bottom line is that as long as we have flawed surveillance criteria defining clinical cases, we are not likely to have a realistic handle on the extent of the problem.*

Patients are often told they couldn't possibly have Lyme because they are not living in an endemic area. Certainly, the chances of contracting the disease are much higher in areas where Bb are endemic. But the logic fails when you consider that in the 21st century: 1) people travel, 2) there is always the first case in an area, 3) the tick habitat is spreading rapidly in all directions, 4) changes in weather allow for ticks to move into areas previously inhospitable to them and remain active for longer periods, and 5) ticks can be transported. Cases of ticks on planes, in cargo, and baggage are common.

> PEARL: *The brown marmorated bug (stink bug) was accidently introduced into eastern Pennsylvania around 1998 after never having been seen on this continent previously. They are now EVERYWHERE, sneaking into your house as you come and go and falling into your hair as you open the door. So far they have not been reported in Indiana. On my last visit to Purdue, when I opened the trunk, three stink bugs fell onto the floor. I dutifully captured them with a tissue and put them into a jar and transported them 800 miles back to eastern PA. Trust me, bugs can be moved across 4 states in 12 hours by the most innocent of carriers.*

The CDC admits that their goal is to decrease the I&P of Lyme disease. They want to curb the Lyme epidemic. One clever way to do that is to not diagnose the majority of true positives. Unfortunately, even if the name is changed and it's next-to-impossible to get an "official" diagnosis, the same number of people will still be sick. If we don't diagnose even when the disease is clearly present, the I&P will obviously drop.

Where are the Lyme cases? Over the years, zones of Bb presence have extended far beyond the traditional Lyme areas. With globalization and weather changes, ticks are now spreading disease into places where 50 years ago they would have been unknown. TBI patients have been reported from every state and 6 continents. From Bulgaria to Japan, the I&P is climbing. Likewise, in North America, Lyme is no longer huddled around Lyme, CT. In the US, the pathogen causing Lyme is most often found in the northeast, west coast, and midwest, but its range is expanding rapidly. Ticks can't read maps.

Lyme is endemic in the northern hemisphere, especially in temperate climates, but is spreading both north and south. More cases are being reported from Central and South America. In some areas Europeans seem to have accepted and addressed the epidemiology around borreliosis more realistically than the US. Europe seems to have a different tick vector than the US with Bb being transmitted by Ixodes *ricinis*. Cases are now being reported in North Africa and Asia, especially Japan, China, Nepal, Thailand, and far eastern Russia. The disease is creeping and cases have been found in Kenya and Mongolia. Who knows how much we have missed and what the real I&P might be? The reporting of cases in Australia and elsewhere may be due to people travelling after tick bites or the ticks being transported in baggage or on clothing.

Cases have now been reported from all 50 states. In the 10 states where the disease is most common there were 31.6 cases/100,000 residents in 2005. About 99% of reported cases come from just 5 regions: New England, Mid-Atlantic, east-north-central, south Atlantic, and west north-central. (Huh? Anyone who thinks those geographic descriptions are clear is deluded. My interpretation is: The Pacific northwest around Washington state, the mid-California coastal area, the northern midwest including Michigan, Minnesota, and Wisconsin, the east coast from Maine to Virginia seeping south, and northwestern Pennsylvania and southwestern New York.) The disease has crept so well into Florida that Lyme is now considered pandemic there, although risk maps have not kept up with the reality.

Urbanization has been implicated in the spread of Lyme. Expansion of suburbs, deforestation of nearby wooded areas, and increased contact between humans and ticks all have contributed to the increased I&P of Lyme. The spread of humans resulted in the decrease in the number of predators that hunt deer as well as reservoir rodents. The more contact and interaction, the more disease transmission.

Whether STARI is a form of Lyme or its own entity, this disease appears to be spreading across the southern US. Overall, probably more than 40% have co-infections. I think that number is MUCH higher in certain geographic locations. I venture that in southeastern PA, solo pathogens are rare. In 2013, we can't know how many people have co-infections because we don't know how many have infections. We're lucky we catch one pathogen, let alone 2, or 3, or more.

LD is most often diagnosed between May and September since that is the active time for the nymphal stage of the tick. Spring and summer tend to have the most tick activity, since fall can be too hot and dry in some areas. Nonetheless, ticks can be active anytime the temperature is warm enough for them to move. Rarely, ticks have been known to mobilize even when the temperatures are below freezing.

There is controversy around whether an increase in the deer population actually is responsible for more Lyme cases. Some authors say that risk does not depend on the number of deer. They believe that if deer herds decrease, the ticks will just move onto rodents. Ron Hamlen and Doug Fearn, from LDASEPA, strongly disagree with this contention. Their work shows that increases in the deer population clearly correlates with an increase in the incidence of LD. The more ticks around that are carrying pathogens, then the more tick bites in both susceptible animals and humans, and ultimately the more disease.

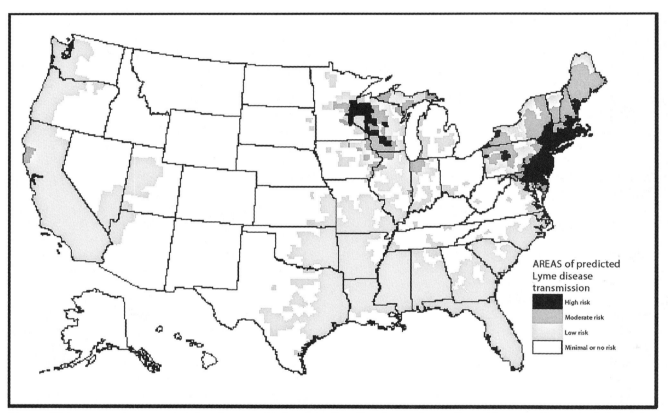

National Lyme disease risk map with four categories of risk
Source: CDC.
Accessed March 2013

Canine Lyme

What is a discourse on canine Lyme doing in the middle of the *Epidemiology* section of the human Lyme chapter? Well, just as we can learn from malaria and syphilis we can also gain insight from reviewing the patterns and distribution of canine Lyme. As I have mentioned repeatedly throughout this text, human HCPs can take a page from the veterinarian's handbook on how to manage borreliosis. Veterinarians appear to be a step ahead in a number of areas including making clinical diagnoses and using diagnostic techniques to support a diagnosis without letting the test result overrule the clinical presentation. Vets seem to be free to treat until the dog is better. They are tuned into co-infections and how these concurrent conditions can impact healing. They have embraced the idea that early treatment can prevent serious and often irreversible sequelae. They do not seem embroiled in a political debate with each case. Wouldn't it be nice to just help the patient? Since we share so much with our pets, including our backyard tick population, we should learn as much as we can from this common pet disease.

LD in dogs is now considered a serious disease that can be fatal if not promptly and effectively addressed. The idea of watchful waiting is passé. If there is a chance that a bitten dog is at risk of disease, treatment is initiated by a number of vets. Still the majority of infected dogs never show signs or symptoms. On necropsy, many more dogs show signs of LD than had displayed signs of illness. Most often, a Lyme synovitis is discovered even in cases where the animal was asymptomatic.

PEARL: Dogs are considered a **sentinel species** *for Lyme. Just like the proverbial canary in the coal mine, the disease is likely to be recognized in canines early-on in a certain area and, only later, does human disease become apparent. Dogs are closer to the tick population and are the first to get recognizable Lyme in an area. Some vets suspect that most dogs in an endemic area are exposed to Bb during their lifetime but only some present with sxs of disease. Hypothetically, some dogs may produce proportionally more antibodies than others.*

In those dogs that die from Lyme the causes are cardiac complications or renal failure, called Lyme nephritis. Just as in humans, dogs can display a number of neuropsychiatric problems due to Lyme. Since LD is now known to be more serious than was realized in the past, the goal is to treat sooner rather than later. Delayed or inadequate treatment can lead to chronic conditions.

Just as with human Bb, once you decide to treat: TREAT. Half-measures can do more harm than good. Most treatment failures are in dogs where the antibiotics were too little, too late. Minimum treatment duration is considered a month but most vets treat as long as the animal is symptomatic plus a cushion.

The earliest sign might be lameness. Just as joint pain can migrate in humans, the lameness seen in dogs can shift from leg to leg. He's probably NOT making this up. (I wonder if there is a Munchhausen by owner syndrome.) Joints can be swollen, warm, and painful. Gait can be stiff with a hunched back. The affected joint might be extremely sensitive to touch and the dog may cry out in pain. Muscles may spasm and rarely there will be the skin target lesion of an EM rash. As might be expected, these can be hard to spot under fur or hair. Appetite usually diminishes. Additional symptoms include lethargy, depression, irritability, fever, GI upset, lymphadenopathy, and neuropsychiatric problems. These NP manifestations can include seizures, vision problems, hypersensitivity, incoordination, anxiety, panic reactions, and compulsive behaviors like chewing fur or licking paws. Just

as with kids, the caretaker might complain, "He's just not himself." In later stages, dysrhythmias and kidney problems might present. Lyme can be fatal in dogs and people.

PEARL: As I was writing this I realized how ridiculous it would be for us to suggest to a dog that he was making up his migrating lameness. That's as ridiculous as suggesting that a 2-year-old is making up her Lyme symptoms.

Doxycycline is the DOC with amoxicillin the back-up option. Doxy is preferred since it might better hit co-infections as well. Common co-infections include ehrlichiosis and RMSF. Babesiosis has also been recognized as a co-infection. There are homeopathic and holistic vets who recommend immune support and there is a canine Lyme nosode made from dead pathogen. Massage and acupuncture have also been used to treat dogs with Lyme.

Canine Lyme vaccines are controversial. Many vets do not believe the benefits outweigh the risks. The canine Lyme immunization has been implicated in initiating a hard-to-treat form of LD in some dogs. There are many AEs associated with the vaccine. Further, protection appears to only last short-term.

PEARL: After my son got so sick, I dutifully scampered off to get my dog a Lyme immunization. Unlike humans, there is a canine vaccine. I didn't know any better and this was a labor of love. About 10 days after the dose he had incapacitating, migrating joint pain where he would pant and scream (if you've never heard a dog scream in pain run right out and get yours a Lyme vaccine) and a week later he had what can only be described as a canine panic attack: extreme anxiety, hysteria, frantic circling, racing, and panting. There were several repeat episodes. Can I say for sure that these symptoms were due to the Lyme vaccine? Of course not. But careful causality analysis as outlined in Chapter 23: Understanding Medicines *made me very suspicious. Believe me when I say NEVER AGAIN! I learned an important lesson from my poor dog. I will be VERY cautious if a human vaccine is ever developed. Note that discussions with Michael Spancake, DVM, has calmed me a little. He has used Lyme vaccines for several years and he believes that reactions like those my dog experienced are rare and may depend on the OSPs used in the formulation. Earlier versions may have presented more risk that those currently available.*

Although the I&P is not well-defined, LD is known in cats, small monkeys, pigs, chimps, other primates, and horses. In fact, every horse owner we know in Chester County, Pennsylvania, has at least one horse with Lyme. Most reservoir animals, in contrast, are infected without being diseased.

V. HISTORY

Lyme disease is named after the town of Lyme, Connecticut, where the first cases were recognized in the mid-1970s. While the connection to ticks was made early on, the pathogen was not identified until 1981 through the intense work of Willy Burgdorfer and the species bears his name. A similar disorder to what we now call Lyme had been described in Europe earlier in the 20th century. But this was by no means the start of borreliosis in humans.

Otzi, a 5300-year-old mummy found in the eastern Alps (where my grandfather was born), was found to have DNA from Bb co-mingled with his DNA. Otzi is now considered the first case of Lyme disease. Unlike many others, Otzi did not die of his LD. He was about 45-years-old when a flint arrowhead shot into his left shoulder likely finished him off. Not only was he the first case of Lyme, I submit he was the first case of chronic Lyme. Lyme has been controversial almost from the beginning and I can imagine some tribal shaman shouting at Otzi, "You do NOT have Lyme!"

Lyme might have been present in North America for thousands of years before we recognized it as such. As the settlers migrated from the northeast to the midwest, the ticks moseyed right along with them. One source that I could not confirm quotes a 17th century visitor to New England named John Josselyn, "…there be infinite number of ticks hanging upon the branches in summer time that will cleave to a man's garments and creep into his beeches eating themselves in a short time into the very flesh of a man." Not too long after these comments were written, the major forests were cut, leaving the ticks to congregate in isolated local pockets until more modern times. Which brings us to Lyme, Connecticut.

In the 1960s Polly Murray and her family began to experience mysterious symptoms that no doctor was able or willing to explain. By the late 60s, eight kids in the neighborhood had been diagnosed with juvenile rheumatoid arthritis (JRA). Several of the kids on the same street recalled being bitten by a tick. In the past doctors had reported that antibiotics had helped in similar cases when the patient also had what came to be called an EM rash.

At about this same time, nearby physicians started to notice a pattern of arthritis, headache, fever, and extreme fatigue in a subset of patients. But UNLIKE juvenile rheumatoid arthritis, these kids had headaches, severe fatigue, and no JRA markers. Treatment with antibiotics made the arthritis go away. Some of these kids also had Strep. They got well if treated early enough.

About this time rheumatologists "took over" the disease, since joint pain was usually part of the clinical presentation. Unfortunately the arthritic component was thought to be the whole of the disease and much early diagnosis was restricted to those who had joint manifestations, ignoring many of the other common signs and symptoms. Even the name "Lyme arthritis," which was used for years, served to limit the focus to joints and away from the various multisystem manifestations. During this period the dermatologists grabbed onto the EM rash and Lyme became a joint and skin disease. While arthralgias are relatively common in Lyme, EM rashes are less frequent. Nevertheless, politics required that the EM rash play a bigger role in diagnosis than the reality warranted.

The rheumatologists were still largely in control. Since the joint pain usually resolved with 10 days of treatment, they assumed that was all that mattered and so a 10-day course of antibiotics became the recommendation. Any residual symptoms were post-infectious and did not need longer treatment. But several practitioners were treating longer and getting better results.

Not to be outdone, the rheumatologists started treating with high dose steroids which certainly got rid of most symptoms QUICKLY, which is the beauty of steroids. Unfortunately steroids are the best suppressors of the immune system, which it turns out the patient might need in order to fight off infection. Suppressing the immune response in Lyme patients, just when they needed it most, set some of these patients up for a lifetime of disease and incapacity. Some of the sickest patients that remain today are a result of the immune suppression caused by the use of steroids in these early cases.

Although they were treating with antibiotics, a number of the rheumatologists were insisting that the causative organism was a virus. Even though antibiotics helped, and viruses are not impacted by antibiotics, an idea once stated seems to merit eternal protection despite evidence to the contrary. Enter Willy Burgdorfer.

Born in Switzerland and with a PhD from the University of Basel, Dr. Burgdorfer specialized in arthropods like spiders and ticks and how they transmit disease. His doctorate was in zoology, parasitology, and bacteriology and his thesis was written on the spirochete that causes African relapsing fever and its tick vector. He was especially interested in how efficient the tick vector was in transmitting spirochetes during feeding. He was also part of the research team that investigated Q fever. When the medical puzzle in Connecticut came around, Willy Burgdorfer was ready. While the relationship between the symptoms and tick bites had been made early on, (mostly because the neighborhood kids and Polly Murray made the association), the underlying pathogen had still not been discovered. Working at the Rocky Mountain Biological Laboratory, while investigating RMSF, Dr. Burgdorfer remembered much of what he had been reading over the past decades:

- Similar disease patterns had been reported in Europe in the 1880s and again in 1902 by Karl Herxheimer. (Remember that name.)

- In 1909, the Swede, Arvid Afzelius described a ring-like rash with expanding borders and clear center appearing on a woman after a bite from a sheep tick. He first called this lesion erythema chronica migrans. The name was later shortened to erythema migrans.

- By 1930, the rash was associated with CNS symptoms, especially meningitis and encephalitis, with the recognition that joints and skin were not the only organs involved.

- The French first started to recognize the neurologic components of the Lyme syndrome including radiculopathies and meningitis. Again a Swede, Sven Hellerstrom first connected the EM rash and the neurologic manifestations. By the 1950s, the tick-related syndrome was being treated with penicillin.

- Rudolph Scrimenti, a dermatologist in Wisconsin observed an EM rash in a patient. He remembered reading a paper by Hellerstrom and so he was able to think to treat the person with penicillin.

- By the time this Wisconsin case was recognized, the disease was nearly a hundred years old in Europe.

- In the mid-1970s Edgar Grunwaldt of Shelter Island off Long Island, New York, saw EM rashes on a number of his patients. He was the first to connect the rash to the tick bite and he recognized that antibiotics helped. Unfortunately, some of the rheumatologists busy treating these patients with high-dose steroids convinced him that the disease was self-curing so Grunwaldt stopped using antibiotics.

In 1982, Dr. Burgdorfer came across poorly staining, long, irregular, coiled microbes that looked like spirochetes. Since he was so familiar with the technical literature, he was able to make the 3-way connection between the ticks and the spirochetes and the disease. Burgdorfer isolated the spirochetes from patients with Lyme disease and confirmed that they were identical to those previously found in the ticks. He was able to show that Bb met all reasonable, defined conditions for causality and proved Bb to be a new species.

CONNECTION! EUREKA!

Willy Burgdorfer is an unassuming, right, jolly gentleman. Read his full history and you will be impressed. He deserves respect as a true scientist. By the way, Dr. Burgdorfer has commented that antibiotic treatment should continue in Lyme patients who remain sick since he believes those patients are still infected with spirochetes. Who better to know?

Finally, here was a pathogen that was known to respond to appropriate antibiotic therapy. In the meantime, astute practitioners were realizing this disease could affect almost any organ and that GI, cardiac, and especially neuropsychiatric problems were common manifestations. Almost all patients complained of extreme fatigue. Joe Burrascano found better outcomes when patients were treated for 6 weeks or more, rather than 10 days. Shorter regimens seemed to result in relapses in a substantial number of patients.

What was not initially recognized was that the pathogen was still present in these persistent cases. When conditions were ripe, the disease would again flare. By blasting with steroids early on, the immune system was suppressed and the spirochetes were able to proliferate and penetrate multiple organ systems. Recently, researchers at the University of California, Davis, found that Bb causes an unusual immune response in the host in some cases. While the body mounts a defense that should be adequate, in some patients this reaction is not STRONG enough to CLEAR the infection. The spirochetes remain and the patient is subject to persistent sxs and flares of the disease. When conditions are favorable, the pathogen will resurface.

When you only look at a multisystem disease through angry rheumatology or dermatology eyes, or restrict the viewpoint to any one specialty, you are going to miss something. Many people take their viewpoint as the perspective of the whole world and that approach is as unfortunate as it is inaccurate. In the case of Lyme, narrow-mindedness has been shown to be damaging.

Soon after the recognition of the pathogen, the history of Lyme became one of controversy and animosity. This on-going conflict is detailed in Chapter 11: *Controversies around Lyme*. The debates continue today. There has been much cherry-picking of the data and intractable positioning. Court orders were ignored as were very sick patients. Begging for help fell on deaf ears. HCPs who did not march in lock-step were targeted for reprisal. Cases that could have been treated early were allowed to progress until the syndrome became much harder to treat and some sequelae became permanent. Patients were stuck in the middle of warring factions. Fortunately, these same people began to talk to one another and strong advocacy groups formed.

PEARL: A few physicians began to say that persistent symptoms were a sham. Small children were accused of pretending to be sick because they were trying to please mothers who wanted to have sick children. How did these little kids manage to conspire to all get sick about the same time? And with a disease that seemed to look a lot like this new Lyme thing that had just started to be recognized? While most doctors had never heard of it, these 4-year-olds were so well versed that they could expertly fake the condition. Why would they scheme to fake such a miserable disease that kept them from playing or going outside? These little connivers were able to coordinate this massive plot against the medical establishment without any help from the Internet or instant messaging or tweets. Fortunately, they selected juvenile rheumatoid arthritis to mimic. Despite not getting JRA exactly right, these counterfeiters were actually quite sophisticated in their pretense. One physician said he wanted to narrow the gate of Lyme so that pretenders couldn't get in. Do you see how ridiculous these conspiracy theories were and are? One Lyme patient was told that her severe headaches were from smiling too much.

The history of Lyme continues to be written. When a chimp mauled a woman in New England, the story stayed in the headlines for years. When the woman had to have facial transplantation, she appeared on Oprah. Interestingly, both local and national veterinarians immediately and appropriately came to the animal's defense saying that his Lyme might have caused him to become aggressive. Yet when a young man in Arkansas shot several people, including himself, and his family said he had significant neuropsychiatric problems ever since he had been diagnosed with Lyme, the ivory tower guys rushed to the media to say that was not possible. One commentator scoffed that Lyme doesn't cause people to kill. The perpetrator had tried to get help but couldn't get the appropriate treatment. There are case reports where TBIs, especially Lyme, Bartonella, and M. *fermentans*, apparently cause or contribute to anxiety, panic, aggression, self-harm, and rage. I find it sad that we can find more compassion for the chimp than for the man, although both deserve our empathy.

The recognition of co-infections is a new chapter in Lyme history. While the presence of additional tick-borne pathogens has made the diagnosis and treatment of Lyme more complicated, their existence is beginning to explain some of the paradoxes we have been struggling to understand.

Even though I told my husband I would brain him if he brought me one more Lyme article, the headline of the *Wall Street Journal* on March 27, 2012 was "Ticks: They're Back Big-Time." Lyme is here to stay, or at least it will remain until we all start working together to eradicate it.

Pam Weintraub reviews the history of Lyme in much clearer detail in her book, *Cure Unknown*. As always, if you want a more comprehensive overview, I recommend reading her work.

As a fitting summation to this history of Lyme section, Ed Masters recognized early on the importance of a rational approach to these complicated diseases. In his book *Bull's Eye*, Jonathan Edlow quotes Masters on the recent history of Lyme saying that the "track record" of the "conventional wisdom" around LD is not very good. "First off, they said it was a new disease, which it wasn't. Then it was thought to be viral, but it isn't. Then it was thought that sero-negativity didn't exist, which it does. They thought it was easily treated by short-courses of antibiotics, which it sometimes isn't. Then it was only the Ixodes *dammini* tick, which we now know is not even a separate valid tick species. If you look throughout the history, almost every time a major dogmatic statement has been made about what we 'know' about this disease, it was subsequently proven wrong or underwent major modifications."

PEARL: I'm jealous. What has taken me hundreds of pages to say, Master's nailed in a paragraph.

VI. PHYSIOLOGY AND PATHOLOGY

Physiology is the study of the normal functions of the body. Pathophysiology is the study of the abnormal processes. When something is amiss with the physiology, you can end up with pathology. I knew that Bb was a complex organism with a highly evolved genetic code. I didn't realize just how complicated until I wrote this section. Multiple mechanisms can be in play simultaneously.

A. The physiology of persistence:

How does Bb survive despite the onslaught of defenses? Let me count the ways.

1. Bb have a complex **genetic** foundation.

   Bb are designed to survive. Of course, they are. We all are. But still, Bb appear to have evolved many tools to help it persist under all kinds of adverse circumstances. If one survival mechanism is not appropriate for the environmental conditions, Bb seem to have many alternatives. Bb persist.

   Barthold, when referring to genetics, said that Bb was the "trickiest, most diabolical microbe" that "can do incredibly complex things." He suggests that it's not the genome that is complex but what Bb can apparently do with the genome. He speaks of "evolutionary intelligence, consistently capable of creating persistent infection and evading host immunity. ..." He suggests that once infection becomes chronic not even the strongest immune system in combination with antibiotics could *guarantee* removal of all remnants of the Bb.

As proof of the persistence, Barthold's group grew the Bb in cultures, measured antibodies in serology, quantified Bb DNA on PCR, and grafted infected skin onto uninfected skin to cause disease in animal models. Even after what should have been effective treatment, most test animals were still PCR + for Bb. A treated mouse was able to transmit living spirochetes to uninfected ticks. Bb persist. Barthold believes that persistence is the norm for Bb.

Even after all signs pointed to cure, the host could become antibody positive again because the pathogen apparently had not been totally eliminated. If the Bb had been killed, an immune-competent host would have gotten rid of the damaged or dead pathogens.

There is considerable evidence that Bb are genetically designed to persist. Liegner reports on a patient who, after very aggressive treatment still had spirochetes cultured from her CSF at the CDC lab. Dog studies by Straubinger demonstrated that antibiotics prevented or cured lameness in 11/12 dogs studied. As they recovered, their antibody titers decreased. Necropsies were done on both treated and untreated dogs. Spirochete load decreased in all treated dogs, but they STILL had spirochetes present. Spirochetes were isolated from three treated dogs and all the untreated dogs. Follow-up studies confirmed the initial results and even though antibiotics decreased the spirochetal DNA in skin tissue by more than a factor of 1000, the spirochetes persisted. Spirochetes persist. Genetically based, they evolved to persist.

PEARL: Does the presence of treated dogs WITHOUT persistent Bb suggest that these cases were cured? Or simply that the methodology didn't always capture what was actually present? Since none of the untreated dogs were Bb-free, I suspect that the pathogen was eliminated in some of the treated animals. I believe that Lyme can be cured with the correct selection of antibiotics, for an adequate length of time. The HCP might need to be as persistent as the Bb.

Nonetheless, these persistent spirochetes are NOT immortal. If their ability to replicate is impeded, they will eventually die. Still, persistence explains the on-going *constitutional* sxs that chronic LD patients experience. Not the obvious, severe signs and symptoms of a flare, but the on-going inflammatory effects like the persistent fatigue and the "I just don't feel good" type sxs. Here again, when critical mass is reached after conditions are more favorable for the Bb, the more distinctive Lyme sxs can flare.

Bb genetics also seem to play a role in how Lyme affects various host organs. Different genes that result in distinct strains of the pathogen might result in alternate disease presentations. Some strains cause more joint problems, while others more often affect the skin or nervous system. The genetics of the strain might be involved in these varying manifestations.

Persistence is programmed into the spirochete in all its many forms. Genetically, Bb know how to free-float, transform into L-forms, encyst, and then reverse all these processes. No matter how bad my environment gets, I cannot form a cyst or change into an L-form. Genetics is the key. Maybe that's why Bb have flattened me so many times. This is what makes Bb so hard to treat.

So for those folks who brag that they were so hearty as to get well without treatment or who only needed a week of doxy to be completely cured, I say, "BE CAREFUL, my friend." Bb could be waiting to pounce in a month or a year – Bb persist. Even a preventive medicine specialist classmate of mine, now employed by the government, told me not to worry when my child was not getting better. After all Lyme was easy to fix with just a little doxy for 10 days. After all it worked for him. NINE TIMES!

The following lists provide some of the means by which Bb use genetics to avoid recognition and survive as well as theories on how Bb actually cause disease.

2. Bb impact the host's **immune system**.

   Remember, just because I list these many Bb activities as though they were separate, all or many of these processes are occurring concurrently. As noted in the work of Barthold and Straubinger, even healthy, intact immune systems have trouble managing Bb with all its tricks. So we would expect impaired or dysfunctional systems to be really vulnerable, especially if the Bb are assisting in the dismantling of the defense. Also, the adverse effects on the immune system seem to increase the longer the Bb are present.

   a. Immune **suppression**: Bb are able to mute the immune response through a number of known mechanisms. Borrelia are known to inactivate parts of the immune system such as decommissioning complement, invading certain white cells, and reducing a number of the host's defensive strategies. By using alterations in gene expression, pathogens like Bb have been shown to change the lymphocytes in terms of structure, function, and the number of subtypes. For example, both autism and Lyme have been associated with a change in the number of NK killer cells.

PEARL: If steroids are given in order to rapidly alleviate symptoms of Lyme, the host's immune system might be suppressed beyond any useful function. Avoid steroids in Lyme patients unless there are no other options in emergency situations. If steroids are critical as in the case of anaphylaxis, antibiotics should be on board ASAP. If possible, get antibiotics in place prior to the emergency steroid use. In non-emergent cases, patients usually LOVE the doctor who gives them steroids because they feel so good so fast – at least until the continued steroid nearly kills them, or they rebound from not weaning off the steroids slowly enough, or they puff up like a watermelon, or...

PEARL: In 2004, Embers et al published the article "Survival Strategies of Borrelia Burgdorferi, the etiologic agent of Lyme Disease" in the Journal of Microbes and Infection. Here the authors discuss the multiple strategies that Bb may employ to enhance survival. For example, Bb have been shown to impede the role of complement by using control proteins and inhibitory factors, thereby avoiding complement-mediated destruction. Bb somehow impact Factor H, which is a control protein involved in the alternative complement pathway, ensuring that the immune response targets the pathogen and not self-tissues. This ability may allow for complement resistance. Further, Bb recruit host proteins to their own cell surfaces so it is mistaken for self. This type of gene transposition or switching was first identified in B. hermsii, the etiologic agent of relapsing fever. In addition, Bb cause hyporesponsiveness of the immune system as seen by a decrease in levels of TNF-α and IFN-γ. Lymphocytes may be less open to the influence of IL-10, thereby increasing the host's susceptibility to Bb damage. For some reason, host antibodies seem able to kill Bb effectively in vitro but not so much in vivo. Theoretically, Bb are somehow impeding the process once inside the host. Bb tie up host antibodies by releasing soluble antigens. Potentially, these false antigens could affect the sensitivity of serologic testing. Phase variation might also contribute to evasion. Bb seemingly can turn their phenotype on and off. Bb are able to vary their phases in response to environmental clues. To orchestrate all these machinations, Bb possess plasmids that help the genotype change the phenotype which is then able to help the genotype survive. Bb may avoid recognition and capture using any or all of these methods. Some of these modalities are clearly evidenced while others are more speculative. Overall, the persistence and survivability of Bb are probably due to a number of these evasive techniques working in tandem. Bb seem to be able to fight back at every level to protect themselves.

PEARL within a PEARL: The genotype is the genetic code that is used to make the phenotype. The phenotype is the set of observable characteristics that are made using that code.

b. B. *burgdorferi* can invade and **kill cells** of the immune system. Most often this is accomplished by lysis of lymphocytes. On autopsies of brains from Lyme patients, MacDonald found spirochetes. Furthermore, Fallon reported lymphocytes and plasma cells throughout the brain tissue indicating a chronic and on-going process. He found inflammation of blood vessels, lesions of the white and grey matter, and cell death in the frontal lobes. Bb can incapacitate the very white cells that are trying to incapacitate them.

c. In those white cells that they do not kill, Bb can inhabit those cells and either diminish their function or use them for their own purposes. Bb can strip away a portal into the B cell, move inside, and burrow within to hide. OR...the Bb have been found to remove part of the B cell membrane and then wear the B cell as a cloak. Either way, the presenting proteins will now be recognized as *self* instead of what they really are: non-*self*. In antigenic "**cloaking**" the host protein is bound to the surface of the pathogen. Think of the invisibility cloak in the *Harry Potter* movies; different MOA but same premise. Likewise, for whatever reason, host proteins might attach to the surface of the spirochete making the pathogen seem like *self*.

d. Bb are thought to be able to **incorporate their gene sequences** into the host cell's genome, tricking the host into thinking that it is *self*. Alan MacDonald reported evidence that in some cases the DNA of the spirochete was combined with human chromosomes. He found hybrid DNA in areas of the brain of Alzheimer's patients where there are often plaques associated with the disease. These plaques may have had cysts in them. These "transfections" could theoretically be an autoimmune trigger. There are many hypothetical transfers of genetic material that could be in play here, but the important point is that Bb have very effective ways to protect themselves from harm.

PEARL: A few terms that may be useful when reading the TBI literature: Transduction is when an infecting pathogen transfers DNA from its protein coat to the host. Use of transduction may render some antibiotics ineffective. Conjugation refers to the passing of genes from one cell to another for mutual benefit.

e. The host seems to mount a different kind of immune defense against Bb than usually seen when combating other bacteria. With Bb the primary response may be from monocytes (macrophages in tissue) rather than the usually expected PMNs. While this may have nothing to do with Bb's survivability and persistence, it just might. We don't understand enough to do more than speculate. What we do know is that this monocytic response may have led us down many wrong paths, looking for things that were not there and drawing incorrect conclusions. My son was told he couldn't have Lyme because he didn't have enough neutrophils in his differential white count. Can natural selection work in favor of one species based on the inadequacies of another? Bb trick humans again.

f. **Antimicrobial tolerance:** Barthold believed that Bb behavior is different in the host before and after the humoral response kicks in. Those persistent Bb that have experienced the immune response are more refractory to antibiotics which usually only target the active, replicating organisms. This is called antimicrobial tolerance. Many pathogens use this mechanism in order to survive. This is not resistance but tolerance. Resistance is due to mutant microbes surviving an antibiotic onslaught, whereas tolerance is an entirely different phenomenon. Antimicrobial tolerance is the ability of a pathogen to resist damage by antibiotics (and host humors) by entering an existence of transient, dormant, non-division. These microbes are then termed **persisters**. They are not mutants, but dormants. By being in the inactive state they survive, whereas their genetically identical cousins are killed by the antimicrobial. The dormant state makes them insensitive or refractory (or tolerant) to antibiotics. When such persistent cells can't be eliminated by the immune system, they are effectively a reservoir from which recurrent infection can develop. As long as the dormant cells have the potential to reactivate into the free spirochete active form, they have the potential to cause the sxs of the disease. Persisters may be the primary cause of relapsing and chronic infections.

PEARL: Read the section just above on Antimicrobial tolerance *again.*

3. Bb probably form **biofilms**.

A biofilm is an aggregate of microorganisms in which cells adhere to one another and sometimes to a host surface. The underlying foundation is made of mucopolysaccharides. These microbes attach forming a bladder-like structure that may be protective of pathogens and allow nutrients and communication signals to pass. This shields the organisms from antibiotics and host immune response. Environmental triggers such as microbial crowding due to high cell density, nutrient depletion, and the introduction of antibiotics might promote biofilm formation. Like a small pathogen community, the biofilm separates the organism from the environment of the host. The pathogen uses the host's resources to build a structure or enclosure around its group. The biofilm provides protection and may even allow for communication between individuals. Biofilms are a way to contain and sequester the microorganisms all at the same time, providing a means to cooperate and interact chemically. The organization is complex and the pathogen takes full advantage of the resources available inside the host. Antibiotic regimens may need to be adjusted with higher spikes to be able to penetrate through the protective film. According to NIH, biofilm formation might be responsible for chronicity in persistent infections.

While there is strong suspicion that Bb form biofilms, which would explain much of their puzzling behavior, the field is too new to draw firm conclusions. Biofilms are frightening. They are very difficult to eradicate once formed. Finding ways to inhibit their formation would be the best option. Unfortunately, we don't know how to do that just yet.

4. Bb are able to **encyst**.

When present in a hostile environment, like when antibiotics are introduced, Bb can go into a cystic form. Here it can remain dormant until conditions are more favorable, like when the antibiotic is stopped or when the temperature or oxygen levels are more conducive to its survival. At that point, the cyst can revert back into the spirochete form

Cysts can help Bb survive and may be responsible for the organism's impressive ability to persist. Inside the cysts, the Bb encapsulate in thick-walled structures that more readily resist unfavorable conditions that would destroy free-floating spirochetes. When Alan MacDonald looked for spirochetes in cadavers he found all kinds of strange shapes and cystic structures. He hypothesized that these cysts protected the Bb when under stress.

And cysts do protect the organism. Cysts make it hard for most antibiotics and immune cells to get to the spirochete. Conventional treatments for Bb like PCNs and CSs do not kill the cystic form. Consider cyst-busters like Flagyl (metronidazole) or Tindamax (tinidazole) to penetrate the cyst capsule. Grapefruit seed extract is also thought to penetrate the cyst. Once the cyst is entered, the Bb can be damaged either by the cyst-buster itself or by the concomitant antibiotics that are able to get to the Bb after the cyst-buster breaks down the door. If the patient is chronically infected, consider metronidazole or tinidazole with one or two other antibiotics. This ensures that all Bb forms are targeted.

Bb are most likely in an L-form when inside the cyst and are thought to be temporarily dormant during that time. Bb will encyst for many of the same reasons that prompt biofilm formation. Once the "coast is clear" the cystic form converts back into the free spirochete. In the meantime, the Bb were safe inside the cyst when times were tough.

Some authorities do not believe in the cystic forms, although there is substantial evidence including images of the cysts. (Never let facts stand in the way of an opinion.) They think that the spirochetal form survives intact under adverse circumstances, even after long and strong antimicrobial treatment, making the cyst an unnecessary step.

When free spirochetes are put into cultures with poor nutrients, their metabolism becomes torpid and cysts form. When these cysts are then transferred to a culture with adequate medium, the thick walls dissolve and spirochetes emerge. A similar study transferred spirochetes to a culture without nutrients and 18 hours later 90% were cysts. Free-floating Bb have also been shown to transform into cysts under other adverse conditions like elevated temperature and increased oxidative stress (secondary to aging, injury, or disease). When mice are inoculated with Lyme cysts, the Bb convert to the spiral form within the mice. The longer the spirochetes had been in cystic form, the longer it takes for them to revert back to the spirochetal form.

PEARL: Eva Sapi's work has been invaluable in providing data demonstrating the various Bb life forms.

Not only must spirochetes form cysts for protection, they must also then be able to reverse the process. Evolutionarily, it serves no purpose if you protect your replicating form by encysting but then can't get back to that replicating form in order to produce offspring. Bb have been shown to do just that. Motile spiral forms have been recovered from tissues from animals inoculated only with cysts. When the Bb are no longer stressed by environmental factors like antibiotics, temperature extremes, or unfavorable oxygen levels, they can come back out again and resume replication, assuming the dormant condition or antibiotics didn't impede their reproductive ability.

Cysts explain a lot about the behavior of Bb and the clinical course of Lyme, such as persistent symptoms, relapses, flares, the need for prolonged antimicrobials

in some cases, and seronegative labs in clearly sick individuals. Theoretically, the Bb inside the cysts wouldn't be accessible to the immune system so they would not generate antibodies as expected if they were free-floating. Cysts provide one reason why a subset of patients have such a hard time getting well and why Lyme so often seems to smolder then explode, or wax and wane, or cycle, or flare.

5. Bb convert into **L-forms**.

    Bb display an altered morphology called L-forms. This version has no cell wall and are called cell wall deficient. Obviously antibiotics that work by harming the cell wall will not be effective against those pathogens that do not have such a wall. (I hate when textbook authors use the terms obviously, clearly, or simply because it is usually NOT obvious, clear, or simple to me, but just this once.) The Bb shed their cell walls to become less-identifiable L-forms. When encysted, the Bb are most often in the L-form in a dormant state.

6. Bb can go **dormant**.

    Dormancy is a time of metabolic slowdown. A survival strategy, dormancy allows an organism to move past a period of external stress. More than one process can be happening simultaneously. For example, Bb may be encysted, dormant, and in an L-form all at the same time. The terms dormant and latent are often used interchangeably.

PEARL: <u>Dormant</u>: Period of time in an organism's life cycle when growth, development, and activity are temporarily stopped. Metabolism slows and energy consumption is significantly reduced. A dormant state is closely associated with environmental conditions. The term dormant refers to the pathogen. <u>Latent</u>: The host is infected but the pathogen does not replicate or grow for a period of time. Latent refers to infection status and the host is asymptomatic during this interval.

7. Bb pursue **protective niches**.

    Some places are just safer for a spirochete than others. Especially secure places where Bb prefer to hide include: inside ligaments and tendons especially in joints, within the CNS, the eye, the GI tract, inside collagen in valves, or on the other side of the BBB.

    A number of factors contribute to what might make Bb gravitate to a specific locale. It's not like the Bb are making a pro and con list. Instead this is all biochemical. While debatable, Bb are thought to prefer areas with less oxygen so they tend to hide in tissue where there are lower levels. This might be tissue where blood flow is less than in other body parts such as joint spaces. If the temperature, viscosity, oxygen level, pH, blood flow, level of nutrients, and other pertinent factors are all perceived to be favorable, the Bb may congregate in that spot.

Once a good spot is located, spirochetes tend to be quite happy in their protective niche. They burrow in and set up a nice retreat. Bb may be encysted, dormant, in an L-form, and in a protected niche all at the same time.

Following the localized phase of infection, Bb may spread to multiple organs. Some sites such as joints, eyes, and the CNS are sometimes considered "immunologically privileged organs" because they contain extracellular fluids such as synovial fluid, vitreous humor, and CSF that do NOT circulate through conventional lymphatics. Sequestration of Bb in such sites, from a physical perspective, could make them less accessible to cells and molecules from the host's immune system.

One niche that is often overlooked is the lymph node. Tunev's group found that Bb migrate to lymph nodes within days of infection. In these patients, significant lymphadenopathy might be present. The body mounts what should be an adequate defense but apparently in some host mice, the response is not strong enough to completely clear the pathogen. Some Lyme patients have significant lymphadenopathy and others have enlargement to a lesser degree. Another subpopulation has barely palpable nodes. Does the degree of enlargement correlate with anything prognostic? Are the Bb free-floating spirochetes or L-forms when present in the nodes?

How well can antibiotics penetrate? Usually a lymph node is thought to be a filter where pathogens can be trapped waiting to meet their demise through the immune response. Perhaps those Bb that are not cleared by the immune response or antibiotics survive in some fashion, only to cause problems later.

8. Bb can hide **intracellularly**.

Bb are often extracellular, free-floating in the circulation. Yet when you try to isolate them, they are notoriously hard to recover. Why? Because, when they detect any unfavorable change in their environment they move into intracellular space to protect their chances of survival. Environmental triggers include changes in temperature, oxygen levels, pH, availability of nutrients, and exposure to antibiotics. The spirochetes can also convert into an L-form or go dormant while in the intracellular niche. HCPs will not be recovering much free-floating spirochete if the Bb are all hunkered down inside cells.

Bb can bind and burrow and hide inside a variety of cells. Common targets include endothelial cells, immune system cells, neurons, glial cells, blood cells, etc. In these safe places, both antibiotics and the host's defending cells have a hard time reaching them. Once sequestered inside a cell, the Bb are shielded from phagocytes and other marauders bent on doing them harm. The spirochete's own antigens are hidden inside the host cell preventing the immune cells from recognizing the Bb as an invader. Bb especially like to hang out in phagocytic vacuoles.

PEARL: There appears to be another advantage to the vacuole hide-away. The environment inside the vacuole is acidic with a low pH. Macrolides can penetrate into the cell but once there, are inactivated in this acid environment. Adding hydroxychloroquine (Plaquenil) seems to increase the pH and allow for more efficacy.

Bb have certain tissues where they especially like to hide. **Organotropism** is the special affinity of pathogens for particular tissues or organs. Bb have several that they really prefer. Whether due to O_2 levels, less blood flow, temperature, the presence of collagen, viscosity, or whatever Bb enjoy, they find good places to burrow and hide. Nerves, endothelial cells, joint spaces, collagen, GI tract, valves – time and again this is where we find them. From initial inoculation, Bb quickly disseminate from the skin into the circulation of blood and lymph and off to its favorite spots where the pathogens soon become intracellular. As much as I want to anthropomorphize and imagine Bb cruising around looking for nerve cells, this process, like all others here, are biochemical and the Bb end up where it is physiologically advantageous for them.

Collagen appears to provide Bb with a safe harbor, especially the collagen in joints, tendons ligaments, and in the valves and vessels in the heart. In mice, even when all signs suggested clinical cure, three months later spirochetes that had been hunkered down in collagen were recovered. This Bb remained infectious and researchers were able to transmit disease to others using these spirochetes. One theory is that there is some quality of collagen that can change the spirochete, making it less susceptible to antibiotics. Collagen is often in obscure locations and since it has no blood supply of its own, antibiotics and immune cells might have a hard time getting to the site of the pathogen. Barthold described Bb sequestration within collagen by non-dividing spirochetes in response to humoral immunity. Humoral response appears to be a critical component of host immunity against Bb and might serve as a signal to the pathogen to hide.

Willy Burgdorfer thought that borreliosis was a disease of the brain. He discovered that the best place to store spirochetes was in the brain of mice. He kept his Bb strains going by feeding brains of infected mice to the next generation."Spirochetes have an organic tropism for the brain that is consistent with the neuropsychiatric nature of patient complaints." Bb can have more than one favorite tissue. Maybe that idea helps explain the multisystem nature of the disease.

Why hang out floating along in the blood stream where you could be swallowed up at any moment by a phagocyte, or assaulted by an antibiotic? Instead you can be safe inside one of the host's cells. If you're hiding in a place where blood flow is low, like a joint or extremity, then fewer immune cells and less antibiotic are going to reach you. Another good place to burrow is brain tissue. Here antibiotics must cross the BBB and not all do. Higher doses of antibiotics may be required and the HCP needs to be careful to select antibiotics known to cross the BBB.

PEARL: Using just doxycycline or another solo agent may inspire the Bb to go intracellular. That's why a combination drug regimen is almost always a prudent choice. Then, if the Bb goes inside the cell, an antibiotic that can penetrate the cell will be there waiting.

Bb have been shown experimentally to penetrate human fibroblasts and live there intracellularly. Edlow demonstrated that when the extracellular milieu contained bacteriocidal levels of ceftriaxone (Rocephin), the Bb went intracellular. This strategy appeared to permit the spirochete to evade normal host defense mechanisms.

PEARL: Chronic infections are highly dependent on intracellular asylum as a mode of persistence. Intracellular pathogens are notoriously difficult to treat and cure.

Now here's the important point. The Bb are not trying to cause disease in the host. Bb do not understand the concept of disease. They are merely trying to survive and procreate. If their life processes get in the way of the normal physiology of the host they are completely unaware. Nevertheless, many of the mechanisms they use to survive inside the host are directly or indirectly the cause of signs and symptoms in the host. Therefore, the ability to go intracellular may be one mechanism by which Bb cause disease. Don't take it personally, although many times it feels that way.

Bb burrow into cells in order to hide, escape, and survive. Once inside the cell, the Bb interfere with normal cell function. How could they not? All of a sudden you have another creature living inside you and taking your resources and blocking chemical and electrical pathways. Bb bind and invade many cell types including endothelial cells, fibroblasts, macrophages, Kupffer cells (macrophages in the liver), and synovial cells. Intracellular survival within synovial cells has been documented for as long as 8 weeks. (A month longer than the maximum 30 day treatment approach endorsed by IDSA. Does that make physiologic sense?)

In a cardiac cell, the presence of the spirochete can interfere with heart function, especially conduction. In the brain, the Bb can reside in glial cells, neurons, and fibroblasts. Muscle pain and weakness can be due to Bb on the premises. Hiding in the bladder or GI tract seems to cause all kinds of problems that often go undiagnosed or misdiagnosed.

PEARL: Glial cells: The non-nerve or supporting tissue of the brain and spinal cord. Fibroblast: Any cell from which connective tissue is formed. Fibroblasts produce collagen, elastin, and reticular protein. Collagen: Strong, fibrous, insoluble protein found in connective tissue in such places as dermis, tendons, ligaments, non-enamel dental tissue, fascia, bone, and cartilage. Connective tissue: Tissue that supports and joins one part of the body to another. Ct has few cells and is comprised mostly of intracellular substance. Ct, except for cartilage, is highly vascular. Blood can be considered a Ct. Bone and cartilage are considered dense Ct.

Once intracellular, the Bb may do nothing, or their mere presence can cause significant dysfunction in the host. The types of signs and symptoms depend on where they settle. Bb in the CNS will cause a whole different clinical presentation than Bb in a joint or in a cardiac valve. Of course, Bb could be in only a few locations or many. Then, of course, this presence can trigger all sorts of secondary activity through initiation of the immune response with white cells coming to the rescue and the humoral cascade releasing all manner of biochemicals that can result in another set of signs and symptoms. Cascade indeed.

As always, remember that more than one process can be occurring at once. Bb may be encysted, dormant, in an L-form, intracellular, free-floating, and inside a protected niche, all at the same time. Intracellular dwelling, niche location, and alternate forms are all potent defense mechanisms.

9. *Bb have evasive mechanisms when **extracellular.***

While Bb often hide intracellularly, even when in extracellular spaces Bb seem to select those places that are safer than the general circulation. They prefer locations where there is less blood flow, like between skin cells. Again, there might not be great blood flow in these locales so antibiotics might have a harder time getting to the spirochete. Bb have it all figured out.

10. Bb have many modes of **resistance**.

First, the term resistance can be used in several contexts that might have nothing to do with one another. Resistance means opposition or putting up a fight. Again, I must refrain from anthropomorphizing, but Bb appear to use a number of strategies to counter the effects of the immune system and antibiotics. The end of Chapter 23: *Understanding Medicines* includes a list of some of the ways pathogens might fight back against harm. These modalities are all forms of resistance. Bb seem to have mastered them all.

One type of resistance is the kind where Bb do NOT happen to excel. This is the kind of resistance that the IDSA uses to argue that LD treatment should be delayed or suspended. They are worried that a certain organism will become resistant to an antibiotic and that drug will no longer be a useful part of the armamentarium against that pathogen. Here, the organism takes advantage of mutations to alter both its genotype and phenotype in order to make the antibiotic or antibody ineffective.

In a large colony of bacteria, antibodies or antibiotics can show up and wipe out most of the population. Certain individual microbes, which have sustained random mutations, might survive the attack. If they are not susceptible to the effect of the antibiotic or antibody for whatever reason, they will live on. Then after the challenge passes, if conditions are favorable, they can resume their reproductive life and make a new generation of resistant bacteria. Their progeny would inherit the mutated genes that allowed them to survive in the first place. Then, they too would be invulnerable when confronted by those same antibodies or antibiotics.

This is a population phenomenon that requires millions of individual cells to generate enough random mutations so that some mutated organisms will survive. Their mutated genes encode different proteins that change the phenotype of the organism. The new phenotype is not vulnerable to the antibody or antibiotic like its ancestors were. Likewise, its progeny will not be susceptible to the old challengers either.

The antibody no longer recognizes the mutated antigen on the cell wall and the Bb are no longer open to the actions of the antibiotic. This may take many generations. After making it through the initial assault, the survivors must live long enough to reproduce or their survival doesn't matter. This is a pure example of natural selection at work. The bacteria adapt to the environment that has eliminated all their siblings.

They were able to survive because mutations gave them an adaptive advantage over the other organisms that were wiped out. This is why it's important to take that next dose of antibiotic on time. Any of the vulnerable microbes who were not wiped out with the first dose should be eliminated on the second round (or third, or fourth, or as long as it takes to get through the reproductive cycle of the population). Perhaps, the survivors will not be able to reproduce sufficiently to repopulate the colony. If they do, the pathogen will live on and the disease will continue. This is one reason why a combination antibiotic approach might be prudent in treating Lyme. If antibiotics that act through different mechanisms are used, when the pathogen is able to dodge one antibiotic, perhaps the other will be able to step in and pick up the slack.

PEARL: Many organisms develop a rapid resistance to Rifampin, so this drug should never be used as a solo agent. There should always be a back-up antibiotic when rifamycin is used.

The best example of antibiotic resistance is seen in the massive quantities of antibiotics fed to millions of cattle (and other feed animals intended for human consumption) as a way to prevent infection in the food industry. When so much antibiotic is used, the only bacteria that can survive are those which have mutated their way out of susceptibility. All others are wiped out. When antibiotics are given to so many animals, they serve as mutation-testing-grounds. The only bacteria coming out the other end of this assembly line would be the mutants that survived the onslaught. When these survivors get out into other ecosystems, the antibiotics they were weaned on will not be useful in treating them. They will be "resistant" to those antibiotics. Bb do not appear to mount much of this "traditional" type of resistance even after very extended courses of antibiotics. Most Bb are still hit by doxy and amoxicillin and azithromycin and ceftriaxone, etcetera, assuming they are used correctly.

PEARL: There is considerable controversy around the mechanism by which microbes become resistant to antibiotics given to livestock. In addition to the survival-of-mutated-pathogen theory already described, there are a number of other hypotheses. Antibiotic is excreted in the urine of dosed animals. Microbes, such as E. coli, *in the soil are exposed and it is these pathogens that then become resistant. Yet another idea is that residual antibiotic in the meat is eaten and the consumer exposes her intestinal flora, which are then the microbes that become resistant. Clearly, there is no consensus around the underlying mechanism. The literature is even unsure about why antibiotics are given in the first place. Some say it is to prevent infection so that the animals don't die in their abysmal, over-crowded surroundings. Others say the antibiotics are to spur rapid growth. I cannot guess by which mechanism additional growth might occur, but farmers have long used antibiotics to fatten up pigs, chickens, and cattle. I guess if they are not sick, the logic follows that they can grow bigger, faster.*

Borrelia do use every other trick in the resistance handbook. A few of the resistance strategies known to be employed by Bb are reviewed below.

a. Bb mounts resistance to the host's **immune response.**

The resistance modalities described above include intracellular location, altered life forms, and protected body sites where the pathogens burrow into safe niches like brain, joints, and eyes. In conjunction with, or as the mechanism underlying those strategies, Bb use additional survival techniques.

i. Antigenic variation and mutation are a spirochete specialty. Bb are masters at changing non-*self* proteins to look like *self* proteins inside the host. Genetic mutations cause new surface proteins to be manufactured so that antibodies cannot recognize pathogens as non-*self*. This is one mechanism responsible for traditional resistance to antibiotics.

Genetic variability may also contribute to an organism's resistance to standard duration of antibiotic treatment. Antigen variation in LD and other diseases is believed to also contribute to resistance to normal immunologic functions such as antibody avoidance, complement evasion, and the lack of detection in diagnostic lab tests.

*PEARL: **Antigenic variation** is a change in surface antigens. **Antigenic variety** refers to distinct serological types, i.e., different strains. To be recognized as a separate strain, the surface antigens must be stable enough to be identified as members of that same strain. Among strains, each one had to have a stable Ag surface protein identifier to be recognized. Diversity at the genetic level of several Bb surface proteins has been detected among different strains.*

ii. Bb can alter **outer surface proteins (OSPs).**

OSPs are proteins located on the outside of the Bb cell. Genes that code for seven distinct OSPs on Bb have been recognized. These are all antigens that can inspire the production of specific antibodies. OspA and OspB are likely the most common, but OspC may be the most clinically significant. OSPs seem to be correlated with virulence.

Bb regulates the expression of antigenic molecules and limits exposure of such molecules on the spirochete's outer surface. In the case of OspC, spirochetes that do NOT express this surface antigen may be able to escape antibody-mediated selection for destruction.

Many OSP molecules are present, but only limited amounts are actually exposed on the outer membrane surface. One theory is that the majority of these proteins are actually subsurface and Bb have mechanisms for translocating the proteins from the cytoplasmic membrane to the outer surface membrane. The antigenicity of the spirochetal cell surface may be weakened by this limited exposure of antigens. All this might be influenced by the location of the spirochete within the host where the ability of the antibodies to penetrate certain tissues can be affected. (Why does Lyme have to be so complicated and the literature so conflicting?)

Bb are able to shift their OSPs making them unrecognizable to the host's immune system. This genetic shift allows for a new generation of spirochetes that aren't susceptible to identification by the antibodies that were made against the original OSPs. The antibodies were produced based on the information they discerned from the original proteins on the Bb.

When first available, those antibodies attacked the original Bb and the host felt the symptoms produced by that inflammatory response. When the antibodies and the rest of the immune system were eventually effective in defending the host, the person responded by feeling better. The fever and other signs of inflammation abated until a new batch of modified Bb appeared causing another immune response and another set of corresponding sxs. This would be perceived as a flare or relapse.

This shift in OSP composition is yet another defensive strategy used by Bb to avoid detection and destruction. The changes seem to be influenced by temperature and other environmental factors, but I believe that full understanding of what triggers and controls these shifts is a long way off. Care must be taken not to anthropomorphize. It's biochemistry, not conspiracy.

An early theory around OspA was that some Lyme patients had a gene for a molecule similar to the antibody made against the spirochetal protein OspA. These individuals were thought to be at higher risk for a severe, inflammatory version of Lyme including bad arthritis and intense neurologic sxs that could damage the myelin sheath protecting the nerves.

PEARL: OspA and OspB are believed to manifest early. OspC is thought to present up to a year later in those left untreated. The true sequence of events remains unclear.

Bb are quite adept at changing their protein coats constantly thus eluding the antibodies that destroy most other germs. As the individual makes antibodies against one set of Lyme proteins, the spirochete cloaks its outer surface with an entirely new set of proteins making it unrecognizable to the immune cells targeting it. So Bb turn into moving targets that can elude the immune system for months or years.

In the journal *Cell*, Norris describes the special segment of DNA in Bb that constantly churns out new gene sequences. These novel genes then direct the production of new proteins. As the proteins (antigens) change, the outer coats of the spirochetes change, making the immune molecules that might once have killed them impotent. Norris comments on "promiscuous recombination" that constructs a vast array of proteins at a rapid pace, potentially producing millions of antigenic variants in the host. Initially Norris believed that the process was random, but in 2006 he reported that the process likely responded to cues in the environment, thereby helping the spirochetes survive as they moved from place to place. The process seemed to increase or decrease with changing temperatures and acidity. The Bb don't necessarily change, but rather they accommodate the change. Bb appear to be able to take advantage of a number of steps in the pathway between a gene and the final outcome to influence the process. Why do Bb seem so much smarter than me?

PEARL: If in serology testing, the antibody from the patient is matched against test antigen that has significantly changed OSP, the odds of getting a positive test could be diminished. (Read: Darn near impossible.)

b. Bb can **resist** antibiotics.

Almost all the ways that Bb resist the immune system can also apply to their fight against antibiotics and vice versa. Resistance to antibiotics can be the type of resistance that one pathogen forms against an antibiotic through mutations, rendering that antibiotic ineffective in the future. One example of this is the *rapid* resistance mounted against Rifampin by many organisms. As detailed above, this type of resistance is the great fear of IDSA. Here, the pathogen mutates and the altered progeny are no longer hit by a particular antibiotic. In fact, Bb do not appear to mount much of this "traditional" type of resistance even after very extended courses of antibiotics. Bb have more tricks up their sleeves. Here are a few of the other ways that pathogens such as Bb "resist" the effect of antibiotics. Bb seem to have mastered most of these methods. The many types of resistance are detailed in Chapters 23 and 24.

i. Bb are slow. In fact, Bb are slow in several ways, all of which provide means to resist the effect of antibiotics.

- Borrelia have long interludes between active phases. Cell wall antibiotics are only effective during active replication. So treatment needs to continue through the longest inactive periods for these antibiotics to work. Microbes not dividing when these antibiotics are in circulation will survive. This detail could help explain why such long courses of antibiotic might be needed to curb a Bb infection. Of course, there are many other MOAs by which an antibiotic can flatten a pathogen aside from harming the cell wall. Bb probably has a way around those as well.

- Actual replication is slow for Bb. Unlike Strep and E. *coli* which can double their numbers in minutes, Bb can take 12 to 24 hours to replicate. In some cases the replication process appears somewhat sluggish. For example, spirochetes that survived antibiotic treatment in mice remained infectious but somehow changed. They had less of an ability to replicate. If they cannot easily replicate, they will be less likely to be impacted by antibiotics that depend on replication for efficacy. For example, ceftriaxone works by hitting the bacterial cells during division. If there is little or no division taking place, ceftriaxone isn't going to have a lot to do. In these cases, there may be just enough spirochete present to resurge another day but not enough to give positive antibody serology results. Further, there may be enough Bb active for low grade inflammatory sxs, but conditions might need to be more favorable before there is sufficient critical mass of Bb to flare.

- Bb are reluctant to grow in culture and overall seem slow metabolically, especially in certain life forms. Bb have a very long generation time with a minimum of 12 to 24 hours and possibly much longer. Some antibiotics are less effective if there is limited metabolic activity. Bb can be considered metabolically sluggish in some phases and can even go dormant, in which case antibiotics will have little effect. This is one reason why so few cultures come back positive.

ii. Bb may be able to kick certain antibiotics out of cells (like TCN and doxy) before the drugs can build up high enough concentrations to eliminate the infection. There are effusion pumps and other modalities at their disposal. Note that the chemical structure of tigecycline does NOT allow it to be pumped out of Bb cells like a number of other antibiotics.

iii. Bb likely enlists many other inherent mechanisms to protect itself and allow for its persistence and survival that we have not yet discovered.

11. Bb resistance may be facilitated by **human intervention**.

We may encourage the hiding of Bb in less accessible areas or their conversion into less vulnerable life forms. Antimicrobial doses that are too low may be sufficient to inspire cyst formation or burrowing of L-forms into safe harbors, while not being high enough to eradicate the spirochete. Too short a duration is a recipe for relapse. Using a single antimicrobial agent without back-up can eliminate one form of the Bb, but leave another untouched. In these scenarios "inadequate" may be just enough to send the pathogen into hiding either burrowing deep into hard-to-penetrate tissue, encysting into a protective L-form, or going dormant. Essentially we are taunting the spirochete with a taste of future harm and pulling back before any real consequences. No wonder they hide. They think we don't know what we're doing. We need to learn to be our own best friend, instead of aiding and abetting the enemy.

12. Bb take advantage of **barriers**.

While Bb are able to cross the placenta and BBB without any problem, many immune cells and antibiotics are held back. The Bb can lurk in tissues protected by these effective barriers. Their unimpeded presence can cause irreparable harm.

13. Bb may be able to **clone.**

Instead of reproducing sexually through exchange of genetic material with each parent contributing information, Bb are thought to occasionally clone. Cloning occurs when the circumstances make this reproductive method the most prudent. Here Bb make replicas of themselves. With complicated processes beyond the scope of this text, the cloning allows for certain mutations to propagate that might otherwise be lost in sexual reproduction (where the "normal" genes usually dominate the mutations). If the mutations involved genes coding for OspC, this occurrence could explain the differences in virulence and clinical presentation from strain to strain. The more invasive strains that may have originated from mutated clones were then capable of genetic exchange with others during sexual reproduction. Luft speculates that the altered structure of OspC is what allows some strains to more easily travel past the skin, burrow into the host, and cause disseminated Lyme disease. See, everything is related. Cloning simply enables more mutations to make it into the general gene pool.

B. Pathogenicity

Bb could not care less about causing disease in animals, although sometimes it seems like they are really out to get us. The organism is just trying to find a safe place to live and replicate. What we call diseases and take so personally are simply the side effects resulting from the organism's attempt to survive. Collateral damage. Many of the processes employed by Bb to survive and persist are the same ones that end up causing the signs and symptoms of LD.

How does Bb cause disease? Let me count the ways.

1. The **direct damage** to tissue can be due to the physical presence of the Bb

Early entry seems to hurt organs most. This initial harm may be due to direct injury to host tissue as the Bb invades cells, organs, and interstitial space. Cells usually don't like having aliens living inside them. This invasion causes disruption of normal processes, using resources that were meant for the maintenance of the host cell. Think of grown kids coming back home to live and eating all the groceries, using tons of energy, making noise, and generally disrupting the normal functions of the household from communication to garbage collection.

The Borrelia life cycle interferes with that of the host. Oblivious to the consequences of their actions, the mechanisms that they use to survive are directly or indirectly the cause of the signs and symptoms experienced by the Lyme patient. As an osteopath, I know one of the basic tenets is that if you disturb structure, you're going to pay with abnormal function. An invading spirochete disturbs the structural integrity of the cell.

Once inside the cell, the Bb interferes with normal cell function. Just taking up space, using resources, and eliminating waste will all have an impact on the normal function of the host cell. Chemical and electrical pathways can be blocked and fluid flow can be inhibited. Soon, the biochemistry will be altered.

Muscle pain and weakness can be due to Bb in the tissue. Hiding in the bladder or GI tract seems to cause all kinds of problems that often go undiagnosed or misdiagnosed.

The spirochete is believed to invade nerve tissue directly which can cause physical damage. Disruption of the white matter in the brain can then affect the grey matter. Neural connections are interrupted or blocked resulting in considerable neuropsychiatric dysfunction including problems with memory, thinking, judgment, emotional lability, and notable disturbance in cognition, coordination, and balance.

The spirochete itself can burrow into brain and nervous tissue which upsets whatever homeostasis was present prior to the invasion. Spirochetes have been isolated from the areas associated with specific symptoms. Bb can get into glial cells and fibroblasts in the brain and neurons. Alan MacDonald found spirochetes in the brains of Lyme patients and was able to associate the Bb with a number of possibly associated conditions.

In the heart, the physical presence of Bb can interfere with electrical conduction. Biofilms containing Bb on heart valves are thought to cause disruption of normal blood flow, decreasing the efficiency of the cardiac pump.

While the actual presence of spirochetes in tissue causes enough problems, this is just the beginning of the problem as the Bb are then responsible for interference with numerous metabolic processes as well as all the aftermath from the chemicals released from the immune response.

2. Impact on various **biochemical and metabolic processes**

   a. **Quinolinic acid** appears to be increased in Bb infection. This molecule is toxic and affects receptors associated with learning, memory, and synapse plasticity. While quinolinic acid is considered a neurotoxin, it is countered by **kynurenic acid** which is neuroprotective. **Tryptophan** is an amino acid that is primarily metabolized in this kynurenine pathway, which has a critical protective effect on neurons. Since tryptophan is a precursor for serotonin and low levels of serotonin are associated with depression, you can see where this is going. Tryptophan, pre-serotonin, is lower than expected in many infections including Lyme and low levels may be associated with depression, anxiety, panic, and OCD. This underlying serotonin pathophysiology might explain the depression often associated with Lyme.

   b. Further, pro-inflammatory cytokines associated with Bb infection can impact the normal pathways causing an imbalance of these biochemicals resulting in a number of other symptoms associated with Lyme and other TBIs. Theoretically, Lyme patients can have excessive **nitric oxide**. Intracellular NO and its metabolites can be toxic to mitochondria. That could explain why low energy and exhaustion are common in Lyme. Nitric acid also promotes inflammation, autoimmunity, and multisystem illness. Consider high NO levels in Lyme patients with a strong neurologic component to their disease. Treatments proposed to deal with high NO levels include CoQ 10, B12, α-lipoic acid, magnesium, and Vitamin D. And, of course, the elimination of the offending pathogen. You can consume all the Vitamin D Walmart has to offer, but if you don't control the causal infection, you won't get very far.

   c. In ways not yet clearly understood, Bb impacts **glutathione** metabolism. Glutathione is a peptide that acts as an antioxidant to protect cells from free radicals. Produced naturally in cells, glutathione neutralizes free radicals and keeps other antioxidants like Vitamins C and E active. This molecule can detoxify a number of foreign molecules and appears to be essential for full immune function. Glutathione helps to regulate immune response and is involved with both the cell-mediated and humoral responses and appears to help regulate apoptosis. The peptide is involved in the synthesis of DNA, proteins, and prostaglandins as well as amino acid transport and enzyme activation. Glutathione affects all body systems, especially the immune response, nervous system, GI tract, and lung. Bb may decrease glutathione levels, resulting in a diverse set of symptoms. In Lyme patients, low glutathione may be a contributor to brain fog.

    d. Lyme is known to impact the **endocrine** system, especially levels of cortisol and catecholamines (NE and epi) which are the primary stress and anxiety hormones. The imbalance of these chemicals is known to diminish healing in a number of conditions. This endocrine effect is thought to be modulated through the **hypothalamic-pituitary-adrenal axis** and would explain a number of the signs and symptoms of Lyme. A disturbance of the HPA is very hard to diagnose and treat, but if associated with Lyme or another TBI, appropriate management of the underlying infection can bring about considerable relief.

PEARL: While cortisol is mentioned repeatedly in this text, a much more likeable molecule is given short shrift, probably because the villain is usually considered more interesting than the saint. **Oxytocin** *is a hormone secreted primarily by the pituitary gland. Long known to be essential for various functions around reproduction and childbirth, oxytocin is now recognized as the nurturing and social hormone. Important for bonding, empathy, and reducing anxiety, oxytocin is sometimes referred to as the love hormone or the comfort chemical. Oxytocin contributes to friendship and contentment. Research has found that compassion causes the frontal lobes of the brain to light up and increases oxytocin levels. In contrast, low levels of oxytocin have been correlated with sociopathy, psychopathy, narcissism, and manipulation. In very stressed children, merely hearing their mother's voice increased oxytocin levels and decreased cortisol. This finding held for late teens and early adults as well as little kids.*

    e. Bb may reduce neurotransmitters or receptors in the CNS.

3. Bb causes disease by impacting the host's **immune system**.

    a. Bb can initiate disease by **suppressing** the immune response.

        While Bb suppression of the host's immune system is crucial for the spirochete's survival and persistence, this suppression can contribute to pathology in the host. Chronic Lyme is known to impede the immune response. The Bb spirochete is believed to affect all major cell types of the immune system, particularly the subset of natural killer cells labeled CD57. Just as in HIV infection, which lowers T cell counts, Lyme reduces natural killer cell numbers as measured by CD57. In Lyme, CD57 counts are sometimes used as a marker of the spirochete's vitality. When Lyme is active, the CD57 count can be diminished. The more active the Lyme, the lower the CD57, and presumably the sicker the patient. Since children make fewer natural killer cells, this measurement may not be as useful in kids as it might be in adults. The patient's clinical status should be included when assessing Lyme activity.

    b. Bb can cause disease through **activation** of an immune response.

        Bb causes the infected host to mount an immune response. The biochemistry of the many humors released as part of the immune cascade can result in a number of the signs and symptoms of Lyme. Certain of the biochemicals associated with aggressive immune response such as the various bad news cytokines (especially some of the interleukins) have been associated with specific manifestations of Lyme, notably the neuropsychiatric signs and symptoms. Fatigue and general malaise may both be increased due to the stimulation of the immune system. Several cells in the CNS are known to secrete IL-6 and TNF-α in the presence of Bb. Cytokine response has been associated with brain fog and cognitive impairment. These biochemical humors can be considered toxins from the host's perspective.

    c. The immune damage theory contends that permanent injury to the immune system is the reason for persistent symptoms in chronic Lyme. While Lyme certainly damages the immune system, in some ways irreversibly, there is overwhelming evidence that active spirochetes are what cause both flares and persistent sxs. Having ONLY the flawed immune system responsible for the waxing and waning of symptoms does not make physiologic sense. Are we to assume that the immune system goes haywire every so often without provocation, attacking us long after the infection is gone? Clearly the spirochetes may be harder to manage now that the immune system is no longer fully functional, but all science points to the presence of living pathogens. Especially since some patients cannot come off antibiotics without having a relapse. Even if the Bb infection initiated an autoimmune pattern in some chronic Lyme patients, that would not account for the symptom patterns or fluctuations in symptoms observed in some chronic Lyme cases.

PEARL: How does the immune damage theory explain cure? With diligent medical care, chronic Lyme patients do get well. Does the irrevocably injured immune system all of a sudden resurrect, Lazarus-like, in time to heal the patient? How does this theory account for relapses? Does the damaged immune system turn on and off? Over-reacting and under-reacting to account for the waxing and waning of the disease? That just doesn't make sense, medical or otherwise.

4. Bb probably release **toxins**.

Bb are hypothesized to produce neurotoxins. These biochemicals may be associated with encephalitis and all the myriad neuropsychiatric signs and symptoms that can present with LD. These toxins are believed to cause on-going inflammation, block hormone receptors, alter cytokine levels, and bring about hormone resistance. Perhaps the sicker the patient is with neuropsychiatric problems, the more neurotoxin is present. Toxins are thought to be stored in fat deposits where they persist. A toxin-binding regimen using cholestyramine has been proposed. When using a binding protocol, remember that good things like medicine, vitamins, and nutrients can also be bound.

Bb toxins are thought to have an affinity for lipids in the brain and NS and around joint cartilage. Toxins can affect neurotransmitters, cell membranes, receptors, enzymes, hormones, Ca channels, and even nucleic acids.

5. Molecular **mimicry**

The human genome is about 90% identical to that of bacteria. Because of this molecular mimicry, when the immune system is assaulted and goes on the offensive, it is understandable that some of the less discriminating defenders might mistake bacterial antigens for *self* antigens. An autoimmune reaction may result where *self* cells are misidentified as non-*self* and are mistakenly targeted for elimination.

Molecular mimicry means that the antigens on the cell walls of the Bb are similar enough to the antigens on the cell walls of the target tissue that antibodies mistake one for the other. For example, in rheumatic fever the target tissues are heart, joints, kidneys, valves, and brain. With PANDAS, the target is primarily nerve tissue. Lyme is thought to display a PANDAS-like syndrome due to antineuronal antibodies producing an autoimmune response from this type of molecular mimicry. This phenomenon may cause damage in other body systems infected with Lyme as well, but the mechanism has not yet been explored.

The autoimmune reaction that results can manifest either with general inflammatory sxs or a more specific presentation. Depending on *where* the host's cells are being mistaken for intruders could define the sxs observed. If cardiac cells are the target, heart problems might be seen. If the kidney cells are mistaken for foreign protein, renal conditions could manifest. If neurons are mimicking bacteria, they will be targeted by the immune response and neuropsychiatric sxs will predominate. The immune system can't go munching on neurons and nephrons without repercussions.

An **antineuronal antibody** is an antibody that attacks the nerve cells of the individual. This *self* destruction might account for some of the wide ranging and intense neuropsychiatric sxs associated with Lyme.

This autoimmune/molecular mimicry phenomenon has been well-described in some patients with remnants of Strep infections. When the body attacks it*self* the signs and symptoms can range from mild to fatal and appear general or specific. Overall, inflammation can seem out-of-control.

6. Autoimmunity

Autoimmunity can manifest for many reasons, only one of which is the molecular mimicry mentioned above. Other explanations include genetics or repeated insults to the immune mechanisms, such as vaccine overload, that might result in a cycle of dysfunction manifesting as autoimmunity.

In autoimmunity, the immune system seems no longer able to distinguish between *self* and non-*self* so healthy tissue could be inadvertently damaged. Under normal conditions, special cells in the thymus and bone marrow educate young lymphocytes and eliminate those that attack *self* antigens in an attempt to avert autoimmunity.

In some patients, Bb appear to be capable of causing a long-term, destructive inflammatory response which is a type of autoimmune condition. Certain patients, especially those with HLA-DR2 and HLA-DR4 markers, can have a tendency toward an autoimmune response to Bb. These patients can appear sicker and achier than those without these specific markers.

In autoimmune responses, the T cell activates the B cell without interruption. The stimuli are continuous whether due to on-going infection or other reasons. Nothing is shutting down. Here persistent Bb infection keeps triggering the immune response. Some keep looking for the autoimmune trigger in Lyme disease and can't find it. The spirochete itself is the likely trigger.

Patients with an autoimmune component to their pathology often are misdiagnosed for years and many are told that their problems are all in their head. Here is a good place to consider the multiple cascades of the immune system and how they may be contributing to what is observed clinically. Autoimmune-complicated Lyme can be especially hard to treat. These patients can be helped by using alternative regimens to address their disease. Adding hydroxychloroquine (Plaquenil) to the treatment seems to help.

7. Bb are able to execute a **rapid dissemination** of pathogens. A spirochetemia develops. The Bb then invade the local endothelium where they cause a low grade disseminated intravascular coagulation and thrombocytopenia. Within the CNS, spirochetes can be found as early as 12 hours after the tick has transmitted the pathogen. This is one reason why the earlier the treatment the better, without halfway measures like low dosing or solo agents. Regimens that include antibiotics that hit both the free-floating spirochete and the intracellular organisms are more prudent. Doses should provide the concentrations necessary to hit the Bb where they live. The more time that passes before treatment is initiated, the more aggressive the treatment will need to be. Better to try to hit hard early, before the pathogens can entrench in multiple forms and disseminate to tissues where they will be hard to pursue.

8. Pathogens like those that cause syphilis and Lyme can **cross barriers** such as the placenta and the BBB. In both the fetus and CNS, these microbes can cause direct physical damage as well as harm from the harsh biochemicals released from the triggered immune response. Not to mention Bb's own toxins. For example, microglia release cytokines, free radicals, and trophic (hormone stimulating) factors that change dendrite length and density, alter dopamine producing cells, impede new neuron formation, stop proliferation of glial cells, and diminish normal white matter function. All this pathophysiology can adversely impact emotional stability, clear thinking, and cognition. Across the placenta, Bb can cause a myriad of devastating problems for the fetus as outlined in Chapter 30.

9. Chronic infection with Bb is thought to increase **oxidative stress**, inflammation, and **mitochondrial dysfunction**. The impact on the energy-making capacity of the mitochondria might explain the debilitating fatigue experienced by so many Lyme patients. Kids experience many of the same pathologic effects as adults with Bb infection, but since many of their organ systems are still developing, the repercussions may be more clinically significant, irreversible, and disabling.

10. Theoretically **cysts** might be especially important in neuropsychiatric pathophysiology. Cysts are one good rationale for why Lyme manifestations wax, wane, flare, relapse and cycle. Cysts explain a lot.

11. Luft hypothesized that the alterable structure of **OspC** is what allows Bb to travel past the skin, burrow into the host, and cause disseminated Lyme disease. Luft thought that just a few of the many Bb strains cause disseminated infection. Likewise, only some of the strains that show a rash can cause invasive disease. Most cannot. Different strains may present very differently in terms of signs and symptoms and clinical course. Some don't cause disease much beyond the rash. I am always asking and wondering what is different about those patients who get the rash and those who do not. Maybe the difference is not with the patient, maybe it's with the strain of pathogen. That would help explain the many faces of Lyme.

We do know that Lyme manifestations can differ from person to person and even within a person. Different strains might be responsible for these distinctions. In each region there can be a different mix of strains. This could be another reason why so many tests are negative and why the symptom patterns are so confounding.

12. Bb get into the **endothelial** cells. Bb invade lots of cells, but the endothelium is especially important. Endothelial cells are the thin layer of cells that line the surface of ALL the blood and lymph vessels. So endothelium is everywhere, from the heart to the smallest terminal capillary. If you want to disseminate, get into the endothelium. Inside the heart, the endothelium is called the endocardium. From the endothelium, the Bb have access to EVERYTHING and this presence helps us understand the multisystemic nature of Lyme disease.

13. Bb may alter the number of **astrocytes.** Astrocytes are also called astroglia since they are the star-shaped glial cells of the brain and spinal cord. They provide biochemical support for the endothelial cells that form the BBB. They also supply nutrients to nervous tissue, stabilize extracellular ion balance, repair brain tissue after injury, release neurotransmitters, facilitate calcium communication channels, and signal neurons. Messing with astrocytes, the Bb are going to cause some kind of trouble.

14. Tunev et al found that Bb **migrate** to lymph nodes within days of infection and this may explain why some people suffer from relapses. Some Lyme patients have significant lymphadenopathy while others have enlargement to a lesser degree. Another subpopulation has barely palpable nodes. Is the degree of lymphadenopathy a harbinger of persistent symptoms or future flares?

C. Lessons from Bb pathophysiology

A number of lessons can be learned from the interminable section above. (If you think it took you forever to read it, think how long it took for me to write. I never thought I'd finish and I had a dozen people asking daily, "Is it done yet?" NO!) Any number of combinations, computations, or permutations of the above factors can be in play at once. Here are the salient points to remember about Bb pathophysiology.

1. Lyme is a multisystem disease.

2. Various strains may make symptoms involving one organ system predominant over others.

3. The physiologic nature of the beast is that some strains of Bb might not respond to short-term antimicrobial regimens. Long-term or open-ended treatment will likely be needed in these cases.

4. While most bacterial infections appear to mount a neutrophil (PMN) defense, Lyme seems to rely on monocytic action, including those monocytes that reside in tissue as macrophages. We may need to adjust our thinking about how the body responds to Bb infection.

5. Co-infections can alter the physiology of Bb and therefore impact diagnosis, clinical course, and treatment.

6. We probably do not recognize more than the tip of the iceberg concerning the physiology around Bb persistence and pathogenicity.

7. Actions taken by Bb to further its chance of survival are often responsible for the signs and symptoms of disease in the host.

8. Bb infection does not appear to confer immunity against subsequent infection.

9. Amazingly, most of the controversies around Lyme can be resolved by looking at the pathophysiology of Bb. This all makes sense if you let it. That doesn't mean it's simple or easy medicine. We still are in the early phase of information-gathering around this pathogen.

10. Each case of Lyme is unique to that individual at a given point in time. My Lyme can be quite different from your Lyme. My Lyme today may present quite a different clinical picture from my Lyme in the past or in the future. This is especially true if I have been reinfected by a different strain of Bb.

11. Here is a practical example of how mulling over the pathophysiology of Bb can lead to real-world applications. Taking all the above information and more into consideration, there are many reasons why someone could have a false negative Lyme test.

   a. Sample drawn before immune response measurable

   b. Antibodies are incorporated into immune complexes

   c. Spirochetes are protected by host tissue, e.g., lymphocytic cell walls.

   d. Spirochetes burrow deep into cells, e.g., fibroblasts, neurons, etc.

   e. Bb are found in blebs in body fluid so no whole organisms are available in test sample. (Blebs are fluid-filled sacs.)

   f. Few or no spirochetes or protein in the sample fluid on the day of a direct detection test

   g. Genetic heterogeneity (Many strains are known and we likely have only begun to count.)

   h. Antigenic variability

   i. Surface antigens can change with temperature, such as that found in a high fever.

   j. Bb use host proteases instead of their own proteases.

   k. Spirochetes are in dormant phase (L-form) with no cell walls.

   l. Recent antibiotic treatment

   m. Recent anti-inflammatory treatment

   n. Co-infection with Babesia may suppress immune response

   o. Immunosuppression or immune deficiency

   p. Lab with poor technique

   q. Lab tests not set up to detect late stage disease

r. Lab tests conducted for investigational use only

s. CDC surveillance criteria not compatible with making diagnoses

t. Lack of standardized control

u. Using only one or a few strains as a reference when others may be involved

v. Encapsulation by S layer glycoprotein which impairs recognition

w. S layer binds to IgM

x. Down regulation of immune system by cytokines

y. WB criteria fails to include most specific Bb bands.

PEARL: An S layer is a surface layer that is part of the covering of a cell made of glycoproteins that provides protection, stabilization, and resistance to adverse environmental conditions like changes in pH. This layer can differ considerably even in those strains that are closely related.

Clearly, the full scope of the pathophysiology of Bb are not yet known. Many of the pieces of the puzzle are still missing and someone will need to put this all together as a cohesive theory. Dr. Burgdorfer, are you busy?

I believe it is safe to say that multiple processes are in play and the presentation in a particular individual may depend on which process is leading the parade on any given day. The diverse and complicated pathology confounds the diagnosis and treatment of Lyme.

PEARL: Run, screaming, from any HCP who believes Lyme is a simple disease that can be managed identically in all cases. Run especially fast when you hear, "It's only Lyme,"... "It's just Lyme,"... "I don't know what it is, but it's not Lyme."...

While Lyme may be straightforward in some cases, the multi-faceted pathophysiology does not lend itself either to cookie-cutter medicine or to a one-size-fits-all approach. Despite all this verbiage about how resilient and tough Bb are, Lyme disease is curable, even in cases previously considered hopeless.

VII. SYPHILIS: Lessons from a similar pathogen

Just as we can learn from studying malaria when we want to understand babesiosis, we can similarly gain insight from studying syphilis when we want to better appreciate the complexity of Lyme.

Syphilis is a multisystem disease caused by the spirochete Treponema *pallidum*. Untreated, syphilis is progressive and can result in on-going infection, chronic inflammation, and permanent sequelae, even death.

A string of PEARLs to help put this comparison in perspective:

PEARL: Just like Lyme, syphilis is an ancient spirochetal disease, plaguing humans for millennia.

PEARL: Syphilis has many aliases. Just like Lyme, both are associated with the geographic locations where they are thought to have originated: Lyme, Connecticut, for Bb and France for syphilis. Neither of these places is the actual starting point, but it makes interesting history. (For the record, the Dutch called syphilis the Spanish disease and the Russians called it the Polish disease, and the Turks called it the Christian disease, and the Tahitians called it the British disease. New world verses old world. East versus west. You get the idea. Everybody pointing a finger - or other body part - at everyone but themselves.)

PEARL: Both diseases are mimics and are routinely mistaken for other conditions. Both have been referred to as the great imitator since misdiagnosis has historically been commonplace.

PEARL: Both diseases are multisystem. Hardly any organ is unscathed from the immune system to the skin to the joints to the heart to the nervous system and most things in between.

PEARL: Diagnostic testing is currently much more reliable in syphilis than in borreliosis.

PEARL: There was a big backlash against Paul Ehrlich as he identified cures for syphilis. In this case, several powerful church organizations opposed treating syphilis because they felt that people would have more sex. In fact, syphilis was deemed an appropriate punishment for having sex at all. I wouldn't believe these outlandish attitudes existed until I turned on the TV and heard certain political candidates saying these very same things a century later. Even today there seems to be a similar attitude against Lyme patients, as if it were somehow immoral to have this disease and they should be punished by withholding treatment.

PEARL: Latent periods with both pathogens can last months or years. This latency can occur before initial sxs appear or between bouts of active disease.

PEARL: Chronic syphilis may have periods of latency alternating with periods of active disease. Failure to eradicate syphilis in some cases, despite what is considered adequate treatment, is well-known.

PEARL: Each of these illnesses has multistage clinical courses which can include acute, disseminated, latent, early, late, and chronic phases. The names of the stages may differ, but the concept is the same.

PEARL: Both can be transmitted gestationally. Gestational transmission can cause severe problems in the neonate. On May 6, 2010, USA Today reported that one baby is born in China every hour with congenital syphilis.

PEARL: Syphilis was once the most common cause of adverse outcomes in pregnancy. We do not want Lyme to assume that dubious honor.

PEARL: Lyme seems to be more genetically and environmentally influenced in terms of severity and clinical course than syphilis.

PEARL: I have to look up how to spell syphilis EVERY time. I have to look up how to spell borreliosis EVERY time. So, they must have important parallels. I think my brain's insistence on two Ls is the problem. Of course, I have to look up parallel EVERY time as well. With that kind of clear logic, I should run for president.

PEARL: Both wreck havoc on the brain. Spirochetes seem to love neurons and surrounding tissue.

PEARL within a PEARL: Tabes dorsalis is a slowly-progressing degeneration of the spinal cord that occurs in tertiary syphilis a decade or more after initial infection. Pathophysiology might include sclerosis of the posterior column of the spinal cord. Sxs include lightening-like pain, lack of coordination, ataxia (wobbliness), dysfunction of optic nerves, instability when eyes closed, staggering gait, incontinence, loss of position sense, and degeneration of joints. Sound familiar? See what spirochetes can do?

PEARL: Both organisms seem to be able to cause sxs directly and indirectly.

PEARL: Both significantly impact the immune system which has a hard time handling them, especially without antibiotics. Both T. pallidum and Bb seem able to elude the immune system in their attempts to survive the onslaught of the host's defenses. After all my research, I would be hard pressed to name a pathogen that does it better than Bb.

PEARL: Currently, syphilis succumbs to antimicrobial treatment much more readily than does Lyme. But this was not always the case. See the next PEARL.

PEARL: Both of these spirochetes are slow dividers. In the 1940s, doctors were stumped by the fact that a short-course of PCN did not always cure syphilis. They assumed that the syphilis was resistant to the PCN. In fact, the T. pallidum was just a slow divider. PCN works by preventing cell wall synthesis, but ONLY in actively dividing cells. So it could only work when the spirochete was dividing. The PCN needed to be at sufficient dose during the ENTIRE replication cycle or the organisms would survive the treatment. The cycle takes at least 12 hours and probably more. So if the concentration of the PCN was below that needed to be effective during the replication period, the bug would live and the infection would continue. Science is based on looking for patterns. You'd think that when we saw these patterns in syphilis, we would logically apply that knowledge to a similar spirochete, Bb.

PEARL: Just as with Lyme, there are cases where the syphilis spirochete is merely suppressed and becomes latent and may not resurface again for years. A cure is assumed when that is, in fact, not the case. Likewise, there is evidence that sometimes antibiotics used for Lyme merely suppress the spirochete but do not eradicate the infection. Further, chronic syphilis may have periods of latency alternating with periods of active disease. This supports the contention that the T. pallidum was simply suppressed rather than eradicated. This outcome was noted despite adequate, presumably effective, treatment. Similar findings have been observed with Bb. Fallon, Schmid, Jacobs, Tierney, and others have all reinforced this point.

PEARL: Both microbes appear to be capable of sexual transmission, although with syphilis intimate contact is the primary conveyor and with borreliosis sexual transmission is thought to be rare. Since syphilis is most often transmitted through sexual intercourse it also has the names Cupid's pox or Lues disease. (My understanding is that Lues means something sexual in French.) Despite the sexual implications, carbon dated skeletons of many medieval monks show syphilitic bone lesions. Pompeii is filled with evidence of syphilis.

PEARL: The history of both diseases has been rife with controversy.

PEARL: While diagnostic false positives are rare in Lyme, false positives can occur when testing for syphilis in the presence of certain viruses.

PEARL: Co-infections can complicate both syphilis and Lyme.

PEARL: Syphilis can have more definitive physical findings and diagnostic test results than Lyme. So it is easier to proclaim, "This patient has syphilis," than "This patient has Lyme." Still, the pioneering physician William Osler didn't pronounce syphilis the great imitator for nothing.

As with Lyme, distinguishing physical manifestations do not appear in all patients all the time.

PEARL: The diagnosis and treatment of both diseases have been subject to political machinations. Today most people agree that treating syphilis is a good idea, while the controversy around Lyme treatment still rages.

PEARL: In the 21st century, treatment for syphilis is usually short-term and effective. In contrast, a significant sub-population of Lyme patients need protracted treatment. Of course, we have been learning about syphilis a lot longer.

PEARL: The list of famous syphilitics include Hitler, Mussolini, Ivan the Terrible, Maupassant, Nietzsche, Al Capone, Manet, Gauguin, Edward Rochester's wife in Jane Eyre, Sydney Carton in A Tale of Two Cities, Napoleon, Keats, Pickfords and Barrymores, Van Gogh, Oscar Wilde, Toulouse-Lautrec, Winston Churchill's dad, Rembrandt, Scott Joplin, Schubert, Paganini, Schuman, Tolstoy, and Lenin. Lyme has George W. Bush.

PEARL: Neither can be contracted from toilet seats. (Although, in some cases, that might be a more appealing method.)

PEARL: Pathogens like those that cause syphilis and Lyme can cross the placenta and the BBB. In both the fetus and CNS, these microbes can cause both direct physical damage as well as harm from the harsh biochemicals released from the immune response. Not to mention the possibility of their own toxins.

PEARL: Just like the Treponema pallidum that causes syphilis, Bb can have many forms: rods, coils, hooks, clumps, granules, and cysts. When Alan MacDonald found these alternative forms, he was told he was looking at artifact even though another spirochete clearly presented in the same way.

PEARL: Until the pathophysiology was better understood syphilis was often treated with remedies like mercury that were often more horrible and deadly than the disease. Of course, if it weren't for the arsenic cure, we wouldn't have War and Peace today.

PEARL: Both syphilis and borreliosis can be fatal.

PEARL: Both spirochetes can cause skin manifestations.

PEARL: Bb seem to be more genetically flexible and adaptable that T. pallidum with more genes and plasmids.

PEARL: Both sets of patients can have significant Herx reactions at the onset of effective antibiotic therapy.

PEARL: Both sets of patients have been subject to unconscionable treatment by the medical establishment. Think about the Tuskegee syphilis study and the rulings against the IDSA in Connecticut. In the Tuskegee study patients were deliberately not treated for syphilis allowing the disease to get so bad that the men had permanent sequelae and even fatal outcomes. The disease was permitted to go into the late stages. The study administrators knew that the men needed treatment but still they withheld any help. A number of wives were infected and, in turn, children were born with congenital syphilis. Withheld treatment. When they knew it was needed. Sound familiar? Despicable. Disgraceful. Shameful.

PEARL: Prevention is the key in both cases.

PEARL: Really understanding the pathophysiology of syphilis could have spared suffering in the Lyme community. But only if we were willing to learn from past misjudgments. We weren't. We didn't. We suffered.

The old saying "To know syphilis is to know all of medicine," can be said of Lyme disease as well.

VIII.   CLINICAL COURSE

In the process of writing this book, I have come across a great deal of what can only be politely termed as malarkey. Nowhere in researching Lyme is the nonsense and misinformation more evident than when sources are trying to describe the clinical course of LD. When authors try to force Lyme into certain prescribed and rigid paradigms, something is either going to be left out or jammed in. Especially when patients are excluded from the elite Lyme club because they don't quite fit, significant harm can be done.

Even though some of the following terms have been shown to be misleading and frankly incorrect, here are a few labels placed on the various manifestations of Lyme in an attempt to define the clinical course: early, late, mid-course, disseminated, localized, chronic, latent, dormant, major, minor, moderate, Stage I, II, III, IV, on-going, persistent, post-Lyme, after-Lyme, life-long, terminal, acute, pre-acute, unsupported, typical (HA!), atypical, traditional, classic, variant, intractable, recalcitrant, unrelenting, waxing, waning, flaring, Herxing, remitting, psychogenic, pre-Lyme, permanent, active, inactive, gestational, congenital, prodromal, false, European, Mexican, intensive, co-morbid, uncontrolled, pretend, asymptomatic, exposed, and interrupted. (What do you think interrupted Lyme might be? Beats me.)

When these terms are used in combination such as in the sentence, "He has late, disseminated, Stage III, minor, migrating Lyme," one can quickly stop being a nice person and turn into a frenetic shrew. One individual told me that his HCP explained that this was the type of Lyme he had, but not to worry. His disease wasn't serious since he only fell into the minor category overall. He died.

Categories should be used to help clarify and organize in a way that allows all players to understand what is being discussed, not to minimize the extent of the problem. Don't be fooled by misnomers. Minor can move to terminal while you stand reading the score card.

In the literature, some classification schemes are thrown about as though the whole world knows what the author is referencing. Only later you learn the guy made the whole thing up himself. As of 2013, I know of no universally accepted staging or categorization that outlines the clinical course of Lyme. Still we need some way to manage this enormous amount of fact, opinion, and misinformation. At least then the HCP and caretaker might be able to get an idea of where they stand.

*PEARL: The **natural history** of an organism takes into consideration how its life normally progresses. The natural history encompasses the creature's life cycle including such things as development, metabolism, behavior, physiology, reproduction, interactions, death, etc. In fact, the term life cycle is almost a synonym for natural history. In turn, the natural history can determine how that organism might cause disease in a host and thereby influence the clinical course of an illness. The **clinical course** is how a pathogen affects a host from exposure, to infection, to symptoms, to signs, to damage, to resolution, to sequelae, to demise. We use what is known about the natural history of a pathogen to **predict** how it might behave inside a host. The best predictor of future behavior is past behavior. Therefore the course is predicated on what we know about how the organism has acted in the past.*

*The problem with all this is that Bb are extremely unpredictable. Or at least we don't know enough about it to make rationale predictions. The clinical course is based on predictable behavior and patterns. The only thing predictable about Lyme is its unpredictability. I still hear case studies where I am surprised at the individual's clinical course. After nearly four years of total immersion in TBIs, I recognize that I can still be way off track in some of these cases. Don't try so hard to make everything fit together perfectly. Although I hesitate to use such a freaky word, go with the gestalt. **Gestalt** is the idea that something is more than the sum of its parts. When all things are considered where does your intuitive reasoning lead you? Gather your information and use rational clinical judgment to make your determinations.*

As in most cases of malarkey, there is usually a kernel of truth. How can we take this contentious mess and make some sense of it? First, stop trying so hard. I am thrilled when a true Lyme case is identified at all. Splitting hairs over whether you have a Stage I or II is only semantics that does not help the patient. Use your clinical judgment to discern how sick the patient is and use your good sense to address the issues for that individual.

PEARL: When I tried to take real cases and categorize their stage based on some of the methods presented in the literature, I had trouble forcing the real people into the artificial models. Using one system, I could not find one patient who fit the proposed paradigm. The best approach might be if we admit that we do not understand enough about LD to etch its clinical course in granite just yet. Then we accept that we still have to move forward taking care of Lyme patients, even when we don't have all the answers.

Still, I have to sort and categorize somehow. I decided to take the most applicable designations and flesh those out in a way that the HCP might be able to get a handle on where their patient stands. I have not included any designations that I consider medically untenable. Here are categories that I felt were as close to clinical reality as I could find:

A. **Exposed:** A tick bite occurs and tick saliva is introduced. The risk of exposure increases with the time of attachment. Do NOT be fooled into thinking that a tick must be attached for 24 or more hours before pathogens can be transmitted. While the risk goes down with shorter attachment times, it does not disappear. In some cases, pathogens have moved into a host in very short order. Further, the tick does not have to be engorged to spread disease. A person has to have exposure to have the disease. You can't have borreliosis without having been exposed to Borrelia from some source. But the patient should not be forced to recall a tick bite in order to qualify for eventual Lyme disease status. I ascribe to the aggressive approach to disease prevention. See Chapter 32 for guidance on what to do after possible exposure.

B. **Infected**: Here the pathogen has been transmitted into the host. There is considerable debate over whether infected means diseased or not. Of course, there are passionate opinions on both sides. One side says if the organism is merely present, without symptoms, then the more appropriate term is colonized rather than infected. I agree. That makes sense. Except that most people who are considering these things are not bacteriologists and don't sling the word colonized around very often. Since many reservoir animals have pathogen present without symptoms of disease, they are often referred to as infected in the literature and in conversation. While they could correctly be called colonized as well, no one I know uses that term. I will not quibble either way. When you read or hear the word infected, make sure you understand the context. For the purpose of this text when I use the word infected I mean pathogen present. To base the term infected only on those who show sxs does not account for the patient with a subclinical presentation or those whose symptoms have waned. Those people would be more than colonized but less than diseased, so let's just call them infected. If there are no symptoms, sometimes the only way a person learns that they had been infected was through the presence of antibodies at a later date.

PEARL: Is there such a thing as a Lyme carrier state where the patient no longer has sxs but the pathogen is still present? Presumably if that person is bitten by an uninfected tick, that tick could then harbor live spirochete that could be passed along to its next host during a subsequent feeding. Most experts don't think humans function as reservoirs, but they don't know everything.

One source speculated that perhaps 12% of infected patients remain asymptomatic. I have no idea how close to reality that guess is. I know of a number of cases where individuals have been infected but did not get sick. There are a number of anecdotal cases of families where all were equally exposed, presumably with the same strains, and some got sick while others did not. Many factors may contribute to who gets sick and who stays well, such as the status of the immune system, overall health at the time of exposure, volume of spirochetes, and bite locations. Of course, some strains are much more virulent, but presumably members of the same family are exposed to the same strains.

Certainly not all infections with Bb cause disease. The common tick hosts such as deer and the white-footed mouse seem to have no problem harboring the organism without subsequent health problems. In contrast, other animals such as humans and dogs can become ill and even die from severe infections. Cats only occasionally get Lyme disease despite many tick bites on countless cats.

C. **Diseased:** Diseased means that the pathogen was able to build a colony of sufficient size (critical mass) to cause signs and symptoms in the host. Of course, we run into the same problem here with the possibility of *subclinical* disease. Where do we draw the line? At least this is where the fun begins. The following list includes possible stages in the clinical course of Lyme disease. These concepts were compiled from hundreds of sources and redacted in an attempt to make sense within my experience with Lyme. Yes, you might have two or more terms applicable at the same time. Sometimes, despite valiant efforts, it is not possible to accurately categorize an individual's disease state. Don't force the process.

1. **Acute:** Sxs appear usually within a few days after the bite. But the gap between bite and sxs may be much longer than that, even months or years. If there is a prolonged interval between exposure and presentation, consider that there might have been an overlooked bite in the interim.

   In usual medical parlance acute is a condition of short duration, the opposite of chronic or persistent. Since IDSA says there is no such thing as chronic Lyme, one would suspect that the definition of acute Lyme would include those signs and symptoms that occur within their 30 day treatment restriction. The difficulty in assigning the label "acute" to Lyme disease is that it may be hard to draw the line between infection, incubation, illness, and on-going disease. The importance in making this distinction is that in a significant proportion of patients, the earlier adequate treatment begins, the less risk of developing intractable disease. Delays can result in a syndrome that is difficult to manage and can progress into a chronic condition.

   I have trouble using the term acute as a descriptor of a stage of LD. Lyme is well-documented to wax and wane and remit, only to flare again at a later date, all from the same tick bite. What is thought to be the end of an acute episode may be just a pause in the action.

2. **Early:** Sometimes acute Lyme is referred to as "early." Again, I am no happier with the label "early" than I am with the term "acute." I find both misleading. Nonetheless, you read a lot about early and late LD. Some signs and symptoms seem to occur more often in the time period just after the bite while others manifest more commonly later in the clinical course. Early symptoms may include fever, headache, aches, joint discomfort, flu-like complaints, brain fog, and malaise. The fatigue may be pronounced. The EM rash may appear early in the course of the disease, as can Bell's palsy. On the other hand, the rash and palsy may not manifest for weeks, if at all, as is the case in the majority of patients. While I have seen early Lyme described as milder than late Lyme, I have seen many exceptions to that general rule. Again, since we rarely know when the exposure occurred, the term early may not be valid in many cases. The primary significance to labeling Lyme as early or acute is that the sooner treatment is started the less likely are intractable sequelae and the easier the condition is to manage and hopefully to cure.

3. **Localized:** The term localized is mostly used to describe a primary EM rash before the patient begins to experience other sxs. Once the sxs become systemic you can assume that you no longer have

localized disease. When localized, the primary EM rash signifies the presence of spirochetes in the area. Once the patient begins to experience systemic signs and symptoms, the spirochetes are likely in transition to a disseminated state.

Usually by the time a patient gets to the HCP, the pathogen has long since disseminated and all those symptoms are trying to tell you the Bb have spread. Again, if you have a patient with only localized disease, POUNCE! Treat before the Bb have a chance to do all those pathophysiologic things that make them so much harder to eradicate once they get around.

After the pathogen is introduced, the Bb microbe reproduces and moves within the skin. In some cases this local movement will result in a primary EM rash. If the spirochetes are not now contained by the immune system, hopefully in conjunction with antibiotics, they can continue to spread throughout the organism. As the pathogen disseminates, the symptoms of Lyme can start to appear.

From initial inoculation, Bb quickly disseminate from the skin into the circulation of blood and lymph and off to its more favored spots where the pathogens soon become intracellular. Locally, the spirochetes invade the nearby endothelium where they might cause some low grade coagulation and inflammation problems but they tend to quickly move on.

Do you consider the closest lymph node local or disseminated? Tunev's work suggests that the Bb migrate quickly to lymph nodes, within a few days of inoculation. Here a broader immune response is triggered. While that response may or may not be sufficient to curb the pathogens, at least the body now knows something is going on. All the immune responders will be called into action and soon the signs and symptoms of general inflammation will be apparent. If the infection was localized before, that state won't last much longer. If there was ever a time to capture a spirochete, it's now, since this is when the free-floating forms are in the circulation on their way to outlying tissues. Unfortunately, the victim usually doesn't recognize that something is going on at this point, so the opportunity is missed. (This is NOT the time to collect serology samples since antibodies against the Bb haven't had a chance to form yet.)

In most cases Bb do not stay local for long. Once the pathogen hits the circulation, the free-floating spirochetes move to more protected locations where they can live long and prosper. While conceivable that some of the early flu-like sxs, and even some of the

initial brain fog, can be due to local infection causing release of inflammatory humors, there is no precise line here. The Bb are transitioning from local to disseminated. The important point is that if you can begin treatment before the pathogen has spread, you have the best chance of curtailing the disease and preventing a more serious illness. Do not "wait and see" what happens. Those are word I have spoken and will always regret. Keep a high index of suspicion.

4. **Disseminated**: To disseminate means to spread or scatter throughout the organism. Now the pathogen is moving through the circulation and reaching tissues and organs. The sxs therefore become systemic as well. A secondary EM rash can indicate the dissemination of spirochetes far from the site of the initial tick bite, but this presentation is quite rare. Migrating joint pain is common and GI, neurologic, and cardiac conditions can manifest. All the while, the early symptoms may or may not persist.

Neuroborreliosis is probably the most common manifestation of Bb dissemination despite being overlooked for many years while HCPs focused on Lyme arthritis and the less frequent EM rashes. Neuropsychiatric problems that can accompany the spread of Bb into the tissue include: palsies, loss of muscle tone, meningitis, encephalitis, severe headache, neck stiffness, sensitivities to light, sound, or touch, radiculopathies, burning and shooting pains, sleep problems, strange sensations, memory loss, mood changes, anxiety, panic, depression, and difficulty with cognition. Occasionally, neuropsychiatric symptoms are the only manifestations apparent in these patients. Brain fog is a common complaint with almost all Lyme cases and especially those that have spread to the CNS.

While dissemination commonly takes days, spread can occur in only a few hours or may take weeks. Disseminated Lyme usually involves one or more organ systems such as musculoskeletal, neurologic, GI, GU, endocrine, immune, or cardiac as the spirochetes spread to distant sites.

Dissemination can occur early or late and in either acute or chronic disease. Even though Bb are notoriously slow replicators, within a few hours enough of the spirochetes can be present to be moving to sites far from the tick bite. Spirochetes have been found in the brain 12 hours after inoculation.

PEARL: In practice, specific sxs that appear early in one case may not manifest until much later in another case, if at all. For instance, the spirochete and its DNA have been isolated from the CSF early in the clinical course. But live spirochetes have also been cultured from the skin years after primary infection.

PEARL: If the joint pain is migratory you likely have migratory spirochetes. If the secondary EM rash is moving you likely have moving spirochetes. Moving spirochetes are living spirochetes, otherwise the immune system would be buzzing around with their cellular Zambonis cleaning up the mess.

There is no need to fret about whether or not the Lyme has disseminated. You want to catch it BEFORE it disseminates. Of course, if you're the HCP, by the time the patient sees you, you're stuck with whatever status presents. Why take chances? If the brain is starting to be affected, consider the possibility that Bb are now invading the neurons and surrounding tissues. Act accordingly, the sooner the better, before they become even more entrenched. Make sure you choose drugs that cross the BBB and that hit both the free-floating spirochete and cystic forms of Bb. When they come out of their cysts, you'd like to have an appropriate antibiotic waiting there for them.

Even months after the tick bite, the spirochetes can continue to spread through the circulatory fluids to the various organs, wherever their biochemistry leads them. Their favorites remain the same: heart, joints, GI tract, GU, eyes, and especially the nervous system. Essentially all tissue can be affected.

Anytime conditions in the host become favorable, the free-floating spirochetal form can emerge. Remember the spirochetal form is the replicating form and all God's creatures are driven to reproduce. While the Bb are safe and secure in their cysts or L-forms, their whole reason to exist is to make baby spirochetes. Replication is only possible in their helical, free-floating persona.

PEARL: George Chaconas, PhD, found that spirochete interaction with and dissemination out of the vasculature was a multi-stage process of unexpected complexity. Spirochete movement appeared to play an integral role in this dissemination. He developed and used high resolution 3D visualization of dissemination of bacterial pathogens in living mammalian hosts. His was the first direct insight into spirochetal dissemination in vivo.

5. **Late:** The term "late stage" is used in several ways in the literature. Either "late" refers to the time within the clinical course far from the initiating tick bite, OR to the severity of the illness such as the end-stage disease of the critically ill. While there are many reasons why a person might develop late-stage Lyme, one likely

explanation is inadequate management of the disease early on. Antibiotics that do not target the organism or are not of sufficient duration or dosage seem to predispose to intractable cases with more permanent sequelae. Solo agents can lead to prolonged problems by stimulating the pathogen to burrow or encyst. Although Bb can be in the brain within hours, later stages of Lyme are thought to be even more likely to predispose to neuropsychiatric problems, since the Bb have more time to cross the BBB, embed in the tissue, and colonize. Damage can be done both directly and indirectly. Although the term "late" is hard for me to pin down, it appears that the general feel is that "late Lyme" disease involves more of the bad stuff like cardiac problems, disabilities, intractable NP issues, and debilitating joint problems, among other things. Unfortunately, in some cases late means too late, since Lyme can be fatal, probably much more often than recognized. Ironically, a patient could conceivably have *early* LD in terms of chronology but *late* LD in terms of the severity of the disease.

PEARL: While late LD can be chronic and chronic LD can manifest as late LD, these terms are not synonymous. There is no need to force labels onto syndromes just for the exercise. The clinical course of Lyme is not so clearly defined as to make this practical or useful for the patient. We're not all singing from the same song sheet yet, so applying labels when they may not be appropriate can only lead to confusion. Remember, my co-worker died from "minor" Lyme disease. What would have happened if he had "major" disease? I shudder to think of it.

6. **Chronic/Persistent/On-going:** By definition, chronic means persistence over time, existing over a long duration, or constant recurrence. The term chronic is used to label several subsets of Lyme patients such as those treated patients who have on-going symptoms after an unspecified length of time. Some say that Lyme becomes chronic after 30 days, while others only allude to the chronic stage of Lyme after a patient has been sick for a year or more. Chronicity can occur in both treated and untreated patients. A long delay before treatment or inadequate treatment can predispose toward chronicity.

To me, chronic is more a "type" of disseminated LD, rather than a date on the calendar. The character of the disease seems different compared to those with a responsive acute presentation. And the disease probably is different in ways we cannot yet explain. Look back in the *Pathophysiology* section above to get some ideas on how Bb might evolve into such an intractable, hard-to-manage pathogen in some cases. Seemingly, delayed or inadequate treatment allows this disease, which should be amenable to antimicrobial intervention, to become a condition that is almost impossible to manage. Chapter 11: *Controversies around Lyme* reviews the disagreement that surrounds the idea of chronic Lyme.

There are many factors that might contribute to persistent Lyme including: higher spirochete load, genetic susceptibility, poor immune defense, co-infections, as well as insipid and inadequate treatment regimes such as solo agents, low doses, and short duration that encourage the Bb to entrench. Some strains appear more virulent and persistent than others.

Chronicity can be hard to define in Lyme since the sxs can seem to recede, only to recur again and again. Where should the line be drawn? What is old and what is new? How often does reinfection account for a new round of sxs? With chronic Lyme you might see many clinical presentations. There can be a steady level of symptoms, or the disease can wax and wane. Symptoms can change midstream or evolve in a way that make them barely recognizable from month to month or year to year. Often discontinuation of antibiotics will cause a flare. There can be long periods when there is no evidence of illness and then the sxs reappear.

While some sources use the term post-Lyme syndrome to be synonymous with chronic Lyme, many ILADS physicians do not believe there is anything "post" about this condition. While some signs and symptoms apparent in chronic Lyme can be due to permanent damage of the immune system, live spirochetes are likely at the root of chronicity. An increasing number of clinicians (including the former president of IDSA who has written a book on chronic Lyme that denounces IDSA's guideline debacle), believe that on-going infection is the underlying cause of chronic manifestations of Lyme disease. While immune dysfunction may certainly contribute to persistent symptoms of Lyme, many HCPs believe that active Bb are at the root of chronic Lyme.

Perhaps a third or more of those treated with supposedly adequate antibiotics continue to have sxs. These sxs can be severe and incapacitating in a small, but significant, number of individuals. The weight of the evidence supports on-going infection in chronic LD. Stricker and Johnson list numerous studies that demonstrate the presence of spirochetes despite antibiotic treatment ranging from 3 weeks to over a year. Yes, in some patients both symptoms and spirochetes seem to go away never to return, but those aren't the cases we're concerned with here.

Chronic Lyme most commonly manifests as progressive rheumatologic, neurologic, psychiatric, endocrine, immunologic, GI, GU, or cardiac disorders. In many cases neuropsychiatric sxs are predominant. Usually there are brief periods of respite followed by recurrent sxs. Longer and more comprehensive treatment usually results in longer periods of relief, but this is unpredictable. Joints usually improve before the brain. Fatigue is often the last symptom to clear. The best chance for these syndromes to resolve is not by treating *only* the troublesome manifestations, but by also attacking the condition at its source with appropriate antibiotics.

The combination of neurologic and rheumatic sxs is probably the most common combination in chronic LD. So often we recognize these characteristic features after the fact. If only we could remember to think of them beforehand more often.

Barthold found that the behavior of Bb is different inside the host before and after the humoral response kicks in. Those persistent spirochetes that have experienced the immune response are more refractory to antibiotics, which usually only target the active, replicating organisms. This phenomenon is called **antimicrobial tolerance.** Many pathogens use this mechanism in order to survive. Antimicrobial tolerance is the ability of a pathogen to resist damage by antibiotics (and host humors) by entering an existence of the transient, dormant, non-dividing state. These microbes are then termed persisters. They are not mutants but dormants. By being in the inactive state they survive, whereas their genetically identical cousins are killed by the antimicrobial. The dormant state makes them insensitive or refractory (or tolerant) to antibiotics. When such persistent cells can't be eliminated by the immune system, they are effectively a reservoir from which recurrent infection can develop. As long as the dormant cells have the potential to reactivate into the free spirochete active form, they have the potential to cause the sxs of the disease. Persisters may be the primary cause of chronic infections. (I realize this wording is identical to what I used earlier to discuss survival techniques used by Bb. But the concept is so important, why not get double duty?)

With the idea of persisters fresh, we still must consider what might be different about the chronic Lyme patient that makes them more susceptible to the long-term torment from the Bb pathogen? Some LD patients have a documented history of frequent illnesses, multiple allergies, or immune conditions like asthma or eczema. All these might make them more susceptible to Bb. In this way Lyme can be considered an opportunistic disease for those with the right combination of genetic and environmental factors. Bb would seemingly pounce when the host was most vulnerable. Who are the ones that get infected but don't get sick? Are they different from the ones that get infected and do get sick? Are they different still from those who stay sick despite aggressive treatment? How are they distinct and how can we take advantage of their singularity to keep the most vulnerable patients from long-term debility? If only we knew the answers to these questions. Hopefully, the second edition of this *Compendium* will have what we all need.

PEARL: Individuals with markers HLA-DR2 and HLA-DR4, as well as those who show bands 31 and 34 in serology testing, may be a subset of "different" patients. These individuals have a tendency to present a more autoimmune-type response to Bb infection. Their clinical picture is also atypical in that they have more achiness and general distress. They do not respond as well to traditional treatment plans. Plaquenil added to their antibiotic panel might help.

Who develops chronic LD? Who knows? Maybe it's genetic predisposition. Some strains may be more persistent. People with strong antibody responses may stay sick longer, showing that while their body is making antibodies, there is something about the response that doesn't allow them to clear the pathogen.

Probably the most prudent course is treating until all signs and symptoms are gone plus a cushion where the patient is symptom-free before discontinuing treatment. The cushion is usually 3 to 6 months depending on how sick the patient was and how long she was sick. If the symptoms return, resume treatment, keeping in mind that you might need to change something in the regimen in an attempt to get complete resolution. We might not have uncovered the best antibiotic combination for chronic Lyme as yet, or the drug that best targets this pathogen has yet to be discovered. We do have to recognize the possibility that the physiology of this pathogen might be such that it will be able to dodge our bullets for a long time to come.

Even the most recalcitrant Lyme seems amenable to treatment and cure if doggedly pursued. Except for the pathology that has been allowed to continue to the point of permanent, irreversible tissue damage, the majority of Lyme manifestations can be tempered and even cured with thoughtful, persistent, targeted case management.

PEARL: An all "R" glossary to help you with the next section: Relapse: Return of sxs after a period of improvement or stability. Deterioration after progress. Reversal in clinical course. Recurrent: Return of sxs after remission or sxs returning once again or repeatedly. Recrudescent: Return after abatement. To break out again after a period of quiescence. Refractory: Not responsive to treatment. Recalcitrant: Stubbornly unresponsive. Often used interchangeably, these terms do have subtle differences.

7. **Relapse:** Just when you thought it was safe to go back in the tall grass, all the progress you made goes out the window. A relapse is an apparent reversal in clinical course with the return of sxs after a period of improvement or stability. The clinical picture deteriorates after getting better. The problem with defining a relapse is knowing the baseline with which to compare. Is it a relapse only when all sxs were previously thought to be gone and then they recur? Or is it a relapse if sxs are on-going and then become noticeably worse? Perhaps that's a flare? Is a relapse the same as a flare or similar to the "wax" in the wax and wane Lyme cycle? Different sources use these terms either synonymously or draw fine lines between them. One author believes that the most common clinical course in Lyme involves an average of three relapses. To me, this means each time the patient believed she was cured, the sxs returned. The feeling most often associated with relapse is disappointment. Right after the denial, "This can't be happening again."

There are several mechanisms that have been proposed to account for the relapse phenomenon. The most logical is the reactivation of the floating spirochete after having been encysted or dormant. Somehow conditions are again favorable for the survival of the free form of Bb. Sometimes the more nurturing environment is due to the cessation of a course of antibiotics that had previously driven the Bb into hiding. Relapse after cessation of antibiotic is common. So now you learn to expect a flare when antibiotics are stopped. Here you have several possible courses of action to consider: 1) Don't stop the antibiotic. Rather, make sure you have a cyst-buster on board. 2) When the Bb stick their curly little heads back out blast them with agents that hit both free-floating and cystic forms. The ability of Bb to encyst and then revert back to a helical form is one mechanism explaining the relapsing and persistent nature of LD.

To me, relapse means the patient was getting the disease under control and then, for reasons hard to pinpoint, the sxs surge again. Relapse sxs can be as bad as they were initially, almost identical to the originals, or totally different. Bell's palsy and meningitis have been reported during a relapse, when they weren't present during the initial manifestation of the disease.

This makes sense when you think about the pathophysiology of Bb. Of course, if the syndrome is so dissimilar to what the patient has experienced in the past, the HCP might want to consider that the patient was reinfected with a different strain of Bb or acquired a co-infection. Here a revised treatment strategy might be needed.

PEARL: A plateau is different from a relapse. A plateau is a state of little or no change after a time of progress. While many Lyme patients are grateful for plateaus compared to what they experienced previously, the sxs persist. This is not a time of waxing and waning but of a fairly stable clinical picture. Patients can plateau with barely noticeable manifestations of Lyme or they can be incapacitated. Practitioners can try to break through a plateau by considering adding medicines, changing regimens, adjusting doses, mulling co-infections, or including ancillary, supportive, or alternative approaches. Continue to pursue cure and you just might achieve it.

Hours to months after the tick bite the spirochetes can spread through the circulatory fluids to the various organs such as the heart, joints, GI tract, and especially the nervous system. Essentially all tissue can be affected. Joe Burrascano has found that relapse often occurs about 10 weeks into the course of chronic Lyme. This recurrence is often triggered by the premature discontinuation of extracellular antibiotics. When the antibiotics are stopped, the encysted Bb come out of hiding. The active spirochetes emerge, allowing the signs and symptoms to return.

Some sources contend that the average Bb infection spawns three relapses. I know relapses are common but I do not know how this number was derived. Come to think of it, I had three relapses. Must be true.

8. **Recurrent:** Recurrence is the return of sxs after remission or an illness presenting repeatedly. Is a recurrence synonymous with a relapse? Usually. Failure to completely eradicate the Bb pathogen is likely the cause of recurrent disease.

PEARL: Even a master diagnostician cannot always tell a relapse from a flare, from a reinfection, from a waxing of sxs. The important point here is that if your patient is experiencing a set of signs and symptoms, active spirochete is the most reasonable explanation. Focus on eradicating the cause instead of selecting the best stage name.

9. **Reinfection:** Here the patient suffered a new tick bite that may have transferred Borrelia of the same or different strain as that which caused the original disease. Reinfection can occur shortly after the first bite or

years into a chronic Lyme infection. Many people who mistook a previous Lyme infection for a cold or flu might not recognize a later infection as a reinfection. They might believe this is the first time they had Lyme. One infection with Lyme does not seem to confer immunity so it can be hard to figure out if the person is infected or reinfected. Nothing about Lyme is simple.

There is not much in the literature about different strains of Bb being concurrently transmitted, although there is mention of Bb and STARI moving into a host together. The only reason this matters is if one strain would benefit from a different antibiotic choice from the regimen currently being used. Fortunately, most Borrelia respond to the same types of antibiotics, although some strains may respond better to different classes of antimicrobials than others.

One reason serology testing has so many false negative patients, who are obviously sick with Lyme, is due to attempting to match one strain of antibodies with a different strain of antigens. Maybe now in "Round 2," we'll finally get lucky and get a true positive for a change. In the summer of my son's big bout with TBIs, serology showed that he had antibodies present from old infection, and we had been unaware. Was this Lyme #2, or #3, or more? (Remember at that time, Lyme was considered easy to cure with short-term antibiotics and a blast of steroids.) The consensus in the literature is that repeated infections appear to result in sicker patients.

10. **Refractory**: Patients who do not respond to treatment are considered refractory or recalcitrant. In the practices of experienced providers, very few patients are permanently refractory. A few teenagers have proven to be especially challenging, but these are kids whose Lyme was ignored by HCPs for a long time before treatment was started. In most cases, the correct antimicrobial combination, in conjunction with appropriate ancillary treatments, can be identified. Never give up. We just don't have the perfect answer YET.

11. **Herx**: Actually the Herx reaction does not belong on this list. Unlike the rest of the stages contained here, which are due to live spirochetes doing damage, the Herx phenomenon is due to a massive kill-off of said spirochetes. I include the Herx reaction here only because it is sometimes hard to distinguish a Herx from a flare, a reinfection, or a co-infection. How can you tell the difference between a Herx due to effective antimicrobials and a flare due to ineffective treatment? Was a different antibiotic regimen recently started? Was a cyst-buster added?

12. **Cured**: A cure is a restoration of health or wellness, the return of lost function, and the ability to resume the AODL. Cure is the recovery from disease with no more signs or symptoms. With Lyme, cure can be elusive. Many times those who are declared cured after short-term treatment are not followed long enough to recognize that the sxs often return. Sometimes the patient or caretaker aren't able to make the connection, thinking they just picked up a new virus somewhere.

As a reasonable working definition, Donta defined **cure** in Lyme patients as an absence of symptoms for a year or more following antibiotic treatment. This definition seems as reasonable as any. As recognized in the *Pathophysiology* section above, in some cases the spirochete is never eradicated. Even in those who never experience another bout, the Bb may still be lurking. It's been more than a year since my last clear Lyme sxs. Still occasionally, I feel something "Lymey" is going on. Am I cured? I wouldn't bet on it. Should I go on another round of antibiotics? Probably.

In the 30% or more who remain symptomatic despite antibiotic treatment, don't expect instant resolution of a long-standing problem. Recovery may be incremental. We are looking for improvement. Whether the progress is gradual or miraculous, we'll take it.

IDSA believes that no further treatment beyond 30 days is needed, whether the patient is still symptomatic or not and whether the discontinuation of the antibiotic causes a flare in sxs or not. Anyone without sxs at the 30 day mark is considered cured irrespective of whether the sxs return in a week, a month, or a year. My public health doctor friend was "cured" nine times in 3 months. What a great way to pad your stats.

Many patients experience a relapse of symptoms soon after the short-term antibiotic is discontinued. Others are only functional when symptoms are muted by antibiotics.

PEARL: IDSA says most Lyme patients eventually recover. How is "eventually recover" defined? If symptoms stop and the patient is designated as a "cure," what then constitutes a relapse? Is it no symptoms for a week, a month, five years? You cannot see what you don't look for. Different periods of time selected to define relapse might provide very different perspectives. Many patients might feel fine for a week or two after treatment stops and then, over time, a number of those considered initially recovered might begin to experience a recurrence of symptoms. While the majority appear to be fully recovered, others can show signs of relapse that range from mild, barely-there symptoms to a syndrome worse than the original presentation. Just monitoring for a brief period will falsely inflate the recovery rate. As I mention elsewhere, a percentage of patients with persistent symptoms leave those doctors who do not try to address their problems. Outcome tracking that does not follow patients over a sufficient time period will give inaccurate relapse data. I relapsed. My husband relapsed. My son relapsed. No one reported any of those relapses. We just thought it was the nature of the beast. Lyme patients have been known to relapse years after they were labeled fully recovered. Donta studied relapse rates in 277 patients and found that recurrence can occur years after therapy is stopped.

Factors that might impact the clinical course of Lyme:

- A higher spirochete load on initial exposure might influence the severity of the illness as well as the clinical path it takes.

- What determines if and when a person gets sick after a bite? The amount of pathogen originally transmitted, the virulence of the organism, whether the immune system is overwhelmed by spirochete load or co-infections, susceptibility of the host due to genetics or other factors, underlying health, vigor of the immune system, wellness of the individual including nutritional status and conditioning, concurrent conditions, etc.

- Incubation is usually one or two weeks, but can be hours or months or years.

- There is speculation that a number of infected patients are asymptomatic. Some sources give percentages. I don't understand how they know this. I guess someone somewhere found positive diagnostic test results in a person who had no signs of illness. I find it hard enough to get patients tested when they are sick as dogs, with a deer tick dangling from their EM rash. I do not know if the asymptomatic patients they refer to are truly asymptomatic, pre-symptomatic, post-symptomatic, in a waning phase, subclinical, etc.

- Late diagnosis and treatment can significantly alter the clinical course of Lyme setting some patients up for protracted illness.

- Bb can enter the CNS within a day.

- Signs and symptoms of Lyme can cycle. The period of these cycles vary in the literature from 3 day cycles, to 4 weeks, to 3 months, etc. There is even discussion of cycles within cycles with temperatures following a pattern within a 24 hour period every 3 or 4 days while the entire symptom complex cycles over weeks. There may be a peri-menstrual cycling of LD sxs. This would likely have less to do with the physiology of the Bb and more to do with how the fluctuating hormones affect the pathogen.

- Some patients become rapidly ill after exposure, while others may experience a gradual, vague onset of symptoms.

- For those who get an EM rash, the estimated average time between bite and appearance of the lesion is between 3 and 7 days. For those who get carditis, signs might present 2 to 4 weeks after the rash, if they have a rash. Arthritis may be the first symptom or may not appear for months, if at all.

- I find it hard to understand how an infectious disease would wax and wane if there were no longer any active pathogen involved. Are proponents of the immune dysfunction etiology theory saying that the immune dysfunction waxes and wanes? If the sole cause is immune damage, then wouldn't the symptoms either stay the same or decrease at some relatively steady rate as the immune problem resolves. The well-documented clinical pattern of waxing and waning associated with LD is compatible with the idea that active, live spirochetes are at the root of chronic Lyme.

- The location of the bite can influence the clinical course. Patients with bites around the head, neck, or axilla seem to have more CNS involvement than those bitten below the waist or on the lower legs. These upper areas seem to give the spirochetes more ready access to the brain. From those sites the Bb appear to go rapidly from the blood to the brain. Bites below the waist manifest differently, perhaps with less CNS involvement.

- Our vague and incomplete understanding of the pathophysiology of LD complicates the design of robust clinical studies. Since the disease waxes and wanes it's hard to select an endpoint, at least until reliable diagnostic markers are developed. Since the target is moving and unpredictable, we need to circumvent the pathophysiology and focus on the patients. In Chapter 11, I discuss a possible study design that avoids these problems.

- Co-infections complicate pathophysiology for all involved.

- Early insult by Bb seems to hurt organs the most. Initial harm may be due to the direct spirochete damage to tissue as it invades cells, tissues, and interstitial areas. Then the biochemical assault from all the immune humors contribute to the pathology as well as the clinical presentation. As the sxs persist, a chronic "feel" to the disease starts to predominate. This presentation can include a low-grade, ongoing inflammation along with sequelae from damaged organs due to fibrosis or humoral damage. Fibrosis is a thickening or scarring of connective tissue usually as part of a healing process. The interstitial Ct can become matted and fixed. Fibrosis can cause many organs like lungs and kidneys to be less efficient in performing their functions. These tissues can also experience excessive cell death through apoptosis. Hypothetically, the physical presence of the spirochete is the trigger for the immune cascade.

- The cyclic nature of Lyme sxs may cause flares in cycles. There is speculation that Bb may have a growth phase about once a month accounting for the cycles. Since antibiotics tend to only kill bacteria in their growth phase, treatment should be designed to bracket one whole generation cycle. A minimum treatment duration is then considered to be at least 4 weeks. If the antibiotics work, flares will lessen in severity and duration, and eventually disappear. The very occurrence of on-going monthly cycles indicates that living organisms are still present and that antibiotics should be continued.

- Herx reactions can occur if the Bb emerge from their dormant state and transform into the spirochete. If antibiotics are then introduced a kill-off will occur and a Herx reaction ensue. Theoretically, the worse the Herx, the higher the germ load must have been and the sicker the patient.

- In those who have been very ill for a long time, consider IV therapy in an attempt to interrupt the clinical course. If on IVs already, consider adjusting the dose or regimen. Both flares and Herxes in these patients can be severe for different reasons. If the Herx is severe, the regimen might need to be adjusted by lowering the dose or altering the frequency of administration. Be careful in stopping the medicine altogether since breaks in antibiotics can result in the need for longer or stronger treatment in the future. Although some authors recommend pulsing antibiotics, in the case of a severe Herx reaction you might want to try to make the Herx tolerable. Except when the MOA and pharmacology of the drug requires (as in the case of artemesia) or when pulsing makes sense in terms of efficacy or tolerability (as is the case with Flagyl and vancomycin), be careful with pulsing.

- The symptom cycle for Babesia is shorter than the Bb cycle. Bb may cycle every 3 to 4 weeks, while Babesia may cycle over 2 to 3 weeks. If a patient has both, which is often the case, trying to discern a cycle pattern can be a thankless task.

- The severity of the LD might be related to the spirochete load. A light load could forecast a mild or asymptomatic clinical course. Higher loads, either from first infection or subsequent infections, can increase the severity of sxs and alter the clinical course.

- Years may pass before sxs appear after a bite. One case reported a longer than 5-year interval. I wonder how they knew there wasn't an intervening bite.

- Winter is thought to be the worst season for chronic Lyme patients.

- Often Lyme, when recognized, is still put off with a "Let's wait and see," approach. If there is a delay in initiating treatment, the disease can become much harder to manage and permanent sequelae may result because of tissue damage.

- At the first hint of exposure the clock starts. Getting treatment quickly can be essential to preventing escalation. In fact, if there is reasonable suspicion of infection, treatment can be started prior to any apparent symptomatology.

- Remember that patients who are infected but remain asymptomatic initially, can still display sxs at a later date.

- Keep a high index of suspicion. If bitten, but asymptomatic, consider prophylactic antibiotics. Some kids who have been sick with Lyme before should go on antibiotics before camp or other risky activities in endemic areas.

- The end of the clinical course of Lyme is the death of the Borrelia. While amazingly persistent, spirochetes are not immortal. If their ability to replicate is impeded, they will eventually die off.

- In those patients not diagnosed for years, many developed chronic, disabling problems.

- Patients with persistent sxs of LD report that they had a longer period of infection before any treatment was initiated, compared to those without a delay. In a chronic Lyme encephalopathy study funded by NIH, the mean number of years between symptom onset and treatment onset for over 3400 patients was 1.2 years.

IX. SIGNS AND SYMPTOMS

A. Foundation for reviewing the signs and symptoms of Lyme disease

A **sign** is an indicator of disease that is observable and that can be measured or documented objectively. A **symptom** is what the patient experiences subjectively. Traditionally in medicine, a sign was considered "real" since it was quantitative and a symptom was considered less valid because it was qualitative, as though the HCP's senses were more reliable than the patient's. Well personally, I care just as much about my symptoms as I do my signs, since

I can feel my headache but not my high blood pressure. People come to HCPs for help with their symptoms and wind up enduring lectures about their signs.

Long ago, I learned from my son that if he said a body part hurt, I better pay attention since something was cooking. I often find kids more reliable historians than adults. They tend to have less of the secondary agendas that plague grown-ups. The child will try to tell you what you need to know.

Lyme is the great imitator. I have trouble conjuring up a sign or symptom, no matter how bizarre or obscure, that has not appeared on someone's list of Lyme manifestations. Everything, and I mean EVERYTHING, has been blamed on Lyme at some point by somebody. With all the co-infections, confounders, and concurrent conditions, parsing out what is and isn't Lyme is a challenge. Soon I will list the major organ systems and include under each category the most common or familiar signs and symptoms, along with a list of other presentations. (EM rash is a *familiar* sign but not necessarily a *common* one.) No, the list is not all-inclusive. The book is too long as it is. If you want the answer to the question, "Has symptom X ever been associated with Lyme?" I can answer that without even knowing what you are asking about. Yes. That does not mean it was caused by Lyme.

Lyme is a multisystem disease that can present with a wide array of symptoms. Some patients have only a few predominant manifestations while others present with a dizzying array of problems that make diagnosing the condition quite difficult. Some of the most common demonstrations of Lyme are similar to dozens of other infections. Most, but not all, start with the indicators of localized, and then generalized, inflammation such as mild swelling and redness at the bite site, fever, headache, general aches, and malaise. Lyme has this presentation in common with just about every infectious disease known to humankind.

As the disease develops, expect diversity, not uniformity. Most Lyme cases present with four or more complaints. Some refer to this type of syndrome as a cluster of symptoms. If you have a patient with only one organ or system involved, keep your differential diagnosis open and gather more information. For example, a patient with only a painful shoulder may have several possible diagnoses as part of the differential. You'd certainly want to consider LD here, but Lyme might not be on top of the list.

Sxs can vary within hours. Some common sxs like joint pain might appear early or not for months. Early features may be mixed with the characteristic manifestations of inflammation. Late sxs can be due to cell damage or fibrosis. Age may influence the presenting sxs, but this is hard to quantify. Perhaps kids have more cognitive and neuropsychiatric sxs, while adults experience more musculoskeletal problems. Commonly involved organ systems are the brain and nervous system, the GI tract, and joints. Fatigue occurs in nearly all patients.

Lack of corroborating physical findings or diagnostic testing does not mean the symptoms were not real. This deficit simply reinforces the limitations of our physical exam techniques as well as the poor sensitivity and specificity in diagnostic testing. Many conditions aside from Lyme have symptoms that are not currently supportable by quantitative measures. Some patients are more symptomatic than others, which may be genetically prescribed.

Lyme tends to dysregulate the whole body, making it hard to parse out the symptoms that belong with Lyme from those that do not. Recognize that LD might be causing what you see, but that doesn't mean everything you see is Lyme. Forcing sxs into the Lyme paradigm is as bad as excluding things which could be Lyme because they don't fit neatly.

Signs and symptoms can vary considerably among individuals and even within the same person at different stages of disease. At first some people hardly seem affected, with barely perceptible illness. Others are flattened shortly after exposure. A flare may manifest identically to the previous round or be quite different. Herx reactions, which are thought to result from a massive pathogen kill when effective antibiotics are used, can also vary in presentation. The sxs of gestational LD are detailed in Chapter 30: *Special Populations* with the most common sign being hypotonia.

Patients can be very sick with Lyme and not meet ANY of the CDC criteria for official recognition of their condition. This explains how so many cases have been left to simmer until the person gets much sicker, the case is harder to manage, and some of the symptoms may then be due to irreversible tissue damage.

The rest of this section is divided into what you might expect to see when a patient presents with Lyme disease, common manifestations, the symptoms that should lead you to put Lyme at the top of your differential diagnosis, quirky Lyme signals, and finally a review of the Lyme signs and symptoms by body system. You will have had enough of Lyme symptoms by then and will need to rest.

B. A patient walks into your office…

The sxs that a Lyme patient may exhibit depend on where she is in the clinical course of LD. Someone presenting soon after infection might show a very different syndrome than a person who is further along the disease path, or someone with chronic Lyme. Lyme can even look quite different in the same individual at the various disease stages.

The first symptoms of borreliosis can be the general signs of inflammation common to most infections. Early sxs may include a flu-like syndrome with headache, general aches and pains, fever, and severe fatigue. Usually there is NO rhinitis, sinusitis, or cough making this distinguishable from flu or URIs. However, there might be lymphadenopathy.

Soon thereafter the patient might complain of on-going fatigue, myalgias, and arthralgias that are often migrating. Arthralgias most commonly involve the big joints like knees, shoulders, hips, and elbows, although smaller joints can also be involved. Do not expect an EM rash. If you see one, you have been given a diagnostic gift. If you do not see a target, bull's eye, or anything else that could be called an EM rash, that is the usual state in the majority of cases. The lack of an EM rash is diagnostically meaningless. GI complaints may start and the neuropsychiatric issues are likely to present early and often in a variety of ways. The nervous system is probably the final one to heal in Lyme. You will see joints get better, and the GI symptoms resolve, and rashes go away and you will think the brain may never get well. Patience. The Lyme brain can be cured, if not left to fester too long.

PEARL: Fatigue is an almost universal complaint in Lyme and can be the last symptom to resolve. While there are fine distinctions made between terms, the following labels have been used to refer to the fatigue associated with Lyme: malaise, exhaustion, tiredness, lethargy, no energy, no stamina, weary, worn out, sluggish, languid, drained, wilted, ready to collapse, listless, lassitude, depleted, unmotivated, and sapped. While most of these are fairly interchangeable, I believe weakness, dizziness, and sleepiness should not be used synonymously with fatigue. Be careful with all these terms and how you use them and look carefully at the context in the literature. Perhaps the author did not choose the best descriptor. When a child says his legs are like jello, which term would you pick? The glossary defines the most common of these expressions.

The following symptoms can be characteristic for Lyme and the patient usually displays more than one: Severe fatigue unrelieved by rest, insomnia, headaches, nausea, abdominal pain, GERD, trouble swallowing, fever, chills, joint pain, dizziness, paresthesias, shakiness, anxiety, fasciculations especially in the face or eyelids, hypersensitivity to sound, light, or touch, and brain fog as manifested by impaired concentration, poor short-term memory, inability to sustain attention, difficulty processing information, problems thinking clearly, diminished ability to express thoughts, impaired reading or writing, feeling overwhelmed, limited decision-making, and confusion. The patient may display uncharacteristic behavior, outbursts, or mood swings. In most cases the patient looks sick and will tell you so. Numbness, tingling, and tremors are common. The combination of fatigue, paresthesias, arthralgias, and brain fog says Lyme.

PEARL: Reread the previous paragraph. It's important.

Remember that all these sxs may occur concurrently with the general sxs of systemic inflammation, such as fever, aches, and fatigue. Also, remember that a characteristic finding in Lyme is that sxs come and go. What is present one hour might be gone the next. Lyme sxs can cycle both short and long-term. This disease is migratory, transitory, intermittent, waxing and waning. With chronic Lyme you may start seeing more tissue damage due to fibrosis, which may be irreversible.

C. **Common signs and symptoms in Lyme**

I smile as I write this section because I have two articles in front of me, one saying drenching sweats are common in Lyme and the other saying that sweats are rare in Lyme. As always, borreliosis is controversial, contradictory, and the truth probably lies somewhere in the middle. In my experience, the drenching sweats associated with Lyme are more likely due to a common co-infection like babesiosis. My point being that even the least controversial topics around Lyme, like whether to expect fever-sweats, is not as straightforward as one might think. With Lyme, all sorts of unexpected sxs may appear and throw you off track. With Lyme, just about anything is possible. Keep an open mind and a high index of suspicion. With that being said, some sxs are more common than others in Lyme cases.

Lyme usually presents with some sort of systemic inflammation including fever, headache, generalized aches and pains, and GI discomfort. These manifestations can wax and wane as the spirochete goes in and out of its various life forms. This inflammatory presentation can be the only thing you're seeing or it can umbrella over the other signs and symptoms of Lyme. Often this is called a flu-like syndrome and LD is frequently misdiagnosed as flu or URI. I also see in the literature the term "off-season" flu which makes me wonder what you call these Lyme-associated sxs when it is flu season. I think this phrase is best avoided for many reasons.

Symptoms essentially universal in Lyme include fatigue, brain fog, and pain. Most LD patients, even very young ones, relate to the idea of brain fog. Whether they knew what they were experiencing when they had it, almost all get that gleam of recognition when brain fog is described to them by a veteran sufferer. Paresthesias would probably be next most frequent. Anxiety, irritability, and joint discomfort are familiar features of Lyme. While EM (especially target or bull's eye) lesions are less frequent than touted (less than 10% in some practices) other rashes can be common. GI complaints are common, especially reflux, nausea, dysphagia, and discomfort. Sleep disturbances are common, but NOT sleep apnea which is in a whole different realm.

Neuropsychiatric complaints are common including any of the manifestations of brain fog. Each symptom can present individually or in any combination: impaired concentration, poor short-term memory, inability to sustain attention, difficulty processing information, problems thinking clearly, diminished ability to express thoughts, impaired reading or writing, feeling overwhelmed, limited decision-making, and confusion. The patient may display a change in behavior or mood swings. Irritability is common as is anxiety and OCD manifestations. Balance is commonly affected.

Most Lyme patients complain of pain or aches usually headache, or joint pain, but bone and muscle pains are common as is neck pain and stiffness. Hypersensitivity to light, sound, or touch is often noted. There are complaints of dizziness. Numbness and tingling especially in the extremities, called paresthesias, should be expected. Twitching or fasciculation, most often of the eyelids, is widespread. Both the paresthesias and fasciculations can be intermittent. Patients often complain of feeling shaky, nervous, or restless. Depression and panic occur more often than reported. Chris had nearly constant eye fasciculations for over a year and we had no idea they could be Lyme-related.

Fatigue, which is sometimes called malaise, lassitude, weakness, or poor stamina is not relieved with rest. The patient may feel the need to nap and she may not be able to perform AODL. Some patients are near collapse after short periods of minimal activity. Lyme can seem to wilt or deflate the person. Fatigue will likely be the first symptom noticed and the last one remaining when all else has resolved. Exhaustion can be crippling. Some patients are too tired to walk or sit up by themselves.

In addition to hypersensitivity there are other problems with the senses. Tinnitus or an underwater feel is common. Eye problems are frequently reported with double vision, trouble with accommodation, and complaints of smeary or wavy vision being the most usual.

PEARL: The most forgotten symptom of Lyme, which is nearly as ubiquitous as fatigue, is irritability.

Lyme joints commonly pop and creak. Neck crepitus is especially common. Kids have called their joints crunchy, crinkly, or clunky. Sometimes you can actually hear the noisy joints from across the room. Lymphadenopathy is frequently found. Hypotonia is the cardinal sign of gestational Lyme.

Over time kids can start to miss developmental milestones. Autism diagnoses have sky-rocketed and it's hard to tell if this is autism or the autism-like syndrome common in Lyme. Interstitial cystitis is a frequent complaint. Abnormalities of the endocrine system are regular findings including fluctuating sugars and abnormal thyroid and cortisol levels.

Please do not buy the hype! A minority of Lyme cases present with an EM rash (maybe 10 to 40% in most TBI-focused practices) and a substantial minority do not have any arthritis or joint discomfort, especially early in the clinical course. Bell's palsy may be a more common sign than the bull's eye or target lesion and even that is infrequent compared to the actual common manifestations. I cringe every time I read a magazine or newspaper saying to look for the EM rash to decide if you have Lyme. Further, more peer-reviewed articles than I care to remember incorrectly indicate that a rash or joint effusion MUST be present for a diagnosis of Lyme. Lyme is a multi-system disease that presents in a variety of ways. If you are waiting for a target lesion or a hot knee to make the diagnosis, you will miss most cases. While an EM rash, within the context of a corroborating history, can be highly suggestive of a Lyme diagnosis (and pathognomonic for borreliosis), the absence of such a lesion is meaningless. Characteristic does not necessarily mean common. Get over the EM rash already!

D. If you see these sxs, put Lyme at the top of your list:

Assuming you have some reason to suspect Lyme, review the following list and if any of these signs or symptoms are present put up your antennae and consider Lyme.

EM rashes, while NOT noted in the majority of cases, unequivocally announce Lyme when present, especially in the company of a tick bite and any corroborating sxs, history, or ROS. In my opinion, EM rashes are pathognomonic for Borrelia, whether Lyme or STARI.

Although much of the information regarding Lyme on WebMD is flawed, the authors do recognize the EM rash as pathognomonic for LD, calling it a "sure sign." STARI can also have an EM rash, so let's just say that an EM rash is pathognomonic for borreliosis.

Although the items on the following list can occur in other conditions, they are strongly suggestive of LD, especially in combinations or clusters: Migrating joint pain, intractable fatigue not addressed by rest, extreme sensitivity to light, sound, touch, and to a lesser degree taste and smell, Bell's palsy, twitching eyelids, paresthesias, Lyme eye or punctated erythema on the conjunctiva, blurred or wavy vision, problems with accommodation, or an autism-like syndrome especially if the manifestations do not appear at an age when autism is usually diagnosed. Be concerned about a child who had been doing well and then starts to miss developmental milestones. Brain fog and any of the listed neuropsychiatric problems in conjunction with these red flags strongly suggest Lyme. A sudden onset of a NP condition, or an increase in intensity of a pre-existing condition, points to Lyme.

When the H&P are supportive, consider neck crepitus, cracking, creaking, stiffness, and popping joints indicators of Lyme. These are often overlooked in making the diagnosis. Likewise, common manifestations like interstitial cystitis and GERD say Lyme more often that we recognize. Hypotonia in neonates is strongly supportive of a Lyme diagnosis.

The European version of Lyme can present with several sxs that are unfamiliar in North American Lyme:

- Acrodermatitis chronica atrophicans: This skin condition is progressive and leads to widespread atrophy of the skin. This manifestation is thought to be associated with problems in the PNS such as polyneuropathy. The skin becomes like tissue paper. Usually the lesions begin in the extremities with a blush-red inflammation and swelling. The clinical course might last for years.

- Borrelial lymphocytoma: A discrete, purple bump, lymphocytoma has been reported on the skin of the ear, nipple, and scrotum.

PEARL: Do not underestimate the potential debility that can come from brain fog, hyper-acute senses, migrating joint pain, and paresthesias. Believe the patient and hope you never have to undergo these symptoms yourself. Even better, hope that your child might never have to experience them. Remember, I used to be a skeptic. Then I got Lyme and my husband got Lyme and my son got Lyme. Experience can be a merciless teacher.

E. Quirky Lyme

Some things about the presentation of Lyme are a tad "quirky" but these extraordinary manifestations are not necessarily uncommon. Unfortunately, we often see them but do not recognize what they might represent and their potential association with Lyme. In my past life, I would never have associated these signs and symptoms with Lyme but I know more now than I did then. Consider the following manifestations as potentially associated with Lyme when there is reason to suspect borreliosis:

• Magnesium deficiency that can manifest as muscle cramps, twitches, and tremors

• More than usual lesions on scalp, such as pimples on the hairline, eczema, or EM rash hidden under hair. "Even my hair hurts."

• Poor visual accommodation

• Bright red tonsillar pillars. One theory is that blood stasis causes petechiae in the back of the throat resulting in red, injected pillars.

• Winter's ear: Pinnae become red and hot. This may be associated with high histamine levels. The ears feel warm to the touch. This phenomenon may increase with activity. The actual temperature of the ears at the time of the reaction is higher than other body tissue. One patient had a 105° temperature on the ear.

• There are multiple and varied NP manifestations and some are not familiar such as bizarre, involuntary movements, atypical sleep patterns, recurrent nightmares, and vocal and muscular tics. Patients can suffer personality changes, wide mood swings, and aggression. Parents will complain, "He's like a different person."

• Tingling of tip of nose or tongue

• Europeans have reported a borrelial lymphocytoma which is a discrete, purple bump appearing on the skin of the ear, nipple, or scrotum. This lesion is not well-known in North American Lyme. Likewise, the acrodermatitis chronica atrophicans noted with some European disease is not a typical manifestation in the US.

• Itch is more common in Lyme than recognized. Could this be the same histamine mechanism that causes Winter's ear? Could the itch be associated with Lyme-induced thyroid dysfunction?

• Lyme patients often complain of a feeling of occlusion in the throat. Some feel like they can't swallow or that there's a golf ball in the way. They have trouble swallowing food and saliva and have the sensation of choking or obstruction.

• Jaw pain

• The term "Lyme shrug" refers to the noisy cracking and popping that occurs in some patients when they move their neck. I was oblivious to this manifestation until I witnessed my son's neck persistent snapping.

• Irritable. Irritable. Irritable.

Speaking of quirky manifestations of Lyme, I wanted to share the sxs that surprised me most in my intense experience with Lyme over the past three years:

1. The migratory nature of the joint pain. Until you've experienced it, it's hard to describe.

2. The density of the brain fog. A number of conditions can cause brain fog but the Lyme fog can be incapacitating. Until you've experienced it, …

3. The intensity of some of the neuropsychiatric sxs. While this can be co-infection or a combination of pathogens, some Lyme patients seem to change personalities overnight. The anxiety, panic, fear, and OCD can frighten even old salts like me.

4. The association between paresthesias and Lyme. The tingling, stabbing, shocking, buzzing, lightening-like sensations that can result from the Bb pathogen are surprising both physically and mentally. Their intermittent nature makes them continue to stun. I never made the connection between my own symptoms and Lyme until I was deep into this book. My neighbor says his Lyme makes him feel like he's had "numb boots" on his feet for years. Paresthesias have also been described as talons or a claw-like sensation, buzzing or vibrations inside the body. PNS involvement can cause sensations of bugs crawling or something stroking the face.

5. The general acceptance of the EM rash. Whether it is due to apathy or laziness on the part of the medical community, we have allowed ourselves to agree to the idea of the near-universal prevalence and even essential-to-diagnosis nature of a sign that is actually less common than we have been led to believe.

F. Specific Organ System Manifestations

• **General Signs and Symptoms**

Lyme can be total body imbalance. This colossal disruption of normal physiology leads to a cluster of sxs that can stump the most astute clinician. Sxs cycle, flare, remit, wax, and wane. There can be good days and bad days and good weeks and bad weeks. The clinical presentation can shift with age, strain of pathogen, concurrent conditions, genetics, co-infections, and underlying wellness. The sxs can even fluctuate within an individual at different stages of the disease. As Tolstoy would have paraphrased if he had Lyme instead of syphilis, "Every unremarkable Lyme case is alike, but each complicated case is different in its own way." Maybe so different that we don't even recognize it as Lyme.

In this *General* section, I will focus only on those signs and symptoms that do not fit better into the other categories below. For example, I have headache listed in the *Head, Neck, Mouth, Throat* section. But head pain would fit just as well in the segment on *Neurologic* manifestations, or even here in the *General* portion. These signs and symptoms can all overlap, adding and detracting from the complete picture.

Once again, Lyme can present with the flu-like syndrome that is the result of the inflammatory response. These general manifestations include fever, pain, and fatigue. Like all Lyme-associated manifestations, the sxs can come and go and cycle. At first some people barely seem sick with vague and subtle discomforts. Others are frankly at the point of collapse, almost from the moment of inoculation.

Most Lyme patients complain of **pain** or aches, usually headache or joint pain, but bone and muscle pains are common as is neck pain and stiffness. This discomfort can range from mild, annoying aches to incapacitating, lightening-like, shooting pains.

Fatigue, which is sometimes called malaise or exhaustion, is not relieved with rest. Some patients are near collapse after short periods of minimal activity. Some authors describe this as deflating or wilting. Fatigue will likely be the first symptom noticed and the last one remaining when all else has resolved. The exhaustion can be crippling. Some patients are too tired to walk or sit up by themselves. Fatigue results in decreased stamina and a limited ability to work, play, and do schoolwork. AODLs are impacted and the person is so tired that he cannot function. He misses sports and other activities that are important to him and that he would really like to do. Lyme fatigue can be horrendous and, along with pain, is largely responsible for the impairment associated with LD.

With Lyme, **fevers** are usually low grade but can occasionally spike quite high. Fevers may follow a cyclic pattern. Sweats do occur in some patients but the question remains whether the sweats are actually due to LD or could be the result of a co-infection such as babesiosis. Lyme fevers tend to be highest in the afternoon. Many Lyme patients have subnormal temperatures the rest of the day but then gradually rise to about 99 by mid-afternoon. Fevers with Lyme tend to be lower than with the other common co-infections. Of course, co-infections complicate the clinical picture.

One of the best indicators of general health is the HCPs first impression of the patient. Irrespective of stage in the clinical course of Lyme, these people can look quite ill. Kids will start falling behind on developmental milestones and can just plain not feel good. They're wilted.

• **Neurologic**

Neuropsychiatric manifestations may be the most common of the signs and symptoms of Lyme. While we have been drilled to expect an EM rash, that rash is not found in the majority of cases. Perhaps 10% to 40% remember an EM rash depending on the practice. Further, perhaps only about 25% to 75% of patients have an associated arthritis, the prevalence of which seems to increase as the clinical course progresses. After general inflammatory-type sxs, some kind of neuropsychiatric presentation is almost universal in Lyme. In fact, in some cases, neuropsychiatric problems can be the presenting complaint. For organizational purposes, I will attempt to separate the neurologic and psychologic. In reality, these Lyme features are hard to distinguish.

Elizabeth Mahoney in the *Journal of American Physicians and Surgeons* listed the most common neurologic signs and symptoms associated with Lyme within her study population: memory loss 81%, fatigue 74%, headache 48%, sensory loss 44%, spinal or radicular pain 41%, depression 37%, sleep disturbance 30%, distal paresthesias 26%, irritability 26%, difficulty finding words 19%, fibromyalgia 15%, and decreased hearing 15%. Overall, just about every conceivable NP problem has been associated with Lyme. Sometimes Bb are to blame, other times it is co-infection, previously undiscovered conditions, or an unrelated co-morbidity. I do not include every NP manifestation I came across in the literature, only those that had multiple mentions and a plausible pathophysiologic basis. Just like the AE sections in drug labels, the inclusion of a specific condition only means that someone at one point made an association with Lyme. That does not mean that Bb caused the condition in the past or will cause the condition in a specific patient in the future.

Neurologic manifestations of Lyme might include: Brain fog, headache, irritability, Bell's palsy, paresthesias (numbness and tingling), pain, autism-like syndromes, hypersensitivity to sound, light, touch, and to a lesser degree smell and taste, sensory integration defect, abnormal senses, sensory dysfunction, sensation ranging from numbness to overly perceptive, touch causing stinging, burning, tenderness, or hyperawareness, shocking, shooting, bolt-like nerve pain that can be debilitating, distal radiculopathies, crawling sensations, buzzing in extremities, encephalitis, meningitis, depression, sleep disturbances, diminished ability to express thoughts, difficulty processing information, unclear thinking, problems reading when there might not have been previously, decreased quality of writing, poor handwriting, bewilderment even in familiar locations and situations, a kind of Lyme-dementia, balance problems, lack of coordination, cognitive deficits, interrupted development milestones, developmental delays, twitches, tremors, fasciculations, personality changes, mood swings, aggressiveness, memory loss, poor short-term memory, problems known to be associated with the CNS, PNS, ANS, and CNs, both upper and lower motor neuron lesions, feeling overwhelmed, difficulty making decisions, confusion, diminished concentration, challenge to focus, forgetfulness, disorientation, getting lost, going to the wrong place, searching for the correct word, hearing loss, tinnitus, dizziness, vertigo, auditory hallucinations, involuntary movements, impaired logic, poor judgment, easily distracted, impulsivity, apraxia, problems with auditory or visual processing, dyslexia, sudden onset of neuropsychiatric symptoms such as OCD, tics, or Tourette's, sensations of stabbing or electrical shock, lightheadedness, fainting, more frequent motion sickness, weakness, peripheral nerve impairment causing neuropathies that might include sensory changes and weakness, muscle atrophy due to damaged innervations, nerve dysfunction that can weaken muscles, radiculopathies, stammers, slow or slurred speech, tongue feels thick or slow, misspeaking, clumsiness, certain seizures, sleep problems including unusual behaviors or postures, inconsistent use or rearrangement of sounds, inability to execute purposeful, previously known acts despite physical ability and willingness, eyelid twitching, inability to perform tasks that they could do before, unable to learn new things, increased intensity of headaches, tendency to reverse numbers and letters when this was not a prior issue, palsies, increased ICP, pseudotumor cerebri, learning disabilities, diminished attention span, feeling shaky or nervous, anxiety, difficulty walking, gait disturbances, decreased facial sensation, and some complain of the need to concentrate hard in order to get their tongue to do what they want. There is some debate over whether there are more of certain kinds of seizures in the Lyme population or not.

PEARL: From caregivers to HCPs, people tend to discount or dismiss neuropsychiatric sxs. I believe this minimization is due to a number of factors. Sometimes parents are embarrassed that their child is not strong enough to overcome the NP sxs. If only the child would try harder. HCPs might overlook these sxs because they lack confidence in their ability to manage them. We all have our prejudices. We wouldn't get angry or frustrated with a patient who developed an EM rash. Why blame them for NP sxs that they can no more control than they can will away a skin lesion?

A description of the most common (or important) neurologic manifestations of Lyme follows.

Brain fog: Brain fog is nearly universal in Lyme. Brain fog is likely due to a number of mechanisms including direct spirochetal impairment of nervous tissue as well as the toxic effects of certain cytokines associated with inflammation. Brain fog is hard to understand unless you've experienced it. Let me try. Brain fog feels like there is a heavy, wet blanket covering your brain. Or like your thoughts are trying to swim through maple syrup. Thick and slow and not getting anywhere. Much of the problem seems to come from difficulty in processing information. A great deal of data is being gathered, but then the Lyme-brain cannot sort or manage the information.

Brain fog can manifest with poor short-term memory, trouble recalling what happened earlier in the day or what is usually done next, impaired concentration, inability to sustain attention, difficulty processing the data that the senses are gathering, trouble thinking clearly, diminished ability to express thoughts, impaired reading or writing (or no desire to do so), feeling overwhelmed, limited decision-making ability, confusion, lack of motivation, forgetfulness, disorientation, getting lost, going to the wrong place, trouble finding the right word, and speech difficulties. The patient might feel like she is under sedation.

The most disturbing thing I found with brain fog is that while I was aware of something being amiss and was wondering about it, I simply DID NOT CARE. I was perfectly content to sit in a recliner and allow Christmas to happen around me. I had no motivation to do anything to discover the cause of my lassitude and apathy. I drove little because I would get to the bottom of the street and not know which way to turn, on roads I had driven a thousand times. I was sensible enough to know that this probably wasn't safe. I covered my dullness with grumpiness and no one was the wiser.

With brain fog, there can be confusion, followed by clarity, followed by apathy. Imagine being in school or at work and having to deal with brain fog – like watching your life story play in slow motion.

PEARL: When I had Lyme-associated brain fog, I had never heard of brain fog or its association with Lyme. I had no idea what was going on. How much better when you know that others have had similar complaints and that you aren't losing your mind. Expect brain fog with Lyme and plan to show compassion.

Headache: Cephalgia or head pain is a very common complaint in LD, as it is in most other infectious diseases. The headache associated with Lyme has been described as a generalized soreness or a pressure, as though the brain is too big for the head. Some say that a Lyme headache is like wearing a helmet that is too small. Lyme headaches are often nuchal and associated with a stiff, painful, crepitant neck. So, it's not surprising that the Lyme headache is similar in nature to those described by syphilis patients.

Encephalitis: A severe inflammation of the brain, encephalitis might present with a sudden onset of fever, headache, vomiting (which can be projectile), stiff neck and back (nuchal rigidity), and signs of neuronal damage such as changes in consciousness, paralysis, malaise, opisthotonos, restlessness, seizures, pupil irregularities, motor dysfunction, involuntary movements, changes in vital signs, ptosis, tremor, increased DTRs, paralysis, paresis (incomplete paralysis), abnormal sleep, behavior changes, nausea, ataxia, and psychoses. Cerebral edema has been observed. After an acute phase, the signs and symptoms may persist for days or weeks. Encephalitis may leave permanent damage and can be fatal. Here the actual brain tissue is affected. The overall syndrome that can accompany brain inflammation is called encephalopathy. When that term is used, it often refers to the cognitive changes and problems the patient with encephalitis might experience.

PEARL: One "expert" told the media there was no such thing as Lyme encephalitis, although meningitis was possible. With a smug and supercilious demeanor, he said Lyme did not contribute to aggressive behavior in one high profile case. Even though the involved individual and his family had been begging for treatment for his Lyme and clearly describing sxs of Lyme encephalitis, the "expert" could not make the connection. Witness for the prosecution! Does his opinion make physiologic sense? If the Bb can get to the covering of the brain as it does in Lyme-meningitis, why wouldn't the pathogen be able to move into the brain itself? The syphilis spirochete is well-known for this type of brain invasion. How else would he explain the Bb spirochetes found in brain tissue on autopsy? With other infectious agents we know that a condition called meningoencephalitis may be more likely than either encephalitis or meningitis alone.

Meningitis: An inflammation of the membrane around the brain and spinal cord is called meningitis. Sxs include headache, stiff neck (nuchal rigidity), fever, change in consciousness, photophobia, phonophobia, irritability, drowsiness, and confusion. Nuchal rigidity is observed in about 70% of cases and Kernig's sign (pain that limits passive extension of the knee) and Brudzinski's sign (flexion of neck causes involuntary flexion of the knees) may be present on physical exam. Most commonly the inflammation is the result of an infection. Therefore, signs of meningitis are initially those of infection: fever, chills, and malaise. As the disease progresses there will be signs of increased ICP such as headache, vomiting, and perhaps papilledema. Soon the signs of meningeal irritation develop, including nuchal rigidity. The PE might also show exaggerated symmetrical DTRs, vision problems, and changes in consciousness. Opisthotonos is a spasm in which the back and extremities arch backwards so that the weight rests on the head and heels. An eye exam looking at the fundus may reveal signs of increased ICP such as papilledema. The meningitis associated with Lyme has been called aseptic but current technology just isn't very adept at recovering the Bb, not that they aren't there.

PEARL: Pseudotumor cerebri is another name for increased intracranial pressure, but doesn't it sound much more impressive? Usually this increased ICP is accompanied by papilledema but that is not always the case. Absence of papilledema does not rule out high ICP. Nevertheless, whenever there is papilledema there can be vision changes. High ICP is often affiliated with headache.

Pediatric acute-onset neuropsychiatric syndrome: (PANS) Recently, a proposal has been made to rename the clinical syndrome called PANDAS to include other pathogens as etiologic agents. The name PANS allows for the possibility of other infectious causes aside from Strep. This symptom cluster is probably an autoimmune response involving antineuronal antibodies and microbial mimicry. There can be a sudden onset of neuropsychiatric symptoms such as OCD, tics, or Tourette's. The basal ganglion seems to be the primary target and this site is responsible for movement and behavior. Some PANS patients display abnormal involuntary movements and various tics that can be predominant presenting signs. PANS can cause a dramatic, almost overnight onset of symptoms with motor or vocal tics, emotional lability, anxiety, OCD manifestations, enuresis, and deterioration in hand writing. Separation anxiety has also been reported.

Paresthesias: Sensations of numbness, tingling, pricking, or heightened sensitivity that can be due to lesions in either the CNS or PNS. Paresthesias are common in Lyme and have been described as burning, shooting, painful, shocking, stunning, and pins and needles. The phenomenon is usually intermittent and can take the patient by surprise. A sharp intake of breath may accompany an unexpected jolt. Sometimes touch will trigger a paresthesia where the contact triggers a burning or stinging sensation. A number of Lyme patients will resist wearing clothing or shoes because of the discomfort associated with the touch of the fabric. While this symptom can be secondary to hyperactive sensitivity, paresthesias have been noted under these circumstances as well.

Pain: Some Lyme patients are incapacitated by pain in joints, head, bones, muscles, or elsewhere. Pain management can be an important component of caring for Lyme patients and can be central in returning the patient to a state of normal function.

Autism-like syndrome: Autism is a spectrum of signs and symptoms that most often include withdrawal, unresponsiveness, and impaired communication. At one point Bb was thought to be the cause of autism. Today autism is thought to be multifactorial and Bb are known to cause an autism-like syndrome which can be hard to distinguish from the autism due to other causes. Chapter 17-N has considerable detail regarding the manifestations of autism and possible means to distinguish between Lyme-induced autism and ASD from other etiologies. This distinction can be important since Bb-caused autism is likely to respond better to treatment if antibiotics are part of the regimen.

Hypersensitivity: People with Lyme often experience excessive sensitivity to any of the senses. There are several hypothesizes attempting to explain why this might be so. Bb may cause direct harm to cranial nerves thereby impeding normal function. This phenomenon could also be due to difficulty processing sensory information, that is, a **sensory integration** problem. If the body cannot process all the sensory data that is gathered then the patient can be subjected to either too much sensory response or too little response to the input. Thereby the patient can suffer a range of sxs from numbness to intense perception of the involved sense. Hypersensitivity can manifest in all senses as well as with pain, but light, sound, and touch are the most common. Some patients exhibit more than one kind of hypersensitivity. We all have preferences, but Lyme-related hypersensitivity interferes with normal life. Neonates with gestational Lyme are especially susceptible. Be cognizant to this possibility since small children cannot explain what's bothering them and we may be torturing them with bright lights and *Barney* reruns.

- Light: Photophobia is an avoidance of light, especially bright or sunlight. Some patients will request a darkened room because even minimal light is too intense. Others might need sunglasses during the day, even indoors. Their intolerance to light can manifest as discomfort or pain in the eyes on even minimal exposure. They may want blinds drawn or lights turned down and might complain that the sun is blinding.

- Sound: Hyperacusis or phonophobia is an oversensitivity to sound. The person will have little or no tolerance for noise or loud sounds and may even feel discomfort with pleasant sounds like music or whispering. These patients cannot bear the usual sounds of daily life and may request sound muting headphones or ear plugs, assuming the touch of these accoutrements is not bothersome. Some want no sound and even soft music is overwhelming.

- Touch: A number of Lyme patients cannot stand any clothing touching them, even the softest cloth. Some refuse all clothes and others cannot tolerate shoes because the touch of the material is too intense. We all know the child who just refuses to have her hair brushed because it hurts. Lyme can compound this hypersensitivity. These individuals may want all the tags removed from clothing and some insist that clothes be washed many times before first wear to stop them from being itchy or scratchy. Some avoidance of certain foods might be due to the texture issues not the taste. In contrast, some kids want more touch and will ask for extra or harder hugs. Some patients are hypersensitive to pain but the pathologic mechanism is probably different.

- Smell: Although olfactory hypersensitivity may be less reported than the overstimulation of the other senses, it does occur in association with Lyme. When I had active Lyme, a smell of cedar trees, which was pleasant to my co-workers, nauseated me. Normally, I love the smell of cedar.

- Taste: We all know picky eaters and sometimes I'm picky myself. Lyme can intensify tastes, turning preferences into aggressive avoidance. Some of these food issues can be textural as well as based on taste.

Often the term sensitivity does not do these symptoms justice. These extreme reactions to even mild stimulation can invade and alter normal life and affect the quality of that life.

Balance problems: Balance is the ability to maintain the center of gravity over the base of support. Damage to the vestibular mechanism in the inner ear as well as problems with CN 8 can alter balance. The patient may wobble, sway, list to one side, have trouble walking in line, or be unable to stand on one foot. The Lyme patient may have difficulty maintaining balance with his eyes closed. Nystagmus may be present on physical exam and coordination and proprioception should also be assessed. Listing to the left or right may help discern which side of the brain is affected.

*PEARL: I had been taking yoga classes for over a year and I was top of the class in balance and flexibility (although yoga is **NOT** competitive). Good yoga practice employs balance in order to help maintain many of the poses. Over time my balance became worse and worse. Eventually my balance deteriorated to such a degree that I had to take a position next to the wall so that I would not topple. The teacher noticed. Of course, I worked myself up for MS and brain tumors before I made the connection. Finally my imbalance, lack of coordination, and poor proprioception made me think Lyme was simmering under the surface.*

Cognitive deficits: Cognition is the ability to think. Lyme impacts clear thinking in every way you can imagine. In order to assess cognitive ability, HCPs look at basic knowledge, vocabulary, analytical ability, problem solving, and the presence of a coherent line of reasoning. Thoughts should be clear, realistic, and follow a logical flow. Tager's work showed that Lyme patients can have significantly more cognitive and psychiatric disturbances than controls. These deficits were still found after controlling for anxiety, depression, and fatigue. Cognition problems in kids can be the primary presenting sign and impaired cognitive function can make it hard to sustain attention, learn new things, and recall information. Cognitive glitches can severely impact developmental milestones. Manifestations of cognitive difficulties due to Lyme might include poor processing of incoming information, plodding thoughts, slow ability to catch on, illogical reasoning, trouble with reading or writing, word searching, limited recall, difficulty in learning new concepts, impaired concentration, confused ideas, and diminished ability to express thoughts. Have a high index of suspicion especially in areas where the child had no prior problems or where there is a sudden, drastic change. While they do not fall neatly under the cognition label, judgment and abstract thought could also be impacted by Lyme.

Delayed Developmental Milestones: Developmental milestones are a set of skills that can be used to assess where a child stands compared to her peers. Usually aptitudes in several areas are observed such as gross motor, fine motor, language, cognition, and social interaction. These skills can be quite variable but documenting milestones can be especially useful in TBI patients because they allow the HCP to see how the child is doing now, compared to past performance. We are not only interested in what the child can do right this minute, but also whether the child improves or deteriorates from visit to visit. This comparative assessment can be extremely important in determining if the treatment plan is working. These developmental markers can be of obsessive concern to parents. They are most useful to the HCP in helping to follow the child over time.

Twitches, tics, fasciculations: Whatever the underlying pathology, Lyme patients seem subject to a wide variety of abnormal movements:

- **Tic:** An involuntary spasmodic muscle contraction usually involving the brief, rapid movement of the face, mouth, head, neck, or shoulder. Tics can resolve for a while, only to return. Tics can be simple or complex and are usually stereotypical and repetitive but NOT rhythmic. Simple tics include things like blinking or repeatedly clearing the throat. Tics often begin in childhood and mimic parts of normal behavior. Complex tics can include both motor and vocalizations and are disabling in some cases. Tics are associated with PANDAS and are common in TBIs.

- **Fasciculation:** A muscle twitch that is a small, local, involuntary muscle contraction visible under the skin. Fasciculations are most common in the eyelid.

- **Tremor:** A tremor is a repetitive, rhythmic movement caused by muscle contractions and relaxations that are described by: 1) pace of the rhythm: slow to rapid, 2) amplitude, 3) distribution or location, and 4) when the tremor occurs, whether at rest or when performing intentional movements. Parkinson's has a resting tremor while cerebellar disease has an intention tremor. Tremors are less common in Lyme than the other abnormal movements.

- **Twitch:** A single contraction of one muscle fiber in response to one nerve impulse. In reality most people use the term twitch to refer to any small, jerking muscle contractions as in, "My eyelid won't stop twitching."

- **Chorea:** Movements that are choreic are brief, purposeless, involuntary movements of the distal extremities. Sometimes the patient can merge these movements into a purposeful action that masks the abnormal motion.

Bell's palsy: While not common in LD, (maybe 10% of Lyme patients develop Bell's palsy), this affliction should be an alert signal for Lyme. Bell's palsy refers to a partial or full paralysis of the 7th cranial nerve, called the facial nerve. Most often the paralysis is one-sided with a sudden onset. Most patients and caretakers are alarmed by this manifestation. Facial expression is distorted and the patient may not be able to control salivation or lacrimation and in severe cases cannot close the eye on the affected side. Very rarely is Bell's palsy bilateral. Occasionally there is associated pain. The nerve is thought to have been injured by inflammation, ischemia, swelling, or trauma. Resolution of symptoms may take months and relapses occur. The presence of Bell's palsy, especially with a history of tick bite, is strongly suggestive of the diagnosis. This manifestation in Lyme suggests that spirochetes have somehow impacted the facial nerve.

Since the facial nerve controls the muscles of the face responsible for puffing out cheeks, raising eyebrows, frowning, smiling, closing the eyes so tight they can't be opened, and showing teeth, half the face will not be able to perform these movements. The victim will have trouble articulating clearly because many of these muscles are important for forming words. CN 7 also provides taste on the forward 2/3 of the tongue. A deficiency of the taste component of the facial nerve will likely go unnoticed since the other half of the tongue will compensate.

PEARL: My friend Greg had to interview for his own job at one of the world's vilest pharmaceutical companies. Because local staff was viewed as incapable of conducting these interviews, bureaucrats from headquarters were flown across the Atlantic. (And you wonder why grandma's medicine costs so much.) Well, poor Greg had a sudden bout of Bell's palsy prior to the interview. Greg salivated and had trouble formulating words throughout the entire meeting. He went through a box of tissues collecting the tears and saliva. The foreign visitors did not know Greg. Even though Greg tried to explain the situation, one interviewer commented that Greg was sadly mentally deficient. This massive company is now failing miserably in the global economy and the world media is appropriately splashing the headlines on countless front pages. Yesterday I read there was a revolt with shareholders demanding all new management. I hope the guy who called Greg mentally impaired is the first to go.

With most of these neuropsychiatric complaints, the rest of the body will heal before the brain. Don't be surprised.

- **Psychologic**

Neuropsychiatric manifestations may be the most common of the signs and symptoms of Lyme. Drawing the line between which manifestations are neurologic and which are psychologic is difficult indeed. Actually, I see no need to set such boundaries. Just as all biology is really chemistry, and all chemistry is really physics, and all physics is really math, neurology and psychology are two sides of the same coin. Nonetheless, the distinction

is long-standing and has been subject to the fallacy that neurologic sxs are more valid than the psychologic and strong willpower or a good kick in the butt will cure all mental health issues. Remember, illness is largely physical or biochemical no matter what organ system is involved. Never overlook, minimize, or underestimate the psychological component of Lyme. These sxs can change a person's life and need to be recognized and addressed. Total emotional dysregulation occurs in some cases. Just when patients are thinking their physical world has fallen apart due to Lyme, they also have to wonder if they have the emotional stamina to deal with the disease.

Lyme-associated psychological issues can be of sudden onset, where the personality seems to change overnight, or can manifest as an exacerbation of a pre-existing condition. The effects can be subtle or earth-shattering. Keep a high index of suspicion that Lyme might be a contributor in these cases. As noted above, Tager's group found that kids with Lyme had significantly more cognitive and psychiatric disturbances than controls. These deficits were still found after controlling for anxiety, depression, and fatigue.

Psychological conditions associated with Lyme include anxiety, emotional lability, increased crying even in older kids and adults, depression, separation anxiety that can be debilitating, change in school performance, trouble processing information, suicidal thinking, self-harm, cutting, GAD, OCD, changes in personality, alterations in mood, panic, irritability, sensation of going crazy, defensiveness, paranoia, sensitivity to criticism or perceived slights, need for reassurance, cries easily, panic, fear, anger, phobias, tics, specific fears like pet getting lost, confusion, trouble concentrating, annoying and easily annoyed, brain fog, disorientation, bad judgment, irrational and illogical reasoning, autism-like presentation, acting out, uncharacteristic behaviors, memory problems, trouble focusing, impulsivity, vocal tics, nightmares, and unusual sleep patterns.

The presence of co-infections can confound the psychologic manifestations of Lyme. Parents will say, "He's not the same child he was a month ago." The personality can seem to be irretrievably altered. Yet, reversals in many of these predominantly psychological conditions induced by Lyme can be orchestrated.

In extreme cases, Lyme has been clearly associated with aggression, hostility, violence, auditory hallucinations, outbursts, bipolar disorders, antisocial behaviors, and psychotic episodes where the individual has lost touch with reality. The mechanism here may be a Bb encephalopathy, Bb toxins, PANS, harmful effects of cytokines, or more likely, a combination of factors in genetically susceptible individuals. The sudden onset of a psychologic episode is a red flag for Lyme. These events can be significant and alarming. Think of TBIs when addressing aggressive and other antisocial behaviors in juvenile offenders.

PEARL: Psych problems can be messy. Patients or caretakers are often embarrassed to admit a mental health issue. Sometimes they keep crucial information to themselves. Since psych conditions can be hard to manage, the HCP may gloss over a complaint hoping to replace it with an easier problem to solve. While antibiotics will likely alleviate or cure the joint pain or rash, psych problems can be more intractable. Never give up.

Lyme can undermine personality, thinking processes, and mood. Underestimate the psychologic manifestations of Lyme at your peril.

- **Musculoskeletal**

The musculoskeletal system is so closely associated with Lyme that some early commentators felt it was solely a joint disease and named it Lyme arthritis. We now know that Lyme is a multisystem illness and the involvement of bones, muscles, and joints makes up only a part of the clinical picture. Arthritis is estimated to be present in between 25 and 75% of cases with the incidence increasing the longer the infection has been present.

Lyme arthritis is most common in the knees, but shoulder pain is well-recognized, and essentially any joint can be affected. A characteristic finding of Lyme is migratory arthritis where one day the shoulder might be achy and the next the opposite knee. The joint may be red, hot, and swollen with effusion. More commonly, they just ache. The discomfort ranges from noticeable to debilitating. Despite my first orthopod telling me that an effusion had to be present for a Lyme diagnosis, that is baloney. Most often an effusion and swelling are not present. Joint cartilage has been eroded by the presence of Bb.

PEARL: A knee joint swollen because of Lyme suggests serious propagation and the clinical course may progress rapidly and vigorously.

Popping joints are common in people with borreliosis. The jaw can pop and the neck can pop and knees can pop. Kids will say their joints are creaky, cracking, crackly, and one kid said crunchy. Lyme patients might constantly be cracking their knuckles, which can pop readily without any help. The neck can be stiff, painful, and crepitant. Ribs are often painful and there can be pain on palpation at the costochondral joints. Point tenderness has been documented on the iliac crest.

Usually arthritis associated with Lyme targets the big joints like knees and shoulders but smaller joints are commonly involved as well. Nevertheless, joints in fingers and toes can be affected and here you might see more swelling. Wrists, hands, and TMJ can be affected. Usually Lyme arthritis starts with monoarticular discomfort that develops into migratory polyarthritis. (That sentence sounds so much more "official" than "First my shoulder hurt, then my knee hurt.")

Borreliosis has been associated with bone pain, carpal tunnel syndrome, tendonitis, myalgia, muscle cramps, spasms, sore soles, chest wall pain, chondritis, jaw pain, chest pain, costochondritis, nerve dysfunction that can weaken muscles, pain in feet, swelling in toes, pain in the balls of feet, burning in feet, shin splints, stiffness in joints beyond the neck, morning stiffness, pain at rest, and inflammatory myopathies. Check for hypermobility which is occasionally affiliated with shoulder subluxation in cases of Lyme. Muscle pain is usually diffuse in Lyme without the trigger point pattern seen in fibromyalgia. Hypotonia is the hallmark of gestational Lyme in neonates.

- **Senses**

Because of Lyme's focus on nervous tissue, the senses would be expected to be a natural target. Again these sxs can be the result of several pathologic mechanisms from spirochetes invading the sensory organ directly, high or low level nerve damage, the effect of toxins, or consequences of powerful immunologic humors. Bb attacks on the optic nerve can lead to decreased vision and blindness. Hypersensation of any of the five senses, as well as to pain, has been described in the *Neurology* section above. Here the focus will be on the effects of Bb on the optic and auditory systems and the potential manifestations.

Sxs of eye problems associated with Lyme: Vision affected by Bb is often blurred or wavy. One patient referred to the visual loss as "smeary." This type of diminished acuity can make it hard to focus on words when reading. Lyme can result in problems with accommodation. ("Do you see one or two?") Astigmatism has also been documented in patients with Lyme, but the mechanism is unclear. Bb may "prefer" the viscous, non-flowing fluid inside the eye.

Eye conditions that have been associated with Lyme disease include blurred vision, hypersensitivity to light, photophobia, floaters, flashes, conjunctivitis, astigmatism, eye pain, dry eyes, papilledema, blind spots, night blindness, peripheral shadows, iritis, anterior uveitis, optic neuritis, eyelid droop, impaired color vision, alteration of colors, double vision, swelling around eyes, eyelid twitching or fasciculations, dark circles under the eyes, change in visual fields, flashing lights, peripheral waves, phantom images at the edge of the visual field, episcleritis, trouble reading because letters run together, general discomfort, gritty feel, extraocular palsies, problems with lacrimation in Bell's palsy, ptosis, cataracts in gestational Lyme, Lyme eye, eye fatigue, tearing, blepharitis, keratitis, and progressive decrease in visual acuity. If the Borrelia impact the optic nerve, blindness can result. Not all these are a direct result of damage to the visual apparatus, but all might be noted during an eye exam.

PEARL: Lyme eye is described as punctated erythema on the conjunctiva.

PEARL: Spirochetes have been cultured from the iris.

<u>Sxs of ear problems associated with Lyme</u>: Tinnitus, or ringing in the ears, is common with Borrelia infection. This tinnitus has been described as an underwater feel, buzzing, ringing, and even screeching. Auditory acuity can decrease and there can be general discomfort in the ears. The patient may experience more earaches than expected. Hypersensitivity to sound causing phonophobia is a frequent manifestation.

PEARL: In Winter's ear, the pinnae are bright red and hot and may be associated with high histamine levels sometimes seen in on-going Lyme. The patient can feel the ears getting hot as they become very red. The intensity increases with activity. The actual temperature of these ears at the time of reaction is higher than the rest of the body's temperature. One patient's ear temperature was 105°F.

- **Skin**

For a time in the history of Lyme disease, the EM rash was thought to be the defining characteristic of the illness. No rash, no Lyme. Even today, the media counsels both HCPs and the lay population to look for the EM rash when making the diagnosis. Well, they're half right. While the presence of an EM rash is pathognomonic for borreliosis, the absence of an EM rash is meaningless. In contrast to popular reports, the EM rash is actually less common in Lyme than we have been led to believe. Estimates vary greatly but perhaps 10 to 40% recall having an EM rash as part of the clinical presentation of their disease. Even less have an EM rash that looks like a target or bull's eye. Certainly there are other rash incidence estimates that are higher. Note that in some studies where the incidence of EM rash was tabulated, patients had to have an EM rash to garner the "official" diagnosis that subsequently allowed them to be in the study that

counted whether or not they had an EM rash. (Phew!) With the possibility of a tick bite, if you have an EM rash you have borreliosis unless proven otherwise. I hope to clarify this EM rash business in the next few paragraphs.

PEARL: In an August 24, 2007, letter to Pat Smith, the president of the Lyme Disease Association, a staff member from a government agency said that his opinion "... reflects the well established fact that the EM rash is not pathognomonic for Lyme disease." His argument was that STARI patients could also present with EM rashes. I think this hairsplitting does a disservice to the patients. I am willing to concede then that while an EM rash might not be pathognomonic for Lyme, it is pathognomonic for borreliosis. See, we can all get along.

Overall, various skin lesions are commonly associated with Lyme disease. These include:

1. **Erythema migrans:** Originally called erythema chronica migrans, this lesion, in the presence of corroborating history and ROS, is pathognomonic for borreliosis. WebMD recognizes the EM rash as pathognomonic of LD calling it a "sure sign." In the SLICE study at Johns Hopkins, the EM rash is used to define a case of Lyme.

But with Lyme, nothing is straightforward. A European study showed definitively that HCPs identified actual EM rashes with less than 30% accuracy. Most could not recognize either the lesion or its name. That's encouraging. Five physicians saw my son's EM rash. Two discounted it because it wasn't round enough. I knew it was an EM rash but didn't know enough to defend it from detractors. One doctor said it was classic and now uses it to illustrate lectures. Another recognized TBI expert agreed that Chris's lesion was certainly an EM rash. The likelihood of determining true incidence of EM rashes is greatly diminished if less than half the doctors can identify the lesion, even in a patient where the H&P and ROS are corroborating, and the deer tick is in a jar.

I get so frustrated with authors who simply repeat the misconception that an EM rash is likely to be seen and only then will you know whether LD is present or not. The majority of patients do not have an EM rash. If you hold the appearance of an EM rash as necessary to have LD, you will be missing half your cases right off the bat. Some practices say that less than 10% of their patients ever had an EM rash.

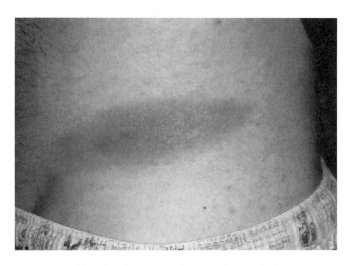

Classic primary erythema migrans lesion
Medical records of Christopher Spreen

Often the offending writers are about to discuss something else in a very enlightened way, but to get to their primary subject matter they just copy and paste the target lesion/bull's eye/EM myth. Then the fallacy gets repeated in every women's magazine on the planet. (A headline in the *WSJ* on March 27, 2012, and WebMD and the Merck Manual, etc.) Get over the rash already! If it's there, it's a diagnostic windfall. If it's not seen, that means nothing in terms of whether this particular patient has Lyme or not. Even when my son had a classic rash with the tick in a jar, it was deemed not exactly right according to the HCP's preconception of what an EM rash should be. Poor Chris did not qualify for the Lyme club. Get over the rash! I know I repeat myself here, but I have a lot of misinformation to rectify.

EM is a fascinating lesion almost like an interactive video with live action pathology on display. The rash itself can have various presentations and can be transient. Sometimes the lesion will only be visible for a very short time. So not only is an EM rash not as common as alleged, it can be a moving target. In some cases it might have been missed because it appeared and then was gone before anyone noticed. Other EM lesions are under hair, in places where no one is looking, or masked by dark skin pigment.

Usually an EM rash has a homogenous red color, but the color can vary from pale to maroon. There can be rings, but rarely central clearing. Very few could be called a bull's eye or target lesion.

We do not know why some patients get an EM rash but the majority do not. Perhaps there is a genetic predisposition. Perhaps there is an autoimmune component. Perhaps there is a genetic predisposition to an autoimmune component. Maybe it's the strain of

Bb responsible in the individual case. We also do not know the prognostic significance of an EM rash. Do these patients get sicker, stay sick longer, have more tendency to a certain clinical presentation, have more autoimmune manifestations? The difference between the haves and the have nots, when eventually uncovered, will explain many things, I bet.

PEARL: Some authors contend that an EM rash does not appear with the first exposure to Bb. They believe that only subsequent contact with this spirochete will cause EM lesions. I do not know how they made this determination and time will tell if this hypothesis is true. Either way the pathophysiology, once delineated, will be fascinating.

An EM rash is a diagnostic blessing. Rarely will you be given such a definitive sign as to what is happening inside a patient. Don't waste your time trying to come up with any possible reason why it is not an EM rash. It is what it is. I call this Lyme avoidance. Right, Lilith[1]?

Many doctors have been drilled that if there is no rash, there is no Lyme. We now know that is not true. Equally damaging is the decision to wait and see if a rash appears. In the majority of patients we would be waiting a long time. I did even more damage to my son. The classic rash was there, the tick was there, signs of inflammation were ringing alarms. Yet, I had been so ingrained that Lyme was no big deal and could easily be cured with a little doxy that I decided to wait and see if he got sicker before doing anything. He got sicker. I was so appalled at my own ignorance that I was compelled to write a book so others don't harm their kids in the same way.

The critical point is that the EM rash is confirmatory, if present. The absence of an EM rash means nothing.

PEARL: If an EM rash isn't borreliosis, what is it? Quick Lilith give me a list of three alternatives in your differential diagnosis. Okay, two.

There are two recognized types of EM rash associated with Lyme:

a. Primary erythema migrans

The primary EM rash is most often a single, homogeneous, red lesion. Usually the primary EM rash presents around the bite site, remaining dark red and possibly slightly indurated. While the outer rim of the lesion remains reddish, the area in between can clear, causing the rash to look like a target or bull's eye. While there may be apparent concentric rings,

1 See Glossary or Introduction for name origin

there is usually no central clearing. (Some sources say the central clearing is missing in over half the cases and it's likely far more than that.) The shape most often observed is an oval, not round. Oval, Lilith[2]. Our desire to make the EM rash into our notion of a perfect target or bull's eye means we must think of it as round. After all, targets aren't oval.

The spirochetes can move in a way that forms visible rings that expand out from the center. EM rashes are called expansive lesions since they can move outward into concentric circles. What is going on here? Actually this presentation makes perfect sense from a physiologic perspective. Spirochetes enter the skin and begin replicating usually near the bite site since that's where they happen to be. As the population increases the microbes move out from the bite spot in all directions. This causes concentric circles which are not always perfectly drawn since some pathogens may move faster and farther than others. (There's an over-achiever in every crowd.) Here the spirochete is present and active and moving and replicating. We know this because Bb have been isolated from biopsies taken at the edge of these lesions. If the biopsy sample is not taken at the periphery of the lesions, spirochetes will probably be missed.

At this point the infection is still localized.

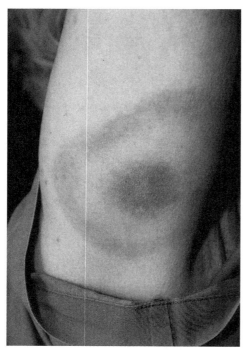

Concentric circles in an EM rash
Source: CDC. Accessed Oct 2012

---

2 See Glossary or Introduction for name origin

But there must be more to life than this. The spirochetes are now moving into the blood, heading out on their way to becoming intracellular inside a variety of organs, and encysting as the need arises. There are plenty of places they like better than skin. Nevertheless, sometimes the Bb are again active near enough to the skin surface to be observed. (Kind of like a creepy aurora borealis, only more elusive.) This brings us to the other recognized EM rash associated with Lyme.

b. Secondary erythema migrans

The secondary EM rash is evidence that Bb are on the move. While primary EM lesions might be referred to as expansive, secondary lesions are more appropriately called evanescent. They provide evidence of disseminated spirochetes. These are usually multiple lesions that appear as a result of Bb migrating through blood vessels and lymph channels. They might look like primary lesions but they come and go quite freely as the floating spirochetes traverse the circulatory system. A lesion, or multiple lesions, seem to pop up briefly, display, and recede.

PEARL: Evanescent means soon passing out of site, quickly fading, and likely to vanish.

A secondary EM rash tends to be multifocal and can appear in any area where the Bb are migrating. By evanescent here we mean quickly vanishing, dispersing, spreading, coming and going, waxing and waning, transient. I have never seen a secondary EM rash but I imagine that they are quite memorable since they are so extraordinary. These lesions are considered pathognomonic for disseminated Lyme. On tissue biopsy, several patients with these types of lesions have been shown to be full of spirochetes. (I have no idea if a secondary EM rash has ever been observed in STARI.)

PEARL: If all this is going on close enough to the surface to be witnessed, imagine the commotion in the tissue where the Bb plan to settle.

Secondary EM rashes are rarely seen and since they are so transitory they can easily be missed. If you should witness this phenomenon ask, "What am I seeing and what should I be doing about it?" I have your answer. You are seeing manifestations of free-floating spirochetes on their way to go intracellular and encyst. Get 'em while they're hot! Soon they will be much less accessible.

PEARL: To sum things up regarding the EM rash, these lesions can be:

- Oval

- Round

- Irregular due to location on skin or unequal movement of Bb

- With concentric circles or without

- Obvious

- Obscure, especially in dark skinned patients, or when the lesion is under hair, or in places not often inspected

- With or without central clearing (Some say that most Lyme EM rashes do not have central clearing, while most STARI lesions do. Or is it the opposite? Who knows?) HCPs questioned about central clearing had very different perceptions on whether or not central clearing was common. Those who saw a lot of Lyme thought only about 20% of EM lesions had central clearing. Those with less experience thought that most EM lesions had central clearing. Where did we get this idea of ubiquitous central clearing?

- Concentric circles can cause a lesion that looks like a target or bull's eye.

- There can be a tiny scab in the center of an EM rash, where the tick chomped.

- Local irritation of the bite site with redness and mild swelling is not an EM rash.

- If you wait for the EM rash to tell you whether there is a Bb infection or not, you could miss 90% of the cases.

- EM rashes are pathognomonic for borreliosis.

2. **Other Lyme associated skin lesions**:

Overall, skin lesions are common in Lyme, it's just the EM rashes that are not as widespread as some commentators would have us believe. There can be redness or a small scab around the tick bite site. This is not an EM rash, but this irritation might persist for several days. Note that this bite mark is most often a tiny scab with minimal surrounding inflammation mostly ON the surface of the skin. The EM lesions are due to spirochetes either IN the skin or IN the circulation. This is a small point that may help you understand why everything red and round is not an EM rash.

Other skin lesions potentially associated with Lyme include multiple flat lesions, raised lesions, blisters, vesicles, eczema-like conditions, purpura, and itchy patches. Lyme patients might complain of more than the usual number of lesions on the scalp such as pimples at the hairline, eczema, hair loss, and extreme sensitivity. "Even my hair hurts." Remember that an EM rash can be hidden under hair (including pubic hair).

All skin lesions concurrent with Lyme should not necessarily be assumed to be Borrelia-driven. A differential diagnosis should be established considering other possible explanations for these skin conditions. Considering the circumstances, you might want to think about insect bites, cellulitis, ringworm (my first Lyme misdiagnosis), and residual tick mouth parts in the skin. When looking for deer ticks, one mom found tiny thorns instead. Chapter 17 B contains an extensive differential listing.

Some patients in Europe have reported a borrelial lymphocytoma which is a discrete, purple bump appearing on the skin of the ear, nipple, or scrotum. Another skin manifestation of Lyme reported in some cases in Europe is acrodermatitis chronica atrophicans where the skin atrophies and becomes like tissue paper.

- **Genitourinary**

The genitourinary system is affected by Lyme. The genitals are impacted primarily because of the significant bearing Bb can have on the endocrine system. The urinary tract can be hit from several directions, including direct injury caused by intracellular Borrelia or the damage to nerves serving the urinary apparatus.

Testicular pain, pelvic discomfort, menstrual irregularity, lactation, and gynecomastia have all been considered associated with Lyme in some cases. Inguinal lymphadenopathy has been documented. Menstrual difficulties have been noted but these can be hard to substantiate since menses is irregular for a time after menarche. Be aware and consider how altered hormone levels might be contributing to the clinical picture.

Lyme is thought to cause problems with urination, occasional incontinence, new onset of enuresis without a family history, irritable bladder, and intermittent loss of bladder control. Kidney failure is one of the principal causes of death in dogs with Lyme.

Interstitial cystitis is very common in Lyme, even though the connection is often missed. IC presents just like any other infectious UTI. This condition is characterized by dysuria, hesitancy, urgency, and frequency. But unlike the

UTIs we are so used to curing with Bactrim for 10 days, here we are surprised when the culture comes back negative. And we're surprised when the culture comes back negative again and again, even though the symptoms persist. The condition does not resolve with traditional antibiotic regimens. Still the dysuria, hesitancy, urgency, and frequency persist. All signs point to a bacterial etiology yet culture after culture does not provide answers. The condition is even referred to as aseptic cystitis. Yet, doctors treat again and again with antibiotics that traditionally hit E. *coli* and other common causes of cystitis with no result. So do you think it's possible that E. *coli* might not be causing the problem? Perhaps the routine culture will not allow growth of the responsible pathogen. Anecdotally, adequate treatment for Lyme has helped resolve the interstitial cystitis in a number of cases. We know that Bb have been picked up with cystoscopy and biopsy of the bladder trigone and supported with PCR findings in a sample of these patients. Perhaps treating the Lyme will resolve these seemingly "aseptic" symptoms.

Chronic pelvic pain has been associated with LD. This pain is defined as discomfort lasting at least 3 months that interferes with some aspects of the person's life. Dr. Deborah Metzger, an expert on chronic pelvic pain associated with inflammatory processes and the inflammation associated with LD, believes that Bb can be responsible or associated with various conditions including allergies, insulin resistance, Candida, and pelvic discomfort. As many as 40% of women with chronic pelvic pain in Dr. Metzger's private practice are positive for Bb.

- **Immune**

  Even though the immune system is regularly overlooked in lists of affected organs, it may be the most impacted system of all. Signs and symptoms associated with Lyme are listed.

  1. Inflammatory reactions can be either acute or chronic and can be manifested by all the systemic indicators of inflammation such as fever, headache, malaise, and aches. This inflammatory response can be subtle or fulminant. Sometimes the only symptom is a general unease where the patient just doesn't feel right. Under other circumstances, the inflammatory response can flatten the person. Cytokines can contribute to brain fog and other symptoms.

  2. Autoimmune reactions seem to be more common in Lyme than originally suspected. Here the body mistakes *self* proteins for non-*self* and inappropriately takes out its own kind. The propensity for this type of response is genetic and those with the markers HLA-DR2 and HLA-DR4 seem more prone to an autoimmune Lyme syndrome. These patients present differently with more achiness and they do not respond as well to conventional treatment regimens. Plaquenil seems to help in these cases.

  3. A subset of Lyme patients appear to present with a syndrome similar to that seen in PANDAS. Here the condition might more appropriately be termed PANS, or pediatric acute-onset neuropsychiatric syndrome. Here through molecular mimicry and antineuronal antibodies the nerve cells are damaged by the patient's own defenses. Symptoms most often associated with PANS include a sudden display of motor or vocal tics, OCD, anxiety, panic, fearfulness, hyperactivity, involuntary movements, enuresis, and emotional lability. The abrupt onset of a PANS manifestation can be stunning to the patient and caretakers since dramatic sxs can appear almost overnight. Anecdotally, several Lyme patients seem to fit this pattern and have displayed aggressive, oppositional, and violent behavior. This presentation likely involves some degree of genetic susceptibility. For the best outcome when PANS is suspected, both the active TBI and the outward display of the syndrome should be treated concurrently.

  4. Lymphadenopathy can be viewed as part of the immune response and can range from barely palpable to grossly swollen. The neck, axilla, and inguinal regions are most often affected.

- **Gastrointestinal**

  I worked in the GI therapeutic area for years and no one was more surprised than me when I learned how significantly Bb might impact the digestive system. GI involvement in the clinical presentation of Lyme is often overlooked. In retrospect, many TBI-focused practitioners realize there have been GI complaints in a high percentage of their patients. These problems may be due in part to Bb's impact on the vagus nerve. The GI tract is also intimately associated with the immune system and the synergy between these two systems may complicate the pathophysiology. Further, the gut is highly innervated and we recognize Bb's affinity for nerve cells and their surrounding tissue.

  The most common GI feature of Lyme is probably GERD. Reflux is associated with burning, substernal discomfort, and spitting up in infants. GERD is a common manifestation of gestational Lyme. Other GI sxs include nausea, vomiting, stomach pain, diarrhea, change in bowel frequency, sense of obstruction, gut palsy, a dull unpleasant sensation, feelings of impending vomiting, vomiting with coughing, distress, bulging, bloating, putty-like stool, constipation, loss of appetite, spasms, 10th rib tenderness, esophageal dysmotility, and intestinal aching. Sxs can mimic IBS or IBD. More than a few patients have experienced difficulty swallowing, which can impede eating. Kids seem more prone to the GI sxs associated with Lyme than adults.

PEARL: Although gallstones are not directly due to Lyme, treatment with certain antibiotics, such as Rocephin, can enable their formation. Cholecystitis might result.

PEARL: Sometimes the only positive diagnostic test for TBIs will come from gut biopsy. Yield is greater than with blood or other body fluid sampling. Both cultures and DNA PCR have more sensitive results with gut biopsies than with many other specimen sources.

- **Endocrine**

Bb are well-known to affect the endocrine system. Lyme pathophysiology is both physical and chemical. The endocrine system produces a collection of powerful biochemicals involved in complex cascades where one event influences another and on and on. So, with Lyme, it is not surprising that hormonal abnormalities might be involved in the clinical presentation.

Simply (if anything about endocrine pathophysiology could be labeled simple), Lyme impacts the hypothalamic-pituitary-adrenal axis, which is involved in steering the whole ship. So essentially all aspects of the body's metabolism can be affected, manifesting in a wide array of sxs.

The thyroid can be damaged with all the associated signs and symptoms including weight changes, feeling hot or cold, changes in skin and hair, and disturbed energy levels.

Lyme affects blood sugars and patients may appear to have diabetes with all its associated sequelae. Here control of the blood sugars may depend on adequately addressing the Lyme as well as treating the blood sugar numbers.

Children with Lyme can have growth problems due to hormonal imbalance. Cortisol is associated with anxiety and dysregulation of this hormone might contribute to the symptomatology of Lyme. Overall, Bb's adverse impact on the endocrine system may be a factor in the debility found in chronic LD.

- **Head, Neck, Mouth, Throat**

A number of sxs attributed to Lyme can be found in the head, neck, mouth, and throat.

Head: Headache is almost ubiquitous in cases of Lyme. The head pain most commonly associated with borreliosis is reviewed in the *Neurology* section above. These headaches are often nuchal and associated with a stiff, painful, and crepitant neck. The pain may be severe and disabling. There might also be head pressure, problems with the hair or scalp, facial fasciculations, paralysis (Bell's palsy), facial tingling especially in tongue, cheek, or nose, facial flushing, and Winter's ear.

Neck: Cervical lymphadenopathy is a frequent finding in Lyme. Also quite common is a stiff, crepitant neck. Movement of the neck can be painful and Lyme-meningitis can cause nuchal rigidity. The term "Lyme shrug" refers to the noisy cracking and popping that occurs in some patients when they move their neck.

Mouth: The TMJ can be one of the joints affected by the migratory joint pain and the jaw can be stiff, sore, and even swollen and warm. There can be soreness and aches around the teeth. Dental issues can be associated with low-grade, chronic inflammation. Gingivitis has been affiliated with the formation of biofilms and Bb likely form biofilms. I wonder…

Throat: Lyme patients have complained of difficulty swallowing or the sensation that something is occluding the throat. (Consider co-morbid HPV.) Also possibly affiliated are injected tonsillar pillars, where blood stasis is thought to be responsible for petechiae in the back of the throat resulting in swollen tissue. Hoarseness has also been reported. (Again, ponder HPV.)

- **Cardiac/Circulation**

If something about Lyme is going to kill you, it very well might be the cardiac manifestations, although Lyme's role in these deaths is usually uncredited. Lyme can affect the heart through several mechanisms including direct invasion of cells and tissues, toxins, biofilms on valves, endocrine imbalances, and interference with nerve function. The affinity of Bb to collagen has been well-established. Tissues around blood vessels and cardiac valves contain a lot of collagen. Do not underestimate the power of Lyme to damage the cardiovascular system. The following list includes the sxs associated with cardiac manifestations of Lyme.

1. **Dysrhythmias:** Bb have been associated with various abnormal heart rhythms including atrial fibrillation, skipped beats, extra beats, premature beats, and flutters. Lyme patients frequently complain of palpitations or fluttering. Abnormal rhythms that result in diminished perfusion or other untoward effects may need to be overridden with pacemakers or medications.

Pacing is required in about a third of these dysrhythmic patients and they may present with chest pain, palpitations, syncope, and dyspnea. If the underlying etiology is Lyme, for goodness sake, treat the Lyme.

2. **Abnormal heart rates** have been linked to Lyme but patterns are not clear.

3. **Heart block**: Common in borreliosis, heart blocks can be due to vagal nerve dysfunction. An EKG will be needed to capture this sign.

PEARL: Lyme has been associated with AV block, 1ˢᵗ, 2ⁿᵈ, and 3ʳᵈ degree blocks, junctional rhythms, and asystolic pauses. Treat the Lyme if you want the overlying cardiac condition to respond.

4. **Valve problems**: Some infections result in the formation of vegetations on the valves themselves which are a combination of pathogen, fibrin, white cells, and other fragments that clog the works and prevent proper operation of the valve. These vegetations can break off as emboli and can damage other organs. There is reason to suspect that Bb may be one of the pathogens that camp on the cardiac valves, perhaps through biofilm formation. Murmurs may be discerned on PE, but ultrasound may be needed to better define the condition and functionality of the cardiac valves.

5. **Inflammation**: Inflammation due to infection or other causes can manifest in various heart locations and can be acute or chronic. Lyme has been known to cause:

   a. **Pericarditis**: The pericardium is the outside membrane around the heart and the base of the great vessels. The patient can present with pleuritic pain that increases with deep inspiration and decreases when position is changed. A friction rub can be auscultated in many cases. Pain can be of sudden onset and continue for days. Usually the pain is substernal to the left of midline and it can radiate to the back or subclavicular area. The discomfort can be mild and superficial or deep and severe. Often the pain is described as stabbing or knife-like. The pain tends to increase with movement and coughing and decrease when sitting up or leaning forward, since the latter position pulls the inflamed pericardium away from the diaphragm and other tissues. Likewise, the friction rub may be less audible under these conditions.

   b. **Endocarditis**: Bb can invade the endocardium, which is the inside endothelial membrane that lines the chambers of the heart, its valves, and is continuous with the lining of the arteries and veins. Inflammation of this membrane can be fatal and there

is significant mortality even if aggressively treated. Endocarditis can cause severe and permanent valve damage, leading to insufficiency and subsequent heart failure. Prosthetic valves are also susceptible. Initial signs and symptoms can be nonspecific, such as weakness, fatigue, weight loss, anorexia, arthralgia, and night sweats. More than 90% have intermittent fever. Sometimes the symptoms can last for weeks. If they resolve, they can recur. Usually a loud regurgitant murmur is heard. Whenever there is a suddenly changing murmur or a new onset murmur in the presence of fever, think endocarditis.

   c. **Myocarditis**: The myocardium is the heart muscle and inflammation of muscle tissue can be acute or chronic and occur at any age. Early symptoms can be nonspecific with fatigue, dyspnea, palpitations, and fever. Here spirochetes invade the muscle cells after dissemination from other locations in the body. The patient may present with a heart beat that sounds weak at the apex, an irregular rapid pulse, dysrhythmias, and tenderness over the precordium.

   d. **Carditis**: A somewhat nonspecific term referring to inflammation of several layers of the heart that can include pericarditis, myocarditis, or endocarditis and might present a complex array of signs and symptoms.

   e. **Pancarditis**: Refers to inflammation of all the structures of the heart and so would include myocarditis, pericarditis, and endocarditis.

6. **Cardiomyopathy** is direct damage to the heart muscle or myocardium due to disease or other modes of injury. The degree of damage will determine the effect on function and the subsequent symptomatology.

7. Children with gestational Lyme can present with a variety of **congenital** cardiac anomalies. Keep a high index of suspicion. Any abnormalities on the cardiac exam or a child who is cyanotic or struggling to breathe should be aggressively evaluated and supported.

8. Additional sxs that may or may not be cardiac have been correlated with the presence of Bb: chest pain, rib pain, cough, SOB, heart failure, and reflux.

Circulation can be significantly affected by Lyme. And why not? The first place the Bb migrate is into the endothelial cells of the blood and lymph vessels. Free-floating spirochetes are the mechanism by which Bb disseminates. At times, Bb seem to be everywhere in the circulation. Their presence can cause Raynaud's, asymmetrical or weak pulses, cold or blue extremities, or vasculitis.

- **Pulmonary**

While cough and SOB have been reported in association with Lyme, it can be hard to determine if these sxs are due to borreliosis or co-infections. Co-morbid respiratory problems appear to increase with Lyme. Further, difficulty breathing may be associated with new onset allergic-type manifestations such as asthma or eczema. Is there an autoimmune mechanism operating here?

PEARL: Children with gestational Lyme may present with tracheomalacia where the cartilage in the windpipe has not properly developed. This can lead to floppy, noisy breathing with high pitched breath sounds.

- **Signs and symptoms in special populations**

Gestational Lyme: Gestational Lyme is the infection of the fetus by active Bb organisms from the mother that occurs between the time of conception and birth. Congenital Lyme disease is present at birth. Chapter 30: *Special Populations* deals in depth with gestational Lyme. The most common signs and symptoms of gestational Lyme include hypotonia, GERD, and extreme sensory hyper-responsivity. Congenital anomalies such as abnormally-formed trachea or cardiac structures have been observed. Later symptoms include irritability associated with impulsivity, cognitive problems including learning disabilities, mood swings, fatigue, lack of stamina, pain, low grade fevers, pallor, arthritis, rashes, GI problems, on-going hypersensitivity to light, sound, taste, or touch, eye problems, and developmental delays. Although only about 25% of these kids have cardiac problems, these can be associated with significant morbidity and mortality. Hypotonia is the cardinal manifestation, occurring in about 90% of cases of congenital Lyme. A hypotonic child presents as limp or floppy with little resistance to passive motion.

Children with gestational Lyme are sick very early on with frequent fevers and increased incidence of ear and throat infections and pneumonia. They are irritable and appear to suffer from joint and body pain. They are often floppy with poor muscle tone. GERD can manifest with spitting up, discomfort on swallowing, and poor feeding behaviors. Some of these children have small windpipes, (tracheomalacia) resulting in audible or high pitched breathing. Others experience eye problems, developmental delays, learning disabilities, and various neuropsychiatric problems. Almost all respond to months or years of continuous antibiotic therapy.

STARI signs and symptoms: Read the Lyme section above. While some sources speculate that the clinical presentation of STARI is more or less severe than that of Bb, I could not substantiate these claims. The medical estab-lishment has enough trouble detailing the signs and symptoms of Lyme, let alone comparing it to another form of borreliosis. Unless there is reason to suspect that strictly distinguishing between these two maladies will somehow benefit patients, energies might be better spent focusing on helping all victims of these spirochetes.

Signs and symptoms of Herxheimer reactions: Depending on the efficacy of the antibiotic, a Lyme patient may experience a significant Herx reaction. Here, after treatment is initiated, the patient feels worse before she feels better. Manifestations can be similar to those experienced with the initial infection or quite different. Since a Herx reaction is due to a massive kill-off of pathogen, many general signs and symptoms of inflammatory response are also present. Nonetheless, a Herx reaction frequently takes on the characteristics of the specific underlying disease probably because the pathogen's toxins are released during their destruction as well as other pathophysiologic mechanisms. Review Chapter 28: *Understanding the Herxheimer Reaction* for additional details.

X. DIAGNOSIS

Lyme is a clinical diagnosis. Not only is Lyme a clinical diagnosis, it will continue to be a clinical diagnosis for the foreseeable future. We do not have the luxury of waiting until someone develops the definitive diagnostic test or biologic marker before we diagnose Lyme. We cannot put off our responsibilities until all controversies have been put to rest. Most of us have allowed too many Lyme cases to simmer and evolve into intractable monsters while we lacked the knowledge or courage to make the diagnosis. The time has come for the rest of us to DIAGNOSE!

Chapter 20: *Making the Diagnosis* provides general background on common-sense diagnosing. In that chapter causality concepts are reviewed including how to take a symptom set and assess it using timing, bioplausibility, challenge/rechallenge, confounders, consistency, and process of elimination. Of course, Lyme is the great imitator and evader, thwarting our best diagnostic efforts at every turn. Further, even those of us who think about Lyme too much have to accept that not everything we see is Lyme. Not even in Chester County Pennsylvania, where Lyme is ubiquitous. Further, more than one pathologic process can be operating at the same time. So do not rest on your diagnostic laurels after you have made one diagnosis. Your job might not be done.

Now is the time to respect your clinical judgment, solidify your knowledge base, and activate your index of suspicion. If you use the CDC surveillance criteria to diagnose Lyme, you will probably miss more than half of the true cases. Estimates vary on the number of cases missed from 30% to 90%. But every true case not diagnosed is 100% lost for that patient. Even the

CDC acknowledges that their criteria were not designed to make the diagnosis in individual cases. Chapters 11, 18, and 19 discuss all the many reasons why the diagnostic parameters issued by the CDC and IDSA result in disproportionate false negatives and missed diagnoses. I will not rehash all that here. Instead, I will attempt to get you from point A to point B and that elusive Lyme diagnosis. You cannot diagnosis what you don't consider, so keep a high index of suspicion.

To diagnose Lyme based on clinical judgment, consider:

1. History or possibility of tick bite. No one should have to PROVE they were bitten by a tick, and that tick was indeed a deer tick, and that it was engorged, and that it was attached for more than 24 hours. That's just silly, not to mention impossible, in most cases.

2. Previous diagnoses of other TBIs

3. Description of cyclical symptoms, waxing and waning, coming and going

4. The first symptoms of borreliosis can be the general signs of inflammation common to most infections. Early sxs may include a flu-like syndrome with headache, general aches and pains, fever, and severe fatigue.

5. As the disease progresses look for on-going fatigue, myalgias, and arthralgias that are often migrating. Arthralgias most commonly involve the big joints like knees, shoulders, hips, and elbows, although smaller joints can also be involved. GI complaints are common and neuropsychiatric manifestations are likely to present early and often in a number of ways. Brain fog with its memory problems, confusion, disorientation, inability to concentrate, poor focus, and dullness is nearly universal. Paresthesias are common. Pain is common.

6. Symptoms characteristic for Lyme: Severe fatigue unrelieved by rest, headaches, nausea, abdominal pain, GERD, fever, chills, joint pain, dizziness, paresthesias, shakiness, anxiety, fasciculations especially in the face or eyelids, hypersensitivity to sound, light, or touch, and brain fog as manifested by impaired concentration, poor short-term memory, inability to sustain attention, difficulty processing information, problems thinking clearly, diminished ability to express thoughts, impaired reading or writing, feeling overwhelmed, limited decision-making, and confusion. The patient may display uncharacteristic behavior, outbursts, or mood swings. Numbness, tingling, and tremors are common. The patient usually displays more than one of the characteristic symptoms.

7. The combination of fatigue, paresthesias, arthralgias, and brain fog says Lyme is likely, but other symptom clusters are also highly suggestive.

8. Do NOT wait for an EM rash, since these are not as common as we have been led to believe. The majority of Lyme patients do not recall an EM rash. Depending on the practice maybe 10% to 40% remember having the characteristic rash. Similarly, do NOT wait for arthritis. Estimates on the prevalence of arthritis are between 25% and 75% depending on the stage of disease. Do NOT wait for Bell's palsy, since it also appears in a minority of patients, although if it is present, you should consider a Lyme diagnosis.

9. In the company of possible tick exposure and any corroboration by H&P and ROS, consider an EM rash as pathognomonic for borreliosis. Consider Bell's palsy and migrating joint pain strong indicators, as well.

10. With persistent Lyme, signs and symptoms might start to become more intractable. In chronic cases, sxs can be due to fibrosis, cell injury or death, or other causes of permanent damage. Lyme's presentation may depend on where the patient is in the clinical course of the disease.

11. Whenever traditional treatment does not impact neuropsychiatric, endocrine, rheumatologic or other systemic conditions, consider that an underlying Bb infection could be complicating the treatment strategy.

12. Lyme is a clinical diagnosis.

To incorporate test results in support of a Lyme diagnosis, consider:

1. NEVER rule out the diagnosis of Lyme based on a single negative lab result. Or two negative lab results, or 12. Why do you keep testing? If the H&P and ROS are so suggestive to make you order the test, don't you think it is time to make the diagnosis based on clinical judgment? As HCPs, we all love it when a test comes back confirming our diagnostic brilliance. "See, I told you!" Instead, have confidence in your clinical judgment.

2. Recognize that current diagnostic methods are not reliable enough to avoid the false negatives that occur with lab testing.

PEARL: According to a published study out of Johns Hopkins School of Public Health, using the recommended CDC two-tiered testing model misses over 80% of the cases. The patients all had EM rashes and confirmatory biopsy results. The strong conclusion was that Lyme is a clinical diagnosis.

3. Lyme is a clinical diagnosis and not one single lab test is *necessary* to confirm the diagnosis. I get exasperated when some of my acquaintances encourage people to, "Get tested. Get tested." When the result comes back negative, they sigh, "At least it wasn't Lyme. I wonder what it could be." It's probably Lyme!

4. When any of the testing methods do come back positive, the patient very likely has Lyme. False positives are rare. (I am not aware of ANY in my experience, although there are some suggestions in the literature.) False negatives abound.

5. With all that being said, what useful information can be gleaned from diagnostic testing?

   • Actually growing the pathogen is the gold standard for Lyme diagnostic support, but culturing can be extremely difficult. Blood culture technology appears to be advancing as outlined in Chapter 18.

   • Biopsy tissue samples are the best choice for attempting to identify spirochetes under the microscope and can also be used for culturing.

   • In terms of serology, NIAID recognizes WB as the most useful method for detecting Bb *antibodies* currently available, at least compared to everything else. ELISA is almost universally panned, except in certain guidelines that were written to appease third parties like insurance companies and realtors. When the Connecticut AG required that these guidelines be reviewed without bias, the agreed-upon process was not followed.

   • Tests such as PCR and FISH are useful when they are positive: You have found Bb. But yield is so low as to be painful. When these tests are negative, the result is meaningless because there are many reasons why the test might not have been able to capture what was being sought.

   • Chapters 18 and 19 review possible diagnostic test choices and provide guidelines on interpretation. Perhaps your money would be better spent on tests such as HLA-DR2 and HLA-DR4, which might actually provide practical help for the patient.

   • If you know how to look at a WB and work around the "official" band criteria, you can use the

information to help figure out what is happening in a specific patient. Know that positive results can be helpful. Know that negative results are meaningless. Recognize that lab findings are just one piece of a much larger diagnostic puzzle. Do not be afraid of making a clinical diagnosis even with a negative lab test sitting in front of you. Treat the patient not the test result. Diagnosing Lyme takes experience, knowledge, flexibility, and courage, not necessarily in that order.

6. What are you so afraid of? In 2013, most of us HCPs have been trained to treat the lab test instead of the person. Life is so much easier when we can rely on a lab result to tell us what the patient has rather than to do the necessary detective work ourselves. Using clinical judgment is half the fun of medicine. Helping the patient get well is the other half. Use your clinical judgment. You might not be as rusty as you think.

7. Lyme is a clinical diagnosis.

Diagnoses in special populations:

1. Gestational Lyme: At birth consider a DNA PCR for Bb as well as Babesia and Bartonella. Take samples from the placenta, cord section, cord blood, and foreskin remnant and send for any appropriate testing. Consider cultures and serology. Hypotonia and hypersensitivity are the key findings in congenital Lyme. Chapter 30: *Special Populations* provides other diagnostic clues.

2. STARI: This borreliosis is a clinical diagnosis. The chances of confirming any tick bite is slim. The chances of capturing the offending Lone Star tick would be nearly miraculous. We might miss even more STARI than we do other borrelioses. Fortunately, just like Lyme, STARI is a clinical diagnosis. If you're worried that you are going to mistake Lyme for STARI, call the condition borreliosis.

3. Co-infections: If diagnosis is hard with one pathogen calling the tune, co-infections definitely complicate the diagnostic challenge. If you are saying, "This is the worst case of Lyme I have EVER seen," this might not just be Lyme. Chapter 5: *The Concept of Co-Infections* will help you navigate this complicated course.

Summary PEARL: Did someone just say that Lyme is a clinical diagnosis? Oh! That was me. While a positive test result is likely positive (good sensitivity), a negative test result is meaningless (lack of specificity). You cannot prove a negative. That is why you should never scream, "You do not have Lyme!" The patient just might have Lyme and your intractable declaration places the patient at risk and makes you look incompetent when the truth finally becomes evident. Rarely is a patient told he has Lyme when he does not. In contrast, patients are commonly told they do not have Lyme when they do. Use your clinical judgment. Gather information and flex your diagnostic intuition. No matter how many cobwebs and moth balls have to be brushed aside, you can resurrect your diagnostic skills. You might surprise yourself with your latent talent. I much more fear the consequences of under-diagnosing than in over-diagnosing. Missing a diagnosis can result in permanent disability and even death. In contrast, the worst outcome that usually occurs with over-diagnosing is a regimen of antibiotics that might be about as long a course as those given inappropriately for a URI virus that hangs on. Probably the duration would be far shorter than the series of antibiotics given for acne or COPD. Keep a high index of suspicion. You cannot diagnose what you don't consider. Do not be afraid to make the call if the signs are pointing you in that direction.

XI. DIFFERENTIAL DIAGNOSIS

Remember that Lyme is the great imitator. Lyme has been misdiagnosed and under-diagnosed probably since Noah accepted that pair of ticks onto the ark, against his better judgment. With Lyme, diagnostic skills will be tested and the differential diagnosis may pose quite the challenge. Most often, Lyme is incorrectly called something else, rather than another disease being called Lyme when it's not. There are many cases of mistaken identity all around.

Chapter 21: *Differential Diagnosis and Concurrent Disease* takes you through the process of rounding up the usual suspects and drawing conclusions. But with Lyme, the usual suspects might not always be who we initially suspect. While Chapter 21 is written to help pare down the possible etiologies that might explain a symptom cluster in any TBI, the material presented there also applies to Lyme.

I don't want to spoil your fun for the up-coming chapters, but you will be gifted with what I humbly refer to as the *Spreen TBI Differential Checklist.* By using this checklist, you will be less likely to overlook some of the more obscure contenders for the correct diagnosis. The checklist is designed to remind the HCP to investigate all reasonable explanations for the presenting clinical picture and answer the question, "What else could this be?" Categories that are included in this differential diagnosis checklist are: infections, inflammation and immune dysfunction, autoimmunity, neoplasms, skin conditions, arthritis, respiratory problems, deficiency syndromes, congenital causes, allergies, toxins, and deficits in the endocrine, neurologic, psychiatric, cardiovascular, sensory, gastrointestinal, musculoskeletal, or genitourinary systems.

With all modesty, this is one fine checklist. I don't think I missed much. If you now review the actual list as it appears in Chapter 21, you will see it looks even better fleshed out and should prove to be not just good looking, but clinically useful.

PEARL: Remember, more than one pathologic process can be active at a time, so more than one diagnosis may be appropriate.

SYNDROMES WITH SIMILAR SIGNS AND SYMPTOMS AS LYME:

Viral infections: Respiratory and gastrointestinal viruses are probably the most common misdiagnoses for Lyme. While they often start with the same general inflammatory signs and symptoms, they generally veer off the Lyme path early on. Usually with Lyme there is NO rhinitis, sinusitis, or cough, making Lyme distinguishable from flu and most URIs. But, of course, this is not always the case. While some Lyme patients get better without any treatment, most will stay sick if the disease is unaddressed, whereas a run-of-the-mill virus would resolve in fairly short order.

Autism: The relationship between Lyme and autism remains unclear. Certainly, in some reports autistic kids seem to have a higher prevalence of Bb. Likewise, Lyme kids can have autism-like presentations. But most pediatric Lyme patients do not demonstrate autistic characteristics. Why some kids do and others don't is unknown. At different points in the history of these diseases, opinion about the degree of causal association has shifted, sometimes 180 degrees. Some practitioners believed that Lyme was the sole cause of autism. Others felt it was one of many factors. The literature also contains articles that strongly state that there is no relationship whatsoever. So perception covers the entire spectrum. Seemingly every month there is a new explanation for autism, from autoimmune mechanisms to genetic predisposition to environmental influences, such as vaccination schedules, mercury derivatives in vaccines, and parenting techniques. Just last week I read a study saying that autistic kids have too many brain cells. How this hypothesis fits into all the other potential contributors and the possible relationship with Bb is far from understood. We are left with the question: "Are Lyme and autism linked always, sometimes, or never?" Lyme and autism seem to hang out together more often than one would expect if the association occurred merely by chance. When dealing with autism-like presentations and the possible presence of Lyme, always consider that there COULD be a connection when formulating your differential. If an autistic kid is not responding to traditional therapies (and unfortunately it can take a long time to discern a response), consider that Bb may be contributing to the clinical presentation. You may never know if Bb CAUSED autism in a particular case or if the two conditions merely coexist, but considering the various possibilities may open up treatment options. When you see one, think of the other and how their interplay may be affecting your patient.

PEARL: Researchers in early 2011 published the results of a study on the possible cause of autism in cases where there was no known family history. These scientists believe that spontaneous mutations at multiple gene sites are responsible. The mutations are thought to be a result of environmental exposure to toxins. Boys needed fewer mutations to present with symptoms than did girls. Since incidence of autism diagnoses is increasing, could some of these toxins be coming from pathogens?

PEARL: Children with autism may also have a high rate of Mycoplasma infections.

Immune reactions: Many diseases, infectious and otherwise, present with general signs of inflammation such as headache, fever, fatigue, and general aches. Discriminating between these almost universal manifestations may be difficult unless the history, or some other more distinguishing signs and symptoms, provide clues. If a patient does not respond to traditional therapeutic approaches consider addressing the possibility of underlying Lyme.

Fibromyalgia: Fibromyalgia most often presents with broad musculoskeletal aches, pain, stiffness, tissue soreness, fatigue, and sleep problems. Common pain sites include neck, back, shoulders, hands, and pelvic girdle. But other body parts can be painful in fibromyalgia as well. Discomfort can be mild to severe and symptoms often flare and regress. Fibromyalgia is frequently misdiagnosed and under-diagnosed. Diagnostic guidelines list widespread pain in combination with tenderness at 11 or more "tender points." More recently, some diagnostic profiles for fibromyalgia have been expanded to include more general pain or aching, persistent fatigue, generalized stiffness, and non-refreshing sleep. At various stages of disease, Lyme and fibromyalgia may present similarly. Do not discount a fibromyalgia diagnosis because a patient has only 10 tender points if other signs are pointing in that direction. I remember a big name neurologist teaching us ways to "trick" fibromyalgia patients to make sure they weren't faking their tender points. This was not in the context of a disability/impairment exam. He just assumed that everyone was making up symptoms for some reason. As if you'd pick the rough life of fibromyalgia if you were going to fake something.

Chronic fatigue syndrome: CFS usually presents with a crushing, disabling, flu-like syndrome with headache, sensitivity to light, widespread pain, and devastating, overwhelming fatigue. Patients are often amazed at the degree of fatigue, if they have the energy to be amazed. Nothing seems to help: not rest, not sleep, not stress reduction, not vacation. Once again, depending on the clinical course, a number of these signs and symptoms are similar to those that can be found

in some cases of Lyme. Bb is often implicated as a cause of CFS. Neither condition has a definitive diagnostic test. A high percentage of CFS patients have tested positive for Bb and in a number of cases, when treated appropriately for Lyme, the CFS sxs appear to recede. A number of other pathogens have been suspected of causing CFS including EBV, other viruses, and Mycoplasma. If Bb is not the sole cause of CFS, it might still contribute to the intensity of symptoms in some patients. In these cases it would be a shame if Bb was not uncovered, when present, so that treatment might be more effective. CFS patients may be a subset of Lyme (or not). Whenever you're dealing with CFS, please consider that Bb may be a cause or a contributor.

PEARL: A number of these syndromes have symptoms in common with Lyme. For example, fibromyalgia, Lyme, and CFS all may have muscle pain, cognitive impairment, and fatigue. You may have to take time to sort through the similarities and differences compared to the actual case you are evaluating.

PEARL: Chronic Fatigue and Immune Dysfunction Syndrome or CFIDS is a new acronym appearing in the literature referring to CFS.

PEARL: The traditional wisdom with CFS was that the patient should rest, but exercise and activity might help more.

Depression: In our society, depression is as common as Kardashians.[3] In my opinion, depression needs to be on every differential from hangnails to trauma. With chronic illness, depression is a common co-morbidity. If the depression is Lyme-related, the patient might not improve as expected with conventional therapies. In these cases, addressing the underlying pathogen has improved outcomes.

PEARL: Virginia Sherr, a psychiatrist in Pennsylvania, discusses her patients who walk in with depression, confusion, obsession, anxiety, and the tendency to lose things. These patients are unaware of the potential for Bb infection. If the HCP does not make the diagnostic connection, chances for recovery can be diminished.

Dementias: Lyme has many neuropsychiatric manifestations, most commonly brain fog, confusion, diminished decision-making, altered judgment, and other manifestations similar to the various dementias. Alan MacDonald found spirochetes in the brains of autopsied Alzheimer's patients and theorized that Bb might contribute to some cases of Alzheimer's, ALS,

---

3 Kardashian is the name of a grossly over-exposed reality-TV family. The patriarch was O. J. Simpson's lawyer and in 2013, the numerous progeny have a half-dozen or so television shows depicting their multiple marriages and other dysfunctional relationships. As far as I know, none of the Kardashians have a TBI, although that might be an interesting premise for a new series.

Parkinson's, and similar syndromes. A number of long-term infections have been identified in Alzheimer's patients including Chlamydia, Bb, Mycoplasma, and HSV. Garth Nicolson, PhD has found chronic bacterial and viral infections in neurodegenerative and neurobehavioral diseases. One theory is that toxins from pathogens may contribute to symptoms. Of course, this may be just one of many contributing factors, but if you are open to various etiologies you might be able to do better assessments and find out what is really going on with your patient.

PEARL: Alan MacDonald is a well-respected pioneer in the field of spirochetal pathophysiology. A phenomenal body of work!

Generalized anxiety disorder: Like depression, anxiety is ubiquitous. Patients with chronic persistent disease may be especially prone to episodic, as well as high baseline level anxiety. Whether the anxiety is Lyme-induced or independent, anxiety should appear on the differential. While anxiety may not be the primary diagnosis, it might appropriately appear on the list. I assure you it should be part of the differential in the parents of chronic Lyme patients.

PEARL: If Lyme is contributing to the presenting syndrome, then consider treating the Lyme, as well as the symptoms, for the best results.

OCD/Panic attacks: Many neuropsychiatric diagnoses may appropriately appear on a differential for Lyme disease. Some may be part of a Lyme (or other TBI) infectious process or can be totally unrelated to the TBD. In cases where a pathogen is contributing to the problem, the patient may respond better if the infection is treated along with the presenting signs and symptoms. Don't assume these conditions are or aren't related to Lyme. Try to find the cause, since the etiology can influence treatment decisions.

PEARL: If a standard diagnosis like depression or anxiety does not respond to traditional therapies, perhaps underlying Lyme is a contributor to the condition. These patients might respond better if treatment for the Lyme is included. If the patient does not improve or is getting worse, would it hurt to consider the possibility of Bb? Improvement has been seen in cases of sleep disturbances and seizures where traditional approaches weren't successful until antibiotics targeted for the Lyme were introduced. If you are treating an ailment and it is not getting better, have a very high index of suspicion as you investigate why a certain condition is not responding when it usually does. You may have the wrong diagnosis altogether or there may be an underlying problem that is preventing healing – this can be a TBI or DM or a number of other things. Until the patient is better, keep exploring various diagnostic and treatment options. If you are treating the signs and symptoms and not treating

the underlying TBI, then you may be tilting at windmills and your patient will have a much harder time recovering.

Multiple sclerosis: MS is a chronic autoimmune inflammatory disease of the CNS. Many patients present with vision changes, muscle weakness, urinary problems, tremors, spasms, cognitive deficits, and mood disorders that can be very similar to the CNS manifestations of Lyme. While MS can progress steadily it can also wax, wane, flare and remit, just like Lyme. During the clinical course, different nerves can be affected and there may be no clear pattern, as with Lyme. Both MS and Lyme can appear as white plaques on MRI of the brain. Take the time to sort this out. The wrong diagnosis can delay appropriate treatment and, in the case of Lyme, lead to permanent sequelae that may have been preventable.

PEARL: Coyle notes the difficulty in distinguishing Lyme from MS in some patients. If antibiotics mitigate the symptoms, Lyme is the likely etiology. Successful treatment of MS using combination antibiotics for a minimum of one year have been reported. The antibiotic choices were quite similar to those often used for Lyme and Chlamydia infections.

Inflammatory arthritis: Lyme can mimic many kinds of arthritis from gout to RA. If joints are involved in a suspected case of Lyme, you might have to go through each manifestation and see how it fits into the various arthritis patterns before attempting a diagnosis. For example, if a child has painful joints you might consider that JRA is a rare, progressive, autoimmune condition with fairly well-defined immune markers, while Lyme is more common with symptoms that can wax and wane. Lyme is many times more common in endemic areas than JRA, which occurs only in about 1 in 100,000 children. JRA is now called JIA.

Systemic lupus erythematosus: Lupus is a chronic, autoimmune, inflammatory disease of multiple organ systems marked by flares and remissions. Polyarthralgias, rashes, fever, malaise, vasculitis, nephritis, and cardiac involvement can all be part of the clinical picture. These manifestations and the clinical course can be similar to that seen in Lyme. However the patient population is usually quite different. Still, just because SLE is not usually seen in male children does not mean it is NEVER seen in male children. Keep an open mind until you have a reason to exclude a diagnosis. If you are asking, "Could this be lupus?" you should also be asking, "Could this be Lyme?" Use of Minocin has been associated with a lupus-like syndrome.

Guillain-Barré syndrome: GBS is an inflammatory, autoimmune destruction of myelin in the nervous system, often showing progressive, rapid loss of symmetrical motor function. The immune response targets parts of the nervous system causing numbness, weak limbs, and in severe cases paralysis. GBS most often occurs after acute viral infection. Paresthesias often precede a loss of motor function that can lead to paralysis. From this description, GBS appears to be easily distinguished from Lyme. Nonetheless, in all cases of GBS that I have observed, the diagnosis was not initially apparent and multiple specialists did not have a clue for days. Sometimes GBS did not even appear on early differentials. The paresthesias may be the confounding sign here that makes the two syndromes hard to distinguish.

Ankylosing spondylitis: AS usually starts with inflammation of the sacroiliac joint and spine in the low back, reaching the neck only late in the clinical course. There is significant decreased ROM with spastic tenderness of the muscles. The patient may need to turn his whole body to look sideways and the neck is often thrust forward. With AS there is chronic degenerative arthritis with increased reflexes and fasciculations. Usually there is no fatigue and the pain may get better with activity. AS is usually diagnosed between the ages of 20 and 40 but signs may begin as early as age 10. One source found that 4 out of 5 patients with AS were also positive for Lyme. I could not confirm this with multiple references but since AS is fatal and miserably progressive, at least consider if Lyme may be contributing to the problem. Ask if antibiotic treatment might help or hurt the patient. A high percentage of AS patients may also be infected with Mycoplasma species. Mycoplasmas are never good news, so concurrent infections with these microbes may be worth exploring.

STARI: Where does STARI fit into the differential diagnosis? Although STARI is viewed by some as a distinct disease, separate from Lyme; this is hard to confirm. STARI, also called Master's disease, seems to have been identified in certain geographic regions primarily in the southern US. Amblyomma *americanum,* the Lone Star tick, is thought to be the vector. Lone Star ticks have been found primarily in the southeastern US, but also north up to Maine and west to Texas. This female tick has a white "lone star" on its back (dorsal aspect). All three life stages are said to aggressively bite humans.

STARI has been reported in regions where Lyme is otherwise rare, such as Arkansas. Pat Smith, the LDA president, received a response from a government staff member insisting that an EM rash was *not* pathognomonic of Lyme because an unspecified number of STARI patients had experienced a similar rash. I could find no solid information on the concurrence of Lyme and STARI although it seems possible since the Borrelia thought to cause STARI has been found in Ixodes ticks and vice versa. I am not entirely convinced that STARI is distinct from Lyme, or if it is, whether that difference is clinically meaningful.

The CDC (and we know they can be inconsistent about Borrelia) describes STARI as similar to Lyme with fatigue, fever, headache, muscle aches, and joint pains. They talk about an expanding red rash around the site of a Lone Star tick bite. The CDC website says this lesion usually appears within 7 days of the bite and can expand to 3 inches or more. (If it's more, why don't they just give the observed dimensions?) There is considerable controversy in the literature around whether or not this lesion has central clearing: often, sometimes, or never. The website says, "Unlike Lyme disease, STARI has not been linked to any arthritic, neurological, or chronic symptoms." (So the CDC admits that Lyme can be associated with chronic sxs?)

Borrelia *burgdorferi* is speculated to not be involved in cases of STARI. Another spirochete, Borrelia *lonestari*, was detected in the skin of one patient and the Lone Star tick that bit him. But study of more than two dozen others have found no *lonestari.* In the STARI cases documented on the CDC website, all symptoms resolved promptly after treatment with antibiotics.

I find STARI to be a conundrum. Just as with Lyme, it's hard to get the straight story from the literature. The published articles are often confusing and contradictory and some authors appear to be in a competition with Lyme vying with STARI for top billing. (I truly believe it's the humans in competition, not the spirochetes.) Please, let's just try to gather accurate information and not start making indefensible claims. The last thing we need is another Lyme war.

Currently, there seems to have been too few confirmed cases to draw definitive conclusions. One example of the confusion is illustrated by a website I accessed. This source definitively declared "Lone star ticks do not transmit B. *burgdorferi*." How do they know this? Have they checked every Lone Star tick? Is there a reason that a Lone Star tick could *not* be infected with Bb if exposed? Is much of STARI actually Lyme? Are they using the same flawed diagnostic testing methods for STARI as have been established for Lyme? The authors continue, "It is highly likely that cases of STARI have been mistaken for LD due to similar symptomatology." "The most common symptom that appears with a STARI rash is fatigue." I am not sure how they believe this is distinguishing. They reinforce that serologic testing for Lyme will not identify STARI. (Heck, those tests don't even identify Lyme half the time.)

Since the EM rash in Lyme is observed in a minority of cases, is it present in a higher percentage of STARI patients? Do all STARI patients get EM rashes? Or are we missing STARI in the same proportions as we miss Lyme because we wait for manifestations that seldom appear? In real clinical practice, who are the HCPs ordering these STARI tests? I'm sure Lilith[4] and her Lyme-averse colleagues at my local hospital would be completely unaware of the possibility.

Finding the infecting tick is rare in any case. How would anyone know to test for STARI, if no tick was found? When I

---

4 See Glossary or Introduction for name origin

tried to show Lilith the tick that bit Chris, she certainly did not inspect it to see if it had a lone star mark on its back. Of course, neither did I.

Some believe that STARI is a milder condition than Lyme, but since Lyme can present in so many ways, with such fluctuating intensities, who is to say? One source said that STARI EM lesions are smaller in diameter and tend to have a central clearing. How would they know this? Lyme EM lesions can be quite variable and overall these lesions can differ in size and intensity. They may be comparing apples and kumquats here. Further, the article said that STARI patients with skin lesions are less likely to report sxs that commonly accompany LD. How did they make this determination? Let me say that certain pertinent information (like how many patients they asked compared to how many patients there are) would have been helpful in making their conclusions more scientifically valid. Who are the STARI patients without skin lesions?

Both conditions are borreliosis that respond to the same treatment regimens, as far as that goes. Splitting hairs is probably not worth our time when so many more important issues need to be addressed. Keep an open mind and do what needs to be done to help the patient. There are many unanswered questions and I think we would all be prudent to refrain from making dogmatic pronouncements until more information is collected. Let's focus on helping the patients irrespective of the type of borreliosis they have. Hopefully, additional information will clear up this confusion in the near future.

Lyme has been misdiagnosed as: Growing pains, autism, URI, flu, mono, many viruses, EBV, ALS, arthritis, depression, anxiety, GAD, CFS, gastroenteritis, dysrhythmia, Bell's palsy, valve problems, OCD, fibromyalgia, immune deficiency, inflammatory arthritis (JIR, JRA), GBS, Asperger's, ADD, ADHD, ringworm, various neuropsychiatric disorders, CFIDS (chronic fatigue), behavior problems, MS, ankylosing spondylitis, Raynaud's, metabolic abnormalities, PANDAS, toxins, heavy metals, mold, allergies, hysteria, panic, Munchausen, Munchausen by proxy, post-Lyme syndrome, Alzheimer's, SLE, Parkinson's, parasites, other pathogens, antiphospholipid syndrome, CIDP, Strep, celiac disease, diabetes, thyroid problems, idiopathic conditions, dysautonomia, neurally-mediated hypotension, 5th disease, B12 deficiency, toxoplasmosis, plague, parvovirus, rheumatic fever, environmental syndrome, hemochromatosis, Giardia, Wilson's disease, alpha 1-antitrypsin deficiency, demyelinating disorders, drug misuse, drug and alcohol addiction, deconditioning, various tics and tremors, anemia, schizophrenia, sleep disruptions, bipolar disorder, Tourette's, dementia, nutrition disorders, GERD, TBI co-infections, hepatitis, nephritis, autoimmune disorders, leaky gut, sensitivity reactions, conversion reactions, vitamin deficiencies, electrolyte imbalances, drug reactions, interstitial cystitis, vasculitis, Gulf War syndrome, normal pressure hydrocephalus, motor neuron disease, sensory disintegration

syndrome, vaccination reaction or overload, multiple chemical sensitivity, and dozens of others. In a number of these misdiagnoses, Bb may have contributed to syndromes that mimicked these diseases or the condition was independent from the Bb. The most common misdiagnosis of Lyme is: "I don't know what it is, but it's **NOT** Lyme."

PEARL: While the CDC wants cases of Lyme to be reported, this almost never happens within the clinical setting. Since Lyme is a judgment call and most states require a positive lab test (or two) for an "official" diagnosis, most HCPs consider it just too much trouble to jump through all the bureaucratic hoops needed to file a report. Some states are purported to require the HCPs to pass an interview, which I have heard rivals an interrogation, before they will accept the case. All the while, the interviewer is trying to talk the reporter out of the reality of the disease. How many times do you think the HCP will call in with a second case under these conditions? Nevertheless, know that Lyme disease is supposed to be reported. Authorities in Chester County, Pennsylvania, will only report a Lyme case if they speak directly to the doctor on the phone. They will try to return a doctor's call twice and then abandon the pursuit. When the LDASEPA intern tried to inquire about the procedure for reporting at the local level no one called her back despite multiple attempts.

In summary, there are many cases of mistaken identity around LD. Of course, the presence of co-infections complicate the process significantly. With TBIs, we may never know when we have identified all possible pathogens responsible for the clinical presentation we are assessing. Put the contenders in the differential diagnosis and go down your list over and over.

One source says that Lyme can mimic more than 300 diseases. While I don't know where that number came from, I do know that there are a lot of misdiagnoses, under-diagnoses, and frankly wrong diagnoses with Lyme. Not everything is Lyme. Unfortunately, some patients, parents, and HCPs can only see through Lyme-colored glasses. Whether this is worse than not seeing Lyme at all is yet to be determined. Keep your mind open in both directions.

XII. TREATMENT

How do you treat Lyme? Let me count the ways.

First, here are some PRACTICAL TREATMENT GUIDELINES that should be considered when treating each patient:

1. Target the individual within the context of the particular case. No cookie-cutter medicine allowed.

2. The duration of treatment should be based on clinical response, as would be the case for any other illness.

3. Individualize the treatment regimen based on age, tolerance, endemic area, primary organ system involved, immune status, HLA profile, stage in clinical course (may need a cyst-buster), overall health, and degree of incapacity.

4. All treatment decisions should be made in conjunction with both patients and caregivers, as appropriate.

5. All options should be on the table.

6. Do a risk/benefit analysis around every treatment decision.

7. Always, always, always treat the patient NOT the guideline. My husband's co-worker was still sick as a dog after his 30 days were up according to the IDSA guideline. He was begging for additional treatment. He was only functional when on antibiotics. I have trouble understanding how an HCP who promised to "First do no harm," could stop his treatment. In her defense, she was young and afraid of the authorities.

8. Always, always, always treat the patient, NOT the lab result.

9. Whichever guideline you choose (and I do have my preferences), it's a guideline not the Ten Commandments. Follow the suggestions that make sense for the specific patient and leave the rest behind. (Why do some HCPs find it so much easier to break any and all of the Ten Commandments than to deviate slightly from certain guidelines? Could reprisal by one professional organization be scarier than the wrath of God?)

10. Make treatment recommendations based on the best interest of the patient, not based on intimidation or fear of retaliation. I know that's easier said than done.

11. Consider probiotics for all patients starting a course of antimicrobials.

12. Set treatment goals (ability to get out of bed an hour a day, desire to sit up, stand up, and walk to the bathroom unaided, resume reading in some capacity, pain control, cure, whatever, as long as the goals are realistic and do not contribute to the already stressful situation). Objectives help you measure progress and keep you from swinging blindly in the dark.

13. The best treatment endpoint: RESULTS! Treat until they are feeling better or functional, or ideally, cured. Do not stop treatment, especially in those who flare when their regimen is stopped, just because an artificial deadline is reached. Ask the patient how she is feeling. Even small children know if they are feeling better. Astute caregivers tend to be very tuned into even subtle changes in the patient's overall condition.

14. Avoid solo agents. Combination regimens help circumvent resistance and more effectively hit all forms of Bb.

15. AVOID STEROIDS! As tempting as they may be to make the HCP look like the hero in achieving almost instant results, RESIST! With that being said, I was part of a group of physicians who discussed using steroids in an incapacitated patient last week. I use steroid eye drops when my vision problems prevent me from working on the book one minute longer. Use steroids when it makes sense to do so, always weighing the risk/benefit of any treatment. Remember, target the individual case.

16. All parties need to be committed to the wellness of the patient. Compliance may be crucial for achieving best outcomes.

17. Don't believe 99% of the hype about new cures, techniques, or regimens. The latest is not always the best. I used to work for the pharmaceutical industry. I know spin and propaganda and fear techniques. I helped create it. Cut through the baloney. Use common-sense. If it's too good to be true, it's probably malarkey. That doesn't mean you don't explore options. But nothing is sadder than to see hopes in Lyme patients build over a new therapy only to realize it's a scam. Although parents grasping at obviously bogus treatment approaches, desperate for help for their children, are sad too. I know because I was one of them. The cons come not only from individual entrepreneurs, but also those big-name, long-respected pharmas. They may be the worst offenders, since they can hide behind skewed science. Caveat emptor.

18. If you decide to treat, treat. None of this half-assed stuff where you give tiny doses of doxy for 5 days so no one can say you over-treated. These tepid, spiritless, cowardly attempts to please everyone without getting in trouble might only make the condition worse. Bb can encyst, and move inside cells, and go dormant only to revive another day with a vengeance. Low-doses for short duration are a good way to spur resistance. If you're going to treat: TREAT!

19. If you cannot bring yourself to make appropriate treatment decisions, send the patient to someone who will. (Sign in medical office building lobby: "If you really cared about the patients, you'd refer them to someone better than you.")

With all that being said, let's take 20 pages or so and see what other nuances make these treatment decisions less clear-cut than we would like. Many factors impact treatment decisions in Lyme disease. ALWAYS target the treatment to the individual using the following considerations to help make your decisions.

LYME TREATMENT OVERVIEW

There are dozens of proposed treatment regimes for Lyme that are detailed in the *Sample Treatment Regimens* section below. Entire books have been written on this topic, as well as two conflicting treatment guidelines. The *goals* of therapy should include: improvement in signs and symptoms, normalization of function, prevention of long-term sequelae, and ultimately cure. To achieve these goals, many possible approaches have been suggested.

FACTORS USED TO DECIDE ON APPROPRIATE TREATMENT STRATEGIES

Some doctors use the primary organ system affected to decide on the best treatment regime. Others try to discern the geographic location of the offending tick. Still others use patient age or stage of disease. Some follow certain practice guidelines so closely that they abstain from all original thought. Consider all pertinent factors and then target the disease in the individual patient.

A. Age/status of patient

1. **Pregnant**: Treatment is critical! Untreated infected mothers have a 50% chance of transmitting disease to their neonates. Those treated with one antibiotic have a 25% chance. Mothers treated with two or more antimicrobials had **NO** chance of a baby born with congenital Lyme disease. Those are pretty good odds. If untreated, the pregnancy can result in miscarriage, stillbirth, or perinatal death. Err on the side of caution. Neurologic problems can become permanent in the fetus if not adequately addressed. Many moms of kids with congenital Lyme wish they had insisted on more aggressive treatment. Most had oblivious HCPs saying that nothing more needed to be done.

   In pregnant Lyme patients, consider the oral options: Amoxil 1000 mg q 6 to 8, OR Ceftin 100 q 12, OR Omnicef 300 to 600 mg bid **PLUS** Zithromax 500 bid. Parenteral options as part of combination therapy include Bicillin 1.2 million units IM 1 to 3 times/week, OR Rocephin 2 g IV pulsed 4 days on and 3 off OR Claforan 6 g either continuous infusion or 2 g IV q 8, pulsed.

Some practitioners use IV for 30 days starting in the 1st and 2nd trimesters and then oral for 6 weeks. The most conservative regimen treats from the time the mother's Bb infection is suspected throughout the pregnancy and all during nursing. After delivery, the mother may experience a flare of her disease due to a lack of the mitigating gestation hormones. With what I understand now, I know which regimen I would choose.

2. **Gestational Lyme:** Chapter 30: *Special Populations* goes into detail on congenital Lyme disease. Hypotonia and hypersensitivity are the cardinal signs. Treatment should be aggressive and for sufficient duration. Kids with congenital Lyme are treated with PCNs, CSs, and macrolides. TCNs are not recommended in children under 8 unless there are extenuating circumstances. Symptoms may not be present or recognized at birth, so be on the lookout well into infancy and beyond.

   Look at the baby. With gestational Lyme you might see hypotonia. The child may be floppy like a rag doll. There may be irritability, trouble feeding secondary to the hypotonia, jaundice, hypersensitivity, or low grade fevers. These kids are often unhappy. Soon after birth, be watchful for a failure to develop. We're not talking failure to thrive here, these children fail to *develop*. These gestationally-infected kids are not good at meeting milestones. Development can be slow. In these cases, consider azithromycin and Omnicef. If they also have Bartonella consider azithromycin and Bactrim. Rifamycin is not often recommended in newborns but sometimes choices are limited. Rifamycin has been used by some practitioners in newborns with success and without obvious untoward effects.

3. **Children**: The treatment information in this text covers newborns to the elderly. With that being said, kids come in all sizes and treatment recommendations can differ considerably from neonates to high school linebackers. Some drugs like the TCNs (doxycycline and minocycline), the fluoroquinolones, and a number of other agents are not recommended in kids. Kids under 8 are not good candidates for TCNs because of potential problems with bones and teeth. Still, sometimes alternatives are limited and some not-recommended antimicrobials are the best choice in a specific case. Chapter 24: *Antimicrobials* reviews all these caveats and discusses options. Each treatment decision should involve a risk/benefit assessment.

   The DOC for borreliosis in kids is amoxicillin. But solo agents are not recommended and the most usual partner is a good intracellular macrolide like azithromycin. Other top picks to be part of combination therapy include Biaxin or one of the cephalosporins like Ceftin or Omnicef. Doxycycline is useful in children > 8 y/o. Note that if the child also has ehrlichiosis, then consider a short-course of doxy in the younger patient. Doxycycline or minocycline has been used for 1 to 2 weeks in these cases. In most cases of short-course treatment there has not been a problem.

4. **Adults**: Many pediatric patients fall into the "adult" designation for drug selection and dosing. The recommended adult doses and usage information is provided in the individual drug sections of Chapter 24: *Antimicrobials*. In general, solo agents are best avoided and combination therapy is encouraged.

B. Stage of disease

As mentioned earlier, Lyme disease has been divided into many categories, some valid, others not so much. When using the disease stage to decide on the course of treatment, realize that these are artificial terms and many overlap. Treat the patient, not the label.

1. **Prophylaxis**: This is a pre-disease state and treatment is used to mitigate the risk of contracting the disease. Chapter 32: *Prevention* reviews the various options. In general, consider azithromycin and Doryx in older kids and azithromycin and amoxicillin or Omnicef in younger kids. Even IDSA concedes that prophylaxis is appropriate in some cases, although their criteria are not always supported by the evidence.

2. **Early or local**: If there is only a single EM lesion with no systemic sxs, this is probably localized disease. Of course, the EM rash is not as universal as we have been led to believe and who is to say that the spirochetes aren't already disseminating as they do in the many cases of LD without an EM rash? There is nothing to say they are required to give us a sign. In up to 90% of the cases they do not. The safest approach is to assume that no matter how quick you were to recognize the infection, the spirochetes are on the move. I'll call it pre-dissemination and say this is the BEST time to treat. Get them as early as possible. Use high enough doses, in combination regimes, for a sufficient duration. Low doses for short periods of a solo agent can drive the Bb into dormant forms, inside cells, that are harder to manage. Actually, the rash itself usually resolves with antibiotics, but don't be fooled.

Spirochetes may have already set up home elsewhere. In cases where there are no additional signs aside from local disease, treat. Treat orally until there is no evidence of infection for at least 4 to 6 weeks. This time frame should bracket an entire Bb life cycle, although

we know that alternative life forms can extend the cycle indefinitely. Usually covering the patient for 3 months after the signs of local infection have dissipated is sufficient. Catching the disease before constitutional sxs begin is a gift. Don't waste it. Treat!

3. **Disseminated**: Once the systemic sxs begin, the spirochetes have probably dispersed. The Lyme disease has spread. Here is where the debate begins over how long to treat. The arguments on both sides of this issue are presented in Chapter 11. Most TBI-familiar physicians treat until the person is well PLUS a cushion. That therapeutic cushion is likely to be between 3 and 6 months depending on the severity of the illness and organ systems involved. Still relapses can occur. Early in the clinical course of Lyme, oral amoxicillin is as effective as doxycycline. Combination regimens are preferred. Note that macrolides may be more effective when combined with Plaquenil.

4. **Chronic**: There is debate over whether chronic Lyme disease exists but the ILADS position is clear. Not only do these HCPs believe that the evidence firmly supports chronicity, most believe that the persistence is due to active infection. So if the invaders continue to cause harm, I support trying to harm the invaders. (Although generally, I am a very peaceful person.) Treat until the patient is better. PLUS a cushion. Chronic infection may require open-ended treatment that must continue until sxs of the active infection have cleared. This might mean IVs for 3 to 6 months or more, followed by months of oral or IM maintenance. If the patient isn't getting better, why not just stop the antibiotics altogether? Because then some get much worse. At least many patients are functional while on antibiotics. These patients stay gratefully on their medicines for months or years. They crash when they come off. The question with chronic Lyme has never been what to do with the majority who find short-term treatment successful. The concern is how to manage those roughly 20% to 50% who fail under this limited treatment approach.

5. **Progressing**: If the clinical picture is obviously getting worse, then it may be time to reassess the treatment strategy. The section below, *When to Change Gears*, provides guidance on when and how to rethink the approach.

6. **Plateau**: What should be done about a plateau? Here the patient is not symptom-free but they aren't getting better or worse either. There is no progress. They may experience low grade signs and symptoms. Here you might consider an overhaul of the entire regimen. Consider a change in antibiotics, adjusting doses,

adding cyst-busters or Plaquenil, or reconfiguring the members of the antimicrobial combination package. You might need to get inventive when you can't get off a plateau. Definitely look for co-infections. Joe Burrascano described a cyclic approach to plateaus. He stopped all antibiotics until the sxs returned, then used high level antibiotics before again stopping until sxs return. He repeats this same cycle until he breaks through. Usually 3 to 4 cycles are needed for effect. The literature contains descriptions of many methods used to overcome a plateau, with varying degrees of success.

7. **Relapsing:** While day-to-day Lyme can wax and wane and come and go, a relapse is usually thought to be a full-fledged return of the disease after a symptom-free period. These are usually occasions of considerable disappointment for patients, caretakers, and HCPs. M. E. Bayer studied 97 patients with sxs of chronic LD confirmed with PCR. Most were treated with antibiotics for extended periods: "It seems to be characteristic for most of the patients in our study that after antibiotic-free periods of a few months, they had again become increasingly ill with neurologic and arthritic symptoms, so that treatment had to be resumed." Many patients with symptoms associated with persistent Lyme improve on antibiotics and then relapse when taken off the treatment. When re-treated, most patients again see sxs diminish.

*PEARL: When antibiotics are resumed after relapse, the neurologist Coyle found that most patients had a favorable response to re-treatment. Since persistent LD symptoms respond to additional treatment with antibiotics, the sxs can only be caused by on-going infection. True **post**-infectious syndromes do not respond to repeated antibiotics. Why would they? Antibiotics are there to damage pathogens and if there are no organisms to hit, they have no contribution to make. When sxs persist, treatment with antimicrobials is generally followed by clinical improvement, because the active pathogens are weakened or destroyed. Some argue that the antibiotics are just providing an anti-inflammatory effect. If this were the case, Advil would have the same effect as a course of antibiotics and it does not.*

For those with persistent or chronic Lyme, treatment with continuous antibiotics may be needed for 3 months to a year or more. Rare cases have been treated for more than a decade. Each time treatment was paused in these long-term cases, the symptoms flared and often the patient became less functional, even incapacitated, and begged for treatment to resume.

8. **Tissue damage:** If the TBI has damaged a tissue or organ permanently, then those cells will probably never go back to the pre-infection state. Usually this occurs when there is a long delay between infection and treatment. Even the best doctor can't turn back time if there is massive fibrosis and apoptosis.

9. **Reinfection:** Is the flare of sxs a reinfection or a recurrence of an old infection? This matters because a new infection could be a different strain that may not respond to the same treatment approach as the previous spirochetes.

C. **Primary organ systems affected**

When I started this book, I had no idea the number of organs involved in the Bb pathologic process and the extent of the potential debility. The systems involved may depend on the primary cell types where the Bb decide to live. If mostly glial cells are the target, you might have quite a different clinical picture than if most of the Bb are on the cardiac valves. This may explain why Lyme is a multisystem disease, since more than one cell type is likely to be targeted by the spirochetes. Further, this explains why one organ system may be predominant whereas the others might have a secondary role. Of course, the strain can have a lot to do with how a case of Lyme presents. Various strains may have different preferred tissue, with some loving joints and others wanting to set up in a nice, juicy neuron. This all makes sense from a natural selection and survival perspective. The organ systems involved should influence treatment decisions.

1. **Neuropsychiatric:** I am not one to hint that you have to go through childbirth in order to be an obstetrician, yet such an experience might broaden your perspective. What I can say is that having witnessed and lived through the NP sxs of Lyme certainly enhanced my understanding of the depth and breadth of the problem. Never underestimate the power of the NP complications of Lyme.

While toxic cytokines can contribute to brain fog and other neuropsychiatric problems, if you see NP sxs assume there are spirochetes present in the CNS. Choose antibiotics that can cross the BBB and that can hit the various forms of Bb.

Macrolides do **not** cross the BBB. Vancomycin does **not** cross. Minocycline does cross the BBB to a limited degree, as does ceftriaxone, and Bicillin. You can have the greatest drug on the planet, but if it can't get to the bugs, it's not going to do much good.

If Lyme sxs are primarily neurologic, treat fast and hard since you want to hit the active spirochete, that is the cell wall form of Bb, when they are still accessible.

Consider Bicillin or Rocephin and also add a good intracellular that crosses the BBB (rifamycin). For an autism-like presentation consider the combination of Flagyl, amoxicillin, and azithromycin. For tics, some HCPs add clonidine 0.1 mg qd.

NP sxs may need longer treatment than any other manifestation. Use agents that cross the BBB and cystbusters. One source noted that doubling the length of IV ceftriaxone treatment from 2 to 4 weeks improved the success rate from 66% to 80%. Neuropsychiatric sxs may need treatment for 6 months or more. One approach is to treat with an IV antimicrobial for 6 to 8 weeks and then IM or oral for as long as it takes. IV Rocephin is said to clear the brain and it appears to be effective in many (but not all) cases.

If you're using doxy or Amoxil make sure they are part of a combination regimen. Consider ceftriaxone (Rocephin) in adults 2 g/day IV and in kids 50 to 75 mg/kg/day IV with a maximum of 2 grams/dose, OR cefotaxime (Claforan) 2 g IV q 8 h in adults and 50-200 mg/kg IV divided tid or qid in kids, with a max of 6 grams per day or 2 grams per dose, OR IV pen G: adult 18-24 million units/day IV in divided doses and kids 200,000-400,000 units/kg/day IV in divided doses given q 4 h with a max of 18-24 million units/day. Bicillin IM 1.2 to 3.6 IM q 3 to 4 days a week has been used with good results. Another successful combination mentioned in the literature to address NP sxs of Lyme is Bicillin and Ketek with Flagyl that is pulsed 2 weeks on and two weeks off.

Even with an appropriate combination drug regimen, resolution of the NP sxs of Lyme can be a long and winding road. If the NP sxs are due to Lyme, they may not respond to conventional therapeutic options such as sleep aids or antidepressants. Often antibiotics need to be part of the mix for the best outcomes.

2. **Skin:** In those patients with an early EM rash, any number of antibiotics seem to be effective in making the rash go away. (That isn't to say that the Lyme is cured, just that the rash is gone.) The rash almost always responds to antibiotic treatment. This can be a mixed blessing. The disappearance of the rash can lead to a false sense of confidence that your brilliant doctoring has cured the patient of all that ails him. If only that were true. If your concern is the rash, several options should lead to the expected result. In kids over 8, consider doxycycline 4 mg/kg bid with a max of 100 mg/dose. The adult dose is 100 mg bid. Or, Amoxil at 50 mg/kg/day divided tid in kids with a max of 500 mg/dose and adults 500 tid. Or, cefuroxime (Ceftin) with the children's dose at 30 mg/kg/day divided bid with a max of 500 mg/dose and adults 500 mg po bid. Always consider combination therapy.

3. **Cardiac:** Along with kidney problems, heart problems in Lyme have high mortality. Of course, all the current cardiac support methodologies should be employed such as pacers and valve repairs. Again, for the best outcome if the sxs are Lyme-induced, antibiotics should be part of the treatment. Antimicrobials found to be effective in cases of cardiac Lyme include doxycycline, amoxicillin, ceftriaxone (Rocephin) with adults dosing at 2 g/day IV and kids at 50 to 75 mg/kg/day IV with a max 2 g/dose, Penicillin G, OR cefotaxime (Claforan) using in children 150-200 mg/kg/day IV tid or qid with a max of 6 g/day or max 2 g/dose or adults at 2 g IV given q 8.

4. **Musculoskeletal**: Early arthritis seems to respond well to a number of antibiotics. (That isn't to say that the Lyme is cured.) Active Bb can lead to joint disintegration. (Just ask my old knee.) Good antibiotic choices include: doxy in high doses bid, amoxicillin, Biaxin, cefdinir (Omnicef), or Ketek. With severe sxs consider ceftriaxone (Rocephin) with adults at 2 g/day IV and kids: 50 to 75 mg/kg/day IV with a max of 2 g/dose or Pen G. Plaquenil (hydroxychloroquine) should be considered when a patient has significant joint problems.

Lyme arthritis also responds well to steroids, but that treatment diminishes the immune response, often to the point of incapacity, allowing the Bb to do all the things it is capable of in order to survive to fight another day. Avoid steroids except in cases of true emergency. Then try to use them only short-term while on concomitant antibiotics.

5. **Endocrine:** As with many Lyme manifestations, the sequelae associated with hormonal imbalances may not respond to traditional treatment methods. Adding an appropriate antibiotic regimen to the treatment protocol may help control blood sugars, thyroid imbalances, and abnormal cortisol levels impacted by Lyme. Bb may be impacting the adrenals, and thereby cortisol levels. This hormone can affect stress, weight control, and fatigue.

6. **Gastrointestinal:** GERD is an especially common manifestation in Lyme patients, especially those born with the infection. A sensation of obstruction or "something stuck" in the throat is also a frequent complaint.

7. **Genitourinary:** Interstitial cystitis and chronic pelvic discomfort have been associated with LD.

8. **Autoimmune and antineuronal antibodies:** Auto-immune-complicated Lyme can be especially hard to treat. These patients can be helped by using alternative regimens to address their disease, such as incorporating Plaquenil in the antibiotic combination. Dr. Cunningham thinks that some Lyme patients might suffer a PANS-like syndrome. In these cases, treatment with IV IgG and plasmapheresis is thought to be more successful when antibiotics against the causative pathogen are part of the treatment strategy. Also, Plaquenil (hydroxychloroquine) might help with autoimmune manifestations associated with Borrelia and appears to kill both the cystic and spiral forms and doesn't affect normal immune function. Patients who test positive for HLA-DR2 or HLA-DR4 or display antibodies 31 or 34 will tend to have an autoimmune reaction to Bb infection. Their clinical picture may display more achiness. Plaquenil might be the best treatment choice for these patients, in combination with other antimicrobial agents.

D. Severity of illness

Most HCPs are influenced in their treatment decisions by the severity of illness. More is sometimes better but the best approach is to use the drugs appropriately in accordance with their pharmacokinetics. Dose doxy high and infrequently to get distinct peaks and troughs. Dose PCNs moderately and frequently in order to maintain a steady blood level. Try to select antibiotics that will hit the pathogen in its predominant current life form based on where the patient appears to be in the clinical course of the disease, remembering that other life forms may be lurking. In critical or end-stage LD, all supportive measures should be employed as indicated.

E. Duration of therapy: Short-term versus open-ended regimens

Imagine with any other disease aside from Lyme saying to a patient, "Even though you still feel terrible, I'm going to stop your medicine now. We both know that soon after we stop, you'll feel even worse. Nevertheless, this arbitrary guideline, which was found by the Connecticut AG to be biased, says I need to stop on day 30. You should 'eventually recover'." The patient would think you were crazy.

*PEARL: Actually one guideline gives 30 days as a **maximum** duration of therapy and shorter courses, with as little as 10 days of antibiotic, are recommended in some cases.*

Chapter 11: *Controversies around Lyme* explores the pros and cons regarding the short versus open-ended treatment recommendations from IDSA and ILADS respectively. I will not rehash those arguments here aside from a few

supportive points. In summary, I believe that overwhelming scientific evidence, as well as clinical experience, support the opinion that chronic Lyme exists, and on-going infection is the underlying etiology. Duration of treatment should be determined by clinical response. Treatment duration should be OPEN-ENDED. Long-term treatment is not mandated, but the option should be available for patients who would benefit from treatment beyond 30 days. Treat until the patient is better PLUS a cushion. Depending on the individual patient, this can be months or years.

PEARL: One study showed that doubling the length of IV ceftriaxone from 2 to 4 weeks improved the success rate from 66% to 80% based on their endpoint criteria.

Continuous, uninterrupted antibiotic therapy until the patient is better or functional has been a successful choice in a number of cases. In fact, short-courses of antibiotics might just cause the Bb to hide, using one of its many survival modes, until the coast is clear. When the pathogen resurfaces in its active form, the sxs of the disease usually resurface as well. Many studies have shown that short-term treatment is related to a high incidence of relapse. Chapter 24: *Antimicrobials* lists all the advantages, disadvantages, as well as possible risks and benefits of open-ended antibiotic use. After all my research, I am much more afraid of the potential damage that can result from not treating Lyme than I am of any risks from long-term antibiotics. I find it interesting that many of the short-term treatment proponents convert to the open-ended approach when they or a family member get persistent Lyme. I can name a few who now demonstrate the zeal of the convert. Lucky for them that as physicians they have access to long-term options that others might not have.

Although estimates vary, disseminated, symptomatic Lyme usually requires 6 to 12 months of antibiotic treatment in order to get the best chance of avoiding relapse. The return of sxs is evidence of the continued presence of Bb, indicating the need for further treatment. Donta defined cure as no symptoms for a year after discontinuation of antibiotics. There is never a guarantee that symptoms will not return.

While some say that treatment over 28 days is unnecessary and costly, they apparently do not consider the costs of relapse as well as the cost of managing the more intractable Lyme that can result from delayed or inadequate treatment. While IDSA worries about resistance and fungus with long-term antibiotic use, they don't seem to have problems with patients using antibiotics for years for acne and rosacea, two conditions with far less significant M&M. Has anyone ever died from rosacea? Believe me when I say I would rather spend my antibiotic credit on treating my Lyme.

F. Regimen options

There are as many ways to treat Lyme as there are practitioners seeing these patients. Of course, for each approach there is an equal amount of controversy and debate. From no treatment to waiting until the patient is at death's door to start therapy, just about every base has been covered. From big guns early to saving your best weapons for last, I think I've heard them all.

Some of these proposals are just bizarre. A few I had to read several times because I couldn't believe what I was reading. Some have no relationship to the physiology of the human being or the pathology of Lyme. One suggested using a new antibiotic every week after the Herx from the previous antibiotic subsided. This makes no sense. If they're Herxing, the drug is probably working, so give it a chance.

Here are several different approaches that merit discussion:

- No treatment or delayed treatment: Some "authorities" recommend not treating at all until you see what happens. I know how that worked out for my son. I didn't want to overreact to such a trivial disease. Most experienced TBI physicians believe that the longer treatment is delayed after the bite the better chance the case will become hard to treat, may become chronic, or could result in permanent sequelae. Inadequate treatment early on makes recovery that much harder. Still there are articles in the literature advocating a "wait and see" approach to treatment. Most TBI-focused practitioners not only endorse treatment asap, as well as prophylactic treatment in most cases, they find the delayed treatment approach unwarranted and potentially dangerous. Who wants Bb milling about burrowing into tissue and encysting? Delay encourages entrenchment and once L-forms and cysts develop, recovery is that much harder. Treatable disease should not be allowed to become intractable.

PEARL: One source from New Haven even said to LET the patient get to an advanced stage before even considering treatment. Even if the patient met the CDC criteria for Lyme there was no reason to treat. (Why'd you waste the money on a test if you weren't going to use the result, Buddy?) Not my kid. Thanks for your advice.

- Pulsing or cycling: Pulse antibiotics in line with the pharmacology of the drug. For example, artemesia MUST be pulsed or it will be metabolized to the point of ineffectiveness. Bicillin is given only several times a week because IM injections act as a depot providing continuous blood levels in line with the metabolism of the drug. Rocephin is used 4 days in a row out of 7. Some drugs such as vancomycin might be better on an interrupted schedule due to safety issues. Pulsing of Flagyl makes sense in line with its work breaking down cysts. Since the spirochetes go in and out of the cystic form, the Flagyl can be interrupted to spare the patient its harsh side effects, and then restarted when the Bb think they are safely back in their cysts. In contrast, do **not** pulse Rifampin so that potential resistance is kept to a minimum. Sometimes a severe Herx will require a loosening of the regimen.

Be cautious if you decide to interrupt antibiotic coverage. Some practitioners believe that the best outcomes result when at least one antibiotic is covering the patient at all times. Although specific antibiotics might be paused or changed during the treatment course, at least one antimicrobial is kept on board continuously. Usually two or more agents are prescribed in order to hit the various Bb forms or to penetrate various tissues. If one agent is paused, the others are there as back-up. With that being said, some well-respected practitioners use pulsing, drug holidays, and treatment vacations with reports of success in their practices, especially in dealing with plateaus and relapses. Use risk/benefit analysis to decide what is best for a particular patient.

PEARL: Pulsing may allow for use of very effective, but potentially more toxic, medicines like vancomycin. This antibiotic can be effective when more conventional medicines have failed. Since efficacy is based on 48 to 72 hours of continuous -cidal levels to kill the spirochete, once that level is reached, you can then pause since it will take longer than the 4 to 5 days between doses for the spirochetes to recover. Then, you can hit 'em again. You spare the patient safety and tolerability risks and still maintain the efficacy inherit in the drug.

PEARL: Pulsing may also tempt bugs out of hiding, where they are then more vulnerable to cell wall antibiotics.

- Saving the big guns for later: In the Christian tradition, Jesus changes water into wine when his hosts at a wedding feast run low. The guests remark that the host saved the best wine for last. This wouldn't make sense. Why would you wait until everyone was drunk to bring out the best tasting wine? That would be equivalent to knowing that one drug worked better against Lyme than other medicines and you still select the less effective drug. The plan in this scenario would be to save the best drugs for later. I saw several variations on this theme, like using all drugs at subtherapeutic doses. I do not quite "get" the rationale here. I am not talking about selecting a less effective drug because it is safer, or easier to administer, or better tolerated, or because the patient was allergic to the more effective medicine. I'm referring to those authors who, with all things being equal, select the less effective drug, saving the potentially more useful options for later. As for the subtherapeutic doses, the spirochetes just smirk and say, "We'll come back out when the coast is clear." Don't save the best wine for later, when the guests are too drunk to appreciate it. Choose the optimum drug combination for the job that needs to be done.

Here's the bottom line on reasonable treatment approaches based on my observations of a number of TBI practices:

- Use combination therapy,

- Continuously, pulsing as appropriate,

- Treating all recognized co-infections simultaneously as tolerated,

- Selecting those antibiotics that seem to fit best with the current picture presented by the patient,

- Choosing optimum doses and routes of administration,

- Fitting the established pharmacokinetics of the drugs,

- Attempting to hit all forms of the pathogen,

- In line with where the patient stands in the clinical course of the disease,

- Considering patient preference, and

- Weighing other options.

Each patient is unique and therapy should be targeted toward that individual using risk/benefit analysis before making any treatment decisions. Does your plan make sense? Is it scientifically logical? This doesn't mean that innovative treatment approaches aren't encouraged, but be careful that your strategy makes medical sense.

G. Tolerability

Sometimes treatment decisions are made for you. For example, an allergy might preclude the use of certain drugs in an individual. Some people can tolerate a "shock and awe" treatment approach and others cannot. One person can endure a savage Herx while the next cannot. Do not torture people in order to treat them. However, in many cases it's prudent to encourage them to withstand what they can in order to get adequate therapy on board. This can be especially pertinent in the case of a bad Herx, where the intensity of the reaction can mean the regimen is working.

If a drug messes with a patient's GI tract, find ways to counter the effects. Does taking with food help? Will that food increase or decrease absorption? It doesn't help to get the medicine in if it can't get to the job site. Does sitting up help? More or less water? Remember to consider probiotics in patients who will be taking antimicrobials. How about a cool compress to an injection site? Or a warm one if that feels better?

Be creative in ways to help the patient tolerate the treatment. I knew that my son would probably tolerate Doryx better than generic doxy, but I saved nearly a thousand dollars on the generic. Chris could not tolerate the generic doxy. A medicine does no good on the outside looking in. Not only did we need to go out and buy the brand drug, we lost the 4 bucks we paid for the generic.

PEARL: Doryx is an enteric-coated doxycycline formulation that is primarily absorbed in the SI, thereby avoiding much of the stomach irritation.

Compliance can be an important issue. If the patient cannot tolerate the medicine consider the alternatives. While treatment pickins may be slim, there is almost always a reasonable substitute.

H. Solo versus combination therapy

"She'll be fine with a little doxy." How many times have those words led to bad things happening in the long-run? Usually, Lyme patients are put on a single drug and sent on their way. To understand the repercussions in using a single antibiotic, we must review the various Bb life forms.

Where the Bb are:

1. Free-floating spirochetes are found in blood and other fluids and also in interstitial space. These helical forms have a cell wall so they can be damaged by cell wall antibiotics.

2. Bb can go intracellular where they especially like vacuoles since they can avoid the antibiotics sent to destroy them. To reach these Bb, the antibiotics need to be able to penetrate into the cells. For this job, intracellular antibiotics such as macrolides should be considered.

3. L-forms (spheroplasts) have no cell wall, so logically cell wall antibiotics can't hurt them. This fact is going to limit the solo use of PCNs and CSs that do a great job with the spirochetal forms.

4. When in a hostile environment (poor nutrients, unfavorable oxygen levels, extreme temperatures, or the presence of an antibiotic), Bb can change from spiral (spirochete) forms into cysts. Most antibiotics have no way to get into these cysts. Inside the cyst capsule, the Bb can stay dormant until conditions are favorable again. To get them where they hide, pick from a few select antibiotics that serve as cyst-busters. These agents include Flagyl (metronidazole) and Tindamax (tinidazole). Plaquenil is thought to penetrate some cysts.

Since Bb can move between these various life forms and locations, we need to have our bases covered. A single agent has trouble performing all these functions. So far no one drug is chemically structured to handle all these roles (except perhaps Tindamax, which has significant tolerability issues). In fact, doxy by itself can signal the spirochetes that adverse conditions are present and now might be the time to hide, burrow into cells, and encyst. Currently, there is no adequately tolerated solo agent that can hit all the life forms and locations.

Of course, some people take doxy all by itself and the Lyme resolves never to resurface. I am happy for them. As always we need to be concerned with those patients who have the recurrent, persistent, chronic type of LD.

Bb can shift among the forms and change locations. We do not clearly understand how all this activity happens, but suffice it to say the Bb understand. This is all a series of biochemical responses used as a means to survive. We must outsmart them.

PEARL: Those that warn against any treatment or suggest delaying treatment misunderstand both the pathophysiology of Lyme and the way antibiotics work. We are targeting a recently discovered pathogen with drugs that are decades old. We must work with what we have until somebody comes up with a better alternative.

Unfortunately, we do not have the one pill that will eradicate Bb at our disposal today. Fortunately, we know how to make do. By carefully assessing the patient status we can select antimicrobial combinations that will cover all we need done. We have ways to go after them when they float by freely, ways to go after them when they hide inside cells, and ways to go after them when they are dormant inside cysts. When they decide it's safe to poke back out, we can be waiting.

*PEARL: Doxy **alone** will not hit Bb that is already intracellular. An intracellular antibiotic will be needed to do that. By driving the free-floating spirochetes into hiding, doxy or other **solo** agents, can contribute to the 10% to 15% of patients who develop intractable, full-blown Lyme that is very hard to treat.*

PEARL: Usually a combination of antibiotics achieves the best result.

For Lyme alone, the most prudent tactic is probably to use two or more agents concomitantly. This way the various life forms can be impacted, cell niches entered, and cysts busted. Further, multiple agents decrease the chance of inefficacy due to resistance. For the most part, rifamycin should never be used without a back-up and should never be paused in the course of treatment.

Some antibiotics perform more than one function. In general, try to select drugs that come at the Bb using different MOAs. For example, a good combination might be a PCN to get the cell walled spirochete, a macrolide to get inside the cells, and an azole to bust the cysts. (That is amoxicillin, azithromycin, and Flagyl.) Of course, combinations get more complicated when all the other factors that impact antibiotic choice are taken into consideration. When co-infections are added to the mix, you might have to juggle and balance to get the right formula. But let's just address combinations based on life forms for right now.

PEARL: Often people will contact me, thinking I am still in practice, and ask if a certain antimicrobial regimen is appropriate. If only things were that simple. I know next-to-nothing about the patient and it takes a long time to factor in all the confounders that could influence a treatment decision. Forgive me for not being more helpful. I just don't have enough information to contribute.

I know you just want the lists:

Cell wall antibiotics: Suitable for use against the spirochetal, free-floating form of Bb: PCNs (Amoxil. Augmentin, Bicillin), CSs (Omnicef, Ceftin, Rocephin, Claforan, Cedax, Suprax), Primaxin, vancomycin, TCNs (doxycycline, Doryx, Minocin), Tindamax. Rifamycin and Plaquenil both might impact the free-floating forms but the mechanism is unclear. L-forms have no cell wall so they are not hurt by cell wall antibiotics.

Intracellular: Macrolides/ketolides (Zithromax, Biaxin, Ketek), Tindamax, rifamycin. Once the pathogen gets inside the cell, doxycycline has less effect, but minocycline may do a little better. Tigecycline can go intracellular.

Cyst-busters: Azoles (Flagyl, Tindamax). Plaquenil is thought to penetrate some cysts.

PEARL: Tindamax likely hits all three life forms of Bb.

BBB status:

Do cross the BBB: Rocephin (ceftriaxone), rifamycin, Bicillin, minocycline to a limited degree, IV doxycycline, Claforan (cefotaxime), Ceftin (cefuroxime), chloramphenicol, Lariam

Do not cross the BBB: Macrolides, oral doxycycline, vancomycin, Mepron, clindamycin

I. Modalities

There are many ways to administer medication, the details of which are provided in Chapter 23: *Understanding Medicines*. For our purposes, we will be mostly interested in the relative advantages and disadvantages of oral, intravenous, and intramuscular administration (po, IV, IM).

Oral administration is often adequate, but thousands of patients have done well on IV and IM regimens. Often patients use more than one modality at a time.

How do you decide if you want IV, IM, or po? Since nothing about Lyme is simple, there are a number of aspects to consider. For every point I make below, trust that someone adamantly disagrees. Do a risk/benefit analysis.

Oral administration (po):

- Many HCPs usually begin with an oral regimen unless other factors suggest differently

- Less costly

- Convenient

Parenteral: Includes any method of administration other than oral. Here parenteral refers to IM or IV.

- Parenteral administration recommended when there are CNS signs, carditis, or complicated Lyme arthritis

- Possibly useful in patients not responding to orals

- Consider if there was prior immunosuppressive treatment while infected with Bb

- May be helpful in patients who have been sick a long time

- Consider when the illness has been present for more than 1 year

- Useful if GI problems

- Consider when unable to tolerate oral meds

- If two meds cannot be taken together orally, parenteral administration solves this problem.

- Possible use when there is active synovitis with a high sedimentation rate

- Consider if there are elevated protein or cells in the CSF

Intramuscular administration (IM):

- Probably second most effective modality for Lyme after IV

- Excellent for achieving steady state levels since injection site acts as depot

- Once injected cannot remove

- Painful

Intravenous administration (IV):

- Consider in those with NP manifestations since the BBB might be circumvented

- For severe sxs IV usually gets everywhere the blood flows

- IV by-passes the GI tract so might avoid some GI side effects

- Considered most effective method of administration

- Parenteral administration recommended when CNS signs, carditis, or complicated Lyme arthritis

- Fastest drug to tissue

- No worries about absorption

- If IV too fast may cause a severe Herx

- Does not eliminate the possibility of a yeast infection

- After oral administration, many then consider IV

- Usually achieves best tissue levels

- Can use IV mode until clear positive response and then transition to orals

- With injection, once injected there's no turning back. Can turn off an infusion

- Can be costly and inconvenient

- Sometimes the only way to get results

The best modality to use is a judgment call which depends a great deal on patient preference and circumstances, as well as the severity of the disease.

J. Pathogen phase

Bb can be spirochetes living and reproducing in the blood, dormant in L-forms, encysted, intracellular, hiding in obscure niches, extracellular, or comfortable in interstitial space. Of course, Bb can be present in several or all these manifestations at once. The more burrowed in the tissue, the less likely the immune cells and antibiotics can reach them and the harder they are to treat. The BBB seems to offer little impediment to the spirochete but considerable barricade to many antibiotics.

The life stage of the Borrelia at the time of treatment can be important to overall success. Ceftin kills Bb only when they are metabolizing. Once threatened by an antibiotic the Bb hide deep in tissue or encyst in hard shells so they are much less accessible. The reproductive cycle of Borrelia is about 4 to 6 weeks. So treatment should then cover several of these cycles to be effective. However, that time frame only takes into account the reproducing spirochetes, not the dormant Borrelia in cysts and L-forms. When treatment stops, Bb perceive they are free to roam and come out of their cysts. Symptoms recur. The spirochetes are back, so now hammer them with a cell wall agent, keeping in mind that you don't want them going back inside cells or cysts. Choose your combination carefully.

K. Hometown of the tick

Carefully consider the **endemic** region where the biting tick originated. (This may or may not be the location where the bite occurred, since both ticks and people travel.) There are many strain differences and that may be one reason why there are so many different presentations of LD. In parts of Connecticut, GI and urinary symptoms along with cognitive problems may predominate. Certain antibiotics work in some of these strains better than others for unclear reasons, but I'm sure biochemistry and genetics are involved somehow. An Omnicef combination works very well in southern Jersey and Pennsylvania but not so much in northern NJ, where a different clinical syndrome predominates. Understand that flexibility may be important in finding the right combination.

L. MOA of drug

Different drugs work differently. Again, we're talking biochemistry and the concept of structure dictating function. Some drugs attack the cell wall. Some drugs attack the cell wall of only those pathogens that are replicating. Some drugs pay no attention to the cell wall. We are talking receptors and markers and all kinds of complicated technical stuff that does not particularly concern us. Better to choose drugs for combination therapy that come at Bb from different angles.

M. Time since tick bite or Lyme diagnosis

Considerable evidence supports the contention that the longer the interval between infection and the initiation of treatment, the more problems could arise. In some patients, the infection evolves from a manageable condition into an entrenched, intractable, refractory entity that becomes quite hard to a handle.

Although the literature refers to the time since diagnosis, this is an essentially meaningless parameter. What we are interested in is the time since infection. Because so few people recall the tick bite, and because the tick they remember may not be the guilty party, we again have little useful information.

There are reports that if the infection is more than 6 months old, the patient is much more likely to require an extended treatment course. Failure to identify and treat early can lead to the patient developing a chronic condition that can lead to infection in the brain, eyes, joints, heart, and other body systems. Sxs can be debilitating and eventually lead to irreversible organ damage. Liegner feels that a delay in the treatment could lead to permanent injury that remains even after the infection is brought under control.

In general with TBIs, the later in the course of the disease that treatment is initiated, the longer treatment will be needed for the patient to improve. Some authors give estimates. I do not know how well these numbers correlate to the reality of the Lyme population but they provide a ball park. If treatment is started when the person has been sick less than a year, the person could take about a year to recover. Those sick longer before therapy begins will correspondingly take longer, more like 2 to 4 years. Some sick for 20 years might take 5 years or more to heal but even they can improve over time. Clearly, delay of treatment makes recovery harder and longer. There are significant risks in postponing an antibiotic regimen.

HCPs who have had personal experience with TBIs tend to "get it" but those who say they just took 14 or 28 days of doxy and all was well, likely caught their infections almost instantly and did not delay their own treatment. They usually don't make their own child wait for treatment either.

My advice is to forget the time from diagnosis, since it is probably longer than you would like anyway, and start treatment NOW, if clinically indicated. Don't wait another minute. The spirochetes aren't waiting for you. They're busy setting up bustling colonies in biofilms and inside tissues. If you do know when the person was infected, use that information to motivate you to take action. Recognize that by the time the individual is seen by an HCP, the Bb will be establishing themselves in all sorts of venues. The clock is ticking. I have enough enmity toward Borrelia that I don't want one more of those spirochetes to replicate before I go after them.

N. Patient preference

While I will encourage the treatment strategy that I think is best for the patient, I will not force. Sometimes it is just too traumatic for some people to get IM or IV medicines when reasonable alternatives are available. Collaborate with patients and caretakers to review the risk/benefit of alternative treatments.

SAMPLE TREATMENT REGIMENS

Although there are other possibilities, here are your choices; Amoxicillin, Augmentin, doxycycline such as Doryx, Minocin, TCN, Plaquenil, Zithromax, Biaxin, Ketek, Omnicef, Ceftin, Flagyl, Tindamax, Bicillin, Rocephin, Levaquin, Primaxin, Claforan, Tygacil, vancomycin, clindamycin, Plaquenil. Each and every one of these medicines is detailed in Chapter 24: *Antimicrobials*. Use the above factors to make your treatment choices. In this section, I will focus on Lyme and provide a few important nuances for you to consider as you weigh the risk/benefit of every treatment decision.

Antibiotics work in conjunction with the immune system to help cure the patient. Treatment response varies with each individual and, while there are a thousand theories, the truth is we just don't understand why some get well and some don't. From all we know so far, it seems that the most treatment success comes when treatment is initiated as early as possible after infection. Using the appropriate combination of antibiotics, in proper doses, for an adequate length of time gives the best chance for positive outcomes.

In all cases the antibiotic regimen should be tailored to the individual patient, the options should be discussed with the patient and guardians, a risk/benefit assessment should be done, and patient preferences taken into consideration. No cookie-cutter or one-size-fits-all medicine allowed.

Antimicrobials are the foundation of TBI treatment and the key to success. I wish this part were as simple as one fly, one swatter. Unfortunately, selection of the appropriate antibiotics will depend on a number of factors both obvious and obscure:

- The pathogen and any number of possible strains
- Potential co-infections
- Co-morbidities
- Allergies
- Tolerance of treatment regimen
- General health
- Stage of disease
- Previous treatment response
- Herx potential
- Age, gender, ethnicity

SELECT INFORMATION ON THE VARIOUS ANTIBIOTICS MOST USED AGAINST LYME

Fundamentals regarding drug class, MOA, dosage, usage, contraindications, adverse events, warnings, and monitoring for problems is included in hideous detail in Chapter 24: *Antimicrobials*. Always consider a probiotic in the patients you treat with antimicrobials. The information provided below is pertinent to the treatment of Lyme.

Penicillins: PCNs work by damaging the cell wall of the pathogen. This MOA makes them ideal antibiotics to use against the spirochetal form of Bb, which has a cell wall. PCNs are not effective against L-forms of Bb, which has no cell wall, and so should be part of a combination regimen. PCNs work best at steady state blood levels so they should be delivered in moderate doses frequently.

- **Amoxicillin** (Amoxil): Amoxicillin is the DOC for Lyme in kids. This is the antibiotic that you build your combination platform on. Especially early in the clinical course of the disease, oral amoxicillin is as effective as doxy. Amoxil combines well with azithromycin. Probenecid 500 mg q 8 h can be added to boost efficacy.

Adults:	1 or 2 grams q 8 h up to 6 g/day
Pregnant:	1 gram q 6 h
Kids:	50 mg/kg/day divided into q 8 doses

- **Amoxicillin plus clavulanate** (Augmentin): This PCN comes with its own efficacy booster. Augmentin can cause savage diarrhea.

- **Benzathine penicillin** (Bicillin): IM Bicillin is a very effective and common treatment for Lyme. In fact, the drug is so good against Bb that a strong, long Herx can occur lasting weeks. Doses may need to be reduced in order for the patient to tolerate the Herx. In Chapter 28, you will be taught to view a Herx reaction as your ally, since it provides evidence of the mass destruction of spirochetes.

  IM dosing allows the medicine to sit in a repository in the muscle and be released at a fairly constant rate, accommodating the steady state blood levels at which PCNs are most effective. Since PCNs need steady state levels for about 72 hours to be effective, the injection need only occur 3 or 4 times a week. This schedule gets around the annoyance of having to take oral PCNs multiple times each day and thereby reduces the risk of skipping a dose. IM Bicillin also avoids all the rigmarole involved in setting up IV administration.

But, alas, IM Bicillin can hurt. A LOT. Doug Fearn from LDASEPA has provided an excellent set of pointers on how to minimize the discomfort of a Bicillin injection, which is included in Chapter 24.

Adults/Preg: 1.2 million units 3 to 4 doses/week

Children: Usually best in kids over 8

Cephalosporins: CSs have a similar mechanism to the PCNs, working to interfere with the cell wall of the pathogen. Therefore, they are effective against the spirochetal form of Bb, but not the L-forms. Like PCNs they are most effective at steady state levels, so they should be administered frequently, several times a day. Since their structures are so close to those of PCNs, patients allergic to one of these drug classes might also be allergic to the other. Consider CSs as part of a combination regimen.

- **Ceftriaxone** (Rocephin): IV Rocephin started to be used for Lyme in the 80s and has one of the best efficacy records. However, there is an increased occurrence of biliary sludge and gallstones associated with its use. Actigall 1 to 3 tablets daily can mitigate the risk. The patient should be screened before use, checking to see if there is a personal or family history of GB trouble, and an ultrasound should be done. Repeat ultrasounds should be conducted monthly during treatment and for about 3 months after Rocephin is discontinued. Patients tend to do pretty well with the IV administration at home. The best ceftriaxone regimens seem to be **4 days** in a row each week with the other **3 days off**.

  Adults/ Preg: 2 g q 12 h, 4 days in a row each week

  Children: 75 mg/kg/day given q 12 h up to 2 g/day, 4 days in a row each week

- **Cefotaxime** (Claforan): IV Claforan has comparable efficacy to Rocephin but much less chance of gallstones. There does not appear to be a risk of biliary complications, although there may be some transient changes in LFTs. Unfortunately Claforan must be administered three times a day or preferably through continuous infusion and that is much less convenient than the Rocephin. Claforan crosses the BBB.

  Adults/Preg: 6 g to 12 g daily - can be given q 8 in divided doses but continuous infusion probably more efficacious. When exceed 6 g /day, consider pulse dosing

  Children: 90 to 180 mg/kg/day dosed q 6 (preferred) or q 8 not to exceed 12 g daily. When exceed 6 g/day, use pulse dosing.

PEARL: If you are choosing between IV formulations consider Rocephin first, then Claforan, then azithromycin, then doxycycline. All have their advantages and disadvantages. Tygacil (tigecycline) is an excellent IV drug and probably quite effective against Lyme, but it is extremely hard to tolerate.

- **Cefuroxime** (Ceftin): This drug may be good in amoxicillin and doxy failures. Useful in EM rashes that are co-infected with common skin pathogens. (Huh? How often does that happen?) Ceftin works nicely for routine skin infections PLUS Ceftin is actually indicated for the treatment of "early" Lyme. The Ceftin package insert, in fact, uses the term "Spirochetes" under which it simply says, "Borrelia *burgdorferi*." The final instruction under Ceftin Tablets (number 8 to be precise) says that these tablets can be used in "Early Lyme Disease (erythema migrans) caused by Borrelia *burgdorferi*." With all empathy to the drug developers at the company, they were just trying to get the indication on the books and get a good performance review. They felt no compunction to understand the disease, since Lyme presents with an EM rash in far less than half the cases. So if you're trying to cure EM rashes, Ceftin is a good choice. If you're going after Lyme, a combination of other agents is probably a better choice. Ceftin crosses the BBB.

  Adults: For Lyme 500 mg to 1 gram bid

  Over 13:   250 mg to 500 mg bid

  Children: Greater than 3 months: 20 to 30 mg/kg per day in two divided doses. This translates to 125 to 500 mg bid depending on weight with a maximum of 1 gram/day

- **Cefdinir** (Omnicef): Sometimes Omnicef in combination with Zithromax is selected as first-line in kids sick with their first bout of Lyme.

  Adults > 13 y/o: 300 mg q 12

  Kids 6 months to 12 years: 7 mg/kg q 12 with 600 mg/day max

- Other CSs: Cedax (ceftibuten), Suprax (cefixime)

Tetracyclines: TCNs are bacteriostatic agents that work best when their blood levels show clear peaks and troughs. Here you want to give high doses less frequently, usually once or twice a day. TCNs can become bacteriocidal at high doses, but these levels are almost impossible to maintain. If good peaks are not achieved the drug might not be effective. Here we need spikes, not steady state. So the best dosing regimen is once a day, but the drug is better tolerated bid, keeping the same total daily dose. TCNs should not be used in pregnancy. All TCNs have associated sun sensitivity and patients and caretakers must be warned. Lyme patients treated with any of the TCNs are likely to Herx because TCNs are effective against Borrelia.

- **Tetracycline**: Old faithful is hardly used at all anymore because of resistance and tolerability issues. Most pharmacies dispense generics. TCN probably works better than either doxy or minocycline for Lyme, but they are much better tolerated. Use in adults only and not in pregnancy.

- **Doxycycline** (Doryx (enteric-coated), Vibramycin): Doxy is great for borreliosis, anaplasmosis, ehrlichiosis, Rickettsia, and perhaps Bartonella and Mycoplasma infections. EXCEPT we are VERY reluctant to use these agents in kids under 8 because of their effect on bones and teeth. In emergencies when a younger child is very sick with Lyme and ehrlichiosis, then a short-course of doxy could be considered. Here doxycycline or minocycline for a limited duration of 1 to 2 weeks should not put these children at undue risk. Most practitioners have not had a problem with these cases. Be careful using doxy as a solo agent. While excellent at hitting free-floating spirochetes, when used alone doxy seems to inspire some of the Bb to go intracellular and encyst, only to resurface another day. Always consider combination regimens, when appropriate.

Chapter 24: *Antimicrobials* has a dosing chart copied from a doxycycline package insert. It is nearly incomprehensible. To paraphrase: For adults 200 mg bid or 400 once daily, if they can tolerate the once-a-day dose, with a maximum of 600 mg/day. Doxy is ONLY effective at high doses. (My 170 pound son was given a trifling 50 bid.) If the patient cannot tolerate the GI side effects consider that the Doryx formulation is usually much better tolerated than the generics. (Of course, it is 250 times more expensive as well. Worth every nickel. No, I am not a spokesperson for Doryx. I don't even know who makes it. I did run into a Doryx sales rep once when I was in a preceptor's office. I asked him why his formulation was so much easier on the stomach than the generics. He had no idea. (That's your big selling point, son!) Otherwise, you may have to consider IV doxy or change drugs entirely.

Note that there is controversy in the literature regarding whether or not oral doxy should be taken with food or not. From a pharmacokinetic perspective, it definitely should NOT be taken with food. But some patients say they can't stand to take it without food. Herein lies the dilemma. Food will decrease absorption, which will lower blood levels, which will diminish the peak needed for efficacy. But if the drug doesn't get taken, there are no blood levels whatsoever. If the patient truly cannot tolerate the doxy without food, consider switching to a different drug or route of administration.

To use IV doxycycline, the patient will need a central line since the material is so caustic. But the IV route is quite effective, probably because you can achieve a nice, distinct peak after a single daily blast of the drug. The high peak level optimizes the efficacy of the drug. Infusion of IV doxy hurts. A LOT.

In children over 8 y/o, consider a loading dose of 200 mg and then give 100 to 200 mg q 12, with a maximum of 600 mg per day depending on the child's size and tolerance. Oral doxy does not cross the BBB so if the patient has considerable NP sxs, think about adding a drug that crosses the BBB or replace the doxy with another agent. IV doxy will travel in the circulation to the brain but it is so toxic otherwise that other antibiotics should be explored.

- **Minocycline** (Minocin): When having to choose an oral TCN, many select minocycline for their patients. Minocycline may cause less sun sensitivity than the other TCNs, but has been associated with vestibular toxicity. A lupus-like syndrome has also been linked to use of minocycline. Minocin may achieve higher brain levels than other TCNs.

  Adults: Loading dose: 200 mg po or IV then 100 mg q 12

  Children:

      Over 8: 4 mg/kg/day po or IV initially then 4 mg/kg daily divided q 12

               Give IV in 500 to 1000 ml solution without calcium over 6 hours

      Under 8: Consider other antibiotics first

- **Tigecycline** (Tygacil): Closely related to the TCNs, this IV antibiotic is used for infection of the abdominal organs and skin. While it's MOA is similar to the TCNs its chemical structure does NOT allow it to be pumped out of Bb cells like a number of other antibiotics. Some sources say it is 100 times more effective against Bb than doxy. Instead of just inhibiting the spirochetes, tigecycline kills them. Rocephin kills them too but it takes much longer to do so. Tigecycline kills them within 24 hours *in vitro*. While that sounds like the description of the perfect Lyme drug, tigecycline can be very hard to tolerate (read next to impossible) for many patients. Some people have found relief if they eat DURING the infusion. Otherwise, they can be miserable. In patients over 18, give an initial dose of 100 mg followed by 50 mg q 12.

Macrolides: Erythromycins do concentrate well in tissues and penetrate cells, so they should be good agents for Lyme and certain other TBIs, but they have not performed as well as might be expected. Bb often resides inside a cell vacuole with low fluid pH. The acid may inactivate the azithromycin or clarithromycin, so consider using these agents in combination with hydroxychloroquine (Plaquenil) to raise the vacuolar pH. Macrolides are good agents to consider in pregnancy. But in Lyme they are not effective alone and should be part of a combination strategy.

- **Azithromycin** (Zithromax): Zithromax is readily absorbed and penetrates most tissues and white cells. For Lyme it is considered an intracellular agent, good for going after the spirochetes in the tissues. In TBI patients, azithromycin is commonly used against Lyme in combination with other agents. Often selected as part of the regimen if M. *fermentans* is suspected. Azithromycin is effective against malaria when used in combination with artemesia and so is presumed to work against Babesia. With Lyme expect a rapid and severe Herx, which may be a sign of efficacy. Zithromax appears quite effective when used IV in Lyme patients.

  Azithromycin is a very common combination drug for Lyme. Some HCPs elect to combine Zithromax with Omnicef in kids experiencing their first Borrelia infection. But this drug also combines well with other cephalosporins, penicillins, tetracyclines, rifamycin, and cyst-busters like Flagyl or Tindamax. Some physicians start azithromycin with a loading dose, while others go directly to the maintenance regimen.

  Azithromycin is pregnancy category B which means it is not expected to be harmful to the unborn baby and is considered the DOC for pregnant women infected with Borrelia.

  Adults: 250 to 500 daily (higher doses up to 1200 mg/day may be considered in certain cases) given twice a day

  Children:

  Less than 6 months: Not recommended

  Greater than 6 months: 5 to 10 mg/kg/day (250 to 500 mg per day)

  Azithromycin seems to be more effective in TBI patients when given IV but must be given through a central line due to the caustic nature of the formulation. IV doses range from 500 to 1000 mg daily in both children and adults.

  Hydroxychloroquine 200 to 400 mg/day can be added to enhance efficacy.

- **Clarithromycin** (Biaxin): Biaxin may be more effective orally than azithromycin but it is harder to tolerate. If the Bb are hiding in cells, Biaxin is thought to have good cell penetration. The oral suspension of Biaxin is the worst tasting stuff on earth, in case you were wondering.

  Adults: 250 to 1 gram q 12.
  Most common dose is 500 bid.
  Children:

  Less than 6 months: not recommended

  Greater than 6 months: 7.5 mg/kg q 12

- **Telithromycin** (Ketek): This drug is the best of the macrolides. Ketek, actually a ketolide, is the most effective of the class so far and probably the best oral agent for Lyme, if tolerated. Because of its superior efficacy, Ketek can produce a long and strong Herx. There is little antimicrobial resistance and less change in GI flora. But some in the FDA despise this drug. I worked on another matter with the congressional investigator who was overseeing the inquiry around deaths due to liver problems associated with Ketek. I got an earful. My son was on Ketek, and while we were vigilant, he had no problems. Be careful when you use Ketek. If you uncover any problems, regroup. Sometimes due to allergies or other contraindications, treatment options are limited, so you work with what you have. I don't think many question the efficacy of this drug. Just be watchful for safety issues. In addition to the potential for liver damage, Ketek can prolong QTc, and be involved in drug interactions. Teens and adults: 800 mg qd.

Azoles: This drug class has a broad spectrum of action especially with anaerobic bacteria and protozoa.

- **Metronidazole** (Flagyl): For some reason, much of my medical education revolved around Flagyl. That was before we were using terms like cyst-busters. Today, Flagyl is a common agent used to treat TBIs in combination with other antimicrobials. In Lyme, Flagyl is often considered when the presentation is predominantly neurologic. Bb are thought to encyst, especially in and around CNS tissue. Flagyl has excellent tissue penetration and is thought to be able to penetrate these cysts, leaving the pathogen vulnerable. Then the Bb can be damaged either by Flagyl inside the cyst or by the concomitant antibiotics that are able to get to the Bb after Flagyl breaks down the door. If the patient is chronically infected, consider metronidazole with one or two other antibiotics. This ensures that all Bb forms are targeted.

  For Lyme, Flagyl is effectively combined with Bicillin, Ketek, or with Zithromax. (That would be a cyst-buster, a cell wall antibiotic, and an intracellular agent – all bases covered.) The combination of Biaxin and Flagyl should hit both Bb and Babesia. In patients who are experiencing a Herx from other antibiotics, an added cyst-buster may be just what is needed to break through to some of the pathogens not reached by the cell wall or intracellular agents.

Flagyl is sometimes part of the **combination** strategy used in the treatment of Babesia *microti*. Since Bb and Babesia are so often found together, Flagyl might be considered when you are trying to hit these two TBIs at once.

In line with the spirochetes coming in and out of cysts, some providers prefer to pulse Flagyl 2 weeks on and 2 weeks off. This allows the drug to do its work, while minimizing the toxicity of the drug. Especially in first time users, Flagyl can be hard to tolerate.

Adults:	250 to 750 po tid translated to 15 mg/kg (loading dose) and then 7.5 mg/kg q 6 hours with a maximum of 4 grams/day
Children:	Use in children only if options are limited. Otherwise not recommended.
	Less than 120 pounds: 250 mg tid
	120 to 150 pounds: 500 mg tid

- **Tinidazole** (Tindamax): Tindamax gets the spirochetal (cell wall) form of Bb as well as all the cell wall deficient variations such as the L-forms found in cysts and inside cells. Tinidazole may be better at penetrating the cyst than metronidazole and may be better tolerated. While Flagyl is used in kids only when other options have been exhausted, Tindamax can be used in children.

PEARL: Comparing Tindamax to Flagyl: Tindamax can be used in kids and hits all three life forms of Bb whereas Flagyl is useful primarily against the cystic form. Both can be hellacious to tolerate, but pulsing may help.

In TBIs Tindamax is often pulsed either in alternate weeks or two weeks on and two weeks off. The regimen varied in the literature. One possible pulsing regimen administers Tindamax on two consecutive days of the week. Be careful. A horrendous Herx can occur which might be best minimized by dosing only one day the first week and then, if the patient can handle that, going to the 2-days-a-week regimen. Still some people must stay with the once per week schedule. Consider dosing on Friday and Saturday since some patients experience extreme fatigue and this is better managed over the weekend than when trying to also deal with work or school. Tindamax is used in combination therapy for Lyme and may be effective against the protozoal agent of Babesia as well.

Children:	While Flagyl is not recommended in children, Tindamax can be given to kids three and older.
Less than 3-years-old:	Not recommended
Greater than 3 years:	50 mg/kg with a maximum 2 g per day in a pulsed regimen

PEARL: Tindamax just might be the "magic bullet" for Bb infections since it appears to hit all life forms even those inside cells and cysts. If only it wasn't so awful to tolerate.

Other antimicrobials effective against Lyme:

- **Rifamycin** (Rifampin): Rifampin has good penetration across the BBB and into the CSF. Its lipophilic nature allows it to penetrate the BBB and so works well against a number of etiologies of meningitis, encephalitis, and other infections involving nerve tissue. Rifampin may be effective against Bartonella, Ehrlichia, and Bb. Rifamycin might also be a good option in those patients where doxy or other first-line choices are contraindicated. Consider that Rifampin has been used as the foundation drug in TBI combination therapy, where the rifamycin remains constant and other drugs are changed around it. In TBIs, Rifampin readily penetrates to the meninges and brain making its way into the cells. This medicine has the potential to act fast against both intracellular and extracellular organisms and reaching dormant organisms lurking in macrophages.

The big problem with Rifampin is resistance. So you NEVER interrupt it and you NEVER use it alone. Do not pulse. ALWAYS use Rifampin in combination with other antimicrobials to decrease the impact of resistance, so if one agent doesn't get the bug, the other will.

This antibiotic is considered a big gun. Some HCPs like to pull this agent out early and try to subdue the pathogen with shock and awe. Others prefer to reserve this type of antimicrobial for the sickest patients and for those showing signs of meningitis or CNS effects. This is a judgment call based on the individual case. If you use Rifampin, this can be the core antibiotic in your combination regimen and you can select complimentary antimicrobials around the Rifampin. While the other drugs can come and go and be interrupted, paused, or changed, the Rifampin would remain steady.

Adults:	300 to 600 mg two times a day
Children:	Less than one month: 5 mg/kg q 12
	Greater than 1 month: 10 mg/kg q 12 with a maximum of 600 mg/day

- **Vancomycin:** As a cell wall antibiotic, vancomycin is probably the best overall treatment for Lyme, but toxicity limits its use. Vancomycin is a good candidate for pulse therapy in order to minimize toxicity. This is one of the few drugs where I would order blood levels. While I do not think therapeutic levels are especially reliable, I want to take advantage of any hint of a problem. Still, this is one of my favorite drugs. In many ways, I think vancomycin has gotten a bad rap. Chapter 24: *Antimicrobials* discusses the history of this drug.

Vancomycin does NOT penetrate the CSF or cross the BBB. Consider combination therapy if there are neuro-psychiatric symptoms.

Vancomycin is an IV drug EXCEPT for its use against C. *difficile*. Oral vancomycin does not cross the intestinal lining at all. It stays right in the GI tract where it can take out the overgrowing Clostridia. Adverse events include red man syndrome and hearing loss.

Intravenous dosing is 15 mg/kg q 12. This dose is recommended for patients with endocarditis and should handle cases where patients are just as sick in other organ systems, except the brain.

- **Hydroxychloroquine** (Plaquenil): What an interesting drug. This jack-of-all-trades has several roles to play in TBI treatment:

1. Macrolides may be more effective when combined with Plaquenil.

2. Plaquenil helps with Lyme-associated autoimmune manifestations. Autoimmune-complicated Lyme can be especially hard to treat. These patients might be helped by using alternative regimens such as Plaquenil to address their disease. Some patients felt that this medicine was the only thing that helped.

3. This antimicrobial likely kills Borrelia in its spiro-chetal form without adversely impacting normal immune function. Plaquenil works best when given with a cyst-buster since it may inspire spirochetes to enter the cell wall deficient stage.

4. Hydroxychloroquine may be a good choice in those patients with significant Lyme-related joint problems. This agent should be considered especially when arthritis is a major presenting component.

5. Patients who test positive for HLA-DR2 or HLA-DR4, or display antibodies 31 or 34 on serology testing, will tend to have an autoimmune-type reaction to Bb infection. Their clinical picture may display more achiness. These patients usually do not respond as well to traditional antibiotic regimens. Plaquenil might be a good additional therapy for these patients.

6. In Lyme arthritis, hydroxychloroquine may have both an anti-spirochetal and anti-inflammatory MOA.

No specific doses have been established for treating Lyme but for rheumatic disorders such as SLE or RA:

Adults:	200 to 600 mg daily (can be in divided doses) with food or milk.
	200 to 400 mg/day can be added to enhance efficacy of macrolides.
Children:	Not established

For long-term use, calculate the best dose to avoid eye toxicity. This dose can be determined using patient height and weight. The manufacturer or pharmacist can provide the formula. Watch for retinal or visual field changes and hepatic dysfunction.

CATEGORIES TO HELP FACILITATE LYME TREATMENT CHOICES

Cell wall antibiotics: Suitable for use against the spiro-chetal, free-floating form of Bb: PCNs (Amoxil, Augmentin, Bicillin), CSs (Omnicef, Ceftin, Rocephin, Claforan, Cedax, Suprax), Primaxin, vancomycin, TCNs (doxycycline, Doryx, Minocin), Tindamax. Both Plaquenil and rifamycin may hit the free-floating forms of Bb, through processes not clearly understood. L-forms have no cell wall so they are not hurt by cell wall antibiotics.

Intracellular: Macrolides/ketolides (Zithromax, Biaxin, Ketek), Tindamax, rifamycin. Once the pathogen gets inside the cell, doxycycline has less effect, but minocycline might do a little better. Tigecycline (Tygacil) can go intracellular.

Cyst-busters: Flagyl, Tindamax. Plaquenil is thought to penetrate some cysts.

PEARL: Tindamax likely hits all three life forms of Bb.

BBB status:

Do cross the BBB: Rocephin (ceftriaxone), rifamycin, Bicillin, minocycline to a limited degree, IV doxycycline, Claforan (cefotaxime), Ceftin (cefuroxime), chloramphenicol, Lariam

Do not cross the BBB: Macrolides, oral doxycycline, vancomycin, Mepron, clindamycin

IV formulations: Rocephin (ceftriaxone), Claforan (cefotaxime), Zithromax (azithromycin), doxycycline, Tygacil (tigecycline)

Primary DOCs for treating Lyme in various populations: (Remember, consider combination therapy!) Choices include: doxycycline for adults, amoxicillin in kids, macrolides in pregnant women, and ceftriaxone for those who need IV therapy, especially with significant NP manifestations. Bicillin is a good IM option. These are the drugs you build your combination regimen around and a combination approach should be pursued in order to hit the various life forms of Bb.

For a child's first bout with Lyme, think about combining amoxicillin PLUS a macrolide (probably azithromycin, Zithromax). Or, consider pairing Zithromax with a cephalosporin (probably cefdinir, Omnicef), depending on the clinical presentation.

> *PEARL: I will do for you what few doctors will do. I will tell you what I would do if it were my kid. If I suspected Lyme **only**, I would **NOT** use a single agent. I would start with a **combination** of amoxicillin and azithromycin. If my child were older, I would replace amoxicillin with doxy. If that didn't seem to do the trick I would look at either adding a cyst-buster (I would do that even earlier if CNS sxs were predominant) or consider IM or IV formulations. I would keep Plaquenil in mind. I am much more afraid of the long-term effects of inadequately treated Lyme than I am of the side effects of antibiotics. (I do not fear vancomycin or clindamycin or Ketek as long as I am aware and careful.) At least with the various antibiotics I can look up what to watch for, carefully monitor in those areas, and be vigilant for side effects. I can control dose and duration and stop any time I think my son is getting into trouble. In contrast, Bb are unpredictable and in charge. I can control the antibiotics. I can only try to manage the Bb.*

ADDITIONAL LYME TREATMENTS

Chapters 25, 26, and 27 provide information on ancillary, alternative, and supportive treatments. Everything from cat's claw to IV γ-globulin is covered. However, many HCPs believe that on-going antimicrobial treatment is the core of Lyme therapy. Still, review these other options and use what might be helpful to your patients.

AVOID STEROIDS! Steroids are contraindicated in active Lyme disease. By suppressing the immune system, steroids diminish the patient's ability to combat the infection, often leaving him with an intractable case of chronic, persistent Lyme. While steroids can seem like the miracle cure in relieving symptoms, they do not get to the root of the problem. Although steroids will tempt you for their rapid action and efficacy, they will make the patient worse in the long-run. Jezebel!

With that warning being aired, don't be a fool and not use steroids when they are clearly indicated. In emergencies such as laryngeal spasm or anaphylaxis, steroids should be used. Steroids can also be used short-term for conditions like croup or asthma. In these cases, try to limit steroid use to 3 to 7 days as the patient regains stability. Many experts believe that if steroids are used in Lyme patients, antibiotics should be used concomitantly.

Treating Lyme is like a chess match. Amazing how often the microbe wins. By keeping in mind the multiple life forms of Bb and the clinical course of the disease and matching these with all the treatments in your armamentarium, you should be able to help your patients. Be creative. Be flexible. Never give up.

MONITORING TREATMENT EFFECT

The best way to see how a patient is doing is to ask, "How ya doin'?" Even little kids have a pretty good idea. Just as you cannot rely on diagnostic testing to tell you if you have Lyme, you cannot count on any test to tell you when you don't have Lyme. This point has been hard to get across. With Lyme, usual indices of treatment success have traditionally been unreliable. Negative serologies, cultures, biopsies, CSF, PCR, FISH: all meaningless. A positive is likely positive, but a negative is not an indicator of anything, except that there was no detectable evidence of Bb in *this* patient, in *this* particular sample, at *this* specific time. There are a dozen reasons why these tests might come back with false negative results. Just as not detected does not mean uninfected, not detected does not mean cured. I KNOW how desperately you wish that were not the case and you hope that a negative test would prove your Lyme nightmare was over. Your disappointment when the symptoms return is hard to witness. If the patient is still sick, she is probably still infected. Bb are still active and the fight continues.

> *PEARL: Repeating a positive test over and over in a symptomatic patient is a waste of money. This practice is incomprehensible to me. What does a negative result in this situation show?*

There are many factors that can influence response to treatment including: co-infection (you might not be treating everything there is to treat), reinfection with a different strain, treatment may have been started late in the clinical course and by now the Bb are present in multiple forms and entrenched in safe niches, the immune system is not effectively helping, the antibiotic regimen is not appropriate to the case, or the underlying physical condition of the patient is not conducive to recovery. If the individual is not improving, all of these possible contributors should be explored and addressed.

Chronic Lyme suppresses the immune system. The Bb spirochete is believed to affect all major cell types of the immune system, particularly the subset of natural killer (NK) cells labeled CD57. Just as in HIV infection, which suppresses T cell counts, Lyme may suppress NK cell counts as measured by CD57. In Lyme, CD57 counts have been used as a marker of the spirochete's vitality. When Lyme is active, the CD57 count is suppressed. The more active the Lyme, the lower the CD57, and presumably the sicker the patient.

Measurement of **CD57** is sometimes used to help determine how active a Lyme infection is, how well treatment is working, whether treatment can be reasonably discontinued, or after treatment ends whether a relapse is likely to occur. Since kids do not make NK cells in the same proportions as adults, CD57 counts might be less useful in the pediatric population.

In chronic Lyme patients the number is usually well below 60. If CD57 levels are drawn as soon as possible in the course of the disease, then they can be used to follow the patient's progress. Some practitioners then recommend a follow-up level about every two months. Subsequently, the results can be used to assess the patient's response to treatment. Here we would want the CD57 to be trending upward or at least not going lower. Steady increases would suggest treatment effectiveness. If the CD57 levels are declining, then the HCP might consider adjusting the therapy.

One CD57 level may provide insight into the patient's clinical status, but a better use of this tool is to follow the levels over time. If on a certain antibiotic regimen the levels improve (rise), then that treatment plan might be considered effective, assuming the patient is also feeling better. In contrast, if the CD57 values are decreasing then adjustments may need to be made. Consider any CD57 results along with the patient's assessment of how he's doing. A CD57 of 244 provides little reassurance if the patient feels terrible.

Some HCPs prefer to continue Lyme treatment until CD57 levels are at least above 60. If antibiotics are discontinued when CD57 is below 60, relapse is considered more likely. Low CD57 might be observed in chronic Lyme or when the disease has been active for more than a year. CD57 can reflect the degree of infection. While CD57 is not a diagnostic test, it might provide corroborating information on the patient's progress.

The actual counts depend on the lab doing the analysis. For a while LabCorp was the only lab performing this testing. Interpretation of LabCorp CD57 results:

Greater than 200	Normal
Less than 20	Severe illness
0 - 60	Chronic Lyme likely
Trending upward	Condition improving
Trending downward	Condition at risk
60 -100	Monitor closely

The best way to see how a patient is doing is to ask, "How ya doin'?"

WHEN TO CHANGE GEARS

If the patient is not getting better, the list of reasons why even solid treatment plans sometimes fail is long and varied:

1. The diagnosis is wrong.

2. Unrecognized co-infections may be preventing recovery.

3. The antibiotic may be inappropriate for the strain.

4. Use of a single agent instead of combination therapy

5. The patient may not be taking the medicine properly or at all.

6. Treatment duration was too short.

7. The dose is too low or administered in a way that does not allow the antimicrobial to be effective.

8. The pathogen became resistant to the antibiotic and there was no back-up.

9. The microbe used evasive techniques: burrowing, encysting, antigen-shifting, etcetera, making it less accessible to antibiotics and immune responders.

10. Poor health habits such as excess alcohol, inadequate nutrition, lack of sleep, etcetera, are not conducive to recovery.

11. Concurrent conditions such as other infections, additional diseases, or outside agents such as allergies, toxins, or molds are present.

12. A Herx reaction caused interruption of treatment.

13. Drugs are interacting or counteracting.

14. The patient does not have enough immune capacity to collaborate with the antibiotic regimen.

15. Additional antibiotics may need to be added to complement the initial drug choices.

16. A different route of administration is needed.

17. The patient was reinfected with different strain.

18. There is an unrecognized immune defect.

19. A genetic predisposition to a poor response is present.

20. There was too much delay between initial infection and eventual treatment.

21. The disease had progressed to a stage where some complications were permanent.

22. Combination of any or all the above

When should you regroup and rethink your current strategy? When the patient is not making the progress you hoped for or expected under the current treatment plan. Consider all possible angles suggested in the treatment failure list above. As the HCP, you may want another opinion on the case. Consult with someone who understands TBIs. A case review with a colleague could provide insight. Maybe you overlooked an important piece of the puzzle. Solicit input from the patient or caregivers. Ask if they think the current regimen is working and what aspects of the plan might be more targeted. Would ancillary treatments or supportive measures help? You do not have to change everything. Try to discern what parts of the current strategy might be working and which might be replaced. Assess whether the patient could benefit from ancillary treatments. Consider the idea of challenge/rechallenge. When a treatment stops, does the patient get better or worse? If the same treatment is restarted does the patient get better or worse?

Plateaus were discussed earlier in this chapter but will be reviewed again. With a plateau, the patient is not symptom-free but they aren't getting better or worse either. They aren't progressing as expected. They may experience low grade symptoms. Consider reworking of the overall strategy. Consider changing antibiotics, altering doses, adding cyst-busters or Plaquenil, or redesigning the composition of the antimicrobial combination. Reconsider co-infections. Dr. Burrascano has used a cyclic approach to plateaus. He would stop all antibiotics until the sxs return, then use high level antibiotics before again stopping until sxs return. He repeats this same cycle until he breaks through. Usually 3 to 4 cycles are needed for effect. The literature contains descriptions of many methods used to overcome a plateau, with more or less success. Some prefer to retain one of the antibiotics in place for the duration and reconstruct the treatment strategy around that core.

With the cyclic nature of LD, with all the waxing and waning and flaring and relapsing, expect to have to change gears more than once in the course of persistent infection. With very sick patients who have been sick a long time with complicated syndromes, lack of progress can be discouraging. Keep trying until you find the right combination for the individual patient. Never give up.

STOPPING LYME TREATMENT

How do you know when to stop treatment? Observe the patient. When the patient feels better, they are usually better. Even very young children get to know their disease pretty well after living with it for a while. They will know if something is still not completely right or if the disease is pretty much all gone.

Some kids who were infected very young or who were born with a congenital TBI don't really know what it feels like to be disease-free. Still, they can provide some pretty solid information about how they are doing.

Many chronic Lyme patients are cured. By cure I mean a resolution of symptoms that do not recur when treatment is stopped. This does not necessarily happen overnight. Sometimes a number of courses of therapy are needed.

Treat until they're better. The signs and symptoms should be gone and there should be at least a period of treatment after symptom resolution to ensure no pathogen is lurking in the shadows waiting to pounce. We know from too much experience that pathogens like Bb can morph into various life forms allowing them to remain dormant while they wait for a more hospitable (antibiotic-free) environment. We accept the fact that TBI cousins like syphilis and malaria can resurface after periods of quiescence, so why not Bb and Babesia? If symptoms return, the logical response would be to re-treat.

PEARL: Treat until they're better PLUS a therapeutic cushion, which can be 3 months or longer depending on the clinical course and intensity of the individual case. IL-ADS says you can try stopping when the patient is symptom-free for 4 weeks. Some prefer a bigger therapeutic cushion than that. Otherwise, re-treatment may be needed anyway.

ILADS does not recommend stopping the antibiotic at an arbitrary point in time, presumably to allow the immune system to pick up the slack. I cannot understand the idea of stopping the antibiotic just because an unsubstantiated and inflexible number of days has passed. Consider discontinuing treatment when the patient is better and a reasonable cushion of antibiotics has been given in order to reduce the risk of relapse.

PEARL: Some authors have suggested that stopping treatment in the presence of persistent sxs is medical negligence since this approach has resulted in additional neurologic injury, debilitation, and death.

Cure is the goal. Nevertheless, recognize that success is not just cure rates. Many of these patients have been so sick for so long that incremental improvement is very welcome. Improvement is the first step. Cure is the goal.

CO-INFECTIONS

Treating Lyme in the presence of co-infections is challenging, but we need to get used to this situation since finding a singular tick-borne disease will become less and less frequent. Co-infections will be the norm. The sickest patients, and those hardest to treat, usually have either multiple infections or an immune vulnerability to Lyme disease. Some have both.

Chapter 24: *Antimicrobials* has a chart that provides suggested drugs that can be used in the case of co-infection. If possible, select drugs that will hit two or more pathogens, so the patient doesn't feel like a walking pharmacopeia. For example, doxycycline is usually not recommended in kids less than 8 y/o. Nevertheless, if the child also has ehrlichiosis then consider a short-course of doxy in the younger kids (doxycycline or minocycline) for 1 to 2 weeks. Doxy is the DOC for treating Ehrlichia and also hits Lyme. Short-course therapy should put these kids at very little risk. You might not be clear about what other co-infections could be present. In some cases doxy will also hit Bartonella and Mycoplasma, but usually doesn't touch Babesia. Since you will be using combination therapy anyway (right?), select your ancillary agents so that you get the most bang for the buck.

As discussed earlier, there are a few authors who suggest treating each co-infection separately, one after the other. They argue over whether Lyme or another TBI should be first. I am quite uncomfortable with this proposition. If you wait for the Lyme to be cured before treating the co-infections, you may never get to the co-infections. In my son's case, treating only the Lyme in the presence of Babesia nearly killed him. Most experienced TBI physicians treat all known co-infections concomitantly as the patient tolerates. If you think I'm going to let some spirochete fester while I focus on the Anaplasma, then you're wrong. I want these invaders out of me. The very idea gives me the creeps. This approach would have all the same adverse consequences as discussed around the problems around delayed treatment. If I know they're there, I'm going after them.

Unfortunately, we probably have not identified all possible co-infections and certainly not all the active strains. Current antibody tests are very species-specific and if we don't even know which species or strains we're dealing with, we are going to have a rough road ahead. As more becomes known, treatment decisions will likely become even more complicated. But at least we might have better explanations for why this has all been so hard to fathom.

ANCILLARY, ALTERNATIVE, AND SUPPORTIVE MEASURES

In addition to the antimicrobial information presented here, review Chapters 25, 26, and 27 for ancillary, alternative, and supportive treatments. Use what is appropriate and leave the rest.

XIII.   PROGNOSIS

If only the prognosis for Lyme disease was known. Are you wondering about the prognosis of acute or chronic forms, early or late, local or disseminated, the true positives or the false negatives? Fortunately, there are a few things I know for sure:

* Some people infected with Bb either don't get sick, spontaneously resolve, have a subclinical presentation, or get well on short-term antibiotics never to be bothered by Lyme again. Their prognosis is excellent.

* Others develop a disseminated borreliosis that causes more severe illness and requires longer-term treatment. After appropriate antibiotics for a sufficient time, they experience resolution of most signs and symptoms. Their prognosis is good.

* A significant subpopulation, for a variety of reasons, develops a persistent, on-going syndrome that can be incapacitating and disabling. Some say this is 10 to 15% of the Lyme population but others speculate that 30% or more of the cases fall into this category. No one knows the actual numbers. These patients have chronic Lyme disease. Without appropriate intervention, their prognosis is fair to poor.

* Morbidity associated with persistent LD is significant, with patients suffering health deterioration equal to that of patients with congestive heart failure.

* Lyme can be fatal.

* Although some believe that Lyme does not result in death, at least 21 research studies have documented deaths associated with LD.

* The three most common causes of death associated with Lyme are probably misdiagnosis, suicide, and cardiac problems. Suicide might be the most common cause of death in Lyme and the least recognized.

* The longer the time from bite to treatment, the more entrenched the pathogen, the harder to manage the case, and the more likelihood of irreversible sequelae. Even the best doc can't fix fibrotic or permanently damaged organs, but she can try to keep them from losing function in the first place. Prognosis depends on when effective intervention was started.

* In all cases, irrespective of the definition of cure, Lyme has been known to recur. Whether this is from the original infection or a subsequent tick bite is difficult to determine.

* In essentially all cases, improvement or cure is possible with HCP persistence. Use flexible, creative, aggressive therapeutic approaches, for as long as it takes to reach the treatment goals. Never give up. While I have no statistics, I believe prognosis is best when the HCP is dedicated to the patient's improvement. I want an HCP who never gives up. I want to be an HCP who never gives up. The path might not be easy, but there's always hope.

We will probably never know the full extent of Lyme and its morbidity and mortality. We can barely identify who has Lyme. Death certificates take the easy way out and list "cardiopulmonary arrest" as the cause of death. Yes, the heart and lungs stopped, as they do in all deaths, but there is rarely information included about Lyme's role. Lyme can be fatal. Currently, because of under-diagnosis and inaccurate attribution of the cause of death, any actual mortality numbers would be speculative. None of the people I knew who died from Lyme had Lyme as their cause of death. In my opinion, Bb contributes to or is the primary cause of death in many more cases than are acknowledged. The actual system failures in Lyme that result in death are usually cardiac and renal.

I am hesitant to quote epidemiologic stats, since we know how grossly inaccurate they have been historically. We know we're missing true positives daily because of lack of sensitivity with the diagnostic testing. This factor, in addition to inappropriate parameters for interpreting results, seems to set us up to miss cases.

Here are some numbers for what they're worth:

1. A few numbers are consistently repeated in the lay press: 27,000 cases in a recent year. Well if we're missing half the cases, the real number would be over 50,000. Even the CDC warns that the I&P numbers are grossly understated. Some sources contend that the numbers should be a hundred times higher. Do we really have 250,000 or 500,000 cases per year? Who knows?

2. Maybe 30% to 70% of patients get well (at least temporarily) with short-term regimens. We do not know the real numbers here, either. The rest might have a less optimal outcome and may require months or years of therapy targeted to their case before they find relief or cure.

3. Falsely high cure rates can be reported from studies where the patients weren't followed long enough to capture relapses. Many patients improve for a time only to relapse at some point in the future. Recurrence is possible weeks, months, or years after the initial illness was incorrectly labeled as cured.

While we might not be able to quote accurate stats on I&P or M&M, there are some measures we can use to try to shift the prognosis from poor (or terminal) to fair or good. Consider:

- Using your clinical judgment to diagnose Lyme

- Treating sooner rather than later

- Remembering that genetic factors (such as HLA-DR2 and 4) may predispose patients to a different clinical presentation. In these cases, adjusting the treatment regimen may get better results.

- Reading Chapter 32: *Prevention* for guidance on ways to avoid both acute and chronic Lyme disease

- Learning from the experience in Europe. Some counties such as Austria and Germany seem to have a healthy respect for Lyme and appear to recognize the risk involved in ignoring the effects of this serious disease. My relatives from northern Italy knew and understood more about Lyme than many HCPs at our local Pennsylvania hospital. The Lyme in continental Europe apparently has much more significant M&M than the North American version. Whether this is due to more virulent strains, superior vigilance, or better acceptance of the realities of the disease, something is different about their attitude. Unfortunately, other countries such as England have a long way to go to in dealing with LD.

- Committing to an optimistic approach with these individuals. If their HCP doesn't believe they can get well, why should the patients? People want to know they are fixable. Most patients want to feel better.

What is the prognosis for the future of Lyme management?

What does the future hold in terms of *vaccines*? There is a significant problem with vaccine development against Bb: In developing a vaccine, life is much easier if you have a clearly identifiable disease so that you can tell if the vaccinated population has less I&P than the unvaccinated. If you have a disease that presents in a 100 different ways, with no reliable biomarker, lotsa luck.

What does the future hold in terms of robust *clinical trials*? I read a lot of gloom and doom about how we can't do clinical trials until there is a reliable biomarker telling us when we have the disease. Poppycock! Perhaps these people have not been doing successful clinical trials as long as I have. There's always a way to design a valid study. However, just like the management of LD, it might take some experimentation, brainstorming, and introduction of a devil's advocate to construct a workable protocol. I'll be the devil's advocate. The bigger problem I see is in clinical research funding. Drug companies won't be interested since they see no blockbuster on the Lyme horizon. Further, generic doxy, amoxicillin, and azithromycin are the DOCs, so a drug company would be hard-pressed to spend millions on a controversial project unless they knew they could beat these stalwarts and earn plenty of profit in both the short and long-term.

PEARL: The SLICE study is currently underway at Johns Hopkins. This trial is looking only at new cases of Lyme presenting with an EM rash.

What does the future hold for the *controversy* around Lyme? As more evidence comes to light supporting the on-going infection hypothesis as the primary underlying mechanism of chronic Lyme, there will be more converts to this way of thinking. Several high-profile IDSA members have already seen the light. Unfortunately, much insight is gained when an individual or his child contracts the disease.

What does the future hold for Lyme in the general *population*? Some local communities are trying hard to curtail the I&P of Lyme. Others, such as those in tick-infested, deer-overrun Chester County, PA, need to get a much better handle on the problem. When I bumped into two game commissioners getting coffee at Northbrook Orchard they agreed, "There sure are a bunch of 'em out there, aren't there?" referring to the deer. They asked me what they could do about them! Further, just as the APA plans to nip the autism epidemic in the bud by calling the condition by a different name and showing that the numbers have gone down, many agencies have tried to reduce the I&P numbers around Lyme by a variety of artificial means. This way credit is doled out for protecting public health while the same number of people are as sick as ever. With the increased potential for interaction between humans and ticks, the real I&P numbers around Lyme are likely to go up.

PROGNOSTIC *PEARLS*

1. *Some authors suggest that certain sxs are prognosticators. For example, dysesthesias (distorted sensation), paresthesias, secondary EM rash, irritability, intractable fatigue, headache, stiff neck, and severe initial illness have all been associated at some point with a worse prognosis than those without these clinical manifestations.*

2. *The best way to shift the prognosis is to treat early enough and long enough. Consider prophylaxis when risk is identified.*

3. *Better understanding of human genetics will eventually affect treatment and outcomes. Specific HLAs may be associated with chronic Lyme, arthritis, autoimmune tendencies, and lack of treatment response. Other genes may eventually be associated with specific manifestations of LD. Understanding the possible genetic contributions to a particularly recalcitrant case or a certain clinical picture may help steer treatment decisions in the future.*

4. *Do not "wait and see." Some of the patients who were denied treatment developed an intractable Lyme syndrome that resulted in disability and in some cases permanent tissue damage. Failure to identify and treat LD early can allow the infection to progress, permitting a treatable acute infection to become a relapsing chronic condition that is less responsive to antibiotics. A European study of risk factors determined that*

the greatest risk came from delayed treatment. The earlier the treatment, the greater the chance for cure. Late disease presents the greatest challenge to success since it may become more and more refractory to various treatment modalities.

5. *Co-infections as described in Chapter 5 may significantly impact the prognosis.*

6. *We do know that suppression of the immune system with steroids gives short-term relief, often followed by long-term disaster. Currently, some of the patients with the worst prognoses are those who were treated early on with a blast of steroids.*

7. *Never give up.*

XIV. CONCLUSION

The treatment of Lyme disease can be a challenge. Why do some get better and some don't? Why do some symptoms resolve without any treatment at all? Why do a number of patients do great on 10 or 14 or 30 days of treatment with an antibiotic like doxycycline? But then why do so many of these same patients relapse and get sick again, often with a clinical presentation that is more intractable and unrelenting than previously experienced? Some only feel well when they are on the correct antibiotics at the right dose. When they go off the medicine they feel sick again. Others get progressively sicker and sicker no matter what the treatment. Some have irreversible sequelae. Some die. Some receive too little, too late. When Martin the Swede, who had the office down the hall from me, had to have a year-long PICC line for his intravenous antibiotic to try to curtail his heart complications from Lyme, why didn't any of us pay attention?

I must say that by the time my son was so sick, I had learned enough from Martin that I knew something was really wrong and that Chris needed an HCP who knew TBI. Some patients get reinfected and some have flares and remissions. Why does one patient act one way and another entirely different? Is it the person's underlying immune system? Is it the state of the immune system when exposed to the organism? Is it the length of time that the organism had to enter? The load of Borrelia at the time of exposure? Are some organisms more virulent? Does solo treatment for too short a time or with a suboptimal dose make things worse for some patients by driving the organisms deeper into the tissue or causing them to encyst? Do treatment decisions predispose for a different clinical course? Does persistence have to do with how long an organism has had to run wild before treatment? We know from treating various body systems that some areas have better penetration of medication than others. Some medicines cross the BBB and others do not. Some medicine easily penetrates joints while others can't get there. No wonder so many HCPs don't want to tackle this monster. So many unanswered questions. Still, we must be at least as persistent as the Borrelia.

I know I constantly encourage HCPs to keep an open mind regarding treatment options and to select the course that is best for the patient. BUT an open mind doesn't mean to be wimpy or non-committal. If you have a sick patient in front of you and you decide to treat, for goodness sake: TREAT! Margaret Thatcher once said, "Standing in the middle of the road is very dangerous; you get knocked down by the traffic from both sides." Unfortunately, here it's the patient who gets knocked down, not you. Use risk/benefit analyses and once you decide to treat, give the patient your best shot. Remember the stories of the local HCP who treated my son with low dose doxy until he was too afraid to continue, leaving Chris in worse shape than when he started. And let's not forget the Maryland clinic physician who was so afraid of prophylactic treatment for Lyme that he would only *whisper* the word Lyme. You are not helping anyone if you do not treat with the correct combination of antimicrobials, in adequate doses, for a sufficient length of time.

Chapter 11

CONTROVERSIES AROUND LYME

If you want an audience start a fight.

Irish proverb

The Controversy: How sad that precious time needs to be spent writing and reading an entire chapter explaining the controversy around Lyme. Instead of all the HCPs involved with Lyme working together, there is conflict and acrimony. The discord has often paralyzed good-faith attempts to treat Lyme patients. The Connecticut legislature had to become involved, unanimously passing a resolution allowing physicians to treat chronic Lyme patients outside certain proscribed "guidelines." Still there are threats and intimidation. Initially, I had planned to go line by line comparing the two predominant sets of conflicting guidelines from ILADS and IDSA. I was not able to do that because I so fundamentally disagree with one group's version. Many of the IDSA recommendations are in direct contradistinction to the TBI experience that I have lived. Since my family was damaged by flawed guidelines and since I naively formed my early views around Lyme when I was "one of them," I feel that I have earned the right to an opinion. From my perspective, the IDSA Guidelines make absolutely no medical sense. I learned a long time ago that trying to force logic onto irrational thinking is a waste of my time. You cannot reason with the irrational.

My career has provided me with hundreds of examples to illustrate standards that make no sense. One 25-year-old-story comes from when I was an occupational/preventive medicine specialist at one of the largest chemical companies in the country. I was in charge of the asbestos medical surveillance program. OSHA had guidelines on how to run these programs and the company had a system they thought was the best in the world. Well, I soon learned that the patients we were screening for asbestos damage in their lungs couldn't possibly have measurable damage because not enough time had elapsed since initial exposure. That's how the disease process works. The employees who were exposed years ago were being ignored. Yet, clearly these were the workers who needed to be screened and identified and helped. Well, as usual, I put up a fuss. Turns out everybody including government agencies, specialists who read the asbestos X-rays, and the upper management of the company all knew that this program made no medical sense. But no one could (or would) do anything about it. As long as the boxes on the checklists were marked off, they were all happy. The company bragged that they had found NO EVIDENCE of medical problems in their screened employees as a result of asbestos exposure. What a source of pride! They failed to mention that they would never find any problems because the population they were screening could not realistically have problems. Personally, I prefer medical common-sense when I can find it.

Once again, Pam Weintraub in *Cure Unknown* does a great job of outlining the chronology of the Lyme controversy and demonstrating how data was often "cherry-picked" to support preconceived conclusions. Since I have been a clinical researcher and a causality investigator for over 20 years and have been trained exhaustively to pick apart bogus science, my research found that Pam was right on target in her conclusions. In fact, in my opinion, she was very kind.

Lorraine Johnson, JD, MBA, and Raphael Stricker, MD, have written several comprehensive articles regarding the controversial issues around Lyme. I cannot hope to match their analytic and historical acumen. I refer you to their work for a more detailed and objective assessment.

For the purposes of this text, I want you to know that significant controversy exists so that you can work around the warring factions to make the best decisions for your patients. I will do my best to present both sides of each issue but I don't pretend to be unbiased. I have lived the Lyme experience as a patient, parent, and physician. Initially, my views were in perfect alignment with the minimalists who do not think Lyme is a serious medical condition and don't believe treatment needs to extend beyond a few weeks, even if a patient is as sick as when she first presented. Several small ticks changed my mind though the school of hard knocks. I had to watch my child suffer and nearly die before I was humbled enough to realize there must be a better way to manage TBI patients.

I formed my revised opinions about the diagnosis and treatment of Lyme from my experience both as a patient and caretaker BEFORE reading the hundreds of articles around the controversy. Reviewing articles from both sides of the issue only re-enforced my adjusted views. I was appalled that some HCPs could recommend ignoring signs and symptoms in sick patients and endorse obviously biased methods of case management.

Yet there is even controversy about the controversy. For many ILADS doctors, Lyme is a clinical diagnosis, which can only be *supported* by lab results. And, you treat a sick person until she's better. You don't stop treatment on a symptomatic person because one biased and flawed guideline says you should. There is an ethical responsibility to face these diseases and not take the easy way out.

There are even arguments about the identity of our biggest argument: is it the debate over chronic infection, is it the lack of a biomarker, is it the controversy about underlying pathophysiology, is it the weak science on both sides, is it the definition of Lyme, is it conflict of interest, is it how to treat persistent symptoms? After months of sorting through the literature, I will attempt to address the fundamental question:

"WHAT ARE THESE PEOPLE FIGHTING ABOUT?"

I will group the controversies by major category and editorialize somewhat about why I think a particular topic is worth debating further or not. I will describe the guidelines that are out there and how you can access them. I will remind you that we are in the infancy of gathering real science on these diseases and we can expect to learn and adjust as time goes on. Healthy debate will benefit us all, especially patients. Vicious, obviously biased, pathetically pandering controversy just keeps people from getting the help they need. As you read, keep an open mind and consider both sides of each issue. I have already struggled through these stages and have landed firmly on one side. Still you have the right to hear both perspectives and I will attempt to give each camp a fair airing. Only by understanding that very different and opposing views exist can you weigh the best options for your patients. Remember each choice you make will have a risk/benefit ratio that should be considered as you move forward.

After seeing TBI patients in preceptorships over several years there is one thing I know for sure. There are very sick people out there desperate for medical care. Most patients can feel better or are even cured under appropriate treatment regimens. If you are an HCP reading this, please mix good medicine with compassion. To those of you who can't bear to admit you have anything to learn I say, "Grow up."

The existence of the multiple debates around LD has caused harm to people and was one of the prime motivators for me to write this book. The founding premise for this text is that readers should be able to take the information they want and discard the rest. That is what the other 33 chapters are for. In this chapter, I do have an opinion. In that spirit, consider the following a debate, remembering that the "other side" is not exactly equally-represented.

There are dozens of controversial issues around all aspects of Lyme disease. I will TRY to be as objective as possible for a person who is clearly biased. I will present a controversial topic and then attempt to present the case on both sides. Sometimes I had great difficulty finding a reasonable counter-argument. Since there are few things I enjoy more than a good debate, I did try. I attempted to gather the arguments on all sides from the literature and I would ask, "Why don't they like that approach?" "What would be their alternative?" What could be the secondary agenda behind that decision?"

In my opinion here are the major controversial issues around Lyme disease.

PRIMARY AREAS OF CONTROVERSY

I. Is there controversy around Lyme?

Controversy is a part of healthcare. Do you think for one minute that there aren't controversies in other areas of medicine? From time immemorial, each branch of medicine has thought it held the magic decoder ring and no one else knew anything. Consider a diagnosis of otitis media on a local level. ENT docs don't think pediatricians know anything about otitis. The pediatricians don't want general surgeons putting in so many ear tubes, who in turn don't think the family practitioners should use long-term antibiotics since antibiotics might result in less ear tube consults. Everyone is mad at the guys in the ER who are treating kids on Saturday nights and therefore taking away business from all the above. When my mother was in the hospital for ulcerative colitis, the GI docs alternated coverage. One doc treated her for constipation and the other for diarrhea. Each would criticize the other's approach in front of my mom, who had no clue what was happening and just wanted to feel better. They refused to talk to each other. We had to get the hospitalist to referee.

On a national and international level, when I did clinical trials on GvHD, I witnessed a fistfight between a transplant surgeon and a hematologist in Italy. They disagreed violently on how to conduct the research. The study coordinator for the site hid under a desk as I tried to break it up since I wanted to go to lunch. For some of these GvHD studies, patients had to be weaned from steroids. I remember Fred Hutchinson Cancer Center would not wean the same way that MD Anderson weaned and Yale would only do it their "special" way. To move the study along I devised a steroid weaning protocol different from all the major transplant centers. Then I lied and told each that I liked their approach best and that I had based the compromise primarily on their method. No one complained. Not a single one of these sites had even read the other methods. They didn't have to. They just KNEW their way was best. Once sufficiently flattered, they were willing to compromise and the study moved forward.

On March 1, 2010, a baby in Brazil died while the two doctors there to perform a C-section started fighting. Instead of taking care of mother and child, fists flew. Which doctor was right? Does anyone even remember who won the fight or what they were fighting about? Was winning the fight worth the baby's life? "We sometimes forget that life is for learning not just for being right," according to Leonard Felder, PhD, in his book *Fitting in is Overrated.* We all need to put aside our chest-pounding hubris and think about what is best for our patients.

With all that being said, controversy is thriving around Lyme and we even argue about who will engage the other side and what we should debate. Unfortunately, LD has evolved into a very controversial issue causing both sides to dig in their heels.

So, expect controversy but do not accept intractability. The problem comes in when, in a paraphrase of Diane Ravitch, an opinion once stated must be forever defended. Take all inflexible proclamations of science with a grain of salt. The more rigid an opinion, the more you should question the agenda of the opinion-holder. In terms of LD and other TBIs, we just don't know enough yet to etch anything in granite.

II. What is the effect of bias in the Lyme controversy?

Bias is a prejudice or inclination in one direction that causes the holder of the bias to maintain one perspective at the expense of equally valid alternatives. In science, bias can come in many forms. Bias can be active, such as when a researcher provides what he thinks the study results "should" be prior to the completion of the study. Alternatively, bias can also be unconscious, which we are all subject to if we are not aware of its potential intrusion into our thinking. An ethical researcher will constantly be checking herself for bias as she grants protocol exemptions or writes amendments to the original study design. Researchers should always be asking how a decision might impact the integrity of the study. Bias can be an important consideration both in clinical decision-making and when gathering and interpreting scientific data.

As I have mentioned a number of times in this text, a researcher can pick through data and find only those things that support preconceived conclusions. Sometimes this happens when the researcher is inexperienced and doesn't know better. One example is when I asked a drug safety tech at a major company to find me all the patients on a certain cardiac medicine who also were found to have abnormal thyroid function. He returned to me so proud that there were no cases. I told him that was impossible since I had personally reviewed several cases. He said he entered the key words for my query in a way that those cases would not come up since he didn't think that the drug should be shown as having caused thyroid problems. He felt he was protecting the drug when he should have been protecting the patients. He didn't understand that a responsible scientist wants to know if there is a relationship.

Bias can involve selection decisions such as asking who should be allowed to participate in a study or who should be excluded. The scientist is attempting to get a homogeneous population that can be used for making comparisons and predictions based on study results. Researchers can also bias studies by saying they never "intended to treat" certain patients and so the data from these subjects should not be included in the analysis. This is a common ploy to get rid of those rude and messy patients who die during a study where including their results might make a drug or treatment look bad. Hopefully, the FDA gets wise to the misuse of these ploys.

Bias can be introduced by improper randomization or flaws in blinding, where a patient is intentionally or accidently placed in a treatment arm in an un-randomized fashion. I experienced this when I was working on a cancer drug and one investigator made sure his favorite patients got what he thought was the better treatment. Thereafter, none of his patients could be used in the study analysis. Who did that help? Bias can occur when a researcher steers the data or result to a preconceived conclusion. This occurred in a major breast cancer study where a researcher so strongly believed his approach was correct that he skewed the study result to his desired conclusion. His intentions were good but his methods were unethical and costly. Always protect the integrity of your study. Once you lose it you can't get it back. If the data looks too good to be true, consider that it is not true. Real data is messy.

Other studies have so many patients dropping out (either because they felt sicker due to the lack of efficacy of their treatment arm or because they couldn't tolerate the side effects of the treatment) that the numbers are no longer large enough to support robust conclusions. Here researchers can try not to count them and only count those who "completed" the study. The definition of completers can be quite variable. Be very aware that horses are often changed in the middle of the stream to make the study results favorable to one side or the other.

Valid science should define parameters for the study, such as inclusion and exclusion criteria, intent-to-treat parameters, completers, and statistical analysis plans BEFORE the study starts. Then, except in rare circumstances, stick by the rules. If half your study population is dropping out there must be a reason and this should be clearly identified in the study report. I cannot begin to tell you how many fights I have had over these issues. When HALF the treatment group in a stroke study dies in the land of the midnight sun and NONE of the placebo group dies, you may have a safety issue here, fellas. And NO we can't wait for you to get back from the archipelago in September to tell the FDA. I witnessed a physician shredding the bad safety results from Pakistani women on hormone therapy. He said since these women were Pakistani the FDA would not be interested in their results. Later, I was told we did not need to collect safety data on drugs in India because Indians don't eat breakfast. (Huh? I do have witnesses.) "We carve out order by leaving the disorderly parts out," said William James.

A simple experiment that we can do right now is to consider how I might be biasing this text. I know this might be hard to believe but I am very cognizant of every word choice in an attempt to be as objective as possible. I believe my integrity is important for the credibility of this book so I try not to make inflammatory choices (at least not without warning). Each word has a flavor and depending on the word I choose, I can influence the reaction of the reader. Consider the word "controversy." Depending on the context, synonyms can include discord, conflict, fight, war, argument, debate, dispute, contest, variance, disagreement, cross-purpose, quarrel, challenge, contention, rumpus, dissent, fuss, wrangle, polemic, squabble, brawl, attack, and many others. While a rumpus and a squabble might be considered cute and inconsequential, a war and an attack would be perceived quite differently. And who even knows what polemic means? But if I choose the word polemic, I will look smarter, but less likeable.

Many times we all engage in both retrospective and prospective cherry-picking. Unfortunately this happens more often if the researcher is motivated by things other than a desire for objective answers (like if she is running for public office or working for the insurance lobby). Especially in retrospective studies, we can select only the data that support our point of view and throw out all the data that doesn't reinforce our desired conclusion. There are a number of ways to accomplish this that even look kosher. I have witnessed every manner of subterfuge. Prospectively, old salts like me can write a clinical trial protocol and pretty much get the results we want. When the first bazillion dollar study on a colorful PPI failed, the company simply hired some vets to rework the study and make sure the next study was positive. By carefully including only select patients and carefully excluding others and choosing endpoints wisely, is it a surprise that the study comes out positive? A hundred million dollars buys a lot of science. (When pharmaceutical trade organizations taut how much money drug companies spend on research, do they mention that a large portion of that money is spent on correcting research mistakes because people had no idea what they were doing, blatant marketing studies, and "support" for the "special" research interests of key opinion leaders? No, all that money they spend does not go to curing kids with cancer. Profits, not patients, often come first.)

Secondary agendas can greatly influence an HCP's perspective on the science. Drug companies have armies of people trained to woo "key opinion leaders," who then are given plenty of contrived opportunity to interact with other HCPs and sway their prescribing habits. Once a KOL has a vested interest in a treatment, she could be suspected of misusing the science in a way that makes the drug seem better than it actually is or that hides safety issues.

I laughed when I read that someone associated with the guideline drafting panel ridiculed the findings of the AG investigation in Connecticut, which concluded there were conflicts of interest with some of the panel participants. He said there could not possibly be any secondary gain for draft team members from drug companies since the recommended drugs were usually old and available as generics. Therefore, kick-back type money would not be likely to flow. Alas, I was schooled by the pharmaceutical industry on how to get by government restrictions and still entice the KOLs. The marketing groups had more people working full time on flattering KOLs than they had physicians developing drugs. The quality of their medicine was NEVER the primary concern. There are so many other ways to compensate an "opinion leader" in the hopes that in his realm of influence he will favorably drop the name of your products over and over and over again. In a number of cases, the cost of a fine is worth it to the company if they get publicity from the hubbub and the eventual sales outweigh the fine.

Let's say that a KOL performs well on a particular issue. There just might be the possibility that the particular KOL could be lead investigator or first author on the company's next big branded product. Or there could be some grant money for personal research. Or how about when one company I worked for rented the palace at Versailles to reward its opinion leaders or when they commissioned an exclusive performance of the Lipizzaner stallions. All expenses paid, naturally. Bring your wife. (One KOL had separate rooms in the four star hotel for his wife AND his mistress.) Tickets to the Super Bowl? No problem. Golf at St. Andrew's? A marketer in each foursome. No secondary gain? I beg to differ.

While there are stricter rules in place now regulating the acceptance of gifts by physicians from companies, there are also many ways to get around these bureaucratic obstacles. Who even knew that you could rent Versailles palace? After all was said and done, the marketers would mock the KOLs because they were so easily put in company pockets, essentially willing to say anything that the industry was willing to pay for. Of course, the KOLs laughed all the way to the bank. You can disagree with me all you want on this point, but I was there and saw it all. Prestige, power, advancement over rivals, and plain ego-boosting all can be as motivating as money.

So, am I surprised that so much of the Lyme data and experience is ignored and contrived? I am only amazed that people are not embarrassed by their continued support of fallacy. Instead of wasting time declaring, "My science can beat up your science," look at what has worked at least in many patients and try to use these successes to help people. Look for bias anywhere and you will find it. Otherwise, you will be vulnerable to the snow-jobs that so often pass for science.

Keep an open mind. Recall from the *Introduction* that I was one of those eye-rolling HCPs when it came to Lyme. I was one of those ER docs who had seen it all and couldn't be told anything even though I considered myself a scientist. Victor Hugo said, "The learned man knows that he is ignorant."

III. My science can beat up your science.

I didn't start out to be a clinical researcher. But, as is often the case for a military doctor, many decisions were made for me. Since I was stationed in places that dealt with chemical and nuclear warfare, I had to develop protocols to manage emergency toxic and radiation injuries. This led me to civilian occupational medicine and eventually drug safety and then drug development. I have written hundreds of clinical research protocols and reviewed thousands (I hesitate to say millions, but it sure felt like it) of data points. I have analyzed results, drawn conclusions, and written many study reports and regulatory submissions. I have had my science parsed by regulators all over the world and by many of the snootiest health care facilities. (I'm talking to you Hutch and Yale.) And I lived to tell the tale. I know how to design a study and select the right population to skew the results in a preferred direction. I know how to select endpoints to get me where I want to be. I have learned by observing many multi-million dollar mistakes. I was begged to return to companies that I had left in frustration in order to clean up other people's messes and help turn out another blockbuster. I have more than a dozen successful NDAs under my belt and I stopped counting the supplemental NDAs and submissions in other countries.

I have tried to remain ethical and not to harm anyone and have refused to participate in activities that I found morally questionable. I hope I succeeded. I have seen companies try to pull every trick in the book in order to hide data and sway results. I have seen compromising results shredded and corporate regulatory directors bragging about lying to the FDA. (I left that company the same day.) One of the few things I know for sure is that anyone who says that all double-blind, randomized, placebo-controlled studies are unbiased simply because they are double-blind, randomized, placebo-controlled studies is a fool. Drug companies hire people because they know how to turn a phrase and to defend that phrase under intense scrutiny.

Anyone who declares that only his conclusion is correct is not speaking scientifically. The entire premise behind statistical significance in science is to determine if two items are associated in a way that is more related than what would be expected purely by chance. Laypeople tend to believe that when you use the word science (or evidence-based medicine) there is no room for interpretation. Science is simply hypothesis testing. You test your hypotheses over and over in order to see if you can start making predictions based on what you have observed. Einstein once said that in science one experiment could prove him wrong, while infinite experiments could never prove him right. The same is true in medicine. Remember, that even though I might be describing various study designs

below, the same basic concepts underscore the diagnosis and management of patients in the clinical setting. Use the following information whether you are designing, participating in, or reading the results of a clinical study in the literature.

Over the years, a great deal of what I learned in medical school has been proven to be only partially correct or totally wrong. In a few areas, we have gone from one idea to another and then completely back again. Be careful in how loudly you proclaim that someone couldn't possibly have Lyme because their target lesion is not quite round enough. You could end up looking inept and worse, causing harm to a patient who would certainly have arranged to have a totally circular bull's eye if it was entirely up to him.

Remember how many times we have been absolutely sure in medicine in the past. Epileptics used to be flogged, and starved, and chained to get the devil out of them. More syphilitic patients were probably killed by the treatments than the disease. Hormone replacement therapy was essentially mandated for perimenopausal women until someone finally looked at the data and discovered that perhaps more harm was being done than good. In recent weeks, sacrosanct ideas in health care like prostate specific antigen testing, mammograms, and breast exams have had their value questioned. When the studies were finally done, we were shocked by the results.

All science is not created equal. Let's take bias out of the equation for the moment and just assume that bias is present in all aspects of science to some degree. How should we view the different scientific methods that provide us with "evidence" on which we make decisions? **Double-blind, randomized, placebo-controlled** studies are the gold standard. Unfortunately these are usually quite expensive, requiring large populations of patients and numerous investigative sites, not to mention considerable staff to run the study. These trials often take a long time from start to result. You usually can't afford to blow it. If you are involved in such a study, make sure the person writing your protocol has written several successful studies before. Get input from all stake holders such as statisticians, data analysts, protocol writers, clinicians, patients, and anyone else you can think of that might care. You don't have to take all the advice, just consider it. Know what you are trying to show. Many protocols are written where the investigators aren't even sure why they are doing the study (aside from the money). In an ideal world, all clinical trials would be **unbiased**, double-blind, randomized, placebo-controlled studies. We do not live in an ideal world.

In assessing which types of studies I think are most scientifically solid, I would subtract one component at a time from the ideal. Maybe you can't randomize, or maybe you can't use a placebo-control for ethical reasons, or the blinding can't be perfect. Still, continue to try to maintain as much of the scientific rigor as you can, considering the disease and the patient population. The study should be sized to allow statistical significance using valid methodology. (Always be cautious when the researcher says he will do his own stats if he is not a *bona fide* statistician with experience in this type of work.) Ensure that any quantified outcomes use *validated* measurement tools.

Prospective studies are usually viewed as more robust scientifically than **retrospective** studies. The variation among the individuals in the study population should be minimized as much as possible. Clearly define your population, eliminating those who would introduce confounders that could compromise the results. But make the study groups as realistic as possible by attempting to mimic the real world. Here you have to balance one objective against the other.

Observational studies are uncontrolled in that the patients are not randomized to a specific study group. Subjects are assigned to a group outside the control of the investigator and then the results are *observed* and documented. Observational studies are often used to draw conclusions about treatment effects. If for some reason the subjects can't be randomized and you are looking for cause and effect, a well designed observational study can be useful.

Population studies look at changes that occur in a defined population after some kind of intervention. We used these types of trials to study vaccines. Essentially all patients in a population that were at risk for the disease were enrolled and vaccinated and then the incidence rate of the disease was compared to the rate in the unvaccinated population.

Outcome studies may eventually prove to be the best choice for studying persistent LD. This type of research is usually designed to measure response to treatment. The findings can be used to help construct practice guidelines that might eventually help improve quality of care. Here, desired outcomes are prospectively described. Examples include the achievement of a particular endpoint such as the lowering of blood pressure by a pre-defined amount, a decrease in mortality, a change in a disease sign or symptom, an alteration in a lab parameter, etc. Once the patient reaches the designated endpoint, that box is checked. The group results can be compared to an untreated population. Outcome research can be used to assess the effectiveness of treatments in the real world by pooling the results from large numbers of patients. Outcome studies might be more practical than controlled trials because the efficacy of an intervention can be assessed in real-world settings. These studies can be difficult, but a well designed outcome study can be a joy to behold.

Anecdotes or **case studies** are perceived as the least scientifically robust. I am not sure why this is so. As long as the facts are documented objectively, a great deal can be learned from a well-written case study. I find anecdotes especially useful if the author describes the logic process used to manage the case and outlines any wrong turns she made as a lesson on pitfalls to avoid. With complex, multifaceted conditions, where "studies" are few or flawed, anecdotes may be invaluable. Remember that several TBIs have only been recently recognized. (Heartland virus is a TBI identified only months ago.) While we have been dealing with syphilis and malaria and consumption for thousands of years we are talking a few decades for some of the TBIs. Case studies may be our best bet in attempting to predict how a patient might respond over time to some of these less familiar diseases. The clinical course of an individual patient may be quite enlightening. Also, when you combine the information from individual case studies, they can pack quite a wallop. The huge data bases that contribute to the safety sections in drug labels are compilations of case reports. Until the 50s when an energetic epidemiologist started to push for controlled studies, anecdotes were pretty much all we had and they took us a long way.

Any of these study types can provide valid scientific evidence if done in as unbiased manner as possible. Actually most studies are a combination of the various types. Do not get on a high horse and only "accept" certain types of evidence. Take all the valid information you can to help you understand the disease and manage your LD cases. Use the information I have provided to read the literature with a more critical eye than you might have used in the past.

Despite all these scientific possibilities, the science around LD is, in my opinion, pretty dismal on both sides of the debate. For a number of reasons, which I will expand upon in later sections, studies on Lyme have been difficult to design and the population has been hard to define. In many cases, retrospective reviews have been forced to compare apples to oranges. Add to this bias, secondary agendas, and inexperience with the scientific method, and you aren't left with much to hold onto in making Lyme management decisions. With that being said, there is some useful information available if you know the limits of the study design being presented.

The pathophysiology and clinical course of LD certainly confounds the science, making study design especially challenging. Remember that the goal of science is to gather data in a way that will eventually allow you to make predictions about future events based on your conclusions. For example, with LD, you might want to look at a set of clinical signs and symptoms and be able to predict which treatment paradigm would be best suited for a specific patient. Do patients with an EM rash respond differently than those who never display a rash? Are CNS symptoms linked with a worse prognosis than musculoskeletal symptoms? Sounds reasonable enough. But as with all things Lyme, the situation is not as simple as it might appear.

Complications in Lyme clinical research: With some diseases you can outline a study design on the back of a napkin in a half an hour. Clearly, Lyme is not one of these illnesses. Studies are usually the most scientifically robust if you keep as many factors as possible controlled and change only one or two variables in order to measure response. Once you get too many variables it is nearly impossible to statistically compare outcomes. With Lyme we are instantly confronted with multiple questions: How do you define the disease? How do you specify an appropriate study population? What should be the inclusion/exclusion criteria? How do you identify valid endpoints? What questions should you be asking? How do you decide which treatments to test? How long do you treat? Are signs and lab results more "valid" measures than symptoms? How do you know when you're done? How do you analyze the data? What conclusions can you draw? How long do you follow up? How do you rescue a relapse?

Remember that LD can wax and wane and relapse and flare and Herx. All these contingencies need to be accommodated in your study plan. You need to think about all these possibilities and make sure your protocol can weather the storm. One way to do this is to design a study and then run "imaginary patients" through the protocol. Come up with all the potential scenarios you can think of and see how your design holds up. Trust me, even if you think of a thousand variations, in the real study something will come up that never crossed your mind that will befuddle you. Yet, if you pre-think as much as possible, your study should hold up to the real world. (This is practical advice in designing practice guidelines as well.)

PEARL: Before you get glum reading all the problems that have plagued Lyme science since the first data was collected, know that after 3 years of contemplation I believe that I have come up with a protocol design that circumvents most of these obstacles. Call me.

Issues in study design: The following material is written for the HCP who might be considering participating in clinical research around LD. However, I am hoping it will also benefit laypersons as they read study reports and try to make sense of the data, since we are all trying to use good science to help TBI patients.

- **Population**: In clinical research, comparable study groups are important if you want to be able to formulate valid conclusions. Because LD presents in so many ways, the difficulty in achieving comparability has impacted the validity of the previous research. There is no lab test that says, "This is Lyme!" Relying on the insensitive, nonspecific, low-yield testing that is currently in place would eliminate the majority of legitimate Lyme patients from study participation. Eliminating valid patients would not represent the real world population that we are ultimately trying to help. At least in 2013, LD remains a clinical diagnosis and there are ways to identify study populations that can be used to test hypotheses. There have been studies successfully conducted in other diseases such as hepatitis C, which also present with heterogeneous populations. Just about any study design conundrum can be overcome with determination, imagination, and flexibility. Refer to the section below for ideas on defining the disease and making the diagnosis.

- **Biomarkers:** Some sources believe that a consistent biomarker is needed to ensure the enrollment of homogeneous, comparable study groups. I think there are good ways around this deficit. While it would be lovely to have a surrogate marker to use in research studies, the arrival of this biomarker does not seem to be on the horizon anytime soon. Should we wait before robust studies are designed and conducted? I don't think we need to delay. There are always ways of designing strong studies if you labor enough over the plan. In good pharmaceutical development teams, we used to force one another to convince the group that one approach was better than another. "Talk me into your way of thinking." This might take hours or days but when all parties have the same goal in mind, you can accomplish a lot. Note that a good, practical, *experienced* statistician can save you a lot of angst. (The first thing I did when starting on any new project, especially if it was a "clean-up someone else's mess" project, was to get a trusted, *experienced* statistician on board.)

- **Variability in clinical presentation:** Like syphilis, Lyme is a great imitator. The previous chapter outlined the almost dizzying array of clinical presentations that have been associated with Lyme. I was reading a women's magazine the other day and they had Lyme listed in a table of diseases associated with inflammation. The symptoms appearing in the tiny little box as representative of Lyme were ones I would have never picked out as being distinctive for Lyme disease: eye twitching, headache, and fever. Well, that clears everything up. No mention of any of the things that you might say are more often associated with LD like fatigue, brain fog, migrating joint pain, neuropsychiatric problems, hypersensitivity, GI complaints, or cardiac manifestations. Where did these authors get this information? I guess they had to fit all the signs and symptoms they thought pertinent into a tiny box. Whatever or wherever, the point is LD can be extremely variable. We just might have to accept the fact that Lyme is never going to fit into that nice box and recognize that we might need to address these variations in the way we design Lyme studies. Why force all patients to have arthritis, or rash, or neuropsychiatric symptoms, or cardiac problems? Should we restrict, like they did in the early days when Lyme was called Lyme arthritis, the acceptable presentation criteria to only some impacted organ systems like musculoskeletal, neurologic, or dermatologic systems? Or do you face the multifaceted disease that often manifests as Lyme? Let patients have their Lyme their way. There are ways we can deal with this variability by measuring *initial* verses *late* manifestations in the individual. This is complicated but feasible. With an *experienced* statistician, miracles are possible.

- **Inclusion criteria:** Know the ramifications of having a patient coming into a study who was just diagnosed (as far as you know) with acute, first-time Lyme versus a patient who has persistent symptoms or multiple previous treatment failures. Depending on what question you are trying to answer, you could get very different results from these dissimilar groups. Mixing these populations might dilute the power of the study to insignificance.

- **Exclusion criteria:** How many treatment regimens will you allow a patient to fail before she is excluded from your study? If the patient has relapsed 2, 3, 4 or more times, should she be excluded from a clinical trial? We know that the longer the interval between infection and treatment the more intractable the disease may be. The longer chronic symptoms persist the harder it is to achieve cure by any definition. Yet you can over-think many of these issues to the point of paralysis. Some of these questions will never be answered and you may have to accept that for now.

- **Endpoints:** How do you tell when you're done? Much of the controversy arising from earlier studies involves how long the treatment should continue before you either declare success or failure. Again, there is no lab test that is going to bail us out here. Outcome or endpoint studies may be the way to go in future testing of LD. Here endpoints can be pre-identified and when a patient achieves that specific endpoint, that result can be tallied. Symptoms can even be used since there are already validated testing tools for a number of Lyme manifestations, such as fatigue, pain, sleep disturbances, and depression. A study could be designed that might assess each patient's top 3 complaints, for example. There is nothing to say that other methodology can't be validated to measure additional parameters as time moves forward. We must get over waiting for the ideal lab test that will make our lives easier. When it comes, I will lead the celebration but in the meantime "Attention must be paid." [1]

- **Length of treatment:** I will expound at length about the duration of treatment debate in a future section, but in terms of clinical trials several points unique to Lyme must be put on the table. First, be careful not to stop treatment too soon without having a follow-up mechanism in place to record relapses or flares. Even if the endpoint is achieved, there must be a way to capture reoccurrence of

symptoms after treatment is stopped. Never let good data go to waste. You can then compare how many relapses occur after a month, two months, six months, or whatever time frame is appropriate. Make sure that Herx reactions are not misidentified as lack of treatment effect and that you give each regimen time to work. If the patient is not improving during the study, you need to decide if he is to be removed from the trial or the treatment schedule is to be adjusted. Keep things simple and don't let the design get so convoluted that you can't possibly figure out what happened. There are a number of ways to accommodate these potential complications. Just remember it is unethical to let a patient suffer or progress in order to save your study. Make sure you build in *rescue* plans so both the patient and the study can be saved.

PEARL: Some HCPs have asked if it isn't unethical to discontinue treatment that might be helping a symptomatic patient for no other reason than "Time's up!"

- **Treatment regimens:** In the past we have just had a gamish of many kinds of treatment plans, from single agents to combinations of two or more antimicrobials and any number of IV, IM, and PO courses of therapy. We have had oral followed by IV and IV followed by oral and IM before, during, and after. No wonder people have trouble making sense of the data. We have had high dose and low dose and doses adjusted to blood levels. (Feel sorry for me, I read all this stuff so you don't have to.) Since treatment should be individualized for each patient, targeting the individual clinical presentation, this problem might be the most challenging. The decisions around the type of treatment will depend on what you are asking of your study. If you are comparing antimicrobials, your plan should be different than if you are comparing delivery systems or length of treatment.

One thing I can guarantee, if you get too many variables you will be glum before the study is over and you will not have robust, usable results. Ensure that the study is powered to handle the questions you are trying to answer. If you do not know what powered means, you might not be the best principal investigator. Make sure you know the main question you are trying to answer. Protect your primary endpoint. Don't allow a whole bunch of secondary endpoints to compromise your principal research goal. If you are looking at length of treatment it MIGHT be okay to use any regimen combination that gets you to an endpoint. Just keep your eye on the prize and keep the design clean.

- **Other confounders:** In 2013, a tick, at least in the northeastern US, is not likely to be carrying just one pathogen. Study patients in certain areas are very likely to be harboring co-infections. Make sure your study design

---

1 Arthur Miller *Death of a Salesman*

accounts for this likely scenario. You can't prove a negative, especially with TBIs, so don't make yourself crazy by insisting that a patient be pure Lyme. We don't have the means to prove solo infection, so you will never know for certain. Just make sure that the patient languishing in front of you isn't near death because of babesiosis or Mycoplasma while you beat on them to respond to Lyme treatment.

Know how you are going to accommodate ancillary and alternative treatments. Certain herbals and other modalities might do something either positive or negative for the patient. Just be careful in how you handle these agents. Decide beforehand how you will respond when a patient won't come into a clinical study unless you let them keep taking their enula or shark fin. If you bend for one patient you need to bend for all, so proceed with caution. When you are designing the study make sure you try to accommodate the practices of the patients in your catchment area. (But don't let the tail wag the dog.)

Clinical research under the best circumstances is a rough row to hoe. Remember that the goal of all research is to eventually be able to make predictions about the future based on your conclusions. Even a solitary case report can be used for this purpose if done objectively. Still with Lyme, the big question becomes who will fund the critical large, prospective trials that are needed to answer the questions that will resolve much of the controversy. Trust me, drug companies will only spend money if they have a reasonable assurance of having a billion-dollar-a-year "blockbuster" result from their efforts. Sometimes they will do a little study on an obscure indication just so they can get their foot inside a much bigger marketing door. Academics might conduct robust studies if they can get funding. There is considerable competition for government money. The CDC, unlike my many previous experiences with them on other issues, has not been consistent from a scientific perspective when it comes to Lyme. NIH has been variable with its understanding of Lyme and TBIs, depending on who's talking.

So far, advocacy groups have not had the type of funding that would be needed to support studies of the magnitude needed to resolve the current conflicts. Time will tell. For the foreseeable future, clinical research around Lyme will continue to be challenging. To paraphrase Bette Davis, this work ain't for sissies.

IV. Who has Lyme disease?

One of the biggest debates around Lyme is who actually has the disease. This controversy is underscored by the lack of a clear surrogate marker that sensitively identifies the disease. Absent that specific biomarker, we are stuck with very questionable supportive testing. While the discovery of that clear biomarker would be ideal, it seems that this development is likely to be sometime in the future. Still patients suffer, so we do not have the luxury of hanging around waiting for a surrogate to tell us when there is active disease. We must make clinical diagnoses based on history, physical, and review of systems.

Blasphemy alert: Until a sensitive and specific marker is identified, I would prefer that HCPs resist the constant pursuit of the positive supportive lab test. I think that false negatives have done far more damage to patients than the good that positive results do in supporting diagnoses that are often clinically obvious. Unfortunately, the HCP needs the courage to admit to the findings gleaned from asking questions and performing an examination. Remember that medicine was practiced for millennia without the crutch of thousands of dollars worth of CBCs and metabolic panels and Western blots. Less testing would spare small children the trauma of being accosted with the phrase, "*You do not have Lyme,*" when all they know is that they don't feel good. Even though we should focus on the patient and not the test result, HCPs constantly order tests that they have no idea how to interpret. So, the controversy thrives. Many other chapters including 10, 18, 19, 20, 21 and all the Chapter 17 subunits provide guidance on how to use your senses to gather the information you need to diagnose with confidence.

But this chapter is about controversy and the supportive diagnostic testing around Lyme provides fertile ground for all manner of discord. In general, the tests used to support a Lyme diagnosis are positive when they are positive, i.e., they identify true positives and are highly sensitive in that regard. Although a few people worry about false positives these are RARELY, if ever, a problem. If you get a positive ELISA, WB, PCR, FISH, or culture for Bb, you are likely looking at Lyme. Still when using WBs, with the band selection being so unscientific, I guess there is potential for some false positives but I am not aware of cases where this has been a problem. Feel compassion for any spirochete that "passes" a 2013 diagnostic panel in any way. That poor little critter has had to jump through so many artificial hoops to be recognized that it must be exhausted.

Note that if you are looking for the most sensitivity, cultures from tissues are probably your best bet. A number of case reviews have shown positive culture results in patients who previously had negative antibody tests. Even though the documented rate with cultures is still low, it's better than other alternatives currently available. And even this most sensitive test is challenging since Bb spirochetes are scarce, tissue bound, and divide slowly making it extremely difficult to culture the organism even using ideal conditions. But you can rest assured that a positive Bb culture is likely a true positive. Likewise, if you are finding evidence of DNA and RNA from Bb, you probably have Bb. The problem is that the yield from this type of testing is dismally low.

Still some continue to recommend ELISA and WB testing for individual case identification even though the College of American Pathologists has said that the currently available ELISA tests are not adequately sensitive to justify the two-tiered approach recommended by the CDC for surveillance. The CAP has a stake in this fight since they are the professionals ultimately responsible for interpreting the test results. Donta has observed that 52% of patients with chronic Lyme are negative by ELISA testing but positive by WB. Since the surveillance criteria recommends that WB testing only be done on those patients with positive ELISA results, half the true positive patients don't even get a chance to have the more specific test. The CDC guidelines have made diagnostic confirmation next to impossible in between 30% and 70% of true patients. One published report estimates an over 80% miss rate. This number may be higher in certain regional hospitals that seem to be determined to reduce the incidence rate of Lyme by selecting test strains that are unlikely to ever be positive in the local population, and by refusing to diagnose on the basis of even pathognomonic physical findings and corroborative history.

While some antigen/antibody testing can provide important information, there can be limitations with antibody tests in general. An antibody response merely reflects past or present exposure to Bb antigen and does not demonstrate active disease. Antibody identification techniques rely on immune response after exposure and will fail if the patient is not producing antibodies at the time the blood is drawn. If the blood is collected just hours after the tick bite you probably will not collect any IgM and almost definitely no specific IgG. IgG may not appear until much later, unless the antibodies collected are from a previous infection. Steroid use may dampen the manufacture of antibodies, or the majority of antibodies may be bound in complexes and not available to bind in the test environment. If the blood is tested at a time when the spirochete is in a cell wall-deficient L-form, the immune system may not be recognizing the pathogen and so antibody formation may be on hiatus. At many different stages in the clinical course of the disease, antibody levels may be low.

Nevertheless, the WB is recognized by the National Institute of Allergy and Infectious Diseases (NIAID, a division of NIH), as the most useful method for detecting Bb *antibodies* currently available, at least compared to everything else. WB can be used to measure both IgG and IgM. With most infections, IgM antibodies appear first and wane after the first few weeks and generally do not recur. These are followed by IgG, which are regarded as the major enduring Ab response in chronic infections. However, LD rarely follows the common path. Here IgM may persist for years, suggesting persistent infection or reactivation of latent infection (which is known to occur in toxoplasmosis, leishmaniasis, and CMV, as well). A number of studies point to the importance of IgM in recurrent or persistent Lyme.

While WB may be the best way to detect antibodies in Lyme, this test is not without significant issues. The bands selected for the testing must represent antigen from the endemic area from which the Bb strain originated. If the antigens selected to test against the patient's antibodies are from a similar strain as the ones to which the patient was exposed, then there is a chance of a positive identification. If not, then binding between antibody and antigen is unlikely. Of course, if the patient was unknowingly bitten by a tick outside the suspected home area due to travel or some other bizarre circumstance, results can be confusing. (Again, don't put all your confidence in test results.)

Clearly, confirmation of active infection is not easy considering the insensitivity of PCR, the low yield of useable results from cultures, and the myriad issues around the antibody tests. In turn, if the tests can't reliably confirm diagnosis, they will not be able to convincingly monitor treatment effect. There is no test that currently demonstrates when a patient is better: either improved or cured. All evidence suggests that a negative test result does not mean absence of infection. Whatever side of the testing debate you fall on, please do not dismiss a clinically plausible diagnosis on the basis of a negative test result, especially when the professionals that read the tests tell you that the current methods do not support valid conclusions. At most, lab results should be supportive not exclusionary, exhaustive, or unimpeachable. The average HCP has no idea of the nuances involved in this type of specialized testing and should be especially mindful of the temptation to view lab results as inviolate. Things we do not understand tend to have more power over us. I shudder to recall all the cases where an obviously sick patient is dismissed because a false negative lab result made an HCP say, "*You do not have Lyme.*"

PEARL: Burrascano and Horowitz have stated that the sicker the patient the less likely she is to test positive. All her antibody is tied up with antigen and not available to bind during testing.

In the CDC's defense, they do make a distinction between criteria used for surveillance versus diagnosis. The CDC, FDA, and NIAID each warn not to rely solely on lab tests for diagnosis of Lyme. The FDA says that lab results should never be the only determinant of the Lyme diagnosis. Even so, many uninformed practitioners insist on positive lab tests before they commit. Trust me when I say that they do not understand all the background around interpretation of these tests. Do not allow misinformation and lack of education harm a patient. Diagnosis of Lyme should be a clinical judgment based on answers gathered regarding potential for exposure, the history of the present illness, and physical exam.

The CDC goes on to say that it is inappropriate to use their surveillance case definitions to make clinical diagnoses, establish standards of care for individual patients, develop guidelines, or provide parameters for reimbursement. Yet, every day the CDC recommendations are used for these very purposes. This issue will be parsed more definitively in the *Guidelines* section below.

An ideal diagnostic test would not only identify active disease, but also allow for the monitoring of treatment efficacy. The NIAID believes that neither the ELISA nor WB is up to this task. A test that is sensitive in identifying active infection, helpful in determining which patients might benefit from antibiotic treatment, and capable of evaluating the effectiveness of said treatment would be superlative. Add cost-effective, noncontroversial, with rapid turn-around, and you would have defined perfection. This test will definitely top the list in my letter to Santa. Such a Lyme biomarker is not currently available and will not likely come our way soon. Whether we like it or not we are going to have to make clinical decisions. Once we accept the fact that a Lyme diagnosis is a clinical judgment we will no longer be a prisoner of the test result, the controversy will have no power over us, and we can get about the business of helping TBI patients.

V. Is there such a thing as chronic Lyme disease?

I submit that the real reason Cain killed Abel was that Abel believed there was a chronic form of Lyme and Cain did not. As a herdsman, Abel would have had more exposure to ticks so he might have known something his brother didn't know. We can only speculate.

To paraphrase a great playwright, if a rose by any other name would smell as sweet, then perhaps a disease by any other name could make you just as sick. My point is that I don't care what you call it, something happens to a significant sub-population of these patients that continues to make them sick. Many are impacted for a prolonged time beyond what anyone would consider an acute phase. In most of the chronic cases, there is overwhelming evidence to hypothesize that this sub-population is suffering from a chronic, infectious form of LD. Whether you call the disease persistent Lyme, chronic TBI, major Lyme, recurrent borreliosis, relapsing Lyme, Stage 4 Lyme, on-going disseminated Borrelia, STARI, or any one of the 100 other names this diverse syndrome has been called, don't just label and run. If the person is sick, do something to make him feel better.

PEARL: Strange that something that doesn't exist has so many names. Recall that even though some can barely squeak out a begrudging acknowledgment that chronic Lyme exists (although rare to them), the CT legislature unanimously recognized the existence of chronic Lyme and allowed HCPs to treat these patients with long-term antibiotics without fear of reprisal.

Advocates of the concept of a persistent form of Lyme must stand up to the bullies who say that chronic Lyme disease doesn't exist, when even they reluctantly admit that it does. We have either experienced chronic Lyme, or worse, witnessed the suffering in our kids. Don't let people with secondary agendas, which have nothing to do with science, make you doubt what you have documented through your own senses and experiences. There are a number of ways to face down a bully, especially one that is much bigger and stronger than you. Usually bullies back off when confronted. Modern psychiatry has determined these folks are scared and attempting to cover their own insecurities with hubris. They only win when their victims cower. Confidence is kryptonite to bullies and those of us who believe in a persistent form of Lyme must stop apologizing for our opinions. The evidence is on our side. Keep reading.

To really get into the meat of this part of the controversy, we have to address the possible pathophysiologic mechanisms resulting in persistent Lyme symptoms. Both sides of the controversy acknowledge that symptoms persist in some patients after a course of antibiotics that should have hit the Bb. ILADS and many TBI-focused practitioners believe the underlying etiology is on-going infection. IDSA thinks that continuing symptoms are a result of damage to the immune system resulting in persistent problems. As you read the many sub-plots surrounding this debate, consider that both pathophysiologic mechanisms can be in play simultaneously. Here are points to consider around this issue:

- If there is on-going infection, why aren't spirochetes more readily observed, cultured, and identified through antibody and nucleic acid testing? Two reasons: First, the technology is not so well developed as to bless us with the most specific and sensitive testing methods. As the science evolves, valid and reliable recognition of Bb will become more commonplace. Second, just as the syphilis microbe and a number of other pathogens are able to elude the immune system in attempts to survive the onslaught of the host's defenses, the Lyme pathogen appears to be a master of evasion. Bb can go intracellular, shed its cell wall to become an unidentifiable **L-form**, go dormant, biofilm, burrow, encyst, and undergo any number of other transformations and machinations in order to avoid detection and destruction. These microbes cause either on-going symptoms or symptoms that resurface in flares when conditions for their active state again become favorable. In fact, spirochetes have been detected reliably many times in patients with persistent symptoms from the early work done by Alan MacDonald to the present day. For example, the spirochete and its DNA have been isolated from the CSF early in the disease process when meningeal signs are present. Similarly, spirochetes have been cultured from the skin even years after primary infection. Spirochetes have been demonstrated over and over with biopsies and PCR. While hard to culture, Bb have been recovered from aspirate, blood, urine, CSF, joint effusions, spinal discs, sputum, skin biopsies, placenta, gallbladder, bladder trigone, nerve tissue, umbilical cord, and various other tissue samples. The difficulty in culturing says more about the limitations of current culturing technique than the lack of pathogen. In the cases of classic symptoms when there is no evidence of live spirochetes, the fault is more likely due to inadequate testing methods than the non-existence of pathogen. Spirochetes are often obvious from the clinical presentation and we simply don't have the tools to detect them.

- If there is on-going infection, why doesn't a blast of Bb-specific antibiotic result in cure in the majority of cases? Just as the IDSA says, many patients are cured with a short-course of appropriate antibiotics. But as we all know, there is a real subpopulation of Lyme patients who do not get well with short-course treatment and, in fact, many suffer for a long time. Others appear cured, only to relapse months or years later. I just walked the 10K component of the Marine Corp Marathon with two sisters from Tennessee who asked the name of the book I was working on. After I disclosed the title, without any prompting, they told me that a third sister had suffered with Lyme and was incapacitated for two years. Why would they think she had persistent problems with Lyme and why would they relay that information to me if it did not happen? If her symptoms were due to damage to the immune system why did her condition improve only after long-term treatment? There was no possibility of secondary gain to them by revealing their story to me. We know that the longer chronic symptoms persist, the harder it is to achieve cure by any definition. Antibiotics, even when appropriately selected and administered, do not always instantly cure Lyme. This failure is likely due to the evasive properties of the Bb in combination with the fact that we have not yet identified or developed the ideal antibiotic regimen to hit the pathogen in all its forms and hiding places. Their ability to survive, along with our inability to effectively target in some cases, have them coming out ahead so far.

- Barthold has developed a theory of antimicrobial tolerance to explain how Bb persist in hosts and are thereby able to cause chronic disease Theoretically, Bb behavior is different in the host before and after the humoral response kicks in. Those persistent Bb that have experienced the immune response are more refractory to antibiotics which usually only target the active, replicating organisms. They endure the antibiotics by entering a state of transient, dormant, non-dividing limbo. They are now called persisters. By being in the inactive state, they survive whereas their genetically identical cousins are killed by either antibiotic or host immune cells. The dormant

state makes them insensitive or refractory (or tolerant) to antibiotics. When such persistent cells can't be eliminated by the immune system, they are effectively a **reservoir** from which recurrent infection can develop. As long as the dormant cells have the potential to reactivate into the free spirochete active form, they have the potential to cause the sxs of the disease. Persisters may be one cause of relapsing and chronic infections.

- If persistent Lyme symptoms are merely manifestations of a dysfunction in the immune system, how do you account for the Herxheimer reaction? I believe that the well-documented Herx phenomenon is one of the best arguments supporting the on-going infection hypothesis. If there were not living spirochetes, resumption of antibiotic therapy should not prompt a Herx reaction. Herx reactions are likely due to the toxins and the inflammation that results from a mass kill-off of pathogen and is a well-documented occurrence with a number of disease-causing microbes, like those that cause syphilis. The Herx sxs that are reminiscent of specific Lyme manifestations are likely due to the release of endotoxins from the dying Bb cells. If this were just an inflammatory manifestation, the sxs would just be those of a general inflammatory response. Instead, many Herx reactions present like a Lyme flare. If there are no active pathogens to die off after the start of antibiotics, what is causing the Herx? When people without an underlying Bb infection take antibiotics that coincidentally hit Bb, they may get diarrhea but they do not Lyme Herx. What could possibly explain the Herx if it is not the demise of previously live organisms responding to antibiotic treatment? With the Herx reaction, antibiotic is started and the patient feels worse. While the mass kill-mechanism is accepted as an explanation for the Herx reaction associated with a number of other conditions, some people have trouble accepting that there could be the same underlying pathophysiology for a similar process occurring with Lyme. There is not a conspiracy by Lyme patients to make up Herx symptoms if they do not have them. Three-year-olds might be clever, but they are not that clever. Why do we accept this model in syphilis and numerous other pathogens and not in Lyme?

- If persistent Lyme symptoms are merely manifestations of a dysfunction in the immune system, why do these on-going symptoms present as though they are due to a specific pathogen and not just signs and symptoms of general inflammation? Migrating joint pain, neurologic problems, and cardiac manifestations are not just everyday signs of inflammation, but indicative of the kinds of sxs more specific to Lyme. Otherwise everyone would just get the standard headache, fever, and generalized aches found in most early inflammatory processes. Persistent symptoms in chronic Lyme are those of Lyme, not garden-variety inflammation, although those nonspecific complaints may occur as well. These pathogens cause either on-going symptoms, or symptoms that resurface in flares, when conditions for their active state become favorable. While there may be permanent, residual damage to the immune system that persists in patients with on-going unremitting signs and symptoms, there is strong evidence that there is continuing infection as well. IDSA uses the argument that persistent Lyme symptoms are just common inflammatory symptoms in the general population and are not specific to Lyme. Well, I have a new knee that begs to disagree with that premise. My husband's recurrence was migratory joint pain and tinnitus. Re-treatment for Lyme resolved his flare. There are many examples of manifestations particular to Lyme.

- Both camps concede that some children are born with signs and symptoms of active Bb infection. How would the child get an active infection if the mother did not have an active infection? I think we can fairly safely assume that the fetus was not bitten by a tick *in utero*. The Bb were transmitted across the placenta in a way that resulted in gestational disease. Live spirochetes have been cultured from tissue samples provided by these children.

- Persistent or relapsing Lyme symptoms often respond to re-treatment either with the same antibiotic regimen that worked previously or with a new Bb-targeted therapeutic approach. Why would an immune dysfunction respond to antibiotic therapy? In contrast, on-going active infection should respond if appropriately pursued. There are many studies demonstrating that persistent Lyme symptoms can respond favorably to antimicrobial re-treatment.

- Just about everyone agrees that many, if not most, microbial pathogens can mount a vast number of defensive mechanisms making them resistant to both innate immune response as well as to antibiotics. Yet some refuse to believe that Bb can be one of these elusive pathogens.

- Some manifestations of Lyme are hard to explain without admitting that some cases of borreliosis are due to on-going infection. Interstitial cystitis is a case in point. If it walks like a duck and quacks like a duck but on repeated cultures there is never any sign of poultry, consider that you might have been looking in the wrong place all this time. Lyme patients have a disproportionate incidence of interstitial cystitis. Yet HCPs keep trying to cure the condition by treating E. *coli*, the most commonly recognized etiology of cystitis. (Now *that* could cause resistance.) The definition of insanity is doing the same thing over and over and expecting a different result. In many cases, addressing the Lyme pathogen has relieved symptoms of interstitial cystitis. This improvement in the clinical condition occurs despite not finding spirochetes in the urine or in the culture or by antibody-binding or nucleic acid identification. Sometimes the priority just has to be the patient and not the test result. I don't know of anyone who treats E. *coli* with doxycycline as the DOC, but if the patient isn't improving on standard treatments for E. *coli* then you might want to consider thinking outside the usual treatment paradigm. Ask, "Why isn't this patient getting better?" Is there a suggestion from the history or ROS that Lyme could be the underlying cause?

- On-going infection is a recognized, legitimate mechanism of disease in cases such as malaria, syphilis, herpes zoster, babesiosis, tuberculosis, herpes simplex, and many others. Just as herpes can remain inactive in the dorsal root ganglia of patients for decades, Bb apparently can remain active or inactive in the tissue of infected individuals indefinitely. Just as with the spirochetal disease syphilis, Bb can be localized, disseminated, or chronic. Many infectious diseases manifest in both acute and chronic forms. Acceptance of the on-going infection model for many chronic diseases should be just as plausible with Lyme as with other pathogens.

- Manifestations of residual immune damage associated with certain types of infections is evidenced by the presence of antineuronal antibodies induced by Strep and probably a number of tick-borne pathogens. In these cases, there is strong support for persistent infection as well. Recovery in these patients does NOT typically occur unless antibiotics are part of the treatment regimen. Intensive immune therapy alone does not usually eradicate these cases of persistent symptoms. Then what accounts for the people who do get well when they are finally treated with an adequate antibiotic regimen? Did the immune pathophysiology suddenly revert to normal? What exactly undid the immune damage? Did the patient detour to Lourdes on the way home? Some patients improve on antibiotics only to have their symptoms recur after the medicine is stopped. Why would the immune system, which was uncomplaining for the time being, suddenly present symptoms of Lyme disease if not re-triggered by pathogen?

- If symptoms were purely an immune malfunction due to prior pathogen damage, signs and symptoms should not be affected by antibiotics, (Yes, I know some antibiotics have a mild anti-inflammatory effect, but not to the degree expressed here.) In the cases of recurrence or relapse, modify the treatment regimen until you find one where the patient can eventually come off antibiotic and remain disease free.

- Lyme affects most body systems. A good way to tell if there is an infectious component to a manifestation that is not usually associated with infection is that the condition doesn't respond to traditional therapies. Examples include sleep problems, high blood sugars, seizures, and other neuropsychiatric issues like anxiety, panic, depression, or OCD. In these cases, the Lyme must be managed for the symptoms to respond. Of course, the clinical picture is complicated if the patient had a propensity for the condition prior to the Lyme infection. So a child prone to OCD because of genetics or environmental factors may be more susceptible to an OCD-like presentation if infected with certain TBIs such as Bb.

- We do all agree that Bb affects the immune system and the immune system affects the Bb. After a long period of illness, we can assume that BOTH an underlying infectious process AND a damaged immune system are contributing to on-going problems. In these cases, addressing all contributing factors in a way that targets the specific case may give the best chance for recovery.

VI. Who makes decisions for Lyme patients and why would this matter?

In my experience, there are a number of "types" of HCPs or scientists who might be involved in health care for Lyme patients. Each of these individuals is likely to be endorsing the perspective most favorable to his or her own niche. Each would be motivated by different incentives and each might make money in a different way. If any were asked, I'm sure all would say that money was not their primary influence. If this is true, then some may be sparked by any number of other factors. They may be in professional competition with colleagues or want tenure or grants or a position on a prestigious panel of a specialty organization. We are all inspired by different things and these might shift our perspective and introduce bias into the best-intentioned individual. Others just can't bear to admit they might be wrong about anything and will defend their position long after it no longer makes medical sense to do so. Whatever the stimulus, the diverse agendas may be contributing to the never-ending controversy. Consider:

A. **The researcher**: These individuals may or may not be physicians and may or may not see patients. If part of an academic system, they may be focused on tenure and grant proposals. There could be considerable politics and competition in their world. A number of researchers were involved in drafting the IDSA Guidelines. Many of these scientists were not actively seeing patients and it is doubtful in some cases whether some had ever been responsible for managing a Lyme case. A number of researchers have affiliations with outside interests or receive grants from third parties. When these same researchers are then entrusted to write practice guidelines, care must be taken to watch for COI, especially when the results of their own research may end up as part of the guideline without adequate balance. Remember that a good scientist is not automatically a good physician and many physicians know next to nothing about the scientific method, trial design, and data analysis. Likewise, high academic credentials do not necessarily correlate with ethical standards or integrity.

B. **The governmental or organizational employee**: More than a few of these HCPs have never seen a patient in the therapeutic area in question and others are not licensed to see patients in any capacity. (Researchers, you might want to check your CRO physicians to see if they are licensed or could even qualify for licensure. You get what you pay for.) There is a difference between going to medical school and being a physician. I appreciate that the physicians at the CDC did concede that diagnosis for surveillance is not the same as diagnosis of individual patients in the clinic. Still, their flawed lab criteria are used in guidelines that grossly limit the diagnosis of Lyme. I appreciate that the FDA has reiterated that Lyme diagnoses should be based on clinical judgment and should not be so dependent on lab testing.

Always consider the source of a recommendation before blindly following. Do not believe that just because it is the FDA, CDC, NIH, Yale, Hutch, Karolinska Institute, or IDSA speaking, everything they say is true. These groups have all the internal squabbles and machinations of any other organization. Many government employees have heavy workloads. Of course, others have little to do. Opinions can be biased. Some folks have secondary agendas, others are bored spitless. Even with the best intentions, lack of personal or patient experience with a condition can limit perspective.

For this book I had the opportunity to re-read one set of diagnostic criteria for PTSD, which because of my professional background, I know something about. If you read these diagnostic criteria, you will see a set of statements that seem to be written by people who might be better suited for excluding others from acceptance into an elite country club than in trying to help identify people who are suffering and may benefit from treatment. There were all sorts of, what seem to be, artificial criteria involved in arriving at the diagnosis. While I do not know for sure, I did not feel that these diagnostic criteria had input either from persons with PTSD or from practitioners with experience and compassion toward these patients.

With guidelines and diagnostic recommendations, as with clinical research study design, put imaginary patients through your criteria and see how they hold up. If no one "makes the cut," perhaps the criteria are too rigid, or unrealistic, or predicated on inexperience. Unfortunately, internal politics plays more of a role than anyone might like to admit. Pharmaceutical company physicians know that Dr. Graham at the FDA is correct about MOST of his safety allegations. They are just handsomely paid to steer in a different direction.

C. **The primary care HCP**: In my opinion, these are the frontline practitioners in recognizing TBIs. Some are quite Lyme-literate but others struggle mightily to do the right thing for their TBI patients. For those who do not see Lyme every day, many are unaware of either of the current treatment guidelines. Others have been exposed to one or the other. A few are firmly in one of the opposing camps. The majority have no idea which side of the debate they are on and they are just trying to get through the day. Some are frankly intimidated by the controversy. When Chris needed scripts for doxy and azithromycin as a preventive measure against a new deer tick bite (since the last one nearly killed him), the physician at the clinic in Maryland was so afraid of doing something wrong around Lyme that he actually whispered the word *Lyme*. I guess he was worried that someone would hear him dealing with a Lyme patient and turn him into the tick police. The lack of sensitive testing and the plethora of false negatives have these first-line HCPs confused and frustrated. They are in the middle of a fight that most don't understand and few have the time to investigate. One of the primary intentions of this book is to help these HCPs cope and, in turn, assist patients who desperately need their considered care.

D. **The infectious disease specialist**: A number of the ID specialists subscribe to the IDSA Guidelines because this is their professional association. I suspect that many have not reviewed the rationale behind the IDSA statements regarding Lyme and take them at face value. They have no reason to suspect secondary agendas. They trust their professional group to process the science for them. While some will treat symptomatic Lyme patients longer than the guidelines recommend, others have stopped treatment while the patients are still sick and begging for continued help. My husband's co-worker was told when his IV Rocephin was discontinued, despite the intense flare of symptoms when the drug was stopped, that he should not have expected to get better with Lyme and that maybe the symptoms would eventually go away some day on their own. Some ID specialists contend that ALL their patients get better after short-term treatment and I am sure that SOME do. However, I submit that the patients who have seen at least a dozen doctors prior to finding one that clicks, have left the practice of those previous doctors who did not address their needs. These specialists are not even aware that the patients have left their practices and gone for help elsewhere. They assume they have cured people who are actually still quite ill. They do not account for the patients who are now under the care of a cardiologist who had to insert a pacemaker because their initial treatment was grossly inadequate. There is usually no follow-up regarding who really got well or who had persistent, progressive, or relapsing disease. The HCPs assume the patients did not return because they were cured. In fact, the sick have just moved on to another HCP more willing to confront their individual problems. Many patients leave when the doc says they aren't sick or that nothing more can be done. I suspect these specialists do not know the full extent of the problem. They say chronic Lyme is rare. That's because they don't see the long-term sufferers. There is no reporting system for treatment failures. No one likes to admit that a subgroup of their patient population is still sick, especially when some are actually incapacitated and sicker than when they first presented.

E. **Other specialists**: There are Lyme-aware practitioners and there are those who scoff at the idea of chronic Lyme. If you are a parent, a patient, or an HCP referring patients, and you are seeking help for a Lyme-related condition, know whether the provider you are consulting is well-versed in persistent Lyme or not. Know if they will target the treatment to the individual case or simply follow the same algorithms for all patients, whether that approach is appropriate in a particular case or not. You will save yourself a lot of agony if you avoid those who tell you that you can't still be feeling sick or that your 3-year-old's symptoms are all in her head. Your local Lyme advocacy group may be able to put you in touch with practitioners who understand the potentially chronic nature of Bb infection.

Some HCPs are only focused on the remission of symptoms during the time period they are involved with a certain patient. Most patients would prefer to eliminate symptoms through permanent eradication of the causal pathogen. Once the patient leaves a practice, the outcome is lost to follow-up. We have no solid data on how many physicians one patient might see prior to finding relief. We do not know how many misdiagnoses are made and actual diagnoses missed and the number of inadequate treatment regimes tried before the proper approach is uncovered. Most patients now going to experienced Lyme-providers have seen many doctors before finding the one who helps. Saying the sick patient is no longer sick is a form of magical thinking that has more to do with the HCP's inability to accept that he might have been wrong than it does with actually curing people. And you wonder why health care costs are out-of-control. You never solve a problem by pretending it's not there.

The IDSA contention that so many of their patients do well with short-course antibiotics does not account for the many patients who go to other physicians for follow-up because they did not get better with the first HCP. Nor does it explain the return of symptoms in weeks or months or years. Some ID docs treat any flares as a new infection, which is possible, but the old infection could also be resurfacing and doing damage as well. They do not account for on-going symptoms that remit when on antibiotics and resurface when antimicrobials are discontinued. When a patient relapses, are we supposed to believe that the immune system that is fine one day suddenly decides to remember it's defective? Why would the immune system unexpectedly present symptoms of Lyme disease if not re-triggered by pathogen? One could argue that the Bb itself is responsible for the suppression and then subsequent revival of the immune system in a particular individual. Bb does impact the immune response but in ways that do not appear associated with resurgence of Lyme symptoms. The recurrence of symptoms seems to be due to return of active forms of pathogen. A majority of patients do recover on short-course antibiotics never to be bothered by Lyme again. But a substantial number do not.

For those HCPs who actually manage the cases of sick 4-year-olds, they know that the symptoms are genuine. Likewise, the resolution of symptoms can be real with proper treatment. Further, the recurrence of problems is just as real if the treatment was not long enough, or strong enough, or if the drugs selected allowed some of the Bb life forms to escape. Come into the real world of chronic Lyme and you will see what we see. Stay in the defensive, convenient peripheral world of Lyme disease and you will have an easier case-load. Unfortunately, you will not be helping the sick people who need you.

Over millennia, science has always prevailed (even in recent political campaigns). As Aldous Huxley mused, "Facts do not cease to exist because they are ignored." Let's hope we don't have to wait a thousand years for resolution.

VII. Which Guidelines should be used?

Currently, there are two accepted guidelines regarding the diagnosis and treatment of Lyme, one from the International Lyme & Associated Diseases Society (ILADS) and one from the Infectious Diseases Society of America (IDSA). Both are considered valid and have been approved and endorsed by various professional and regulatory groups. Both are evidence-based and peer-reviewed. They are readily accessible on the Internet through www.ilads.org and www.idsociety.org. They are quite different in their approaches to the diagnosis and treatment of Lyme.

In my opinion, I think both sets of guidelines split too many hairs on things that are not so important in the overall scheme of things. When my son was lying on the floor unconscious, quaking with rigors, I wanted the doctors to use any set of guidelines that allowed him to survive. I didn't care if they were scrawled on the back of an envelope as long as someone did something productive. Frankly, the ER personnel were so misinformed about TBIs that I am fairly certain that they hadn't read anybody's guidelines on anything.

I wanted Chris to be treated with respect and not have to endure the Lilith[2] eye-roll. He had dared not follow some bogus algorithm that had nothing to do with his individual case. By adhering to guidelines that had no basis in medical reality, the first several HCPs nearly killed him. As Thoreau said, "Any fool can make a rule," but actually contemplating the best course of action takes both expertise and courage.

When researching Lyme when Chris first got sick, I soon realized that there was a colossal disconnect between some of the literature and the reality lived by a number of the patients. I came across one Lyme classification system defining the major and minor symptoms categories. Even though I knew next to nothing at that point, I understood that these categories did not fit the profile of ANY of the many people who I knew with Lyme. These arbitrary classifications are both ridiculous and dangerous and have little relationship to real patients. Thank goodness my former co-worker from Sweden didn't have any *major* symptoms when his Lyme disease killed him. Should we wait until we have all the answers perfectly before we move to help suffering people? What would happen if we did that in the cases of cancer or syphilis or pneumonia? Or high blood pressure or diabetes or rheumatic fever or schizophrenia? Or…?

The proof is in the pudding. Is the child getting better or not? If the patient is still sick, what is plan B? Tell the individual it's all in his head? That there is a vast, short-wing conspiracy of 4-year-olds trying to deceive the medical establishment?

I hope the following section clarifies some of the options around managing Lyme disease. By recognizing what the fight is about, you might be able to better collaborate with your patients in making the best decisions regarding their disease.

A. The guideline perspectives are different because the authors are different.

Each of us is influenced by what we perceive to be the best path for us. Many people see the boundaries of their experience as the boundaries of the whole world. Therefore the differences in the guidelines might be explained by the differences in composition of the drafting teams. Many of the IDSA panel were academic researchers with established views. In contrast, the ILADS group was comprised largely of primary care clinicians who focus on TBI patients. The ILADS panel also included other stakeholders such as patients, researchers, and community-based HCPs. One source said that 11/12 authors of the IDSA Guidelines were researchers with little or no experience in the clinic. Persons who do not have the face-to-face responsibility to alleviate patient suffering may not understand the full complexity of LD and the serious repercussions of their decisions.

---

2 See Glossary or Introduction for name origin

My understanding is that attempts by ILADS to initiate dialogue with their IDSA counterparts have been rebuffed. IDSA also historically declined to participate in providing information when asked by legislative bodies to do so. This intractability does not portend well for the resolution of the controversy anytime soon. How strong is your argument if you fear questions or transparency?

The good news is that IDSA has become the poster child for how NOT to construct useful guidelines. Many professional organizations have called for reform of the guideline drafting process. The Institute of Medicine says that many guidelines are based on weak, mixed, or no evidence. Further, much of the information used to support some guidelines does not match the reality of the patient population. The IOM recommends that guidelines be formulated by panels of diverse stakeholders who review a broad base of evidence and solicit input from all those who might be affected by the panel's recommendations. When I worked for a company based in the Asian subcontinent, I could never understand the fear of the data. The data just is what it is and should be managed without trying to ignore or revise it in order to satisfy ulterior motives. Knowing the limits of your data and how it was collected is important, but fear is unnecessary. I have never seen a case where hiding from or burying data came out good in the end. For some reason, regulatory agencies take a dim view of that.

Drafters of documents that affect public health should remember that the goals of research and clinical case management are quite different. Like surveillance, the goal of research is to define a homogeneous population. Outliers, real though they might be, are excluded to keep the data clean and manageable. Better to compare apples to apples. Still, diseases like chronic Lyme do not present in a homogeneous way in a homogeneous population. Diversity and mimicry is the norm. The real-world clinician does not have the option to see only those cases who present inside the box. Treating Lyme is a messy business and because of the heterogeneity in presentation and population, each individual case must be assessed and addressed on its own merits. If only each Lyme patient could be squeezed back inside the cookie-cutter, how simple life would be. Many researchers do not have to face the patients or parents of kids in the throes of an ongoing severe illness that is impacting their hearts, their joints, or their nervous systems in ways that potentially disable them in daily life. The IDSA approach excludes the majority of chronic Lyme patients. The fact that the disease can progress and result in permanent incapacity is not of concern to those who don't have to worry about seeing the sick person again in a few weeks. In the clinic we want to be erring on the side of over-diagnosing in order to decrease M&M. The question of "What's the worst that could happen if we over-diagnose or over-treat?" will be addressed in later sections.

B. There are numerous conflicting opinions between the ILADS and IDSA Guidelines.

   Controversies include the approach to Lyme diagnosis, the prevalence of chronic Lyme, and use of lab testing. These issues are covered elsewhere in detail.

C. There is a short-term treatment approach and an open-ended treatment approach.

SHORT-TERM OR IDSA RECOMMENDATIONS

Description: IDSA recommends standardized short treatment of 30 days *or less* even if the individual remains unwell at the end of this treatment course. Treatment is stopped regardless of patient response unless there are reliable measures of relapse (presumably by the same flawed methods depended upon to make the initial diagnosis). Response to treatment could be slow but antibiotics beyond 30 days are not recommended. IDSA endorses either IV antibiotics for 2 to 4 weeks or oral for a maximum of 4 weeks for all LD and "eventual recovery" is expected in most patients.

Pros:

- Palliative treatment is permitted for residual symptoms. (Please give me credit for all the opportunities I had to be sarcastic that I chose not to take.)

- IDSA says there is not convincing data to prove that repeated or prolonged antibiotics are effective.

- There could be less drug resistance when shorter courses of antibiotics are used.

- IDSA believes that with a maximum of 30 days of treatment most patients "eventually recover."

- What does that mean? "Eventually recover." I want better odds than that. No one is worried about the more than half of Lyme patients who do get better on short-courses of antibiotic. We need to be concerned about the 25% to 50% who have residual, progressive, or relapsing problems. IDSA does not talk about those patients, except to say that they are rare. What should you do while you wait to "eventually recover"? What do IDSA members do as they wait to "eventually recover"? A better question is: "What do they do while they wait for their children to 'eventually recover'?" Do they sit by and not treat as the pacemaker is inserted into their own child? I would bet big money on what they do. I want one to honestly say to me, "I allowed my child to be incapacitated with pain and fatigue while heart, joint, and neurologic problems progressed. I confidently and patiently waited for her to 'eventually recover'." What would that prove? Would anyone really do that?

- IDSA says that long-term use of antibiotics puts patients at risk of infection by super bugs without improving their underlying condition. They believe that symptoms commonly attributed to chronic or persistent Lyme could be any number of other conditions and are common in the general population and so not likely to be Lyme. How do they KNOW?

- There is a perceived cost-saving to insurers in terminating treatment, even if the patient remains symptomatic, especially if the treatment includes the more costly IV protocols.

Cons:

- The evidence is clear that the longer that chronic symptoms persist, the harder it is to achieve cure by any definition. If the cause is underlying, on-going infection and the problem is not addressed adequately, we might be dooming the patient to permanent adverse sequelae. So in the words of the old cliché: the operation was a success but the patient died. I know of innumerable cases where the symptoms were allowed to progress to pacemakers or knee replacements or incapacitating neuropsychiatric problems. Here the end-organ problems were treated and the underlying etiology was ignored because it just couldn't be Lyme. Failure to identify and appropriately treat LD early can allow the infection to progress, permitting a treatable acute infection to become a relapsing chronic disease that becomes less and less responsive to antibiotics. The earlier the treatment, the greater the chance for cure. Late disease presents the greatest treatment challenge and may develop into a condition refractory to various therapeutic modalities. Some HCPs feel that termination of treatment in those patients who still feel sick constitutes negligence that may result in avoidable neurologic injury, debilitation, and even death.

- There is no provision for the complications introduced by co-infections.

- There is no recourse if for some reason an inappropriate antibiotic was selected or the drug was administered in an inadequate dose.

- When drug resistance occurs, the resistance can develop in courses of 30 days or less as well as with longer courses. With some antibiotics, resistance can appear within hours and other measures must be taken to combat the resistance. In these cases, you will need to address the possibility of resistance whether the short-term or long-term treatment course is selected.

- Although it is hard to prove a negative, there is no evidence that spirochetes are NOT present after the 30 day antibiotic course. Since Bb are so difficult to culture and otherwise prove, this evidence is not likely to be available anytime soon. I don't expect the IDSA to go spirochete hunting to prove their own premise incorrect. There are numerous published reports of spirochetes present in patients long after treatment was discontinued.

- Johnson and Stricker cite a number of studies that have found treatment failures ranging from 24% to 50% using the short-term antibiotic regimens.

- There are no prospective human trials proving the effectiveness of the 30 days or less regimen. However, animal studies show that while this limited duration may reduce the bacterial load, it does not usually eradicate the Lyme organism.

- These guidelines tend to be inflexible, with weak, if any, evidence supporting the recommended duration of treatment. There are minimal provisions allowing adjustment of the regimen to accommodate individual variation.

- Where did the number 30 come from? Why not 35 which would be 5 weeks or 28 which would be 4 weeks? What is magic about 30? I am unaware of any studies that compared 30 days with any other regimen in terms of safety or efficacy. Actually, 30 days is the upper limit of treatment length in the IDSA Guidelines. They are happy with 10 days in certain cases but they have no provision to follow who might relapse after such a limited antibiotic course.

- Continuation of treatment is allowed only if evidence is available from lab testing known to be flawed according to the CAP, FDA, CDC, and NIAID.

- Many patients experience a relapse of symptoms soon after the short-term antibiotic is discontinued. Others are only functional when symptoms are muted by antibiotics.

- How is "eventually recover" defined? If symptoms stop and the patient is designated as a "cure," what then constitutes a relapse? Is it no symptoms for a week, a month, five years? You cannot see what you don't look for. Different periods of time selected to look for relapse might provide very different perspectives. Many patients might feel fine for a week or two after treatment stops and then, over time, a number of those considered initially cured might begin to experience a recurrence of symptoms. While the majority appear to be fully recovered, others can show signs of relapse that range from mild, barely-there symptoms to a syndrome worse than the original presentation. Monitoring for just a brief period will falsely inflate the recovery rate. As I mentioned earlier, a percentage of patients with persistent symptoms leave those doctors who do not try to address their problems. Monitoring that does not follow patients over a sufficient time period will give inaccurate relapse data. I relapsed. My husband relapsed. My son relapsed. No one reported any of those relapses. Lyme patients have been known to relapse years after they were labeled fully-recovered. Donta studied relapse rates in 277 patients and found that recurrence can occur years after therapy is stopped. As a reasonable working definition, Donta defined **cure** as an absence of symptoms for a year or more following antibiotic treatment. While that timing model isn't perfect, it provides a place to start.

- Essentially all patients seen by the high tier TBI specialists have tried the IDSA limited treatment regimens and have failed. If the short-term treatment worked, these experts would have no patients instead of long waiting lists. They don't see the patients who get better on short-term antibiotics because they don't need to be seen. They're better. They see those who did not get well on short-term therapy. If these regimens worked in all people, they would work in all people. Many treatment paradigms for other medical conditions contain provisions for treatment failure. The IDSA guidelines do not.

- The view set forth in the IDSA guidelines, that treatment be withheld from patients with on-going symptoms who have been previously treated, results in a mini-clinical trial to which the patients have not consented. Without knowing there are valid alternative treatments, the patients lose their right to be involved in their own medical care decisions. Those who are still sick, who are lucky enough to know that options exist, often prefer not to experiment with their health and find HCPs who will treat them as individuals.

- The short-term approach which expects a percentage of patients to NOT be well at the end of the treatment course forgets that the goal of all intervention is improved health or wellness. If measures of treatment success do not include the possibility of on-going symptoms, the measure is artificial and invalid. Chronic Lyme patients, who rank their incapacity the same as that of chronic CHF patients, do not consider themselves well by any stretch of the imagination. Wellness is best addressed by asking the patient if she is well. IDSA guidelines attempt to define wellness by excluding subjective symptoms. Ignoring what the patient is trying to tell you does not make the patient well.

- IDSA does not track treatment experience including failures that might result from its short-term approach.

- The next section discusses the importance of the medicolegal aspects of patient preference, individual autonomy, and the need to disclose the availability of alternative approaches to Lyme treatment. IDSA short-course approach undervalues the clinical picture, discounts response variability, and ignores patient preferences and the existence of options. When a patient is begging for a continuation of treatment, the HCP might safely assume he might want a continuation of treatment. I do not recall my son being offered alternative treatments from his initial HCPs. Nor was I presented with options even when my knee joint was destroyed, presumably by Lyme. These legal implications are detailed below.

<u>**Potential risks of this approach**</u>:

- Patients continue to suffer and some are incapacitated by on-going disease.

- Evidence suggests that the later in the clinical course that the Bb infection is adequately managed, the more chronic and progressive the disease can become.

- A manageable acute disease can progress to an intractable, chronic condition.

- Lyme is a serious disease that can lead to permanent sequelae, disability, and death.

- There are ethical and legal issues around allowing a serious multisystem disease to progress without attempting to curtail its effects.

<u>**What's the worst that could happen with this approach?**</u>

Continuing infection could lead to permanent severe sequelae including heart, nerve, and joint damage as well as on-going problems in other organ systems, gestational transmission, daily incapacity, diminished QOL, behavior problems, and death. While some IDSA members insist this is rare, they do not have valid (let's say any) data to support this contention. When it's your child affected the incidence is 100%.

<u>**What's the best that could happen with this approach?**</u>

If the patient is asymptomatic at the end of treatment, then this short treatment regimen can be counted as a success. But if no system is in place to count recurrence or relapse, then no one is the wiser. If symptoms persist or recur, then this approach is a failure that can result in significant M&M, including permanent problems. When you are five-years-old, permanent is a long time. Some "experts" may be willing to risk their own children, but I do not believe they should have the right to risk yours and mine.

OPEN-ENDED OR LONG-TERM ILADS RECOMMENDATIONS:

Description: The ILADS approach is targeted to the individual case and depends on clinical response. If clinically indicated, treatment beyond 30 days is considered reasonable and medically necessary. The goal of treatment is improvement of symptoms to the point of desired function or complete cure.

Pros:

- Stricker and Johnson list multiple studies and case reports where long-term antibiotics have helped patients with persistent symptoms. More than 1300 peer-reviewed studies were presented to IDSA in support of the flexible, open-ended treatment approach based on clinical response.

- Straubinger has repeatedly demonstrated persistent Bb, with isolation of the spirochete, in canine studies examining 25 tissue samples per dog after what was considered adequate antibiotic treatment. This work supports the need for longer therapy in those cases where symptoms persist.

- Work by Donta showed that in patients with persistent symptoms, the longer the course of antibiotics, the more improvement could be documented. Oksi's work reinforces these conclusions.

- ILADS allows for longer term treatment but does not *require* longer therapy if not clinically indicated. Therefore, the ILADS approach is more flexible and targeted to the individual case. ILADS believes that duration of therapy should be OPEN-ENDED.

- While the results of several long-term studies show conflicting results, these studies tended to have apparent design flaws. One lead investigator revealed to the press what he thought the study result should be before the data was analyzed. This is the primal red-flag in clinical research and essentially eliminates the possibility of an unbiased conclusion. The validity of this study was impeached before the data base could be locked.

- Laboratory testing is viewed as ancillary to clinical judgment and not essential to confirm the need for continued treatment.

- The ILADS recommendations for the duration of treatment are based on individual clinical response and patient preference.

- Burrascano, Liegner, Bransfield, Stricker, and other TBI experts believe that if antibiotics are stopped before the

predominant Lyme disease symptoms have cleared, a relapse is more likely.

- Lyme is a complex disease and ILADS understands we are still early in the information-gathering phase. We simply do not know enough to etch treatment paradigms in stone, especially when patients continue to feel sick. Treatment should be targeted to the specific case, in line with the desires of the patient.

- The reality of heterogeneous patient populations and multi-organ presentations suggests that individualized treatment rather than rote, inflexible interventions may be more effective. Until a better method comes along, the patient's actual clinical response is the best measure of treatment effect.

- Prolonged antibiotic regimens are accepted for a number of chronic infectious diseases such as TB, malaria, and leprosy. Why not Lyme? Teens spend years on antibiotics for acne and adults are prescribed antibiotics for decades to treat rosacea in doses more conducive to resistance without all the fuss. Kids are prescribed daily antibiotics for years to prevent recurrence of otitis media because their infection resurfaces every time they come off the medicine. Many COPD patients are on long-term antibiotics to lessen the chance of bacteria settling in their susceptible lungs. Why bring up arguments in Lyme treatment that are ignored with conditions with less M&M? The biggest cause of antibiotic resistance is widespread use of antibiotics in animal feed to increase profit, not the treating of sick patients with Lyme. Antibiotics are given out like candy to patients who the HCP is well aware have a viral URI. Americans have been conditioned to call their doctor at the first inkling of a sniffle so they can get their Z-Pak called in. (I'm not innocent. I have called in a few Z-Paks in my day. Anything to stop the whining, including my own.) These patients often request refills so that they can keep taking antibiotic as long as their slightest symptoms persist. "I just can't seem to get rid of this cough." Their cumulative use of antibiotic may be longer than the 30 day limit imposed by IDSA in sick Lyme patients. Many people are quite happy that the doctor thinks they are sick enough to get antibiotics for their cold. "I told you I was sick."

- ILADS guidelines respect the role of clinical judgment when different treatment options exist. In general, the more complex the disease the more targeted, individualized treatment is needed. With Lyme, the discretion and good sense of the HCP is critical.

- Cost savings, which may result from terminating therapy after a short-course, may evaporate in the long-run as the still-sick patients go from doctor to doctor in an attempt to find relief. The short-course approach in patients with persistent symptoms may be penny wise and pound foolish. I would like to see data comparing the cost of both approaches, but I would want to make sure the data collection is unbiased. I would be happy to volunteer my services to review that protocol.

- ILADS has maintained a database to track the efficacy of its approach.

Cons:

- Antibiotic resistance is possible with the use of long-term antibiotics. In fact, depending on the specific drug, resistance can occur within hours. Therefore, 31 days or more is not going to be much different from shorter courses in terms of resistance. The type of low-dose, long-term antibiotic used in acne is more likely to result in bacterial resistance than are appropriate doses of targeted antibiotic in a Lyme patient. It's ridiculous to blame antibiotic use in Lyme for global antibiotic drug resistance. We really need to put things in perspective.

- IDSA says there are no convincing published data to prove that repeated or prolonged antibiotics are effective. Of course, there are also no convincing published data to prove that short-term antibiotics are effective especially in the significant percentage of patients with persistent or relapsing Lyme. IDSA fails to consider scores of studies evidencing persistent infection and the 1300 studies presented by ILADS to the IDSA guideline review panel. Of course, a narrow panel might have a narrow perspective.

- Adverse events such as diarrhea and GI upset can occur with antibiotic use. In fact, most GI problems associated with antibiotic use resolve as the intestinal flora adjusts to the changes caused by the antibiotics. Use of probiotics probably reduces the possibility of loose stools even further. In some cases, C. *difficile* may be more associated with the type of antibiotic than the length of treatment.

- Antibiotics can cause fungal overgrowth. Yup. After 24 hours or 24 days.

- Solo antibiotics can cause Bb to encyst, hide, encapsulate, or otherwise go dormant. Yes, many pathogens are known to morph or go dormant in order to survive. Pathogens use any mechanism available to them to avoid their own demise. Don't you? These defensive measures occur reflexively when the pathogen detects a detrimental change in its milieu. This occurs under both short and long-term treatment conditions. The pathogen has no idea how long you plan to treat so it goes on the defensive as soon as it senses something bad is happening. The shingles virus is a case in point where the herpes can remain dormant,

sometimes for half a century, until conditions are favorable for reemergence. Fortunately, there are ways to circumvent the tricks of the elusive Bb. When symptoms recur that suggest that the spirochete is active once again, try to hit it with a targeted antibiotic regimen that covers all forms (i.e., hits the cystic, intracellular, and spirochetal forms of the creature), in a high enough dose to penetrate all areas of interest from the BBB to the joint spaces, for long enough that they have no choice but to die or at least remit. Combination therapy usually is the key.

- Superbugs. The IDSA is worried about superbugs. This fear falls under the fear of drug resistance. Yes, resistance can occur and is a common manifestation with antibiotic use. But resistance is more likely to occur with low dose antibiotics than those used at appropriate levels. Resistance is more often associated with the type of antibiotic than the length of treatment. Clearly resistance can occur within hours with some drugs and within 30 days in others. I know of no data that shows that for the antibiotics most commonly used for treatment of Lyme that superbugs result more often in 31 days than in 30 days. Try to focus your concerns around resistance in areas where they are more likely to cause harm, like ubiquitous antibiotics in animal feed and the never-ending low dose treatments of conditions like viral URIs and rosacea.

Potential risks of this approach:

While fungal overgrowth, loose stools, and drug resistance are all possible, the risks are essentially the same for both long and short-term regimens. I may be missing something, but I see no down-side of attempting to address on-going illness with on-going treatment. If the treatment is not working, then the plan may need to be re-thought and re-structured. If it were my child, not treating would not be an option. Lucky for me that I have options that others may not.

What's the worst that could happen with this approach?

According to IDSA, superbugs perpetuated by antibiotic resistance are the biggest concern. I am not aware of a super-Bb that has resulted from treatment of Lyme. I am very aware of the potential for permanent sequelae that results from not treating persistent Lyme.

What's the best that could happen with this approach?

Continuing treatment may preclude permanent sequelae, allow the person to function day-to-day, and lead to cure.

Clearly we do not yet have all the answers. Hopefully we will soon identify the best anti-Lyme antibiotic combinations, at the ideal dose, and better understand the optimum length of treatment.

PEARL: Surveys show that nearly 60% of responding physicians treat persistent LD for 3 months or more. Fallon notes that for over 3400 patients at Columbia, the mean duration of IV treatment was 2.3 months and mean duration of oral treatment was 7.5 months. In still another survey, half the responders considered using antibiotics for a time greater than a year in symptomatic seropositive LD patients. Almost the same number would extend therapy to 18 months if clinically appropriate. I think this disregard for the IDSA treatment guidelines has to do with having face-to-face responsibility for the sick person sitting on the exam table. If you don't have to look the chronically ill in the eye, it is much easier to claim there is no problem. If short-term therapy doesn't work, then an alternative might be both ethically and medically prudent.

VIII. Medicolegal issues

The Lyme controversy, also called the Lyme war, is steeped in medico-legal issues. The situation became so outrageous and skewed that the AG of Connecticut stepped in and investigated the guidelines provided by the IDSA from an antitrust and abuse-of-power perspective. As detailed below, the guidelines were determined to be biased and, as part of the settlement with the IDSA, their recommendations had to be reviewed. Also in Connecticut, the legislature and governor enacted a law to protect HCPs treating chronic Lyme patients, allowing for the use of long-term antibiotics without reprisal. (My dog has been on long-term antibiotics for an infected gland. Every time he comes off the medicine, the symptoms recur within 3 days. Should I have my vet arrested for trying to help my sick, old dog?) I always prefer the separation of medicine and state but when people are being hurt by medical arrogance, I appreciate the legal system acting in patient defense.

Works by Johnson and Stricker provide a comprehensive examination and chronology of the medicolegal aspects of the Lyme controversy. While laws may differ from state-to-state, the concepts listed below provide the minimum you should recognize as you begin to explore the controversial Lyme world. Education can help keep you out of trouble.

Because Lyme is such a contentious topic, I felt it was important to have access to some of the basic background regarding the legal issues around Lyme. Knowledge is your best defense. Take from this section what you can use.

Medicolegal history of the Lyme controversy

Dr. Stricker provides an excellent overview of the recent history of the Lyme controversy in several of his published works. Along with Lorraine Johnson, he has the best understanding of the events leading to the current impasse. I will attempt to briefly summarize the history so that you have a better appreciation of how things got so messy, and how patients may have

been sacrificed on the altar of hubris. As I summarize the story, know that I do have bias, but I will attempt to let the facts speak for themselves. As you read, remember that physicians promise to "First, do no harm."

In 2000, IDSA published guidelines for the diagnosis and treatment of Lyme disease. These recommendations came with the disclaimer that the guidelines were not meant to dictate practice and were not intended to be mandatory. Practitioners should use clinical judgment in diagnosing and treating Lyme. However, the IDSA doesn't acknowledge any other Lyme management options aside from what they present in their guidelines.

With the guidelines in place, the IDSA soon began to testify against physicians who were not following their recommendations. Seemingly, a number of Lyme patients were transferring to HCPs interested in treating them as individuals by addressing their specific needs, as opposed to slavishly conforming to guidelines that did not remotely fit their clinical presentation. Selected practitioners were targeted with threats of revocation of hospital privileges, limitations on state licenses, and medical board procedures. Because the IDSA guidelines were so rigid and made so little medical sense in real world medicine, it was easy to fall outside the recommendations and become a target of this medical inquisition. The IDSA was interested in HCPs that they felt were out of compliance with their Lyme guidelines. A number of high-quality practitioners either stopped seeing Lyme patients or left practice altogether. Insurers were denying coverage and patients were having a hard time finding physicians who could address their persistent symptoms. IDSA actively opposed state legislation designed to protect competitors from medical board action for what they labeled as unprofessional conduct based on the use of other guidelines.

In response to these limits on physician judgment and patient preference, ILADS developed a set of guidelines in 2004 that was peer-reviewed, evidence-based, and accepted by the NGC.[3] The ILADS recommendations were more flexible and driven by individual case presentation and clinical response to treatment. Both sets of guidelines are considered valid and, although diametrically opposed in many areas, both represent legitimate options in the standard care of Lyme patients.

Some IDSA members began to see their role as gate keepers and preservers of their holy writ. IDSA associates would testify against those not towing the party line and sought action against physicians through state medical boards. Since IDSA is a large professional organization, their "experts" can label a doctor with the vague term "unprofessional" and thereby do a great deal of harm. The motivation for the vitriol was hard to understand.

---

3   *NGC is the National Guideline Clearinghouse which is a database of evidence-based clinical practice guidelines maintained by the Agency for Healthcare Research and Quality as part of the US Department of Health and Human Services.*

PEARL: The acronyms ILADS and IDSA are very close in letters if not philosophy. The shorter acronym refers to the organization that endorses the shorter treatment course. The acronym with the L prefers the longer treatment option if indicated. Took me a year to figure that out.

Because the IDSA Guidelines clearly restricted case management and limited the discretion of the attending physician, 19 members of Congress sent a letter to the CDC requesting review of the guidelines that effectively eliminated the existence and treatment of chronic Lyme disease. IDSA would not recognize any valid alternative therapies. By restricting physician discretion and patient options, IDSA opened itself up to legal proceedings since their actions effectively served to decrease competition.

Since guidelines are intended to influence medical practice and may be used to eradicate competing viewpoints, there is potential for conflict of interest and the possibility for secondary gain. By suggesting (or in this case requiring) the use of certain lab tests or preferring one treatment regimen over another, there is the real opportunity for commercial benefit. Gain is not always monetary but can be meted out in terms of panel chairmanships, career advancement, or promises of being a corporation's KOL on its "next big thing." All you need to do is witness the machinations of KOLs competing for most favored status to understand how motivated these people can be. When I was in the pharmaceutical industry, I could get a dozen calls from competing KOLs in the course of a day. At professional meetings, I would hide behind potted plants.

In the meantime, insurers had been given a gift that keeps on giving. By making the diagnostic hoops almost impossible to surmount, the "official" diagnosis of Lyme would remain elusive for many patients who were continuing to suffer. Patients had difficulty finding physicians who were willing to risk taking care of their on-going disease.

Over time, members of CALDA[4], along with other advocacy groups, felt that IDSA might be using its power to control medical practice. They considered the possibility of using antitrust laws to address the tight control imposed on clinical judgment imposed by the IDSA guidelines. The Attorney General of Connecticut, Richard Blumenthal, launched an antitrust investigation. Antitrust laws are concerned with the abuse of power by those in authority in ways that suppress competition. Here there were questions about the fairness and integrity of the guideline development process and how those guidelines were subsequently used to suppress options around the management of Lyme disease.

During the investigation, a number of interesting details were exposed. First, the panel charged with drafting the initial

IDSA guidelines was tainted with many conflicts of interest. Conflict of interest is a situation where an official's decisions might be influenced by personal agendas. The conflicted person is in a position where a professional or official role could be exploited for her own benefit. Both groups and individuals have multiple interests, and focus in one area could potentially corrupt impartial action in another area. COI does not automatically mean wrong-doing, just the potential for such. Conflicts can only exist if the person is in a position where impartiality may be important or where the person is trusted to act without bias. Some commentators feel that "self-policing" is the highest form of COI. This gives the artificial perception that COI has been eliminated when it has actually just been formalized.

When the IDSA investigation concluded, many improprieties had been uncovered and a settlement was reached where IDSA agreed to revisit its guidelines. The IDSA was to avoid bias and conflicts of interest, accept all submitted evidence for review, and hold public hearings. Each recommendation would be reviewed and the determination made whether the statement was medically sound. Revisions were expected to be made based on impartial evaluation.

Interestingly, IDSA convened essentially the same conflicted panel members as were involved with the first set of guidelines. Again, few of the many interested stakeholders were allowed to participate. When patient advocates complained that one interest group would essentially be speaking for all, the concerns were not heeded. IDSA eliminated participation by any HCP who earned more than $10,000 per year treating Lyme. This meant that no one who knew anything about Lyme could provide input. The AG had to step in and remove one panel member because the COI was blatant. The 1300 peer-reviewed studies and 300 pages of analysis submitted by ILADS were largely ignored and the primary compiler of the ILADS submission was not allowed to testify. The IDSA panel refused to hear certain information. The panel representatives then lied and said the panel was full when the membership was later increased with members who again had clear bias. When the deck is stacked, there can be the false appearance of unanimity and consensus.

Time for input was halved from two days to one. Some data presented as scientific evidence was actually compiled by an actuarial firm contracted by insurance interests. When one topic under review ended in a tie vote (astounding in itself since all members were selected for their parallel thinking), the voting rules were changed midstream in direct contradiction to the settlement agreement AND the internal rules previously established by IDSA. So, while IDSA has trouble accepting that not everyone wants to follow their guidelines, they seem comfortable discarding court directives and even rules they established to govern themselves. The panel sidestepped that issue by saying that the controversial item was

---

[4] *CALDA is now Lymedisease.org*

a *statement* and not a *recommendation* so that it did not fall under the settlement provisions that they review their *recommendations*. (I don't make this stuff up.)

This was the ultimate example of self-policing. How can you review 69 items and find NOTHING that could benefit from the slightest improvement? Obviously, perfection had been achieved and this from documents that had been determined to be so flawed that the drafting body was required to assess the validity of the entire original work. Not one item was found to need revision. This result came from guidelines determined to be so restrictive and potentially damaging that the Connecticut state legislature unanimously passed a law protecting HCPs who practiced outside their purview.

Before I examined the history, I had read the IDSA revision document, simply because I had run across it in the course of my research. On my initial reading I honestly didn't know the difference between ILADS and IDSA and that there was a blood feud between two sets of guidelines. I read this document totally cold and unbiased. I learned quickly. Fortunately, I had done enough examination of data over the years to know that something was fishy with the IDSA review. Here are the notes I wrote upon my initial assessment of the IDSA analysis:

For this book, I read page after page of IDSA guideline reviews. In Chapter 19 of this text, I counsel readers repeatedly to look for patterns and trends. Well, the IDSA documentation of their guideline review shows a distinct pattern. After each guideline statement made in the IDSA revision record, there is a section called "Discussion." The discussion is always the same. The panel has reviewed its own findings and found them to be correct. After reading the exact words over and over after each point, I had to chortle. Quite reassuring to see that the panel members agreed with themselves. I can think of no human interaction in the history of the cosmos where everyone agreed with everything in all cases. In my experience with groups attempting to reach consensus, or even simple majority, it is hard to reach agreement on where the bathrooms are, let alone a controversial point of contention. I don't agree with myself that consistently. Not one of the 69 statements was seen to be in need of any adjustment whatsoever. Personally, I don't find that intractability to be a testament to infallible science, but rather an inability to discern important nuances. Since patient welfare is at stake, I find the obstinance frightening. How much stronger their overall position would be if they had found even the most trivial improvements that could be made on the original document.

According to multiple media sources and court documents, many questionable decisions were made by IDSA during the review process. AG Blumenthal found that IDSA had represented certain items as independent scientific work when it was the work of the same panel members who had made

dubious contributions to the construction of the first set of guidelines. (Now THAT'S hubris!) The AG repeatedly expressed concern about COI and changes in voting procedures midstream. He said that the IDSA panel violated not only the settlement voting rules but also their own internal voting process. When questioned, one panel member was affronted at the allegations of COI, saying that since treatments were recommended using old drugs there could not be any possible monetary gain. In other sections I talk about the many ways to reward opinion leaders that do not involve immediate exchange of funds but are quite advantageous in the long-run. For example, if you play your cards right, you just might get the chair position of the same panel convened to review the work of the panel that you chaired (and compromised) in the first place. You could be the head fox in the hen house policing your own work that is the subject of such controversy. What an opportunity to vindicate yourself. To quote Diane Ravitch again: "An opinion once stated is by necessity an opinion forever defended." Notice that patient welfare has not been a big part of the IDSA argument at any juncture. In the end, the IDSA concluded that all 69 guideline recommendations were found to be "medically and scientifically justified in light of all the evidence and information and required no revision."

So, currently the contents of the original IDSA Lyme guidelines, which had been found to be flawed by numerous professional organizations as well as the state AG, remain inviolate. Today, when reading the IDSA original guidelines or their subsequent review document, the reader would be completely unaware that an alternative, valid guideline exists. An unsuspecting HCP just looking for some practice advice could assume that the management of Lyme is as clear and unambiguous as the IDSA makes it appear. Fortunately, the CT state government unanimously passed the legislation protecting HCPs from the restriction. There can be no retaliation for those HCPs who choose to manage Lyme patients with their own medical discretion. Of course, there are many ways to get back at heretics. I find it astounding that, in the case of Lyme, politicians are more reasonable about medical practice than a large physician-based medical organization. But what if you are sick and you don't live in Connecticut? I wonder if all IDSA members agree with the IDSA guidelines or are they just as embarrassed for their specialty as the rest of us? Perhaps they are unaware of the background story. Imagine the state having to pass a law to protect physicians from the work of a medical society. Imagine seeing a Lyme patient and not knowing there were valid alternatives aside from the IDSA guidelines. Imagine being that sick child and being told you aren't really sick and there is nothing more to be done for your complaints.

Although the AG in Connecticut initially pursued the case, recognizing the bogus review process, he moved on to higher office. Remember, I admitted to being biased.

The definitions provided below are not intended to be "legal" definitions since those differ from jurisdiction to jurisdiction and I wouldn't know how to write that way anyhow. Rather, I tried for brief explanations of terms that might be useful to Lyme HCPs, patients, and caretakers. Might come in handy if you want to read the antitrust judgment against IDSA.

Medicolegal terms common in Lyme references

Standard of care: The SOC is usually determined to be the level at which the average, prudent provider in a given community would practice medicine or how a similarly qualified HCP would manage a patient's care under similar circumstances.

In the past, SOC used to be based solely on physician judgment. No one would even consider questioning Marcus Welby on his medical decisions. He defined the standard of care. Today SOC is more often defined by the consensus of professional judgment in a given community. SOC is *not* defined by which guidelines are used. Rather the actual practice of HCPs in a locale is taken into account.

The SOC for managing a specific condition is determined by the manner in which practicing physicians actually treat patients. A practitioner in Toledo is judged compared to other physicians in Toledo and a practitioner in Coral Gables is measured against those nearby. Most jurisdictions recognize that more than one SOC may exist around a given medical condition, but many doctors do not.

With Lyme we have a conundrum. What if you are the physician setting the standard? What if your fellow HCPs have not yet evolved to your higher level of care? What if no one in the community is similarly qualified? What if you adhere to the guideline that is not in favor by the ruling party? I guess that is when the government has to pass laws to protect you from restricted medical practice and initiate antitrust investigations. Still, not everyone lives in a state where she is protected.

Lyme disease has split the medical community, or, at least, split those who are aware enough to know there is a controversy. In all legal matters thus far where persistent Lyme has been an issue, both the IDSA and ILADS guidelines have been recognized.

In cases where two or more valid guidelines might influence the SOC, the HCP must use her best judgment, in line with the patient's preferences, to select the best course for the individual. Here, the HCP can provide care within the provisions of either standard. The choice remains with the patient. Of course, informed choice can only take place if the patient is aware of the options. If the patient is presented with only one option, when the HCP is aware of two or more, is that ethical practice? Even if that choice later turns out to have been the wrong one or is in conflict with the choice preferred by another faction, the right to make that choice remains.

Community standard: Community standards are local norms defining acceptable conduct. Community standards can be used to judge everything from medical care to obscenity.

Antitrust: Antitrust legislation exercises control over monopolies with the intention of promoting fair competition. These measures can apply to all areas of business and are designed to protect competitors from unlawful restraints, controls, and unfair practices. I was encouraged by the ingenuity of the CALDA group (Lymedisease.org) and the Connecticut AG in recognizing the unfair playing field that existed around Lyme disease that was potentially harming patients.

Evidence: Evidence is the available body of facts or information supporting whether a proposition or belief is valid or true. Evidence can be helpful in forming a judgment or opinion and is offered to sustain a point or to provide foundation for a belief.

PEARL: IDSA contends that there is not enough evidence to support treatment of persistent manifestations of LD. Do we wait to treat diabetes, seizures, hypertension, or anything else until we have all possible information? As the patient experiences a repeat grand mal seizure do we say, "Since the medical community doesn't know all there is to know about seizures, we should hold off in diagnosing and treating this patient until we know everything there is to know. Since there is much muscle spasm and incontinence and altered consciousness in the general population, this might not really be a seizure and since it could be something else we should postpone doing anything since the patient is likely to eventually recover." Others in medicine and society would think we were delusional, in denial, or just plain daft.

Even if all the evidence says A causes B 99.9% of the time, you may have that one patient who is the outlier and that patient will need to have individualized attention. Besides, the strongest science does not absolve the HCP from responsibility to the patient and her unique case.

Evidence-based medicine: EBM is the integration of clinical experience with the best external evidence available to make sound medical decisions. Although EBM is touted to be the "new wave" in medicine, the idea first evolved in the mid-1950s when epidemiologist Archie Cochran tried to incorporate randomized, controlled studies as the gold standard for clinical research.

EBM is the use of current best evidence in making decisions around the care of an individual patient. The **best** evidence may not be the best science and you may only have *available* evidence to help you formulate a practical case management plan. While the term EBM is sometimes used as a synonym for good medical decision-making, that is not always the case. Plenty of abysmal medical decisions have been made while standing atop a stack of "evidence." To be worth anything in medical practice, evidence must be meshed with experience and common-sense.

Traditionally the premises around EBM did not include patient input. More recently, EBM proponents are encouraging the combination of science with patient participation to determine which option best suits the individual case. You can have all the swell, solid science on the planet, but if the patient doesn't want that particular approach, then that is her right. EBM requires on-going review of the science (which most docs have no idea how to do and even fewer have the time) or the reliance on others to digest the science for them. If those "others" have secondary agendas, interpretation of the science could be biased. Science must be incorporated with the clinician's training and experience, along with active involvement by the patient, to make the best decisions.

PEARL: For years drug reps with sandwiches and presents provided the only scientific exposure for most physicians. No possibility of COI there. A former colleague would only meet with the female reps and the meetings were private. We would look to see if Evie came out of the meeting with her pony tail on the same side of her head as when she went into the office. Other reps provided him with greens fees and concert tickets and amusement park passes. He never even listened to their biased sales pitches since he felt he knew all the latest science and he didn't have the time since he wanted to finish his latest Louis L'Amour novel before his afternoon patients. He did use their drugs plenty, whether they were indicated or not. Heartbroken, he was discouraged when the reps couldn't find a way to pay his daughter's private school tuition.

The practitioner has the responsibility not to be paternalistic and to provide valid alternatives. Likewise, the patient (or guardian) has the responsibility to be an educated consumer, understanding the options and weighing the risk/benefit. The best decisions are made in collaboration.

Unfortunately, EBM in some quarters has evolved into permission-not-to-think, cookie-cutter medicine. This type of medicine is detailed in Chapter 34: *Friendly Advice*. Optimally, EBM describes the best combination of all good facets of medicine. But at its worst, EBM results in HCPs screaming at 2-year-olds who dare not fit into their preordained boxes. Since anything outside the paradigm will require thought on the part of the HCP, some practitioners resent that intrusion on their time.

With Lyme and other recently discovered conditions, science lags behind the need to act. Even the most enthusiastic

proponent of EBM wouldn't require sick people to go without treatment until stronger science is amassed. Can you imagine what would have happened to the AIDS population if this were the thinking? Instead, HIV patients eventually had strong advocacy support campaigning for their care. If we were required to know everything about a condition before we could progress, no one would ever get treated for anything. Someone would always be insisting that the evidence that was available was not enough. When you're sick do you say, " I'd really prefer to do nothing until all the evidence is in." Just as the urologist at Fort Dix gave the trainees only Tylenol for THEIR kidney stones until he was whimpering for morphine for HIS kidney stone, perspectives change when it's you or your child who is sick.

In real life, Hitt estimates that only a small portion of actual practice is evidence-based. Most common practices have little to support them from controlled scientific studies. That is why so many clinical traditions that we thought were inviolate are now under scrutiny. When I was in medical school and at army basic training for physicians, we had to practice CPR on recording manikins until perfect. After many hours, our lips would bleed and we didn't even think about pathogen transmission back then, so we exchanged a lot of slobber. Well, all that mouth-to-mouth stuff for cardiac arrest was recently eliminated in one fell swoop. I never would have believed that there would be such a 180 degree turn. All gone. No more. So if you believe there will be no more changes in how you practice medicine in the remainder of your practice life, prepare to be disappointed. Of course, if some of these pronouncements run true to form, we will switch back just when we have all the books revised to accommodate these initial changes. Ordering mammograms or PSAs or colonoscopies in certain patient populations anytime soon? Well, if you do, you might be at odds with EBM.

EBM has been used as a shield to cover bad medical decisions. The HCP in a malpractice case or a chair of a guideline review panel might throw the term EBM around freely as though it justifies not taking good care of a patient.

In many actual cases there is good evidence for a particular intervention that has absolutely no practical value. With other therapies, there is little evidence but excellent value for a specific patient. Many innovations in surgery and trauma have come from the battlefield where there was no time to read the randomized, controlled clinical trials. These new methods were often pioneered by impressive medics on the front lines who wouldn't know a clinical trial report from a *Sports Illustrated*. Don't become an evidence snob. An objective anecdotal report can be as valuable to a similarly-presenting patient as a 10,000 patient trial. Use what might be helpful to your patient. Trust someone who has looked at data for the last 20+ years; you don't have time to parse each study. Consider what makes medical sense. Don't be a marionette. If an intervention works, you just had a successful experiment. Consider writing a case report. Then you will be part of the evidence-base.

Do not automatically value the quantitative over the qualitative. Remember that many of the gigantic, bazillion dollar, blinded, randomized, placebo-controlled clinical trials were conducted in a way that gives the best chance for a certain result. We are all naive to start. Many times the news media reports a medical breakthrough that we had uncovered in clinical trials 10 years ago or that are so obvious that one wonders why millions were spent proving what grandma had been saying since 1930. In fact, in a number of serious conditions, controlled studies can be unethical if there is a well-established, effective, treatment and part of the study population would be denied this known treatment in order to be randomized to a placebo arm. With Lyme, due to the complexity of the disease and the heterogeneity of the population, don't expect robust clinical trial results soon. You may not have much more than you currently have to work with for a number of years.

Most medicine is practiced in an arena of uncertainty. If the outcome of every decision was 100% guaranteed prior to implementation, a robot could and should practice medicine. We do not have the luxury of waiting until more, or better, or all evidence comes in, especially in an area where you know there is not a large, robust, prospective study in the offing. When you are the HCP responsible for the patient sitting nearby, you have a different perspective on evidence than those who see patients only on paper.

Good EBM is simply what clinical practice always should be: the combination of science, continuous learning, experience, training, and good sense. Add the patient and a dash of compassion and you have good medicine.

Consensus: Consensus describes an opinion reached by a group as a whole. Consensus seeks consent, not necessarily agreement. I could never get that point across to my Swedish colleagues who were obsessed with consensus. They were not satisfied with your consent but wanted to spend days getting you to UNDERSTAND their point of view even after you had surrendered to their plan a week ago. Consensus is a commonly agreed position or conclusion arrived at after resolution of any important disagreements. Consensus usually builds group solidarity and commitment to a plan. Majority opinion is different from consensus since majority rule implies winners and losers and is competitive rather than cooperative. Consensus can build on compromise. Be careful, desire to build consensus can lead to coercion.

Medically necessary: As with many health care concepts medical necessity is in the eye of the beholder. I believe birth control is a medical necessity and Rick Santorum does not. Some believe that Viagra is a medical necessity but most

80-year-old women that I have seen in the clinic do not. ("If you give him that stuff, I'm going to flush it down the toilet.") After I had a bad fall and most of my face remained on Haines Mill Road, I had a different opinion about the medical necessity of cosmetic procedures. I was getting skin grafts and laser treatments to put me back together again in a way that my wounds would not scare small children. I was not getting procedures to make me cuter or younger or sexier. This distinction had to be clearly made to the insurer. Third party payers use the term "medically necessary" to describe what they *will* cover after they have justified the intervention as reasonable or appropriate (necessary), based on evidence-based SOC. Medical necessity can apply to the diagnosis and treatment of illness or injury or to the need to improve function. In my experience, multiple appeals may be needed before *your* medical necessity becomes *their* medical necessity. Of course, there are opportunities for abuse. Not all approved users of medical marijuana have a legitimate medical need.

Guidelines: The term guideline comes from a line or rope used to aid travelers over a difficult point. If only that were the case in the current medical use of the term. Guidelines are guides, not laws or regulations. They are recommendations for practice that should allow both discretion and leeway in their interpretation, implementation, and use. Guidelines have a number of functions. For some practitioners, like me, guidelines save time and provide a quick clue on how to handle a case that I might not see every day.

More than a few HCPs have no idea that there are any guidelines available for anything. In clinical research, I used them for insight into protocol writing and study design. I suspect that, as with most clinicians, I would have no idea that more than one guideline might be available for a particular disease. Guidelines are just *there* and I never considered where they might come from or that political and personal bias might enter into their construction. If you see TBI patients daily you will be very familiar with the existence of a guideline from both ILADS and IDSA. If you see one Lyme patient a month, you will not likely know the depth of the guideline conflict or the potential repercussions of choosing one approach over the other.

I know from working with a company that sold a generic amoxicillin in a new formulation, a number of physicians can be aware of a guideline for something like OM and choose not to follow the recommendations because it does not fit into their practice experience. They toss the recommendations even farther out the window when their own child has AOM. I know of no colleague who considers a guideline a mandatory way for them to practice medicine. A general practitioner would have to quit practice in order to find time to read and essentially memorize all the guidelines she could reasonably be expected to use in a family practice if guidelines were mandatory.

While guidelines can provide useful "Cliffs Notes" for the HCP, they cannot replace the fundamental basic knowledge that is required to make real medical decisions. Especially with a complex, multifaceted condition, nothing can replace experience and training in the therapeutic area.

While the potential for guidelines to be used for the greater good exists, there are pitfalls to recognize. As we have learned the hard way, guidelines can restrict patient care, enhance third party interests, diminish competing viewpoints, and limit clinical judgment due to inflexibility. Stolberg estimates that between 72% and 90% of contributors to practice guidelines have undisclosed COIs. Be aware of these numbers. Even if Stolberg is only half correct, would that be any less outrageous? Even one entrenched contributor could potentially bias the entire process.

While ILADS acknowledges the existence of another guideline, IDSA does not. Not knowing the availability of alternative methods restricts patient choice and autonomy. Rigid guidelines where HCPs have to fear reprisal for non-compliance give the impression that an organization has more power than it really has, and implies that they somehow regulate this area of medicine, which they do not. Still guidelines can be used to discredit an HCP in front of a medical review board.

The IDSA Lyme guidelines discount the role of the history, physical, symptoms, clinical course, and response to therapy. Unproven symptoms are totally left out of their recommendations. We all know it is difficult to quantify the subjective. However, that does not mean that the qualitative is not real. IDSA requires objective measures that they know are not currently available or are so flawed as to be dangerous. Yet, the history and other qualitative parameters are critical points of evidence available in real time. Their guidelines discount the experience of the HCP. There are many medical conditions that lack biomarkers or other quantitative measures and HCPs must rely largely on symptoms for diagnosis. Sometimes IDSA practitioners elect to ignore demonstrable signs as well, such as the tick in a jar and the bite scab sitting inside an EM lesion.

The goal of guidelines should be to improve patient care both for individuals and groups. Better outcomes should come from better guidelines. How convenient not to keep track. The goal should not be to control medical practice at the expense of provider discretion. Feeling coerced to go down a treatment path in direct contradistinction to the clinical picture in front of you, would make most reasonable HCPs nervous. Any provider with compassion would be affronted. Yet, fear of reprisal is very powerful and quite understandable. No wonder my son's clinic physician in Maryland whispered the word *Lyme*. As clever and determined as the chronic Lyme community is, someone will soon latch onto this possibility and previously unexamined legal avenues could be explored.

Inflexible guidelines create a false regulatory environment. This environment is open to abuse from all sides. Guidelines that attempt to dictate rather than inform eliminate the decision-making role reserved for HCPs and patients. The guideline authors have no hands-on responsibility for the outcome. How much easier to ignore suffering that you never have to witness.

Recent reviews of guidelines from various medical sources show that most do not meet basic quality standards. Many are of little value and look as though no one had a cousin who could proofread. (My editors will make me take that phrase out for being mean, but you should read some of this stuff.)

Trust me, nothing would have delighted me more than if the IDSA recommendations of short-term treatment would have worked for my son. He would have gotten better, we would not have gone through hell for months, and I would not have felt compelled to spend years of 18-hour days writing this book. If only the IDSA guidelines did what they are advertised to do. Yes, Chris did "eventually recover" but only after aggressive long-term treatment. What possible kick-back do I get from stating those facts? I have no secondary gain. Bad guidelines can hurt people. First, do no harm.

At best, guidelines provide a succinct compilation of research and accepted practice. For the HCP too busy to read all the literature himself, especially if there are thousands of articles and hundreds of books pertinent to the condition, guidelines should be lifelines for the practitioner. Unfortunately, guidelines can be used to ration health care and undermine autonomy of both doctors and patients.

When IDSA says there is no compelling evidence to change their guidelines, what do they mean? If they mean controlled clinical trials they are right. Equally true is the lack of compelling evidence to support their position. In fact, conclusions from controlled trials are rarely used to set the SOCs for the majority of conditions. Why is there a different standard for Lyme?

In my exposure to the staff of the local ER, I have another complaint about questionable, rigid guidelines. Both the ER doc and Lilith[5] seemed empowered by misinformation. They were very rote, disrespectful, and condescending to my son and the other TBI patients within ear shot. Were they emboldened by guidelines that enabled them to dismiss the critically ill children in front of them? Their arguments were circular and illogical: We should be satisfied that he was already being treated for Lyme, which they swore he didn't have. Yet it must be Lyme, since Lyme could present with fevers over 105, but the EM rash at the bite site and the deer tick in hand did not in any way suggest Lyme. His symptoms could NOT be anything else aside from Lyme, but they could NOT be

_____

5 *See Glossary or Introduction for name origin*

Lyme. He turned out to have lab-confirmed Lyme, babesiosis, and ehrlichiosis. Bartonellosis was also diagnosed later. My head was spinning. Which is more frightening, that the guidelines inspired this ineptness or that they are seeing numerous TBI patients each day without knowledge of either guideline?

An appropriate use of guidelines is to provide information especially around the risks and benefits of alternative approaches to care. But guidelines that drive medicine in one direction, when there are equally legitimate alternatives, do not take the responsibility from the attending HCP. Automatic decisions based on guidelines instead of the specifics of the case can get you in trouble and, besides, it's just not the ethical path.

Partially inspired by the cry for reform of the guideline formulation process, the Institute of Medicine has national standards for guideline development. IOM weighed the evidence/consensus balance that goes into drafting guidelines and came forward with recommendations including review of a broad body of various types of evidence and input from diverse stakeholders. Further, organizations like the American National Standards Institute have a due process mission and could potentially have a role in overseeing a balanced guideline-development process. Some neutral and fair parameters might be that all stakeholders can participate and give a position and have that position considered. There should be ability to appeal, open dialog, lack of dominance by one faction on the committee or during discussion, balance, confidential votes, consideration of divergent views, patient input, recorded comments on negative votes, and agreement on procedural matters, such as voting, occurring *before* the panel convenes. Independent monitoring during the IDSA guideline review might have helped produce a less biased result. Instead we had the fox providing security at the hen house. An impartial review of the final product might keep all parties aboveboard.

Guidelines can be useful time-savers, but they do not remove the responsibility to know the underlying medicine. Take from the guidelines what will benefit your patients and be aware of all options for both your sakes.

Informed consent: Patients must have sufficient information in order to make reasonable decisions. This means a clear appreciation and understanding of the facts, implications, and potential consequences around an action. The concept of informed consent becomes more complicated when dealing with children and their guardians. Either way, informed consent involves communication between the HCP and patient or legal representative.

I recall no informed consent with my son with his initial HCPs, but plenty of intimidation. Any questions resulted in an eye-roll and were taken as an affront to their medical acumen. When we tried to provide a piece of information that we thought might help solve the puzzle, we were met with derision since the piece didn't fit neatly into some preconceived algorithm. We were never informed that there were two schools of thought on Lyme or that options were available. My son was given a huge dose of acetaminophen in the ER (probably higher than that recommended in the acetaminophen-in-the-ER guidelines) and then we were told that he ONLY had a 102 fever not over 105 as we had said, as though we had embellished in order for him to appear sicker. Guidelines written by St. Luke himself cannot make up for plain old bad medicine.

Lyme can be a serious condition that can progress to permanent injury and even death. Assume that most patients would like to be informed about the existence of alternative treatment, especially if the approach currently in use is not working.

Legitimate informed consent should allow for questions since consent implies that the patient wants to move forward with the proposed plan. Informed consent law varies considerably from state to state. The paternalism allowed in the past is not as accepted by courts today. Be aware that providing the patient with appropriate balanced information is the best way to go from any perspective.

> *PEARL: Except in emergencies, consent is obtained prior to a course of treatment. During consent the patient is given the information necessary to be able to make informed decisions in the selection of treatments. Usually the pros and cons are discussed as well as the risks of not undergoing the treatment. The probability of success is reviewed as well as alternative approaches. With balanced information the patient or caretakers can weigh the risk/benefit and come to an informed decision.*

Conflict of interest: Conflict of interest is a situation where an individual's decisions might be influenced by personal agendas. The person is in a position where a professional or official role could be exploited for her own benefit. Both groups and individuals have multiple interests and focus in one area could potentially corrupt impartial action in another area. COI does not automatically mean wrong doing, just the potential for bias. Conflicts can only exist if the person is in a position where neutrality may be expected or where the person is trusted to act without prejudice. Some COI is obvious while other conflicts are not so apparent. "Self-policing" is a form of COI that gives the perception that all is objective when the bias has just been sanctioned. Most conflicts are associated with health care companies, insurers, or other commercial enterprises. When I worked with companies in Asia and the subcontinent, COI was referred to as bribes and was frequently encouraged (as was smuggling). Dr. Bransfield has speculated that there would be no Lyme controversy at all if money wasn't involved.

Patient preferences: There is actually a journal called the *Journal of Patient Preferences and Adherence*. Who knew? A medical preference is a choice made by a person after considering the options. The patient may regard one treatment useful and another not so much. She may prefer one delivery method over another. In some cases the patient may decide the risk is not worth the benefit. What is the patient willing to tolerate? While patient opinion should always be respected, the sicker the person, perhaps the more important to consider her preferences.

Traditionally, patient preferences took a back seat to physician paternalism, since the patient was not considered capable of making decisions in his own best interest. Clearly, the best medical decisions are made in a collaboration between patient and HCP.

> *PEARL: One of my pet peeves is the practitioner who, after presenting the options, then takes absolutely no role in assisting the patient in making the decision. I am not talking about the type of guidance where the HCP assumes you are too simple-minded to make your own choice and therefore steers you to only one possible conclusion. The information available, much of it conflicting, can be overwhelming to most patients. In the case of children, you have one person too young to input and panicked parents too distraught to reason objectively. The compassionate, technical input of the HCP would be appreciated right about now. Here is what I would like my HCPs to say to me: "Here are the pros and cons of Choice A. Here are the pros and cons of Choice B. Ultimately, the decision will be yours but I will help you weigh your choices. Knowing what I know about your case I think that Choice A might be better for you and here are my reasons. If this were my child, I would favor choice A over B because of the specifics of the case. Let's tackle any questions you might have before you make your decision" I had one practitioner tell me that if I didn't agree to do everything her way with my son she would not see him. He was so sick I would have agreed to anything.*

Respect for patient autonomy is a fundamental part of medical ethics. Having spent too much time over the past 3 years sitting in hospitals with in-patient relatives, I realize that most patients have no idea that they can say no. The doctor is still sacred. I had to preach forever to my mom that it was better to tell the nurse that she despised Metamucil and was throwing it away as soon as the nurse left the room, than to let the staff think she was taking medicine that wasn't working. Once she confessed, we were able to bring in her fiber from home and she was happy as a clam. She told me she didn't think she was allowed to say no and that she didn't want to hurt the doctor's

feelings. HCPs need to respect patient preferences and not take a "no" personally. Patients must realize that they do not need to accept everything thrown in their path and they can refuse. If you are the declining patient, all decisions should be carefully considered since you don't want to put your HCP in the position where she has to cajole you every step of the way. Both sides might need to give a little.

Where the patient is in the clinical course of her disease can influence her preferences. The more seriously ill patients may have a different view than those with a milder presentation. Others who have been sick for a long time may see things differently than those who are just recognizing they have a TBI. Whether the patient sees herself as progressing and getting worse or improving and getting better may influence her decisions. One patient may be able to tolerate drug side effects much better than another who physically cannot stand a certain treatment. For some the QOL and functionality issues are paramount. Some patients may change their mind during the course of treatment. More than once. Make sure that the patient is not declining treatment because they are too depressed to agree to anything. A patient who has been unsuccessfully treated in the past may weigh his choices differently from a relapsing patient who had been responsive to antibiotics previously. Individualize the treatment approach based on the specifics of the case and patient preferences.

If you do not tell the patients about options you curb their autonomy and their ability to make reasoned decisions. The AMA reviews these concepts in their Code of Medical Ethics. The AMA prefers that the physician disclose and discuss with the patient, not only the risk/benefit of the proposed treatment, but also the availability of options regardless of cost or insurance coverage.

Sadly, some HCPs see the same conditions over and over and over all day long. They take for granted that the patient already knows all the options and all the pros and cons. They assume the decision has been made in favor of the approach they feel is best. No matter how obvious the decision is for them, the patient has the right to ask questions and input into their own treatment plan. I recall the first orthopod I went to for my Lyme-decimated knee. The nurse took my history. The doctor came in and said not a single word to me and then told the nurse to schedule me for surgery and walked out of the room. So much for options.

IDSA implies that short-term treatment is the only option when, in fact, another option exists that would allow for continued therapy. By failing to recognize alternative management plans for persistent LD, the IDSA does not consider patient preference and this is a paternalistic approach. Patient choice is crucial since the patient knows best what has been occurring and what he might be able to accept in his particular case. The greatest treatment plan on earth has

NO chance of being effective if the patient is non-compliant. Only the patient knows what he is willing to tolerate. Usually the patient is motivated to act in his own interest. In pediatrics, the parents I saw were desperate for options and to do the best they could for their child. Paternalism assumes the patient or guardian is too mentally feeble to make a reasonable choice and must be protected from himself in order to prevent a bad decision. Under ideal circumstances, paternalism can be viewed as compassionate, but often it is used as a means of control and a way to coerce the patient to go down a path they might not choose for themselves. My husband's co-worker was begging for additional treatment. He was not given a choice.

Paternalism: The term paternalism refers to those in medical authority acting like a father or parent. Benign paternalism is great if you're someone's dad but from a medical perspective in 2013, it's not a compliment. Paternalism allows people in authority to restrict and control the behavior of subordinates. The underling has no freedom or responsibility. That works if you're 2-years-old, but for adults and older kids, the concept is insulting. How many women have been told not to worry their pretty little heads over an important issue, even when that issue was their own health?

A father provides for the child's needs without her input. All is done "in the child's best interest" for her own good. The parent can use his power to control, protect, punish, and reward in return for obedience and loyalty. Until very recently the tradition in health care has been paternalism, which has also been used to justify slavery and child abuse. Paternalism is rooted in the idea that the almighty doctor is always correct and the patient is too naive to take action on her own behalf.

In 2013 in the US, patients have the right to input into their own medical decisions and say no to any procedure or plan that they feel does not meet their health needs. Without repercussion. Still, often the knowledge gap is so great between HCP and patient that the patient (including me) can be easily manipulated to go in the direction that the HCP steers. The caretakers of Lyme patients that I observed in preceptorships had educated themselves to such a degree that they were able to combat the previous paternalism and find their way to a helpful HCP. Still, many patients do not have the same opportunity.

Medical decision-making: My son is a slow decision-maker, as are many of his contemporaries. He is often astounded that I am able to make decisions so quickly. I tell him that is from years in the ER, where you are required to act before all the information is in. Sometimes we had to run two codes at once. That was just how life was a few years ago. You did the best you could with what you had. Actually, we did pretty well even though we never had the option to wait for all the data to be on-hand before we had to respond.

With Lyme, decision-making is complicated by the existence of the two guidelines. Physicians aware of the controversy and the possible repercussions against HCPs not following the IDSA paradigm may feel intimidated to choose the guidelines from the more powerful organization. This type of decision-making has nothing to do with the science that is supposed to support the recommendations. As one of my physician friends said, "All I know is that a couple of weeks of doxy and he'll be fine." This is not decision-making but rote recitation of unsubstantiated medical lore. By the way, he wasn't fine.

Most HCPs recognize that the more complicated the case, the more you must target the treatment to the individual patient. Just as one drug manufacturer touts the idea on TV that each individual with RA has a unique presentation, this individualized approach must be considered in the complicated Lyme patient. The more the therapy needs to be targeted for the specific case, the more important are collaboration and clinical judgment in arriving at a treatment plan.

In managing Lyme, as with other conditions clouded with therapeutic uncertainty, HCPs must decide if they are going to be conservative and risk under-treating or aggressive and risk over-treating. My son was so sick that I didn't think he was going to live. Guess which approach I would select. Damn the potential for superbugs, save my kid! Yes, I understand the responsibility I have as a physician for the health of the general population, but I have seen no evidence that long-term treatment for Lyme has resulted in highly resistant pathogens that will adversely impact the rest of humankind.

Medical decisions must take many factors into account: What are the pros and cons of the various options? How significant is the possible morbidity and mortality? Are permanent sequelae possible? How is the patient functioning day-to-day? What is the risk of bad outcomes or side effects? Will the treatment selected make a difference? Will delaying treatment help or hurt the patient? What is the worst that can happen if you're wrong?

A high percentage of malpractice cases are filed because of perceived missed or delayed diagnoses so that treatment was postponed or not done. These misses and delays resulted in adverse outcomes that may have been preventable had the problem been addressed sooner. Collaborative decision-making is the best way to prevent discord later. Of course, if the shared decision-making is not documented, it is assumed to have not happened. I recall writing the following note in a family practice patient chart: "Pt is still v concerned @ skin lesion she perceives to be present on abd. Despite (-) cultures, (-) fungal testing, (-) bx results, & a derm consult which found nothing of concern, pt remains anxious. She'll RTC 1 month for re-exam and to plan f/u if needed." While this may be overkill, when the patient returned in 4 weeks she was satisfied that her problem was resolved and I documented that as well.

I often hear complaints about delayed diagnosis and treatment. Recently my friend's grandson was taken to his PCP and the ER repeatedly for what was diagnosed as growing pains and various viruses. Four weeks after the initial visit he was diagnosed with leukemia. Treatment was delayed a month because of the classic, Lilith[6], cavalier brush-off. With his type of leukemia, that month would have been priceless to have back. I have never heard a single patient complain that a doctor was overly concerned, listened too much, or decided to treat when treatment wasn't really warranted. I often hear, "He didn't do anything." Antibiotic treatment can always be stopped if it's no longer indicated. But, time lost in waiting to treat or electing not to treat can never be regained.

The HCP's role in decision-making is to provide information including the availability of options. Using her knowledge and experience, the HCP then works with the patient (and family as appropriate) to arrive at the best course of action for that individual. The doctor neither takes over the process nor abandons the patient in the middle of the course. There usually isn't just one right approach. The risks and benefits must be weighed. What is the patient's goal for her treatment? How do you get there from here?

What if the patient or family decides to proceed in a way that you, as the HCP, totally oppose? I believe there is nothing wrong with reiterating your views and trying to steer in the other direction. But, do not assume that your values are their values or that your acceptable level of risk is identical to theirs. Do not coerce or intimidate, or (as I have witnessed both personally and professionally) threaten. Regardless of the HCP's views, the final decision among options belongs to the patient. I have seen doctors pout. As long as the patient has had a balanced hearing of the options, you must let him decide. For goodness sake, document the discussion and your advice that alternative paths might be considered.

While the patient benefits from good medical decisions, he also suffers from the bad ones. This is why open communication and collaboration is essential. The HCP role here is to provide the patient with all the information and tools she needs to decide wisely. The HCP inputs his experience and knowledge. The best way to review risk/benefit of the various options is together. You can't do that if you do not reveal all the options. All decisions, medical and otherwise, involve trade-offs and juggling the risk/benefit ratio. Make a pro and con list. There may be more than one "right" answer.

Treatment Options: Where two SOCs exist most jurisdictions recognize the obligation to provide treatment that abides by *either* standard. Still, patient choice is important. To be able to make a reasonable choice, the patient has to be aware of the options. There is no reason to think that all Lyme patients realize the existence of two guidelines. The HCP would

be expected to provide that information in a balanced way. The HCP is expected to outline alternatives, not be paternalistic, and not deride opposing views. The patient or guardian must be allowed to make an autonomous choice.

Since the patient is usually in the weaker position in terms of knowledge and experience regarding a particular condition, the doctor must be aware of the possibility that the patient is overwhelmed or intimidated or scared. Parents of very sick kids are usually terrified and dazed and the HCP should be careful not to take advantage of their weakened state to impose his values or biases on them. Consider what you would do if this were your child. Do not take a refusal of a particular approach as a personal affront. It's not always about you.

With Lyme, stopping treatment when the patient is still sick can result in significant adverse sequelae which can be permanent. Although most death certificates do not list Lyme as an underlying cause (it's more politically correct to just say cardiopulmonary arrest), people die from Lyme more often than necessary. Patients should have the option to select which of the two valid approaches to select. Of course, if you are discussing treatment options with an ILADS physician, you can go either way. If you are working with an IDSA physician, you might have to change HCPs if you want longer treatment. That reality in itself can be seen as restricting patient options. Most patients do not like to get into a contest with their doctor. They are not equipped for the debate. Even as a physician, I did not feel competent to argue in a field I knew little about. Each time I mentioned a fact that did not seem to fit into the rigid model they were embracing, I was shot down (rudely). At least at the onset of my son's illness, I just didn't know enough to present a rational case or realize there were alternatives.

Depending on the HCP, the patient might not be aware that a whole other avenue is available to address chronic Lyme. Further, without knowing the options, the patient may not realize that a decision was made for her. Whether the patient would have approved of that decision or not, never seems to enter the equation. Remember that without a specific restrictive clause in the insurance contract, the choice usually remains with the patient if the treatment is within the SOC.

My husband came home concerned that his co-worker was cut off from long-term treatment for his Lyme, even though his symptoms repeatedly flared when his medicine was discontinued. I told my husband to inform his friend that he may have options that were not disclosed to him. He had no idea that there was another valid, approved treatment approach. It didn't sound like his HCP knew either. She was reciting right off the IDSA manifesto. She was young and seemingly interested in helping her patient, but felt her hands were tied. Oh, the damage that can come from hubris.

---

6 *See Glossary or Introduction for name origin*

Economic factors and the impact on patient preference: Without the possibility of secondary gain, in all its glorious manifestations, there would not likely be such a vehement Lyme controversy. For third party payers, there are economic incentives to restrict access to care. Some authors believe that managed care deliberately sets up obstacles to encourage the chronically ill to leave their program. Other literature documents the repeated disapprovals for certain interventions and recommend numerous appeals before surrender. (My personal experience is that 4 or 5 appeals may be needed to get results. Make it more costly for them to keep reviewing and denying than it would be for them to pay your request.) Of course, some people take advantage. I remember in the early 80s when I was a medical student, HCPs would send in a half dozen patients after office hours for a 3 or 4 day hospital stay just to increase revenues. Families would send grandma to the hospital for the weekend when they wanted to be free for a little holiday. I appreciate prudent use of healthcare, but a systemic and automatic program of denials may need to be confronted when the care is legitimate and medically necessary.

Although some payers have jumped on restrictive guidelines as a way to control costs, guidelines do not dictate SOC. Managed care groups are supposed to provide the reason for denial. Initial denials are often on form letters that are automatically issued. "Telephone contact is not covered" or "Your treatment was not determined to be medically necessary." Medical necessity is supposed to be based on physician discretion. Many HCPs do not have time to deal with the repeated appeals and their staffs try to deal with the payers. Supposedly the unique presentation of each case is to be taken into consideration.

PEARL: I remember one managed care gate keeper telling me that I had to send a critically ill patient (Stevens-Johnson syndrome) to Philadelphia or New York since their plan had no dermatologists in Delaware since Delaware was not a state. What do you say to that? "What does Delaware's statehood have to do with a shocky patient who has sloughed off all his skin on my exam table? Delaware is not only a state, it is the FIRST state!" She then tried another approach, "Oh, Dr. Spreen you are so smart, you can handle this case and that patient doesn't need a specialist." I said, "If I tell you I can't handle it in the office, I can't handle it. If he dies, your name will be listed as the cause of death on his death certificate." I have a million of these stories. How about the guy that the managed care company transferred by ambulance from Philadelphia to me in Wilmington (70 miles roundtrip) because his donor kidney was en route *to the transplant hospital? As his listed PCP, I was required to do the pre-op clearance physical prior to the surgery, which was to take place in a few hours. Only I would do. The dozen specialists who had been taking care of him for the last month as an in-patient could not clear him for surgery. He showed up at my office at about 5 p.m. on a Friday afternoon unannounced and fortunately*

I was still there to see him. He had tried to tell them this was a silly waste of money, but they would not listen. I was the PCP of record. What was I going to do, deny his kidney transplant because he had a bunion? What were these people thinking?

Dr. Liegner wrote about a case in 2002 describing a Lyme patient who died within one month of being denied further insurance coverage for IV antibiotics. While this case was documented ten years ago, we still struggle with the same issues. The case of my husband's co-worker detailed above, who was still sick when his treatment was discontinued, and who historically flared to the point of incapacity each time his antibiotic was stopped, is too familiar. Bob Dylan should have been talking about Lyme when he asked, "When will we ever learn?"

Expert opinion: An expert is a specialist in a subject who has gained more than the usual expertise through experience or training. Today we hear a great deal about expert opinion in both the judicial and medical arenas. In these cases, an expert witness is called upon to present an opinion that might have impact on a decision or influence behavior in others, like prescribing a certain drug or adhering to a certain practice guideline. Usually an "expert" is recognized as such by peers in the field or "made" by corporate endorsement. Physician proficiency in an area is often considered based on how many similar cases they have seen.

PEARL: As I type, I see in the background on my muted TV the face of Dr. Conrad Murray. His case around the SOC of Michael Jackson underscores the important point that experts can be bought. There were articulate experts providing opinion on both sides of the aisle in this case. All the testifying experts had lists of credentials a mile long. Having worked a bit on propofol in a past life I had an inkling on who knew what they were talking about. I worry more about a cardiologist who asks the patient's kids and staff if anyone knows CPR than his misuse of propofol. Further, experts can be made. In the pharmaceutical industry I would return the calls from wanna-be KOLs that I liked and ignore for months those I did not. This had nothing to do with their expertise in the given field. If they were arrogant, pompous, and entitled, they were going to be waiting a while.

How do I know so much about experts and KOLs? Because I was trained in the pharmaceutical KOL sycophant school. There were entire departments devoted to KOL relationships. We even had internal meetings to decide who the up-and-comers were so we could mold them to suit our purposes. When we needed "expert" testimony at the FDA or in court, we could pick from a long list of "appropriate" candidates already bought and paid for – two factions using each other with the money made from selling drugs at exorbitant rates. Even groups were part of this quid pro quo. If a professional organization would agree to like our drug best, we would pay for TV ads saying that patients needed a medical procedure performed primarily by that specialty group to make the diagnosis of the condition treated by our drug. Starting to see how this works?

I may have mentioned the "expert" in the women's health field from the UK who was thought to be the "top of his field." He drove his $200,000 car hundreds of miles to a meeting on the continent. He bragged that he averaged over 100 mph. He had his girlfriend in the car (his wife was home) and he was drunk to the point of lapsing consciousness. The girlfriend had to take over the driving after arguing with him heatedly about his ability to stay behind the wheel. When we got to our thatch-hut restaurant meeting, he nearly started the place on fire by knocking over several candles. He continued to drink all through dinner on the corporate tab. The next day at the professional meeting where he was to present all the reasons why a particular drug was much better than the competition, he passed out at the podium. When he came to, he staggered over to the competitor's seminar and spoke there.

Experts are paid to take all sides of an issue. My expert can beat up your expert. This has little to do with science and more to do with charm and finesse. I recall a story of a KOL from Australia when I was working on PPIs. I was at one company working on a certain PPI and had worked with this KOL. When I moved to another company and was working on a different PPI, this same guy was again one of the investigators. When I had to contact him regarding a study patient, he was going on and on about my old drug. " Hi, Kathy, so good to hear from you. At the meeting next week, I hope the FDA approves the new indication because your drug is the best PPI on the market." On and on, I finally broke in to tell him I was now working at the competitor company. He actually gasped, "Oh good, because that drug is really the best on the market. By far superior." He was tripping over himself and stammering trying to back-pedal. Actually the drugs were essentially identical and as the product physician for both, I would be hard pressed to find clear distinctions between them, but this guy was able to change his loyalty and passion on the drop of a dime (literally). I learned over the years that the opinion leaders' convictions are based mostly on the size of your checkbook. For a fee you can get experts to say anything. Like politicians they will gladly contradict themselves next week if it suits their agenda.

When there is weak or minimal science, experts are sometimes used to fill the gap. Expert opinion is not necessarily evidence. Some experts stake their careers on one particular theory and then resist any challenge to their authority, even long after new data has shown them to be incorrect.

There are many ways to compensate a KOL that do not involve actual cash crossing palms. Drug companies want to influence prescription writers and formulary compliers and guideline developers through their use of KOLs. So, before

you get too enthralled by the credentials of some of the experts, look at their ties to the insurance and pharmaceutical industries. Many have been paid handsomely for their "objective" opinions.

Patient autonomy: Medical autonomy is the right of patients to make decisions about their own care without undue influence on those decisions. Autonomy is self-determination in personal matters. However, true autonomy requires being aware of the options. Keeping patients from knowing that there are two accepted sets of guidelines removes their autonomy. HCPs must respect a patient's right to choose and thereby steer their own path to health and wellness.

The existence of two distinct guidelines with different risk/benefit ratios for each patient makes patient preference an even more critical part of the equation. What is right for one patient may be detrimental to another. Patients need to understand that they have the right to choose and refuse. Yes, we have all talked a reluctant child into holding still for the blood test that she doesn't want or to swallow medicine she would rather give to the cat. This is not what we are referring to here. In pediatrics, the caretakers are the ones whose autonomy must be protected. This doesn't mean the tail wags the dog and the HCP is expected to bow to unreasonable treatment plans formulated by laypersons. Communication and collaboration are key.

The patient (or guardian) has the right to leave a medical relationship at any time but the HCP needs to be careful he doesn't abandon the patient without all the recommended warnings. Is it abandonment to stop treating a patient that is still sick and asking for continuing treatment? I don't know, but I'm acquainted with several people who do. Patients, who leave one HCP, may have trouble finding another who has even heard of TBIs or the controversy around chronic manifestations. There are doctors who don't know anything about Lyme and there are those who don't want to take on the responsibility of a complex, chronic, potentially incapacitating disease – especially in the middle of intense controversy, where there might be punishment for selecting one guideline approach over another. There are plenty of other "easy" diseases to occupy the day. Why invite trouble?

If options aren't provided and patients don't realize they have a choice, there is no autonomy. Respect for autonomy is the legal basis for informed consent.

Ethics: Ethics are the moral principles that govern behavior and can apply to either individuals or groups. In medicine, one application of ethics is putting the needs of the patient first. Additional definitions of ethics include doing the right thing when no one is watching and never doing anything that you wouldn't do in front of your grandmother. If someone asks how to tell what the right choice is, tell them that people always know, they just don't want to admit it.

IX. The future of the Lyme controversy

The Lyme controversy makes doctors scared. In our litigious society after reading what happened to the good guys treating TBIs, people are scared. The controversy will likely continue until the primary adversaries are no longer active. Many could have a lot of face to save. While even IDSA is now grudgingly admitting that *a few* patients might have on-going infection, more years will be required for the thinking to evolve. Still, certain individuals persist in not seeing the writing on the wall, while thousands of patients continue to suffer.

As long as special interests like pharmaceutical companies, insurers, and realtors benefit from minimizing the impact of chronic Lyme, the controversy will persist. Would you buy a house on a lot where the tick population and subsequent disease caused the previous owners to flee? I did. I didn't know any better. I later learned that local political machinations allowed developers to not disclose the presence of an endemic Lyme area. During one of my preceptorships, one parent was a local realtor. He explained everything. He no longer lives in endemic areas, but he still sells houses there. Guess which topic usually doesn't get introduced. HCPs, like me, change our perspective when our own children get sick. Bb are changing the nature of the debate, one sick child at a time.

How do you practice medicine in this controversial world where good people are pilloried? Unfortunately, a number of HCPs have left practice or had their licenses threatened. First, you read the friendly advice in Chapter 34. Then you practice medicine in a way that does no harm, targets the individual patient, and stays with each case until the person improves. You take what's good about evidence-based medicine and you move beyond it, as appropriate. You never allow what is purported to be science-based guidelines to restrict your thinking, or judgment, or responsibility to your patients. If you want to see Lyme patients, you must be willing to think and protect your patients from rigid posturing by outside influences trying to force your patients into boxes where they don't belong.

Medical students are now taught to follow preset algorithms and practice guidelines in the form of decision trees. The sooner the student can plug a person into a rigid checklist, the sooner he can stop thinking and no longer be held accountable. Jerome Groopman in *How Doctors Think* reinforces the need to think outside the yes and no boxes especially "when symptoms are vague, or multiple and confusing, or when test results are inexact." Algorithms "discourage physicians from thinking independently and creatively. Instead of expanding a doctor's thinking, they can constrain it." Don't become a slave to the check list. Don't let the process become more important than the patient. Groopman quotes Dr. Myron Falchuk, "And once you remove yourself from the patient's story, you no longer are truly a doctor."

You can't reason with the irrational. You can remain optimistic that the truth will eventually prevail.

X. Interesting insights

While I believe that I have made some quite sensible arguments in this chapter, clearly supporting one point of view, will I change any minds? Probably not. An article by Chris Moody in the May 20, 2011, issue of *The Week* magazine explains why. Here is my interpretation of Moody's points:

- Beliefs are rooted in emotion so the facts are often irrelevant.

- While we think our conclusions are logical and devoid of emotion, pre-existing beliefs hold more weight than any new "facts" in forming our thoughts and opinions.

- "Motivated reasoning" explains why groups become so polarized over issues where the evidence is clear and unequivocal. He uses the issues of global warming, Obama's birth certificate, and the exact date for the end of the world as examples.

- If you expect people to be swayed by the facts, you will be disappointed.

- Reasoning is completely submerged in emotion.

- We cherry-pick information, hanging on to any tidbit that confirms our already held beliefs and dismissing any ideas that may challenge our thinking. Arthur Lupia, from the University of Michigan said that we apply "fight or flight" reasoning to data as well as to predators as a survival skill.

- What we call reasoning, might actually be rationalizing preconceived notions.

- Jonathan Haidt from the University of Virginia said that we think we're being scientists when we're actually being lawyers.

- We reason only so far as our pre-determined conclusion.

- We will rationalize anything to win our case.

- Confirmation bias is the act of giving more credence to the ideas that support what we already believe.

- We spend disproportionate energy refuting opposing views.

- While modern science evolved from an attempt to diminish subjectivity, current science is very prone to selective understanding.

- Giving a fanatic ideologue data that can be used to make his case causes bliss.

- Giving a fanatic ideologue data that can be used to refute his case causes blinders.

- Partisans often label opposing theories immoral, unethical, or illegal.

- A passionate advocate of a point of view will say the other side is conspiring, or their experts are not credible, or they don't really understand the issue.

- The best way to persuade someone to your point of view is not through facts, which might make her just hold on more tightly to her own views.

- Monica Prasad from Northwestern University conducted an experiment to determine how hard someone would hold onto a belief after it has been clearly refuted. She used the idea that Saddam Hussein and al Qaida worked together to orchestrate the 9/11 attacks. The 9/11 Commission provided clear evidence refuting this claim and even George W. Bush said this idea was false. Only 1 of 49 study subjects changed his/her mind. The other 48 countered or rationalized these "facts."

- Groups become more divided as facts become stronger and more unequivocal.

- Education has little to do with these intractable and irrational opinions. Unsophisticated people tend to just dismiss opposing views while sophisticated people will try to come up with "good arguments" to sway others to their side and to defend their opinions.

- When you are smart enough to devise arguments, you tend to become more entrenched in your opinions, no matter what evidence is presented to the contrary. Zealots devise a belief system that they think is irrefutable.

- If you want to persuade someone to your way of thinking present your views in a way that does not make the listener defensive or emotional. (Advice I didn't exactly follow above!)

- Dan Kahan at Yale Law School said the best way to frame an argument is to do it in a way that allows the audience to fit the new idea into their overall world-view. Don't lead with the facts, lead with the values. Fit the facts to the audience. Conservatives may be more likely to accept a fact as valid if presented by a religious leader or businessman.

Unfortunately, you are likely to leave this chapter with the same opinion with which you came. After reading Moody's ideas, rescan the points and counterpoints above and see if it makes a difference.

Conclusion: Most patients and many HCPs don't even realize there are options in the diagnosis and treatment of Lyme disease. If you are an HCP, educate yourself on the alternatives. If you are a patient or caretaker ask, "Are there any other choices?" When all is said and done, one side will prevail, as in all cases of previously controversial illnesses that were said to be fabricated. Just like me, as soon as one of the detractors or his family suffers from a chronic manifestation of Lyme, he becomes one of us. Sorry, if your child had to get sick to get you here but, welcome aboard.

PEARL: Burton A. Waisbren Sr., MD FACP FIDSA, is a founding member of the IDSA. His book Treatment of Chronic Lyme Disease: Fifty-One Case Reports and Essays in Their Regard was published in 2011 by iUniverse. In the introduction Dr. Waisbren writes that based on his 55 years of training in infectious diseases, medical literature, and clinical experience, he has concluded that "...there is an epidemic of chronic Lyme disease occurring in the US that warrants more attention than it is getting from the government and the academic medical establishment. It is hard for me to believe that the 51 cases of what I call chronic lyme disease syndrome is a figment of my imagination." He recommends the 200 peer-reviewed references in the associated summary articles. He laments "a conundrum why a group of respected physicians who are members of IDSA have not recognized this and have instead written a guideline that essentially denies that the syndrome exists. This guideline has resulted in literally hundreds of patients being unable to be treated for chronic lyme disease." He then refers to the multitude of rebuttals of the IDSA guidelines provided in the literature.

Chapter 12

OTHER RECOGNIZED TBIs

The world now produces more information in 48 hours
than it did throughout all human history to 2003.
Claim made by James Gleick and Claude Shannon

The co-infections of Lyme disease seen most often in clinical practice are babesiosis, ehrlichiosis, bartonellosis, and the complications of Mycoplasma *fermentans*. Each of these conditions has earned its own chapter. The diseases in this chapter are even murkier in terms of clear scientific information. Since much of the data that could be gleaned from the TBI literature are contradictory and confusing, only the bare essentials will be provided here. Simply put, not enough is known about several of these maladies to expound at length. We don't even know if they are separate diseases or overlap onto two or more other TBIs. We also don't know if they ever exist by themselves or always ride the rails with other co-infections. We don't know their incidence or prevalence, but it's a safe bet that all are grossly underreported.

Please note that the information below is a compilation from many sources, anecdotes, and chatter. These diseases are not documented sufficiently for me to guarantee that all the information provided is 100% accurate. I just don't know. Authors may be talking about one disease in their article when they were actually looking at another in their practice. The information provided here should allow you to keep an open mind when assessing TBI patients and to provide alternatives that you may not have otherwise considered. If you want to pick through this chapter and say, "She said symptoms usually occur in 3 to 5 days and I know of a case that presented in 2 days," feel free. I spent hundreds of hours trying to reconcile loose "facts," and I can assure you that splitting hairs is not worth the time.

If you are struggling with the next step in the management of a TBI patient, consider the directory below, always remembering that there are probably a hundred more where these came from. The conditions below are in no particular order. I don't know which is the most severe, or the most common, or the most interesting. I did the only reasonable thing—I alphabetized them.

- **Colorado Tick Fever (CTF)**

    Aliases: American tick fever, mountain tick fever

    Pathogen: Colorado tick fever virus (genus Coltivirus also called Orbivirus)

Vector: Rocky Mountain wood tick (Dermacentor *andersoni*)

Distribution: Identified in the western US and Canada, primarily in high mountain areas like Colorado and Idaho. Reported primarily from March to September with a peak incidence in June. This disease appears to be seasonal with infections occurring mostly at altitudes from 4,000 to 10,000 feet, predominantly in campers and young males.

History: First isolated in humans in the 1940s

Pathophysiology: CTF virus affects the red blood cells and can live for an undetermined time in the blood stream. The involvement of RBCs explains how it is inoculated through tick bites and can be transmitted through blood transfusions, although this is thought to be rare. There is no evidence of person-to-person transmission, but this might be because we have not yet observed such a transmission, not that it is impossible. The organisms are thought to live in the blood for around 120 days so this capacity should be kept in mind when coming in contact with blood from an infected patient or during transfusions.

Clinical course: After a recognized tick bite, clinicians have found that symptoms of CTF can begin within 3 to 6 days, but there may be a long delay. Manifestations have appeared 4 months after a tick bite. Of course, other bites may have been missed. Usually there is a bout of fever which resolves only to recur again. The initial fever can last about 3 days, then there is resolution followed by a return of symptoms for another 3 to 6 day run.

Signs and symptoms: Patients complain of high fever, severe headache, chills, fatigue, muscle pain, back pain, pain behind the eyes, generalized malaise, a flat or pimply rash, light sensitivities, abdominal discomfort, nausea, vomiting, and diarrhea. The second phase of symptoms may be more severe.

Diagnosis: As with all TBIs, clinical signs and symptoms should be the strongest indicator. Laboratory confirmation may be useful including complement fixation to Colorado tick virus or immunofluorescence for the Colorado tick pathogen. Findings of leukopenia, thrombocytopenia, and mild elevation of LFTs can support the diagnosis. Detection of antibodies can be considered. As with all TBIs, diagnostic labs should be undertaken with prudence. Contact a lab you trust and ask exactly which tests to order and how to collect the samples. If you do not order these tests routinely, make sure you ask for guidance on how to interpret the result. There is no shame in asking for help, only in not taking full advantage of the expertise of others.

Treatment: Currently, no specific treatment is available. Make sure the tick is completely removed. Supportive measures may help with the fever and discomfort. I could find no documentation of the use of antivirals in these cases.

Prognosis: Colorado tick fever can be especially serious in children. Some will require hospitalization. Rare complications include encephalitis, aseptic meningitis, and hemorrhagic fever. Some of the literature suggests that one infection by Colorado tick fever virus provides immunity from future infection, but I could not find confirmation. The best recommendation is to avoid reinfection.

- **Powassan Viral Encephalitis (POW)**

    Aliases: Powassan encephalitis, tick-borne meningoencephalitis, tick-borne encephalitis, Powassan fever

    Pathogen: Powassan virus, a flavivirus (or arbovirus). This is the only known tick-borne arbovirus in the US and Canada. (Does that mean anything to you? Me either.)

    Vector: Woodchuck tick (Ixodes *cookei,* not cookie) primarily, also deer tick (Ixodes *scapularis)*

    Distribution: Found in eastern Canada and US, especially New York. While not common in humans, both Maine and Vermont have reported several cases recently. In the 40 years from the late 50s to the late 90s, about 30 cases have been reported in North America. A similar flavivirus-borne illness called Kyasanur Forest disease is known in India. POW may be related to the Eastern hemisphere's tick-borne encephalitis viruses. There are anecdotal cases in the western US.

    Hosts: POW is not a common disease in humans.

    History: First recognized in the small town of Powassan, Ontario, Canada in 1958

    Pathophysiology: This virus is thought to readily invade the brain.

Clinical course: Symptoms are thought to appear within 7 to 10 days of infection.

Signs and symptoms: The hallmarks of this infection are fever and CNS involvement. Other reported symptoms include headache, nausea, pain behind the eyes, light sensitivity, lethargy, muscle weakness, partial paralysis, and coma. Since the virus invades the brain, symptoms can progress to brain inflammation including meningoencephalitis with disorientation, seizures, and paralysis, all of which can lead to coma and death.

Diagnosis: The diagnosis is based primarily on history and physical with serology used for support. If you suspect POW, call a lab you trust to receive guidance on proper tests to order and how to gather samples.

Treatment: Since POW is a viral disease, there is no specific treatment and no vaccine. Supportive care is used. Consider antivirals if early in the clinical course.

Prognosis: Half of all cases result in permanent neurological damage. There is a 10% to 15% death rate. Serious illness can cause residual neurological problems in those patients who recover.

- **Q Fever**

    Pathogen: Coxiella *burnetii* is a Rickettsia which are considered an "almost bacteria." From an evolutionary perspective, they are somewhere between the mitochondrial organelles found in eukaryotic cells and the organisms we consider bacteria. Fortunately, they respond to antibiotics in a way that is similar to traditional bacteria.

    Vector: Brown dog tick, Rocky Mountain wood tick, and Lone Star tick are all known vectors.

    Distribution: Q fever has been diagnosed throughout the US and the world. Coxiella is not only transmitted by ticks but also by inhaling contaminated dust, drinking unpasteurized milk from infected animals, or handling animals that are reservoirs for the pathogen. Q fever is reportable in the US, but since many human infections are not apparent, the incidence is likely grossly underestimated.

    Hosts: This Rickettsia is found in cattle, sheep, and goats which are common hosts for the pathogen. A wide variety of other animals including domestic pets harbor Coxiella *burnetii*. These animals usually do not show signs of illness. Organisms are excreted in milk, urine, and feces of infected animals and in high numbers during birth in the amniotic fluids and placenta. Rickettsia are also maintained in nature through the animal-tick cycle. Humans most often get infected through inhalation of the pathogen, but tick inoculation is becoming more recognized.

History: The term Q comes from the word *query* since the etiology was initially unknown.

Pathophysiology: Coxiella *burnetii* is resistant to heat, drying, and common disinfectants, so these organisms can survive for long periods in hostile environments. Humans are very susceptible and there does not need to be a big load of these pathogens to infect. Transmission by tick is rare, but may become more common (or just more recognized). There have been rare reports of human-to-human transmission.

Clinical course: Presumably, only about half of those infected with Coxiella *burnetii* ever show signs of infection. The fever lasts 1 to 2 weeks. The incubation period depends on the pathogen load at the time of infection: the more organisms, the shorter the incubation period. Usually, the victim gets sick 2 to 3 weeks after infection, long after the actual vector has been forgotten. The incubation period is from 9 to 28 days with an average of about 18 to 21 days.

Signs and symptoms: Unfortunately, the manifestations of Q fever are similar to those of many other TBIs. The patient may present with acute fever, chills, sweats, headache, malaise, myalgia, anorexia, confusion, sore throat, cough, nausea, vomiting, chest pain, and other symptoms. Weight loss can occur and persist. Suspect Q fever in TBI patients with pneumonia and abnormal liver function.

C. *burnetii* can cause a non-productive cough and pneumonia. X-ray evidence of localized pneumonitis can develop in the 2nd week. Between 30% and 50% of those with symptomatic infection will develop pneumonia. If symptoms persist, the alveolar linings can swell and plasma cells can infiltrate the lungs. The alveoli can become cluttered with cellular debris.

Unlike other rickettsial diseases, Q fever is NOT associated with a rash. Fevers of 104 or 105 can persist for 1 to 3 weeks. If the clinical course is prolonged, about a third of these patients will develop hepatitis. Chronic endocarditis has been documented.

Diagnosis: Because the presentation of Q fever is similar to many other infectious diseases, the diagnosis may be missed or overlooked. To make this diagnosis, the HCP must have a high index of suspicion. While routine lab results can suggest transient thrombocytopenia or abnormal LFTs, support for the diagnosis includes serologic testing to detect antibodies to Coxiella *burnetii*. Q fever antigens can be especially diagnostic. Antigen IFA (indirect immunofluorescence assay) is most reliable and most often used. Coxiella *burnetii* can also be detected using immunohistochemical staining and DNA detection.

C. *burnetii* can be isolated from blood complement fixation and agglutination antibodies in convalescence. Agglutination is often more sensitive than complement fixation. Fluorescent antibody tests can be useful. Antibodies against Coxiella *burnetii* usually can't be found in the acutely infected, but later when they are detected, they may suggest chronic disease.

An experienced practitioner should be consulted to help interpret the tests if you are not familiar with this type of testing. Coxiella *burnetii* has two antigenic phases that are very different in terms of diagnosis. Acute disease and chronic disease may show opposite test results. Understanding this difference can help determine where a patient is in the course of the disease. Looking at levels of specific antibodies may be a more accurate assessment than looking at IgG alone. Combined levels of IgM and IgA, in addition to IgG, expands the specificity of the assays and improves diagnostic accuracy. IgM is helpful for identifying recent infections, while increased IgA and IgG are thought to suggest impending endocarditis. Liver biopsy will sometimes show diffuse granulomatous changes in those with liver involvement.

Signs and symptoms of Coxiella *burnetii* are easily misidentified as manifestations of other TBIs, various viruses, and bacteria, especially the Chlamydial cause of psittacosis. The differential diagnosis should include tuberculosis, influenza, salmonella, malaria, hepatitis, sarcoidosis, histoplasmosis, brucellosis, tularemia, and syphilis. Mycoplasma also should be considered. The key to a diagnosis of Q fever may be the association with animals, especially goats and their by-products. While a tick bite can steer you toward TBIs, and away from illnesses such as tuberculosis, it will not help distinguish between Coxiella *burnetii*, Mycoplasma, Borrelia, and tularemia. Always remember that more than one pathogen can be operational.

Treatment: Both tetracyclines and chloramphenicol are effective against Coxiella *burnetii*. Doxycycline is the treatment of choice for those in whom it is not contraindicated and the medicine is most effective when started within 3 days of infection.

One source recommends 100 mg of doxycycline bid for 15 to 21 days in those over 8-years-old. Other sources have used the following regimens:

Tetracycline 250 mg po q 4 to 6 hours. Preferred in adults and those with endocarditis

Doxycycline 100 mg bid until asymptomatic at least 5 days

Chloramphenicol 50 mg/kg daily in 4 divided doses given q 6 hours. Chloramphenicol can be considered in kids who can't use TCNs.

Quinolones are also thought to be effective.

Restart antibiotic therapy if symptoms reappear.

Chronic Q endocarditis is much harder to manage. If antibiotics do not resolve the symptoms of endocarditis, valve replacement may be considered. Two treatment combinations have been suggested for Q endocarditis:

1. Doxycycline plus quinolones for those 4 years and older

2. Doxycycline with hydroxychloroquine (Plaquenil) for those 1.5 to 3 years. This regimen gets less relapses, but regular eye exams are needed to check for accumulation of chloroquine. Also, there are always the caveats surrounding the use of doxycycline in kids under 8 but remember you are dealing with endocarditis here.

A vaccine was available in Australia for a while and recommended for those in frequent contact with pregnant sheep.

Prognosis: Treatment hastens recovery but most patients will recover after several months without treatment. (Who wants to be sick for several months waiting to find out? Give 'em some antibiotic already.) Some patients develop a chronic form of Q fever lasting more than 6 months, and this presentation can be a much more serious illness. This chronic form may develop as soon as 1 year after initial infection or as long as 20 years later. A serious complication of chronic Q is endocarditis, and this can be especially problematic for those who had pre-existing valve problems. Patients with cancer, kidney disease, or transplants are at greater risk of developing chronic Q fever. As many as 65% of persons with chronic Q die. Those who recover fully may have immunity, but who knows? For those with acute Q only, the mortality rate is about 1% to 2%. One final thought: A recent article discusses the exceptional potential for Coxiella *burnetii* to be used as a bioterrorism agent. GREAT!!

- **Rocky Mountain Spotted Fever (RMSF)**

Aliases: Tick typhus, tick fever, spotted fever, Tobia fever, Sao Paulo fever, febre maculos, feibre manchada, black measles

Pathogen: Rickettsia *rickettsii,* a type of bacteria

Vector: Ticks such as the American dog tick and the Rocky Mountain wood tick (Dermacentor ticks) and some Ixodes species, such as I. *pacificus*. The wood tick is the principal vector in the US. Ticks serve as both vectors and hosts for Rickettsia *rickettsii*, and disease may be spread through bites as well as contact with tick feces and crushed tick fluids. (Just when I was getting used to tick spit.) Male ticks may be more involved here than with other TBIs since males appear to be able to transmit the pathogen to the female tick in sperm. Once infected with the Rickettsia *rickettsii,* the tick may harbor the organism for life. The tick is believed to need about 24 hours of attachment to transmit RMSF, but we know how wrong these estimates have been in other TBIs. One source says that only a small percentage of ticks carry R. *rickettsii* even in areas where the most cases have been reported.

Hosts: Ticks, rabbits, and other small mammals. Humans are accidental hosts and not otherwise involved in transmission.

Distribution: Despite its name this pathogen is now believed to be in every state except Alaska and Hawaii. The range seems to be expanding. There are about 800 cases reported in the US each year and less than half of the patients recall the tick. RMSF seems to be only in the western hemisphere so far. The disease is diagnosed primarily from May to September when the adult ticks are most active and when people are often in infested areas for work or recreation. Cases in southern states have been reported all year round. The incidence is higher in kids younger than 15 and in males. Currently, most cases are being reported from the eastern and southern US. There does not seem to be person-to-person transmission even when cough particulates are inhaled. Certain populations appear to be at greater risk of death or complications including the elderly, males, blacks, alcoholics, and those with G6PD deficiency. There is a high proportion of severe RMSF in the G6PD population which affects about 10% of African Americans. For these patients RMSF can be rapidly fatal, but this is a rare combination.

History: Howard Ricketts first established the role of Rickettsia in disease and realized the association with tick bites. He began to understand the complex cycle involving ticks and mammals. RMSF was first recognized in

1896 in Idaho in the Snake River Valley. The disease was feared by locals because it killed so many people before treatment was available. Dr. Ricketts died of a rickettsial disease in Mexico in 1910 (typhus).

Pathophysiology: Rickettsia *rickettsii* invades the cells lining the heart and blood vessels. The endothelial cells of the small vessels are the site of the most damage. The vessels can be blocked by thrombi, producing a vasculitis. This vasculitis can be seen in the skin manifestations of the disease. However, just because you can't see what is going on inside doesn't mean the endothelial cells inside the body are not just as affected. Damage occurs in the skin, subcutaneous tissues, lungs, CNS, heart, kidneys, liver, GI tract, and spleen. Because the endothelial cells in the vessels are the hardest hit, damage can occur anywhere there is circulation. The more circulation, the more the organ system could be impacted. Further, disseminated intravascular coagulation (DIC) may develop in the very ill.

Clinical course: Since only a small percentage of those eventually diagnosed with RMSF recall a tick bite, the incubation period is not well-defined. For those who do recall a tick encounter, symptoms usually appear after a week or two. The rash is interesting in that it usually starts on the extremities and moves to the core. Incubation averages 7 days, but the disease has been known to present as early as 3 days and after 2 weeks. The shorter the incubation period, the worse the illness. Rarely, if ever, does RMSF become chronic.

Signs & symptoms: Within a few days of infection, the patient may present with the abrupt onset of a high fever of 103° to 104° accompanied by a severe headache, especially behind the eyes. The fever may persist for 2 or 3 weeks, although there may be some relief in the mornings.

As the disease progresses, an annoying, unproductive cough may manifest. In the first week of fever, most patients develop a petechial rash on their palms, soles, wrists, ankles, and forearms. This rash then extends to the face, axilla, buttocks, and trunk. Warm water or alcohol compresses tend to bring out the rash. Initially, the lesions blanch when compressed. The lesions start as small, non-itchy, pink macules, eventually becoming darker and more raised. After about 4 days, the rash can become petechial with bright red pinpoints which may coalesce to form large hemorrhagic patches. These lesions could later ulcerate. The presentation of the rash on the soles and palms can be highly suggestive of RMSF, but don't forget that other pathogens like Coxsackie viruses can also start out this way.

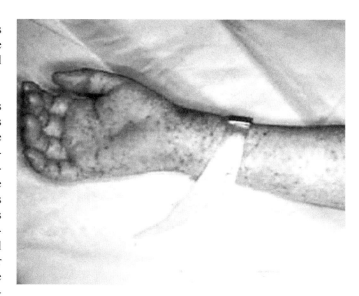

Petechial rash of RMSF
Source: http://en.wikipedia.org/wiki/File:Rocky_mountian_spotted_fever.jpg. Accessed March 2013

Additional symptoms can include severe pain behind the eyes, nausea, emesis, lack of appetite, abdominal pain, joint pain, bleeding problems, and muscle aches. The initial presentation of RMSF can be nonspecific and similar to many other TBIs, leading to much misdiagnosis and delay in treatment.

Some authors write about a "classic triad" for RMSF consisting of fever, rash, and a history of tick bite. This is of great help AFTER the diagnosis is made. Very often, the patient cannot recall a tick bite, a nonspecific fever is present in hundreds of infectious diseases, and the rash does not provide its clues until well into the first week of symptoms. Keep a high index of suspicion, since treatment should be started as soon as there is reason to consider RMSF. Compassion suggests that treatment not be held until a rash presents or until lab tests support the diagnosis.

In fact, the characteristic spotted (petechial) rash of RMSF does not appear for several days, and it may not look at all like the distinctive pin-spot rash we have seen in textbooks. This rash occurs only in about 35% to 60% of patients and of those, the palms and soles are involved in about 50% to 80% of the cases. Further, 10% to 15% of confirmed patients never develop a rash at all.

RMSF may cause abnormal lab results such as thrombocytopenia, hyponatremia, and elevated LFTs, but none of these are diagnostic. Patients who remain sick with Rickettsia *rickettsii* may experience neurological symptoms such as persistent headache, restlessness, insomnia, delirium, and coma: all indicative of encephalitis.

Hypotension occurs in severe cases, as well as localized pneumonitis. Hepatomegaly can manifest, but jaundice is rarely seen. Circulatory collapse with oliguria, anuria, abnormal electrolytes, and azotemia leading to shock has been described. Shock can lead to brain and heart damage and death.

Patients with long-term disease that was considered life-threatening and those with protracted hospital stays are subject to permanent sequelae including paralysis of the legs, gangrene, tissue necrosis, hearing loss, incontinence, movement disorders, and language problems.

Diagnosis: RMSF can be difficult to recognize early in its course, even with very experienced HCPs. When present, the spotted rash can be useful in the differential diagnosis. Unfortunately, the rash may not come into sight for a week or more and then its appearance may further confuse the diagnosis by not looking the way we have come to expect. Be prepared to treat based on clinical judgment since lab confirmation and more distinctive physical signs may not present until after treatment needs to begin.

If you do not diagnose RMSF routinely, contact a trusted lab and ask for guidance on which labs to order and how to gather the samples you need. Rickettsia *rickettsii* can be isolated and identified from blood or tissue samples. Support of the diagnosis of RMSF has been successful using tissue from the biopsy of skin lesions.

Antibodies to RMSF, usually IgM, do not appear until the second or third week of symptoms. The timing of measurable antibodies may also be skewed if antibiotics were started early.

The serologic patterns of RMSF are distinctive for two types of specific complement fixation antigens: 1) the soluble fraction which is common to most rickettsia, and 2) the purified fraction which is specific to the individual rickettsiae. RMSF may be identified by type-specific washed rickettsial-body antigen.

Immunofluorescence (IFA) is the standard test now for RMSF with sensitivity over 90% and specificity of nearly 100%. One source recommends three samples: one the first week, one the second week, and one between weeks 4 and 6. If the clinical picture is suggestive, do NOT wait for a positive result to begin treatment.

PCR can be used in early identification of Rickettsia *rickettsii* nucleic acids with moderate sensitivity. With the lag time in processing the samples and getting the results, these tests will not be of much use in making early treatment decisions. However, they may be valuable if the patient is not getting better on their current treatment regimen. Results might help you know what the patient probably doesn't have. You may need to reassess.

RMSF rarely becomes chronic, so with good response to available antibiotics some HCPs do not order lab testing. Treat on first suspicion and don't wait for support by antibody or other testing.

RMSF can increase CPK levels. This finding is nonspecific and I wouldn't rely on its usefulness in tipping the differential diagnosis one way or the other.

Treatment: The sooner treatment is started in RMSF, the faster the patient will improve and the shorter the duration of fever. Before the use of antibiotic therapy for RMSF in the 1940s, more than 30% of patients died. Antibiotics have greatly decreased both morbidity and mortality. Remember that patients may be so ill that they will need both antibiotics and aggressive supportive care. If you suspect a patient might have RMSF, and the rash appears before you have started antibiotics, you are late. In untreated RMSF, the patient could die or suffer irrevocable sequelae before lab tests confirm your suspicions. Be careful every time you say, "Oh, it's just a little virus." Treat when you have good reason to suspect.

Once started on antibiotics the patient usually improves within a day, with the fever breaking in 2 to 3 days. Nonetheless, despite timely and appropriate treatment, 3% to 5% of patients will die. You may need to be quite aggressive.

Recommended regimens include:

1. Doxycycline is usually considered the treatment of choice. The dose of doxycycline in adults is 100 bid (every 12 hours). For kids (under 100 pounds) consider 4 mg/kg in 2 divided doses. Doxycycline can be given po or IV. As always, use caution in children.

2. Chloramphenicol is an alternative. Load with 50 mg/kg, then use the same amount daily in divided doses q 6 or 8 hours. Chloramphenicol is most often given IV, and depending on which day of the week you are reading this, oral preparations may not be available on the legitimate commercial market. Use of chloramphenicol requires careful monitoring such as vigilance regarding aplastic anemia.

3. Tetracycline is also occasionally used if doxycycline is not an option.

Extensive details on the use and caveats of these medications in kids is provided in Chapter 24: *Antimicrobials.*

Both doxycycline and chloramphenicol are rickettsiostatic not -cidal. Continue treatment until the patient is afebrile and essentially asymptomatic. Allow for a therapeutic cushion. Most sources suggest a total of at least 10 days of treatment and continuing the medicine for at least 3 days after the fever subsides. Treat longer if the patient is severely ill or the case is complicated. Failure to respond to antibiotics suggests the diagnosis may be incorrect. Consider other options. Use IV antibiotics when the patient is too sick to take orals. Do not fluid overload since capillary permeability can cause pulmonary and cerebral edema and electrolyte imbalances. Patients near death have been treated with steroids in an attempt to stabilize.

PEARL: I could find no reliable information on the co-infection rates of RMSF and Lyme. So while I label RMSF a co-infection, this might not be a common event. RMSF might be a TBI that usually flies solo.

There is no vaccine so far. Attempts have been made to control the rickettsia-bearing ticks by controlling small mammals in endemic areas.

Prognosis: RMSF is not a disease to dismiss lightly. More than 30% will die if left untreated. Even with appropriate, early treatment, there is still a 3% to 5% mortality rate. Untreated, half will develop permanent neurologic problems. RMSF almost always requires hospitalization. A high index of suspicion and early initiation of antibiotics can prevent serious sequelae. Half the deaths from RMSF in children occur within 9 days of the start of symptoms.

The disease can be difficult to diagnose in the early stages, and without prompt and adequate treatment, can be fatal. Rickettsia *rickettsii* is the most lethal of the rickettsial diseases, but early treatment is thought to significantly decrease mortality. Once you ask, "Could this be Rocky Mountain spotted fever?" follow up with, "Should I already be treating?" Early treatment prevents most complications.

- **Tick Paralysis**

Vector: American dog tick, Rocky Mountain wood tick, deer tick, Lone Star tick. In Australia Ixodes *holocyclus*

Pathogen: The agent for tick paralysis is a neurotoxin associated with certain tick species and not a separate pathogen (unless we just don't know the pathogen, as yet). Apparently, some ticks secrete a toxin that causes a progressive paralysis in the host which is reversed when the tick is removed. Tick paralysis is responsible for the deaths of thousands of domestic and wild animals annually. So far, scientists have not been able to isolate a pathogen.

Distribution: Tick paralysis is caused by a number of tick species throughout the world, including at least five species in the US. In Australia, I. *holocyclus* is found along the populated eastern coastline and is called the paralysis tick. Common hosts include koalas, bandicoots, possums, and kangaroos. Human and dog bites are common with I. *holocyclus.*

PEARL: On August 25, 2010, Ixodes holocyclus *was named "Parasite of the Day." Who knew?*

Pathophysiology: A neurotoxin excreted from the salivary gland of the American dog tick, the Rocky Mountain wood tick, and the Lone Star tick, among others, is thought to cause tick paralysis. The paralysis is a toxic reaction to the saliva of female ticks which seems to reverse fairly rapidly after the tick is removed. Why some ticks excrete this toxin in their saliva, but the vast majority of ticks do not, does not seem to be well understood. Maybe some hosts are susceptible to a universally present toxin, but most are not. For a toxin to be so powerful as to paralyze the victim within hours and yet dissipate so quickly after the tick is removed also seems physiologically puzzling to me.

Clinical course: Most of the anecdotal literature describing tick paralysis consists of case studies after-the-fact. In general, a paralyzed patient was found to have had a tick bite, and the symptoms resolved soon after the tick was removed. For the most part, the paralysis was progressive, beginning in the legs and spreading throughout the body within hours. Symptoms appeared to resolve quickly after the tick was gone. I could not find any mention of how this condition might overlap with other TBIs or the consideration that these symptoms might be a manifestation of another illness, as yet unrecognized.

Signs and symptoms: Symptoms begin with fatigue, followed by flaccid paralysis, loss of function of the tongue and facial muscles, and progressive paralysis beginning in the legs and moving over the rest of the body within hours. Convulsions and death have been reported.

Treatment: Remove the tick completely. Do not squeeze or break the tick. If you do, you could be injecting additional neurotoxin. No one (except the most bizarre) tries to break the tick during removal, but it happens. When removing ticks from a paralyzed patient, gently express a small amount of bloody fluid from the site before moving on to the next tick or the next step. If symptoms do not start to resolve after proper tick removal, consider that more than one thing might be going on with your patient, or more than one tick might be present.

Prognosis: Symptoms of tick paralysis seem to reverse fairly quickly after the tick is removed. While I could not find much definitive information on this condition, know that it exists and can be fatal. Remove all ticks (look in all the nooks and crannies) and always consider that something else may result from this tick bite. Be vigilant.

- **Tick Relapsing Fever**

  Aliases: Tick-borne relapsing fever (TBRF), typhinia, TRF

  Pathogen: Spirochetes of the genus Borrelia. In the US, Borrelia *hermsii* is tick-borne, and Borrelia *recurrentis* is transmitted by a louse. (Note that Lyme's pathogen is B. *burgdorferi*, and all these are spirochetes, as is syphilis.) A number of other Borrelia species also cause recurring fevers, including B. *parkeri*, and B. *duttoni*, and these may be responsible for several of the African relapsing diseases. There could be co-infection with B. *burgdorferi*, but I could not find substantiation of this possibility.

PEARL: Should TRF be listed here or in Chapter 10 with the other Borrelia? I went back and forth with this. Because Chapter 10 had to deal with STARI, the book organization started to get messy so I left TRF here. This disease is as much of a borreliosis as Lyme. I want no pathogen to feel disenfranchised.

Vector: TBRF is carried by the relapsing fever tick, also called the Washington tick of the genus Ornithodoros. Relapsing fever is more often recognized as a louse-borne disease, but this book is a *Compendium of Tick-Borne Disease*, so we will focus on the tick. A number of Borrelia species cause relapsing fevers and use rodents as reservoirs via tick vectors. The soft-bodied African tick is generally responsible for carrying the relapsing fevers found in Africa. Louse-borne disease may be more severe than the tick-borne variety, but this is hard to quantify.

This type of tick feeds for only a short period of time (an hour or so) and the Borrelia spirochetes are thought to be inoculated within minutes. This is in sharp contrast to the pronouncements by certain groups regarding B. *burgdorferi*, where they insist that the spirochete can only be transmitted if the tick is attached for at least 24 hours and fully engorged before infection can occur. Transplacental transmission of relapsing fever has been reported.

Distribution: TBRF caused by B. *hermsii* is diagnosed primarily in the western US. Other Borrelia-relapsing fevers are transmitted by the African soft-bodied tick which is responsible for much of the relapsing fevers found in south, central, and eastern Africa. B. *hermsii* is the most common etiologic agent in the US. Cases of relapsing fever have also been reported in Spain, Saudi Arabia, Asia, and certain areas in Canada. An occasional traveler to the US presents with a louse-borne relapsing fever.

Overall, there seem to be few cases of the tick-borne relapsing fever in the US, but of course, there may be considerable under-reporting. Cases are reported sporadically with a dozen counties producing half the cases. Most reports occur in the late spring and summer in western mountain states, with a few cases in Texas and the northwest. There is a slight predominance in females for the louse-borne disease, whereas the tick-borne variety is somewhat more prevalent in males. This may be due to more exposure to ticks through work and recreation. Clusters of cases have been reported in groups of campers who shared rustic facilities infested with rodents on which the ticks dine. Cavers and those who have played around in decaying wood piles have also reported disease. There is a trend to more pediatric than adult case reports.

History: The characteristic pattern of remission and relapse in TBRF has allowed for some differentiation from other febrile illnesses since the 1840s. Relapsing fever *may* be the etiology of a series of plagues in late medieval and early renaissance England. At that time the disease was referred to as sweating sickness. These plagues have not recurred in epidemic form since the 16th century.

Pathophysiology: Regardless of the mode of transmission, a spirochetemia develops. Borrelia then invade the endothelium where they cause a low grade disseminated intravascular coagulation and thrombocytopenia. One hypothesis to explain the relapsing nature of the fevers is that Borrelia are readily able to shift their outer surface proteins, making them unrecognizable to the immune system. This genetically engineered shift allows for a new generation of the pathogens that are not susceptible to destruction by the originally manufactured antibodies. The first antibodies produced were directed against the earliest infecting organisms. Those antibodies attacked the initial pathogens that helped cause symptoms along with the released cytokines. As the antibodies and overall immune response were successful in defending the host, the person responded by feeling better. The fevers and other inflammatory signs abated until a new batch of modified clones multiplied sufficiently to cause another immune response, manifested by the symptoms of relapse. Tick-borne disease tends to have more relapses (average of 3) compared with louse transmission (usually one or two relapses).

PEARL: Spirochetal gene transposition or switching was first identified in B. hermsii, *the etiologic agent of relapsing fever. These genetic machinations appear similar to those found with Bb.*

Clinical course: TBRF presents with high fevers that spontaneously abate and then recur. This characteristic pattern of remission and recurrence logically resulted in the name relapsing fever. B. *hermsii* and B. *recurrentis* cause very similar diseases, although they may cause different numbers of relapses if untreated. B. *recurrentis* tends to have longer febrile and afebrile intervals and a longer incubation period than B. *hermsii*. Patients do not usually experience symptoms until about 5 to 15 days after they were bitten by a tick. Symptoms of fever, chills, aches, nausea, and rash generally continue for 2 to 9 days before they disappear. Just when patients believe they are well, the symptoms recur. This pattern may continue for weeks if not treated.

The primary febrile episode usually ends after 3 to 6 days. Sometimes these febrile events end in crisis that can result in fatal shock. About 7 to 10 days after the initial manifestation subsides, the first relapse can occur abruptly. Subsequent relapses tend to be less severe. As many as ten relapses have been reported.

PEARL: The time frames here are a compilation from multiple sources and are inexact. Case reports usually were recorded after-the-fact with the patient "remembering" what happened. The goal here is to provide a frame of reference. Don't get locked into a particular number of days.

Signs and symptoms: Patients present with cycles of high fever, sudden chills, eye inflammation, cough, jaundice, muscle and joint aches, nausea, headaches, and petechial rash. The symptoms are in full force for an average of 3 to 6 days before resolving. After a transient asymptomatic period, the clinical picture recurs and these relapses can occur on average from 2 to 4 times depending on the pathogen. Treatment appears to interrupt the cycle. The onset is abrupt and the pulse can be rapid in proportion to the fever. This tachycardia may be helpful in distinguishing relapsing fever from typhoid fever.

Headache is almost universal with 95% of patients complaining of head pain. Similarly almost all experience myalgias and chills. Other reported signs and symptoms include: arthralgias, weakness, anorexia, weight loss, dry cough, nausea, vomiting, upper abdominal pain possibly due to liver and spleen involvement, abdominal tenderness with hepatosplenomegaly, tachypnea, tachycardia, rales, rhonchi, hypotension, petechial or maculopapular rash, nuchal rigidity, lymphadenopathy, jaundice, iritis, and iridocyclitis. (If you know what that is without looking it up, I am impressed, but no prizes will be given. Iridocyclitis is an inflammation of the iris and ciliary body.)

Neurologic findings are more common in louse-borne disease but can present in tick-borne infection as well and include: cranial neuropathy especially Bell's palsy, hemiplegia, meningitis, seizures, and coma. Adult respiratory distress syndrome (ARDS) has recently been reported in several North American cases.

Of course, fever is universal in these patients. Unfortunately, when a patient initially presents, you probably will not know that the fever will eventually be recurring if left untreated. The fever has to come and go a few times before the pieces are put together and you realize the fever keeps relapsing. This can impede diagnosis.

Diagnosis: While cycles of high fever can suggest the diagnosis of relapsing fever, many other infections also present with high fevers followed by transient resolution. Nonetheless, when clear fever patterns are observed, TBRF should at least be in the differential along with babesiosis. Most are misdiagnosed or unreported. Always consider the potential for co-infection, including B. *burgdorferi*.

Physical findings are not diagnostic and TBRF can be mistaken for any other TBI, other spirochete-induced conditions, typhoid fever, etc. For example, the dry cough found in TBRF, is also common in typhoid. Note that if treatment is started within the first cycle of fever, you may never know if the fever is actually relapsing, but that's okay, you don't need to know everything.

Blood can be tested for the pathogens and antibodies that cause TBRF. If you feel the need to confirm the diagnosis, call your trusted lab and ask for guidance.

Treatment: Antibiotics are usually effective in interrupting the relapsing cycle. Doxycycline, tetracycline, and chloramphenicol have all been successfully used. No consistent regimen could be found in the literature, but treatment plans that have been effective for RMSF and Lyme might also be useful in these cases. Patients usually improve within 24 hours of the start of antibiotic therapy. Most are treated for at least 1 to 2 weeks.

Usually tetracyclines have been the most effective antimicrobial for tick relapsing fever but these drugs may induce a significant Jarisch-Herxheimer reaction. Over 50% of the TBRF patients treated with TCNs have experienced a Herx. This reaction produces apprehension, diaphoresis, fever, tachycardia, and tachypnea. Although there may be an initial pressor response (increased BP), this can be followed by rapid hypotension. Recent studies have shown that tumor necrosis factor-α (TNF-α) may be partly responsible for the Herx reaction. In general, patients with Herx reactions feel just terrible, and they may want to stop therapy. Usually signs of a Herx reaction suggest that the therapy is working. More information is found in Chapter 28: *Understanding the Herxheimer Reaction.*

Prognosis: Complications and death are rare for *treated* relapsing fever. In untreated victims of the louse-borne disease mortality is high with 30% to 70% dying. Mortality falls to 5% for louse-borne disease and less than 1% in TBD if appropriate antibiotics are used. Many of the louse victims are in refugee camps and have numerous other problems, such as malnutrition, that contribute to the high mortality rate.

- **Tularemia**

  Aliases: Rabbit fever, Deer fly fever

  Pathogen: Tularemia is a bacterial disease caused by the small, non-motile, aerobic bacillus, Francisella *tularensis.*

  Vector: Tick vectors include the American dog tick, Rocky Mountain wood tick, and the Lone Star tick, although other insects such as deer flies may be involved. Many wild and domestic animals can be infected, although the rabbit is most often involved in human outbreaks. The most virulent pathogens appear to like rabbits and rodents best. Interestingly, Francisella *tularensis* has been found in water and aquatic animals, although it is not clear what role these might play in disease transmission.

  Distribution: Tularemia is named for Tulare, California, where the disease was first recognized. There are many routes of exposure besides the bite of an infected tick including exposure of the skin or mucus membranes to the blood or tissue of infected animals, contact with fluid from deer flies or ticks, consumption of insufficiently cooked rabbit, ingestion of contaminated water, inhalation of dust from contaminated soil, or handling infested pelts. Those most at risk include hunters, butchers, farmers, fur handlers, and lab workers. In winter, most cases come from skinning rabbits, while in summer, infections come from tick bites or handling contaminated animals. Person-to-person transmission has not been documented.

  Tularemia is distributed throughout the US, although it is considered rare. For example, Illinois records about five cases per year. Although reports are received all year, the highest incidence for adults is in early winter during rabbit season and for kids in summer when ticks and flies abound.

  Pathophysiology: Francisella *tularensis* enters the host by ingestion, inhalation, inoculation, or contamination. While the patient can be quite systemically ill, no toxins have been identified. The bacteria can penetrate unbroken skin or enter through microlesions. Entry points are surrounded by monocytes and fibroblasts, which are themselves surrounded by lymphocytes.

  Clinical Course: Symptoms of tularemia usually start from 1 to 14 days after an infectious event, with the average onset being 3 to 5 days after exposure. These numbers vary greatly in the literature to the point where they have little meaning. Signs and symptoms vary considerably for each individual. Incubation has been noted to be anywhere from 2 hours to 3 weeks. Keep an open mind and a high index of suspicion. Symptoms may come on suddenly.

  The following is a list of possible clinical manifestations of tularemia:

  1. Ulceroglandular is the most common type of tularemia with a skin ulcer that forms at the site of infection, often an insect or animal bite. The patient experiences swollen and painful nodes, fever, chills, headache, and exhaustion.

  2. Glandular is exactly like ulceroglandular except there are no skin ulcers. HCPs, this looks like a good board question to me.

  3. Oculoglandular affects the eye and can cause eye pain, redness, swelling, and discharge. An ulcer may form on the inside of the eyelid.

  4. Oropharyngeal usually occurs after eating poorly cooked wild animals or drinking contaminated water. It affects the GI tract with vomiting, diarrhea, fever, and sore throat.

  5. Pneumonic tularemia affects mostly the elderly with a pneumonia-like presentation of cough, high fever, extreme exhaustion, vomiting, diarrhea, large spleen, hepatomegaly, and pneumonia.

  6. Combination of any or all the above except that #1 and #2 cannot coexist, by definition.

  Tularemia varies from a mild condition to acute sepsis which is a serious infection of the blood and other tissues. If untreated, the temperature may remain high for 3 to 4 weeks and symptoms resolve very gradually. In many victims, progressive weakness precedes a dry cough and pneumonia. F. *tularensis*-induced pneumonia can cause chest pain, bloody sputum, and trouble breathing, leading to death.

  Signs & symptoms: Patients with tularemia usually have headache, chills, vomiting, aches, and fever. Many have an ulcer at the bite site and lymphadenopathy which becomes painful. Symptoms may vary depending on the source of infection. If you ate contaminated food, the symptoms may be primarily GI. If you were inoculated by a tick, there may be more skin and generalized signs. With inhalation of F. *tularensis* there is likely to be a more pulmonary presentation.

The disease may have a sudden onset of fever, chills, headaches, diarrhea, muscle aches, joint stiffness or pain, dry cough, and weakness. Skin lesions can appear near the onset or at any time during the disease.

Other possible symptoms include:

Skin – Just about anything goes with the possible skin manifestations of F. *tularensis* including ulcers, abscesses, and even a nonspecific, spotty, roseola-type rash that can appear over the body at any time during the clinical course. Most characteristic, however, is a single ulcer usually at the invasion site. This lesion often starts as a papule, which can become purple and inflamed and which occasionally is pustular. Later this lesion can evolve into a clean crater ulcer with a small amount of thin, colorless discharge. Usually the lesion is close to the entry location of the infection and if a tick is involved, this would be the bite site. But some patients have skin lesions other places on the body such as the fingers, arm, eye, or the roof of the mouth. Some of these lesions are painful and most are very slow to resolve. Some report a single ulcer near the bite site and multiple lesions elsewhere. Scattered necrotic lesions have been documented from 1 mm to 8 cm with a white-yellow appearance.

HEENT – Much eye involvement is reported including inflammation, ulcers, severe exudative conjunctivitis, pain, redness, swelling, and discharge. An ulcer may form on the inside of the eyelid which can be extremely slow to heal. Other areas of the head and neck can be involved with periauricular and cervical adenopathy, stomatitis, pharyngitis, and tonsillitis. Mouth ulcers are notoriously indolent.

Systemic - Generalized symptoms include painful and swollen lymph nodes, fever, sore and stiff joints, muscle aches, dry cough, chills, fatigue, and nodes on the spleen, liver, and kidney. Fever is often between 103 and 104 with recurring chills and drenching sweats. Patients present with severe prostration, weakness, tiredness, and persistent weight loss. Adenopathy can be painful and can be local, regional, or generalized.

GI – Gastrointestinal symptoms seem to be worse if the pathogen is ingested, but can occur whatever the method of transmission. Signs and symptoms include diarrhea, vomiting, abdominal discomfort, hepatosplenomegaly, and perisplenitis (an inflammation of the peritoneal covering of the spleen).

Respiratory- Pulmonary manifestations are common including pneumonia, atypical or otherwise. Imaging studies have shown nodules, consolidation, and abscesses on the lungs. F. *tularensis*-induced pneumonia can cause chest pain, bloody sputum, dry or productive coughs, retrosternal burning, shortness of breath, and trouble breathing. Patients may have reduced breath sounds or rales on exam. Respiratory failure has been known to lead to death.

As patients get sicker they can develop a number of complications such as meningitis, pericarditis, osteomyelitis, pneumonia, lung abscesses, respiratory failure, mediastinitis, delirium, and other signs of significant bacteremia. Rhabdomyolysis, which is a breakdown of muscle fiber leading to a spill of myoglobin into the blood that can damage the kidneys, is known to occur in tularemia. Death has been reported.

Diagnosis: With tularemia, the history may be your only friend. While the appearance of a primary skin lesion may be extremely useful, you cannot always count on a characteristic ulcer to be around when you need it. A history that could account for exposure, a sudden onset of symptoms, and the appearance of the primary skin lesion would suggest Francisella *tularensis.*

Routine labs will at most show a leukocytosis, but total WBCs may be normal with a disproportionate amount of PMNs. Of course, these same findings can be seen in dozens of infectious diseases.

You will have to deal with the sick patient in front of you long before any diagnostic lab tests can be processed. This one can be hard to differentiate. Unless the patient comes in covered in ticks and ulcers and dangling a raw rabbit from his jaw, I defy the best HCPs to get this right the first time. In the differential consider: other TBIs, anthrax, cat-scratch disease, mono, plague, and typhoid.

Note that this pathogen can be viable in tissue and blood specimens and is highly infectious. Lab technicians handling the specimens must be protected. Even with today's knowledge, lab workers remain one of the most at-risk populations. They should be using gloves, masks, and protective hoods, and they should exhibit extreme caution in handling infected tissues and swabbed culture materials.

Agglutination tests can be positive after ten days (but almost never before day 8). A rising titer supports the diagnosis. Brucellosis may also react positively to F. *tularensis* antigens but in lower titers. Be aware.

If the patient is at risk for tularemia take a careful history, examine her, do diagnostic testing as appropriate, and treat. Not necessarily in that order.

Treatment: Several regimens have been used with success:

1. The drug of choice is streptomycin.[1] In adults consider 0.5 g IM q 12 hours until temperature is normal. Thereafter use 0.5 g/day IM for at least 5 days.

2. Gentamicin 3 to 5 mg/kg/day IM or IV in 3 divided doses may also be effective.

3. Chloramphenicol has shown positive results.

4. Tetracycline 500 mg po q 6 hours until temperature is normal and then 250 qid for 5 to 7 days has been tried, but relapses have been recorded with this approach. (Maybe they should have tried higher, less frequent doses, if tolerated.)

5. F. *tularensis* has been shown to be susceptible to third-generation cephalosporins *in vitro*. Some recommend the use of a cephalosporin when the diagnosis is unclear. Consider cefotaxime (Claforan) 1 to 2 grams IV q 8 hours or ceftriaxone (Rocephin) 1 gram q 12 hours. Cephalosporins have been used effectively in combination with streptomycin or gentamicin.

Supportive care is often appreciated. Wet saline dressings may soothe ulcers. Draining large abscesses may provide relief. (Careful, there may be viable organisms in the pus!) Warm saline compresses and dark glasses may ameliorate eye discomfort.

Prognosis: Untreated cases can progress to severe illness, complications, and death. About 6% of the untreated patients die from overwhelming infection, pneumonitis, meningitis, or peritonitis. Mortality is almost non-existent in treated cases. The initial infection *may* provide immunity, but there is considerable mention of relapse and recurrence. I would not risk it and would take all precautions after an initial bout of tularemia to avoid reinfection.

Several sources were especially helpful in their prevention recommendations. We are counseled to cook rodents

thoroughly. (Yes, indeed, count on me.) Tularemia is also considered a good agent for bioterrorism since inhalation of the infectious agent would likely cause severe respiratory problems.

PEARL: Dr. Eva Sapi from the University of New Haven has conducted a number of "tick drag" studies for local municipalities in Connecticut. She then identifies the types of tick and the pathogens present. She has found many potentially pathogenic organisms in addition to those listed here. In addition to the "usual suspects," she has identified Chlamydia pneumoniae, Mycoplasma pneumoniae, EBV, and CMV. She has found potential pathogens with and without Bb present. How do we know what might be co-infections, what might be concurrent disease, and what was transmitted by a tick or through other routes? Right now, we don't. Dr. Sapi's work should prove invaluable as the broader picture of TBIs comes together. Rumor has it that Dr. Sapi responds to critics by sending them free tickets to her scientific symposia.

References: I don't know a single expert who has encountered all of these potential co-infections. Bits of information were gleaned from literally thousands of articles and put together in as coherent a way as I could manage. Trust me; you do not want to sift through all this yourself. Much is contradictory and I spent months compiling this information. Anything that is not accurate or complete is because I could not substantiate the inference, or the conflicting reports cancelled one another. Use the material above as a general guide, not as the definitive, last word on anything.

---

1 *Aminoglycosides are a class of antibiotics rarely indicated for treatment of TBIs although they are sometimes used to treat tularemia. However, if given for other reasons in TBI patients they might increase the risk of kidney damage. They include: gentamicin, tobramycin, amikacin, kanamycin, streptomycin, and neomycin.*

Chapter 13   **OVERALL PATIENT EVALUATION – Detailed chapter contents**

Chapter 13

OVERALL PATIENT EVALUATION

No passion in the world is equal to the passion to alter someone else's draft.
H. G. Wells

As I observed clinicians during preceptorships, I wanted to learn to gather information in an efficient and productive way. Of course, this level of expertise comes only after years of clinical experience and intense study. The purpose of the following chapters is to introduce a practical approach to patient evaluation. The format should allow the book to be used both as a handbook for practice as well as a reference book to be able to "just check one thing" before you move on. So if you have a patient with violaceous striae and you want to see which TBI might manifest with violaceous striae you will have several places to check: Chapter 17-B: *Physical Examination* in the section *Common skin manifestations in TBIs*, or you can also check the *Bartonellosis* chapter, the *Differential Diagnosis* chapter, the *Glossary*, or the *Index*. So there will be many opportunities to find what you need. But before you can evaluate your findings, you have to interact with the patient. That takes organization. This chapter will help you follow a common sense approach to patient assessment.

Patients with TBIs take time. With some preceptors, I witnessed so many inefficient practices that the patient was paying more for the HCP's disorganization than expertise. Do as much organizing behind the scenes as possible. This way the patient gets your undivided attention when you are together.

In writing the five *Patient Evaluation* chapters, I am assuming you are seeing patients with complications of TBIs: acute, disseminated, unresolving, recurrent, or chronic. These next chapters may contain more information than required for some cases. Use what you need and set aside the rest. Since this book is targeted not only to HCPs, but also to high level lay readers some definitions and explanations may be basic. That's okay. When I think back to my own practice over the years, I am amazed at how much I didn't know and how inept I might have been with some examination techniques. Did I really hear that murmur or see that optic disc? Did I know what I was observing if I did happen to notice?

The following chapters will err on the side of the conservative and contain history-gathering recommendations and assessment guidelines that are quite broad. Of course, they cannot be all-inclusive because of time and space constraints, but they should provide sufficient foundation for you to conduct a productive TBI assessment.

As you become more adept at evaluating TBDs, you will become more efficient, and thereby faster. Although some HMOs restrict you to six total minutes per patient, this will not be viable for patients with TBIs. Trust me, you will serve yourself, your staff, and your patients better if you arrange for more time than you need rather than try to squeeze in one more patient. I know this is hard. Once people find out you are working with these types of complicated cases, your waiting list will overflow. You will be torn between helping a very sick kid who has already seen twelve unhelpful HCPs and doing a more comprehensive assessment on the patient already sitting in your office. I hesitate to say this but, "Charge what you need to in order to buy the time necessary to give patients the attention they require." If you're a decent TBI doc, we want you to stay in business.

Experienced HCPs know when to dig deeper in a specific area and when they have all the information they need and can move on. This skill takes years and I am not sure I will live long enough to garner this type of expertise. For this reason, I tend to gather and examine more than might be absolutely necessary. Remember, an extensive baseline will allow you to make comparative judgments over time that will not be available to you unless you record them now. If you don't make yourself some kind of note you WILL forget. I have never regretted gathering too much information. On the contrary, I have kicked myself many times when I did not document an abnormality. Where was that liver edge six weeks ago in the kid I would never forget? I don't remember.

Consider yourself a compassionate medical detective. As I said, most of these patients have seen many doctors. With each HCP they have probably been told a different theory (including that a three-year-old is just acting sick to annoy them). Many of these patients have had dozens of tests (often tests that were not specific or sensitive enough for their condition) and most have been told to just "buck up." To help these people is going to take more than six minutes. If you are thinking that you will never be able to make a living this way, let me give you this compensation: There will be immeasurable gratitude. The patients and parents are often so thankful for even the smallest improvement. They will reward you over and over again. You might never be the master, but you can reap these kinds of rewards. (Warning: Do not look in this book for financial advice. I am *not* the person to ask.) Set up your practice in a way that you can allocate enough time to the patient and still pay your electric bill.

You need to pace yourself so you don't burn out. Competent TBI docs are hard to find. Hopefully through this book, these patients will soon have other knowledgeable HCPs to see about their TBIs. They will have you.

On that note: Do not panic when you see the length of some of the patient assessment chapters. The sample forms will provide you with history forms that can be filled out in advance and physical forms that hopefully will help you save time and energy. You can adapt these forms in ways that better accommodate your personal style and the nature of your practice. The rest of this chapter provides you with suggested content for various patient interactions.

Organization will be the key to your success and provide the patient with the best chance of getting well. There's no time like the present.

Focus on the patient. Continuously gather information. Talk to the person. Make eye contact with the patient early and often. Talk to parents, spouses, siblings, and grandparents. While this may seem to be friendly chatter, it is all part of gathering pertinent information. Does a child "get" age appropriate jokes? When does the patient laugh? How does he interact with his family? Was a child able to sit still? Could he listen to a complete sentence? Did he laugh at the joke meant for his older sister? Did he not get the joke thrown to his younger brother? Always engage the individual. You will garner a great deal of information.

Initial contact

A patient, parent, or caregiver will contact your office and speak to someone on your staff. If you are seeing people who have been abused by the traditional health care system, your staff should try to be kind. Nothing can be more aggravating to your staff than handling a distraught, desperate person pleading for an appointment. Patients who I have talked to on the phone are often crying and literally begging. No one on earth needs more tolerance and empathy than these folks. Please ask your staff to have the patience of Job and the wisdom of Solomon. They will need it.

Also, as you get a better feel for how TBI cases fit into your practice, build in some cushion time. Some people do need to be seen fast (and they have already been to the emergency room). If the person sounds as if he needs help before the

next available open appointment, please talk to the patient or caretaker yourself and assess the situation. Be careful to weigh the hysteria of the caregiver against the nonchalance of the overworked HCP. These folks are not trying to annoy you; they are simply trying to get help. (As an experienced ER physician, I know that I was treated abominably by some of the staff and HCPs that my son saw early in the course of his disease. Soon I, too, was screaming into the phone.)

When the staff first speaks to the caregiver, please ask them not to lead with money talk. I recall a receptionist's first words to me: "We don't take insurance. Cash or check only and you must have a picture ID. We charge $50 for any bounced checks." (Try not to care so much.) Of course, the responsible person can be told the cost of the visit up front. Although I do not give pricing advice, know that many insurances will not cover extensive assessment or testing for TBIs so the patient or caregiver may need to pay out-of-pocket. Your staff should know your payment program. (Just some advice that I have no credentials to give: If you are not seeing only TBI patients in your practice, you may want to charge based on how long this patient will take compared to how many routine patients you usually see in this time period. You can't help anyone if you don't stay solvent. Please consider these financial considerations as you begin to see complicated TBI cases.)

Make sure that the person answering the phone has an idea of how to judge the urgency of the appointment request. If not, ask the office nurse to speak to the caller.

Please try to be reachable. An answering service is fine if they answer and the caller does not have to push 124 buttons to reach a human. I know the service company tells you that their automated system is just as good as a person, but it's not. Remember that when the recording tells the caller to go to the ER if they have a "true" emergency, they probably already have. Forgive callers for being a little hysterical. They may have been trying to get help for their sick kid for hours or days or…

Consider that you might construct a website that provides information. On the website, have ALL contact information. Do not make it as hard as possible to find or reach you. If you say you can be reached by e-mail, read your e-mail and ensure that a response is sent in a timely manner. Because of confidentiality issues, e-mail may not be a good place to discuss specifics of a case but it can be great for scheduling times to talk on the phone or for making an appointment.

Once an appointment is made, have clear directions to your office available. Patients come from all over the place and clear directions are essential. Don't just print out something from MapQuest. Make sure someone actually tries the directions and that they are viable. Add landmarks if possible. According to Gandhi nothing is more aggravating than calmness, but Gandhi never dealt with TBIs. Nothing is more aggravating than getting close and then not being able to find the office.

These directions should be available by phone, by e-mail, and hard copy. Since patients may be coming from far away (there are not many TBD literate HCPs out there) know a local, reasonably priced hotel for them to use in case they must stay overnight. Know the local parking situation.

> *PEARL: Have directions to the office posted over the phone so that the clerical staff can read them. Don't have them rely on memory. This saves time and is especially helpful for new staff members. You would be surprised at how many people answer the phone and don't seem to know what city or state they are in let alone how to get there. Make sure the answering service has a copy of the directions.*

Review the cancellation policy. Tell the caller they may have to wait in case you get behind. Explain how long the visit will last. If they know up front that there might be a LONG wait, they are usually okay with it and they can prepare. Also, they may be more patient if they know that the visit they are waiting for is worthwhile and that they will get the same individual attention when it is their turn. Most patients are so grateful to be able to see a competent TBI clinician that they are willing to walk across hot coals and then wait as long as necessary. Unfortunately, many of us have not yet earned that kind of reputation. Have a staff member reassure folks in the waiting room that they have not been forgotten and that it takes time for a comprehensive evaluation especially if surprises intrude on the schedule. A child you thought was a routine follow-up could be much sicker than expected. Everyone gets behind. My mother would insist on arriving at any appointment an hour early and then get furious because she had to wait even BEFORE her scheduled time. Buddha said that expectations lead to disappointments. In the case of TBI practices, getting in close to on-time is a gift.

Arrange to send the patient all forms you will need to have filled out prior to the initial visit including HIPAA release, any payment or insurance forms, medical release forms for other doctors, informed consent or disclaimer forms, demographics form, and history forms (including history of TBI, general history, and ROS). Sample forms are presented throughout the text. Mail the forms as soon as reasonable. If possible, have the caretaker mail the completed forms back to you. (They should keep copies: forms do get lost in the mail in an inverse relationship to how long it took to fill them out.) This way the staff has time to organize the chart and you have time to review the patient's situation.

If the patient had previous lab work or other tests, or was seen by other HCPs for TBI, see if those records are available.

Usually the authorized guardian will need to sign a release form to obtain these records. Send several release forms along with the initial information packet. Have this information sent directly to your office to save time. This material can then be incorporated in the chart and reviewed prior to the visit. Previous records can save considerable time and money. At least they might show you what didn't work. Sample Form IV: Release of Information is presented in the *Sample Form Gallery* at the end of this chapter.

> *PEARL: I once worked in an office where the HCP charged $50 for each bit of information he sent out for a patient. He took this money under the table and the IRS found out. I was gone from that practice by then, but rest assured, I smiled. Remember, while the physical chart belongs to the practice, the information belongs to the patient and he has a right to it. My former co-worker soon learned that you cannot hold medical information hostage. While it may be appropriate to charge for materials and copying, this guy was running a tax-dodging scam.*

You and your staff should not make promises you can't keep. If you tell the patient you will meet her in the ER, meet her in the ER. Do not promise her that and then after seven hours of inane assessment, tell her it would be inconvenient for you to come in this late. (She came to the ER only because YOU told her to!) Most parents are at the point that they will do anything you say, so just give them the straight story.

If you see non-TBI patients, you may occasionally find yourself with a patient you thought was coming in for an earache and was therefore scheduled in one of your 6-minute slots. You learn by minute 2 that the child probably has a complicated TBI. This leaves you in a bind because you know that a full work-up will take hours.

Likewise, with many TBI kids, when the family finally gets to your office from Arkansas, you see that one of the kids accompanying the patient is sicker with TBD than the one who was scheduled. If possible, try to build into your daily schedule time to accommodate modern medicine's little surprises. If the child is not seriously ill and lives nearby, put him on the schedule in the next day or so to handle the TBI issue. In the meantime, try to provide some relief for the chief complaint. Unfortunately, this might mean coming in early or staying late. Welcome to medicine in 2013.

Refer patients to the ER if they have an emergency that needs to be addressed immediately and you cannot handle the problem in your office. But recall that ERs do not do well with TBIs and the child and her family may have to wait half a day only to be told she is annoying and faking and to pay the co-pay before she leaves. Show as much compassion as you can and hope that someone will do the same for you when you need some understanding.

PEARL: Be careful. There are a few caretakers out there who will take advantage of your compassion. I remember once seeing four siblings of a child with an earache. Each kid looked sicker than the last one. This meant that in the middle of my exam with the scheduled child, the staff had to make charts and take histories and get vital signs on four more separate patients. I spent an hour that night documenting these cases. Of course, the mother felt that this all should be charged as just one office visit. After all, she only came in once. A good motto is: If they can sue separately, then they need to pay separately. Further, a scheduled TBI visit is not the best time to work-up Abigail's scar from last year's dog bite, even if you completely understand the dog's motivation. Schedule separate appointments for problems that are clearly unrelated such as camp physicals, tattoo removal, etc.

Prior to first visit

If you are going to be seeing a lot of TBD, get organized now. Know how you want your charts set up. Know where in the chart the HIPAA forms go and the informed consent and the basic demographic cover sheet. The chart should reflect your working style so that you can flow from page to page without flipping back and forth all the time. You need to be able to find what you need when you need it. Make the chart work for you. Run a tight ship when it comes to meticulous maintenance of your records.

Construct as much of the chart as possible before the first visit. You may want to have a standard chart checklist to ensure that everything is in its place and there is a place for everything. These cases get complicated. Sample Form I: Chart Checklist is located at the end of this chapter in the section titled *Sample Form Gallery.*

Note that the visits, contacts, updates, and instructions can be placed in chronological order from oldest to most recent for easy access. Each * corresponds to a sample form presented in this chapter or the following chapters. All forms in this text are for your perusal, adjustment, and use. They should be adapted to your practice. They are not all-inclusive and are not intended to dictate practices of medicine. With the rapidly changing field of TBIs, the content will likely need to be updated regularly. In fact, some items may no longer be the latest thinking. Use what is pertinent for you and your patients and leave the rest.

Demographics are the basic identifiers for the patient. The Demographics Form is Sample Form II presented in the *Sample Form Gallery* at the end of the chapter. Likewise, a sample Informed Consent or Disclaimer form can be found there.

Many practices dealing with TBIs include what could be called an "Informed Consent" or "Disclaimer" form. Usually these forms describe the options around managing TBI cases and the alternatives regarding testing, diagnosis, and treatment. The purpose of these documents is to minimize the risk of lawsuits for malpractice, negligence, or any other reason to pursue a legal claim. Many experienced TBI practitioners include some type of "Informed Consent" or "Disclaimer" form as part of the patient registration packet. The document might outline the different approaches to the diagnosis of Lyme including mention of both the ILADS and IDSA guidelines, treatment options, and the potential benefits and risks of alternative approaches. Since I do not know the scope of your practice, a sample outlined by me is not practical. With that being said, this is not a document that you write by yourself. If you elect to include such a disclaimer, get experienced legal counsel to help you draft the text. Please know that the lawyer may have you sign an informed consent saying that the document she drafted is no guarantee against law suits that can come at any time, from anyone, from anywhere. Some states have laws that say patients cannot sign away their right to sue. Check what is true in your state and never believe that a signed informed consent is insurance against lawsuits. A determined adversary can find a way to come after you. Make sure your charts protect you.

A sample Informed Consent form is available at www.lyme-disease.org and a description is located in the *Sample Form Gallery* as Sample Form III at the end of this chapter.

First visit

Patients with TBIs take time. Forget that the average HMO is proud that they allow only 6 minutes per patient. You will need about two hours for an initial visit and an hour for each subsequent visit. Please take this into consideration as you schedule patients and make sure your staff understands. It's not fair to get angry at a patient or rush a patient because you did not plan properly. I am telling you these patients are complicated and they take time. Even after you get all your forms in order and your visits hum like a well-oiled machine: expect two hours for an initial visit and an hour for each subsequent visit.

PEARL: Last night I spent two hours answering an e-mail question about Lyme from a relative. The question was simple and straightforward. Still, the response took me two hours. Do not underestimate the time involved.

Since there is a lot of ground to cover, you will want to use your time as wisely as possible. In my work over the years, I have witnessed so much wasteful medicine that I hope to provide insight into how to make your patient visits efficient and effective. I am a great advocate of documentation. I believe if you don't document, you forget. I believe if you don't document, it never happened. Document.

With that being said, it is a waste of time to write the same things over and over and over. For example to write the word *musculoskeletal* three times as you record the history, the review of systems, and the physical is just eating time you do not have. I would rather pay my money for you to think about the patient than to write the word musculoskeletal over and over again. I have seen this so many times in all the major medical centers. While dictating and electronic record keeping may solve these problems in the future, those HCPs currently using these on-line systems seem to spend a lot of time being confused about the software with their eyes glued to the screen, rarely glancing at the patient. We ain't there yet.

Make your chart work for you. Use checklists to assure that nothing falls through the cracks. Chapters 15, 16, and 17 contain long, detailed H&P recommendations that were written to instruct, not necessarily to put in the chart. But, sample forms for the history, physical, and ROS, along with a sample form for follow-up visits that combines the information from all three of these data-gathering exercises are also included. While this 3-in-1 form may be very different from the "progress notes" you are used to putting in your charts, consider giving it a try or modifying it into a style that works for you. Hopefully, this form will help make follow-up visits more time-efficient. I constructed this form after watching several preceptors document their data. The time wasting was often painful to see. Time is limited. Use it wisely. Develop forms that work for you, remembering that there should not be many reasons to gather the same bits of information over and over. Sample Form VIII: The 3-in-1 Follow-up Visit Form is presented in the *Sample Form Gallery* at the end of the chapter.

When the patient is in your presence, look at the patient. Study the chart BEFORE the patient comes into the room and if possible document most of the details AFTER the person leaves. Make sure your scheduling and charting and billing are set up in a way that allows your practice to survive.

Remember that this patient may be new to you but not new to the TBI world. Most TBI patients have seen more than a dozen HCPs in their quest to get well. Their caregivers come in with reams of paper and files. As part of their history, see what they've already had done. You may find some valid reports that will save time and money now. Old negatives are no more valid than new negatives. While a positive test result may support a diagnosis, a negative test result merely says there was no evidence of the pathogen in this ONE sample, using the particular testing methods of a certain lab, on a specific day. The tests may not have been sensitive or specific enough to register a positive on this patient. Negative means not detected, NOT uninfected.

Things to do on the first visit:

> Meet the patient
>
> Meet the family

Review old records

Review history of TBI

Review general history

Conduct comprehensive ROS

Perform physical examination

Discuss initial impressions

Decide on lab or other testing

Consider treatment options

Involve the patient and caregivers

Formulate a path forward

Review instructions

Answer questions

Discuss next contact

Complete all charting

On the first visit, depending on what you suspect, here are some tests you might consider:

> For Lyme: ELISA (only if forced for insurance purposes), IgM & IgG Western blot. Consider Bb blood culture as delineated in Chapter 18. This culture developed by Advanced Laboratory Services is best drawn BEFORE the start of antibiotics.
>
> For ehrlichiosis/anaplasmosis: HME and HGA titers, blood smear
>
> For babesiosis: Blood smear, or select from IFA, PCR, or FISH
>
> For bartonellosis: IFA or PCR
>
> For Mycoplasma *fermentans*: IFA or PCR
>
> Depending on the clinical presentation and history also consider: chronic fatigue panel, EBV, CMV (IgM and IgG), Chlamydia screen, HHV-6, HHV-8, Strep testing (cultures, titers, antibodies), screening for M. *pneumonia*
>
> Routine studies for baseline pretreatment and diagnostic clues: CBC with differential, metabolic panel with BUN, creatinine, calcium, albumin, magnesium, LFTs such as alkaline phosphatase, ALT, AST, and bilirubin. You probably do not need a routine glucose or chloride or CO_2, but it is usually cheaper to order a panel than to try to NOT get these tests. Routine panels of more than about a dozen components are usually overkill.

Depending on the clinical picture, consider thyroid functions and anti-thyroid antibodies. Some do a variety of additional hormonal testing including cortisol ratios.

If there is a suggestion of autoimmunity, consider an immune panel. Chapter 18: *Ordering Appropriate Tests* reviews the options that might be appropriate for your patient. Consider ordering HLA-DR2 and HLA-DR4 testing on most Lyme patients with on-going sxs to check for their proclivity towards an autoimmune response to Lyme. Many of the other tests in the immune panel are nonspecific, qualitative assessments of inflammation. If you already know the answer to the question, you might want to hold off on some of these tests. Remember these people are already mortgaging the house to pay for this work-up. Some docs order tests just because they can. Some order the test to show they know more than you. Really. Some are afraid they don't know enough and if they order everything off the menu they are bound to hit some correct choices. Really.

PEARL: I just heard of a case where the HCP kept ordering "Lyme tests" since results from several labs kept coming back <u>*positive*</u>*. He was hoping to get a* <u>*negative*</u> *result. Please tell me how that would have changed the patient's clinical condition. If nothing else, this story inspires me to write faster since apparently many HCPs need a little guidance.*

Some sources recommend baseline CPKs. Others recommend tests that I couldn't figure out even after I researched for days. Ask yourself, "Do I really need this test result? What will I do with it when I get it? Can I get my answer another way?"

Discuss what you are thinking. Explain why you are recommending certain tests. Review the pros and cons of various treatment options. Make a plan together.

As a parent of a TBI patient, I know that the instructions given to us were often overwhelming and incomprehensible (and I'm a physician who studied like a rabid dog for each appointment). I needed written instructions. If you will be seeing a number of TBI patients, you may want to make an instruction sheet to fill in and hand out to the parent/patient, so nothing falls through the cracks. A sample is included as Form V in the *Sample Form Gallery* at the end of the chapter.

This Patient Instructions Form should be in duplicate, one for the caregiver and one for the chart. Use this form during the next visit to assess progress. Of all the work I have done on this book, this form has had the most positive response. Caretakers have told me that "if only" they had this

form when their child was sick... Give it a chance. Further, the HCPs who have reviewed the document feel that it is comprehensive and will help prevent important aspects of the treatment plan from being overlooked. When so much information is flying back and forth, it is easy to inadvertently skip something. This form serves as a checklist and review of the material you have already discussed. If your handwriting is abysmal, make small label sheets of your most commonly used orders and stick them in place on the form. For example, "Alternate ibuprofen and acetaminophen for fever over 102." Some HCPs like to have a standard "one-size-fits-all" instruction sheet for their patients. These can be quite valuable. But in broad medical practice with all the different ages and nuances and the many possible co-infections and concurrent conditions, the Patient Instructions form may allow for more flexibility and a means to target the needs of a particular patient. The instruction sheet can also serve as the conversation-starter at the next patient visit.

The more TBI patients you see the easier these instructions will flow off your tongue. But for the caretaker/patient this all sounds like Klingon no matter how many times they have heard it. All the work you have done in assessing the patient and making a treatment plan will be for naught if the caretakers do not know what to do when they walk out the door.... Or if they do things incorrectly..... Or don't do some things at all.

HCPs familiar with TBIs will often rattle off species and lab test results and medications, leaving the patient or caretaker in the dust. Just because you know these things, does not mean the patient or parent will know them (even if they are HCPs). Although I remembered a little from medical school about some pathogen killing cattle by making them pee blood, when my son was diagnosed, I had to look up Babesia right quick when I got home. (Babesia were Piroplasma when I was in school.) Then before the next visit we practiced sounding it out in the car before we got to the office so we wouldn't look like nincompoops in front of the physician. (Bab EEE See O sis)

This is a patient population that has been to a dozen HCPs, is still sick to the core, and is about to spend thousands of dollars on lab tests and medicines, so you might want to communicate with them with some frequency. Generally a telephone contact with each new patient within two weeks is prudent. Tell them to call the office any time if there is a problem before the scheduled follow-up.

<u>Follow-up visits</u>

Follow-up visits can be done by phone or in person. Since some of your patients may live far away, the follow-up may need to occur over the phone.

Things to do on a follow-up visit:

    Greet the patient and know who else is on the phone

    Review the Status Update form*

    Discuss any lab or test results

    If this is an in-office visit, examine patient

    Review previous Patient Instructions form*

    Discuss current status and next steps

    Revise previous diagnoses and treatment plans if needed

    Order more testing if appropriate

    Consider ancillary treatments, supportive measures, and need for consultations

    Involve the patient and caregivers in formulating a path forward

    Fill in a new Patient Instructions form*

    Answer any questions

    Decide on next contact

    Attach one copy of the Patient Instructions form to chart and mail/fax/hand the other to the patient

    Finish charting.

At each follow-up visit use a new Patient Instructions sheet and a new Status Update form and incorporate these documents into the chronological notes in the chart. This way you know what happened last time and you know the specific issues you want to address and follow-up during this contact visit. A sample Status Update form is Sample Form VI in the *Sample Form Gallery* at the end of this chapter.

Telephone contacts

Usually office staff handle in-coming calls regarding administrative issues. For medical questions or concerns, the nurse might be able to handle the issue. If needed, the physician can review the question to determine when she can talk to or see the patient. These contacts can be documented on Sample Form VII: Telephone Contact found at the end of this chapter.

Telephone communication can be used:

- As follow-up

- To discuss intermittent issues such as change in symptoms or adverse drug effects.

If the telephone is used to follow-up, take advantage of both the Patient Instructions form and the Status Update form to document the interaction. For example, if you are using a phone contact as follow-up two weeks after an initial visit, write on the phone contact sheet that this is a follow-up contact. Use the previous Patient Instructions sheet to direct the conversation and fill in the new Patient Instructions form. Send a copy of the new Instructions sheet to the patient and keep one in the chart.

General Advice for a Productive Visit:

1. Before each visit, review the chart.

2. Recognize that these diseases can be confounding. The more organized you are, the clearer your thinking.

3. Don't just go down the checklist like a robot. Let the patient express concerns.

4. End each encounter with HEAVY encouragement. TBIs can be a rough road, especially for a sick kid and overwrought caretakers.

5. Make sure the patient and caretakers have time to ask their questions.

6. When assessing a patient make sure that she is stable before proceeding.

7. There will be assessment areas where you are strong and others where you are weak. When you are out of your depth, consult.

8. When working with consultants, don't lose your patient. Someone has to coordinate the overall management of the TBI. That coordinator should be you.

9. There is a lot of ground to cover at each visit. Remember you can be gathering information from many sources simultaneously.

10. While the sample forms may look quite different from "the way we've always done things around here" try them to see if they might make your visits more efficient.

11. The recommended approach in the following chapters is geared to TBIs. You may need to expand your knowledge base if you are dealing outside this therapeutic area.

12. Don't have Lyme tunnel vision. Every patient doesn't have Lyme or any TBI for that matter. We are so outraged that our TBIs were ignored or mistreated that we tend to overcompensate.

13. When doing the H&P, remember that a patient can have two or more different disease processes going on at once. Just because they have acute otitis media does not mean

that they can't also have hearing problems due to a TBI. Just because they have one kind of arthritis does not mean they cannot have two. This is especially true with neuropsychiatric manifestations.

14. Do not be too quick to dismiss signs and symptoms by saying "Oh, that's all part of his Lyme." More than one thing can be happening.

15. Have an open mind and a high index of suspicion and see how all the pieces of the puzzle fit. Do not cherry-pick where you focus only on those findings that support a preconceived diagnosis and dismiss those that could lead you down a different path.

16. If you need more time to better assess the patient, take more time. You do not have to be better than the masters, just learn from them.

17. Address all affirmative responses made on the history and ROS. Don't have a child tell you that his stomach always hurts after he eats and then you let that go into the ether.

18. If you stop worrying about how behind you are you can actually enjoy patient care. Especially when you are just beginning to see many TBI patients, allow yourself plenty of scheduling cushion. As you get more comfortable in this field, you will get faster and more efficient. If you are constantly behind, you will be perpetually stressed and annoyed. That's no fun and not especially healthy for you.

19. Keep your eyes and ears and all remaining senses on the patient. I once had an ophthalmologist at Hopkins do my entire exam, except for a few seconds looking at my fundus, with her back toward me. When she dictated the note, still with backside prominent, she had the wrong chief complaint, history, and ROS. Attempting to correct her got me nowhere. Her diagnosis had nothing to do with why I was there and her treatment plan was to use OTC saline drops. Think she enjoys her work?

20. A number of the physical assessments can be done concurrently. Every area is a smorgasbord of information. When evaluating an extremity, you can be assessing the skin, joints, movement, circulation, ROM, coordination, demeanor, as well as the nervous system with reflexes, sensation, and pain distribution. When examining the back look at the skin, ribs, kidney, spine, ROM, and tenderness. You don't want to examine the right leg for reflexes and then go do something else and then come back to the right leg to check pulses and then do something else and then come back and check the range of motion in that knee. Find a style that flows effectively for you.

21. Always be observant for any hint that will cause you to target an area more specifically. Each step in the H&P should guide you to where you need to go as the exam progresses.

22. Many of the questions and techniques listed in the next chapters apply to both children and adults. Nevertheless, kids are not just short adults and infants are very different from teenagers. While the older a child gets the more adult-like she becomes, it is equally true that recent studies have shown that a 24-year-old may be more like an 18-year-old than she is like a 30-year-old.

23. You know what you know, but it is equally important to admit what you don't know. When you are out of your league, refer to a specialist but don't lose your patient. You need to follow both the TBI as well as the condition that needs specialty assessment. If the condition is related to the TBI then there is much less chance of a successful outcome if the underlying TBI is not adequately addressed. In fact, an unresolving symptom might have led someone to consider TBIs in the first place.

24. Each HCP must find the techniques that work best for her. The sample forms presented are not intended to be used exactly as outlined but to be adapted for the most efficient use in your practice. The forms can help ensure that you don't forget anything as you move through the exam. Modify them to suit your style and practice.

25. The assessment information provided in the following chapters cannot be all-inclusive because of time and space constraints. Nonetheless, the text should provide sufficient foundation for you to conduct a productive TBI assessment.

Since I had no idea where in the text to include the 3-in-1 form, I decided to put it in the *Sample Form Gallery* at the end of this chapter. The forms designed to capture the initial visit History, Physical, and Review of Systems are long and detailed and hopefully present a broad view of what is happening with the patient. In contrast, the 3-in-1 form works off only those items pertinent to that individual. By not re-inventing the wheel at each visit, your practice should become more efficient. Use a version of Sample Form VIII during follow-up visits.

Sample Form VIII: 3-IN-1 Follow-up Visit is presented at the end of the chapter in the *Sample Form Gallery*. The 3-in-1 Follow-Up Visit form is designed to allow the HCP to quickly move through the information in the pertinent history, review of systems, and physical exam without going over the same material again and again. The patient or caretaker fills in the demographic information on the top of the form and then completes the history and ROS. The HCP then adds comments as appropriate to those sections and completes the PE section. This form serves as a checklist so that nothing falls through the cracks. Since *only* positive findings are recorded, the form allows for a rapid sweep of the information so the HCP can focus on the important issues for the specific patient. If the patient or caretaker can complete portions of the form before they are in the doctor's office, much time can be saved since each question does not need to be asked individually. This way the visit can concentrate on those items that are important to the particular case. While the 3-in-1 form will take much of the repetitiveness out of the information gathering during the follow-up visit and save considerable time, the HCP will still need to write a visit note outlining any conclusions and plans associated with the patient contact.

SAMPLE FORM GALLERY

SAMPLE FORM I: CHART CONTENT CHECKLIST

CHART CONTENT CHECKLIST

__	1.	HIPPA form
__	2.	Insurance information
__	3.	Demographics sheet or Cover sheet*
__	4.	Informed Consent or Disclaimer form*
__	5.	History of the Patient's TBD form*
__	6.	General Patient History form*
__	7.	ROS form*
__	8.	Physical Examination form*
__	9.	Follow-up visit update form*
__	10.	Lab results
__	11.	Test results
__	12.	Consultation reports
__	13.	Visit/Contact notes
__	14.	Patient Instructions*
__	15.	Telephone contacts*
__	16.	Old records
__	17.	Miscellaneous: School or work notes, etc.

SAMPLE FORM II: DEMOGRAPHICS FORM

DEMOGRAPHICS FORM

Last name: _____ Today's date: _____

Full name: _____ DOB: _____ Age today: _____

SSN: _____

Address: _____

Phone: _____ Alternate Phone: _____

School: _____ School Phone: _____

Pharmacy: _____ Phone: _____ Fax:_____ E-mail:_____

Father: _____ Phone: _____ E-mail:_____

Mother: _____ Phone: _____ E-mail:_____

Guardian: _____ Phone: _____ E-mail:_____

Caretaker: _____ Phone: _____ E-mail:_____

Primary HCP: _____ Phone: _____ E-mail:_____

Insurance: _____ Phone: _____ E-mail:_____

Additional insurance information: _____

_____

Other contact information: _____

_____

ALLERGIES: _____

_____

SAMPLE FORM III: INFORMED CONSENT or DISCLAIMER FORM

INFORMED CONSENT or DISCLAIMER FORM

Many practices dealing with TBIs include what could be called an "Informed Consent" or "Disclaimer" form. Usually these forms describe the options around managing TBI cases and the alternatives regarding testing, diagnosis, and treatment. The purpose of these documents is to minimize the risk of lawsuits for malpractice, negligence, or any other reason to pursue a legal claim. Many experienced TBI practitioners include some type of "Informed Consent" or "Disclaimer" form as part of the patient registration packet. The document might outline the different approaches to the diagnosis of Lyme including mention of both the ILADS and IDSA guidelines, treatment options, and the potential benefits and risks of alternative approaches. Since I do not know the scope of your practice, a sample outlined by me is not practical. With that being said, this is not a document that you write by yourself. If you elect to include such a disclaimer, get experienced legal counsel to help you draft the text. Please know that the lawyer may have you sign an informed consent saying that the document she drafted is no guarantee against law suits that can come at anytime, from anyone, from anywhere. Some states have laws that say patients cannot sign away their right to sue. Check what is true in your state and never believe that a signed informed consent is insurance against lawsuits. A determined adversary can find a way to come after you. Make sure your charts protect you.

A sample Informed Consent form is available at www.lymedisease.org

SAMPLE FORM IV: RELEASE OF INFORMATION FORM

Many patients have seen multiple HCPs prior to their first visit. Past records can provide important information or at least tell you what has already been tried and perhaps establish some baseline values. To have the records released requires permission from the responsible party.

RELEASE OF INFORMATION REQUEST

Patient Name: _____   Date: _____

Birthday: _____   SSN: _____

Please send copies of all available medical records for _____ to:

(Patient Name)

_____

(Name of HCP requesting records)

_____

(Address of HCP requesting records)

_____

_____

Signature of person authorized to release records: _____

Printed name of person authorized to release records: _____

This form will need to be delivered to the site retaining the records.

SAMPLE FORM V: PATIENT INSTRUCTIONS FORM

PATIENT INSTRUCTIONS

Patient name: _____ Date: _____

To best help you until our next contact, I recommend the following:

1. Medications:

    Start: _____

    Stop: _____

    Continue: _____

    Change:_____

    New OTC: (Vitamins, Supplements, etc.) _____

2. Diet: (For almost all patients I recommend minimizing sugar, white flour, and processed foods.) Drink water. Also, consider: _____

3. Exercise (For almost all patients, I recommend daily activity, recognizing that a TBI may impact ability.) Also, consider: _____

4. Testing (You may need an order slip for these.) _____

5. Lab tests (You should have a slip for these unless they were drawn here in the office.)

    _____

6. School or work note: (Attach copy to chart or reproduce here.) _____

7. Referrals: _____

8. Other: _____

9. At your next visit please bring: _____

10. Any questions? _____

Our next contact is: _____Office appointment: _____Telephone contact: _____

Date and time:_____

Given a copy of Status Update Form to be used at next contact. _____YES

If you have any questions or problems, please call: _____

_____

Signature of provider

SAMPLE FORM VI: STATUS UPDATE

STATUS UPDATE

Name: _____   Date: _____

Birthday : _____   Age today: _____

Allergies: _____

Since your last visit:

- Are you better? Worse? The same? _____

- What has changed? _____

- Have you changed any medicines? _____

- Have you had problems with any medicines? _____

- Has another doctor given you any treatment? _____

- What is bothering you the most? _____

- If you could eliminate one symptom it would be: _____

- Anything else you want us to know? _____

_____

Signature of person taking information

SAMPLE FORM VII: TELEPHONE CONTACT

TELEPHONE CONTACT

NAME: _____ AGE: _____ DATE: _____

Allergies: _____ Phone #: _____

Problem:

_____

_____

_____

_____

Discussion:

_____

_____

_____

_____

Instructions:

_____

_____

_____

_____

Was told to call back if any further problems.

_____

Signature of contact

SAMPLE FORM VIII: 3-IN-1 FOLLOW-UP VISIT

3-IN-1 FOLLOW-UP VISIT

NAME: _____ Birthday: _____ Age today: _____

Allergies: _____

Current medications: _____

_____

_____

Measurements: Height _____ Weight _____ Other _____

Vital signs: Temp _____ (Circle: Oral, Rectal, Forehead, Axilla)

RR _____ HR _____ BP _____/_____

Chief complaint today: _____

_____

Check YES only if there is an abnormality or problem:

Parameter	History		Current ROS		Physical Exam	
	Yes	Describe	Yes	Describe	Yes	Describe
General						
Fever						
Demeanor						
Energy levels						
Skin						
Rash						
Nails						
Hair/Scalp						
Head						
Bell's palsy						
Eyes						
Ears						
Nose						
Mouth						
Tongue						
Teeth						
TMJ						
Throat						

Neck					
Nodes					
Thyroid					
Back					
Chest					
Breasts					
Axillary nodes					
Lungs					
Cough					
SOB					
Heart					
Rate					
Rhythm					
Sounds					
Circulation					
Pulses					
Cold limbs					
Bleeding					
Abdomen					
GI problems					
Rectal Area					
Groin					
Pulses					
Nodes					
Genitals					
Tanner stages					
Pelvis					
Urinary sxs					
Bones					
Muscles					
Strength					
Tone					
Motion					
Joints					
ROM					
Effusion					
Heat					
Fainting					
Weakness					
Numbness					

Dizziness					
Seizures					
Mental status					
Cranial nerves					
Reflexes					
Balance					
Gait					
Coordination					
Motor/movement					
Sensation					
Cold					
Hypersensitivity					
Pain					
Speech					
Tics					
Tremors					
Spasms					
Mood					
Anxiety					
Obsessions					
Compulsions					
Suicidal					
Thought processes					
Relation to reality					
Paranoia					
Aggression					
Anger					
Passivity					
Focus					
Distractibility					
Impulsivity					
Judgment					
Depression					
Panic					
Irritability					
Social interaction					
School issues					
Family					
Home life					
Sleep					

Activities					
Outlook					
Eye contact					
Age appropriate					
Cooperation					
Lability					
Oppositional					
Repetitive behavior					
Cooperation					
Developmental milestones					

Chapter 14

HISTORY OF PRESENT TICK-BORNE ILLNESS

An appeaser is one who feeds a crocodile, hoping it will eat him last.
Winston Churchill

While cognizant that any number of problems could be brewing in your patient, I focus here on the tick and the presumed reason for the office visit. In practice, this history of the current TBI can be incorporated into the larger patient history form. The history of the possible TBI is best illustrated with a sample form.

SAMPLE FORM IX: HISTORY OF THIS PATIENT'S TICK-BORNE ILLNESS

HISTORY OF THIS TICK-BORNE ILLNESS

Last name: _____ Date: _____

Full name: _____ DOB: _____ Age today: _____

Tick Bite Risk:

Live in known tick area   Yes__ No__ Describe:_____

Outdoor activities: Yes__ No__ Describe: _____

Pets that go outside: Yes__ No__ Describe: _____

Recent travel: Yes__ No__ Describe: _____

Bite: No recollection of bite does **NOT** mean there was no bite.

Do you remember a tick bite? _____

What did the tick look like? _____

Was the tick attached? _____

Was the tick swollen? _____

Estimate how long the tick might have been attached? _____

What is the most likely geographic source of the tick? _____

How was the tick removed? _____

Were all tick parts removed? _____

After the bite:

Did you get a rash after the bite? _____ Yes? When? _____

Where? _____

Describe: _____

Were you seen by a doctor? _____ Yes? Who? _____

Any lab work done? _____ Where? _____

Results? _____

Any treatments given? _____

Current treatment? _____

TBI History:

Have you been bitten by ticks in the past? _____

Have you been diagnosed with a tick-borne illness in the past? When? Check all that apply.

Lyme (Borreliosis)	☐ When? _____		STARI (Borreliosis)	☐ When? _____		
Babesiosis	☐ When? _____		Ehrlichiosis/Anaplasmosis	☐ When? _____		
Bartonella	☐ When? _____		Mycoplasma *fermentans*	☐ When? _____		
RMSF	☐ When? _____		Other	☐ When? _____		

Current Illness:

What is your chief complaint today? _____

When did you first notice a problem? _____

Looking back, did you notice anything unusual before you thought there was something wrong?

_____

What other symptoms do you have? _____

What is your worst symptom? _____

What is your strangest symptom? _____

What makes you feel better? _____

What makes you feel worse? _____

ROS:

Do you have pain? __ Severity? _____ Where? _____

Describe: _____

Do you have fever? Chills? Sweats? _____

Do you have fatigue? Weakness? Sleepiness? _____

Do you have any rash anywhere? Describe. _____

Upset stomach, diarrhea, constipation, nausea, vomiting, heartburn, problem urinating?

_____

Shortness of breath or cough? _____

Do you have joint or muscle pain? Stiffness? Cramps? _____

Do you have any twitching, tremors, tics, numbness, stinging, burning, paralysis, sensitivity?

_____

Vision or hearing problems?_____

Are you having trouble with balance or coordination? _____

Are you having trouble thinking, concentrating, feeling confused, or using poor judgment?

_____

Is your neck stiff or cracking?_____

Are you overly emotional, feeling angry, irritable, sad, suicidal, violent?_____

Sleeping too much or too little? _____

Current Treatment:

List all current medicines including vitamins and OTC products. Include doses and how long you have been taking these treatments.

_____

_____

_____

_____

Medicines you have tried in the past for this problem but stopped. Why did you stop?

_____

_____

Have you had any bad reactions to any of these medicines?

_____

_____

Did your symptoms seem worse after starting treatment?

_____

_____

Anything else we should know? _____

_____

_____

ALLERGIES: _____

Chapter 15

PATIENT HISTORY

What would be the use of immortality to a person who can't make good use of a half hour?
Unknown

The patient history records the answers to the questions: "Did you EVER have____?" and "Did anyone in your family EVER have ____?" The form as it might be adapted in your practice is presented below. Some of this material is targeted to pediatric patients. Convert the form to meet your needs.

SAMPLE FORM X: PATIENT HISTORY

PATIENT HISTORY

Patient Name: _____ Date: _____

Birthday: _____ Age today: _____

CHIEF COMPLAINT: _____

ALLERGIES:

      Medicine: ____ Yes _____

      Animals: ____ Yes _____

      Latex: ____ Yes _____

      Foods: ____ Yes _____

      Pollens: ____ Yes _____

      Molds: ____ Yes _____

      Other: ____ Yes _____

GENERAL HISTORY:

      Historian: (check) ____ patient ____ caregiver ____ parent ____ guardian ____ other

      Other current HCPs: _____ Phone: _____

                           _____   _____

                             _____   _____

      Identifying demographics:

      DOB: _____ Age today: _____ Gender: _____ Ethnic group: _____

DETAILS OF PREGNANCY:

Complications during pregnancy: _____

Was mother known to be infected with any TBI during pregnancy or ever? _____

Term, early, or late delivery? _____

APGAR: First score _____ Second score _____

Did the attendant mention any problems? _____

Did the mother think there was anything wrong? _____

Breast or formula fed? _____

Jaundice at birth or soon after? _____ Increased bilirubin? _____ Treatment with lights? _____

Kept in hospital after birth for any reason? _____

GROWTH HISTORY:

Length at birth _____ Weight at birth _____

Current height _____ Current weight _____

Has there been a change in growth pattern recently (spurt or halt)? _____

Has child stayed at the same growth percentile? ___ yes ___ no

Has child ever moved more than two growth lines between visits? __ yes__ up __ down

Why? _____

VACCINATION HISTORY:

On schedule as given by primary care provider? ___ yes ___ no

Were any vaccinations skipped and had to be doubled up on next visits? ___ yes ___ no

DEVELOPMENTAL HISTORY:

Attach Weight/Height charts if appropriate.

Known congenital problems: _____

Milestones:	Early	On-time	Delayed
Bonding			
Held head up			
Rolled over			
Sat up			
First words			
Sentences			
Crawled			
Walked			

Toileting			
Dry bed			
Reading			
Printing			
Writing			

PATIENT'S CHILDHOOD ILLNESSES Check all that apply.

___ Chicken pox   ___ Meningitis   ___ Whooping cough   ___ RSV

___ Mononucleosis   ___ Strep   ___ Earaches   ___ Rheumatic fever

___ Scarlet fever   ___ Urinary infection   ___ Cold sores   ___ Mumps

___ Frequent URIs   ___ Dental problems   ___ Measles (any variety)   ___ Fifth's disease

OTHER: _____

_____

SURGICAL HISTORY: _____

_____

INJURY HISTORY: (Accidents, broken bones, etc.) _____

_____

HOSPITALIZATIONS: _____

_____

TRANSFUSIONS: _____

_____

ABNORMAL X-RAYS OR OTHER TESTS: _____

_____

ABNORMAL LAB RESULTS: _____

_____

HISTORY OF PATIENT'S TBI: Collected on separate form.

SOCIAL HISTORY:

HABITS:

HAVE YOU EVER:

- Smoked? ___ yes ___ tobacco ___ marijuana

  List amount and frequency: _____

  Last use: _____

- Drank alcohol? ___ yes

  Type: _____

  Usual frequency and amount: _____

  Last use: _____

- Used recreational drugs of any kind? Sniffing? Snorting? Ingesting? Inhaling? Prescription or over the counter medicines? Herbs? Smoking? Injecting? Include anything you used to alter your consciousness. Add usual frequency and amounts.

  _____

  _____

  Last use: _____

- Consumed caffeine? Consider any source: coffee, tea, chocolate, energy drinks, NoDoz, energy bars, stimulant pills. ___ yes Describe: _____

  EATING HISTORY:

  HAVE YOU EVER:

  - Had an eating disorder? (Check all that apply.)

    ___ Compulsive overeating?

    ___ Addictive eating?

    ___ Binge eating?

    ___ Emotional eating?

    ___ Purging?

    ___ Anorexia?

    ___ Bulimia?

- Had a bad reaction to food?

   Name the food: _____

   What happened? _____

- Had a weight problem? ___ overweight ___ underweight

SLEEP HISTORY:

   HAVE YOU EVER: (Check all that apply.)

   ____ Had a problem sleeping?

   ____ Had nightmares?

   ____ Been found sleepwalking?

   ____ Performed unusual acts while asleep?

   ____ Experienced odd behaviors while asleep: strange positions or inability to move?

   ____ Fallen asleep at inappropriate times?

   ____ Snored?

   ____ Had trouble breathing while asleep?

   ____ Have you ever taken a medicine to sleep? What happened?

   ____ Had trouble falling asleep?

   ____ Had trouble staying asleep?

EXERCISE HISTORY:

   HAVE YOU EVER: (Check all that apply.)

   ____ Exercised regularly?

   ____ Considered yourself fit or athletic?

   ____ Been injured so that you had to stop exercising?

   ____ Had physical limits on what you could do?

   If you do not exercise, what limits you? _____

   At what exercise have you done your best? _____

   What exercise have you liked best? _____

HOME LIFE:

HAVE YOU EVER:

Lived in a house where there was abuse? __ Physical __ Emotional __ Sexual

Lived in a house where the family dynamics were unstable? __ Yes?
__ Divorce __ Prison __ Job loss __ Frequent conflict

Aside from your current illness, have you lived where there were major stressors like money problems, alcohol or drug abuse, school or work issues? ___ yes Describe:

_____

_____

_____

Lived in a house with:

___ Lead paint

___ Copper pipes

___ Mold

___ Asbestos

Been exposed to mercury or other heavy metals? __ YES:
Dental fillings__ Broken thermometer __ Free mercury __ Other __

Have you ever lived near a landfill or waste holding site? ___ yes

SIGNIFICANT FAMILY HISTORY:

Has anyone else in the house had a similar illness? ___ yes _____

Has a pet been sick? ___ yes _____

AUTOIMMUNE HISTORY:

The following is a list of possible autoimmune diseases. Check whether the patient or family member EVER had this problem. If you don't know what the condition is, that's okay, just move to the next item. Some diseases are listed twice under different names.

Condition	Patient	Family	Condition	Patient	Family
Addison's Disease			Infertility		
Adrenal Disease			Inflammatory Bowel Disease		
AIDS			Kawasaki's Disease		
Alzheimer's Disease			Lou Gehrig's Disease		
ALS			Lupus, SLE		

Ankylosing Spondylitis			Meniere's Disease			
Antiphospholipid Dis			Meningitis			
Aplastic Anemia			Miscarriage			
Arteritis			Multiple Sclerosis			
Arthritis			Myasthenia Gravis			
Asthma			Myositis			
Atopic Dermatitis			Narcolepsy			
Autism			Organomegaly			
Behcet's Disease			Pancreatitis			
Cancer			PANDAS			
Cardiomyopathy			Pemphigus			
Celiac Disease			Polymyalgia Rheumatica			
Chronic Fatigue			Psoriasis			
Cirrhosis			Raynaud's Syndrome			
Cogan's Syndrome			Reiter's Syndrome			
Connective Tissue Dis			Rheumatic Fever			
CREST Syndrome			Rheumatoid Arthritis			
Crohn's Disease			Sarcoid			
Cushing's Syndrome			Scleroderma			
Diabetes			Seizures (certain types)			
Dressler's Syndrome			Sjogren's Syndrome			
Eczema			Still's Disease			
Encephalitis			Thymus Dysfunction			
Evan's Syndrome			Thyroid Problems			
Fibromyalgia			Transplant Rejection			
Glomerulonephritis			Ulcerative Colitis			
Goodpasture's Myositis			Vasculitis			
Graft vs Host Disease			Vitiligo			
Guillain-Barré			Wegener's Granulomatosis			
Hepatitis			Wilson's Syndrome			
Hughes Syndrome						

OTHER PERTINENT FAMILY HISTORY:

Aside from the current health problem, has the patient or anyone in the family EVER had any of the following problems? Check only for yes responses and briefly describe.

Condition	Patient	Family	Describe
Allergies			
Arthritis			
Autoimmune Disease			
Birth Defects			

Tick-Borne Disease			
Frequent infections			
Trouble w/ blood sugars (high, low, DM)			
Hormone problems			
Thyroid disease			
Infections (Egs: TB, hepatitis, herpes, HIV)			
Cancers			
Eye problems			
Ear problems			
Throat conditions			
Dental problems			
Problems with head, hair, scalp			
Skin conditions			
Heart conditions			
Lung problems (asthma, infections)			
Digestive problems			
Urinary conditions			
Kidney concerns			
Liver dysfunction			
Reproductive problems			
Blood disorders			
Weight control issues			
Cholesterol or lipid problems			
Difficulties w/ muscles, joints, bones			
Neuropsychiatric problems:			
Fainting			
Weakness			
Numbness			
Dizziness			
Seizures			
Headaches			
Chronic pain			
Learning problems			
Dyslexia			
Tourette's			
Tics, tremors, spasms			
Decision-making issues			
Confusion			
Personality disorders			
Poor judgment			

Psychosis (loss of reality)			
Depression			
Anxiety			
Nervous breakdown			
Panic			
OCD (obsessive/compulsive)			
Sleep problems			
Aggression			
Anger			
Irritability			
ADHD			
ADD			
Autism			
Mood swings			
Self-harm			
Suicidal thoughts or actions			
Developmental delays			
PAND or PANDAS			
Oppositional disorders			

OTHER: _____

ANYTHING ELSE YOU WANT US TO KNOW ABOUT YOUR HISTORY? _____

_____

After all that, here are a few PEARLS to help patients fill out the History form and HCPs review the answers:

- Most people do not recall APGAR scores and they should not agonize over this. These scores might provide useful information with regard to gestational Lyme or other congenital problems. Usually there are two APGAR scores done at 1 minute and at 5 minutes. The score after birth is useful in determining if there were significant problems with the newborn that may still be impacting the child's health. The assessment of muscle tone might be especially enlightening. The highest score is a 10. Scores of 4 or less indicate that the child likely needed resuscitation and 7 or less indicate there may have been neurologic deficits. Ask if they know why scores were low and what was done to revive the child.

- In reviewing the vaccination history, see if the patient has any signs or symptoms of Asperger's or any of the autism spectrum disorders including PDD, autism, Asperger's, Rett syndrome, or CDD. While the most recent word is that there is no relationship between vaccinations and autism, there are numerous anecdotes describing post-vaccination syndromes after multiple concomitant immunizations of military personnel going to the Gulf War. Since this topic remains controversial, be cognizant of the possibility of unlikely associations if the child has an unusual immunization history.

- Be cognizant of any Strep history. Strep infections are associated with PANDAS.

- Recreational drugs are often dismissed as unimportant by patients. These drugs in all their forms and variations can impact healing. Make sure the patient understands that you are not there to judge his use, but rather to ensure he is giving his body every chance it needs to recover.

- Adequate sleep is probably more critical to wellness than we currently recognize. Patients are often unrealistic in estimating the real quality of sleep either grossly under or overestimating.

- Since I live in the Penn State catchment area, I am very tuned onto the issues around abuse. Chronically ill kids may be at higher risk so do not skim these topics because you are uncomfortable. The beauty of a comprehensive form is that the checkbox can introduce the topic. Recognize that the patient may need privacy to discuss all that is on her mind.

Chapter 16

REVIEW OF SYSTEMS

There is a fine line between fishing and standing on the shore like an idiot.

Stephen Wright

The *Review of Systems* is another way of asking the patient, "What's happening with you **NOW**?" While the *History* deals with things that have happened in the past and cannot be changed, the ROS is current. The review includes a series of detailed questions that prompt the patient to recall the range of signs and symptoms that have been occurring recently.

Of course, the events do not need to be happening right this second. In general, if the patient is answering your questions, he is not actively seizing, bleeding, or comatose. So the ROS should document things that have been happening in the recent past, say a month. More leeway is appropriate if the signs or symptoms are associated with the chief complaint. A febrile seizure that happened 8 years ago would be part of the history. A tonic-clonic seizure that happened last week would be part of the current ROS. (Although the patient would also have checked yes to the question, "Have you EVER seized?" on the History form, as well.) You are trying to capture the essence of the current health status of this patient.

The ROS should help put things into perspective in terms of the patient's present state of health or disease. BUT… just because something is happening now doesn't mean it is part of the TBI you are evaluating. This patient may not even have a TBI. The ROS will provide information that will help you make that determination.

A current symptom could be from a co-infection, concurrent disease, congenital problem, pre-existing condition, or adverse drug reaction. The ROS just gives you a big bunch of data and you will still have to sort through the morass. I prefer that the ROS be done as a comprehensive questionnaire rather than a list of questions rotely asked by the examiner. This way the HCP cannot "lead" the patient by asking a question in a certain way or go off in a tangent that leaves many questions unanswered or given short shrift. The allotted time passes quickly, so it needs to be managed efficiently.

Usually, the ROS is done in some sort of systematic fashion asking questions about one body system then another. I prefer to have the patient or caretaker fill out a very detailed and broad-based ROS form which can then be used to focus on the positive responses. I have seen HCPs go over every single question on the list (sometimes three times as they ask the same questions over and over and over). "Have you EVER been constipated?" No. Five minutes later, "Are you NOW constipated?" No. Two minutes later. "What are you doing to keep from getting constipated?" Please STOP. The patient told you three times already. If on PE you find evidence of constipation, by all means bring it up again. But if he says he's not constipated, believe him and save his precious visit time. Focus on the stuff he says is bothersome.

This chapter contains a comprehensive ROS form. I recommend that the patient or caregiver fill out this form as part of the packet they receive by mail or in the waiting room before you sit down together. Ideally, this information is mailed or faxed back to you prior to the visit so you know where to focus. If the person says he has no joint pain or problems, that doesn't mean you ignore the joints during the visit, it just means you make sure you closely target those issues most important to the patient. If the patient says her heart has skipped beats in the past and now sometimes feels like it is racing, pay attention. Get over the darn constipation and look at the patient in front of you.

The detailed ROS should then become part of the chart. Use it to help target your investigation. Do not be a slave to its list of questions. The list is just there to make sure that nothing is missed, not to limit your patient focus. Make your forms work for you. Use the detailed form to help make your notes during the initial visit.

The integrated 3-in-1 Follow-up form presented at the end of Chapter 13 allows the history, ROS, and PE to appear in parallel columns on the page. This form can be used for subsequent visits. That way the patient can answer "Did you EVER?" and "Do you NOW?" on one side of the page and then the HCP can make notes from the interview and PE on the other. The HCP can address these issues either by more in-depth questioning or by documenting physical findings. A full ROS is outlined below and is appropriate for the first visit. On follow-up visits the shorter ROS is available in the 3-in-1form found as Sample Form VIII at the end of Chapter 13.

The ROS provides perimeters within which you can develop your list of potential diagnoses. This is where you get to play medical detective and it's kind of fun. I do a similar, but not identical, ROS exam if I am working up a child for seizures versus a deviated septum versus TBIs. All have many of the foundation questions in common. Yet, each has aspects that the other conditions do not share that you should explore further. Since TBIs affect so many organ systems and can be associated with numerous co-infections and co-morbidities, a comprehensive ROS should prove useful in developing the differential diagnosis.

If possible have the patient or caretaker fill out these forms BEFORE the visit or in the waiting room. Then address all positive responses. Confirm any negative responses if that specific item is of particular importance for this patient.

The following form is for your perusal or modification.

SAMPLE FORM XI: REVIEW OF SYSTEMS

REVIEW OF SYSTEMS

Patient Name: _____ Date: _____

Birthday: _____ Age today: _____

Person(s) filling out this form: ___ patient ___ parent ___ caretaker ___ other

General Health:

What is bothering you most today? _____

What other symptoms do you have? _____

What makes you feel better? _____

What makes you feel worse? _____

What treatments are you currently taking? (There is a place to list all medicines below. Here put general treatments like antibiotics, vitamins, heat, physical therapy, etc.)_____

_____

In general, aside from this problem, how has your health been? _____

Demographics:

List all persons and types of pets in household: _____

_____

Current health status of family members: _____

Significant relationship: ___ Girlfriend ___ Boyfriend ___ Spouse

Recent HCPs names and contact numbers. Check if you do NOT want them contacted.

    Name: _____ Phone: _____ Do not contact: _____

    Name: _____ Phone: _____ Do not contact: _____

Considering any recent symptoms associated with your chief complaint and anything you have experienced in the past month, answer the following questions. Answer only if the answer is yes. Leave blank if the answer is no or you do not know.

DO YOU **NOW** HAVE?

ALLERGIES: List all known. Otherwise leave blank.

Medicine: ____ Yes _____

Animals: ____ Yes _____

Latex: ____ Yes _____

Foods: ____ Yes _____

Pollens: ____ Yes _____

Molds: ____ Yes _____

Other ____ Yes _____

GENERAL CURRENT HEALTH:

DO YOU **NOW** HAVE?

Check only if yes. Leave blank if the answer is no or you do not know. Describe if asked.

Abnormal energy levels? ____ Yes _____

    Any recent change? ____ Yes _____

Too high? ____ Yes _____

    Unable to sit still? ____ Yes _____

    Fidgety/Restless? ____ Yes _____

    Foot or hand tapper? ____ Yes _____

Too low? ____ Yes _____

    Sleepy? ____ Yes _____

    Weak? ____ Yes _____

    No energy? ____ Yes _____

    No desire to do anything? ____ Yes _____

    Poor stamina? ____ Yes _____

Other? ____ Yes _____

Fever? ___ Yes

    Describe fever pattern: _____

    How long? _____

    When did fever start in relation to tick bite? _____

    Chills? ___ Yes _____

    Severe chills (rigors)? ___ Yes _____

    Can't get warm? ___ Yes _____

    Other? ___ Yes _____

Swollen glands (lymph nodes)? ___ Yes

    Where? _____

Weight problems? ___ Yes _____

    Any recent weight change? ___ Yes _____

    Other? ___ Yes _____

Do you have pain? ___ Yes

    Where? _____

    Describe: ___ sharp ___ dull ___ throbbing ___ shooting ___ other

    How bad is it? On a scale of 1 to 10 with 1 being noticeable and 10 intolerable: _____

    The pain is: ___ constant ___ comes and goes

    Other? _____

Recent travel? ___ Yes Where? _____

Recent trauma or accidents? ___ Yes Describe: _____

CURRENT MEDICINES:

List all current medicines including vitamins and OTC medicines, doses, and length of treatment:

Name	Dose	Directions and dura-tion
1.		
2.		
3.		
4.		
5.		
6.		

Continue on back of form if needed.

Other medicines you have tried in the past for this problem but stopped. Why did you stop?

Name	Reasons stopped
1.	
2.	
3.	

Have you had any bad reactions to any of these medicines? ___ Yes _____

Did your symptoms seem worse after starting any of these medicines? ___ Yes _____

Have you ever had a Herx reaction? ___ Yes

Do you think you are having a Herx reaction now? ___ Yes

SYSTEM REVIEW:

DO YOU **NOW** HAVE PROBLEMS WITH ANY OF THE FOLLOWING SYSTEMS?

Check only if yes. Leave blank if the answer is no or you do not know. Describe if asked.

<u>Skin</u>:

Sensitive to touch?		___ Yes
Striae or stretch marks?		___ Yes
Changes in moles?		___ Yes
Rash?		___ Yes

Describe: _____

Where? _____

When in relation to tick bite? _____

Did you see what looked like a target or bull's eye?		___ Yes
Blister?		___ Yes
Pus?		___ Yes
Bad odor?		___ Yes
Itch?		___ Yes
Dryness?		___ Yes
Thickening?		___ Yes
Lumps?		___ Yes
Unusual color?		___ Yes

Discomfort? ___ Yes

Has the rash changed over the time of this illness? ___ Yes

Slow healing wounds? ___ Yes

Frequent or severe diaper rash? ___ Yes

Allergic rash? Hives, wheals, streaks? ___ Yes

Other? _____

Hair:

Breakage? ___ Yes

Pulling? ___ Yes

Loss? ___ Yes

Sensitive scalp? ___ Yes

Scalp lesions? ___ Yes

Dandruff? ___ Yes

Other? _____

Nails:

Thickening? ___ Yes

Discoloration? ___ Yes

Easily breaking? ___ Yes

Other? _____

Head:

Soft spot: bulging, sinking? ___ Yes

Asymmetry? ___ Yes

Scars? ___ Yes

Face drooping on one side? ___ Yes

Scalp nodules? ___ Yes

Painful scalp? ___ Yes

Even hair hurts? ___ Yes

Other? _____

<u>Eyes</u>:

Problems with vision? _____ Yes

Blurred? Wavy? Smeared? _____ Yes

Double? _____ Yes

Rings or halos? _____ Yes

Blind spots? _____ Yes

Flashing lights or spots? _____ Yes

Floaters? _____ Yes

Trouble seeing at night? _____ Yes

Glasses/contacts? _____ Yes

Discomfort? _____ Yes

Dryness? _____ Yes

Discharge? _____ Yes

Redness? _____ Yes

Itching? _____ Yes

Tearing? _____ Yes

Twitching? _____ Yes

Problems with lids or lashes? _____ Yes

Trouble closing one or both lids? _____ Yes

Eyes do not move equally or together? _____ Yes

Sensitive to light? _____ Yes

Yellow whites? _____ Yes

Other? _____

<u>Ears</u>:

Trouble hearing? _____ Yes

Can hear sounds loud enough but cannot tell what is being said? _____ Yes

Ringing or buzzing? _____ Yes

Underwater feel? _____ Yes

Pain?   ___ Yes

Discharge?   ___ Yes

Excess wax?   ___ Yes

Ears often red or hot?   ___ Yes

Sensitive to sound?   ___ Yes

Persistent or intermittent redness?   ___ Yes

Other? _____

Nose/sinuses:

Sensitive to smells?   ___ Yes

Postnasal drip?   ___ Yes

Clearing throat often?   ___ Yes

Hay fever?   ___ Yes

Stuffy nose?   ___ Yes

Nasal voice?   ___ Yes

Snoring?   ___ Yes

Pain?   ___ Yes

Bleeding?   ___ Yes

Other? _____

Mouth:

Overall dental status:

Problems?   ___ Yes

Hygiene?   ___ Yes

Odor?   ___ Yes

Gum issues?   ___ Yes

Bleeding?   ___ Yes

Teeth grinding?   ___ Yes

Jaw problems?   ___ Yes

Tongue abnormalities?   ___ Yes

Coated?   ___ Yes

Sores or blisters? ___ Yes

Mouth breather? ___ Yes

Other? _____

Throat:

Pain? ___ Yes

Soreness? ___ Yes

Hoarseness? ___ Yes

Trouble swallowing? ___ Yes

Tonsils? ___ Yes

Spots or pus? ___ Yes

Hot potato voice? ___ Yes

Voice changes? ___ Yes

Redness? ___ Yes

Postnasal drip? ___ Yes

Feeling of throat closing off? ___ Yes

Other? _____

Neck:

Problems moving? ___ Yes

Pain? ___ Yes

Limits on movement? ___ Yes

Creaking, cracking? ___ Yes

Lumps? ___ Yes

Swollen glands? ___ Yes

Other? _____

Chest:

Pain? ___ Yes

Movement? ___ Yes

Breast problems? ___ Yes

Lumps? ___ Yes

Discharge?   ___ Yes

Other? _____

Heart:

Pain over heart?   ___ Yes

Racing?   ___ Yes

Skipping?   ___ Yes

Swollen ankles?   ___ Yes

Murmur?   ___ Yes

Blood pressure abnormal?   ___ Yes

Other? _____

Respiration/Lungs:

Trouble breathing?   ___ Yes

Air hunger or feel like you can't get a satisfying breath?   ___ Yes

Short of breath?   ___ Yes

Easily out of breath with activity?   ___ Yes

Snoring?   ___ Yes

Extra yawning or sighing?   ___ Yes

Coughing?   ___ Yes

Pattern?   ___ Yes

Does anything come up when you cough?   ___ Yes

Describe: _____

Blood?   ___ Yes

Other? _____

Gastrointestinal/Digestion:

Abnormal appetite?   ___ Yes

Loss of appetite?   ___ Yes

Frequent use of laxatives?   ___ Yes

Frequent use of antacids?   ___ Yes

Food allergies?   ___ Yes

Lactose intolerance?   ___ Yes

Discomfort after eating?   ___ Yes

Pain in upper right side?   ___ Yes

Heartburn/Indigestion?   ___ Yes

Reflux?   ___ Yes

Acid taste in mouth?   ___ Yes

Feel of food sticking in throat?   ___ Yes

Trouble swallowing?   ___Yes

Nausea?   ___ Yes

Pattern? _____

Vomiting?   ___ Yes

Pattern? _____

Blood?   ___ Yes

Bowel movements abnormal?   ___ Yes

Usual pattern: _____

Recent changes?   ___ Yes

Abnormal color?   ___ Yes

Loose stool?/Diarrhea?   ___ Yes

Hard?/Constipation?   ___ Yes

Blood?   ___ Yes

Black tar?   ___ Yes

Straining?   ___ Yes

Hemorrhoids?   ___ Yes

Stomach or abdominal pain?   ___ Yes

Where? _____

Describe: _____

Sharp?   ___ Yes

Dull?   ___ Yes

Nature of pain:___ occasional ___ frequent ___ constant

Excessive burping? _____ Yes

Excessive gas? _____ Yes

Yellow skin or whites of eyes? _____ Yes

Other? _____

Urinary:

Usual pattern: _____

Blood? _____ Yes

Cloudy? _____ Yes

Unusual odor? _____ Yes

Pain, burning, or itch on urination? _____ Yes

Change in urinary habits? _____ Yes

Regression in toileting/bed wetting? _____ Yes

Difficulty passing urine? _____ Yes

Discomfort? _____ Yes

Going more often? _____ Yes

Getting up at night? _____ Yes

Hard to start? _____ Yes

Hard to stop? _____ Yes

Leaking? _____ Yes

Other? _____

Genital/Reproductive:

I would like to discuss with the doctor privately any history of sexual activity, abuse, birth control, safe sex, pregnancy, and sexually transmitted diseases, as it pertains to my current condition. A chaperone will be available. _____ Okay _____ No need

Female:

Age of menarche: _____

Period cycle: _____

Regular? _____ Yes (Regular cycles not expected for 1 or 2 years after menarche.)

Length of periods? _____

Amount of bleeding: ___ light ___ moderate ___ heavy

Spotting?   ___ Yes

Discomfort? Cramps?   ___ Yes

Mood changes with period?   ___ Yes

Discharge?   ___ Yes

Itch?   ___ Yes

Sores?   ___ Yes

Known STDs?   ___ Yes
List: _____

Pregnant?   ___ Yes

Birth control?   ___ Yes

Sexual problems?   ___ Yes

Concerns about sexual development?   ___ Yes

Other? _____

Male:

Discharge?   ___ Yes

Sores?   ___ Yes

Hernias?   ___ Yes

Lumps in testicles?   ___ Yes

Pain?   ___ Yes

Known STDs?   ___ Yes

List: _____

Concerns about sexual development?   ___ Yes

Sexual problems?   ___ Yes

Other? _____

Musculoskeletal:

Bones:

Pain?   ___ Yes

Deformity?   ___ Yes

Bumps? ___ Yes

Hurt to touch? ___ Yes

Nodules along tibia or other bones? ___ Yes

Other? _____

Joints:

Pain? ___ Yes

Swelling? ___ Yes

Heat? ___ Yes

Popping? ___ Yes

Stiffness? ___ Yes

Back pain? ___ Yes

Neck pain? Cracking? ___ Yes

Redness? ___ Yes

Limits on motion? ___ Yes

Pain in soles especially in the morning? ___ Yes

Other? _____

Muscles:

Cramps? ___ Yes

Twitches? ___ Yes

Pain or soreness? ___ Yes

Hurt to touch? ___ Yes

Recent strains or sprains? ___ Yes

Development? ___ Yes

Nodules along triceps or elsewhere? ___ Yes

Weakness? ___ Yes

Other? _____

Glands:

Diabetes or trouble with high or low sugars? ___ Yes

Trouble with heat or cold? ___ Yes

Fidgeting? ___ Yes

Lethargy? ___ Yes

Flushing? ___ Yes

Excess sweating? ___ Yes

Excessive thirst? ___ Yes

Increased urination? ___ Yes

Dry hair or skin? ___ Yes

Brittle nails? ___ Yes

Change in hair growth? ___ Yes

Lump or swelling on front of neck? ___ Yes

Other? _____

Blood/Circulation:

Cold extremities? ___ Yes

Easy bruising? ___ Yes

Recent transfusions? ___ Yes

Bleeding? ___ Yes

Clotting problems? ___ Yes

Leg cramping? ___ Yes

Weak pulses? ___ Yes

Anemia? ___ Yes

Hemophilia? ___ Yes

Sickle cell? ___ Yes

Pale? ___ Yes

Weak? ___ Yes

Other? _____

Neurological:

Unstable balance? ___ Yes

Lack of coordination? ___ Yes

Changes in consciousness? ___ Yes

Memory loss? ___ Yes

Problems with gait? ___ Yes

Flat expression? ___ Yes

Recent concussion? ___ Yes

Recent loss of consciousness? ___ Yes

Problems with senses? ___ Yes

More or less sensitive to:

    Light? ___ Yes

    Touch? ___ Yes

    Sound? ___ Yes

    Taste? ___ Yes

    Smell? ___ Yes

    Temperature? ___ Yes

Other? _____

Abnormal speech? ___ Yes

    Hesitant? ___ Yes

    Stammer? ___ Yes

    Stutter? ___ Yes

    Lisp? ___ Yes

Other? _____

Trouble processing what is said? ___ Yes

Dizzy? ___ Yes

Room spinning? ___ Yes

Fainting? ___ Yes

Blackouts? ___ Yes

Can't follow directions? ___ Yes

Memory problems? ___ Yes

Tics? ___ Yes

Tremors? ___ Yes

Twitching? ___ Yes

Seizures? ___ Yes

    Describe: _____

    Muscles spasm rhythmically? ___ Yes

    Gestures? ___ Yes

    Postures? ___ Yes

    Absence? ___ Yes

    Staring? ___ Yes

    With fevers only? ___ Yes

    Frequency? _____

    Pattern? _____

    Aura or signs that a seizure may be coming on? ___ Yes

    Other? _____

Headache? ___ Yes

    Describe: ___ sharp ___ dull ___ shooting ___ throb ___ other

    Location: _____

    Pattern: _____

    Timing: _____

    Recent increase in severity or frequency? ___ Yes

    Triggers: _____

    Aura or signs that a headache may be coming on? ___ Yes

    Describe: _____

    Nausea? ___ Yes

    Other? _____

Developmental milestones:

    Caretakers concerned about not progressing normally? ___ Yes

    In what ways? _____

    Recent regression on developmental milestones? ___ Yes

    Describe: _____

Involuntary loss of a body function w/o a good reason?   ___ Yes

Describe: _____

Other? _____

<u>Psychiatric</u>:

Recent visit to psychologist, counselor, or therapist?   ___ Yes

Don't feel like doing anything?   ___ Yes

Can't stop talking?   ___ Yes

Hallucinations: hears, sees, or smells things that aren't there?   ___ Yes

Paranoia? Everyone out to hurt you?   ___ Yes

Tapping?   ___ Yes

Fidgeting?   ___ Yes

Poking?   ___ Yes

Compulsive behaviors?   ___ Yes

Poor eye contact?   ___ Yes

Limited attention?   ___ Yes

Easily distractible?   ___ Yes

Unable to focus?   ___ Yes

Unable to sit still?   ___ Yes

Behavior not appropriate for age?   ___ Yes

Anxiety?   ___ Yes

Easily stressed?   ___ Yes

Panicky?   ___ Yes

Mood problems?   ___ Yes

Recent changes?   ___ Yes

Too happy?   ___ Yes

Too sad?   ___ Yes

Mood swings?   ___ Yes

Depression?   ___ Yes

Threats of self-harm?   ___ Yes

Suicidal thoughts?	___ Yes
Suicidal Actions?	___ Yes
Aggression?	___ Yes
Violence?	___ Yes
Inflexibility?	___ Yes
Lack of cooperation?	___ Yes
Won't follow directions?	___ Yes
Personality problems?	___ Yes
Only thinks of self?	___ Yes
Lacks compassion?	___ Yes
Harmed animals, pets, friends, or family?	___ Yes
Ever been in a physical fight? ___ siblings ___ others	___ Yes
Obsessive thoughts?	___ Yes
Compulsive actions?	___ Yes
Repetitive motions?	___ Yes
Repetitive actions?	___ Yes
Poor interactions with others?	___ Yes
Rebellious?	___ Yes
Disobedient?	___ Yes
Sassy?	___ Yes
Disrespectful?	___ Yes
No sense of humor?	___ Yes
Limited traditional intelligence?	___ Yes
Limited emotional Intelligence?	___ Yes
Lacks social skills?	___ Yes
Can't read social cues?	___ Yes
Talks of dark things?	___ Yes
Self-harm?	___ Yes
Cutting?	___ Yes

Feels emotionally numb? _____ Yes

Poor self-image? _____ Yes

Troubled by nightmares? _____ Yes

Just plain mean? _____ Yes

Oppositional? _____ Yes

Defiant? _____ Yes

Trouble with authority figures? _____ Yes

Has damaged property or set fires? _____ Yes

General attitude pessimistic? _____ Yes

Intense fears that impact daily living? _____ Yes

Other? _____

CURRENT HABITS:

Do you NOW, or have you in the past month, engaged in any of the following behaviors?

Substance Use:

Smoke? _____ tobacco _____ marijuana

List amount and frequency: _____

Drink alcohol? _____ Yes

Type: _____

Usual frequency and amount: _____

Use recreational drugs of any kind? Sniff? Snort? Ingest? Inhale? Prescription or over the counter medicines? Herbs? Smoke? Inject? Include anything you use to alter your consciousness. List along with usual frequency and amounts.

Substance	Method	Amount	Last use

Consume caffeine? _____ Yes. Consider any source: coffee, tea, chocolate, energy drinks, NoDoz, energy bars, stimulant pills. How much? _____

Eating Habits:

Do you have any problems with food? _____ Yes

Have a weight problem? ___ overweight ___ underweight ___ Yes

Addictive eating? ___ Yes

Compulsive overeating? ___ Yes

Binge eating? ___ Yes

Emotional eating? ___ Yes

Purging? ___ Yes

Anorexia? ___ Yes

Bulimia? ___ Yes

Do you think you are too fat? ___ Yes

Other? _____

Usual eating pattern:

Meals per day: _____

Snacks per day: _____

Take a multivitamin? ___ Yes

Eat all kinds of foods including fruits and vegetables? ___ Yes

Eat junk food (cookies, candy, chips, soda) daily? ___ Yes

I do not eat: _____

I am: ___ vegetarian ___ vegan ___ on a restricted diet

Other? _____

Sleep Habits:

How are you sleeping now? ___ fine ___ okay ___ some problems ___ terrible

What kinds of problems do you have sleeping? _____

On a typical night how many hours do you sleep? ___ hours

What keeps you awake? _____

Do you exercise or use caffeine near sleep time? ___ Yes

Do you have trouble finding a quiet, secure place to sleep? ___ Yes

Do you:

Sleep too much? ___ Yes

Sleep too little? ___ Yes

Have trouble going to sleep? ___ Yes

Have trouble staying asleep? ___ Yes

Have nightmares? ___ Yes

Sleepwalk? ___ Yes

Do unusual things while asleep? ___ Yes

Assume odd positions or find you can't move? ___ Yes

Fall asleep at inappropriate times? ___ Yes

Snore? ___ Yes

Have trouble breathing while asleep? ___ Yes

Take medicine to sleep? ___ Yes

Is what you feel when awake:
___ sleepiness, ___ tiredness, ___ weakness, ___ fatigue ___other

Other? _____

Exercise habits:

Exercise regularly? ___ Yes

How often? _____

What keeps you from doing things:

___ Don't feel well enough to exercise

___ Get too tired

___ Get short of breath

___ Don't like it

___ Too sick

___ Too much pain

___ Injured

Has ability to exercise changed after onset of illness? ___ Yes

Do you over-exercise? ___ Yes

Do others think you exercise too much? ___ Yes

Upset if can't exercise? ___ Yes

Play one or more sports? ___ Yes

Physically fit for age? ___ Yes

Participate in gym class?   ___ Yes

Joints or muscles hurt during or after exercise?   ___ Yes

Trouble walking?   ___ Yes

Unstable balance?   ___ Yes

Lack coordination?   ___ Yes

Other? _____

Life habits:

Brush and floss daily?   ___ Yes

Shower, bathe, or wash regularly?   ___ Yes

For age, able to care for self: ___ teeth ___ wash ___ feeding ___ toileting

Problems with toileting?   ___ Yes

New onset of bedwetting with no family history?   ___ Yes

Typical day: Rises: _____ Bedtime: _____ Naps: _____

Spends day: ___ home ___ with relative ___ day care ___ school ___ job ___ other

Home life:

Age of current building? _____

Possibility of exposure to ___ lead ___ copper ___ mercury ___ mold ___ asbestos

Do you live near a landfill or waste holding site?   ___ Yes

Home life unstable?   ___ Yes

Financial problems?   ___ Yes

Conflict?   ___ Yes

Alcohol or drug abuse?   ___ Yes

Single parent household?   ___ Yes

Discord over chronic illness?   ___ Yes

Constant tension?   ___ Yes

Divorce or separation?   ___ Yes

More than one residence?   ___ Yes

Abuse?   ___ Yes

    Physical?   ___ Yes

Emotional? ___ Yes

Sexual? ___ Yes

CURRENT SOCIAL INTERACTIONS:

<u>School</u>: (Check all that apply.)

___ Full time

___ Part time

___ Home schooled

___ Special education

___ Tutors

___ Advanced abilities

___ Learning disabilities

___ ADD/ADHD

___ Autism spectrum

___ Speech or language support

___ Interaction with guidance counselor

___ 504 plan for student with disabilities

___ Special accommodations

___ Held back

___ Disciplinary problems

___ Detention

___ Suspension

___ Difficulty with more than one teacher

___ Other

Grade level: ___

___ Grades:

    ___ Excellent

    ___ Good

    ___ Average

    ___ Fair

___ Poor

___ Failing

Happy with current school situation? ____ Yes ____ No

Friends:

Status of friends:

___ too many

___ several good confidants and companions

___ few acquaintances

___ alone mostly

___ solitary

Demeanor:

___ too friendly

___ outgoing

___ courteous

___ shy

___ restrained

___ prefers solitude

___ secretive

Has personality changed since illness?   ___ Yes

How? _____

Hard time making friends?   ___ Yes

Current: ___ Girlfriend ___ Boyfriend ___ Spouse ___ Children

Relationships with significant other: ___ usually stable ___ frequent change ___ conflicts

Problems getting along with others? ___ Yes

Happy with current situation? ___ Yes ___ No

Other? _____

Activities:

Currently participates in:

___ clubs

___ sports

___ organizations

___ play groups

___ hobbies

___ pets

___ spontaneous neighborhood play

___ religious affiliation

Usually: ___ leader ___ follower

Jobs: ___ full time ___ part time ___ occasional ___ military

Work problems: ___ tardiness ___ sleepiness ___ inattention

___ conflict ___ disciplined ___ fired

Spiritual:

___ Believes in God or religious tradition

___ Attends services within community

___ Finds support or solace in religion

___ Participates because family participates

___ Not interested

Problems:

Recently: ___ picked up by police ___ criminal charges ___ jail ___ violent behavior ___ other

Satisfied with current life situation? ___ Yes ___ No

IS THERE ANYTHING ELSE YOU WANT US TO KNOW ABOUT YOUR CURRENT HEALTH STATUS?

_____

_____

_____

Here are several PEARLS to help with the completion of the ROS evaluation:

- I like the idea of a very comprehensive ROS form. Here the patient can focus on the issues important to her rather than the ones the HCP steers her toward. As an HCP, I must confess that we all steer sometimes. There is a fine line between trying to gather additional, pertinent information and leading a patient in a way that will make their complaints "fit" into your preconceived diagnosis. Just be aware of this possibility as you gather data and review what the patient checked as important to her.

- Those of us who have been treating patients for a number of years know that adults who have problems with alcohol tend to grossly underestimate their drinking. In contrast, middle schoolers and high school kids can grossly overstate the amount they drink in order to appear cool.

- Often the distinction between neurologic and psychologic symptoms is difficult to make. Don't worry about the category, just be careful to capture the essence of what is going on with the patient. Many misguided HCPs, parents, and laypeople believe that neurologic signs are "real" while psychologic conditions are fake, or made-up to get noticed. If the patient would just "buck up" these symptoms would go away. The patient just isn't trying hard enough. She is only seeking attention. Skeptics obviously don't understand the power of biochemistry, especially biochemistry affected by a pathogen.

- In the *Genitourinary* section there is a statement that might seem odd:

  I would like to discuss with the doctor privately any history of sexual activity, abuse, birth control, safe sex, pregnancy, and sexually transmitted diseases, as it pertains to my current condition. A chaperone will be available. ___Okay ___ No need

  A few children might request this opportunity. I have been in offices when patients did want to discuss these topics and I served as chaperone. Here, I want the person to feel she can discuss any issue she believes to be impacting her health. In pediatrics, most of these forms will be filled out by the guardian, so I suspect that there will not be many discussions in this regard. However, teens who fill out their own forms may have issues to talk about. As I have mentioned, these forms should be adapted to your practice.

Chapter 17

PHYSICAL EXAMINATION

We're drowning in information and starving for knowledge.

Rutherford D. Rogers

The physical exam begins when you first set eyes on the patient and continues for the duration of the visit. Gather information throughout your entire encounter. See how the person holds his head and adjusts his balance and makes eye contact. Look at skin and hair and demeanor. Evaluate dental health while conversing and watch eye-hand coordination as a child reaches for your stethoscope. Take every opportunity to assess.

Unfortunately since many of us do not see patients of all ages with any frequency and since TBIs can present in so many ways, this section might be more basic than you require. Many definitions and lists of age-specific normals are included. While you might not be called upon to see newborns, the information is available. Hopefully, this chapter will help prepare you for most contingencies.

In all cases, ensure that the patient you are examining is physically and mentally stable before proceeding. While you may see people with *acute* TBIs, often you will be assessing for *long-term* disease complications and co-infections. Even if the acute process is due to a TBI, ensure that the person is not compromised and is stable before you continue with the more in-depth assessment. Don't ignore an acute abdomen or fulminating pneumonia because the person paid for two hours of TBI work and they're going to get it.

Much of the physical exam information gathering can be done through multitasking. For example, when you are asking about vision problems you can be looking in the eye and asking what the person is planning later in the day. When you are examining a leg, examine several systems at a time (musculoskeletal, neurologic, circulatory, skin) while you're there, instead of doing all the reflexes and then coming back later and doing all the pulses, and later examining the skin.

You may do the PE in a totally different order than presented here and each HCP needs to find a flow that works for her. Take the time you need to do a thorough exam, but do the exam efficiently as described previously in Chapter 13: *Overall Patient Evaluation.*

Note that the more experience you have the smoother the exam will go. This actual physical exam takes an experienced TBI clinician about 15 to 20 minutes and me about 40 minutes. But remember to gather information for the physical assessment from the time you greet the patient until s/he is ready to say goodbye. I am not yet that polished in evaluating TBI patients. As you become more proficient you will better know what information you want to gather and how to dig deeper when indicated. I still follow the checklist.

Know what you don't know and consult as needed. But, don't lose your patient in the system. **You** are the TBI doc and the patient needs your opinion and advocacy.

The following *Physical Examination* outline is designed with a TBI focus. This is not a comprehensive physical. If you are the PCP for this patient, you are going to gather and assess more information than I have listed here. I tried to confine myself to physical findings pertinent to TBIs. However, since TBIs can affect essentially all body systems, there will be a lot of ground to cover. This chapter was not written to be an all-inclusive exam. Of course, you do not ignore non-TBI abnormalities that you come across in the exam. Depending on your role, you address them or refer them.

Document everything but do NOT write everything down for each patient for each visit. Do yourself a favor. No one knows your practice style like you do. Take some initial time and adapt the sample forms provided in this text to your needs. Appropriate use of the forms will allow you to target important information for that patient. You can design forms that allow for simple checks for negatives and items that are WNL so you do not have to write as I used to "No abdominal pain on palpation or percussion. No rebound or guarding. No masses or organomegaly. Normal BS t/o." Adapt the sample forms to your practice.

There are many physical findings here that do not appear to be applicable for TBIs. They are included either to allow you to make sure the patient is stable prior to a full TBI work-up or because these conditions should be considered as part of the differential diagnosis in evaluating a TBI. For example, an early appendicitis might mimic the kinds of physical findings you could see in several TBIs. Also, patients who are sick with TBIs get appendicitis, too. Don't miss an unrelated thyroid mass because you are so focused on the TBI.

This chapter deals with physical findings but does not include the full diagnostic work-up for things like pancreatitis or housemaid's knee. I tried to provide enough information to help you build a reasonable differential diagnosis. In fact, Chapter 21: *Differential Diagnosis and Concurrent Disease* will refer you back to this chapter frequently. More than one thing can be going on at a time in every single patient. Just because they have acute otitis media does not mean that they can't also have muted hearing due to a TBI. Just because they have one kind of arthritis does not mean they cannot have two. Hopefully, some of the distinguishing physical findings listed here will help sort through possible concurrent illnesses as well.

The sample physical exam form is not especially intimidating, just long. The rest of the *Physical Examination* chapter will be divided into manageable sections, categorized by body system, and include considerable information about examining TBI patients with an eye toward differential diagnosis and co-morbidities.

This text includes both this individual physical form and the 3-in-1 Follow-up Visit form (combining HX, ROS, and PE) for your perusal or modification. The full physical is best for the initial visit, while the 3-in-1 form is suited for subsequent visits. The following form is designed to make the exam as easy as possible to conduct without the HCP worrying about missing anything, while still capturing all pertinent information.

SAMPLE FORM XII: PHYSICAL EXAMINATION

This form is designed for the initial physical with a new patient. On subsequent visits the PE can be documented, along with the History and ROS, on the 3-in-1 Follow-Up Visit form. This PE form is designed to have only essential marks on the paper. Any parameter not examined is checked NE. Everything else is presumed to be negative or normal unless the Abnormal or Present box is checked. If checked, there is space to describe the abnormality. For example, a patient with a primary EM rash, a hot right knee, and large axillary lymph nodes would have 3 checks in the Abnormal or Present cells. No other boxes need to be checked unless the rectal and any other exams were deferred, in which case NE would be marked in the appropriate places. On the next visit, your eyes can review this form in seconds so that you know which areas to address during the visit.

PHYSICAL EXAMINATION

Name: _____ Date: _____

DOB: _____ Age today: _____

Photographs taken of the following areas: _____

Vital Signs: HR _____ RR _____ BP ___ / ___

Temp_____ (rectal, oral, axillary, ear, forehead) Time of last fever medicine_____

Measurements:

Height/length ____, ____% ile Weight ____, ____% ile Head circ ____, ____% ile

Other: _____

General Appearance: _____

Any listed area not examined is labeled NE.
All other examined parameters were within normal limits unless otherwise indicated.

Feature	NE	Abn or Present	Describe
Skin			
Texture	—	—	_____
Turgor	—	—	_____
Hypersensitivity	—	—	_____
Color	—	—	_____
Moisture	—	—	_____
Hair pattern	—	—	_____
Birthmarks/moles	—	—	_____
Lesions			_____
EM rash primary	—	—	_____
EM rash secondary	—	—	_____
Violet striae	—	—	_____
Nodules	—	—	_____
Other	—	—	_____
Nails			
Lesions	—	—	_____
Fungus	—	—	_____
Other	—	—	_____
Hair/scalp			
Lesions	—	—	_____
Other	—	—	

Head			
Shape	—	—	_____
Symmetry	—	—	_____
Evidence of injury	—	—	_____
Signs of Bell's palsy	—	—	_____
Other	—	—	
Eyes			
General	—	—	_____
Pain	—	—	_____
Redness (conjunctival/sclera)	—	—	_____
Hypersensitivity	—	—	_____
Lids	—	—	_____
Signs of Bell's palsy	—	—	_____
Acuity	—	—	_____
Gross	—	—	_____
Measured	—	—	_____
Color Sight	—	—	_____
Astigmatism	—	—	_____
Eye Movements	—	—	_____
Strabismus	—	—	_____
Pupils	—	—	_____
Light reaction	—	—	_____
Accommodation	—	—	_____
Field of Vision	—	—	_____
Fundus	—	—	_____
Other	—	—	
Ears			
Outer Ear	—	—	_____
Skin	—	—	_____
Morphology	—	—	_____
Color	—	—	_____
Temperature	—	—	_____
Lesions	—	—	_____
Pain	—	—	_____
Discharge	—	—	_____
Mastoid	—	—	_____
Middle Ear	—	—	_____
Canal			_____
Discharge	—	—	_____
TM	—	—	_____
Hearing	—	—	_____
Gross acuity/hypersensitivity	—	—	_____
Measured acuity	—	—	_____
Inner Ear	—	—	_____
Balance	—	—	_____
Other	—	—	

Nose			
Patent	—	—	_____
Septum	—	—	_____
Turbinates	—	—	_____
Discharge	—	—	_____
Lesions	—	—	_____
Other	—	—	_____
Mouth			
Lips	—	—	_____
Mucosal color	—	—	_____
Lesions	—	—	_____
Salivary glands	—	—	_____
Evidence of Bell's palsy	—	—	_____
Fungus	—	—	_____
Other	—	—	_____
Tongue			
Symmetry	—	—	_____
Motility	—	—	_____
Involuntary movements	—	—	_____
Lesions	—	—	_____
Coating	—	—	_____
Other	—	—	_____
TMJ			
ROM	—	—	_____
Pain	—	—	_____
Malocclusion	—	—	_____
Inflammation	—	—	_____
Audible or palpable click	—	—	_____
Other	—	—	_____
Teeth			
Hygiene	—	—	_____
Pain	—	—	_____
Pattern	—	—	_____
Gums	—	—	_____
Inflammation	—	—	_____
Other	—	—	_____
Throat			
Redness	—	—	_____
Pus	—	—	_____
Odor	—	—	_____
Lesions	—	—	_____
Tonsils	—	—	_____
Other	—	—	_____
Neck			
Nodes	—	—	_____
ROM, Cracking	—	—	_____

Signs of inflammation	—	—	_____
Trachea	—	—	_____
Masses	—	—	_____
Pulses	—	—	_____
Other	—	—	
Thyroid			
Symmetry	—	—	_____
Nodules	—	—	_____
Masses	—	—	_____
Other	—	—	
Back			
General structure	—	—	_____
Skin	—	—	_____
Motion	—	—	_____
Curvature	—	—	_____
Pain	—	—	_____
Kidney (CVA)	—	—	_____
Other	—	—	
Chest			
Symmetry	—	—	_____
Skin	—	—	_____
Breasts	—	—	_____
Lesions	—	—	_____
Discharge	—	—	_____
Gynecomastia	—	—	_____
Tenderness	—	—	_____
Developmental stage	—	—	_____
Other	—	—	_____
Axilla	—	—	_____
Nodes	—	—	_____
Pulses	—	—	_____
Masses	—	—	_____
Lesions	—	—	_____
Other	—	—	
Lungs			
Rate	—	—	_____
Respiratory pattern	—	—	_____
Breath sounds abnormal	—	—	_____
Cough	—	—	_____
Rub/rales/rhonchi	—	—	_____
Sputum	—	—	_____
Other	—	—	
Heart			
Rate	—	—	_____
Rhythm	—	—	_____
Heart sounds	—	—	

Murmurs	—	—	_____
Rubs	—	—	_____
Other	—	—	_____
Circulation			
Arteries	—	—	_____
Pulses	—	—	_____
Symmetrical	—	—	_____
Intensity	—	—	_____
Veins	—	—	_____
Enlarged	—	—	_____
Stasis changes	—	—	_____
Lymph	—	—	_____
Edema/mode	—	—	_____
Extremities	—	—	_____
Temperature	—	—	_____
Color	—	—	_____
Signs of phlebitis	—	—	_____
Other	—	—	_____
Abdomen			
General appearance	—	—	_____
Bloating	—	—	_____
Gas	—	—	_____
Fluid	—	—	_____
Abdominal respirations	—	—	_____
Skin	—	—	_____
EM rash	—	—	_____
Striae	—	—	_____
Lesions	—	—	_____
Percussion	—	—	_____
Auscultation	—	—	_____
Palpation	—	—	_____
Organomegaly	—	—	_____
Masses	—	—	_____
Pulsations	—	—	_____
Umbilicus	—	—	_____
Hernias	—	—	_____
Signs of acute abdomen	—	—	_____
Pain	—	—	_____
Diffuse	—	—	_____
Point	—	—	_____
Other	—	—	_____
Rectum			
Anal region	—	—	_____
Redness	—	—	_____
Lesions	—	—	_____
Skin	—	—	_____

Rectal Exam	—	—	
Blood	—	—	
Prostate	—	—	
Other	—	—	
Groin			
Hernias	—	—	
Pulses	—	—	
Nodes	—	—	
Lesions	—	—	
Other	—	—	
Genitals			
Male	—	—	
Developmental Stage	—	—	
Lesions	—	—	
Testes	—	—	
Scrotum	—	—	
Discharge	—	—	
Masses	—	—	
Signs of fungus	—	—	
Other	—	—	
Female	—	—	
Developmental stage	—	—	
Lesions	—	—	
Pain	—	—	
Organomegaly	—	—	
Signs of fungus	—	—	
Discharge	—	—	
Masses	—	—	
Pelvic exam	—	—	
Other	—	—	
Urinary Tract			
Kidney	—	—	
Abdominal Assessment	—	—	
Back Assessment	—	—	
CVA pain	—	—	
Masses	—	—	
Other	—	—	
Bladder	—	—	
Percussion	—	—	
Palpation	—	—	
Masses	—	—	
Pain	—	—	
Spasm	—	—	
Other	—	—	
Bones			
For each bone check:	—	—	

Deformities	—	—	_____
Nodules	—	—	_____
Point tenderness	—	—	_____
Shin pain	—	—	_____
Metatarsal pain	—	—	_____
Masses	—	—	_____
General pain	—	—	_____
Asymmetry/unequal length	—	—	_____
Compared to other bone, if paired	—	—	_____
Normal characteristics for specific bone	—	—	_____
Other	—	—	_____
Muscle			
For each muscle check:			
Tone (Hypotonia/Hypertonia)	—	—	_____
Tendons	—	—	_____
Nodules along tendons	—	—	_____
Spasms	—	—	_____
Mobility	—	—	_____
Flexibility	—	—	_____
Strength	—	—	_____
Pain to palpation	—	—	_____
Achilles pain	—	—	_____
Calf pain	—	—	_____
General tenderness	—	—	_____
Nodules	—	—	_____
Masses	—	—	_____
Development	—	—	_____
Symmetry if paired	—	—	_____
Other	—	—	_____
Joints			
For each joint check:			
Heat	—	—	_____
Redness	—	—	_____
Swelling	—	—	_____
Effusion	—	—	_____
Stability	—	—	_____
Ligaments	—	—	_____
ROM	—	—	_____
Boney enlargement	—	—	_____
Creaking, cracking	—	—	_____
Compared to other joint, if paired	—	—	_____
Normal characteristic for specific joint	—	—	_____
Specific Joint:	—	—	_____
Neck	—	—	_____
Back	—	—	_____
Costovertebral	—	—	

Costochondral	—	—	_____
Shoulders	—	—	_____
Elbows	—	—	_____
Wrists	—	—	_____
Hands	—	—	_____
Fingers	—	—	_____
SI	—	—	_____
Hips	—	—	_____
Knees	—	—	_____
Ankles	—	—	_____
Feet	—	—	_____
Lesions	—	—	_____
Infections	—	—	_____
Fungus	—	—	_____
Warts	—	—	_____
Anomalies	—	—	_____
Nails	—	—	_____
Plantar fasciitis	—	—	_____
Sole Pain	—	—	_____
Heel pain	—	—	_____
Toes	—	—	_____
Other	—	—	
Neurologic			
Mental Status	—	—	_____
Consciousness	—	—	_____
Affect	—	—	_____
Orientation	—	—	_____
Mood	—	—	_____
Interactions	—	—	_____
Cognition	—	—	_____
Abstract Thinking	—	—	_____
Judgment	—	—	_____
Memory	—	—	_____
Reflexes	—	—	_____
Deep	—	—	_____
Superficial	—	—	_____
Cranial nerves	—	—	_____
CN 7 Facial	—	—	_____
Symmetry	—	—	_____
Motion	—	—	_____
Lid closure	—	—	_____
Show teeth	—	—	_____
Balance	—	—	_____
Proprioception	—	—	_____
Gait	—	—	_____
Coordination	—	—	_____

Motor			
Tone	—	—	_____
Strength	—	—	_____
Movement	—	—	_____
Abnormal movements	—	—	_____
Motor tics	—	—	_____
Sensation	—	—	_____
Touch	—	—	_____
Hypersensitivity to touch	—	—	_____
Temperature	—	—	_____
Position	—	—	_____
Vibration	—	—	_____
Discrimination	—	—	_____
Pain	—	—	_____
Speech	—	—	_____
Vocal tics	—	—	_____
Developmental Milestones	—	—	_____
Appropriate for age	—	—	_____
Other	—	—	_____
Psychologic Exam			
Mood	—	—	_____
Suicidal attitudes	—	—	_____
Anxiety	—	—	_____
Obsessions	—	—	_____
Compulsions	—	—	_____
Thought processes	—	—	_____
Disorganized	—	—	_____
Rigid	—	—	_____
Irrational	—	—	_____
Relationship to reality	—	—	_____
Paranoia	—	—	_____
Aggression	—	—	_____
Anger	—	—	_____
Personality issues	—	—	_____
Passive-Aggressive	—	—	_____
Evidence of anorexia	—	—	_____
Evidence of needle use	—	—	_____
Social interactions	—	—	_____
Recent change in mental outlook	—	—	_____
Other	—	—	_____

_____

Signature of examining HCP

Well, I wanted to write a book that would allow me to examine a TBI patient effectively. I hope I have. After spending 4 months writing this chapter, all I can say is you have to know a helluva lot of stuff to be a good TBI doc.

Section 17-A

General, Vital Signs, Dimensions, and Pertinent Differential

There is no satisfaction in hanging a man who doesn't object to it.
George Bernard Shaw

I. GENERAL APPEARANCE

Look at the patient. By engaging the person, you can gauge her fundamental health status fairly quickly. You can tell if she has pain by the way she moves her body. Is she acutely ill or chronically debilitated? These first impressions provide considerable information. Is the individual clean and well-groomed? Is she glassy-eyed, sweating, shaking? What is her demeanor? How does the patient interact with the caregivers present? Is she age-appropriate? Are there obvious signs of disease?

Examine a child with underwear or diaper on and look inside the covering only during that specific part of the exam. An older child or adult can wear an exam gown. Be careful to keep the room temperature comfortable for the person with the least amount of clothing. Some little kids love to be naked and that is okay. Allow for as much modesty as the patient prefers.

PEARL: Some patients, especially those with neurologic manifestations of Lyme, are extremely sensitive to touch and do not like to have anything in contact with their skin, even the softest cloth. Sometimes it is hard to keep clothes on Lyme kids.

PEARL: Almost all Lyme patients have a lower than normal activity level. Many are frustrated and sick of being sick. Some present with an incapacitating or debilitating fatigue. Lyme kids can appear to deflate before your eyes. Terms found in the literature to describe this dwindling phenomenon associated with Lyme include: sag, fade, wilt, melt, turn limp, cave, collapse, etc.

PEARL: Lyme patients sometimes have been described as having an excess of visceral symptoms such as swallowing, burping, coughing, or vomiting. Look at the person's overall habitus.

PEARL: The presenting signs of gestational Lyme include hypotonia, irritability, fatigue, lack of stamina, wilting, pallor, and as they get a little older, dark circles under the eyes.

II. VITAL SIGNS AND DIMENSIONS

In young children, growth and development measures may be the best way to track progress, both improvement and deterioration. Growth charts are useful in TBIs to see if a child falls outside their normal range and how they compare to population standards. The more data points charted the better, since you can see how the child was trending and how the new data fits into his usual pattern. If the parents are tiny and the child has always been in the lower percentiles on a growth chart, this would be expected for this particular child. If on the next visit, the child falls off the charts or jumps high into territory where he has never been before, you have reason to look for an explanation. Growth charts for height, weight, and head and chest circumference can all be printed off the Internet. Vital signs provide data point information about the individual's current condition. These can be followed in order to uncover any changes that might need to be addressed.

Height

You don't actually measure height in infants as much as length. To measure a supine infant you will be measuring from crown to heel. Don't think you can do this by yourself. With one person holding the child with legs extended, the other person handles the measuring tape. Children who can stand still should be measured using a regular scale with an attached measuring arm. The child should be in stocking feet. Document the height on the growth chart and follow the child over time. One data point will allow comparison with the population ranges. Several data points will allow you to follow the specific child.

PEARL: Despite a savage limp, I was unaware that I had lost significant leg length unilaterally due to damaged knee cartilage. An astute podiatrist attributed this finding to spirochetes munching away on my person. Other people lose height due to disc space disruption or vertebral disintegration.

Weight

Weigh an infant on an infant scale if available. If none is handy, an infant can be held by another person and that person's weight subtracted. All clothing should be removed from the infant (not the holder). Older children can be weighed in underwear.

There may be a growth problem if the child is above the 97th percentile or below the 3rd percentile. Look at the parents to see if these extreme measurements are consistent with the genes the child is carrying. If not, consider why the child may be at either end of the spectrum. If you have access to previous growth charts, any change (up or down) from the usual pattern deserves exploration about why this might have happened.

PEARL: Steroid use in young kids can significantly stunt growth. This includes steroids in diaper rash creams. Steroids in skin creams penetrate the dermis easily and can get into the general circulation. Prolonged use of steroids on baby skin will cause it to thin and look smooth and transparent. This is a good time to consider stopping the steroid cream.

Head circumference

In babies the head circumference should be documented every time you see the child until age 2. Continue with this measurement beyond that time if there has been any question about growth or development. Measure at the broadest part of the head starting by putting the tape around the frontal area (forehead), around the side above the ear, and around the back at the broadest point. Problems with the size of the cranium can impede the growth of its contents such as the brain. Since there can be so many developmental and neurologic complications of Lyme, it's important to determine if there may be alternative explanations for problems. If the head circumference is small, look to see if sutures are prematurely closed. If the baby's head appears too large, or there has been an abrupt change, consider a mass, hydrocephalus, or hematoma.

PEARL: Supine is the patient tummy-up like a bowl of soup. (Get it? Soup-ine?) Prone is tummy down.

Chest circumference

With the infant supine, pass the tape around the chest at nipple level and take the measure halfway between inspiration and expiration. The only reason to look at this measure is if there is a problem with the head circumference. Generally, the head circumference is greater than the chest circumference until 2-years-old and smaller after that.

Temperature

The documentation of fever can be particularly important in TBIs. Some HCPs encourage daily or more frequent measures of temperature to see if an underlying pattern will help make the diagnosis. In general, bacteria and protozoa cause higher temperatures than viruses, but this is one rule that often finds exceptions. Usually the temperature is higher in the evening than in the morning. When looking for fever patterns make sure you document the time of the last antipyretic medications in relation to the time of the measurement of temperature. Acetaminophen will mute the fever for about 4 hours and ibuprofen for 6 to 8 hours.

If fever is one of the complaints, the most accurate measure is a rectal temp especially in young kids who can't put up much of a fuss. Otherwise the order of preferred location is ear, under tongue, axillary, and forehead. Note the location used on the chart. Oral temps can be difficult to get in kids under 3. To get a rectal temp lay the child prone or on her side on a table or lap. Using a lubricated rectal thermometer, enter the anus and aim for the belly button about one inch into the rectum. Allow the thermometer to remain in place until the temperature has had a chance to stabilize.

The younger the child the less well regulated the temperature. Rectal temperatures are higher in infants than in older kids. Rectal temps are not usually below 99 in kids under 3. At 18 months the average rectal temp in a healthy child is 100. In an individual, non-febrile child the temperature can vary by 3° in the course of 24 hours, with the temp highest in late afternoon. That is why a temperature of 102 may indicate more severe illness in a 12-year-old than in a 2-year-old. Extremely high temps in young kids are not unusual up to 105. As the child gets older these high temps can mean more significant illness. Conversely, if a child is approaching sepsis, the temperature can be normal or low. Don't be fooled.

PEARL: Dr. Burrascano uses fever patterns to narrow the differential diagnosis. A low-grade fever in the morning can mean active Bartonella. Subnormal morning temperatures, with low-grade afternoon elevations may be more indicative of active Lyme.

Heart rate

A measure of actual heart rate is preferred to pulse in younger children. Directly auscultate the heart to get the number of beats per minute. In older kids use the radial pulse. HR in kids is more variable than in adults and more affected by illness.

Birth:	140
Up to 6 months:	130
6 to 12 months:	115
1 to 2 years:	110
2 to 6 years:	104
6 to 10 years:	95

The normal HR for healthy kids can range 30 to 50 beats above or below average:

The average heart rate continues to decline then into adulthood where the average BPM is 72. Athletes can have normal bradycardias into the 40s. Fevers tend to raise HR. Beyond the neonatal period a heart rate above 180 usually suggests PAT (paroxysmal atrial tachycardia).

Blood pressure

BP in babies is rarely taken in a routine exam or even in the ER. Other vital signs tend to provide more information. BPs can usually be taken after the age of 3. Width of the cuff should be about 1/2 to 2/3 the width of the arm (or a leg can be used). The cuff should completely encircle the limb. A cuff that is too small will artificially increase the reading. In adults, the diastolic reading is made when the heart sound is no longer heard in the stethoscope over the artery. This is not always so clear in children or the elderly. In cases where the pulse sounds are not heard with the stethoscope, the radial pulse can be used to determine the BP. Here the point where the pulse is first felt is the systolic pressure, which will be somewhat different from what would be measured using the stethoscope. The diastolic BP will not be able to be obtained.

Systolic normals:

@ 50 mm Hg	at	birth
60	at	1 month
70	at	6 months
90	at	1 year
100	at	6 years
110	at	10 years
120	at	16 years

Diastolic normals:

Diastolic rises to about 60 mm Hg at 1 year and then gradually increases throughout childhood to @ 75.

BP can vary with exercise, crying, or anxiety. Patients can have abnormally high BPs due to kidney disease, atherosclerosis, renal artery disease, coarctation of the aorta, and pheochromocytoma. Today, older kids are getting HTN for the same reason as adults: obesity, diabetes, and vessel constriction.

Hypertension without a clear reason should be monitored over time, by you, if that is your role, or by a HTN specialist. Pharmaceutical companies, with their direct-to-consumer advertising around hypertension, allow us to conveniently forget that many elderly people are overmedicated for their formerly high blood pressure to the point where **hypo**tension becomes the biggest concern.

PEARL: A neurally mediated hypotension has been described in association with Lyme.

Respiratory rate

You can tell if a patient is in respiratory distress as he is coming into the room. If there is any compromise, assess the respiratory condition immediately. Do not be a slave to your forms or checklists and allow a person to deteriorate in front of you. This tends to make parents especially nervous and I have witnessed it with my own child. Any patient with rapid breathing or respiratory distress, who looks sick or compromised, should have the breathing problem addressed immediately. The acute condition should be stabilized before you continue the assessment for TBI, even if a TBI is the underlying cause of the acute illness.

In neonates and infants the RR is more variable and more influenced by illness than in older kids or adults. Exercise and anxiety can affect the rate as well. Average respiratory rates in healthy people:

Newborn:	30 to 80
Young children:	20 to 40
Late childhood:	15 to 25
After age 15:	12 to 20

Premature infants and full term newborns may have variable rates from rapid respirations to short periods of apnea. Respiratory rates over 100 are associated with lower respiratory tract diseases such as bronchiolitis, asthma, RSV, or a number of other problems that need to be assessed. These people may need to go to the ER, and the TBI assessment postponed until later.

In infants, count the abdominal respiratory efforts rather than the chest movement. Abdominal retractions in neonates and infants are a sign of respiratory distress and are signaled by sucking in of the accessory muscles in the chest and abdomen with each breath.

A number of TBIs can cause pulmonary signs and symptoms. Remember, that more than one problem can manifest at a time and confound the clinical picture. Concurrent illness can make the TBI symptoms worse and vice versa. Aside from some cases of babesiosis and some of the Mycoplasma pathogens, respiratory problems are not usually the primary presenting symptom in TBIs, at least not early in the clinical course. Nevertheless, allergic reactions are a common reason for respiratory compromise.

Because TBIs can compromise the immune system, patients can present with more overall respiratory problems in addition to any pulmonary issues that may be due to the TBI. These include any number of infectious and allergic type conditions.

Here are a few underlying causes of respiratory compromise that should be stabilized prior to further routine evaluation:

- Respiratory syncytial virus (RSV) is a lower respiratory tract infection that can be fatal in infants and young kids. By causing the formation of cell masses connected by syncytium, RSV can result in pneumonia and bronchiolitis. Hard to diagnose early, this condition can confuse many differential diagnoses. Most cases occur in winter and early spring and present with dyspnea, cough, wheeze, and fever. Severe signs and symptoms may require hospitalization before the diagnosis is made.

- Croup is a viral respiratory inflammation characterized by stridor on inspiration and respiratory distress. The child may present with a barking cough often at night, seeming suffocation, retractions, long inspirations, and distress. The airway can spasm. Presenting mostly in kids 6 months to 3-years-old, fever is present in only about half the cases. Intense hydration and humidification can alleviate symptoms and the child may need to be hospitalized.

- Epiglottitis can be an emergency. Inflammation of the epiglottis can be life-threatening with symptoms including cough, hoarseness, difficulty swallowing, and signs of upper respiratory tract obstruction. A lateral X-ray view of the neck may be needed to confirm the diagnosis.

- Bronchiolitis is inflammation of the bronchioles in the lower pulmonary tree, usually caused by viruses such as RSV. The child presents with what appears to be a URI but then quickly deteriorates to respiratory compromise with wheezes, crackles, tachypnea, expiratory obstruction, tachycardia, hacking cough, circumoral cyanosis, and retractions. Bronchiolitis is most often diagnosed in children less than 18 months. They usually have no fever, but can be quite lethargic.

- Pneumonia is an inflammation of the lower respiratory tract due to infection or chemical irritation. Pneumonia can affect an entire lobe of a lung or just a section. With bacterial pneumonia, the patient may be more acutely ill but may respond more rapidly to treatment than viral etiologies. On PE, there may be a section of the lung area with no or diminished breath sounds. The Mycoplasma genus, which can be tick-borne, can cause atypical pneumonias. X-ray can show a white-out of the affected area due to increased fluid and immune molecules at the site. The X-ray may lag behind the clinical picture by hours. So treat the person, not the picture. Patients with chronic TBIs and those who are bedridden or in late stages of disease can present with pneumonia due to opportunistic secondary infections. Tularemia, Q fever, and the Mycoplasma genus have all been associated with pneumonia.

- Aspiration pneumonia: Pneumonia caused by inhaling into the lungs gastric contents (vomit), food, saliva, mucus, or other substances. Patients who lose their gag reflex due to CNS depression, as in alcohol intoxication, are especially prone to aspirate. Newborns can inhale any manner of fluids during the birth process including meconium.

- Asthma is becoming a more frequent diagnosis, especially in kids, and can be associated with infection, allergies, and irritants. We used to think that if the patient wasn't wheezing then he couldn't have asthma. Now we know that asthma can present with cough or no obvious symptoms aside from shortness of breath. We also used to say that no one ever died from asthma. Unfortunately, that assertion has also been disproven. A susceptible airway is triggered by a stimulus to constrict in paroxysms usually causing wheezing, which can progress to significant dyspnea. Kids are most vulnerable to asthma attacks and the symptoms can come on slowly or quite suddenly. School age kids seem to be the most affected. If triggered by allergens, the asthmatic response can be mediated by eosinophils and IgE. Boys are about twice as likely to have asthma as girls, but that ratio becomes more equitable as they get older. As many as 10% of kids will have some degree of asthmatic symptoms during childhood. If the individual already has inhalers or other methods to manage the symptoms, the situation can be stabilized and the routine assessment continued. Otherwise, the person may need to go to the ER for stabilization.

- Obstructed airway is a common reason for respiratory distress and may be the most pertinent to TBI patients due to allergies from medicines and other sensitizers. Airway obstruction from allergies causes the respiratory tract to swell, eventually occluding the passage way. This presentation can be a part of an anaphylactic reaction. Symptoms may build gradually or can be surprisingly rapid. This is a medical emergency and is most often treated with epinephrine, steroids, and bronchodilators. Airway obstruction can also be due to a foreign body which can be dislodged acutely by the Heimlich maneuver or through other removal techniques. Masses can also obstruct the airway but these cases usually have a gradual onset of symptoms. If the obstruction appears to have been caused by an allergic reaction, try to identify the allergen. Review medication lists and make sure the person does not get another dose of the suspected medication. Identifying the causal agent is not always as easy as we might hope.

Section 17-B

Skin and Pertinent Differential

"Even if I knew that tomorrow the world would go to pieces, I would still plant my apple tree."
Martin Luther King, Jr.

SKIN

Rashes can be an important part of the diagnosis of TBIs. Because there is so much controversy around rashes in Lyme disease, it is imperative to be as accurate as possible in describing any skin lesions found on physical exam. Precise documentation could help with the differential diagnosis and aid in defining the stage of disease. Changes in these lesions in subsequent visits can help assess efficacy of treatment. Describe the lesion along with its size and location. Take photographs when appropriate.

The overall examination of the skin includes:

- Texture is the visual or surface characteristics of the skin. How does the skin look and feel? Is it rough, smooth, wrinkled, taut?

- Turgor is a measure of normal pressure or tension inside a cell. A dry plant can droop over its pot looking limp and lifeless. After watering, this same plant can reinflate in minutes due to a normalization of its turgor pressure. Children and the elderly can dehydrate easily. Look for tenting by gently pinching up a small tag of flesh on the forearm or leg and see how quickly this skin snaps back to flat. Rapid return indicates normal hydration. Slow resolution or visible tenting of the skin indicates dehydration. Skin can also have too much turgor. Generalized swelling can occur in kidney problems, heart conditions, and electrolyte imbalances.

- Moisture can refer to either how lubricated the skin is with oils or how much water is present. Is the skin dry and flakey or greasy and flakey? Is there a visible sheen or a powdery residue? Is perspiration abnormal? Is the sweat due to a skin condition or a systemic infection?

- Hair pattern over skin can suggest endocrine abnormalities. Too much hair can indicate high levels of certain hormones. Too little hair can suggest diabetes or ischemia.

- Birthmarks should be documented since they can mask pathologic lesions.

- Moles can come in all shapes and sizes and their numbers can vary with age. Usually moles are defined as discolored spots elevated above the surface of the skin. Most are harmless if not irritated. Skin cancers are often dismissed as moles and any changes in the shape of a mole or an irregular surface area should be investigated. Some people have dozens of moles and others never have a single mole throughout life. A mole is also called a nevus.

- Freckles are hyperpigmented areas where the body sends out melanin to protect the skin from UV rays. We used to think freckles were cute on kids. We still refer to the "freckle-faced" kid as the epitome of wholesomeness and health. That is, until we made the association between sun exposure and skin cancer. Teenage girls are more likely to use sunscreen if told that the sun will make them wrinkle than if they think it causes cancer. Freckles are most common in Caucasians but can occur in any race or ethnic group.

- Color in healthy persons ranges from albinism with no skin pigment to black.

  Abnormal color:

  Yellow: Consider liver problems including increased bilirubin levels. Yellow discoloration usually first appears in scleras, then mucous membranes, and finally general skin locations.

  Yellow brown: May be chronic renal disease and may not involve the sclera or mucous membranes

PEARL: Chronic uremia (toxins in the blood due to kidney failure) will cause yellow/brown skin color, which may be generalized, but does not include sclera or mucous membranes.

  Orange: Can mean too much Vitamin A, problems in the hypopituitary, or diabetes

  Pink or red: Usually means sunburn. Many of the antibiotics used in TBI patients, especially the TCNs, can cause extreme sensitivity to UV light. The importance of sun protection must be emphasized in these patients. Tanning beds are never encouraged. Skin can also be temporarily red from flushing, which in some cases can indicate a hypersensitivity or histamine reaction.

Dark patches: Can be DM, Addison's, or Cushing's with excess cortisol

PEARL: Bartonella can have a rash that looks more like a bruise because of neovascularization. This lesion can appear like a purple patch. Bartonella is also responsible for violaceous striae.

Decreased color:

Pallor or paleness most often suggests anemia and in these cases the conjunctiva and oral mucosa will also tend to be pale.

Acquired pigment loss:

White patches can be due to vitiligo which is an acquired skin disease manifested by white patches surrounded by normal colored skin. Vitiligo has been associated with thyroid problems, diabetes, anemia, Addison's disease, and Candida. The actual cause is unknown. While more prevalent in blacks, this condition is not uncommon in other races. Vitiligo can also remove pigment from patches of hair.

Lightened patches are often due to a fungus such as tinea versicolor which presents as yellow or buff colored patches on the skin. Tinea versicolor most commonly appears on the chest, upper back, and neck and usually responds to antifungals.

Albinism is a genetic variation and not a disease. Albinism can affect the skin, hair, and eyes and can be partial or total. Albinism can be accompanied by astigmatism, photophobia, and nystagmus because the eyes are not sufficiently protected from light. Mention of albinos with TBIs appears in the literature more often than you might suspect. Since an EM rash has nothing to do with pigmentation, the presentation of this lesion in an albino would be just like it might be in a person with any other pigment status. The lesion may stand out more because of additional contrast.

- Lesions should be described in the chart as accurately as possible and the location documented. While you are certainly not going to count every petechiae in a patient with RMSF, try to detail the lesions as much as possible. This will help you recall how the skin looked during the next visit. How else will you know if the lesion got better or worse? In these cases, a photograph might be your best friend.

PEARL: Better to take a photo that you never need than to desperately wish you had one when you need it. As a technophobe, even I find it hard to make excuses with all that cell phones can do today. Date the photo.

A **lesion** is defined as an area of pathology in tissue and can refer to an injury, irritation, wound, infection, or any other abnormal process in the skin or any other tissue. Rash is a general term used to refer to a skin eruption that can be temporary, long-term, or chronic.

Considerable confusion has been generated in TBIs by the interchangeable use and misuse of these dermatologic terms. What a mess the authorities have made of this! Do the best you can to be as clear as possible in your descriptions of these conditions. The more we all sing from the same song sheet and standardize our language, the better for the patients in the long-run. What follows are descriptions and definitions of the most common lesions found in TBIs.

A. **Non-palpable or flat lesions:**

Macule: A small, flat lesion up to 1 cm (e.g., freckles, petechiae)

Patch: A lesion larger than 1 cm (e.g., vitiligo)

B. **Palpable or raised lesions**

Papule: A raised lesion up to 0.5 cm such as a nevus or pimple

Plaque: A larger than 0.5 cm lesion, which can have both flat and raised regions such as a grouping of papules

Nodule: A bump, knot, knob, protuberance, swelling or cluster of cells. A nodule is a small node usually up to 0.5 to 2 cm. Nodules are often deeper and firmer than papules. Subcutaneous nodules can be found along the legs and triceps in Bartonella infections. Nodules under the skin can also suggest RA or rheumatic fever.

Tumor: A lesion larger than 1 to 2 cm. The term tumor does not mean cancer. Tumor means lump or growth, some of which are cancerous. Most are benign.

Wheal (hive): Irregular, often round, skin reaction that occurs in response to allergies and insect bites (even in those bites not associated with allergy). A wheal is a swollen bump that can be red with a white area in the center. A wheal can be isolated or can be disseminated over large skin areas and in those cases the reaction is often called urticaria. Usually wheals are quite itchy. Scratching often results in more wheals. Generally, wheals are transient, but some forms of urticaria last for years.

PEARL: Sometimes vasculitis is mistaken for a wheal.

C. Miscellaneous Lesions:

<u>Erosion</u>: A loss of epidermis often seen after rupture of a superficial blister or chicken pock that does not bleed or scar

PEARL: A pock is a scar left by a pox. Had I not written this book I would have never known that.

<u>Ulcer</u>: A deeper loss of skin surface that is likely to bleed and scar

<u>Fissure</u>: A crack in the skin often seen with fungus in the foot or in the mucous membranes near the anus. Fissures can develop in chapped lips or hands. Fissures in the tongue are characteristic of Sjogren's syndrome.

<u>Crust</u>: Dried blood, serum, or pus as can be found in impetigo infections caused by Staph or Strep

<u>Scale</u>: Exfoliated skin with thin flakes as seen with dandruff, psoriasis, or severe dry skin

<u>Hemangioma</u>: A benign tumor of dilated blood vessels, not uncommon in Lyme and Bartonella infections. These may appear as small bright red, raised dots.

<u>Cyst</u>: A closed sac or pouch with definite boundaries that contain fluid or other materials. A cyst is an abnormal structure caused by infection or obstruction of ducts. As much fun as it might be to poke a cyst, this doesn't usually get your anywhere. First, they are hard to hit and second, they just refill within a few days or hours with the same stuff that was in there in the first place. To get rid of a cyst, the sack usually has to be removed. Sometimes an infected cyst will remit and shrink without intervention. Cysts are common over the sacrum (pilonidal cysts) or in cystic acne.

PEARL: Note that the term cyst is also used to refer to a structure formed by certain pathogens where they are enclosed inside the cyst capsule and become inactive until environmental conditions are more favorable.

<u>Keritosis pilaris</u>: Little bumps on the upper arms or thighs are common in kids with about 40% of kids noticing the lesions at some point, especially in teens. OTC lactic acid lotion can be helpful.

<u>Atrophy</u>: A wasting away of the skin caused by many mechanisms including cell death, resorption, diminished replenishment of cells, ischemia, pressure, poor nutrition, or hormone changes. The skin will appear thin, shiny, and translucent with decreased furrows. Repeated local steroid use can cause atrophy.

PEARL: Steroids in skin creams can penetrate the skin easily and can get into the general circulation. Prolonged use of steroids on baby skin will cause it to thin and look smooth and transparent. This is a good time to consider stopping the steroid cream. Better to limit steroid use in the first place. Steroids should be avoided in Lyme patients except in cases of emergency.

PEARL: Acrodermatitis chronica atrophicans has been associated with Lyme in Europe. This skin manifestation is progressive and leads to widespread atrophy of the skin. The condition has been linked to problems in the PNS such as polyneuropathy. The skin becomes like tissue paper. Usually the lesions begin in the extremities with a blush-red inflammation and swelling. The clinical course might last for years.

<u>Excoriation</u>: An abrasion or scratch. Sometimes patients with intense itching will excoriate their own skin.

<u>Scar</u>: Replacement of damaged tissue with fibrous material leaving a less flexible healed area. Initially a scar will be a red or purple mark that eventually becomes white. A keloid is a hypertrophied scar more common in dark-skinned races. Multiple scars, especially of different ages can suggest abuse. We suspect that chronically sick people may be at higher risk for abuse, so be aware. Multiple scars on knees could mean the person is falling more than usual and might lead you to examine gait, balance, and coordination more carefully.

<u>Fluid-filled lesions</u>:

<u>Vesicle</u>: A small elevation of skin with free fluid in the skin layers such as those that occur with friction blisters or herpes simplex

<u>Blister</u>: A collection of serous or other fluid under or in the epidermis. Never underestimate a blister. We had several soldiers die at Fort Dix from toxic shock due to improperly treated blisters. Blisters can be due to friction or inflammation.

<u>Bulla</u>: Large (greater than 0.5 cm) lesions filled with serous fluid. A good example is a 2nd degree burn.

<u>Pustule</u>: A blister filled with pus such as those seen in acne and impetigo

Acne: Inflammation of sebaceous glands and follicles in the skin characterized by comedones (whiteheads and blackheads), papules, and pustules. Acne can be cystic and leave scars and nodules.

Milia: White-headed, pin-point, sebum-plugged glands that can be found on the face and trunk of newborns and usually disappear within a few weeks (Three hyphens were used and it's not even a complete sentence.)

Broken vessels:

Petechiae: Spots of blood outside the vessels. These lesions are usually small and purplish and do not blanch with pressure. Petechiae can be associated with severe fevers. I have never had a good experience with petechiae. They can be a significant finding in toxic shock syndrome and DIC and in these cases can be quickly fatal. Petechiae are often seen in the rash of RMSF.

Bruising: Also called contusions or ecchymoses. Blood is released from the vessels usually due to trauma, but can also be seen in bleeding disorders.

Purpura: Bleeding into the skin with various presentations and probably as many etiologies. The red/purple discoloration turns into yellow/green and then brown before resolution. The bleeding can be into skin, mucous membranes, internal organs, and other tissue. The discoloration usually disappears within 2 to 3 weeks. There is no blanching on pressure. Purpura can be allergic, autoimmune, or due to vascular inflammation. Most purpura is idiopathic especially in the very young or very old. While the term idiopathic sounds very sophisticated and technical, it means we have no clue what is going on.

Common skin manifestations of TBIs:

Sensitivity: Many Lyme patients are exceedingly sensitive to touch. They do not want anything touching their skin, even the softest cloth. Some reports of similar sensitivities have been noted in patients with babesiosis, M. *fermentans*, and bartonellosis. In these cases it is difficult to tell if the hypersensitivity is due to one of these co-infections, to Lyme, or to a combination of problems. Could autoimmunity be a factor?

Striae: A line formed on the skin where the connective tissue has been stretched. This streak is a different color and texture than the surrounding normal skin.

White striae: Stretch marks are common in persons whose skin has been stretched beyond its ability to rebound such as the stretch marks found in pregnancy or with significant weight loss.

Violaceous striae: Purple or violet marks found commonly in patients with Bartonella infections. B. *henselea* is believed to create new vasculature and new blood vessels form in tissue where the pathogen is lurking. These purple streaks are called violaceous striae. While they resemble the white stretch marks that appear during pregnancy and after significant weight loss, these are definitely violet in appearance and may not follow the skin planes like mechanical stretch marks tend to do. Further, these violet marks can appear in patients where there has been no extreme stretching of the soft tissue. Usually the purple striae appear as violet snakes on the back, abdomen, flanks, thighs, and occasionally under the axilla and over the breasts. Some may look more like a bruise or purple patch. I know of no other condition that presents with violaceous striae, so in assessing TBI patients these striae should be considered pathognomonic for Bartonella *henselea*. Pink striae can accompany Cushing's disease.

PEARL: I write here of B. henselea *as though that's the microbe we are dealing with when referring to the causative agent of tick-borne bartonellosis. That is probably NOT the case, since BLOs are likely responsible.*

Subcutaneous nodules: Subcutaneous nodules can be palpated and sometimes visualized under the skin and most often present along the extremities, outer thighs, shins, and occasionally along the triceps. These nodules may be a manifestation of neovascularization in bartonellosis.

Raynaud's: Both Lyme and bartonellosis have been associated with Raynaud's phenomenon. While not a skin condition, the skin can appear purplish due to vascular constriction. The extremities will be cold and blue.

Erythema migrans rash:

Literally translated, erythema migrans means moving redness. There are so many misconceptions about these lesions that it's hard to know where to begin. First, EM rashes ARE pathognomonic for borreliosis. I can think of nothing else that causes an EM rash. Despite an excitable government worker telling the president of the LDA that EM was not pathognomonic for Lyme because STARI patients could have it too, EM pretty much equals Lyme. But to keep all parties calm, I will surrender and say EM means borreliosis. Before you can split another hair, let's clear up a few more fallacies. Most EM rashes are oval, not round, most do not have central clearing, and most do not look like a target or bull's eye; although EM rashes can present all those ways upon occasion. And the biggest myth buster of all: EM rashes are not as common as professed. Pathognomonic does not mean common.

If you see an EM rash, you're dealing with Borrelia. But most often you don't see an EM rash. The majority of Lyme patients do not ever notice an EM rash. If you hold the appearance of an EM rash as necessary to have LD, you will be missing half your cases right off the bat. Depending on the practice perhaps 10 to 40% recall an EM rash. Only a small percentage of those lesions have anything that looks like a target or bull's eye. Last night, my husband interrupted me to tell me they were showing EM target rashes on the nightly news because 2012 was going to be such a big tick year. The perpetual touting of the bull's eye is misleading. This causes both the public and HCPs to think they only need to worry if they see a target lesion. The concept of no rash, no Lyme, was dispelled ages ago, but refocusing on the rash resurrects this myth.

The presence of an EM rash is a diagnostic blessing, a gift. You have evidence of Lyme. You do not need to do anything else to confirm the diagnosis. You might be able to scoop out a few spirochetes if you biopsy the periphery of the lesion. But why? The EM rash says it all. Be grateful. Treat the Lyme and make sure your excitement is not masking a co-infection.

Usually an EM rash has a homogenous red color, but the color can vary from pale to maroon. There can be rings and occasionally there is said to be central clearing. We do not know why some patients get an EM rash but the majority do not. There may be a genetic predisposition or an autoimmune factor, or perhaps the Bb strain determines who gets the skin lesions. The critical point is that the EM rash is confirmatory if present. The absence of an EM rash means nothing.

In reality, we should worry even less about the presence of EM rashes since a study of European doctors has demonstrated that most docs wouldn't know an EM rash if they fell over it. Only 30% could correctly identify such a rash. Unfortunately with LD, myth is often stacked on legend which is added to fallacy. In the past, doctors were told not to treat unless there was a classic EM rash. This idea is dangerous not only because an EM rash, in the experience of some clinicians, develops in perhaps only 10% to 40% of Lyme patients, but also because doctors don't know an EM rash when they see one. That means that 70% of the visible rashes will be mislabeled by the HCPs and since many of the patients don't have the rash in the first place, that's a lot of untreated cases of Lyme.

There are two recognized forms of EM rash associated with Lyme disease. This concept is important and few get it right.

> **Primary erythema migrans:** Originally called erythema chronica migrans, this lesion, in the presence of corroborating history and ROS, is pathognomonic for borreliosis. This skin manifestation usually appears near the location of the tick bite and suggests

localized disease. The rash usually appears as a single, flat, non-palpable, homogeneous, oval, discolored, red patch most often on an extremity, trunk, thigh, buttock, axilla, or just about any skin area where a tick can bite. There is often a tiny scab or bite mark in the center of the lesion where the tick was attached. These lesions can be harder to discern in dark-skinned individuals or when they appear under hair or in areas not easily visualized.

Usually the primary EM rash presents around the bite site, remaining dark red and possibly slightly indurated. While the outer rim of the lesion remains reddish, the area in between can clear, causing the rash to look like a target or bull's eye. While there may be apparent concentric rings, there is usually no central clearing. Central clearing is missing in most of these cases.

EM lesions can vary in size but often get quite large up to a foot in diameter. An EM rash can be very brief or can last for weeks. More might appear than are observed since they can sometimes fade and flare. Other EM lesions can be under hair, in places where no one is looking, or masked by dark skin pigment.

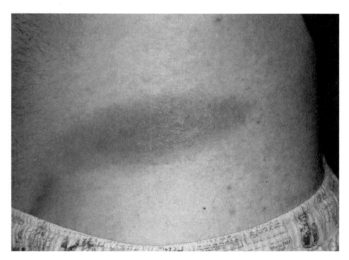

Classic primary erythema migrans lesion
Medical records of Christopher Spreen

In the photograph above my son displays the most common appearance of a primary EM rash: homogenous, oval, with a small scab slightly off-center where the tick bit him.

The EM rash can be a moving target. In some cases it might have been missed because it appeared and then was gone before anyone noticed. Likewise, sometimes there is slight central clearing around the bite mark and sometimes not.

These photographs are from the personal records of Christopher Spreen illustrating a primary EM rash. These images are used in lectures as examples of a classic primary EM rash.

Usually primary EM lesions respond quickly to antibiotics but they can persist through antibiotic therapy. They can reappear during relapses and have been observed during Herx reactions. (The presentation during a Herx might be the spirochetes scrambling to get back into hiding in order to escape the massive kill-off caused by antibiotics.) EM rashes can present within hours of a tick bite or as late as 6 months later (but these late bloomers could be due to a subsequent unrecognized bite).

PEARL: In all cases, take a photo of the EM rash. Date the photo. When the lesion changes, take another picture.

The lesion can clear between the rings that expand out from the center. EM rashes are called **expansive** lesions since they sometimes move outward into concentric circles. Spirochetes enter the skin and begin replicating usually near the bite site since that's where they happen to be. As the population increases the microbes move out from the bite spot in all directions. This causes circles which are not always perfectly drawn since some pathogens may move faster and further than others. Here the spirochete is present and active and moving and replicating. We know this because Bb have been isolated from biopsies taken at the edge of these lesions. If the biopsy sample is not taken at the periphery of the lesions, spirochetes will probably be missed.

The following primary EM lesion is the less common clinical presentation. Here you can almost visualize the spirochetes heading out to safer ground, running (or flagellating) in all directions from the inoculation site. (Again, it's hard not to anthropomorphize.)

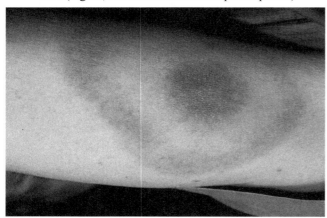

Concentric circles in an EM rash
Source: CDC. Accessed Oct 2012

At this point the infection is probably still localized. But the spirochetes are now moving into the blood, heading out on their way to becoming intracellular inside a variety of organs, and encysting as the need arises. Nevertheless, sometimes the Bb are again active close enough to the skin surface to be observed. This brings us to the other recognized EM rash associated with Lyme. ...

Secondary erythema migrans:

The secondary EM rash is evidence that Bb are on the move. While primary EM lesions might be referred to as expansive, secondary lesions are more appropriately called **evanescent**, which means not permanent or of short duration. They provide evidence of disseminated spirochetes. These are usually multiple lesions that appear as a result of Bb migrating through blood vessels and lymph channels. They can look like primary lesions but they come and go as the free-floating spirochetes traverse the circulatory system. A lesion, or multiple lesions, seem to pop up briefly, display, and recede.

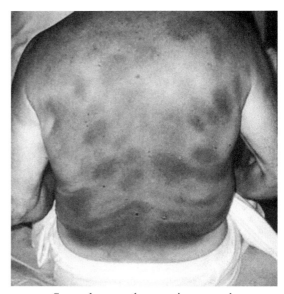

Secondary erythema migrans rash
Source: http://en.wikipedia.org.Accessed Oct 2012
Accessed March 2013

A secondary EM rash tends to be multifocal and can appear in any area where the Bb are migrating. By evanescent here we mean quickly vanishing, dispersing, spreading, coming and going, waxing and waning, transient. Secondary EM rashes are rarely seen and since they are so transitory they can easily be missed. You are witnessing manifestations of spirochetes on their way to go intracellular and encyst. While spirochetes are often on the move inside a host, the opportunity to observe them is exceptional.

PEARL: Take a photograph of the secondary EM rash. Date the photograph. You may never witness this again.

As the spirochetes disseminate by way of the blood vessels, they move through the body including distant areas of the skin. The term migrans means migrating or moving and these lesions often expand as the Bb move, appearing in other body locations far from the original bite site. These lesions indicate dissemination or distribution of the live spirochetes throughout the system. When visible, the secondary rash can be amorphous with some coming as others are going. They appear for 3 to 4 seconds or up to a minute or so and can be distributed across many areas. The most common sites where secondary EM rashes are observed are the back, trunk, abdomen, and thighs. There can be numerous simultaneous and sequential migrating lesions. Dozens can be present at once and these patients are usually found to be filled with spirochetes.

The Bb spirochetes can certainly spread without the presence of either type of erythema migrans. While a secondary EM rash provides evidence of dissemination, the presence of signs and symptoms compatible with systemic infection also suggests general distribution of the pathogen.

Biopsies might demonstrate the Bb spirochete, but the biopsy MUST be done at the periphery of the lesion or no spirochetes are likely to be recovered. They are hard enough to capture as it is. Since the periphery is the site of spirochetal replication, the biopsy tissue must be excised from this area to have the best chance of recovering any organism. Invasive biopsies are not done frequently anymore since observation of the rash itself gives the answer that you would be trying to uncover with the biopsy: presence of spirochetes. Bb are difficult pathogens to isolate and the percent recovered on peripheral biopsy is probably between 50% and 70%. (This isn't bad, considering some of the numbers we get with other testing.)

PEARL: The CDC has a staging scheme that says the primary EM rash is Stage 1 Lyme disease and the presence of a secondary EM rash is Stage 2. This staging scheme is artificial and not consistent with clinical experience. A person can have cardiac, joint, CNS, and other system involvement, indicating systemic disease in a clearly disseminated presentation without ever showing an EM rash. The primary EM lesion can persist or recur into long-term disease. Some HCPs could be confused by this inaccurate staging scheme. Why base a staging method on something that is not consistently present? That's like basing horse breeds on unicorns. Aside from this mention, I do not include staging contrivances that do not have a relationship to clinical reality as it is experienced by most Lyme patients.

PEARL: Is an EM rash pathognomonic for Lyme? Yes, if the history and clinical impressions support a diagnosis of Lyme. Absence of an EM rash does not rule out Lyme. Certainly not for the majority of Lyme patients who do not present with any form of EM lesions. In some practices this can be more than 90% of the patients.

PEARL: Certain people may be genetically predisposed to the development of an EM rash. Some authors think EM rashes might be strain related. Others think that EM lesions do not appear on first exposure but only after subsequent infection. We just don't know.

Other skin lesions associated with Lyme: While the EM rash is pathognomonic for borreliosis, it is certainly not a universal manifestation of Lyme. A number of other rashes have also been noted with Bb infection. Various macules and papules, not always in any identifiable pattern, have been discernible in Lyme cases. These rashes may not be seen immediately but can appear after a few weeks or even later in the clinical course. Some patients in Europe have reported a borrelial lymphocytoma which is a discrete, purple bump appearing most often on the skin of the ear, nipple, or scrotum. Some TBI patients complain of itchy, peeling skin. Acrodermatitis chronica atrophicans is a progressive skin atrophy associated with some Lyme cases in Europe.

Tick bite site lesion: As with any insect bite there can be redness around the bite mark. This is not an EM rash. This bite mark can persist for several days. Tick saliva can also cause an allergic reaction locally and perhaps systemically. This would result in more swelling in the area and perhaps some itching. This is not an EM rash. Also the tick may leave a small scab in the area where she was so unceremoniously pulled from the buffet table.

RMSF rash: The rash in RMSF is so important that it's part of the name. In the first week of fever, most patients develop a rash on their palms, soles, wrists, ankles, and forearms. This rash then extends to the face, axilla, buttocks, and trunk. Warm water or alcohol compresses tend to bring out the rash. Initially, the lesions blanch when compressed. The lesions start as small, non-itchy, pink macules, eventually becoming darker and more raised. After about four days, the rash can become petechial with bright red pinpoints which may coalesce to form large hemorrhagic patches. These lesions could later ulcerate.

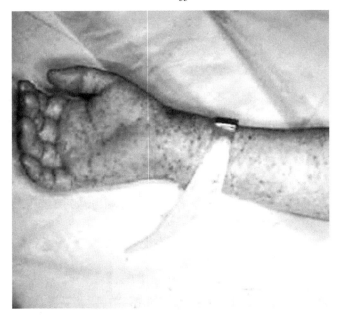

Petechial rash of RMSF
Source: http://en.wikipedia.org/wiki/File:Rocky_mount-
ian_spotted_fever.jpg. Accessed March 2013

Special pediatric skin considerations:

When assessing newborns with possible TBIs, the normal neonatal condition is useful to know. Newborn skin is unique: soft and smooth. The neonate can be flushed red for the first several hours, after which the child should be pink. A slight blueness of the hands and feet may be normal for 24 hours. The bluish color dissipates in the hands before the feet. If the color does not resolve, start looking for other reasons. If the baby is cold, the skin may look mottled or dappled (a reticular pattern) especially in premature infants and those with Down syndrome. If the newborn is generally pale this should have been reflected in the APGAR scores. If the pallor remains, the problem can be low oxygen and the child might have a slower heart rate. In anemia, the HR will be rapid. Black newborns are often not very black except in the scrotal area and sometimes at the base of the fingernails. (This fact seems to cause considerable angst on the *Jerry Springer Show*.)

Newborns may have Mongolian spots, which are blue-black areas especially over the butt and lower back. These spots are more frequent in black, Asian, or Native American children. They gradually fade and usually disappear.

Most newborns are covered with fine hair, like bird down, called lanugo, especially on the shoulders and upper back. This fuzz can be variable in density and distribution and may be considerable in premature babies. Head hair in newborns is not an indicator of overall health.

At birth the skin can be flaking and even whole areas of skin can shed in large sheets. Babies from vaginal births often have edema because of the pressure and the fluid can be present in the face, limbs, or pubic area. The excess fluid begins to dissipate soon after birth. Newborns may have edema and bruising at the back of the head, or swelling over the cranial bones, which does not extend across a suture.

PEARL: If you are not an expert in taking care of very small children but you are approached to assess for a congenital TBI, consider asking a colleague to share the patient.

Common skin conditions in newborns:

*   Milia are white pinpoint-sized areas on the face caused by sebum plugging sebaceous glands. These may be present at birth or appear within the first weeks. They spontaneously resolve.

*   Milia rubra, or red milia, can be due to the obstruction of sweat glands and may cause reddened milia or tiny blisters on a red base.

*   Red nevi or hemangiomas are small, round, bright red, bumps over the back of the head, on eyelids, and elsewhere that may be enlarged capillary beds. Bartonella has been associated with hemangiomas.

*   Hydration status in infants can be assessed by examining the skin. Pinch (without pain) a small amount of skin and lift it gently away from the body. In normally hydrated kids, this skin will immediately snap back to the level of the other skin. If the child is dehydrated, the skin will tent upward and the slower it rebounds, the drier the child.

*   Jaundice is common in neonates. About half of newborns will have a mild physiologic yellowing that appears after about 48 hours and often disappears in the first week but may persist longer. Jaundice that appears earlier could suggest hemolysis. Yellowing that lasts beyond two weeks could be an obstruction. At any time during the infant period jaundice could mean infection so be vigilant.

Skin conditions in older patients:

*   Older kids who appear yellowish may be eating a disproportionate amount of yellow and orange foods. This condition can be mistaken for jaundice but here the yellowing is primarily in the palms, soles, and around the nose. In assessing a yellow child who is suspected of having a TBI, consider both an underlying disease and the potential effects of treatment drugs on the liver.

- People with high histamine levels may present with bright red ears called **Winter's ear**, although some believe the mechanism could be blood stasis. Maybe both?

- **Eczema**: Found in all age groups, eczema is a cutaneous inflammation that can include redness, papules, vesicles, pustules, scales, crusts, or scabs. Eczema can be wet or dry in presentation and can itch and burn. Secondary infection can cause pus formation and oozing. The etiology has not been determined but eczema can be aggravated by irritants, allergens, infections, extreme temperatures, and stress. Persons with dry, thin skin are more susceptible.

- **Psoriasis:** A chronic skin disease with red papules that coalesce to form plaques with distinct borders. Progression leads to silver-white scales and new lesions form at sites of irritation or trauma. Psoriasis can be found at any location but can frequently be seen on the scalp, knees, elbows, belly button, and genitals. The clinical course varies and there can be periods of remission but no one knows why the symptoms come and go when they do. In about 5% of cases there is an arthritis with joint involvement occurring after the skin eruption. Symptoms may be due to an accelerated cell cycle with psoriatic cells turning over much faster than normal. There seems to be a genetic component but infection, some medications, climate, and hormones may play a role. Treatment includes softening and removing scales. Steroids are often used as a primary treatment and you must be careful that treatments ordered by other HCPs do not work against your goals. People with this problem may need considerable support around self-image.

PEARL: What's the difference between eczema and psoriasis? Both are chronic skin conditions that cause red, scaly lesions and tend to involve some of the same body parts like the scalp. Psoriasis is often thicker than eczema and is usually dry. Eczema tends to be more moist and oozing. Psoriasis involves the back of the elbows and front of the knees (the extensor surfaces), while eczema hits the back of the knees and the front of the elbows (flexor surfaces).

Section 17-C

Nails, Hair, Head, and Pertinent Differential

It's not that I'm so smart, it's just that I stay with a problem longer.
Albert Einstein

I.   NAILS

I am unaware of specific TBI issues, but nails can provide clues to overall health. Lyme is thought to impact normal endocrine function and thyroid problems can cause brittle nails. Look for:

Signs of infection: pus, swelling, redness, tenderness

Signs of biting, breaking

Signs of fungus (thickening, crumbling, weakening, yellowing)

Signs of poor circulation in surrounding tissue

Common nail findings:

Paronychia is an inflammation, often with infection, of the tissue near the nail. The soft tissue becomes red, swollen, tender, pus-filled, and warm. Paronychia are common in kids.

Clubbing: The angle between the nail and base flattens and then the nail base becomes swollen with an increased angle. Clubbing is usually associated with long-term hypoxia but is also seen in IBD and endocarditis. Endocarditis can be seen in cardiac involvement in Lyme.

Spoon nails are present when the nails bow up like little spoons and can be associated with iron deficiency anemia.

Nail lines are transverse depressions in the nail often associated with severe illness. Linear streaks can be non-specific. White transverse lines can be associated with a history of nail bed trauma. Transverse lines from side to side suggest severe, acute illness with fever. When horizontal lines, sometimes called Beau's lines, are noted, ask what happened to the patient in the previous 3 months. These lines are linked to significant physical or metabolic trauma including stress.

Pitting can be seen in psoriasis.

Black spots can mean trauma.

Separation of the nail from the bed is usually traumatic but can also indicate thyroid dysfunction.

White nails suggest liver problems, CHF, DM, thyroid problems, or malnutrition. Nails that are white at the bed and brown at the tip can mean kidney issues.

Pale nail beds: Anemia such as that seen with babesiosis

II.   HAIR

Lyme has been associated with thinning and broken hair. Whether this is due to the direct action of the spirochetes, or indirectly through compromise of the endocrine system, is speculative. Lyme could impact thyroid function causing unhealthy hair.

Look for:

Breakage

Thinning can suggest thyroid problems

Thickening can indicate endocrine problems

Don't miss nits

Skin lesions under the hair that may be easy to miss

Scalp lesions:
Dandruff, suggesting fungus

Eczema

Scalp sensitivity

Sores

There may be an increased incidence of scalp complaints associated with Lyme. In TBIs look for scalp sensitivity and rashes. Some patients with Lyme can barely stand to have their scalps touched.

III.   HEAD

In general look for:

Skull symmetry

Forehead size and shape

Signs of previous injury such as scars or broken nose

Circumference (if age appropriate)

Facial asymmetry

Bell's palsy is paralysis of one side of the face, which can be found in Lyme. A partial paralysis might tempt you to dismiss this clear sign of LD. The presence of Bell's palsy, especially with a history of tick bite, is strongly suggestive of Lyme. Bell's palsy is unilateral facial paralysis, usually of sudden onset. Frequently, the patient cannot control salivation or lacrimation and in severe cases cannot close the eye on the affected side. Facial expression is distorted probably due to inflammation and swelling of the 7th CN. Manifestation in Lyme suggests that spirochetes have somehow impacted this facial nerve. Bell's palsy then becomes a clinical sign that we can readily document. It's hard for people to fake unilateral paralysis. The mechanism by which Bb cause the paralysis can be from direct physical interference, intracellular disruption of neurons, or the biochemical onslaught that accompanies the inflammation and the toxic cytokines that are released. Unfortunately, if a patient comes to the ER and the only finding is Bell's palsy, Lyme is rarely considered, even in endemic areas. Most often the cause is said to be idiopathic. While incidence rates vary, this type of paralysis occurs in about 10% of Lyme patients and may be more common than the infamous EM rash in some populations. Sometimes painful, recovery is variable and if the eye cannot close it will need to be patched with a moisturizing ointment. Be careful, in the non-Lyme world Bell's palsy is commonly treated with steroids. If the underlying cause is Bb, these patients could get worse.

PEARL: Not all facial paralysis is Lyme. If the palsy is partial or subtle, determine if the asymmetry was present prior to the tick bite, if possible. Examining a photo taken before the tick bite might be useful!. Of course, most patients don't recall the tick bite so we again have a Catch-22 situation.

Age-specific issues:

The soft spot in infants is the area where the bones of the skull are separated by sutures (non-bone tissue). The places where these sutures come together are called fontanelles (anterior fontanelle and posterior fontanelle). The sutures feel like ridges while the soft spots themselves are slight depressions. The anterior fontanelle is about 2 to 3 inches at birth and closes between 4 and 24 months, with the majority closing between 7 and 18 months. The posterior fontanelle is usually less than an inch at birth and closes by about 2 months.

A bulging or full anterior fontanelle may simply be due to crying, vomiting, or coughing but may also be a sign of increased intracranial pressure. Dilated scalp veins suggest long-standing increased pressure. While decreased ICP will cause a sunken fontanelle, the cause is more likely dehydration. A persistently tense or bulging fontanelle suggests problems and in terms of assessing for TBI, consider infections in the CNS as the possible cause.

Chapter 17-D

Eyes and Pertinent Differential

When in doubt, make a Western.
John Ford

EYES

Visual problems are very common in TBIs, especially Lyme, bartonellosis, and tularemia. Examine eyes carefully. Bb can cause inflammatory changes and direct damage all along the visual pathway including the optic nerve and retinal tissue. The processing of visual information by the ophthalmic nerves can be impacted. This section is not designed to make you into an ophthalmologist. Rather, you should know enough to recognize if there is a problem and to consult when necessary. Abnormalities thought to be associated with TBIs that are beyond your expertise will need a referral. Consider an ophthalmologist, rather than other eye professional since the patient could need medical intervention. Choose a physician who has some understanding of TBIs. As always, do not lose your patient. You are still in charge of managing the TBI. Select someone who will work with you.

Eye conditions that have been associated with Lyme disease include blurred vision, hypersensitivity to light, photophobia, floaters, flashes, conjunctivitis, astigmatism, eye pain, dry eyes, papilledema, blind spots, night blindness, peripheral shadows, iritis, anterior uveitis, optic neuritis, eyelid droop, impaired color vision, alteration of colors, double vision, swelling around eyes, eyelid twitching or fasciculations, dark circles under the eyes, change in visual fields, flashing lights, peripheral waves, phantom images at the edge of the visual field, episcleritis, trouble reading because letters run together, general discomfort in eyes, gritty feel, extraocular palsies, problems with lacrimation in Bell's palsy, ptosis, cataracts in gestational Lyme, Lyme eye, eye fatigue, tearing blepharitis, keratitis, and progressive decrease in visual acuity. If the Borrelia impact the optic nerve, blindness can result. Not all of these are a direct result of damage to the visual apparatus, but all might be noted during an eye exam.

PEARL: Lyme eye is punctated erythema on the conjunctiva.

ASSESS:

1. Eye contact and appearance:

The patient should look the examiner in the eye for intermittent periods. Eyes should move in tandem. The eyes may seem to protrude in hyperthyroidism.

2. Eyebrows:

Movement

Symmetry

Hair health

3. Lids:

What is the relationship between the lid and the eye? Bulging or retracted lids can suggest thyroid problems.

Swelling?

Color?

Crust?

Trouble closing lid?

Twitching or fasciculations?

Pale mucosa inside the lower lid can mean anemia.

PEARL: Lid lag and poor convergence can be seen in hyperthyroidism. Lid lag is present when the upper lid lags behind the upper edge of the iris as the eye moves downward. So when the gaze shifts from the upper to the lower field of vision, the lid should follow without lagging behind. Normally, the lid slightly overlaps the iris throughout this movement.

4. Tear apparatus:

If difficulty with the lacrimal apparatus is suspected, raise the upper outer lid and ask the patient to look away and down. If there is inflammation, you should see a swollen gland between the eye and the lid.

Bell's palsy is noted in perhaps 10% of Lyme patients. Lacrimation can be affected. If the eye cannot close it will need to be patched with a moisturizing ointment. Be careful, Bell's palsy is commonly treated with steroids. If the underlying cause is Bb, these patients could get worse.

5. Lashes:

Scarce or patches of loss?

Crust could mean allergies or infection.

6. **Conjunctiva:** The visible membrane covering the sclera
    Is the Conjunctiva injected?

A pterygium is a bunching of the conjunctiva visible over the sclera. Usually unsightly, but benign.

Lyme eye is conjunctival punctated erythema.

7. **Sclera:** The white part of the eye

Broken vessels can mean trauma or pressure.

Color: Yellow or brown color can mean liver problems especially with the metabolism of BR. Yellow discoloration usually first appears in the scleras, then mucous membranes, and then general skin locations. Orange coloring can mean too much Vitamin A from orange foods.

8. **Cornea:** The transparent front cover of the eye

The cornea is often the site of scratches. While these heal quickly, they are often uncomfortable and may cause considerable tearing and blinking. They are usually treated with a patch and moisturizing ointment. Under the cornea, you see the iris or colored part of the eye with the pupil in the middle.

> *PEARL: Uveitis and iritis are common in Lyme. The iris is the colored part of the eye. Inflammation of the iris, or iritis, is also called anterior uveitis. The uvea is the middle layer of the eye that provides blood to the retina. Inflammation of these areas can be an autoimmune response and can be associated with RA or ankylosing spondylitis. Symptoms often appear after an acute infection. Distinguishing between the two may be tricky since both present with irritation, swelling, pain, redness, photophobia, blurred or cloudy vision, and haziness. There may be white floaters in the anterior chamber consistent with white blood cells in the area. Uveitis may also display dark floaters as you look at the fundus.*

9. **Cataracts:**

A cataract is the clouding of the lens which can obscure vision. These present as opacities in the lens behind the cornea. Cataracts have been noted in congenital Lyme cases.

10. **Astigmatism:**

Astigmatism is the inability of the eye to focus incoming light on one focal point in the retina. Usually in astigmatism, the cornea has an irregular curve so that the image spreads out over the retina, resulting in a blurred view. This is a problem that even little kids get and can occur from infancy on with the I&P increasing throughout childhood. About 3 in 10 kids between the ages of 5 and 17 have astigmatism.

Caretakers usually first notice squinting. Older kids may complain of blurred vision at all distances. They may see one part of a picture more clearly than another. Mild astigmatism may go unnoticed but more significant cases can cause eye discomfort, headaches, and fatigue. While astigmatism is not inherited, the tendency to develop astigmatism is. Therefore trauma, scarring, and a number of pathologic conditions such as DM can influence the occurrence of astigmatism. While epidemiologic data is not available, astigmatism may be more common in Lyme. Seemingly, Bb LOVES collagen and much of the cornea is made of collagen.

Astigmatism is not the same as diminished visual acuity although they can be concurrent. Having 20/20 vision on the wall chart does not rule out astigmatism. There are a number of ways to test for astigmatism including an astigmatic dial where a series of lines radiate out from a central point. If the patient sees some of the lines more clearly than others or the entire image is blurred, consider astigmatism. Progressively worse astigmatism over time may mean that something is continuing to affect the cornea or lens of the eye. Treatment is usually corrective lenses or weighted contacts called toric lenses. Surgery may be useful in some cases. Ben Franklin made the first spectacles to correct for astigmatism in 1784.

11. **Extraocular eye movement:** Abnormalities can indicate CN damage or muscle weakness.

We need 6 muscles and both CNs 3 and 4 to control eye movements. This means we have to check for full and symmetrical movements up, down, and to the right and left. To accomplish this, ask the patient to look up and down and from side to side or have the patient follow your finger. If one of the muscles is impaired, the eyes will not work together in a normal conjugate manner. Normal eyes will move in tandem. Ask the patient to follow the test object as you move it to the bridge of her nose. This is called tracking movements. If the eyes do not work symmetrically together, there is abnormal tracking. Asymmetry suggests a congenital deficit or nerve or muscle dysfunction. If a child is too young to follow directions use a toy to attract the gaze in the various directions.

In young children, check for *strabismus*. Since so many neurological problems are associated with TBIs and since strabismus is common in non-infected kids, you will need to keep on top of any abnormality. Strabismus occurs when the two eyes cannot focus on the same object at the same time. Strabismus is caused either from a problem with the EOMs or from neurologic or ocular disease.

If the eye crosses constantly, the patient should be assessed as soon as possible after it is discovered. If the problem is intermittent, evaluation should take place at least within a few months of notice. If crossing seems to be occurring more rather than less often, assess ASAP. Never ignore deviating eyes because you think the child will outgrow it. *Amblyopia* (reduced vision) can occur in association with strabismus.

There are a number of ways to check to see if a child's eye is crossing. The child should be asked to fix on a light held in the middle of the examiner's forehead. Then as the HCP covers and uncovers one of the child's eyes, he can detect if that eye shifts when it tries to refocus on the light. The eye will either turn in or out to refix if strabismus is present. To prevent permanent vision loss, the strabismus generally needs to be addressed before age 4.

Nystagmus is the rhythmic fine pulsing of the eyes. They appear to oscillate or beat. A few beats is normal but beyond that, nystagmus is abnormal. Nystagmus is an involuntary, constant, rhythmic movement of the eye and can be present in any direction. Nystagmus is seen in a variety of neurologic conditions.

Nystagmus is easiest to assess if the patient is looking far left or right. Nystagmus can be congenital and may present as a mild condition inapparent to the patient. In contrast, the pulsations can be so great that it is hard to understand how the patient can focus to see at all. Nystagmus can be from inner ear problems or any number of neurologic diseases. If significant nystagmus presents when not previously observed, investigate.

12. **Fields of vision:** Visual fields are the areas in space where the fixed eye can see.

To assess visual fields, have the patient cover one eye without pressure. You should be directly in front of the patient. Bring your finger or other small test object into the visual field and ask the patient when he can see it. A normal person when staring ahead can see objects at almost 90 degrees to the side except for the temporal fields. In the temporal locations the test object (finger) must be placed far behind the expected visual field. Do this testing slowly enough so that the patient has time to see the object. Repeat with the other eye.

Visual fields can be done in fairly young kids with their eyes initially looking in front of their face. Bring a finger or small object from behind, below, and above. If the child turns the eyes in the direction of the invading object she can likely see it.

PEARL: Quinine and derivatives such as chloroquine and hydroxychloroquine can cause retinal and visual field changes.

13. **Visual acuity:**

Visual acuity is the sharpness or clearness of vision. Have the patient read or identify objects with each eye individually. If significant loss of acuity is suspected ask the patient how many fingers you are holding up.

If appropriate, use eye charts specifically designed for little kids who might not yet know letters. Older kids can be tested with the standard eye chart. This tests their ability to read letters of various sizes at a specified distance from the chart. The result is given as a ratio such as 20/20 meaning that the patient has the ability to see from a distance of 20 feet what a normal eye would see at 20 feet. If the result is 20/200 then the person has the ability to see at 20 feet what the normal eye would see at 200 feet.

Children are more often nearsighted than farsighted. Nearsighted means they can clearly see only those objects close to the eye. Farsighted means they can see things far away but not up close. Having good visual acuity does not rule out astigmatism.

14. **Pupillary reflexes:**

Light directed into the retina causes pupillary constriction of that eye (direct light reflex) and of the other eye (consensual light reflex) and involves the 3rd CN.

PEARL: Many TBI patients have extreme sensitivity to light. Many must stay in a darkened room during the day because the discomfort from even minimal light is too great.

A red glow in the pupil is called the red reflex. No red reflex suggests an opaque lens such as that seen with cataracts. To assess: Set the ophthalmoscope on zero diopters and aim for the pupil from about a foot away. In normal people, a red color will reflect back. Many significant eye problems can cause an abnormal red reflex. If you are not proficient at eliciting the reflex, recheck or refer before you panic.

Normal pupillary reflexes, along with adequate accommodation, are often documented with the acronym PERLA meaning pupils equally reactive to light and accommodation.

PEARL: Anisocoria is inequity of the pupils. Ask if the individual has always had unequal pupils. Like Lady Gaga they might just be born that way. If the disparity is new onset, look for a cause.

15. **Accommodation:**

Eyes adjust so that clear vision is maintained when the gaze is shifted from far to near. By changing the curve of the lens, the eye can correct for varying distances so that it can focus an image onto the retina. The eyes are accommodating adequately if clear vision is retained when the stare moves from distant to close-up. Ask the patient to look in the distance and then at your finger about 2 to 4 inches from the bridge of his nose. The pupils should constrict and the eyes should converge (come toward the same point).

PEARL: Poor accommodation is associated with Lyme. Have the person follow a finger or pen with her eyes. Ask, "Do you see one or two?"

16. Fundal examination:

The fundus is the back of the eye that you can see looking through the pupil with an ophthalmoscope. Once you focus, follow the vessels centrally to the disc which is a yellowish oval or round area. The arterioles are red and the veins are darker. If you can't find the disc, start over, following a vessel centrally until you locate it.

The optic disc (disk) is the head of the optic nerve (CN 2) where the nerve cell axons exit the eye to form the optic nerve. More than a million neurons converge there to form the nerve. In the disc there are no light sensitive tissues (rods or cones) so the actual disc is blind.

There is a central depression in the disc called the optic cup, which should reflect a little brighter than the disc. The color of the disc should be a yellowish-orange to pink. A pale disc indicates disease. Look at the size of the cup in relation to the entire disc. Look for a clear demarcation of the disc edge, although the nasal side can be slightly blurred. There may be some normal rings or crescents near the disc. Look for swelling of the disc which can indicate elevated ICP, also called papilledema, which is a common finding in CNS inflammation. Look for notching or other damage, since the disc should be a smooth, roundish, little plate. The optic disc is paler in infants and the retinal vessels are not as well developed as in older individuals. If you are looking for papilledema as an indicator of increased ICP, you will not likely find it in infants. Until the child is past age two, the sutures will still separate enough to prevent papilledema.

PEARL: Know enough to recognize if there might be a problem so you can consult when appropriate.

In the remainder of the fundus, look at the blood vessels. Arterioles and veins should cross clearly. Look for hemorrhages, exudates, patches, or debris. Examine the listed areas carefully.

a. **Retina**: The retina is the inner part of the eye that contains the rods and cones needed to see. Here the light waves come into focus. Normally, the retina is red but it will be pale in anemia.

b. **Macula:** This yellow spot in the center of the retina is close to the optic nerve. To examine the macula, have the patient look directly into the light or direct the light laterally. You should see a tiny bright reflection from the fovea which identifies the broader-based macula area.

c. **Fovea:** The pit in the center of the macula is where the retina thins to a layer of tightly packed cones. The fovea is the area of the most acute vision.

Age-specific issues:

Because a neonate closes his lids so tightly, it is almost impossible to examine a newborn's eyes. During the first few days of life, the baby may have searching nystagmus. The doll's eye phenomenon will show up if there is any problem with some of the EOMs. Here the child will not move his eyes when his head is turned and the eyes will remain in the starting position. Normally when the head is rotated quickly from one side to the other the eyes will move TOGETHER to the opposite side. If this doesn't happen there may be brainstem or oculomotor damage.

In slightly older kids, you can see EOM, irises, pupils, and sclera by holding the baby up with your arms extended and rotating the baby. When rotated, he will turn his eyes in the direction he is being turned. When the turning stops the baby will look back in the opposite direction. He may have a few beats of nystagmus in the first few days of life but this should be gone within several days. If nystagmus persists, consider that vision might be impaired.

After birth, conjugate eye movements develop rapidly. However, neonates cannot reliably follow an object for several weeks. There may be small amounts of bleeding in the sclera, retina, or conjunctiva of a newborn due to the pressures encountered in the birth canal. If retinal bleeding is substantial, consider that there is a problem with oxygen exchange or clotting.

A neonate should blink and flex his head back when faced with a bright light. If he does not, he might not be seeing the light. The pupils may not respond equally initially but if this inequality persists, consider that there may be other problems with the eyes or nervous system.

Neonates may have a chemical conjunctivitis from the antibiotic drops placed in their eyes immediately after birth, with swelling and inflammation of the conjunctiva and lids and possible discharge. (Makes for lovely family photos.)

Babies with Down syndrome will have enlarged epicanthal folds and a possible upward slant of the eyes. They may also have white specks scattered linearly in the iris.

The only assessment of vision that can be done reliably in newborns is the checking of reflexes. If pupils constrict in response to light individually and consensually, then there is likely some degree of vision. The child should also blink when a light or object is moved rapidly toward the eyes.

Carefully assess the eyes in kids with suspected TBIs. In some cases once a problem progresses, the damage is irreversible. Careful examination often finds abnormalities. Some problems are obvious and some very subtle. No HCP is an island. If you suspect that a vision problem is due to TBI, consider joining forces with an eye specialist to work together in assessing the etiology and the best corrective actions.

PEARL: Optic discs are paler in infants and the retinal vessels are not as well developed as in older individuals.

A first fundal exam can usually be done at around 4 months, but this will depend on the child. If you have reason to suspect that a fundal exam is needed earlier, or you cannot get a good exam when one is indicated, refer.

Ears and Pertinent Differential

The person with the new idea is a crank until that idea succeeds.

Mark Twain

EARS

- <u>Outer or External Ear and the External Auditory Canal</u>

The outer ear is the part of the ear composed of the auricle and ear canal and separated from the middle ear by the tympanic membrane. Look at the color, shape, and size of the outer ear. Bright red ears can indicate abnormally high histamine levels. Look for cysts and psoriasis and other skin lesions. In the ear canal, observe the degree of wax and if the cerumen is impacted, a condition that can significantly decrease hearing. With congenital Lyme, the pinna can be altered, deformed, or absent.

Discharge from the canal can indicate an external otitis which is an infection of the outer ear. This condition also presents with tenderness to pressure in both the front and back of the ear. Also called swimmer's ear, these puppies can really hurt. Often the canal is so swollen it's hard to get the medicine drops inside. Sometimes there is unilateral cervical lymphadenopathy.

PEARL: Moving the external ear is painful in acute otitis externa but usually not in otitis media.

PEARL: A nodule in the canal can be an osteoma which is a nonmalignant overgrowth of tissue. This growth can obscure the drum.

PEARL: Red, hot ears are commonly observed in Lyme.

PEARL: Congenital Lyme can have an alteration of the pinna which can be absent or deformed.

- <u>Middle Ear</u>

The middle ear begins with the tympanic membrane and includes the three tiny bones or ossicles (malleus, incus, and stapes) that transmit the vibrations from the drum to the inner ear.

The middle ear has three areas where it can potentially communicate with other locations: 1) The TM or ear drum which, except when perforated, is closed, 2) The mastoid cells and bone posteriorly which is also usually closed, and 3) The eustachian tube which remains open unless occluded by fluids or swelling. The eustachian tube forms an open channel between the middle ear and the nasopharynx. Blowing the nose too hard or suppressing a sneeze can force fluids from the tube up into the middle ear. With the fluid can come any pathogens that were milling about as well.

PEARL: The Valsalva maneuver can be used to attempt to "clear" the ears and the eustachian tubes, especially when changing altitude abruptly like during air travel. The person holds the nose and mouth shut and exhales or swallows. This should be done gently.

Inspect the entire drum. Examine the cone of light. Look for redness, dullness, bulging, fluid lines, air bubbles, holes, and scars. A normal drum is pearl grey and with a good cone of light you can see the ends of the bones of the inner ear. If pathology progresses, the landmarks become obscured and, if the problem is infectious, the drum will become red, even scarlet.

One of the banes of early childhood is otitis media, also called middle ear infection, OM, or earache. This condition has almost as much controversy as Lyme disease with arguments that have lasted decades over how to diagnose, best treatment plans, high dose versus low dose antibiotics, ten days or a month, to prophylax or not, broad spectrum or targeted, and whether there is both an acute and chronic form. We have learned from otitis media that many kids do well while on antibiotics but as soon as they come off the medicine, the symptoms return.

I have kept tabs on this area because I recently worked on antibiotics to treat OM. Over the years I have read many opinions that OM needs no treatment at all and that the condition will resolve in about a week. Interesting that I never see these same authors touting this claim after their child has her first ear infection. While many will improve in about a week, it is a week of suffering, screaming through the night, possible broken ear drums, and agony for both parent and child. What purpose does this torture serve? Oh, I forget that antibiotic resistance might develop. One of the reasons that there is so much resistance today from the most common pathogens causing OM is because we listened to the "experts" in the first place.

For years they said low dose amoxicillin for ten days would do the trick. We ordered the low dose amoxicillin. When that didn't work, the parents came in begging for something stronger. They would actually say, "The pink stuff doesn't work for Bootsy. She needs the bigger guns." We ordered the bigger guns. When that didn't work, we went on to the next gorillacillin until Bootsy felt better and the exhausted family finally got a night's sleep. The next time Bootsy got an ear infection we started with gorillacillin.

Now we learn that the problem with the amoxicillin was not that it didn't work, but that we were not giving it in high enough doses for a long enough time. Does this sound familiar to anyone?

I find it cruel to not treat ear infections in kids. In my experience, symptoms seem to resolve much faster than they do in kids who are not treated. I think I may have told you my story about the Fort Dix urologist who used to treat the trainees with kidney stones with Tylenol until he had his first kidney stone. He came into the ER whimpering for me to give him morphine. Treat the patient as you would want to be treated.

PEARL: The child with Bb infection may have more frequent earaches. Whether this increased incidence is due to impairment of the immune system or more direct damage to the middle ear is speculative. Probably a combination of factors are to blame.

On exam, acute otitis media shows a red or dull drum which may be bulging into the canal with fluid. Sometimes there will be a discernible fluid line. They used to insist that we measure pneumatic pressure with a little bulb and a puff of air. If the drum moved, then the person could not possibly have acute OM since he could still equalize pressure on either side of the drum. Treat the person not the test results, especially since none of us knew how to do the test properly anyway.

Do not panic if the external canal is filled with smelly pus. The drum may have broken. This is not the ideal situation but it is also not the end of the world. The patient probably feels better since the pressure behind the drum is gone. Just be careful that you do not get water from the bath or shower in that ear and that you use ear drops that should not move beyond the perforation. Wait until the perforation heals to immerse the head so we don't have water from the swimming pool communicating with the 8th cranial nerve.

Occasionally you will see an actual hole in the drum from where past perforations never completely healed or scarring from where there was healing. Scarring is fibrous tissue that is not as flexible as normal tissue, so it cannot vibrate and transmit sound as well. Too much scarring and there will be a reduction in auditory acuity. We learned that from the generation now in their 80s and 90s. While some of their hearing loss may be from exposure to loud noises, a great deal may also be due to the considerable amount of scarring after years of

untreated ear infections. Hearing loss can remain for several months after an episode of acute otitis.

- Inner Ear

The inner ear consists of the cochlea, shaped like a snail shell, that contains the organ of Corti, which is the actual organ for hearing. Also, in the inner ear are the vestibular organs and semicircular canals, which have receptors for equilibrium and sense of position. Stimulation moves to the acoustic or 8th CN that has both a hearing branch and a vestibular branch. TBIs can have many ramifications on both hearing and balance including hypersensitivity to sound, decreased auditory acuity, tinnitus, and stability problems. Carefully evaluate balance and equilibrium, as well as a hearing.

HEARING

The usual pathway to hearing is through sound waves moving through the air-filled external ear, vibrating the TM and ossicles, stimulating the organ of Corti in the cochlea, and sending the stimulus to the cochlear branch of the acoustic or 8th CN. Another pathway by which sound can be transmitted, if the usual pathway is impaired, is through bone to the inner ear and is called bone conduction. This pathway can be useful in assessing auditory acuity. Air conduction is normally more sensitive than bone conduction.

Diminished hearing can be due to a number of reasons: impacted cerumen, fluid behind the drum, impairment of any of the structural components, infections, toxins including some medications, autoimmunity, damage from pathogens, and neurologic compromise. Auditory processing may actually be the main problem. The patient can hear the sound but the brain can't understand the meaning. The person may always be asking others to repeat what they say and even then may misconstrue the meaning.

PEARL: TBI patients often complain about extreme sensitivity to sound. Some of these patients are intolerant of even minimal noise.

Acuity can be grossly assessed in several ways. You can ask the patient to repeat words or phrases or answer questions spoken while the HCP is facing away. Another possible assessment is to occlude one ear. From about two feet away, where the patient cannot read your lips, whisper 2 digit numbers and see if the patient can repeat them. Can the patient hear an audible watch ticking?

In infants, gross hearing can be assessed by checking to see if the eyes blink in response to a sharp, sudden sound. Ensure that the blinking is not because air from a clap or snap caused the child to blink. Between 3 and 4 months of age the eyes and head may turn to the sound.

A more accurate measure can be done with a properly calibrated audiometer and a trained technician. These results can be compared from visit to visit.

If hearing loss is present then try to distinguish between sensorineural deafness and conduction deafness using tuning forks:

> Lateralization Weber test: Place a lightly vibrating tuning fork firmly on the patient's head or forehead and ask where he hears the sound. Does he hear the vibration on one or both sides? This can suggest a problem on one side compared to the other. A normal test is heard equally on both sides or in the midline. If the patient has unilateral hearing deficit due to a conduction problem, the sound will be louder in the bad ear. If the deficit is neurosensory then the sound is louder in the good ear.

> Compare bone and air conduction using the Rinne test. Place the vibrating tuning fork on the mastoid process behind the ear until the patient can no longer hear it. Then quickly place the still vibrating fork NEAR the ear canal on the same side. Can the patient still hear it? Usually the patient can hear it longer through air than through bone.

PEARL: As a medical student on a pediatric rotation at Walter Reed, I was scheduled to cover a well baby clinic with a student from the Air Force. I can't remember if his first or last name was Brooks. Instead of initiating the vibration of the tuning fork by striking it on the heel of his hand, he smacked the baby directly in the middle of the forehead. Well, the vibration started all right. The child was stunned. I will never forget the look on the face of the attending pediatrician. The mother screamed. While some believe that all people are redeemable, I think Brooks might be the exception to that rule. That kind of obtuseness is incurable. I wonder where Brooks is practicing now or if he is on any committees that issue practice guidelines.

Helen Keller said that hearing loss was worse than blindness and muteness. Hearing deficit can be quite frustrating for the caretaker, as well. A surprising number of people with hearing deficit do not think they have a problem. They complain that the rest of the world mumbles or that restaurants have too much background noise. Denial has been shown to be a big issue with some of the hearing impaired. Many teens also don't see the harm in loud music or machines. Nothing bad will ever happen to them. Care must be taken to avoid ototoxic drugs, since these can cause the most damage in those who already have an underlying deficit.

PEARL: Quinine and derivatives such as chloroquine and hydroxychloroquine can cause hearing changes.

TINNITUS

Tinnitus has been reported in many cases of Lyme. Tinnitus is the sensation of ringing or buzzing in the ear. Feel very sorry for people with tinnitus. Tinnitus not only impacts the ability to hear, it's annoying and its constant presence can lead to anxiety, depression, and suicide. Hearing aids generally are of no help. Nonetheless, there are many unscrupulous vendors trying to sell ineffective treatments. There are some legitimate classes in university settings and established hearing centers that help teach patients to live with their tinnitus. Counseling may be helpful. Never dismiss tinnitus as just a non-fatal inconvenience. If the underlying cause is a TBI, you can do the victim no greater good than to appropriately manage that condition.

BALANCE

Balance is the ability to maintain the center of gravity over the base of support. Balance can be impacted by a number of physical parameters including muscle strength, coordination, and damage to the vestibular mechanism in the inner ear or to CN 8. A patient with nystagmus should have balance checked very carefully. Imbalance is not the same as dizziness. The person with Lyme may experience additional motion sickness. Check balance very conscientiously since this capacity can be greatly impacted by Lyme and other TBIs. With a young kid, check balance by putting her head forward, then back, and next tilting left and right. Observe her ability to remain stable and not tip. For children old enough to walk, have them stand on one foot, then walk with one foot in front of the other. After that ask them to stand with eyes closed and assess the degree of wobble. With eyes still closed, see how well they do on each foot alone. A positive Romberg test occurs when the person can keep her balance when the eyes are open and the feet are close together, but sways and falls when the eyes are closed. With each of these tasks, there will be slight instability even in healthy people. Patients with impairment will have considerable difficulty.

PEARL: When a patient presents with balance problems, an unsteady gait, or a history of streptomycin use, test vestibular function with a cold water test. Flush water at about 65°F into the external auditory canal. This should produce nystagmus within half a minute in a normal person. No nystagmus could mean drug toxicity, meningitis, tumor, or labyrinthitis.

Section 17-F

Nose, Sinuses, Mouth, Tongue, TMJs, Teeth, and Pertinent Differential

It's illegal to mispronounce Arkansas in Arkansas.

I. NOSE/SINUSES

Examine:

Nares: Nostrils should be patent without crust.

Mucosa: Signs of scabs could mean dryness or picking. Picking is the chief cause of nose bleeds in kids (and adults. I'm watching you.)

Discharge: Is it clear, suggesting allergies or virus? Is it purulent, suggesting bacterial infection or foreign body? A nose "stuffed" with discharge can be annoying and impede the senses of smell and taste.

Septum: Holes in the septum suggest inhaled drugs such as cocaine. Deviation can be congenital or due to trauma. Assess whether deviation is impacting air flow.

Turbinates: Should be pink and plump without occluding the passageway. You may see polyps especially in individuals with a history of allergic rhinitis.

Sinuses: Apply gentle pressure over the maxillary and frontal sinuses. Infection will usually elicit tenderness. Frontal sinuses can be percussed. Dullness suggests these sinuses are full of fluid, which may mean sinusitis. If you suspect infected sinuses, attempt to transilluminate the frontal or maxillary sinuses by shining the light through the sinus space in a fairly dark room. For transillumination of the frontal sinuses, place the light above the eye against the supraorbital ridge. For maxillary sinuses, place the light inside the mouth with the tip against the hard palate, and look for the light to shine through to the opposite side. If there is no transillumination, then the sinus may be filled with fluid (infected?) rather than air. An infected sinus is usually painful to firm pressure.

Age-specific issues:

Newborns breathe though their noses and blockage of the nose could impede respiration. Keep that nose open. A blue bulb aspirator can be used for this purpose.

Nasal speech can mean large adenoids occluding the back of the throat.

PEARL: In June, 2011, scientists announced a startling finding: Whining is the most annoying sound on earth, as though every parent didn't already know that. This was found to be true in all examined cultures everywhere. That same week, other researchers discovered a previously uncontacted tribe in the Amazon. I am sure that they feel the same way about whining as the rest of us. Add a nasal component to the whining and I believe you will have complete solidarity among parents all over the world.

II. MOUTH

The mouth is the opening on the face between the cheeks, bordered by the lips, containing the tongue, teeth, and salivary glands. The mouth is the aperture into the throat and is partially divided from it by lymph tissues called tonsils. In case you're ever on *Jeopardy*, the little thing that dangles in the back is called the uvula. The palate forms the roof. The frenulum is the small piece of fibrous tissue attaching the tongue to the floor of the mouth cavity. Inspection of the mouth can provide a good synopsis of overall health.

Take a look around. The mucosa should be pink and moist. There should not be a foul odor. While the tongue may have a thin white coating, this coating should not be thick or discolored. There should not be vesicles or breaks in the mucosa. There should not be masses, nodules, or other lesions on the inside cheeks, on the mucosa, or under the tongue.

The lips should be a pink-beige without cracks, splits, fissures, or vesicles. Minimal chapping is common. Unlike skin, lips do not have a mechanism to self-moisturize. Severe chapping sometimes occurs with strips of skin flaking off and bleeding. Kids' fingers are like magnets to metal with chapped lips and they will pull off strips until blood runs down their chins. This is not recommended. A moisturizing lip balm may help. Caution, a few contain steroids.

Openings of the salivary ducts can be seen on the buccal mucosa and under the tongue. These should appear as small openings and should not be red, swollen, painful, or hard.

Make sure all structural features are midline and not deviated by masses or neurologic defects. The mouth can droop on one side with Bell's palsy or stroke.

Selected pathology of the mouth:

A. Bell's palsy may be more common in Lyme than the over-promoted EM rash. With Bell's palsy the mouth will droop on one side. This deficit is more noticeable when the patient smiles. Since this condition affects the 7th cranial nerve, the patient may have trouble puffing out one cheek and taste and salivation may be impaired. The person may have difficulty forming some words clearly, since the musculature can be affected.

B. Vesicles on the lips are usually herpes simplex. Also called cold sores or fever blisters, these lesions can be solitary or erupt in clusters and develop crusts. Some HSV lesions can form inside the lips. When I see a cold sore, I consider that something is taxing the immune system, allowing this virus to manifest. What else might be going on with this patient? A number of other viruses can cause vesicles on the oral mucosa such as the Coxsackie virus that causes hand, foot, and mouth disease.

C. Aphthous ulcers, which may be viral or due to excess acidity or other irritants, are small white ulcers surrounded by red that appear on the buccal mucosa and can be painful. These aren't so painful that the tongue will not be drawn to them like a politician to a lie. Kids will use their tongues to fiddle with these ulcers until they disappear in a few days.

D. Trauma can result when the mouth has been hit, after falls, or when the tongue or cheeks have been bitten.

E. Koplik's spots are rarely seen today in the US. These are a prodromal sign of measles (rubeola) and look like grains of salt on individual red bases throughout the mouth. Subsequently, the generalized macular-papular rash of measles usually appears within 24 hours.

F. Erythema in the mouth can be due to a number of etiologies. The palate may be erythematous after a burn from too hot food or drink. Usually this is painful but resolves fairly quickly. Some mucosa may slough off a day or so after the burn. Viral pharyngitis can cause considerable redness in the back of the mouth and throat. Bacterial pathogens also cause redness but they tend to present with more exudate. But, of course, that rule has many exceptions.

PEARL: With Lyme the tonsillar pillars may be bright red or scarlet, possibly due to blood stasis or histamines. Petechiae may be present.

G. Dark lines along the gums can suggest heavy metal ingestion. Look especially at kids living in old housing.

H. Pale gums and mucosa suggest anemias.

I. Patchy pigmentation may be present on the buccal mucosa in patients with dark skin.

J. Bacterial infection in the mouth often presents with white exudate on tonsils or pillars. Strep is a common bacterial agent but there are others. There can be thick white, grey, black necrotic tissue in the posterior mouth on and around the tonsils or in the area where the tonsils have been removed. As you might imagine, this smells terrible and the odor is quite distinctive. Mononucleosis can present similarly. Diphtheria results in a gray film and can be indistinguishable from Strep and mono. Cultures and other testing may be needed.

K. Fungal monilia or candidiasis is also called thrush. Fungal overgrowth can involve all or only parts of the oral mucosa. Usually the caretaker will notice white clumpy patches and initially mistake them for milk curds. You can't just rub these off like you would milk debris. If you rub hard enough to remove them there can be irritation or even a little bleeding. Thrush can also look more like a lacy white material with a red base. Thrush is common in infants either from contact with fungus in the birth canal or from overgrowth after antibiotics.

L. Mumps is a viral infection of the salivary glands particularly the large parotid glands. Both parotids can be involved although one may swell and almost resolve before the other becomes enlarged. Mumps incidence has increased since parents backed off vaccinations in the past decade. Any salivary gland can be involved including those under the tongue. Salivary glands can also get stones which can be palpable in some cases. Here the inability of the saliva to leave the gland can cause swelling and discomfort. In mumps, the angle of the jaw is usually obscured by the swelling. In males past puberty, an orchitis can follow mumps.

M. Smokeless tobacco places users at a higher risk of mouth cancers.

N. In newborns, petechiae are possible in the soft tissues of the mouth after birth. Epstein's pearls are tiny whitish round bumps along the center of the hard palate near the back that disappear a few months after birth. Newborns can be tongue-tied, where the thickened frenulum under the tip of the tongue inhibits full extension. This is usually not a problem unless restriction causes difficulty nursing.

III. TONGUE

The tongue is a very interesting muscle that lies on the floor of the mouth and back into the entryway of the throat. The tongue functions to move food around for chewing and swallowing, helps form words in speech, and is largely responsible for the sense of taste. The tongue is covered with papillae, many of which contain taste buds. Not only is the tongue sensitive to taste, but also touch, temperature, position, and pressure. Humans are quite "tongue aware." Unlike a healthy shin, earlobe, or pinky, we have a pretty good idea what our tongue is up to at any given time. People who have lost their sense of taste for neurologic or other reasons report that this deficit is more debilitating than they would have thought. With LD, extreme hypersensitivity to certain tastes and textures can impede feeding.

Problems:

A. Motility: The tongue is a strong voluntary muscle which should be able to extend out of the mouth and then move left or right, up and down. Abnormal motion of the tongue can cause problems with eating and speaking.

- Restricted motion in babies can be due to a short frenulum, the fibrous tissue that attaches the bottom of the tongue to the floor of the mouth. Make sure the frenulum is not interfering with nursing. Older kids used to be called tongue-tied if the short frenulum interfered with speech. The frenulum can be released.

- Tremors or fasciculations in the tongue can be due to meningitis, alcoholism, prolonged weakness, neurologic conditions, or hyperthyroidism.

- Tardive dyskinesia is a slow, rhythmic, involuntary movement of the tongue or other muscles that can occur with use of certain medications. This condition is often irreversible.

- Paralysis can cause the tongue to deviate to one side or the other depending on the location of the lesion.

- Spasms of the tongue can occur in MS, stuttering, or general weakness.

B. Moisture: A dry tongue is often due to mouth breathing or dehydration. Excess salivation is not the tongue's fault. In this case, look at the salivary glands or for neurologic deficits.

C. Deviation: Asymmetry may indicate problems with CN 12 (the hypoglossal nerve). Paralysis of the 12th CN can cause atrophy and fasciculations on half of the tongue. When the tongue is extended it will deviate to the affected side. The tongue may protrude outside the mouth in toxemia or in advanced illness. Problems with CN 7, the facial nerve, such as the pathology found in Bell's palsy, might also affect the tongue, but this is primarily sensory.

D. Color: The normal tongue is pink. A tongue that looks like a strawberry with whitish papillae, protruding from a red base is likely due to Strep-induced scarlet fever. Strep is a common co-morbidity with TBIs. Some medications, foods, or drinks can temporarily discolor the tongue. A black tongue is found in dysentery and is not a good prognostic sign. The yellow of jaundice can be seen under the tongue. A blue tongue suggests impaired circulation, respiration, heart function, asthma, or cyanosis. A pale tongue could mean anemias.

E. Texture: Papillae cover the tongue and should be visible throughout. Some larger papillae in the back of the tongue are also normal. (I just confirmed this in the mirror.)

A smooth tongue is abnormal and suggests vitamin deficiencies such as B12, niacin, or iron. Sometimes allergies will smooth the tongue. The loss of papillae makes the tongue look reddish and slick.

A hairy tongue is typically comprised of long papillae and is usually benign. If fungus overgrows, the papillae can mix with fungal fibers and there can be a yellow-brown to black discoloration. This is unattractive and more common after antibiotics.

A geographic tongue has red patches and areas denuded and smooth. Some areas are raised and rough in sharp contrast to those areas that are smooth. The tongue looks like a relief map. The etiology is unknown and the condition is considered benign.

A white furred tongue can be seen in almost all fevers.

F. Coating: A normal tongue is slightly coated. This thin white coating is epithelium, bacteria, and food debris. Mouth breathing will increase the coating as will dehydration. A thick or discolored coating suggests fungus, which is common after antibiotic use.

G. Size: The tongue may be large in hypothyroidism, amyloidosis, or inflammation. A small tongue suggests anemia or emaciation.

H. Pain: Lesions on the tongue like viral or aphthous ulcers can hurt. Fissures, trauma, and pernicious anemia can all cause a painful tongue.

I. Tongue swallowing: No one ever "swallows" their tongue during seizures or unconsciousness. The tongue can lax backward over the airway, partially obstructing it. This is best handled by positioning. My preference is to turn the person on her side with her chin toward the chest and the mouth facing down. In this position, the tongue cannot easily relax over the airway and the patient is not as likely to aspirate vomit or saliva. Another position that helps prevent obstruction is to raise the shoulders slightly and extend the neck. I have seen so many wooden tongue blades snapped by well meaning people trying to prevent tongue swallowing. I have seen tongues impaled by splinters and more than a few bloody fingers. Position is the key here.

J. Abnormal taste: Medicines like clarithromycin can cause a bad taste in the mouth for days after the last dose. Also, pus and blood can have distinctive tastes. Diminished or absent taste is most often caused by a muted sense of smell from a congested upper airway as with URIs and allergies. Less common but more pertinent with TBIs is a neurologic lesion. Some Lyme patients complain of hypersensitive taste.

K. Lesions

> **Fissures** are furrows in the tongue epithelium which seem to be more prevalent in the elderly. The etiology is unknown and they may be normal although they seem to be more common in people with liver disease and DM. Fissures may be prominent in Sjogren's syndrome.

> **Varicose veins** are large veins under the tongue that can be alarming to both the patient and the HCP if they are not familiar with them. They are usually not a problem.

> **Leukoplakia** is a thick white patch on the mucous membrane like dried paint, which can be pre-malignant.

> **Carcinoma**: When present, cancers are mostly found under the tongue. Any ulcer or nodule that fails to heal is suspicious. Induration around any lesion could suggest malignancy.

> **Vesicles**: Vesicles on the tongue or oral mucosa usually indicate viral infection.

> **Nodules**: Nodules under the tongue can be normal.

PEARL: Kids are fascinated with the ability of some people to curl their tongues into a U shape. This is genetic and means nothing either way, although I have heard children try to convince others that it is a sign of intelligence or royalty. This ability has nothing to do with TBIs.

IV. TEMPOROMANDIBULAR JOINTS

The two TMJs are synovial joints that connect the jaw (mandible) to the temporal bones of the skull. The TMJ should be checked for motion, stiffness, alignment, and discomfort. Fingertips of two or three fingers of each hand are placed on the joint articulation and the patient is asked to open and close the jaw. A normal TMJ will move smoothly, without noise, and the two bones will slide together.

Problems:

- Mumps will obscure the angle of the jaw and stiffen motion. Swelling at the jaw angle due to parotid obstruction or tenderness in the parotid gland can be due to mumps or obstruction. The swelling may be palpated above the jaw angle or in front of the ear.

- TMJ syndrome is a significant aching pain in the joint. Chewing makes the pain worse. Motion is limited and a click is often audible. Inflammation of the joint and trauma are the primary causes.

- The TMJ has been known to be painful in Lyme and is actually a common location for migrating arthralgia.

V. TEETH

Teeth are hard projections in the jaws that chew the food. The teeth sit in the gums. Recent work on oral hygiene has shown that dental health plays a bigger role in overall wellness than previously thought. Gums should be pink and neither retracted away from the teeth or hypertrophied. Dental problems can be the source of chronic inflammation. On-going work on biofilms and infected gums and their association with heart disease have changed the perspective on the importance of good dental hygiene.

Examine:

> Appropriate number of teeth for age?

> Appropriate loss/permanent tooth pattern?

> Hygiene?

> Lesions on teeth or gums?

PEARL: Some kids are born with teeth and others don't get their first tooth until they are well over a year old. I can remember going on a date in high school and losing a baby tooth.

Problems:

- Most of us have a pretty decent idea about good dental health. Plaque between teeth, redness and swelling of gums, bad odor, broken and missing teeth, and obvious decay are signs that you are not brushing and flossing with regularity. Gingivitis causes redness and swelling of the gums, which may bleed on slight contact. Infection can harbor in decaying teeth and infected gums and TBI patients don't need any more pathogen repositories.

- Periodontal disease is also called pyorrhea or gingivitis and can lead to inflammation of deeper tissues around the teeth. The gums recede and debris soon fills in any gaps. Pus can collect. Teeth may loosen and fall out. This needs to be dealt with by a dental professional and vigilance with oral hygiene. Gingivitis can mask other conditions so it must be treated early and aggressively. Inflammation in the mouth has been associated with chronic low-grade systemic infection.

- Treatment with certain anti-epilepsy drugs such as Dilantin can cause gum hypertrophy.

- Pain in the teeth and gums has been reported by Lyme patients.

Section 17-G

Throat, Neck, Thyroid, and Pertinent Differential

When you win the game, get off the field.

Unknown

I. THROAT (PHARYNX)

The pharynx is a passageway for air, food, and sound. The top part of the pharynx is above the soft palate. The eustachian tubes, from below the middle ears, open into this area. The middle throat opens into the mouth and the lower throat opens into the larynx anteriorly and the esophagus posteriorly. The throat is a few square inches of intense activity and so an area of potential problems. The opening into the throat is surrounded by lymph tissue which is good and bad. The lymph nodes, adenoids, and tonsils collect pathogens and accumulate white cells to identify and destroy them. They provide a first-line of defense for the body against infection. Unfortunately, these filters get considerable exposure and the tissue can become red, sore, and swollen. Escaping pathogens can enter the eustachian tubes and move into the ears and sinuses, into the respiratory tract over the voice box, and onto the GI tract by way of the esophagus. This is one reason why people with upper respiratory infections get symptoms affecting all areas that communicate with the pharynx such as hoarseness, sore throat, cough, and queasiness.

Ask the patient to say "Ah" or yawn. This raises the soft palate and tests CN 10. If the vagal nerve is impaired, the soft palate on the affected side will not rise when the person says "Ah." Little kids will not be able to follow this instruction. I have found that they usually will open their mouths quite wide at some point in the exam and you can either take a quick look if you have your light ready or you may need to use a tongue blade for an adequate view.

> *PEARL: Lyme patients often complain of a feeling of occlusion in the throat. They feel like they can't swallow or that there's a golf ball in the way. They have trouble swallowing food and saliva and have the sensation of choking or obstruction. In most cases there is nothing found on PE. In these cases consider co-morbid HPV on the larynx.*

The uvula should be midline. A bifid uvula is a normal variant. The soft tissues should be pink, not red or pale. Look for pus, lesions like vesicles or ulcers, bad odor, or anything that could cause occlusion of the airway.

Problems with the throat:

A. Infections: The throat is a common local repository for infection. Cultures or other testing may be needed to identify the causative agent. Any of these throat infections can be concurrent with TBIs and can either mask or enhance the signs and symptoms of the co-morbidity.

- Viral etiologies are probably the most common cause of pharyngitis with mild to moderate redness, exudate, difficulty swallowing, hoarseness, swelling of the pillars, enlarged lymph nodes, and fever. Tonsils and surrounding tissues can be involved. In general, viral pharyngitis is thought to be milder than bacterial infection but this is not always the case. Many viruses can infect the throat and these infections do not respond to antibiotics. One viral pharyngitis that can present with considerable swelling, exudate, adenopathy, and foul odor is mononucleosis.

- Bacterial infections of the throat include Strep pharyngitis which presents with redness, white or yellow exudates, distinctive foul odor, lymphadenopathy, swelling of the tonsils and pillars, hot potato voice, and difficulty swallowing. If suspicious, do Strep cultures. Strep usually responds well to appropriate antibiotics.

PEARL: A history of Strep infections, as well as TBIs, has been associated with the development of a symptom complex referred to as PANDAS or pediatric autoimmune neuropsychiatric disorders associated with Streptococcal infections. PANDAS appear to be responsible for a wide variety of signs and symptoms from anxiety and OCD to oppositional and aggressive behaviors. Be vigilant.

PEARL: I anticipate the name PANDAS will be modified, removing the "AS" in order to open the door to the possibility of other infectious etiologies. Also I expect that someday these syndromes will be confirmed in adults as well. TBIs such as Lyme, bartonellosis, and M. fermentans are suspected of causing PAND-like syndromes.

- Fungal infections of the throat, for our purposes, are usually due to fungal overgrowth secondary to antibiotic use.

B. Enlarged tonsils can be present in all ages but are more common in children. The size of uninfected tonsils usually has no relationship to disease.

C. A peritonsillar abscess can be a medical emergency. An abscess is a localized collection of pus in the tissue usually due to infection by pyrogenic (pus-forming) bacteria, often Staphylococcus *aureus*. The sore throat gets progressively worse on one side with fever, pain, hot potato voice, neck discomfort, large, tender lymph nodes, foul odor, and difficulty opening the mouth fully. The uvula may be displaced. Swallowing is very painful and there may be referred ear pain. On exam the abscess is visible as it encroaches into the throat. This is reason for hospitalization and usually requires surgical drainage of the abscess along with antibiotics to target the bacteria. George Washington is thought to have died from treatment for a peritonsillar abscess. (Of course, George Washington is said to have died from just about everything except Lyme disease. Did you know that as a youth George Washington had sandy, *red* hair? I confirmed this with Mt. Vernon after I ran into a second-grade doubter.)

D. Nasal speech can be due to large adenoids occluding the back of the throat.

E. A number of Lyme patients complain of hoarseness or vocal changes.

F. Allergies or URIs can cause postnasal drip to run into the throat. Sometimes PND is visible in the back of the throat.

G. Persistent hoarseness can be a sign of human papilloma virus.

H. Obstructed airway can be due to swelling from infection, anaphylaxis, or a foreign body. When choking is due to a foreign body the obstruction can be removed by using the Heimlich maneuver in kids big enough to get a partial fist in position to apply subdiaphragmatic pressure. If the person is talking, breathing, or coughing the maneuver is not needed. Reassure the patient and encourage them to keep coughing. In babies and small kids, place the victim head down on your forearm with the head lower than the thorax. Using the heel of the hand apply 5 or more firm, distinct back blows in an attempt to dislodge the foreign body. Chest thrusts can also be used. If you are not well-versed in these procedures, a formal class is recommended and these are available in many venues.

I. The epiglottis is a bit of cartilage just behind the root of the tongue that covers the opening of the airway. When a person swallows, the epiglottis prevents food and liquids from entering the airway. Inflammation of the epiglottis can be life-threatening. Symptoms of acute epiglottitis include cough, which can be croupy, hoarseness, difficulty swallowing, and signs of upper respiratory tract obstruction. This is an emergency. Do not cause the patient to gag here since that will totally obstruct the airway. Occasionally, in looking in the back of the mouth, you might see a swollen, red epiglottis, but don't count on it. When you call the ambulance, specify a transport with a tracheotomy kit available. The person will need to be taken to a location where the obstructed airway can be managed immediately. Tell the ambulance who they will be transporting and alert the ER. A lateral X-ray view of the neck may be needed to confirm the diagnosis.

PEARL: Anecdotally, bright red tonsillar pillars might be indicative of Lyme infection. Petechiae in the back of the throat may also suggest Lyme and could be due to blood stasis, but this is speculative.

II. NECK

The neck supports the head on the shoulders and is a concentrated area of bones, joints, nerves, lymph nodes, and blood vessels. Neck pain and restricted motion are common features of Lyme and other TBIs. When examining the neck look for:

A. Lymph nodes: Normal nodes are barely palpable and fairly symmetrical in size bilaterally. The most familiar nodes are the cervical strings on either side of the neck. But there are also tonsillar, submaxillary, submental, posterior cervical, superficial cervical, deep cervical, and supraclavicular nodes. Whenever there is a potential inflammatory or infectious process, palpate for nodes and describe any abnormalities so that comparison can be made at future visits. When one node is enlarged look "up the chain" of the lymphatic system to see if other nodes are also large. Identifying an abnormal region can help isolate areas of inflammation or infection. Single, nontender nodes are common in normal exams. Tender nodes suggest inflammation, while hard or fixed nodes suggest malignancy.

PEARL: Tunev et al found that Bb migrate to lymph nodes within days of infection and this may explain why some people eventually suffer from relapses. In these cases the hypothesis is that the body mounts what should be an adequate defense but apparently in some host mice the response is not STRONG enough to clear the infection, accounting for recurrent or persistent symptoms. While other things might explain this phenomenon, these findings make me wonder. I am constantly commenting about whether the EM rash somehow correlates to the state of the immune system at the time of infection and whether the EM rash portends anything about the severity or duration of the disease. Well, what if I am curious in the wrong direction? Some Lyme patients have significant lymphadenopathy and others have enlargement to a lesser degree. Still another subpopulation has barely palpable nodes. How are these groups different from one another? What if the lymphadenopathy is the omen that serves to identify those who will have persistent symptoms or flares? What if the more Bb a person has sequestered in nodes, the more likely the Lyme will manifest as a chronic condition? What if those patients whose Bb are not lurking in the nodes are more easily defended by the immune system? What if antibiotics cannot reach the Bb as readily when they are in the nodes? What if the Bb can remain hidden but not effectively removed in the nodes allowing for relapse? What if....? I will rejoice when someone finally puts this all together.

B. Full range of motion: The neck is the most mobile part of the spine and can move forward and back, laterally, and rotate to about 70 degrees on either side. In a normal exam, the patient should be able to:

- lateral bend by touching each ear to the shoulder

- rotate by touching the chin to each shoulder

- put the head back in extension

- touch the chin to the chest in flexion

The inability to move the neck, either actively or passively, can strongly suggest either structural problems or CNS disease, especially meningitis. Cradle the head of the supine patient in the hands. Support the head and then move in all directions to assess the ease of movement and suppleness. If the meninges are inflamed this will be difficult or painful, especially on flexion. In older kids ask the child to sit on the exam table with legs extended. Then ask her to touch her chin to her chest. In meningitis, the child will not be able to remain upright and touch the chin to the chest. If the patient cannot flex the chin to the chest due to pain or new onset stiffness, be sure to rule out meningitis if the person has signs of infection. Meningitis is a well-established manifestation of Lyme.

PEARL: Sometimes the first sign of an on-coming URI is a structural lesion in the neck or upper thorax. While it is hard to determine which came first the URI or the "crick" in the neck, when you experience one, look out for the other.

PEARL: Cracking, popping, or crepitus in the neck is a frequent complaint in Lyme patients and significant neck pain has been documented with babesiosis.

C. The trachea should be midline. Masses or pathologic respiratory conditions can cause the trachea to be skewed from midline.

D. The neck can be the site of much cracking and popping of joints in Lyme.

E. Carotid pulses should be equally strong bilaterally since the carotid arteries supply blood to the head and brain. A bruit over the carotid can sometimes be heard in older kids with a neck space large enough to place a stethoscope. This bruit is a murmur or blowing sound that indicates some compromise in blood flow due to narrowing or other pathology. Examine the pulse on one side at a time. Do not lean across the trachea to take the pulse on the other side, like they do in the movies.

F. Torticollis occurs when the sternocleidomastoid muscle of the neck spasms, causing a painful shortening of the neck to one side, a bending of the head to the contracted side, while the chin goes in the opposite direction.

PEARL: Surprisingly, the skin of the neck can be a site for HPV lesions that appear like translucent bumps.

III. THYROID

Lyme is commonly associated with having a significant impact on endocrine function, especially thyroid and adrenal performance. Because fatigue is a hallmark of both TBI and thyroid disease, careful attention should be paid to the thyroid. Just because the patient has one condition does not mean she cannot have the other. Thyroid problems are an important part of the differential diagnosis in this population. Missing this condition in a potential TBI patient is embarrassing. Examination of the thyroid is easier in older kids than in babies with small neck space and not a little fat.

Inspect the neck for obvious enlargements or asymmetry. While palpating ask the patient to swallow. The thyroid tissue rises on swallowing. To examine the thyroid: Use the index and middle fingers to feel below the cricoid cartilage for the thyroid isthmus. Feel the isthmus rise up under the fingers. The thyroid, along with the trachea and Adam's apple (laryngeal protuberance) rise on swallowing. Nodes do not.

Check for lumps, nodules, and asymmetry. Assess hardness of any nodule and matting to surrounding tissue. Inquire about a history of rapid enlargement. Multiple nodules are suggestive of a metabolic problem but remain suspicious until cleared for malignancy.

PEARL: The physical examination of the thyroid can be completely normal and yet thyroid function can be quite abnormal. Put the entire picture together before reaching a conclusion.

Section 17-H

Back, Chest, and Pertinent Differential

Friendship is born at the moment when one person says to another,
"What! You too?" I thought I was the only one."

C.S. Lewis

I.   BACK

The back is the dorsum of the trunk from the neck to the pelvis. Back pain is one of the most common reasons for seeing a doctor and is a frequent complaint in Lyme patients.

Examination of the back includes an assessment of:

* Skin: Look for all the usual suspects. The back is a common site for shingles and the vesicular streaks of poison ivy and the wheals of urticaria from allergic reactions. The back of the neck is a possible area for subtle wart-like lesions from HPV. You will miss these translucent clusters if you don't think of it. Remember that a secondary EM rash can appear anywhere and not just at the site of the tick bite. If you don't visualize the skin, you cannot see the lesions. The back is a good place to observe the skin without all the complications of noses and nipples and belly buttons obscuring the view.

* Structure: The back should be examined when the patient is standing equally on both feet and again when the patient is prone. The bottom of the scapula is at about the 7th rib. The most prominent spine is usually cervical 7 but can be thoracic 1. The top of each lung lies about 2 to 4 cm above the inner clavicle. One scapula should not be protruding or predominant. Fingers run down the spine from the base of the neck to the lower lumbar regions should trace an essentially straight line.

  The anterior-posterior curvature of the spine changes with age. Babies are fairly flat and curves develop as the child matures. Note the concave cervical curve, convex thoracic curve, concave lumbar curve, and convex sacrum. The younger the child the less curvature there will be in the spine. In newborns the spine has little AP curvature at all.

  From behind, inspect for any lateral curving. Notice any difference in the height of the shoulders and iliac crests. Unequal heights of the iliac crests or a pelvic tilt suggest unequal leg length.

* Movement: The spine is a mobile structure and restrictions of movement can cause pain and impede the optimum function of internal organs such as the restriction of lung expansion. Pain on motion of the back can significantly impact activities of daily living.

  Have the patient bend forward at the waist toward the floor. Hold onto the patient's pelvis and ask her to bend forward, backward, and to each side. Normally the patient should be able to flex to almost 90 degrees, back bend (extend) to about 30 degrees, rotate at the waist 30 degrees on each side, and side bend laterally at the waist about 30 degrees on either side of the spine.

  As the patient flexes forward to touch the toes, note symmetry. Flexibility can be grossly assessed by the distance the fingertips are from the floor. Some patients are much more naturally flexible than others. Lack of flexibility does not necessarily mean pathology. Has there been a change in the person's flexibility? Is the family relatively inflexible? Lack of movement due to illness or bed rest can leave a temporary limitation on flexibility. ROM exercises and stretching can keep the back supple and less stiff and constricted.

* Lungs can be percussed from the back for high fluid levels in the bases and auscultated across the back.

Problems with the back that may be pertinent to TBI patients:

A.   **Pain**: Back pain can be due to congenital problems, structural mal-alignments, muscle spasm, nerve inflammation, disc disease, lower lung pathology, arthritis, kidney problems, or a combination of factors. I once read an article called the hundred causes of back pain. Whatever the reason, if it hurts, the patient is not going to want to move it. As movement declines then other problems set in, including risk of clots and fluid stasis. The pain cycle leads to other pathology. The less the area moves the less it can move. If TBIs are part of the underlying cause of the pain, aggressively address the TBI. (If only it were that simple.) Tenderness over the vertebral column can be inflammation, arthritis, or an osteopathic lesion. Muscles in spasm can also be tender. In a chronic spasm, the muscle will feel tight and will be sore to movement and palpation. If the pain is due to arthritis, there could be spot tenderness over the affected joints. TBI patients often complain of severe back pain that can be incapacitating.

PEARL: Tenderness to palpation of the costovertebral joints is common in Lyme.

B. **Scoliosis** is an abnormal curvature of the spine and kyphoscoliosis refers to a lateral curve that can be deforming. Curvature is best assessed by having the patient bend forward at the waist and watching for asymmetry and unilateral protrusion of structures such as the scapula. The fingertips will trace a curve when run from the neck to the pelvis. Depending on the severity of the curvature, lung capacity can be compromised and intestinal organs compressed. A significant curve can result in an AP hump. Curves can impede flow of fluids, air, and nerve conduction. While TBIs do not cause scoliosis, the pathology from both conditions can work in tandem to make the patient feel worse and complicate the case.

PEARL: When bending over, scoliosis will accentuate if it is due to curvature of the spine. If the problem is due to unequal leg length, the curvature will disappear.

PEARL: When looking for scoliosis, have the patient bend forward and if there is any question, use a marker to mark each spinous process.

C. **Arthritis:** Arthritis is an inflammation of a joint. The spine is composed of multiple joints. Lyme, of course, can affect the joints and the spine is no exception. If when bending, the patient cannot remove the lumbar concavity and if the spinous processes do not separate when moving forward, consider arthritis of the spine. Arthritis usually presents with pain, swelling, and often structural changes. Arthritis is sometimes treated with immunosuppressants, which may not be the best choice in Lyme patients.

D. **Herniated disc:** A ruptured disc is a herniation or protrusion of the cushion between the vertebras most often in the neck or lower back. A herniated disc usually causes pain on the side where the disc is bulging. If the patient complains of LBP or sciatic pain, straight leg raise one leg until the pain is reproduced. Then dorsiflex the foot. On the straight leg raise, the hamstrings will normally pull behind the knees because of the stretching of muscle not used to moving that far. But increased pain on dorsiflexion of the foot indicates pressure on nerve roots which suggests a herniated disc.

PEARL: There may be an increased incidence of disc problems and herniations in Lyme disease. A Lyme patient who had surgery to repair a damaged disc insisted that the tissue be tested for Bb. The sample was filled with spirochetes. The surgeon who initially refused to order the test because "It couldn't be Lyme," was amazed and contrite. I wonder if he now routinely considers Lyme in patients with a suggestive history.

E. **Spondylitis** is an inflammation of the spine joints. The chest cannot expand as much as normal if there is significant spondylitis.

Ankylosing spondylitis is a chronic progressive condition involving the joints of the spine, the costovertebral joints, and the sacroiliac joints. Sclerosis (fibrosis or scarring) of the SI joints is a hallmark sign. The changes here are similar to those seen in RA. Ankylosis (stiffening, immobility) may occur, giving rise to a stiff, straight, immobile back. Usually ankylosis starts in the SI joints and low back, reaching the neck only late in the clinical course. This condition, depending on the underlying etiology, can cause significant decrease in ROM and spastic tenderness of muscles. The patient may need to turn the whole body to look sideways and the neck thrusts forward. Ankylosing spondylitis should be part of the differential diagnosis when assessing joint involvement in Lyme disease.

PEARL: HLA-B27 is one of thousands of identifying markers found on cells. This particular antigen on the cell surface is associated with ankylosing spondylitis. About 6% of the Caucasian population has the HLA-B27 marker which is associated with back pain including ankylosing spondylitis and IBS. These people tend to have more general achiness and arthralgias. Not everyone with HLA-B27 has ankylosing spondylitis but essentially everyone with AS has the B27 marker.

F. **Sacroiliac joint pain:** The sacroiliac joint is the articulation between the sacrum and the innominate bone of the pelvis. Even though this joint normally has very limited motion due to interlocking surfaces, the joint can be the site of much discomfort. I forget if it was Moe or Curly who constantly complained, "Oh! My aching sacroiliac." On assessment, palpate the SI area for tenderness.

G. **Structural lesions:** As an osteopath, I am aware of the possibility of somatic lesions throughout the spine that can restrict movement and therefore impede function. To an osteopath, proper structure allows for optimum function. Somatic lesions can cause discomfort and restricted movement. Structural manipulative therapy can resolve these complaints and allow for better fluid flow and nerve conduction in the area. I am a good doctor, but a terrible osteopath. Some people are naturals like Ruggsy in my study group in med school. He would have fellow students lined up a mile for his structural manipulations. There are excellent osteopaths and many Lyme patients have found considerable relief after treatment with osteopathic modalities.

PEARL: Some Lyme patients have reported point tenderness at rib articulations 8, 9, and 10.

PEARL: Many people think an X-ray will clearly identify the cause of acute back pain. Unless there is trauma or significant arthritis, back films are not especially enlightening. Some can hint at muscle spasm or misalignment but usually they don't tell you any more than you already learned from the physical exam. Nonetheless, just like chest X-rays, many people feel much better after the film is taken, even before they know the result. I once spent two hours giving a brilliant talk to union reps about why routine chest X-rays in asymptomatic workers were not the best way to use their health care dollars. They agreed with everything I said and thought I was the smartest doctor ever. But they would not give up their chest X-rays even in favor of tests that had a much better PPV of disease in the population.

II. CHEST

Also called the thorax, the chest lies between the neck and the diaphragm. The bones enclosing the chest include the sternum or breast bone to the front, the spine posteriorly, and the ribs. Be aware of the xiphoid process at the tip of the sternum when positioning to do chest compressions in CPR. Between the ribs and the sternum is the costal cartilage. Point tenderness in this area can help distinguish inflammation of the cartilage from other conditions such as GERD and cardiac ischemia.

PEARL: Bb appear to have a preference for tissue containing collagen including connective tissue, skin, tendons, ligaments, fascia, bone, and cartilage.

In examining the chest look for:

A. Symmetry: The chest should inflate on inspiration symmetrically, without effort or discomfort. Injured ribs can cause splinting where the patient tries to prevent pain by restricting motion on the injured side. Persistent coughing can cause pain that restricts motion and wears the patient out.

B. Skin: Chest skin should be examined looking for lesions and discolorations.

C. Breasts: Adults reading this text will likely think of breast exams in terms of early detection of cancer in grown women. The concerns are different in kids and cancer of the breast in children is exceedingly rare. Since hormones are greatly affected by Lyme and certain other TBIs, mention of the pediatric breast exam is warranted.

Many neonates have small palpable breast buds right after birth. These are common in both males and females and they spontaneously dissipate as the influence of the maternal hormones lessens. Likewise, a clear or milky fluid, sometimes called witch's milk can be discharged from the nipples of neonates. This again is due to mater-

nal hormones and will diminish along with the palpable breast bud over a few weeks or months.

Of more concern is a discharge that is unilateral and bloody. This condition is usually secondary to a transient growth of ducts under the nipple and usually resolves spontaneously. Keep an eye on these kids. Sometimes a patient with fever and a sore swollen breast has mastitis, a bacterial infection that responds to antibiotics. Most neonatal breast conditions spontaneously resolve, respond readily to antibiotics, or are otherwise benign.

Later in childhood a girl might get a blockage of a small duct near the nipple which can cause enlargement into a small lump which usually spontaneously resolves. Tanner stages of breast development are described in the *Genitals* section. Although a reason for considerable angst in grown women, one breast is almost always larger than the other.

Gynecomastia is enlargement of breast tissue in males. This enlargement occurs most often during three periods in the male's life: transiently at birth, beginning at puberty and then declining during the late teens, and in older men. Most often this condition is due to a hormonal fluctuation but can be associated with a number of clinical conditions, endocrine problems, obesity, or the use of certain drugs including marijuana, antidepressants, and steroids. Temporary gynecomastia is actually common in puberty.

The need for treatment will depend on whether the condition is pathologic and, if so, addressing the underlying cause. Usually gynecomastia regresses spontaneously, but the condition can be the cause of considerable distress in the patient. Since Bb are so closely associated with endocrine function, the presence of gynecomastia should prompt consideration of Lyme as a factor, if the history is supportive.

Occasionally, a person of either gender will have clear discharge from a nipple. Again, spontaneous resolution is usually the outcome. For the record, adult males do get breast cancer. Rare but real.

PEARL: In the world of hormones, anything is possible. When I worked on the development of an aromatase inhibitor that prevented the synthesis of estrogen, we requested a special exemption from the FDA to be able to use the drug prior to approval in children with inappropriate breast development. These were rare and sad cases in kids of both sexes, where hormonal imbalances resulted in breast growth. One pre-school girl had essentially adult sized breasts and had begun to menstruate. Older boys and men had begun to show sexual interest in her and she was scared. A small boy had already had to have a bilateral mastectomy because his adipose tissue continued to pump estrogen. One corporate marionette was opposed to giving these children the drug because use could result in adverse events that might hurt the commercial development of the product. PLEASE. Fortunately, the FDA agreed with the more compassionate individuals and a number of children were helped. If you find a problem, investigate. There may be something you can do about it.

D. Axilla: The underarm, or armpit, should be examined for skin lesions, enlarged or sore lymph nodes, and masses.

E. Palpation of the chest can provide information about the etiology of pain. Point tenderness in costochondral areas can suggest costochondritis or inflammation of the cartilage. The presence of costochondritis does not rule out cardiac or GI etiologies for chest pain. I learned the hard way that a chest pain patient can have more than one thing happening at a time. Lyme patients may have a greater incidence of costochondritis.

F. Auscultation of the chest is conducted in order to examine the heart and lungs and the techniques are discussed in later sections. Percussion can be done to look for fluid levels.

Fremitus is the name given to vibrations that can be felt through the chest wall when the patient is speaking or coughing. If both hands are placed on either side of the chest the vibrations on one side can be compared to the other side. Alternatively, a stethoscope can be used to auscultate fremitus. Fremitus decreases in pleural effusions, emphysema, lung collapse, edema, or with large masses. Vibrations may be more noticeable when there is obstruction of one bronchus. Ask the patient to repeat the number "99" to evaluate fremitus.

Percussion of the chest wall helps the HCP to decide if underlying tissue is air-filled or fluid-filled (as in pneumonia). Chest percussion is not good for identifying deep-seated problems. Usually the examiner uses the middle finger of one hand to tap the middle finger of the other hand over the area to be percussed. This is a direct, firm strike which is repeated as the fingers are moved across the area to be examined. The percussion note will be dull when the area below is fluid-filled (such as in pneumonia) and tympanic over air. Hyperresonance will be heard in areas of overexpansion such as found in the overextended lung of emphysema. High dullness is suggestive of lung tissue filled with fluid or a pleural effusion.

G. Gastroesophageal reflux disease (GERD) is the result of acid back flowing from the stomach into the esophagus. While the stomach is designed to handle the caustic acid, the tissue of the esophagus is not. Reflux is due to either a laxity of the sphincter at the entry way into the stomach or abnormal pressure forcing contents backward. The acid in the esophagus often results in a substernal burning sensation after eating, commonly called heartburn. The pain can mimic cardiac ischemia. There are usually no physical findings and diagnosis is made based on history and ROS. Of course, spending a few thousand dollars on an endoscopy will confirm what we already know.

PEARL: There are multiple mentions in the literature of GERD associated with Lyme disease. In fact, GERD is one of the most common manifestation of gestational Lyme. GERD is not found on PE but is described as part of the ROS. Could it be the hypotonia that allows the reflux?

Lungs, Respiratory, and Pertinent Differential

The secret of managing is to keep the guys who hate you
away from the guys who are undecided.

Unknown

LUNGS/RESPIRATORY

A lung is one of the two spongy organs that are used for respiration, which involves the exchange of the gases oxygen and carbon dioxide. The trachea splits into two bronchi which subsequently divide into numerous bronchioles. These terminal bronchioles further subdivide into smaller and smaller pieces until they conclude in the alveolar sacs where the work is done. This branching from tree trunk to twig allows for the immense surface area needed for gas exchange.

The base of the lung rests on the diaphragm, the domed muscle that separates the chest cavity from the abdomen. The right lung has 3 lobes and the left has only 2 since the heart is taking up space on the left side. The right lung descends slightly lower than the left.

The job of the lung is to bring air and blood into such close contact that oxygen can be added to the blood and wastes can be removed. Therefore, the lungs are highly vascular. In the alveoli, the blood and air are separated only by the thin cell walls of the alveoli and its adjacent capillary. This area is a physiologist's dream where all kinds of complex biochemistry allows for gas exchange. The old saying repeated when trying to revive someone, "In with the good air and out with the bad," applies to the lung. (I can't remember if that was the mantra used in *Popeye* cartoons or on *The Three Stooges* but I've had worse medical sources.) Usually the lung goes about its business without any thought required. But, of course, this wouldn't be a very interesting book if numerous things couldn't go wrong. Efficient respiration can be impacted in a number of ways:

1. Structural problems impeding air flow

2. Mechanical problems not allowing for proper breathing

3. Obstructions

4. Constrictions

5. Poor oxygen level in the environment

6. Not enough RBCs to carry oxygen

7. Impedance of gas exchange through:

   a. Scarring

   b. Loss of elasticity

   c. Fluid presence due to inflammation, irritation, or infection

   d. Over-inflation

   e. Poor or shallow inspiration

   f. Ineffective expiration

   g. Collapse of lung tissue

8. A number of other mechanisms less pertinent to TBIs

Respiration can also be altered because the lungs are trying to compensate for pathology elsewhere.

Unlike the cardiac, musculoskeletal, and nervous systems, lung tissue does not seem to be a primary target of Lyme. Even with babesiosis, where respiratory signs and symptoms are more common, these are secondary to the underlying pathophysiology of RBC damage due to pathogen infiltration and edema. In most cases, respiratory failure is a prelude to disease-driven fatalities.

PEARL: You would think there would be more lung pathology associated with Lyme because of the extensive vasculature. Maybe the oxygen level is too high for Bb's comfort.

Physical examination of the lungs includes:

A. Inspection:

You can learn a lot about a patient's respiratory status just by watching her come into the room. Observe the respiratory rate and pattern of breathing. Which muscles is she using to breathe? Note the depth of the breath and effort required. The inspiration should be somewhat longer than the expiration. Is this balance maintained or is one phase prolonged or needing more effort? Look for retractions or use of accessory muscles in the neck and abdomen.

Is the trachea midline? Look for symmetry, splinting, or increased anterior-posterior diameter. Is the patient in apparent respiratory distress? Some findings apparent on inspection include:

- Barrel chest is an increase in AP diameter seen in emphysema or chronic overexpansion.

- Kyphoscoliosis can compromise breathing.

- Signs of respiratory distress include rapid breathing, nasal flaring in infants, use of accessory muscles, retractions, and bluish tinge. All these signs are readily observable.

- Retractions are a sign of respiratory distress and are seen mostly in compromised babies. The skin between each rib, below the sternum, and above the collar bones is sucked in on each inspiration.

- If accessory muscles are in use, the person is expending more than normal effort to breathe. Usually, use of upper chest and neck muscles come into play only under physical stress. Aside from infants who make good use of their diaphragms when they breathe, older patients should not be using muscles in the epigastric area or neck to help them suck in air.

- A baby repeatedly extending her head may be signaling respiratory compromise.

- Signs of choking are usually apparent. Airway obstruction causes prolonged forceful expiration and pursed lips.

B. Palpation:

By touching the back and chest, considerable information can be gathered regarding the respiratory condition. Palpate any areas of tenderness or deformity. To assess expansion and symmetry, place hands on the patient's back with thumbs together at the midline. Ask the patient to breathe deeply. By putting your hands on the person you can feel sensations such as fremitus which are palpable vibrations and crepitus which is air in the subcutaneous tissues.

C. Percussion:

By assessing the resonance heard over the lung fields, the HCP can discern air versus fluid versus solid tissue. Using the middle finger of one hand, place the distal end firmly against the patient's chest or back. With the end of the opposite middle finger, flick the wrist to strike the finger in contact with the patient. The anterior chest can be percussed from the collar bone to under the breasts. Percuss from side to side and top to bottom, except for the areas covered by the scapula. A normal chest should be resonant throughout, meaning there is air in the lung space as there should be. Compare the sides. You should find the dull sounding diaphragm on both sides. The lungs are slightly asymmetrical with the right side lower than the left. Remember this when assessing fluid levels.

If there is fluid present, percussion will be dull or flat sounding suggesting consolidation or fluid such as in pneumonia or a pleural effusion. Hyperresonance suggests too much air such as with emphysema or pneumothorax. With bronchitis, the lung should sound normal on percussion since there is no fluid in the lung tissue.

D. Auscultation:

Auscultation of lungs is used to assess airflow, presence of fluid, mucus, obstruction, and the condition of the pleura. Using the diaphragm of the stethoscope, listen to both the chest and the back. Use a small diaphragm when examining babies since you can better localize abnormalities using the smaller tool. The best way to assess the lungs is with the patient sitting up. Have the person take big breaths in and out through the mouth. These breaths should be deeper than normal. In a crying baby, listen between cries when the child inspires. Compare symmetrical areas left and right. Listen to one full breath in each location.

Normal breath sounds should be heard throughout the lung fields. Vesicular (normal) breath sounds are low pitched and heard across the lungs, front and back. BSs are the sound of air flowing and the larger the airway, the louder and more high pitched the BS. Tracheal BS are highest pitched. Inspiration is usually longer than expiration.

BSs will be diminished when normal air-filled lung tissue is displaced by an even higher concentration of air. There will be little sound of air moving in the case of emphysema where the lungs are overinflated and it is hard to exhale. There will be no BS over the area of pneumothorax where there is free air in the pleural cavity. Where lung tissue has collapsed, little air will be moving. Areas with fluid or consolidation in the lung tissue will also have few or no BS such as localized pleural effusions or pneumonias. BS shift from normal vesicular to bronchial when there is fluid in the lung tissue that is not consolidated, such as in bronchitis. Here the sound of rhonchi might be bad, but rhonchi are better than the non-existent movement of air found in pneumonia. Many abnormal BS can be heard when there is pathology including rales, rhonchi, and wheezes all described below. Extra sounds are called adventitious. They are always abnormal but not always clinically significant, and include fremitus and crepitus. Morbid obesity can mute breath sounds.

Findings in a normal pulmonary exam:

Normal respiration should demonstrate symmetrical effort with inspiration somewhat longer than expiration. The chest should raise slightly on inspiration and regress on expiration. Normal BSs over lung tissue are low pitched overall but slightly higher on inspiration and less intense during the shorter expiration phase. Normally, unless there has been recent extraordinary exertion, there is no need for individuals to use accessory muscles in the neck or abdomen to breathe. In contrast, infants will show a lot of abdominal movement when breathing normally.

Vesicular breathing is another way of saying normal breathing. Why not just say normal breathing? Apparently, the term vesicular breathing came about when the experts thought that breath sounds came from the air moving in the small alveolar sacs or vesicles. They don't. So a name derived under false pretenses lingers, despite the fact that we now know better.

Terms, signs, and symptoms associated with lung pathology:

Absent breath sounds: No sound indicates no air is moving, not that no air is present. In fact, in emphysema little air is moving because the lungs are over-expanded with air. Air will also not move through collapsed lung or fluid-filled lung.

Air hunger: Air hunger is a sensation that one cannot get an effective breath. The breathing does not feel adequate or satisfactory. The patient may not be able to sigh sufficiently. Air hunger can range from mild discomfort to respiratory distress. Air hunger can occur with acute babesiosis. Lyme patients have also complained of air hunger but I wonder if they aren't experiencing the effects of a Babesia co-infection.

Apnea: A period with no breathing with a pause of greater than 10 seconds is called apnea.

Atelectasis: Incomplete expansion of lung tissue that can result in collapse. There is no oxygen to be had in the area of atelectasis since there is no air there. The blood moves through and there is less and less O_2 to pick up on each pass. Breath sounds will progressively diminish and there will be a haziness progressing to white-out on X-ray since space that was previously filled with air is now deflated lung tissue. Atelectasis results in a shrunken or airless state that can affect all or part of a lung. This condition can be acute or chronic. There are a number of reasons for atelectasis including obstruction due to plugs of mucus or other foreign bodies, strictures, compression from masses or nodes, pressure from effusion or pneumothorax, or loss of surfactant. Rapid occlusion due to aggressive pneumonia or FB obstruction can cause massive collapse on the affected side with dyspnea, cyanosis, drop in BP, tachycardia, temperature elevation, sometimes leading to shock. Percussion of the atelectic area is dull or flat. Both the trachea and the heart can deviate to the affected side, especially if the area collapses.

Biot's breathing: Several short breaths followed by long, irregular periods of apnea. Biot's breathing is seen in cases of significant increases in intracranial pressure.

Bradypnea: A slow respiratory rate is called bradypnea and can be seen in end-stage disease, increased intracranial pressure, diabetic coma, and drugs that depress respiration.

Cheyne-Stokes respiration: Cheyne-Stokes breathing is a cyclic pattern where bouts of deep breathing alternate with periods of apnea and is not uncommon in children.

PEARL: Not all respiratory compromise is due to pulmonary problems. Intracranial lesions can cause Cheyne-Stokes and Biot's respiration.

Clubbing: The enlargement of the distal finger phalanx and the loss of the nail bed angle due to chronic pulmonary problems. Clubbing can be seen in infants with congenital disease and in other chronic respiratory conditions.

Consolidation: The coalescence of fluid in the lung instead of air in the air sacs

Cough: A cough is a sudden explosive expiration designed to clear the airway. There are many kinds of coughs from acute to chronic, barking to wheezy, dry or rattling, and those filled with secretions. Plus the cough caused by the annoying tickle in the back of the throat. Asthma and allergies are both common causes of coughs. Some asthmatics present only with a cough and SOB, no wheezing. Of course, URIs are the primary reason that people cough. On PE, if the patient is complaining of cough, listen both before and after a cough to see how the cough might have changed the lung sounds.

PEARL: Throat clearing and coughing have both been observed as tics in neuropsychiatric disease, including those resulting from on-going infections. These coughs are not due to underlying pulmonary conditions.

PEARL: I believe coughing is your friend. I like it when patients move mucus out of the airway. The more mucus

moves out, the less chance it has to consolidate in lung tissue. The more mucus around, the more chance of secondary bacteria taking up residence. I do not believe in cough suppressants unless the cough is so intense and continuous that the patient cannot sleep or rest. Otherwise, I like coughing.

PEARL: Some of the "new" mucus-moving drugs promoted endlessly on TV are just VERY old drugs with new names. Don't be fooled. Marketing is usually driving medicine.

Crackles: Also called rales, crackles are high pitched, discontinuous sounds almost like the noise made by the crinkly plastic bubble wrap used by the post office.

Cyanosis: The blue coloration of the skin or mucous membranes indicating there is not enough oxygen in the blood for some reason. Fingers, toes, and lips are common sites of blue color.

Dyspnea: Unpleasant sensation of shortness of breath where the person feels as though he is not getting enough oxygen. We are not talking here about the feeling everyone gets when they exert themselves past their usual comfort zone. While that feeling isn't fun, it's not worrisome since the person recognizes that breathing will go back to normal shortly. There are a number of reasons for SOB including fevers, infections, high altitude, heart problems, and underlying lung disease. Dyspnea can be exhausting and as the body realizes it needs more oxygen it begins to compensate with use of accessory muscles, retractions, faster respiratory rate, increased heart rate, and nasal flaring. The patient will perceive that more oxygen is urgently needed and may experience a tight chest and feel the need to rest.

PEARL: The SOB experienced with a panic attack is due to a flood of "flight or fight" hormones, including epinephrine, and does not signify underlying lung disease.

Flaring: Infants (and all age groups) in respiratory distress will unconsciously flare their nostrils in an attempt to get more air into the lungs.

Fremitus: Sometimes called a thrill, fremitus is the vibration that can be felt through the chest wall on palpation when the patient is speaking or coughing. If both hands are placed on either side of the chest, the vibrations on one side can be compared to the other side. Alternatively, a stethoscope can be used to auscultate fremitus. Fremitus decreases in pleural effusions, emphysema, lung collapse, edema, or with large masses. Vibrations may be more noticeable when there is obstruction of one bronchus. Ask the patient to repeat the number "99" to evaluate fremitus. Make sure the examining hands are

exerting the same pressure on both sides of the chest for accurate comparison.

Friction rub: A rub is the crackling heard when two rough or dry surfaces chafe together. Sometimes rubs are described as squeaking, grating, or the sound of walking on crunchy snow. I don't happen to think that the rubs I've heard sound like any of those descriptions but we all hear different music. To me it sounds like two things that should be moist, but aren't, moving against each other. Rubs are heard in pericarditis, pneumonia, pleural effusions, and pleurisy. Here the pleura lining the lung is rubbing against the pleura of the chest cavity. Since the rubbing occurs each time the pleura moves, the rub is heard on both inspiration and expiration. Rubs occur when membranes are inflamed and lose their lubrication. A rub does not usually change after a cough.

Grunt: A grunt is a quick, harsh sound of forced expiration against a closed glottis. A grunt temporarily halts expiration and is seen in pneumonia, pulmonary edema, and painful ribs. A newborn with atelectasis will grunt. Infants in respiratory distress may grunt as the body tries to keep air in the lung and keep up the O_2 level. Female tennis players grunt.

Hemoptysis: Blood in the cough product may be from the respiratory system, oral cavity, GI tract, or pulmonary tree. If from the lung, the blood and mucus may be frothy. Try to determine the source. Blood in the pulmonary tree can be infections, due to bleeding disorders, or can be coming from the GI tract. The source may be hard to uncover and here the history and ROS might help.

Hyperpnea: Rapid, deep breathing found after exercise, anxiety, metabolic acidosis, or hypoxia. Deeper than normal breathing is common after exercise. Hyperpnea is seen with pain, respiratory disease, fevers, cardiac problems, certain drugs, hysteria, and high altitude. Hyperpnea is a compensatory measure, trying to get things back to normal. The difference between hyperpnea and hyperventilation is that hyperpnea is an <u>appropriate</u> response to the patient's metabolic state while hyperventilation is an <u>inappropriate</u> response. Hyperpnea is fixing the problem, while hyperventilation is causing the problem.

Hyperventilation: Increased ventilation which results in blowing off CO_2 that may result in hypocapnia. Patients can hyperventilate in cases of asthma, acidosis, anxiety, pulmonary embolism, or pulmonary edema. Treatment involves slowing the rate of CO_2 loss such as breathing only through one nostril or rebreathing the CO_2 you just exhaled by breathing into a paper bag. The difference between hyperpnea and hyperventilation is that hyperpnea is an <u>appropriate</u> response to the patient's metabolic state while hyperventilation is an <u>inappropriate</u> response. Hyperpnea is fixing the problem while hyperventilation is contributing to the problem. I think I just said that above.

Hypoxia: Low oxygen in the blood

Obstructive breathing: When there is a barrier in the airway there will be prolonged expirations because the chest gets overfull (air trapping).

Periodic breathing: Periodic breathing is a normal variant in infants where the child will breathe rapidly for a few breaths and then have a short pause and then resume breathing.

Pleural effusion: An excess of fluid in the pleural space is called a pleural effusion and is the result of increased production of fluid or decreased removal. Normally, the pleural space has just enough fluid to keep the surfaces slippy. For some reason, there is a fluid imbalance and a pressure differential that allows fluid to be forced into the pleural space between the lining of the lung and the lining of the chest wall. A significant effusion can crowd the lung and restrict full expansion, decreasing the efficacy of respiration. The patient may complain of shortness of breath and chest pain. Percussion may find fluid at higher levels than anatomically normal. There will be no breath sounds in the area of effusion because there is no air moving there. An effusion may need to be "tapped" in order to allow the lung to completely reinflate.

Pulmonary edema: Here there is fluid in the lung tissue which may present with a cough productive of frothy, blood-tinged foam. While the problem appears to be in the lung parenchyma, the real trouble lies with ineffective pumping by the heart. If the pump is broken, fluid will back up into the lung and swelling may occur elsewhere in the body. Patients with weak hearts can develop pulmonary edema as can people who have heart damage secondary to infections.

Rales: Also called crackles, rales signify interstitial lung disease. Rales are discrete, non-continuous breath sounds most audible on inspiration. This crinkling noise can be heard in CHF, bronchitis, near-pneumonia, and with fibrosis. Rales are higher pitched than rhonchi.

Respiratory rate: The average RR is about 44 per minute in infants and 16 to 20 in adults. Anything over 60 in infants is considered rapid. The RR will increase for a number of non-pathologic reasons including crying, exercising, and overheating. Fevers can increase the breathing rate. The RR slows when sleeping.

Retractions: Retractions of the soft tissue of the chest during inspiration indicate some degree of respiratory distress and should not be ignored. Babies born with babesiosis can be struggling to breath and be retracting. Retractions include the sucking in of the intercostal muscles, upper abdominal muscles, those below the sternum, and above the clavicles.

PEARL: Abdominal retraction during breathing usually indicates some type of respiratory compromise but can also accompany cases of meningitis, pericarditis, and abdominal pain. There will be greater abdominal movement with breathing in cases of pleurisy and pneumonia.

Rhonchi: Secretions in the moderate and large airways can cause rhonchi which are loud, coarse, gurgling, almost snore-like sounds that are due to a partial blockage of the tube. Rhonchi are usually low-pitched and sonorous. Since they demonstrate only partial obstruction, they can be heard on both inspirations and expirations. Rhonchi can also be caused by swelling and masses. Rhonchi can change after a cough since the fluid can shift.

Shortness of breath: Dyspnea or SOB is defined above.

Sibilant breath sounds: Sibilant sounds are hissing noises like a persistent "s" or "sh."

Sigh: A sigh is a deep inspiration followed by a slow audible expiration. Pathologic sighing as a sign of incomplete respiration is found in babesiosis.

Sonorous breath sounds: A sonorous sound is a deep, resonant, snore-like noise heard when there is fluid in a bronchus like the breath sounds heard in bronchitis. Rhonchi can be sonorous.

Sputum: While I love pus, sputum is my least favorite body fluid. Nonetheless, sputum needs to be defined and discussed. Sputum is the slippy material that is expelled by coughing or clearing the throat. Sputum can contain many things: mucus, cellular debris, blood, pus, and pathogens. Cheesy or caseous material is found in infections like TB. If sputum is available, look at it and collect a sample for testing, such as a smear under the microscope, plus culture and sensitivity. The general rule is the more colorful and foul smelling the sputum, the higher the likelihood of bacterial infection. If there are squamous cells present, the specimen came from high in the respiratory tract above the larynx. This will not yield reliable results. A "good" sputum sample has macrophages from deep in the alveolar sacs. The presence of eosinophils indicates allergies or parasites. Neutrophils suggest infection since they are the primary component of pus. Gram stain might help categorize the pathogen.

PEARL: To help a child get a "good" productive cough have him take several deep breaths and then cough. Kids often say they can't get anything up but they often do when using this technique.

PEARL: Bb are difficult to identify from sputum and rarely grow on a sputum culture.

Stridor: A somewhat musical sound audible without a stethoscope and most predominant during inspiration. Stridor means there is some obstruction of the upper airway. Similar to a wheeze, the two can be hard to distinguish. Stridor is thought to be louder and primarily audible on inspiration. Heard closer to the larynx than the lower chest, stridor can be associated with epiglottitis. Even though distinction may be difficult, it is important to try to tell if you are hearing a wheeze or stridor since treatments are quite different. The stridor of epiglottis can be mistaken for croup.

Tachypnea: Rapid, shallow breathing, with the definition of rapid depending on age

PEARL: Do not make yourself glum by splitting the hairs between tachypnea, hyperpnea, and hyperventilation. If the respiratory rate is increased and does not seem to be trending toward normal, and the patient seems to be in any level of distress, investigate what is going on.

Wheeze: To create a wheeze, air flow must be obstructed at some level. Wheezing is commonly associated with SOB. Asthma is the most common cause of wheezing, although allergies and URIs are close behind. Generally the wheezing heard in these three cases is audible throughout all the lung fields. Sometimes you will put a stethoscope on an asthmatic kid's back and hear absolutely nothing as the child is struggling to breathe. Treatment should be initiated stat. Here the sound of wheezing is welcome. A monophonic wheeze over a single location indicates localized obstruction like a tumor or FB. Wheezes often start high-pitched and treatment usually lowers the pitch of the wheeze to the point where the lung sounds more like rhonchi than wheezes.

PEARL: Usually an inspiratory wheeze is indicative of high airway obstruction and an expiratory wheeze suggests low airway obstruction.

PEARL: In crying babies, listen between cries. Inspiration is the best time to hear a wheeze when options are limited. Be glad the child has enough air moving to cry.

PEARL: New-onset allergies can cause wheezing and have been reported in Lyme patients.

Yawn: A yawn is a normal involuntary action where a large slow breath is inspired usually in association with fatigue or sleepiness. Some speculate that yawning is an attempt to increase the oxygen levels in the individual. The only reason yawning appears on this list is because yawning has been documented as a muscular tic in cases of neuropsychiatric manifestations of other conditions, including PANDAS, and because air hunger in babesiosis can manifest as frequent yawns.

Problems with respiration that can present as part of the clinical picture of a TBI, as a co-morbidity, or that should be in the differential diagnosis include:

NOTE: I apologize for redundancies. Several of the conditions listed below also appear in Chapter 17-A under Respiratory Rate, *discussing the importance of recognizing and managing any emergency situations before conducting the full PE.*

1. **Asthma** is becoming a more frequent diagnosis in all age groups and can be associated with infection, allergies, and irritants. We used to think that if the patient wasn't wheezing, then he couldn't have asthma. Now we know that asthma can present with cough or no obvious symptoms aside from shortness of breath. We also used to say that no one ever died from asthma. Unfortunately, that assertion has also been disproved. A susceptible airway is triggered by a stimulus to constrict in paroxysms usually causing wheezing, which can progress to significant dyspnea. Kids are most vulnerable to asthma attacks and the symptoms can come on slowly or quite suddenly. School age kids seem to be the most affected. If triggered by allergens, the asthmatic response can be mediated by eosinophils and IgE. Boys are about twice as likely to have asthma as girls, but that ratio becomes more equitable as they get older. As many as 10% of kids will have some degree of asthmatic symptoms during childhood. They are normal between attacks.

   On PE, usually there will be wheezing and some rhonchi throughout all lung fields. The less you hear, the worse the attack. Expiration will be prolonged as the patient tries to get the air out through the constricted airways. Sometimes the wheeze can be heard without a stethoscope.

2. **Bronchiolitis** is inflammation of the bronchioles in the lower pulmonary tree, usually caused by viruses such as RSV. The child presents with what appears to be a URI but then quickly deteriorates to respiratory compromise with wheezes, crackles, tachypnea, expiratory obstruction, tachycardia, hacking cough, circumoral cyanosis, and retractions. Bronchiolitis is most

commonly diagnosed in children less than 18 months. They usually have no fever, but can be quite lethargic.

3. **Bronchitis** is an acute inflammation of the tracheo-bronchial tree which can be due to infections or irritations like dusts or fumes. Bronchitis is usually preceded by the signs and symptoms of a URI such as coryza (inflammation of the nasal passages with profuse clear discharge), malaise, mild fever, chills, aches, and sore throat. The beginning of the cough is probably the onset of the bronchitis. The cough starts dry and non-productive but soon sputum might be raised. The more colorful and purulent the sputum, the more likely a bacterial etiology. There may be mild pain in the chest which is aggravated by coughing. A moderate fever around 101 to 102 might continue for a few days. The patient feels bad for 3 to 5 days, but signs may last longer. Persistent fever and illness might suggest pneumonia. While acute bronchitis is usually viral, secondary bacterial infection can settle into the secretions in the pulmonary tract. With deeper penetration, infection can invade the lung parenchyma. Pneumonia is a common complication.

4. **Chronic obstructive pulmonary disease:** COPD is long-term airway obstruction. There are a number of possible underlying causes, but the most common is smoking. COPD is divided into two primary presentations: chronic bronchitis and emphysema, but most patients have aspects of both. Both types of COPD present with dyspnea on exertion (DOE), hypoxemia, and abnormal PFTs.

   a. **Emphysema:** The lungs of an emphysema patient are chronically inflamed and enzymes destroy tissue. Scarring and fibrosis result. The lungs lose their elasticity and become overinflated and the patient has a hard time exhaling the old air out of his lungs so that fresh, O_2-rich air can replace it. DOE gets gradually worse. Smoking cessation will halt the disease progression but much of the damage is irreversible. The patient will have a chronic cough and need to use accessory muscles to breathe. SOB is the primary symptom. The patient can lose weight and usually looks bad enough to end up as the face on the cigarette package. Often these patients have a barrel chest which is an increased AP diameter due to chronic hyperinflation of the chest cavity. There is hyperresonance on percussion because there is more air than tissue present. There are markedly decreased BSs and prolonged expiration.

   b. **Chronic bronchitis** causes hypertrophy of mucus glands with damage to the cilia lining the respiratory tract. As with emphysema there is chronic inflammation. There is almost always mucus in the airways with a severe ventilation/perfusion imbalance. There is a frequent productive cough and exertional dyspnea. These patients can gain weight due to edema. On physical exam, there may be cyanosis, rhonchi, wheezes, neck vein distension, and pedal edema. The exam will likely be interrupted with productive coughing.

5. **Croup** is a viral respiratory inflammation characterized by stridor on inspiration and respiratory distress. The child may present with a barking cough, often at night, seeming suffocation, retractions, long inspirations, and distress. The airway can spasm. Presenting mostly in kids 6 months to 3-years-old, fever is present in only about half the cases. Intense hydration and humidification can alleviate symptoms and the child may need to be hospitalized.

6. **Epiglottitis** can be an emergency. Inflammation of the epiglottis can be life-threatening with symptoms including cough, hoarseness, difficulty swallowing, and signs of upper respiratory tract obstruction. A lateral X-ray view of the neck may be needed to confirm the diagnosis.

7. **Obstructed airway** is a common reason for respiratory distress in kids and may be the most pertinent to TBI patients due to allergies from medicines and other sensitizers. Airway obstruction from allergies causes the airway to swell, eventually occluding the passage and this presentation can be part of an anaphylactic reaction. Symptoms may build gradually or can be surprisingly rapid. This is a medical emergency and is most often treated with epinephrine, steroids, and bronchodilators. Airway obstruction can also be due to a foreign body which can be dislodged acutely by the Heimlich maneuver or through other removal techniques. Masses can also obstruct the airway but these cases usually have a gradual onset of symptoms. If the obstruction appears to have been caused by an allergic reaction, try to identify the allergen. Review medication lists and make sure the person does not get another dose of the suspected medication. Identifying the causal agent is not always easy.

8. **Pleurisy** is inflammation of the membranes lining the chest cavity and the lungs. There can be sharp, stabbing pain that increases with respiration and can significantly limit the movement of the chest on the affected side. The patient will complain of SOB. On exam there will be a pleural friction rub, which is a coarse, creaky sound heard during late inspiration and early expiration. Over the area of inflammation, coarse vibrations can be felt.

9. **Pneumonia** is an inflammation of the lower respiratory tract due to infection or chemical irritation. Pneumonia can affect an entire lobe or just a section. The actual lung parenchyma is involved including the alveoli and interstitial tissue. With bacterial pneumonia, the patient may be more acutely ill but may respond more rapidly to treatment than with viral etiologies. On PE, there may be a section of the lung area with no or diminished breath sounds. The Mycoplasma genus, which can be tick-borne, can cause atypical pneumonias. X-ray can show a white-out of the affected area due to increased fluid and immune molecules at the site. The X-ray may lag behind the clinical picture by hours. So treat the person not the image. In patients with chronic TBIs, those who are bedridden or in late stages of disease can present with pneumonia due to opportunistic secondary infections.

- **Aspiration pneumonia**: Pneumonia due to aspiration is caused by inhaling into the lungs: food, saliva, mucus, gastric contents such as vomit, or other substances. Patients who lose their gag reflex due to CNS depression, as with alcohol intoxication, are especially prone to aspirate. Newborns can inhale any manner of fluids during the birth process including meconium.

Pneumonia can be bacterial, viral, fungal, or irritant-induced. Common bacterial etiologies include:

- Strep, also called Pneumococcal pneumonia, is probably the most common.

- Staphlococcus

- Haemophilus *influenzae* is a relatively common cause of bacterial pneumonia. Unfortunately H. *flu* got its name when it was mistaken for the viral cause of flu in the pandemic of 1889.

PEARL: Just as the many medical errors that have been made in the past, someday the misinformation around Lyme will be just a sad footnote in the history of medicine.

- Mycoplasma *pneumoniae* is the most common pathogen causing pneumonia in 5 to 35-year-olds. M. *pneumoniae* starts off looking like flu and then increases in severity. The patient presents with purulent, blood-streaked sputum. Unlike a number of other pneumonia-causing pathogens, M. *pneumoniae* progresses slowly. Symptoms can persist and there can be numerous extra-pulmonary complications including anemias, emboli, polyarthritis, neurologic syndromes such as meningoencephalitis, myelitis (inflammation of the spinal cord), peripheral neuropathies,

and cerebellar ataxias. PE may be unimpressive compared to how bad the person feels. Pneumonia due to M. *pneumoniae* is often called atypical pneumonia. Maculopapular rashes present in 10% to 20% of these patients and some display erythema multiforme. Recent tick drags have shown that M. *pneumoniae* can be found in ticks along with its cousin, M. *fermentans*.

Pneumonia can occur in TBIs including Q fever and tularemia.

10. **Pulmonary embolism:** An embolus is an obstruction of a blood vessel by a clot or other substance. There is a sudden lodging of a blood clot in a pulmonary vessel with a resulting loss of blood supply to the lung tissue. Most often a thrombus breaks off from a DVT in the leg. Clots can form in patients at bed rest or other state of immobility because of the static blood. Signs and symptoms include: SOB, pain, tachycardia, cough, tachypnea, pleural friction rub, gallop, and rales. A pulmonary embolism can be hard to diagnose early on because the signs and symptoms can be non-specific and vary in intensity. Symptoms can present within minutes, although an infarct due to an embolus may take longer to manifest. A scan to compare the ventilation to the perfusion may be needed to make the diagnosis.

PEARL: Many TBI patients have limited mobility because of severe fatigue and prostration. This would increase the risk of clotting. Also, the possibility of DIC in the end-stages of any of the TBIs would increase the chance of coagulopathies and possible clots.

11. **Respiratory failure:** In respiratory failure, gas exchange is hindered to the point of impending compromise and is seen at the end-stage of nearly every disease. The complexities of the condition is beyond the scope of this book and involve hypoxia, hypercapnea, hypoventilation, and acid/base imbalances.

12. **Respiratory syncytial virus** (RSV) is a lower respiratory tract infection that can be fatal in infants and young kids. By causing the formation of cell masses connected by syncytium, RSV can result in pneumonia and bronchiolitis. Hard to diagnose early, this condition can confuse many differential diagnoses. Most cases occur in winter and early spring and present with dyspnea, cough, wheeze, and fever. Severe signs and symptoms may require hospitalization before the diagnosis is made.

Lung problems associated with specific TBIs:

a. Babesiosis

While air hunger is not necessarily common with Babesia infection, when it occurs Babesia should be included in the differential diagnosis. Air hunger can be subtle or intense. If you do not have enough functional RBCs in the circulation you might begin to feel hypoxic. Likewise, if excessive fluid is present in the lung tissue, gas exchange could be compromised.

Air hunger can range from excessive sighing and yawning to the inability to take a satisfactory deep breath. Eventually frank shortness of breath and respiratory distress could ensue. SOB can become serious quickly and the patient may need hospitalization for respiratory support. B. *duncani* might affect the lungs more than B. *microti*. Babies born with babesiosis can be struggling to breathe from the onset. Their problem is not underlying pulmonary disease but not enough working RBCs to carry oxygen. Their hypoxia needs urgent attention.

PEARL: My son had obvious signs of air hunger in association with babesiosis before we had ever heard the term. He had no evidence of anemia. Another teen male patient with no signs of anemia, clearly described his air hunger to me in conjunction with his babesiosis. Without prompting, both complained of frequent inefficient yawning and sighing and the sensation of not being able to get a good breath. The pathophysiologic mechanism here was likely mild lung edema from B. duncani *instead of anemia induced air hunger which is more likely associated with B.* microti.

b. Tularemia

Tularemia is caused by Francisella *tularensis,* a bacterial pathogen. Pulmonary manifestations are common including pneumonia, atypical or otherwise. Imaging studies have shown nodules, consolidation, and abscesses in the lungs. Francisella *tularensis*-induced pneumonia can cause chest pain, bloody sputum, dry or productive coughs, retrosternal burning, shortness of breath, and trouble breathing. Patients may have reduced breath sounds or rales on exam. Respiratory failure has been known to lead to death. In older populations, pneumonic tularemia presents with cough, high fever, extreme exhaustion. vomiting, diarrhea, enlarged liver and spleen, and localized pneumonia. Tularemia can affect many body systems and respiratory signs and symptoms occur most often in patients who inhaled the infectious agent.

c. Q Fever

Coxiella *burnetii*, a tick-borne Rickettsia, can cause a non-productive cough and pneumonia. X-ray evidence of localized pneumonitis can develop in the 2nd week. Between 30% and 50% of those with symptomatic infection will develop pneumonia. If symptoms persist, the alveolar linings can swell and plasma cells can infiltrate the lungs. The alveoli can become cluttered with cellular debris.

d. Lyme

The effects of Lyme on the respiratory system are usually secondary and incidental to more pressing problems. Maybe the theory that Bb avoids areas with high oxygen concentrations is true. I did find numerous vague references to pneumonitis, cough, and difficulty breathing but these manifestations could have been due to co-infections or co-morbidities. Of course, end-stage disease in any TBI will involve pulmonary compromise.

Ancillary tests:

While the ROS, history, and PE will provide considerable diagnostic information, in some cases additional testing will be needed. In the case of pulmonary problems consider:

- Chest X-ray: Distinguishes fluid from gas. Can see collapsed tissue (atelectasis), effusions, fluid levels, air in the thorax, lesions, some masses, structural shifts, and edema. In acute processes like pneumonia and CHF, the X-ray may be hours behind the clinical picture and give a false sense of security that nothing really bad is happening. More definitive scans may be needed to get a better handle on the clinical picture.

- Sputum: Look at color, quantity, and odor. Consider stains and cultures to identify pathogens and cytology looking for malignancy. Remember that Bb do not easily culture in the lab so you cannot rule out Lyme based on a negative sputum culture. If you get a positive, immediately call the Vatican because you have witnessed a miracle.

- Pulmonary function tests: PFTs provide information on volumes, flow rates, and tissue compliance. These results can be compared over time. I was once tasked to write a guideline on interpretation of PFTs for occupational medicine physicians. What a miserable month that was.

- Bronchoscopy involves using a scope to visualize into the pulmonary tract. For example, this test could show HPV lesions on the larynx as part of the differential diagnosis.

- Arterial blood gases: ABGs are used to assess gas exchange by measuring levels of O_2, CO_2, and pH. If you are ordering an ABG on a TBI patient, you have a sick kid in front of you and you may need to step back and regroup.

- Lung scans: CAT scans, MRIs, and ventilation/perfusion (V/Q) scans might be used to uncover information not necessarily related to TBIs but important from a co-morbidity and differential diagnosis perspective.

Section 17-J

Heart, Circulation, and Pertinent Differential

You won't find a solution by saying there's no problem.

William Rostler

HEART

When patients die from Lyme it's often because of associated heart problems. No amount of writing in this textbook is going to turn any of us into cardiologists. The point of this chapter will try to get you comfortable with what is normal so that you can discern abnormalities and refer as needed.

If Lyme is the underlying cause of the cardiac problem, the *Lyme must be treated,* and not just the sequelae of the Lyme. I hear so many stories here in Southern Chester County, PA, of parents who are so grateful to the cardiologist who saved their Lyme child by putting in a pacemaker. With all due respect, if the infectious disease doc had treated the Lyme appropriately in the first place, maybe the kid would not have needed the pacemaker. Make sure the cardiologist you partner with understands this concept. Do not lose your patient. If active Lyme is the underlying cause of cardiac complications, the person cannot be expected to improve if the etiologic agent is still in business.

Auscultation of the normal heart:

Some people got it and some people don't. I am a visual learner. No matter how many hours I spent listening to recorded heart sounds in med school, I never had the auditory acuity or the patience to differentiate the subtle sounds. Nonetheless, there were days when I had to listen to too many heart sounds. I survived, and so did most of my patients, because I learned to discern what was normal. Anything beyond that was under suspicion. I don't think I was worse than the average doctor. I think most lie like crazy about what they might have heard. When the attending would say, "Did you hear that click?" we would all stand mutely. As he walked away, we would shake our heads and shrug indicating that not one of us had heard a thing.

The **bell** of the stethoscope is best for low-pitched sounds like some mitral murmurs and the S3 sounds of heart failure. The **diaphragm** filters out those low pitched sounds and is better for the higher pitched 2nd heart sound, clicks, and aortic murmurs. Consider using both. The patient can be supine or sitting up. Auscultate at the apex, at the base, and in the areas to the right and left of the sternum.

You should hear:

1st heart sound: Lub or S1 is heard just before the carotid pulse. S1 is louder at the apex and low pitched.

2nd heart sound: Dub or S2 is auscultated just after the carotid pulse and is louder at the base and higher pitched.

A regular rhythm without skips, pauses, extra beats, flurries, or fluctuations. Rate should be within the range for the patient's age, taking into account any extenuating circumstances such as crying or fever.

A measure of actual heart rate is preferred to pulse in younger children. Directly auscultate the heart to get the number of beats per minute. HR in kids is more variable than in adults and more affected by illness.

The normal HR for healthy kids can range 30 to 50 beats above or below average:

Birth:	140
Up to 6 months:	130
6 to 12 months:	115
1 to 2 years:	110
2 to 6 years:	104
6 to 10 years:	95

The average heart rate continues to decline into adulthood where the average BPM is 72. Athletes can have normal bradycardias into the 40s. Fevers tend to raise the HR. Beyond the neonatal period a heart rate above 180 usually suggests PAT (paroxysmal atrial tachycardia).

You should not hear:

Murmurs: A murmur is an abnormal heart sound associated with turbulent blood flow usually originating at the site of one of the heart valves. Apparently there is enough disruption either through stenosis (constriction) or back flow (regurgitation) to make some noise. While murmurs are often classified as physiologic (benign) or pathologic (abnormal and potentially problematic), with Lyme patients proceed with caution before you too quickly dismiss a murmur. What are heart valves made of? Collagen. What do Bb love? Collagen. I have learned the hard way not to underestimate Bb. Although I have no published evidence of this, I think it might be possible that a child with a benign physiologic murmur could be more susceptible to valve involvement by Bb than a child with no underlying condition. Whether that theory has any scientific merit or not, it is always prudent to remember that two things can be happening at once and, in the case of the cardiac manifestations of Lyme, err on the side of the conservative.

Murmurs are defined by where they are best heard, corresponding to the location on the chest over the valve that is most likely to be involved. There are many terms used to describe them including: soft, blowing, loud, booming, early, late, contraction, relaxation, systolic, diastolic, crescendo, decrescendo, flow, holosystolic, sloshing, stiff, variable, high frequency, harsh, rumbling, regurgitant, and mid-phase. They can be labeled with more than one of these monikers at a time. Different murmurs can be heard in different parts of the cardiac cycle. Murmurs can change intensity with inspiration and position. Of course, the description and the grading lies in the ear of the beholder.

Murmur Grades:

1. Faint

2. Quiet

3. Moderate

4. Loud with palpable thrill (vibration from the murmur felt on palpation)

5. Very loud with thrill and can be perceived with stethoscope partly off chest

6. Very loud with thrill detected without stethoscope

While many murmurs will be of no consequence, in TBI patients retain a high index of suspicion.

PEARL: Murmurs Grade 3 or more may suggest heart disease and should be evaluated further. About half of all kids have benign heart murmurs. Unless you are an expert in this area and confident in your assessment, murmurs should be assessed by a pediatric cardiologist. Most murmurs in kids are deemed innocent or functional. Non-benign murmurs can either be congenital or secondary to acquired dysfunction. In the past, the most common cause of acquired heart diseases causing a murmur was rheumatic fever. RF is much less common now in the US since we aggressively treat Strep. Cyanosis in the presence of a murmur is significant and needs urgent assessment.

Gallops: Extra, or adventitious, beats that sound like a horse galloping. Usually a third sound constitutes a gallop, although sometimes an S3 and S4 combine.

S3: In the case of an S3 gallop the examiner will hear S1, S2, and then S3. Sometimes called the Kentucky gallop because to some (not me) the beats sound like ken tuck y. Benign in kids, athletes, and some pregnancies, later this ventricular gallop can mean heart failure. Lyme has been associated with heart failure.

S4: This atrial gallop is rare and in keeping with the horse theme is called the Tennessee (Tenn ess ee) gallop. At fast rates, S4 is hard to distinguish from S3 and sometimes this garnish is termed a summation gallop or S7.

Clicks: Clicks are short high-pitched sounds that may be associated with abnormal valve motion and are often associated with mitral valve disease.

Splits: S2 sometimes splits normally during inspiration due to a decrease in intrathoracic pressure. A wide split can be associated with pathology like right bundle branch block or pulmonary stenosis.

Snaps: Snaps can be the cracking sound of abnormal valve movement.

Rubs: A scratching, creaking high-pitched noise, a rub is the result of two surfaces moving against each other. Here the pericardium is inflamed and the friction of the layers chafing together can be heard. There can be rubbing if there is not enough lubricant or if there is too much swelling or fluid in an area. Patients with pericarditis or pleural effusion may present with audible rubs. Rubs are dependent on body position and can change frequently and rapidly.

Thrills: A thrill is not exactly a heart sound but rather the palpable vibration associated with loud murmurs.

Cardiac problems potentially associated with TBIs: (Here I am mostly talking Lyme.)

- **Dysrhythmias** are abnormal heart beat patterns. Usually the heart beats in a normal sinus rhythm, where the electrical stimulus is initiated in the sinus node and continues throughout the heart in the flow that nature intended. Many things can alter the electrical conductivity and cause the impulse to either originate elsewhere or impede the normal conduction. The list is long and varied and can include congenital problems, some medications, inflammation, infection, and multiple underlying disease states. Our focus here is Lyme. Bb have been associated with various abnormal heart rhythms including atrial fibrillation, skipped beats, extra beats, premature beats, and flutters. Lyme patients frequently complain of palpitations. A palpitation is a perceptible fluttering of the heart. In contrast, many dysrhythmias occur without the individual ever being aware. We all experience short episodes of inconsequential dysrhythmia.

*PEARL: **Rhythm** is the regularity with which something occurs such as the beating of a drum, the pacing of a bass, or the timing of a heart beat. **Rate** is how fast something goes in time.*

PEARL: A pet peeve of mine is the use of the word arrhythmia when clearly dysrhythmia is meant. Although, these two terms are often used interchangeably, the "a" in arrhythmia means without and the "dys" in dysrhythmia means abnormal. Same number of syllables, and equally difficult to spell, why not just use the correct term? I've waited hundreds of pages to get that off my chest.

Abnormal rhythms that result in diminished perfusion or other untoward effects may need to be overridden with pacemakers or medications. If the underlying etiology is Lyme, for goodness sake, treat the Lyme.

PEARL: A Holter monitor is a device meant to be worn for an extended period in order to better capture abnormal heart rates and rhythms that might elude capture during the short timing of an EKG.

- **Abnormal heart rates** occur for many reasons, not all of them pathologic. Trained athletes and meditating monks often have resting heart rates in the 30s. I don't know about athletic monks. Exercise, excitement, and crying will appropriately raise the rate. Medication can alter rates and many abnormal rates are the result of pathology in other organ systems not directly attributable to the heart. Bradycardia is a rate that is too slow for the individual and the circumstance. Tachycardia is a rate that is too fast for the individual and the circumstance.

PEARL: While the PE will provide useful information about the heart rate and rhythm, an EKG might be more definitive. While not perfect in identifying ischemia, EKGs can give a good idea about rate, rhythm, blocks, and abnormal beats. If there is any question about a cardiac component to a patient's Lyme, do a baseline EKG. Further, if the antibiotic selected is one that could impact the QT interval or otherwise impact the heart, a baseline EKG is prudent. This EKG can then serve as a basis of comparison during the therapeutic course.

- **Heart block**: The term heart block refers to an impediment in the normal electrical conduction. Many things can interfere with normal impulse transfer including structural changes, ischemia, hypothyroidism, digitalis toxicity, K imbalance, infarct, vagal nerve dysfunction, mitral valve problems, heart failure, and hypoxia. We

have clear documentation that Lyme can be involved in a number of these pathophysiologic processes.

Lyme has often been associated with various heart blocks. Cardiac problems associated with Lyme often include conduction system problems. The most common site of blockage is thought to be at the AV node. Pacing may be needed in about a third of these patients and they may present with chest pain, palpitations, syncope, and dyspnea. Keep a high index of suspicion.

PEARL: Lyme has been associated with AV block, 1ˢᵗ, 2ⁿᵈ, and 3ʳᵈ degree blocks, junctional rhythms, and asystolic pauses.

PEARL: Treat the Lyme if you want the overlying cardiac condition to respond.

PEARL: What is the mechanism by which Bb perform their cardiac mischief? Many ideas have been postulated. First, Bb are known to affect the systems that influence the heart such as the endocrine and nervous systems. Also likely is the possibility that spirochetes do direct damage to the heart tissue itself. As I have mentioned once or twice, Bb seem to gravitate to high concentrations of collagen and there is considerable collagen in the valves and blood vessels inside the heart. Probably a combination of factors is involved. Remember, it doesn't matter how the elephant got on the road, as long as we get him off.

- **Valve problems:** A valve is a flap of tissue found in a hollow organ or passageway that is designed to keep fluids flowing in one direction. The GI tract and the circulatory systems have many valves so that flow goes only one way. This makes their function much more efficient. Once things start going the wrong way, problems arise. The cardiac valves keep blood going in the direction it's supposed to. Problems can occur when valves weaken or stiffen or otherwise allow back-flow. One reason for impaired valvular function is infection. Infections such as Strep can result in RF with significant cardiac manifestations. Some infections result in the formation of vegetations on the valves themselves, which are a combination of pathogen, fibrin, white cells, and other fragments that clog the works and prevent proper operation of the valve. These vegetations can break off as emboli and can damage other organs. There is reason to suspect that Bb may act in similar fashion, but the mechanism is still poorly understood. Ultrasound may be needed to better define the condition of the cardiac valves.

- **Inflammation:** Inflammation due to infection or other causes can manifest in various heart locations and can be acute or chronic. Structures of interest to TBI patients include the pericardium which is the membranous sac around the heart, the myocardium which is the actual heart muscle, and the endocardium which is the lining of the chambers, valves, and blood vessels. Any or all of these structures can get inflamed. Sometimes it is hard to tell one from the other. The literature is lax in mixing the terms and in making distinctions when sometimes none are warranted. For our purposes, it is important that you recognize when something is amiss and partner with a cardiologist who understands Lyme. Bb have been implicated in all the following inflammatory processes:

Pericarditis: The pericardium is the protective membrane that covers the heart. Inflammation can be due to a number of causes including infection and can be acute or chronic. The underlying pathophysiology can be fibrous or effusive with purulence or blood in the pericardial sac. Chronic forms are mostly due to constrictive formations like scarring that can thicken the pericardium. RF with cardiac manifestations can cause pericarditis with friction rub. The patient can present with pleuritic pain that increases with deep inspiration and decreases when position is changed. Pain can be of sudden onset and continue for days. Usually the pain is substernal to the left of midline and it can radiate to the back or subclavicular area. The discomfort can be mild and superficial or deep and severe. Often the pain is described as stabbing or knife-like. The pain tends to increase with movement and coughing and decrease when sitting up or leaning forward, since this position pulls the inflamed pericardium away from the diaphragm and other tissues. Likewise, the friction rub may be less audible under these conditions.

PEARL: There are lessons to be learned from rheumatic fever. RF is a systemic inflammatory disease of childhood that can be recurrent and is associated with a Strep infection. RF can impact many organ systems. Rheumatic heart disease is the set of cardiac manifestations attributed to RF. Early heart problems can occur, with chronic valve problems developing later. Damage is often permanent. Systemically, the patient can present with migratory joint pain or polyarthritis with swelling, redness, and effusion in the joints. There may be skin lesions and a small percentage may display red lesions with blanched centers called erythema marginatum. Subcutaneous nodules on or near joints and on the scalp and hands might be observed. Early neuropsychiatric symptoms include irritability, decline in legible writing, and inability to concentrate which can progress to chorea with purposeless, non-repetitive, involuntary muscle movements, along with problems with coordination and muscle weakness. Some type of carditis develops in about half of the RF patients. With pericarditis there may be an audible friction rub. A myocarditis can develop with Aschoff's bodies which are small nodules composed of

pathogen and white cells found in the cardiac tissue. There can be cellular swelling and fragmentation of collagen leading to fibrosis and scarring of the valves. The valve leaflets can swell and erode. Debris and deposits can form bead-like vegetations in and on the valves. These can break off as emboli and affect other organs. Endocarditis from RF affects the mitral valve most in females and the aortic valve in males and the tricuspid can be affected in both genders resulting in a cacophony of loud murmurs.

Long-term antibiotics are an accepted treatment for chronic cardiac manifestations of RF.

Endocarditis: The endocardium is the endothelial membrane that lines the chambers of the heart, the valves, and is continuous with the lining of the arteries and veins. Endocarditis is inflammation of this membrane. This inflammation can be due to infection or immune processes. Infectious etiologies are usually bacterial but fungus is found in some cases. As unappealing as this may sound, there are often vegetative growths comprised of fibrin, pathogen, platelets, white cells, and other debris that aggregate on valves and vessels. These vegetations can break off and embolize to other organs such as the spleen, kidneys, CNS, or lungs. These emboli do not dissolve entirely with anticoagulants as thrombotic emboli might. They lodge in the end-organ and can cause ischemia and infarction. Vegetative endocarditis has been reported with Bb but in several cases the vegetations were too small to be detected with an echocardiogram. The vegetations may contribute to relapses since they could act as a repository for the spirochetes. Their physical presence can affect the valve and cause the subsequent murmur. Endocarditis can be fatal and there is a significant mortality even if aggressively treated. Endocarditis can cause severe and permanent valve damage leading to insufficiency and subsequent heart failure. Prosthetic valves are also susceptible. Initial signs and symptoms can be nonspecific such as weakness, fatigue, weight loss, anorexia, arthralgia, and night sweats. More than 90% have intermittent fever. Sometimes the symptoms can last for weeks. If they resolve, they can recur. Usually a loud regurgitant murmur is heard. Whenever there is a suddenly changing murmur or a new onset murmur in the presence of fever, think endocarditis.

Myocarditis: The myocardium is the heart muscle and is the middle layer of the heart. Inflammation of the cardiac muscle is myocarditis. Bb are thought to get inside the cardiac cells and cause conduction problems. Myocarditis can be acute or chronic and occur at any age. Early symptoms can be nonspecific with fatigue, dyspnea, palpitations, and fever. Often myocarditis comes from an infection that started elsewhere in the body and became systemic. The originating pathogen can be viral, bacterial, and occasionally fungal. Other etiologies include autoimmunity, RF, radiation, heat stroke, chemicals such as alcohol, and numerous parasites such as helminths. The patient may present with a heart beat that sounds weak at the apex, an irregular rapid pulse, dysrhythmias, and tenderness over the precordium.

Carditis: A somewhat nonspecific term referring to inflammation of several layers of the heart and can include pericarditis, myocarditis, or endocarditis. In one reported case, white cell infiltrate of the myocardium had a substantial concentration of macrophages and we are learning that monocytes/macrophages may be the primary immune responders to Bb infection.

Pancarditis: Pancarditis refers to inflammation of all the structures of the heart and so would include myocarditis, pericarditis, and endocarditis.

PEARL. My Swedish co-worker died from cardiac manifestations of Lyme. He had struggled with cardiac Lyme for several years. His ID doctors treated the sequelae with pacers and cardiac meds but never adequately addressed the Lyme. His death certificate listed cardiopulmonary arrest, which is what we all ultimately die from, and is the fall-back on every certificate filled out by apathetic house staff. We will never know the full extent of the impact of Bb on the heart unless we have accurate record-keeping and list Lyme when appropriate. This subterfuge helps no one and public health suffers.

PEARL: Some articles on Lyme carditis would be laughable if the condition were not potentially so serious. The authors often try to minimize the importance of the condition, stressing that the majority of cases, probably as many as 90%, survive. The 10% would beg to differ, if they could. Such perky prose is best left to teen tabloids, rather than used to encourage HCPs to make light of a potentially fatal complication.

- **Cardiomyopathy** is direct damage to the heart muscle or myocardium due to disease or other modes of injury. Cardiomyopathy can impede the normal, effective contraction of the heart. Damage to the muscle can lead to fibrosis which can restrict motion. The sequelae can include metabolic malfunctions that impair normal efficiency. The degree of damage will determine the effect on function. Lyme is theorized to cause direct harm to the heart muscle in some cases. Here you would want to curtail the pathogen as much as feasible in an attempt to circumvent more destruction.

PEARL: Some of the literature suggests that cardiac problems associated with Lyme can ONLY occur early in the clinical course. I know patients where the onset was quite delayed after the implicated tick bite. If the cardiac symptoms start late, should they be ignored and declared to be non-Lyme related? What purpose would be served? Keep a high index of suspicion and don't believe everything you read.

PEARL: There are many kinds of congenital heart anomalies and some can have serious repercussions. Any abnormalities on the cardiac exam, or a child who is cyanotic or struggling to breathe, should be aggressively evaluated and addressed. Lyme is thought to be associated with some congenital heart conditions. Refer as needed, always keeping in mind your responsibility to manage any underlying TBI.

PEARL: Chapter 30: Special Populations *reviews the congenital cardiac anomalies associated with gestational Lyme. Kids infected* in utero *have presented with palpitations, PVCs, septal defects, murmurs, MVP, cavernous hemangiomas, and structural deformities.*

CIRCULATION

Circulation is the movement of fluids such as blood and lymph. In general, we usually think of blood, but lymph must also be considered. Arteries move blood away from the heart, under pressure that can be felt as a pulse. Veins move blood toward the heart with the help of skeletal muscle and valves. Lymph sloshes to its own drummer, although there are vessels in the lymphatic system eventually connecting with the venous circulation.

When assessing circulation on physical exam check pulses for symmetry and extremities for abnormal temperature and swelling.

Pulses

A pulse is the palpable tap that can be felt by the expansion and relaxation of arteries as the blood moves through under pressure. Pulses are assessed by rate, rhythm, and intensity. The thumb should not be used to check a pulse since it has a slight pulse of its own. Also, one should not reach across the windpipe as they do on TV to check a carotid pulse since this maneuver could potentially compromise the airway. Usually people do not assess pulses long enough and if you discern any abnormality, check again for at least 30 seconds. Check all pulses for strength and symmetry.

A normal pulse should just come out to meet you with a tap on the exam finger, neither mousy nor obnoxious. While a pulse can be felt at any place where an artery is close enough to the surface of the skin to be perceived, the most common pulse points include: radial at the wrist, carotid in the neck, brachial under the arm, femoral in the groin, popliteal behind the knee, and dorsalis pedis on the top of the foot.

Large, intense, bounding pulses can be due to hyperkinesis, anxiety, exercise, fever, anemia, or hyperthyroidism. A thready pulse is weak and barely perceptible. A small, weak pulse can mean decreased stroke volume like that found in heart failure, shock, or obstruction of left ventricular output as found in aortic stenosis.

Vasculature

Look for enlarged or broken vessels, varicose veins, spider veins, bruising, petechiae, and purpura. Finding such lesions can indicate problems with the small vessels, inflammation, or clotting disorders. Cavernous hemangiomas have been associated with congenital Lyme. These dilated tangles of blood vessels can be anywhere, but are most often recognized in the brain. They can be asymptomatic or cause problems. These are not found on PE but usually uncovered with scanning.

> PEARL: The excess inflammation that is associated with some TBIs can cause a mild hypercoagulability which is associated with stickier blood.

> PEARL: Vasculitis, especially cerebral vasculitis, can contribute to vascular headaches. In some cases this inflammation has been detected on SPECT scans.

Temperature

Assess the temperature in the extremities. If cold, is the condition one sided or bilateral? Are the digits blue? Is there a hot swollen area?

Swelling

Swelling can be localized or general and occurs when there is too much fluid in places where you normally would not find it. Is the swelling free fluid in a joint space or dispersed throughout the tissue? Is the area also hot, red, or tender?

Problems with the circulatory system pertinent to TBIs:

1. **Shock**

   Shock in many cases can be referred to as circulatory system collapse. For one of many reasons the tissues are not getting adequate perfusion and so they become hypoxic. Usually, either the pump (heart) is failing or there is not enough fluid to pump. In shock, patients will present with a small, weak pulse and hypotension. There may be a narrow pulse pressure, decreased sensorium, tachycardia, rapid shallow breathing, decreased urine output, and

cold, pale, clammy skin. Metabolic acidosis and DIC can occur and shock represents the end-stage of many terminal diseases. The extremities may be cold. Shock is an emergency and patients will soon have altered consciousness and, if not adequately addressed, the patient will deteriorate quickly. Shock can be a serious complication of many conditions from traumatic hemorrhage to myocardial infarction. There can be irreversible tissue damage including injury to the kidneys, brain, and heart. Sepsis from overwhelming systemic infection can cause shock.

2. **Swelling/Edema**

   Edema can be localized or general and occurs when there is too much fluid in the tissue. This fluid usually accumulates because it is oozing from capillaries, the heart is not pumping effectively, the lymphatic system is obstructed, fluids are imbalanced from kidney problems, water is retained from high salt intake, electrolytes are disturbed, there are allergic reactions involving histamine, toxins from pathogens are drawing fluid, or hormone disturbances are causing problems. Fluid often gathers in dependent areas such as the ankles or the base of the lungs. With edema, the body is either making too much fluid or getting rid of too little. What could be causing the excess? Is the disposal system broken?

3. **Unequal pulses**

   Pulses can be discerned when an artery lies close enough to the surface of the skin to be felt. Aside from the aorta, most arteries are paired and the pulses should be compared right to left. If one is greater than the other, what could be the reason for this discrepancy? Look up the chain to see if you can identify the problem. If both pulses are weak or otherwise abnormal, what is the explanation? Bilateral bad pulses in the extremities suggest that something is hindering arterial flow. Is the problem mechanical, structural, or metabolic?

   > PEARL: In infants, discrepancies between the femoral pulses compared to the radial pulses can indicate severe heart problems. Explore this finding further.

4. **Lymphadenopathy**

   Enlarged lymph nodes suggest that the body is mounting a defense against an infectious agent and both white cells and pathogen are being trapped in the nodes. Since the spleen is essentially a bigger lymph node with some additional responsibilities, this organ can also be enlarged in acute or chronic infections. Chapter 2: *Gentle Immunology* contains more detail on the role of the lymphatic system.

Lymphadenopathy is a common finding in TBIs. The location of the large nodes might help localize the distribution of the pathogen. In many infectious processes, the nodes can remain large for months. Some kids seem to have giant nodes throughout their entire childhood. Is the large node mobile or fixed? One sided or bilateral? Tender? One hypothesis is that nodes serve as spirochete repositories in some cases of Lyme.

5. Aneurysms

An aneurysm is a localized defect in a blood vessel, most commonly an artery. The defect can pooch out like a bubble in an inner tube. In fact, an aneurysm can occur in any artery but the most common sites are the aorta and arteries in the brain. The defect can dissect, meaning the blood gets between the layers of the artery wall and spreads. A broad pulsing mass in the abdomen could be an aortic aneurysm. A bruit located over a pulse point suggests a flow problem. If you hear a bruit, look up the chain to see if you can hear it higher. For example, if you hear a femoral bruit, make sure the noise is not actually coming from an abdominal bruit.

6. Raynaud's

The term Raynaud's is used to describe at least two conditions, one fairly benign and one not so much. Raynaud's can be a spastic disorder of the arteries. The vessels can undergo episodic vasospasm of the smaller peripheral arteries, which seems to be precipitated by cold or stress. This condition is bilateral and affects primarily the hands but sometimes the feet, which might present with cold, pale, blue, cyanotic digits. Raynaud's is most often seen in females in puberty and young adulthood. Here's the rub: Some Raynaud's can be associated with autoimmunity and connective tissue diseases like lupus and scleroderma. This type seems to be progressive. So, while some of the literature presents Raynaud's as a benign condition of nervous teenage girls, others see it almost as prodromal to more serious conditions.

PEARL: Raynaud's is observed in a number of TBIs including Lyme and bartonellosis and may be due to the presence of pathogen in the endothelial cells. Inquire about sxs consistent with Raynaud's and examine for it.

7. Varicose veins

Varicose veins are distended, swollen, or knotted vessels. These enlarged veins are twisted and superficial and can occur in any part of the body, but are most common in the lower legs and esophagus. A hemorrhoid can be considered a varicose vein. There can be a genetic predisposition to develop these varicosities, but pressure and other strains can also increase the incidence.

PEARL: Ruptured esophageal varices can bleed like crazy and lead to shock and death. A haunting image from my internship is of a nurse who stayed up all night administering ice water irrigation to an unconscious alcoholic with bleeding esophageal varices. She saved his life and he never knew it. She quit the next day.

8. Impaired circulation

A cold extremity suggests a problem with an artery especially if the coldness is one-sided. Remember that diabetes is largely a disease of circulation. Chronic high sugars damage small vessels which in turn cannot oxygenate the nearby nerves. The tissue dies leading to gangrene and amputation. Lyme can significantly alter blood sugar control.

PEARL: You can garner considerable information about the circulation through a careful examination of the feet. Circulatory compromise shows up first where vessels are smallest and farthest from the heart.

9. Thrombophlebitis

A thrombus is a blood clot. Phlebitis is the inflammation of a vein. In phlebitis there is pain along the course of the affected vein. The area is usually red, firm, and swollen. No one knows why a particular vein gets inflamed but incidence appears to be higher after systemic infection or with long periods of stasis. Because certain locations easily congest, blood can become static in the area creating ideal conditions for clot formation. The most commonly affected veins are those in the calf. On exam, there will be significant discomfort in the calf, especially on dorsiflexion of the foot. These clots can be superficial or deep (deep vein thrombosis). Now we have a problem. Once formed, pieces of the clot can break off causing thrombotic emboli to circulate in the blood. These clots can land in the lung, causing a pulmonary embolus, or in the brain causing a stroke. There are anecdotal reports of patients with Lyme suffering strokes, so have a high index of suspicion.

Section 17-K

Abdomen and Pertinent Differential

Headline April 17, 2011, "Could a jelly bean that resembles Kate Middleton fetch 500 pounds?"

ABDOMEN

The abdomen is the part of the body between the thorax and the pelvis and is bounded by the diaphragm on top and the pelvic bones on the bottom. Many major organs are found in the abdomen including the bottom of the esophagus, the stomach, intestines, spleen, liver, gallbladder, pancreas, rectum, and bladder. Some reproductive organs are also present in the lower abdominal cavity. A membrane called the peritoneum lines the abdomen and many, but not all, of its organs. The kidneys lie within the abdominal cavity but outside the peritoneum.

We are just beginning to recognize that GI complaints are common in Lyme. Sometimes the gastrointestinal tract is the only system involved. Reflux is especially common and children with gestational Lyme can have severe colic. Bb seemingly can invade GI cells causing Lyme-associated complaints, but the pathophysiology can also involve the nervous system. Bell's palsy of the gut has to do with impairment of the vagus nerve. The most common GI feature of Lyme is probably GERD. Reflux is associated with burning, substernal discomfort, and spitting up in infants. GERD is a common manifestation of gestational Lyme. Other GI sxs include nausea, vomiting, stomach pain, diarrhea, change in bowel frequency, gut palsy, a dull unpleasant sensation, feelings of impending vomiting, vomiting with coughing, GI distress, gastritis, colitis, cramps, periumbilical pain, bulging, bloating, putty-like stool, constipation, loss of appetite, spasms, 10th rib tenderness, esophageal dysmotility, and intestinal aching. Sxs can mimic IBS or IBD. More than a few patients have experienced difficulty swallowing, which can impede eating. Gastroparesis has been reported. This condition decreases the ability of the stomach to empty its contents even though there is no blockage. Also called delayed gastric emptying, gastroparesis is a partial paralysis that makes the patient feel bloated.

Kids seem more prone to the GI sxs associated with Lyme than adults. Until recently, few HCPs made the connection between Lyme and the GI tract. I was in the GI therapeutic area for years and was quite surprised by this association, and I focused on pediatric GERD.

Further, often the only positive diagnostic test will come from samples taken for GI biopsy.

Just about every infectious disease manifests with some type of GI sign or symptom. Mycoplasma, Babesia, and Bartonella have all been associated with GI complaints. Treating the underlying infectious process appears to relieve symptoms better than treating the symptoms alone. With TBIs there are many GI complaints and careful examination of the abdomen can provide a wealth of information. The most common GI symptoms associated with TBIs include nausea, vomiting, reflux, constipation, and diarrhea. Since a number of treatments for TBIs can result in diarrhea, GI upset, anorexia, and even gallstones, examine the abdomen carefully for clues as to what is happening. Never forget that sick people get sick, too, and there may be more than one pathologic process active at any one time.

Usually the abdomen is examined in 4 steps:

A. **Inspection:** Look at the abdomen. This is best done with the patient lying supine with knees slightly bent. A normal abdomen should be symmetrical with no apparent bulges, pulsations, or discolorations. In kids, the tummy is usually more prominent than the chest.

General symmetrical enlargement can be fluid (ascites) or distension from gas. Asymmetrical swellings can be tumors or organomegaly. Hernias of the umbilicus or at a surgical site are often apparent on inspection, while hernias in the groin can be more subtle.

The abdomen may be persistently retracted due to eating disorders or starvation. Abdominal retraction during breathing usually indicates some type of respiratory compromise but can also accompany cases of meningitis, pericarditis, and abdominal pain. There will be greater abdominal movement with breathing in cases of pleurisy and pneumonia.

Striae should be noticeable on inspection. Silver-white stretch marks are most often due to pregnancy or from rapid weight change. Pink striae can be associated with Cushing's disease, while violaceous striae are a hallmark of the TBI, bartonellosis.

Look for scars and hernias around incision sites. Discoloration can come from bruising, bleeding, or skin manifestations of disease such as an EM rash or kidney or liver disease.

B. **Auscultation**: Listen to the abdomen in all 4 quadrants. Although a stethoscope is used to auscultate the abdomen, an ear to the belly can provide information in a pinch. In general, there should be air moving in the parts of the abdomen that should have air, and no air in the parts of the abdomen where there should not be air. If your stethoscope is over the liver, and you hear bowel sounds, something may be amiss. Check this abdomen carefully.

Listen *before* you palpate since both percussion and palpation may alter the dynamics in the abdomen. A bowel sound more or less every 15 to 20 seconds is normal. Listen not only for the frequency of sounds but also the pitch. This is certainly not an exact science but some possible interpretations include:

- No BS: obstruction, impaction, paralysis, peritonitis, perforated bowel, ileus. Before you say there are no bowel sounds you must listen at least two minutes.

- Minimal BS: ileus (a stoppage of intestinal movement or peristalsis), impending peritonitis

- Increased BS: obstruction especially early in the pathology. A diet high in processed carbs will make the person "gassy."

- High pitched BS: obstruction or ileus, sometimes described as tinkling

PEARL: While diminished or no BSs is the most common manifestation of ileus, don't be fooled. You may hear an increased amount of sound as the intestinal contents try to get by the blockage. As everything stops, the sounds will stop.

Bruits are vascular noises that sound like a murmur. Bruits might suggest aneurysm.

C. **Percussion**:

Percussion uses the fingertips to tap the body firmly to determine the size, position, and consistency of underlying structures. A good percussionist can tell fluid from air from solid. The experienced examiner can tell by the different tones and resonances what might be underneath.

Many HCPs have their own percussion style. One approach is to start under the xiphoid process and percuss down the midline, including over the bladder. Then move laterally to percuss both sides of the abdomen. Some HCPs use one finger only, tapping gently but firmly over each area of interest. Others use two or three fingers, and still others prefer to lay the fingers of one hand on the abdomen and hit them with the fingers of the other hand.

Do a few hundred abdominal percussions and you will develop your own style.

There should be perceptible differences as you percuss over the stomach compared to the intestine compared to the more solid liver and spleen and the ever amorphous pancreas. There are many nuances to this modality and it may take much practice to become proficient. For example, the resonance over the urinary bladder will depend on whether the bladder is full. There should be a small area of splenic dullness to percussion. An aneurysm is usually dull or flat. Fluid from a right pleural effusion can be mistaken for an enlarged liver. Gas high in the colon may produce the tympany of gas and cause an underestimation of liver size. Free air under the diaphragm can be from a perforated portion of the GI tract.

You don't master percussion overnight, but using this technique can provide one more piece in the diagnostic puzzle. Some examiners are virtuosos in this regard but for many of the newly trained, percussion is a lost art. Why touch a patient when you can order an MRI?

D. **Palpation**:

Palpation is the use of touch to examine the body in order to gather information about the structures beneath the skin and procure evidence of disease. Auscultate before you palpate so that your manipulation of the abdomen does not alter the findings. Of course, you can always auscultate again after you palpate to see if the touch has had any effect.

Have the patient lay in the supine position with the head slightly raised and knees bent. The head should be supported in order to relax the abdominal wall. Using the fingertips, palpate the abdominal cavity. Start abdominal palpation with a light touch. Deeper palpation will be needed for organs and masses.

PEARL: If a person is too tense or ticklish for an exam, first put your hand over his and use that as the examining hand until he is comfortable. Ask him to point to the place that hurts.

For each organ assess the size, position, and consistency, the presence of tenderness, irregularities, or masses. Are masses fixed or movable? Boggy used to be a common descriptor when I was a student and was used to refer to any organ that was softer and spongier than expected, as though you stepped into a bog and it was hard to get back out. Back then everything was boggy. I didn't really know what it meant then and I don't know now. Fortunately, we now have scans and MRIs to help us clarify the situation.

Ascites is free fluid in the abdomen usually from liver disease. If the patient turns on his side and the fluid shifts to the new low point, you have free fluid present and now you have to figure out why.

Describe any abnormalities in the chart. Note the size of the organ, location of any masses, and descriptors such as pulsating or matted. Palpate each of the following areas:

1. **Epigastrium:** Area just below the xiphoid in the upper midsection where the stomach enters into the SI. This area can be quite sore in gastritis, ulcerations, or secondary to irritation from medications.

2. **Liver:** The liver is the largest organ in the body and is located in the upper right quadrant of the abdomen just under the diaphragm. The liver lies level to the bottom of the sternum. The underside of the liver is like an umbrella over parts of the stomach, some intestine, the tops of the kidneys, and the adrenals. The liver edge should be smooth. To best palpate the liver, have the patient take a deep breath in. Tenderness suggests inflammation, as with hepatitis. You can usually palpate the liver and spleen edges in kids. The liver should be a cm or two below the right ribcage. More than 2 cm and the liver is considered enlarged. The liver can be fatty where the organ is large without specific abnormal structural findings.

3. **Gallbladder:** This organ is a pear-shaped sac on the underside of the right lobe of the liver. Here bile made in the liver is concentrated by removing water. When stimulated, the gallbladder releases bile into the duodenum where it emulsifies fats and aids in digestion. Since bile is concentrated by removing water, any time the conditions are such that cholesterol and various salts cannot remain in solution, they can precipitate out forming gravel and stones. Stone formation is twice as likely in females. Gallstones can sit without causing any problems for years. Symptoms can be prompted when a stone obstructs a bile duct, in cases of dehydration, or after a particularly fatty meal. Then inflammation occurs with colicky pain due to spasms of the tubes of the biliary system. Pain can be intense and radiates into the back and right shoulder. Symptoms can resolve and then recur again after the next meal. On exam there will be pain on palpation in the region of the distended gallbladder. Stones are not common in kids except under certain conditions and one is the treatment of Lyme with Rocephin. Patients undergoing treatment with IV Rocephin should be examined and ultrasounded regularly. Treatment with agents to prevent and dissolve stones has been useful. See Chapter 24: *Antimicrobials* and Chapter 25: *Ancillary Treatments*.

4. **Spleen:** The spleen is an oval organ in the upper left of the abdomen slightly behind and below the stomach. The normal spleen is usually barely palpable. The spleen contains numerous white cells and stores red cells. The organ can rupture with trauma, causing considerable blood loss. In infection, the spleen can enlarge greatly and become congested with white cells and various immune molecules. The pathogen is trapped, recognized, and targeted for destruction in the spleen. This activity can greatly enlarge the spleen. Ask the patient to take a deep breath in and hold it. Attempt to palpate the spleen. Release the breath. If the spleen of an adult is palpable, it is enlarged. A massive spleen can extend over the midline. Expect the spleen to be enlarged in TBIs since this organ is a prime filter of the lymph system.

5. **Pancreas**: Behind the stomach is the pancreas. Lying almost horizontal, the head of the pancreas is attached to the duodenum of the SI and its tail reaches to the spleen. The pancreas is both an exocrine organ, making digestive enzymes, and an endocrine organ, making insulin. When inflamed with pancreatitis, these patients are SICK. Symptoms can be a sudden onset of severe epigastric pain, nausea, vomiting, and prostration. Palpation causes significant discomfort. Hospitalization is often required. By whatever mechanism, Bb are well-known to raise havoc with insulin metabolism and the balance of blood sugars. Pay attention to the pancreas in all cases.

6. **Intestines**: The intestines are the tubular portion of the alimentary canal that extend from the pylorus of the stomach to the anus.

   a. **Small Intestine (SI)**: Receives chyme from the stomach, bile from the liver and gallbladder, and digestive enzymes from the pancreas. Considerable digestion and absorption occurs in the SI. In the lower right quadrant of the abdomen the SI empties into the LI. The SI secretes a number of hormones. Unlike the stomach where the pH is strongly acidic, the SI is basic. On auscultation, BS should be audible from the SI in the upper quadrants and midline. Depending on contents, percussion should show a mix of air and fluid. Tenderness on palpation can be experienced with duodenal ulcerations or irritations and with gastroenteritis.

   b. **Large Intestine (LI)**: The colon extends from the ileum of the SI to the anus. The LI absorbs water, vitamins, and minerals and eliminates undigested matter through defecation. Originating in the RLQ, the colon rises up the right side of the abdomen crosses over the top, and then descends down the left side into the rectum ending in the anus. In the RLQ, the appendix is attached to the cecum as the SI and LI join. On auscultation BSs from the LI can be heard in these regions. BSs will be increased in cases of diarrhea and dampened when motion is slowed or stopped as in ileus or paralysis. Cases of obstruction can increase the BSs initially or raise their pitch as the contents of the intestine try to pass by the occluded area. Eventually, as the obstruction shuts things down, the BSs will cease. On percussion, there may be more solid findings than in the SI, but there can also be more gas. A full colon will sound dull. Palpation of a normal LI should find soft, non-tender tissue. Hard stool may be palpable in cases of constipation or obstruction. Hard feces can feel like a tumor and is more often noticed in the descending colon. Attempt to distinguish abdominal organs from intestinal masses. Pain on palpation of the intestine can occur in appendicitis, diverticulitis, diarrhea, obstruction, and toxic megacolon. All are described below.

7. **Aorta:** The aorta is the main artery of the body carrying blood from the heart to all areas by way of its many branches. The aorta can be palpated in the abdomen just cephalad to where it divides into the two iliac arteries in the pelvis. The aorta is usually distinguished from other organs and masses in the abdomen because it is pulsing.

8. **Umbilicus:** The belly button is the scar that forms at the former attachment point of the umbilical cord to the fetus. After infancy the umbilicus is a small depressed area in the middle of the abdomen. The umbilicus is a common site of herniation.

9. **Kidney:** One of a pair of organs situated in the back of the abdomen outside the peritoneum, each kidney is just lateral to the spine. Palpate the kidney through the abdomen, but assess kidney pain from the back. A technically expert examiner can palpate cysts or masses on the kidney through the abdominal wall.

10. **Bladder:** The urinary bladder is a sac holding urine and is located in the anterior part of the pelvis and can be palpated through the abdominal wall. The bladder cannot be palpated when empty. When filled with urine, the round superior margin is easily discerned. Take your chances palpating a full bladder in a little kid. Usually smooth and oval, the bladder can also be assessed by percussion. The nearby intestine will sound tympanic, while a full bladder will be dull. Sometimes masses and spasms can be palpated. Since a tumor can feel like a full bladder, consider additional testing if there is any question.

Age-related abdominal findings:

Infants usually have a protuberant tummy because of undeveloped muscles. (That is also my excuse.) The cord should be uninfected and healing. A newborn with a sunken abdomen should be examined for a diaphragmatic hernia and the examiner should check to see if the abdominal organs have been displaced. Infants are prone to hernias. About 10% of newborns have a curious finding on abdominal exam that bears watching.

Specific abdominal problems:

Before you continue with the physical examination make sure any abdominal complaints are not due to an acute abdomen. An acute abdomen is an emergency and needs to be addressed prior to resuming routine evaluation. Lyme can be especially hard on the digestive tract, as can treatment for Lyme and other TBIs. Since GI complaints are common in most infections, and since any patient can have more than one pathologic process active at any given time, consider the following list as you move through your differential diagnosis. There are hundreds of diagnoses associated with abdominal complaints. These are a few you should be aware of in TBI patients:

- **Acute abdomen:** If the patient is complaining of abdominal pain, rule out an acute abdomen. By definition, an acute abdomen presents with a sudden onset of severe pain, often with other symptoms such as fever, guarding, and rebound tenderness. This is an emergency that must be addressed immediately and may need surgical intervention. The most common causes of an acute abdomen include: appendicitis, peritonitis, perforation, obstruction, aneurysm, bleeding, sickle cell crisis, and incarcerated hernia. Know enough to recognize an acute abdomen and refer the person in cases that you cannot manage. On examination, an acute abdomen may present with:

  1. Guarding: Guarding occurs when the patient voluntarily tries to protect the sore spot by tensing the abdominal muscles.

  2. Rigidity: Rigidity is the involuntary contraction of abdominal muscles and the abdominal wall can be board-like.

  3. Localized discomfort: Sometimes an acute abdomen starts out with generalized aches but then the pain settles in a more specific location.

  4. Rebound tenderness: On examination, rebound tenderness is noted when pain is increased with the sudden release of firm pressure. Rebound suggests peritoneal inflammation.

- **Hernia:** Also called rupture, a hernia is the protrusion of an organ or part of an organ through the wall of the cavity that normally contains it. A hernia can become an emergency when the contents become incarcerated or strangulated. In all cases, make sure the contents of the hernia are not suffocating and becoming necrotic. In these situations, the hernia cannot be replaced manually and ischemia and gangrene can result. Since TBIs are often associated with abdominal signs and symptoms, make sure the problem is not actually a hernia.

Common hernias include:

1. Umbilical: The belly button is the scar that forms at the former attachment point of the umbilical cord to the fetus. After infancy the umbilicus is a small depressed area in the middle of the abdomen. The umbilicus is a common site of herniation, especially in babies of African-American descent. These hernias may be 2 or more inches in diameter and may protrude from the abdominal wall. Most disappear by age 1. An umbilical hernia usually needs no intervention. In infants this type of hernia is centrally located, but as the child gets older the hernia may move above the umbilicus.

2. Inguinal: Protrusion of the hernia sac into the groin is called an inguinal hernia. Since inguinal is a synonym for groin, these hernias will be detailed in the *Groin* section below.

3. Incisional: Surgical hernias occur when there is poor healing at the surgical site or the wound splits. Watch for strangulation and infection in these cases.

4. Abdominal: The hernia sac protrudes through the abdominal wall, due to a separation of musculature or other mechanical defect.

5. Diaphragmatic: Here the abdominal contents move into the thorax. Most often the GI contents move up through the opening in the diaphragm where the esophagus goes through to meet the stomach. These hernias can go undetected or, if there is considerable herniation, the hernia contents can crowd the lungs and heart in the chest cavity. Symptoms can include: respiratory distress, irritation of the covering of the heart, reflux, discomfort, or strangulation of the parts of the intestine that squeezed through. Examination with percussion, auscultation, and palpation might suggest that there is alimentary canal where there should be air-filled tissue.

6. Femoral: A femoral hernia occurs when there is a gap where the artery runs through the tissue that is big enough to allow part of the peritoneum or bladder to go through.

7. Diastasis recti is a separation of the two halves of the rectus abdominis muscle of the abdomen. This is not a hernia but a split between two superficial muscles caused by pregnancy, obesity, or other strains. When supine, raise the head and shoulders and the separation will produce a midline bulge. In kids, diastasis recti can be due to weak muscles or congenital problems.

PEARL: To elicit the defect at the linea alba that defines a diastasis recti, lift the legs <u>together</u> and the defect should be apparent.

- **Cholecystitis**: Inflammation of the gallbladder can be acute or chronic. Described earlier, the gallbladder is a pear-shaped sac on the underside of the right lobe of the liver. Here bile, made in the liver, is concentrated by removing water. When stimulated, the gallbladder releases bile into the duodenum where it emulsifies fats and aids in digestion. Since bile is concentrated by removing water, anytime the conditions are such that cholesterol and various salts cannot remain in solution, they can precipitate out, forming gravel and stones. Gallstones can sit without causing any problems for years. Symptoms can be prompted when a stone obstructs a bile duct, in cases of dehydration, or after a particularly fatty meal. Then inflammation occurs with colicky pain due to spasms in the tubes of the biliary system. Pain can be intense and radiates into the back and right shoulder. Symptoms can resolve and then recur again after the next meal. On exam, there will be pain on palpation in the region of the distended gallbladder. Stones are not common in kids except under certain conditions and one is the treatment of Lyme with Rocephin. Patients undergoing treatment with IV Rocephin should be examined and ultrasounded regularly. Treatment with agents to prevent and dissolve stones has been useful.

An acute gallbladder attack often occurs after a fatty meal when the bladder would be releasing its bile. Here is where a stone can get stuck, causing colicky pain. This pain is due to spasms in the ducts as a stone tries to pass through. The patient can have fever and mild jaundice if there is obstruction of the bile flow. Most of the symptoms are localized in the RUQ. Ask the patient to take a deep breath in. Then press a thumb under the right costal margin. A sharp increase of pain when the inflamed gallbladder is touched by the examining thumb is called Murphy's sign and indicates acute cholecystitis. The patient may also have muscle rigidity and rebound tenderness but not always. Sometimes the pain can awaken the patient in the middle of the night. Clay-colored stools may occur if the problem is recurrent. The hallmark of chronic cholecystitis is intermittent recurrence of colicky pain. If a Lyme patient is on Rocephin and experiencing any of these symptoms, refer to Chapter 25: *Ancillary Treatments*.

- **Pancreatitis**: Inflammation of the pancreas can be acute or chronic. In adults, pancreatitis is often due to chronic alcoholism but can also be associated with ulcers, trauma, endocrine problems, or biliary disease. Steroids can affect pancreatic function and infectious agents such as Coxsackie viruses, mumps virus, and certain Mycoplasma strains also seem able to damage the pancreas. Bb are often associated with digestive and blood sugar problems and pancreatic function should be watched in Lyme patients.

Pancreatitis can start with steady epigastric pain close to the umbilicus. While the person may feel like vomiting she rarely gets relief from doing so. The sicker the patient gets, the more signs of inflammation appear including: escalating pain which may become severe, persistent vomiting, abdominal rigidity, malaise, and restlessness. Never underestimate how sick these people can be. The more damage to the pancreas, the less stable the insulin supply and the less reliable the production of digestive enzymes. Many other body systems can be affected. When I was an intern the patients with pancreatitis got little attention, since they were often alcoholics and we were so self-righteous. How sad. In the case of TBI patients, be vigilant. Life without a fully functioning pancreas is miserable and supportive therapy may be needed.

Acute pancreatitis can present with the sudden onset of intense epigastric pain, nausea, vomiting, rigidity, rebound, and tenderness over the umbilicus. Early in the course, constipation may predominate, but later diarrhea can be present. A slow pulse and sometimes jaundice can occur. In severe cases the pancreas can bleed and ooze pus which can result in necrosis and gangrene. These patients are SICK. Palpation causes significant discomfort. Hospitalization is often required. Additional findings may include elevated white count, high glucose levels, and increased levels of amylase and lipase. High amylase levels confirm the diagnosis, but these can return to near normal after a few days even though the patient is still quite sick. Then look to the lipase, since these levels take longer to increase and may stay high longer in the clinical course. Serum calcium may be low and affect heart function.

Chronic pancreatitis is usually due to scar tissue, leading to permanent loss of function. Pain can radiate into the back and diarrhea, jaundice, and weakness can occur.

- **Ulcerations**: GI ulcers are open lesions in the mucosa of the lower esophagus, stomach, or duodenum caused by chemical irritation from acid or base. The bacteria, Helicobacter *pylori* are now known to be a contributing agent in a high percentage of gastric ulcers. In these cases, the patient is treated with both an antacid agent like a PPI and an antibiotic regimen. The chances of recovery are much lower if only the symptoms are treated without the antibiotics to hit the underlying infectious etiology. (This scenario should sound familiar.) Symptoms include heartburn, indigestion, bloating, and mid-epigastric pain. Food can relieve the discomfort in some cases but symptoms can recur a few hours after eating. Consumption of acidic or irritating materials such as aspirin, some NSAIDs, alcohol, or acidic juices can trigger an acute episode. Exacerbations come and go. Ulcers can bleed and the patient can quickly destabilize. Bleeding can cause peritonitis, anemia, and shock. I kept a photograph taken during an endoscopy of a clinical trial patient showing an aspirin sitting on a bleeding ulcer.

- **Omental trapping**: The omentum is a double fold of peritoneum attached to the stomach and draping over a number of abdominal organs. Abnormalities in the omentum can sometimes be palpated and occasionally a mass is found. Dr. Oz on TV is obsessed with the omentum and has been known to drag an especially portly omentum onto the *Oprah Show* to demonstrate what happens when we get fat.... as if we didn't know. Normally the omentum seems to float over the surface of the intestines. The omentum has a role in fat deposition and can also serve to isolate infection by cordoning off the infectious process. Milky spots on the omentum are macrophage collections that may function in immune response. The free flow of the omentum can be impeded by adhesions and entrapment by hernias. Omental trapping is thought to be a common cause of abdominal pain in Lyme. A few sit-ups every day seems to help realign the abdominal contents if the omentum appears to be contributing to discomfort.

- **Appendicitis**: The appendix is a small piece of tissue attached to the cecum at the junction of the small and large intestines. No one knows the original purpose of the appendix, although there are some wild theories. Removal of the appendix does not seem to have any untoward consequences. The appendix may play a minor role in maintaining normal gut flora but this is unproven and inconsequential either way. The appendix becomes inflamed when it is obstructed or infected or traumatized. Appendicitis is most common in kids older than 10 and throughout the teen years.

Appendectomy is the most common emergency abdominal surgery. Symptoms often start with epigastric or RUQ unease, which gradually localizes to the RLQ, at McBurney's point. Early on there may be anorexia, nausea, and some vomiting. The patient may develop guarding, rigidity, and rebound tenderness. There may be a low grade fever and a moderately elevated white count. Sudden cessation of symptoms may not be a good thing. The appendix may have burst, in which case it doesn't hurt anymore and we'll soon be dealing with peritonitis.

Even today, acute appendicitis is misdiagnosed with some frequency. When the surgeon opens what she thought was an acute abdomen she finds a happy, un-inflamed organ, minding its own business. She removes it anyway. So often in the ER, I saw the surgeons struggling to decide if they should operate or not. They are torn between going in and finding that the signs and symptoms were due to something beside appendicitis or waiting and risking that the organ will burst.

There are a number of ways to support the diagnosis of appendicitis on physical exam. Look for:

1. Point tenderness in the RLQ at McBurney's point

2. Guarding

3. Rebound tenderness

4. Rigidity

5. Positive psoas sign: Because an inflamed appendix can rest near a part of the psoas muscle, movement of the muscle will cause pain in the inflamed site. Place the patient on her side with knees extended. Then either by passively extending the thigh or asking the patient to actively extend the thigh, the psoas test is performed. A positive psoas test elicits pain on movement. A negative test does not cause pain.

6. Positive obdurator sign: The inflamed appendix may be in contact with a portion of the obdurator muscle. Moving the muscle in a way that touches the appendix should cause discomfort if the appendix is inflamed. The test is done on each leg in succession. The patient should be supine with hips flexed at 90 degrees. The examiner holds the right ankle with one hand. Using the left hand, the hip is rotated by moving the right knee inward. Since the obdurator must stretch here, if the appendix is inflamed, it will hurt.

7. Positive signs of peritoneal irritation: Have the patient lie on his back and then have him try to raise his head while the HCP pushes down on his forehead. Even slight effort will cause discomfort if the peritoneum is inflamed.

Reportedly, the longest appendix ever removed was 26 cm (over 10 inches) from a patient in Croatia. How do people know these things?

- **Diverticulitis:** Also called left-sided appendicitis. Diverticuli are little out-pouches of tissue in the colon, like bubbles on an old inner tube. They remain asymptomatic until they become inflamed. Acute cases are similar to the presentation found in appendicitis and care must be taken that a diverticuli does not rupture, leading to peritonitis. Chronic problems with flares can lead to worsening constipation, mucus in the stool, and intermittent episodes of gripping abdominal pain. Since most people do not want to have a repeat episode, they are advised to eat a diet high in fiber, consume non-irritating foods, and drink plenty of water.

- **Diarrhea:** Loose stools are discussed in detail in Chapter 25: *Ancillary Treatments.* On physical exam, bowel sounds may be loud and rapid. Percussion may show considerable air and fluid. Palpation may result in generalized discomfort, but not specific localized pain. Frequent, loose stools are common in TBI patients, either as part of the disease process or as a side effect of antibiotic therapy. Look also for signs of dehydration. With diarrhea due to C. *difficile,* address the issue immediately and remain vigilant for complications like megacolon.

- **Aortic aneurysm:** An aneurysm is a widening or dilation of a blood vessel, usually an artery, due to a weakening of the vessel wall. An abdominal aortic aneurysm is a wide pulsating mass located about midline near the back of the abdomen. The more the pulse of the aorta is felt laterally, the more likely that what you're feeling is an aneurysm. On auscultation, a bruit may be heard which sounds like a murmur and suggests turbulent blood flow as found in an aneurysm. A radiating cardiac murmur can be mistaken for an abdominal bruit. Symptoms can be hard to distinguish until it is late: vague, generalized abdominal pain, low back pain unaffected by movement, a sensation of fullness, sudden lumbar discomfort, pain radiating to the flank or groin, an escalating pulsating mass in the periumbilical area, and mounting systolic bruit over the aorta. Aneurysms can be present but asymptomatic. While the primary cause of aortic aneurysm is atherosclerosis, infections can also be an etiologic agent and infections are what this book is all about. Infections like those caused by the spirochetes that cause syphilis. I know two cases in the last year where the patient died from an aneurysm and both the PCPs and ER docs were shocked. Have a high index of suspicion.

- **Toxic megacolon:** An acute distension of the colon can become very dilated, hence the term "mega"colon. While some types of megacolon are congenital, here we are referring to the dilation that is a complication of conditions like inflammatory bowel disease or the sequelae of C. *difficile* overgrowth and pseudomembranous colitis. Toxic megacolon can present with fever, pain, and tenderness.

A key finding is an accompanying tachycardia. Toxic megacolon can lead to sepsis, shock, and death. Perforation can lead to significant blood loss. Colonoscopy is contraindicated if megacolon is suspected. With an acute abdomen secondary to toxic megacolon, the risk of rupture is high and mortality is 50%. This is an emergency and needs to be addressed immediately.

- **Bleeding**: Blood loss from the GI tract can be due to bleeding anywhere from the mouth to the anus. Sometimes blood can be seen in vomit or stool. The blood can be visible or occult, which means not visible to the eye but detectable on lab tests. The bleeding can seep over time leading to weakness and anemia or can gush to the point of being life-threatening. A bleeding ulcer or ruptured varices (varicose veins) can be fatal if not appropriately addressed. Bleeding from high in the GI tract will result in black, tarry stool, while red blood in the stool means the source is likely the rectum or anus. These variations are sometimes discernible on the rectal exam glove. On physical exam, slow bleeding may result in pallor, difficulty breathing over time, lightheadedness, dizziness, weakness, and loss of consciousness. Rapid, voluminous bleeding will quickly lead to respiratory compromise. Pain over the bleeding site can occur and diffuse discomfort over the entire abdomen can evolve if the bleeding has caused peritonitis. If this bleeding is not stopped the patient could go into shock and die. With TBI patients, medicines like NSAIDs can result in GI bleeding.

- **Peritonitis:** An inflammation of the peritoneum which can be caused by irritation from exposure to pathogens or intestinal contents, infections, rupture in the female reproductive tract, surgical penetration, or sepsis. Peritonitis is an emergency requiring immediate attention. If any of the physical findings listed above for an acute abdomen are observed, peritonitis could be present. Signs include involuntary rigidity, rebound, guarding, or spasm of abdominal muscles. These are all indications of peritoneal inflammation and very bad news indeed. Peritonitis is the very thing we are trying to prevent with all these other conditions. Get busy. Refer to hospital care.

- **Bladder conditions**: The urinary bladder is able to be examined through the abdominal wall with percussion and palpation. Spasms can be felt as firm muscle cramps. Stones can cause colicky pain as they move down the ureters into the bladder and then out the urethra. Bladder infections cause painful urination, urgency, frequency, and hesitancy. UTIs are common and can be due to poor hand washing habits or wiping from back to front. These infections are much more common in females, since the E. *coli* which are the most commonly implicated pathogens have a much shorter distance to travel to the urethral meatus in females than males. In usual infectious UTIs, pathogens can be cultured and respond readily to antibiotics.

Interstitial cystitis is very common in Lyme and presents just like an infectious UTI characterized by dysuria, hesitancy, urgency, and frequency. The difference is that with interstitial cystitis cultures are routinely NEGATIVE and the symptoms do not resolve with traditional antibiotic regimens. Perhaps we have not been looking for the right pathogens. In these patients, Bb have been picked up with cystoscopy and biopsy of the bladder trigone and supported with PCR. Perhaps treating the Lyme will resolve these seemingly "aseptic" symptoms.

PEARL: The irritability associated with the bladder in a number of chronic Lyme patients may be due to damage to the autonomic nervous system.

PEARL: Speculatively, IC may be more common in perimenopausal women because the decrease in estrogen might make it harder for normal bacteria to flourish allowing pathogens to survive.

- **Kidney stones or infection**: Kidney stones are said to be one of the most painful experiences imaginable. The pain is an intense colicky spasm as the stone moves through the urinary system. Crystals precipitate out of solution and form stones anywhere along the route. When the stone is moving things are bad enough. The real problem occurs when the stone gets stuck when it would prefer to be moving. Excessive intake of Vitamin D and calcium may predispose to stones. Bacteria can also serve as the nidus for stone formation. Pain is the key symptom here and, unlike other types of abdominal pain, the pain of kidney stones is distinctive. Some patients can point to the stone as it passes along their flank. Dehydration can be a factor in stone formation. Pain usually travels from the back near the junction of the rib and vertebra to the flank and then into the pubis. Nausea and vomiting can be present and there may be blood in the urine. Jagged stones can damage the tissue, making it ripe for secondary infection. In these cases there may be white cells in the urine and fever, chills, and distension. Here the history and review of systems makes the diagnosis, confirmed with diagnostic testing. PE takes a back seat.

Pyelonephritis is a bacterial infection of the kidneys, commonly due to E. *coli* but Staph, Strep, and Pseudomonas are also common etiologic pathogens. The microbes spread from the bladder and up the ureters. Diabetics are more prone to infection as are those who cannot completely empty the bladder. Symptoms may develop rapidly over a few hours and include fever, chills, pain on urination, frequency, burning, urgency, and nocturia.

Recurring infection can cause a chronic pyelonephritis with scarring of the kidney.

PEARL: Strep-associated kidney infections (glomerulonephritis) are relatively common sequelae to inadequately treated Strep throat or skin infections. Most cases occur in boys from about ages 3 to 7. Most fully recover with treatment. A good reason to treat Strep throat is to prevent glomerulonephritis.

- **Enteritis**: When you have TBI patients who are chronically ill for extended periods, you are going to run into basic enteritis at some point. This inflammation of the intestines causes abdominal discomfort, increased BSs, and diarrhea, and is common in all age groups. There is no point tenderness on palpation, just vague general discomfort. Add nausea and vomiting and you have **gastroenteritis**. The etiology is almost always viral with a common agent being norovirus (as seen with the continual outbreaks hitting cruise ship passengers in recent years). Unfortunately, the ailment is often referred to as stomach flu, when the disease usually has nothing to do with influenza. Nonetheless, viral pathogens like H1N1 can have significant associated enteritis.

- **Hepatitis:** Inflammation of the liver, which is most commonly due to viral agents, is also caused by bacteria, parasites, and chemical irritation from drugs, alcohol, or other toxins. Clinical findings include an enlarged liver and jaundice. Usually a prodromal stage presents with malaise, fever, anorexia, nausea, vomiting, muscle aches, fatigue, headache, dark urine, and clay colored stools. The condition then progresses to an icteric stage where jaundice worsens and other signs and symptoms progress. Pruritis can occur and the liver is large and tender. Lab tests including antigen and antibody screens and elevated liver enzyme levels support the diagnosis. Hepatitis is common and is often part of the differential diagnosis in TBI cases. Many conditions will involve inflammation of the liver as part of the clinical presentation. There may be more than one thing going on in a patient at the same time.

- **Problems with reproductive organs**: Many abnormalities palpable through the abdominal wall can relate to the reproductive system. Know the anatomy of the region before you perform the physical examination. Know enough to recognize abnormalities for which you might need to refer. Even though these conditions can be rare in the pediatric population, there are many teens with TBIs who can present with abnormal findings on exam. It's embarrassing to miss an ectopic pregnancy because you did not think of this as a possible diagnosis in a 14-year-old. On physical exam you may come across:

1. Ovarian cysts are usually benign and asymptomatic but may be felt as an enlarged area in the region of the ovary. Torsion or rupture of an ovarian cyst can result in an acute abdomen.

2. Pelvic discomfort upon palpation is a common finding in Lyme patients.

3. Endometriosis is the presence of endometrial tissue outside the lining of the uterus and presents with constant pain in the lower abdomen that may increase with palpation. The pain is usually cyclic with the menstrual cycle.

4. Ectopic pregnancy is the implantation of a fetus outside the womb. There may be considerable pain to palpation and a ruptured ectopic pregnancy can result in an acute abdomen and shock with all the associated clinical signs.

5. An undescended testicle is occasionally discernible in a child who has an absent testicle in the scrotal sac.

- **Bowel obstruction**: Intestinal obstruction is a mechanical or functional blockage of the intestine that prevents normal movement of the products of digestion. The blockage can be at any location within the intestine. This is an emergency. Signs and symptoms depend on location and duration. In general, there is abdominal pain and distension, vomiting (sometimes of fecal material), diminished BSs, and constipation. X-rays can show distinct air-fluid levels. Vomiting can lead to dehydration and electrolyte imbalances. Distension of the abdomen can press up on the diaphragm and compromise respiration. The most serious complications include ischemia and perforation. (Did I mention death?)

SI obstruction: Small bowel obstruction presents with colicky pain with intermittent cramping. The spasm can last a few minutes. There is central and mid-abdominal pain. Patients will not like having the area touched. Vomiting usually occurs before constipation. Causes of SI obstruction include: adhesions, hernias, IBD, strictures, tumors, intussusception, volvulus, and foreign bodies including gallstones. In babies, atresia is a common cause of bowel obstruction. Neonates can have a meconium obstruction. "Never let the sun set on a small bowel obstruction."

PEARL: Atresia is the absence, restriction, or closure of a normal body opening or tube. Atresia can be congenital, surgical, traumatic, or metabolic.

LI obstruction: With large bowel obstruction, pain is present lower in the abdomen and spasms last longer than with SI obstruction. Constipation begins earlier and there is less vomiting. Causes of LI obstruction include: tumors, hernias, IBD, volvulus, adhesions, constipation, fecal impaction, atresia, strictures from diverticuli, and endometriosis. Occasionally, a hard fecal mass is palpable.

In partial obstruction there can be anorexia, vomiting, and tenderness to palpation. Here bowel sounds can be diminished OR they can be high pitched and tinkling as the fecal material tries to move past the blockage. There can even be intense diarrhea in partial obstruction as the feces tries to escape around the obstacle.

Prolonged obstruction can lead to high fever, absent bowel sounds, shock, and death. Manage the obstruction.

Although the term **ileus** is often used interchangeably with obstruction there is a subtle difference. While obstruction refers to blockage, ileus is a problem with the normal motility in the GI tract. Material can no longer be propelled forward. There is no more propulsion. Ileus can be due to inflammation or infection and is often found in cases of acute pancreatitis. After surgery, ileus is common and a light diet is recommended until the bowel starts to move again. Drugs like opioids cause a whopping ileus. Neurologic problems or injury can cause a paralytic ileus with atony. Paralytic ileus need not be total, but if sufficient to prevent passage of the digestive material there can be problems. Ileus usually causes constipation, bloating, diminished bowel sounds, diffuse discomfort, excess belching, no flatulence, and nausea and vomiting after meals. Risk factors for ileus include abdominal surgery, GI procedures, electrolyte imbalances, hypothyroidism, diabetic ketoacidosis, narcotics and some other medications, spinal cord injury, peritonitis, and severe illness with inflammation. Any of these conditions can cause decreased motor activity leading to ileus.

- **Adhesions**: Fibrotic scars, most often in the abdomen and pelvis, can bind organs which are not normally attached. On palpation sometimes the abdomen can feel stiff, immobile, and unnatural. Adhesions can cause discomfort and in some cases obstruction and loss of function. Adhesions often occur after surgery as the tissues scar as part of wound healing. They are also common after infection, inflammation, or trauma. Adhesions can present as an acute abdomen. If pain is intractable, or the adhesions cause obstruction, they may need surgical intervention. The problem with using surgery to release adhesions is that the surgery usually results in more adhesions.

- **Masses**: Even the word *mass,* causes people to panic. However, most tumors are benign. When I first started medical training, I did a pediatric rotation at Walter Reed Army Hospital where they transported complicated cases from all over the world. I thought every other child had a Wilm's tumor or neuroblastoma, since we saw so many cases. When I got back to Wilmington, the pediatrician who I worked with had seen one Wilm's tumor in his 50-year career and had never seen a neuroblastoma. Of course, cancer is only rare if it is not happening to you. The one thing that Lyme does *not* seem to be associated with is a higher incidence of cancers. But, as always, more than one thing can be happening. TBIs, like Lyme, have such a significant impact on immune response that perhaps cancers can more easily manifest. Maybe the cancer is better able to grow if the Bb inhibits the body's defenses. In contrast, perhaps some cancers are suppressed due to the immune response being on high alert to combat the TBI. The immune system might be overwhelmed by either the cancer or the TBI, allowing the other condition to express itself more apparently. There is no data. If you find a mass, work it up or send the patient to an HCP who specializes in that type of investigation, never forgetting that there could be co-morbidities.

PEARL: Bb appear to be attracted to areas of tissue damage or loci of abnormal cells such as malignancies. While Bb do not seem to cause cancer, they have been found in tumor tissue especially gliomas near the brain.

- **Sickle cell crisis**: Abnormal red cells in sickle cell patients can obstruct blood flow and lead to ischemia, causing severe abdominal pain. In some sickle cell patients there can be sequestration of both red and white cells in the spleen and liver causing engorgement. In other patients there can be an essential "autosplenectomy" where the spleen is so damaged by fibrotic scarring that it is shrunken and impalpable.

- **Intussusception**: The telescoping of a part of the bowel into a distal portion of the intestine is most common in boys under age 2 and may be the result of viral or other infections. Usually the lower right quadrant is the most commonly involved location. A tender distended abdomen with a palpable sausage shaped mass is noted. The child may have intermittent severe colicky pain which causes him to scream and draw up his legs. He may turn pale, sweat, and grunt. At first he may vomit stomach contents and later bile or fecal material. Current jelly stools are a combination of blood and mucus. This is an acute abdomen and needs to be addressed immediately. Otherwise, intussusception can be fatal within 24 hours. A **volvulus** is the twisting of the intestine which can result in compromise of blood flow. Here there is marked abdominal distension along with severe pain. A mass may be palpable. Volvulus can also be fatal.

- **Irritable Bowel Syndrome**: (IBS or spastic colon) IBS is another one of those diseases where the medical establishment insists that the patients are making it up instead of admitting they don't know what's going on. Clearly, IBS is just another vast conspiracy to annoy academics with a group of young, otherwise healthy people plotting and scheming to make themselves physically miserable in order to exasperate researchers. Often when vague intestinal signs and symptoms occur and no other diagnosis is found, the patient is said to have IBS. Symptoms include chronic abdominal pain, general GI discomfort, bloating, and alternating bowel habits. There are usually no definitive findings on PE or diagnostic testing. Either diarrhea or constipation can be dominant in the clinical picture. Some patients alternate between extremes. Some find that symptoms are relieved by having a bowel movement. IBS may start after an infection, stressful event, or the onset of puberty. An incomplete differential diagnosis includes malabsorption, lactose intolerance, celiac disease, parasites, and IBD. Patients may be more sensitive to certain stimuli like some foods, changes in the gut flora, and hits to the immune system. Some hypothesize about miscommunications between the nervous system and the GI tract. The frequent trips to the bathroom can be wearing and IBS with its subsequent fatigue is a common reason for missing school and work. There may be associations with thyroid dysfunction and bacterial or fungal overgrowth. IBS patients have a higher incidence of certain co-morbidities such as depression, CFS, fibromyalgia, headache, endometriosis, interstitial cystitis, and various chronic pain syndromes. On exam, there may be alterations in BS depending on the predominant symptoms, vague tenderness on palpation, and general exasperation with the situation. Whatever the pathophysiology, there is no question that IBS affects QOL and some patients request special accommodations at school or work.

- **Inflammatory Bowel Disease**: IBD is a group of inflammatory conditions of the intestine, the most common of which are **Crohn's disease** and **ulcerative colitis**. These two present similarly, the difference being the location and nature of the inflammatory changes in the gut. Crohn's can impact any part of the GI tract from mouth to anus in what are called **skip lesions.** UC affects the colon and rectum. Both can involve body systems outside the alimentary canal such as the liver, joints, skin, and eyes. Crohn's is thought to be autoimmune, while the consensus is still out on UC. Both may be associated with cytokine response. Both present with diarrhea, abdominal discomfort, and cramps. Symptoms can be incapacitating and affect the ability to go to school and work.

Of course, having been around the block a few thousand times, I have done clinical studies on IBD over the years. These were some of the most difficult trials to design.

Individual presentation varies considerably and signs and symptoms wax and wane. Patients were always very reluctant to come off any anti-inflammatories that were working and who can blame them? Diagnosis of IBD is made by colonoscopy and biopsy.

Common signs of Crohn's are abnormal soft, fatty stool, fever, fistulae, weight loss, and both ileal and anal involvement. Deep snake-like ulcerations and granulomas manifested as a series of skip lesions are seen on endoscopy. Patients with Crohn's are more likely than UC patients to have nutritional deficits due to problems with absorption.

Common symptoms of UC are mucus and blood in the stool, frequent bowel movements, tenesmus (anal spasm), with fever present only in severe disease. The colon is always involved and usually the rectum as well. The bile duct has been involved in some cases. On endoscopy, there is often a *continuous* area of inflammation with contiguous ulceration. Lesion depth is superficial. Colon cancer risk may be higher in UC patients.

I thought I would NEVER finish this section. I can't tell you how I am looking forward to moving onto the rectum.

Rectum, Groin, Genitals, Urinary Tract, and Pertinent Differential

One man in the right will finally get to be a majority.

R. G. Ingersoll

I. RECTUM

There is an old story that still goes around medical schools about the anus being the most important part of the body since if the anus is not happy, nothing else matters. This is probably true. The rectum is the lower part of the large intestine and contains the centers for the defecation reflex. The rectum collects the final waste material which is then expelled through the anus. The anus controls the elimination of feces and contains a series of sphincter muscles. A sphincter is a circular muscle that constricts an orifice or opening. The sphincter contracts to close the orifice and relaxes to open the orifice. In the anus, the internal sphincter is made of smooth muscle and is not under voluntary control. The external anal sphincter is made of striated muscle and is under voluntary control.

The rectal exam is not a favorite of adults and should be done only if indicated in kids. The exam can be traumatic if not done gently and with consideration of the patient's privacy. In an adult, I would not hesitate to do a rectal exam on any routine screen and as part of any work-up that involves the GI tract. In kids, the invasive nature of the exam probably outweighs the information that can be collected. You can still do a thorough exam of the area, including the anus, without causing discomfort or distress. Adult exam fingers can be awfully large for little kids. Of course, in some cases, there is no alternative and a rectal exam is indicated. First, see what you can glean in children without a full rectal.

When I was in medical training at Walter Reed, one of the assignments was to go to the VA and do hundreds (or was it thousands?) of rectal exams on the veterans. We were screening for prostate cancer. After a few dozen exams, you get your own rhythm. When you are on the military assembly line, you usually have the patient stand and flex forward at the waist and the exam is done quickly and efficiently. With a hundred other guys waiting in line, you don't have much choice. We were thrilled to have exam gloves. This is NOT the technique I would recommend in other circumstances.

Gentle rectal technique: Have the patient lie on her side. The knees should be flexed in close to the chest. Examine the external area quickly and systematically for the lesions described below. Then using water based lubricant, insert the exam finger. If doing the rectal as part of a gyn exam the patient can be supine with knees bent and relaxed toward the sides of the table. There is no requirement to use stirrups. Initially aim for the belly button to have easy entry. Run the exam finger down the floor of the rectum as far as you can without causing discomfort. Then curve the exam finger 180 degrees in one direction and then repeat in the other direction. Ensure that your finger covers the entire surface of the rectum. Assess if any organs outside the GI tract seem to be infringing on the rectum. If a mature male, run the exam finger over the caudad floor of the rectum and the finger should ride over the prostate gland. Always be looking for evidence of damage from trauma, blood, masses, enlarged veins, nodules, strictures, warts, abnormal texture, prolapse of other organs into the rectal space, fistulas, fissures, impaction, and cysts. This is a get-in-there-and-get-the-information exam. Do not lollygag while you consider what you should have for lunch. Once the exam finger is withdrawn, if there is not obvious blood, use a quick occult blood kit to check for blood that is not visible. Use a tissue to gently clean the gel off the patient.

PEARL: If you cannot do a pelvic exam without stirrups, I recommend a short stint of work in a third world country where a pile of cardboard is your exam table. You will be helping people and you will learn to use your medical skills again without the reliance on modern technology.

During the rectal and external exam of the anus and perineum look for:

A. Hemorrhoids: Varicose veins of the rectum. The dilation and enlargement can be extremely painful, hot, and swollen, making it difficult to sit. The dilated veins can be internal where they are not easily seen or external where they protrude from the anus. Hemorrhoids may be due to straining and are common in pregnancy and in athletes. Straining due to constipation or internal pressure from diarrhea can dilate the vessels, as can long periods of standing or sitting. More common in the teen years as kids start to lift heavier weights, hemorrhoids can appear earlier in children who are routinely constipated and strain to pass stool. These can be quite painful and cause bright red blood on the toilet paper which scares kids. Sometimes a clot or thrombus forms in the dilated vein and this too causes pain manifesting as a large, firm lump. Care must be taken to clean the perineal area well when hemorrhoids are present. Itching can occur which can be unpleasant and socially inconvenient.

B. Perianal skin tags are common and not significant.

C. Fissures: A fissure is a crack, tear, or furrow in the lining of the anus. At the onset, there is a tearing or burning pain, usually after a bowel movement. There can be blood in the water or toilet paper. The sphincter may spasm in protest. A fissure may heal without sequelae but some re-open and cause scarring which can impede defecation. On physical exam you should be able to visualize the fissure on the anus.

D. Abscess: A collection of pus can form due to inflammation and infection of the soft tissue near the rectum or anus. This abscess can result in the formation of a canal in the tissue that allows the pus to drain. This fistula may open to the outside skin or inside into the rectum. An abscess may be the result of a secondary bacterial infection after mild trauma such as the slight injury caused by an enema tip or the passing of fish bones or eggshells. Abscesses in this area can result from infections in nearby tissue as well.

E. Fistulas are abnormal tubes that form allowing communication between two areas that are usually not connected. Fistulas connect one cavity to the outside surface or to another cavity. For example, an infected anal abscess may form a fistula to the outside skin surface allowing the pus to drain. (With the multiple procedures on my face after a bad fall, fistulas formed at the suture sites.)

F. Atresia or strictures: Atresia is the absence or closure of a normal opening, while a stricture generally refers to a narrowing or tightening. The lumen of the rectum can be diminished congenitally or from scarring, inflammation, or laxative abuse. With strictures the patient may need to strain excessively to defecate and might never feel as though the bowel is fully evacuated. Pain, bleeding, and itch may result.

G. Blood: If not doing a full rectal exam you can use a cotton swab to gently go inside the anus to the rectum to get a sample to test for occult blood.

H. Impaction: A hard solid mass made of feces can compact in the rectum secondary to chronic constipation. This mass may be palpable through the lower abdomen. Impaction can happen to constipated patients and in those taking opioids for pain. Symptoms can include pain, bloating, and loss of appetite. If left untreated the tissue can ulcerate and necrose. Paradoxically, diarrhea may present as stool overflows around the impaction. See Chapter 25: *Ancillary Treatments* for ideas on how to manage impaction.

I. Masses: Malignant growths are occasionally found in the anorectal area of older patients. If a mass is discovered on PE, conduct further evaluation.

J. Skin lesions: Remember that obscure skin can be hiding lesions like an EM rash that you will miss if you don't look.

K. Warts: If you recall in the *Introduction*, I mentioned that I was traveling for business in September of 2001. This was the trip where I realized I had Lyme disease. I was in Brazil to attend the international HPV conference and to set up clinical research sites for HPV studies. I know my warts. I still have the tee shirt. The anal region is a very common site for warts caused by human papilloma virus. These warts can be large and cumbersome and interfere with defecation. If the patient has HPV warts, check for other STDs.

PEARL: HPV warts in one area can mean HPV warts in another area. The larynx is a common site. In the pediatric population, kids can contract HPV from the birth canal of an infected mother. For kids who have immune compromise, HPV warts can be a recurrent, debilitating problem. Chronic hoarseness, without URI, might signify HPV.

L. Rectal prolapse: Part of the rectal mucosa can fall down through the anus. Prolapse can occur at rest, but is more likely after defecation or long periods of walking. The rectum can feel full and there may be bloody diarrhea and pain in the lower abdomen.

M. Pilonidal cysts: Cysts over the coccyx area in the gluteal fold are most common in older teenage males. These cysts can contain hairs and become infected producing abscesses and a draining sinus or fistula. They can be irritated by pressure in the sacrococcygeal area, excessive heat, and constrictive clothing. The cyst is present and dormant until aggravated. If provoked, the inflammation can cause local pain, tenderness, swelling, and draining. If the cyst progresses, then fever, pus, headache, chills, and malaise might occur. The opening of a pilonidal cyst is seen above the gluteal cleft near the coccyx and can be inflamed or infected and draining.

N. Prostate problems: On exam, if the finger tip running along the floor of the rectum bumps into a rounded mound, the prostate might be enlarged. Note that the finger only explores one side of the prostate and the side that cannot be palpated can be undetectably large. Be aware of masses and asymmetry. Tenderness can mean inflammation. In acute prostatitis, the gland is swollen and tender. If chronically inflamed, the prostate can be somewhat enlarged, tender, and boggy. The prostate can be scarred with fibrosis.

II. GROIN

Inguinal is a synonym for groin. The groin is a busy place with skin, pulses, and lymph nodes to assess. When examining the groin, look for:

A. Hernias: A hernia is the protrusion of an organ or part of an organ through the wall of the cavity that normally contains it. A hernia can become an emergency when the contents become incarcerated or strangulated. In these situations the contents of the hernia cannot be replaced manually and ischemia and gangrene can result. Inguinal hernias are a protrusion of the hernia sac into the groin.

An inguinal hernia is reducible when the contents can be manipulated back where they belong without too much difficulty. In irreducible hernias, manual maneuvering cannot return the hernia to its rightful place and care must be taken to ensure that the contents do not strangulate. Usually with inguinal hernias, there is a lump noticeable when the patient stands or strains. The lump often disappears when the patient is supine. Older kids or athletes will complain of a sharp or catching pain when lifting.

To assess for an inguinal hernia, have the patient stand where the examiner has easy access to the groin area. Insert the index finger up into the inguinal ring, using the loose skin of the scrotum to allow entry. Have the patient cough. The hernia sac will be forced down with the pressure from the cough. The examiner will feel a tap on the tip of the finger with an indirect hernia and on the side of the finger with a direct hernia. Strangulation produces severe pain in the groin. These hernias can be direct or indirect.

- Indirect hernias are due to a weak internal ring and the sac descends through the canal into the scrotum or labia. This type of hernia is very common in infants. While indirect hernias can occur at any age they are most common in boys less than a year old. In an infant, an inguinal hernia often coexists with an undescended testicle or hydrocele.

- With direct hernias, the sac protrudes through the abdominal wall because of weakness of the fascial floor of the inguinal canal.

B. Pulses should be symmetrical on both sides of the groin. If there is a disparity, look up the line to see what might be affecting the flow.

C. Nodes are plentiful in the inguinal area. Assess for enlargement and tenderness. Compare sides.

D. The skin in the groin should be examined since an EM rash could be missed if no one bothers to look.

III. GENITALS

The examination of the genitals might provide useful information in TBI patients because Lyme can so greatly impact the endocrine system. However, an internal exam in females is unnecessary unless clearly indicated and there is no other means to gather the necessary information.

PEARL: Since Bb can so powerfully influence hormones, it might be difficult to determine what is underlying co-morbidity and what is Lyme-influenced. The following sxs have been reported with LD: testicular pain, pelvic discomfort, menstrual irregularity, chronic pelvic pain, lactation, gynecomastia, inguinal lymphadenopathy, and menstrual difficulties.

In both males and females examine the skin in the genital region for lesions. Assess lymph nodes and pulses. Be on the look-out for any discharge or odor. Tanner staging may help you follow your TBI patient over time and provide a frame of reference.

Tanner stages are part of a scale of physical maturation in children and teens. This scale uses primary and secondary sexual characteristics to determine where the individual is on the maturation timeline. Development of pubic hair, male genitalia, and female breasts are the staging criteria. Due to natural variation individuals pass through Tanner stages at different rates that depend on genetics, nutrition, and general health status. This scale is useful in determining where an individual stands when compared to others in the same age group in reaching the various stages. Tanner stages can be useful in Lyme patients to see how the patient is progressing in areas governed by hormone levels which can be significantly impacted by Bb.

Pubic hair (male and female):

Tanner I: None (< 10 y/o)

Tanner II: Small amount of downy hair with minimal pigmentation on the penis and scrotum in males and labia in females (10 to 11.5 y/o)

Tanner III: Hair more coarse and curly and extends laterally (11.5 to 13 y/o)

Tanner IV: Adult-like hair extending across pubis (13 to 15 y/o)

Tanner V: Hair to medial thighs (15 +)

Genitals (male):

Tanner I: Prepubertal with undeveloped testicles and penis (< 9 y/o)

Tanner II: Testicular volume increases, scrotal skin thins, reddens, and enlarges, and penis grows (9 to 11 y/o)

Tanner III: Testes, penis, and scrotum enlarge (11 to 12.5 y/o)

Tanner IV: Testicular volume increases, scrotum enlarges and darkens, penis increases in length and circumference (12.5 to 14 y/o)

Tanner V: Adult testicular volume, scrotum, and penis (14+)

Breasts (female):

Tanner I: Prepubertal with no gland tissue and the areola follows contours of skin (<10 y/o)

Tanner II: Breast bud with small glandular tissue, areola widens (10 to 11.5 y/o)

Tanner III: Breast elevated and extends beyond areola which widens (11.5 to 13 y/o)

Tanner IV: Breast increases in size and elevation, areola and papilla project from the contour of the breast (13 to 15 y/o)

Tanner V: Adult size projecting papilla from areola (15 +)

Genital issues that might affect TBI patients:

MALE:

- The meatus is not always in the center of the penis. Hypospadias is not uncommon with the urethral opening found on the ventral surface of the penis.

- Check the foreskin for adhesions, retractability, swelling, or redness. Ensure that any circumcision site is healing. Circumcised foreskin should always be considered as a sample for pathogen testing as part of a TBI work-up.

- Hydroceles of the testicles and cord are common in babies and can sometimes be associated with inguinal hernias. A hydrocele is a collection of serous fluid in the scrotal sac. Hydroceles will transilluminate and will not reduce, whereas hernias usually will reduce and do not transilluminate. Most cases occur in kids between years 2 and 5 and the hydrocele is usually a sequela of localized inflammation.

- In infants, testes may be undescended and the scrotal sac will be empty. An undescended testicle remains in the inguinal canal or abdominal cavity instead of moving into the scrotum where it belongs. The testis may be undescended at birth or discovered later. On examination, one or both sides of the scrotum will be empty.

- The contents of an inguinal hernia can descend into the scrotum.

- Fungal infections are common over the scrotum and between the legs.

- A varicocele is the presence of varicose veins in the cord and presents like a "bag of worms."

- If the scrotum is filled with serous fluid the sac will transilluminate. If blood or tissue is present, the area will not easily transilluminate.

- In a number of STDs, males can be asymptomatic. If discharge is present, culture. Culture if there is a reason to suspect.

- Additional detail regarding the PE of the male genitalia was provided earlier in the *Groin* section of this chapter.

FEMALE:

- Dysmenorrhea is painful menstruation with cramping. The most common physical finding here is mild lower abdominal discomfort on palpation.

- A common finding in women with LD is chronic pelvic pressure or discomfort.

- Ovarian cysts can sometimes be felt through the abdominal wall if they are large. These most often are benign sacs of fluid that can start to appear at puberty. Usually ovarian cysts are asymptomatic but on those occasions when they twist or rupture they present signs and symptoms of an acute abdomen.

- Vaginal yeast infections due to antibiotic use can present with itchy, thick, white discharge.

- Endometriosis is the presence of endometrial tissue outside the uterine lining. This ectopic tissue usually remains in the pelvis but can show up in various body locations. This is functional tissue and will go through all the tissue changes that the endometrium inside the uterus will undergo. Discomfort will be cyclic. There may be pain to palpation in the lower abdomen. Severity of the pain does not correlate with the extent of the disease.

- Pelvic inflammatory disease or PID is an infection of the internal reproductive organs and adjacent tissue and can result in permanent damage and infertility if untreated. Usually bacterial, PID can lead to an acute abdomen, septicemia, and shock. Physical findings will show progression to an acute abdomen.

- Ectopic pregnancy is the implantation of a fertilized ovum outside the uterine cavity, most often in the fallopian tube. At first, an ectopic pregnancy can present like a regular pregnancy. But, invariably things go wrong. If ruptured, an ectopic pregnancy is life-threatening and can present as an acute abdomen.

- Premenstrual syndrome (PMS) consists of a wide range of symptoms that occur a few days prior to menses and usually stop at the onset of bleeding. PMS may be due to changes in hormones and we know Lyme can affect hormone balance. PMS includes physical, behavioral, and emotional signs and symptoms: bloating, cramping, breast tenderness, changes in bowels, changes in eating habits with cravings, less tolerance for noise or light, moods swings, difficulty concentrating, annoyance, fatigue, anxiety, edginess, forgetfulness, irritability, hostility, anger, poor judgment, sluggishness, and lethargy. Some of these signs and symptoms overlap with those of LD.

- PMDD or premenstrual dysphoric disorder can cause severe depression, irritability, and tension prior to menses. PMDD is considered more severe and potentially disabling than PMS.

- Females can have irritation to the external genitalia from a variety of causes including fungal rashes and contact dermatitis from soap or bubbles.

- Cysts and inflamed glands are not uncommon.

- If an internal pelvic exam is critical in a child, you might want to defer to a pediatric gynecologist unless you are very comfortable with this type of exam.

- Menstruating girls can and do get pregnant. In these cases, both the fetus and mother need to be treated for the TBI if indicated.

COMMON TO BOTH GENDERS:

- Nits can be present. A nit is the egg of a louse. Small, itchy, red maculopapules with nits indicate lice. Equally delightful are scabies which are skin mites. Here you will likely see excoriations from scratching.

- Both genders are susceptible to fungal infections. Chapter 25: *Ancillary Treatments* details all about fungus. The antibiotic regimens prescribed for many of the TBIs can allow fungal overgrowth. Fungus can cause a raised, red, itchy, uncomfortable (even painful) rash in both males and females.

- Genital warts are caused by HPV. The genital/anal region is a very common site of warts caused by human papilloma virus. These warts can be large and cumbersome and interfere with defecation. If you find warts here, consider there may also be lesions on the skin elsewhere and on the larynx.

- Cysts and inflamed glands are not uncommon on the genitals of both sexes.

- Common STDs include GC, genital herpes, and genital warts, but there are many others. Lab testing looking for co-morbidities might include HSV, which can present as ulcers or vesicles. If you find one STD, look for others. There may be discharge but in many cases of GC, males will be asymptomatic. If indicated, get a culture or refer to someone who can do all the indicated testing.

- HPV can look like traditional warts with small, irregular vegetations or they can present as translucent bumps. HPV is the most common viral STD and there are many subtypes, some associated with a higher risk of cervical cancer.

- Always be cognizant of the possibility of sexual abuse.

- Sexual concerns: Sexual problems are beyond the scope of this book. Still, TBIs can significantly impact all manner of hormone levels. This might complicate the clinical picture especially at puberty and other times of significant hormonal shifts such as pregnancy and menopause. STDs can impact the immune system as can TBIs. Remember that the causal pathogens of Lyme and syphilis are cousins. Concurrent disease may exacerbate or mask symptoms. In the US, syphilis is less common but not unheard of these days, and we certainly don't want to be dealing with two spirochetes at once. Prevention of pregnancy is a topic of interest to many patients but from the TBI perspective, the HCP needs to make sure that the patient is not pregnant. If so, then the fetus would need to be protected with appropriate antibiotic therapy of sufficient dose and duration. In the chapters dealing with specific pathogens, pregnancy regimens are discussed. The patient should be given the opportunity to speak to the HCP alone if desired. Chaperones should always be available and used as appropriate.

- Hernias can manifest in both genders. A description of the hernia exam is detailed in the earlier *Groin* section.

IV. URINARY TRACT

The urinary tract consists of the kidney, ureters, bladder, and urethra. The kidney can be palpated through the abdominal wall, but look for pain at the costovertebral angle (CVA) of the back to gather additional information about kidney infections and stones.

Lyme is thought to cause problems with urination, occasional incontinence, new onset of enuresis without a family history, irritable bladder, interstitial cystitis, and intermittent loss of bladder control. Kidney failure is one of the principal causes of death in dogs with Lyme.

Palpation of the kidney through the abdominal wall has its limitations. A technically expert examiner can palpate cysts or masses on the kidney through the abdominal wall in some patients. Imaging studies tend to provide much more detail, when indicated. Considerable insight can be gathered by examining the kidneys from the back. The top of each kidney is at about the 12th thoracic vertebrae and the bottom extends to about lumbar 3. Symptoms of kidney problems often include lower back pain. A firm blow with the side of the fist at the costovertebral angle can elicit pain and suggest inflammation of the kidney.

The urinary bladder is a sac holding urine that is located in the anterior part of the pelvis and can be palpated through the abdominal wall. The normal bladder cannot be palpated when empty. When filled with urine the round superior margin is easily discerned. Usually smooth and oval, the bladder can also be assessed by percussion. The nearby intestine will sound tympanic, while a full bladder will be dull. Sometimes masses and spasms can be palpated. Since a tumor can feel like a full bladder, consider additional testing if there is any question.

Renal disease affects all body systems so check the skin for abnormal color and turgor. Kidney malfunction can be one reason for edema. Renal disease can be associated with hypertension. A patient may hyperventilate in an effort to blow off CO_2 to compensate for a metabolic acidosis due to kidney problems. The high blood sugars in uncontrolled diabetics are notorious for damaging the kidney. While there are many signs and symptoms associated with urinary problems, the most common will be frequency, urgency, flow problems, nocturia, dysuria, pain in the flank or over the bladder, pyuria, blood, and incontinence.

The kidney is the primary site for drug elimination and should be monitored carefully. The kidney is also susceptible to toxins whether it be from drug molecules or pathogens. There can be immune and autoimmune reactions affecting the kidney. In the case of Strep (and possibly Bb), several pathologic mechanisms can be in play at once.

PEARL: The pain of a kidney stone is exquisite, right up there with natural childbirth on the unbearable scale, and beyond.

Terms and conditions associated with the urinary tract that may be pertinent to TBI patients:

Polyuria: Too much urine

Oliguria: Too little urine

Azotemia: Presence of nitrogen compounds, like BUN, in the blood. Increasing azotemia suggests decreasing renal function.

Enuresis: Bedwetting is normal up to about 3 y/o and can be due to delayed neuromuscular maturation. Genetics is a factor. Ask the parents how long they wet the bed. Bedwetting associated with Lyme may be due to spirochete damage to the bladder or other organs or pathogen impact on the ANS.

Urinary Tract Infection: UTIs can affect the upper part of the urinary tract (kidney and ureters) or the lower segments (the bladder and urethra). Lower UTIs are one of the most prevalent bacterial diseases in kids.

Pyelonephritis: An infection of the kidney is called pyelonephritis and this illness can present with flank pain, bloody urine, fever, and chills. These patients can rapidly become SICK. Bacterial kidney infections usually respond quickly to appropriate antibiotics. Nonetheless, some cases become chronic which can lead to fibrosis and compromise of kidney function.

Cystitis: Cystitis is an infection of the bladder that is more common in females since the E. *coli* pathogen, which is often the causative agent, has a shorter distance to go from the anus to the urethra in girls. In contrast, the pathogens would need to traverse the length of the penis to infect the bladder in boys. Some common signs and symptoms include urgency, frequency, painful urination, bladder spasms, nocturia, and enuresis. Persistent symptoms can lead to mild fever, low back pain, malaise, and nausea. There may be tenderness to palpation over the bladder.

Urethritis: An infection of the urethra can be a part of a UTI or an STD. The meatus in both sexes can be red and inflamed due to mechanical irritation, or chemicals. Do they still make Mr. Bubble? Such products irritated many a meatus over decades. Urethritis caused by STDs can result in purulent discharge, but lack of discharge does not rule out an STD.

Interstitial cystitis: This condition presents exactly like a bacterial UTI except no bacteria is ever recovered on routine cultures. Interstitial cystitis is very common in Lyme patients and presents just like an infectious UTI characterized by dysuria, hesitancy, urgency, and frequency. The difference is that with interstitial cystitis cultures are consistently NEGATIVE and the symptoms do not resolve with traditional antibiotic regimens. Perhaps we have not been looking for the right pathogens. In these patients, Bb have been picked up with cystoscopy and biopsy of the bladder trigone and supported with PCR. Perhaps treating the Lyme will resolve these seemingly "aseptic" symptoms. The common UTI antibiotics are not the best choices against Bb.

Acute renal failure: ARF is loss of kidney function which can have many causes including diabetes, diminished circulation, obstruction, drug reactions, toxins, or autoimmunity. If not treated ARF can lead to progressive loss of kidney function and end-stage disease. Early signs are oliguria and azotemia. Chronic renal failure can impact other body systems especially GI, CNS, skin, CVS, and respiratory function. Watch the BUN and creatinine.

Neurogenic bladder: The term neurogenic bladder is used to refer to any of the myriad problems that can come from interruption of normal innervations to the bladder including incontinence or retention. Neurologic problems can be spastic and hypertonic or flaccid and hypotonic. Signs and symptoms will depend on the underlying cause and the extent of ANS involvement. Some complaints include retention, incontinence, trouble with the process of micturation, and inability to completely empty the bladder. In these cases, the residual urine can make the patient more prone to infections and stones. Neurogenic bladder can be due to congenital anomalies, injury to nerves, spinal cord damage, or brain injury. Certain pathogens, like Bb, which can alter the ANS, have been implicated.

Streptococcal glomerulonephritis: This autoimmune type reaction is a bilateral inflammation of the glomeruli which are the business units of the kidney. Symptoms present in association with Strep infection of the throat or skin such as pharyngitis or impetigo. Most common in boys 3 to 7 y/o, SG can occur at any age. Most patients recover if appropriately treated. About 5% develop long-term renal problems. Glomerulonephritis can become chronic with inflammation and scarring and progressive failure. Usually symptoms begin 1 to 3 weeks after an untreated sore throat. Signs and symptoms include edema, proteinuria, azotemia, hematuria, coffee-colored urine, oliguria, fatigue, HTN, and electrolyte imbalances. CHF from fluid overload can lead to pulmonary edema.

PEARL: There are a number of parallels between the clinical course of Strep and that of Bb. Mechanisms of disease that have shown to be pathophysiologic for Strep should be considered as a possibility for Bb.

Section 17-M

Joints, Musculoskeletal, and Pertinent Differential

I do the very best I can. I mean to keep going. If the end brings me out all right, then what is said against me won't matter. If I'm wrong, ten angels swearing I was right won't make a difference.

Abe Lincoln

JOINTS/MUSCULOSKELETAL

Early in the history of Lyme disease, the condition was called Lyme arthritis. If there was no joint involvement, there was thought to be no Lyme. We now know that there are many ways for Bb to present itself. Still the examination of the joints and the overall effects on the musculoskeletal system are especially important in evaluating TBI patients.

The musculoskeletal exam can be taking place throughout the initial interview and all through the PE. See how the patient walks, stands, sits, gets up, lies down, grasps, pinches, and leans over. Observe the person in various positions: from front, from behind, with feet together and apart, walking, bending forward, and touching toes while standing. Be aware of any person with a limp. That limp could be hiding a lot of Lyme pathology. On exam, a Lyme patient might be able to kneel but then not be able to get back up. They might have a hard time climbing stairs or difficulty lifting and carrying.

As always, examine the overlying skin for lesions, rashes, and discolorations. Assess pulses and lymph nodes. Although the *Neurologic Exam* section in the next chapter will detail the examination of reflexes, strength, and sensation, all of these parameters can be assessed at the same time as the musculoskeletal system during an actual exam.

For each bone check:

>   Deformities
>
>   Nodules
>
>   Point tenderness
>
>   Masses
>
>   General pain
>
>   Asymmetry
>
>   Compare to other bone, if paired
>
>   Normal characteristics for the specific bone

For each joint check:

>   Heat
>
>   Redness
>
>   Swelling
>
>   Effusion

>   Stability
>
>   Ligaments
>
>   ROM
>
>   Boney enlargement
>
>   Compare to other joint, if paired
>
>   Normal characteristics for the specific joint
>   (The knee should not be expected to rotate.)

*PEARL: A **ligament** is a strong fibrous band connecting bone to bone. A **tendon** is fibrous connective tissue that connects muscle to bone. I looked that up so you didn't have to.*

For each muscle check:

>   Tendons
>
>   Spasms
>
>   Mobility
>
>   Flexibility
>
>   Strength
>
>   Pain to palpation
>
>   General tenderness
>
>   Nodules
>
>   Masses
>
>   Development
>
>   Symmetry, if paired

Individual bones:

Each bone has a characteristic shape. Palpation of the bones, even point pressure should not hurt. Inspection should tell you most of what you need to know. If you find an abnormal shape, prominences that should not be there, or bone pain on physical exam, investigate further. For those of you who are counting PEARLS, consider each of the following bullet points to be a PEARL.

Bone PEARLS:

- Unequal leg length can impact gait, balance, and coordination and may result in a noticeable limp.

- Infection in the bone is a very big deal and should be aggressively treated. **Osteomyelitis** is a pyrogenic bone infection that may be acute or chronic. This infection can occur after trauma, resulting in a hematoma in the bone with subsequent blood-borne spread of infection elsewhere in the body. Osteomyelitis can remain local, but might also disseminate systemically. With chronic infection, draining sinus tracts might find their way to the surface, most commonly at the lower end of the femur, but also the humerus, tibia, and radius. Acute osteomyelitis causes sudden pain, tenderness, heat, swelling, and limited movement. Associated systemic manifestations include fever, nausea, and malaise. Staph *aureus* is a common etiologic agent. Chronic infection can persist for years with persistent drainage of pus from pockets in old sinus tracts.

- Bone cancers do occur in all ages.

- The clavicle or collar bone is a common fracture site.

- Broken or bruised ribs can result in point tenderness and cause splinting to avoid pain. This discomfort can restrict respirations and result in shallow breathing and suppressed coughs. Even without trauma, the ribs of Lyme patients are often tender to touch.

- The H&P may not reveal everything. With bones, X-rays and other diagnostic modalities can be especially useful.

- Shin splints can be hard to distinguish from the sharp shin pain of Bartonella.

- Shin pain occurs in some cases of Lyme.

- One arm hanging lower than the other may suggest transient growth asymmetry in the boney structure, which has been observed in Lyme patients.

- **Exostosis** is exaggerated bone growth at the point where bone typically grows and can be normal. Exostosis is seen in growing kids and adolescents. Often painful at first, the discomfort diminishes as the outgrowth blends in with the normal skeletal architecture. Often these enhanced growth areas are of no significance unless they press on the adjacent nerves, tendons, and muscles causing pain. They are most commonly found in the phalanges and occasionally need to be removed.

- Bone pain in Lyme is most common in the tibia, ribs, iliac crest, sternum, and clavicles.

- Heel spurs can be due to repetitive injury to the calcaneus

Individual muscles:

Muscles are tissues composed of contractile fibers that allow for movement. The unique characteristic of muscle is its ability to contract. There are three types of muscles in humans 1) smooth muscle which includes the involuntary muscle of the viscera, 2) cardiac which is the heart muscle, and 3) striated muscle which is the voluntary skeletal muscle. Here we are focused on physical examination of skeletal muscle.

Muscles should be fairly symmetrical, although they are often slightly more developed on the dominant side. Muscle tone is usually recorded as normal, spastic, or flaccid. Muscles are the main conveyors of strength and coordination. Toned muscles help to protect joints. Is the muscle development age appropriate? Are there suggestions of steroid use?

Muscle hypotonia is the cardinal manifestation of gestational Lyme. Features of hypotonia include: arms and legs hanging by sides, decreased DTRs, little resistance to passive motion, diminished muscle tone, delay in gross and fine motor skills, excess flexibility, drooling, speech difficulties secondary to decreased muscle strength, rounded shoulders, and leaning.

PEARL: Use of fluoroquinolones (ciprofloxacin, ofloxacin, levofloxacin) has been associated with rhabdomyolysis (muscle wasting), tendonitis, and tendon rupture. Be careful to monitor muscle health when using these drugs.

PEARL: In LD, muscles may be stiff in the morning and weak and painful at rest.

Individual joints:

With TBIs, joints are prime targets. Begin by looking at the patient's overall habitus. Habitus means the combined physical characteristics with the learned set of attitudes, dispositions, skills, and actions acquired through AODL. How do they carry themselves? How do they move? Many patients are hypermobile at baseline and this could predispose them to more joint problems over time. Other people are naturally inflexible, which will limit their ROM on exam. Consider their baseline prior to the disease.

Joint PEARLS:

- A thick warm synovial area suggests rheumatoid arthritis.

- In infants the joints should move symmetrically and be equally active.

- Redness of the skin over a joint can suggest infection or gout or rheumatic fever.

- Boney enlargement at a joint suggests degenerative disease.

- Creaky and cracking joints can suggest Lyme.

- Noisy popping and cracking of the neck upon movement is sometimes called the "Lyme shrug."

- Joint pain is one of the most common findings in Lyme, especially at the shoulder and knee.

- Lyme can have migratory joint involvement.

- Jaw pain due to Lyme damage to the TMJ is not uncommon.

- Bb are known to cause pain in the SI joint.

- Arthritis associated with Lyme may not appear for months.

- Check carefully for hypermobility which can predispose a patient to joint problems.

- Bb can find its way into the fibroblasts of joints. Since the fibroblasts are involved with the synthesis of collagen, connective tissue, and cartilage, the entire structural foundation of the joint might be impacted. I think my old right knee might confirm that.

To fully examine a joint you need to take the joint through its full ROM. Unfortunately, this means you need to know the ROM of each joint. Trying to move a joint through a motion that is not anatomically possible is not only unpleasant for the patient but also clues her into the idea that you might not know what you're doing. Remember, many motions have reciprocal motions, for example, flexion is the opposite of extension. Most functional movement requires a combination of motions. You will need to remember a few basics before you begin the structural exam.

Common terms that describe motion:

Flexion	Movement that DECREASES the angle between two parts such as bending the elbow or clenching the fingers into a fist. At 90 degrees, as when sitting, the knees are flexed.
Extension	Movement that INCREASES the angle between two parts. When shaking hands, the fingers are fully extended. At 180 degrees, as when standing, the knees are extended.

Abduction	Motion that pulls a part AWAY from the midline of the body. Spreading the fingers apart is abduction. Raising the arms out to the side is abduction.
Adduction	Motion that pulls a part TOWARD the midline of the body. Dropping the arms to the sides, bringing the knees to touch each other, and pulling the toes together are all adduction. Think of "adding" a part to the whole.
Rotation	Motion that occurs when a part turns on its axis. The head rotates on the neck when a child shakes her head "no." Rotation can be internal (medial) or external (lateral), but no one reading this really cares.
Elevation	Movement in a superior direction as when the shoulders shrug
Depression	Movement in an inferior direction as when the shoulders unshrug
Medial	Direction TOWARD the midline
Lateral	Direction AWAY from the midline
Pronation	Motion of forearm that leaves palm facing down
Supination	Motion of forearm that leaves palm facing up (like holding a bowl of soup)
Apposition	The ability to put two parts in contact. Opposable thumbs allow humans to place the thumb in touch with the fingers of the same hand and separate us from camels on the evolutionary tree.
Dorsiflexion	Movement of the entire foot TOWARD the head as though you were going to scratch your eyebrow with your toe
Plantar flexion	Movement at the ankle that takes the foot AWAY from the head as though pushing on the gas pedal
Eversion	Movement of the sole of the foot AWAY from the body midline
Inversion	Movement of the sole of the foot TOWARD the body midline. Hyperinversion is usually what occurs when an ankle is sprained.

The prefix *hyper-* before a motion such as hyperextension means the joint is moving beyond what is normal and this excessive motion may stress the joint.

Common terms that describe joint pathology:

Sprain: A stretch or tear of a joint capsule or a ligament connecting <u>bone to bone</u>. A sprain threatens the stability of a joint.

A sprain often occurs after a joint is forced beyond its normal ROM such as a twisted ankle. Symptoms include pain, swelling, and difficulty moving.

Strain: A stretch or tear of a tendon connecting <u>muscle to bone</u> occurs when the muscle is stretched and then suddenly contracts. This can occur when running or jumping. An acute strain causes pain, spasm, or tightness, diminished strength, and decreased ROM. Chronic strain can develop from overuse or repeat stress such as the tendonitis of tennis elbow.

Bursitis: Inflammation of a bursa. A bursa is a sac or cavity lined with a synovial membrane and filled with synovial fluid which has the consistency of raw egg whites. The bursae provide a cushion for the joint and decrease friction allowing for free movement. Bursae can become inflamed due to stress on the joint, irritants, or infection. The most common sites of bursitis are the shoulder, knee, and elbow.

Tendonitis: Inflammation of a tendon

Chondritis: Inflammation of cartilage has been associated with Lyme. Cartilage is a preferred tissue for Bb. Lacking blood vessels and nerves, cartilage is often used as a safe refuge for the spirochete. Once there, the Bb can release toxins that can damage and inflame the cartilage. The most commonly affected sites are the ear, nose, and costochondral joints.

Effusion: An effusion is an escape of fluid into an area where it is not normally present in such amounts. A joint effusion is increased fluid in the joint space. The fluid can be comprised of synovial fluid, inflammatory fluids, blood, serum, or pus. An effusion in a joint can be due to trauma, infection, or inflammation such as arthritis. My first experience with Lyme in my knee presented with effusion, the second did not. One orthopod told me that a joint wasn't a Lyme joint unless it presented with effusion. That's not true.

Arthritis: An inflammation of the joints. There are more than 100 forms of arthritis but we will focus on those that may be pertinent to TBIs. Several of the TBIs, especially Lyme, inflame joints and are the primary etiologic agents of the associated arthritis. Remember that more than one pathologic process can be active at a time. TBI co-infections can combine to hammer away at the joints. To treat infectious arthritis, appropriate antibiotics will be needed. The following list is provided to give clues on what to look for during the physical exam. Use the list as you are working your way through the differential diagnosis. Hopefully, if you have a patient with significant joint signs, this list will help you discriminate one type of arthritis from another. Assume that all forms of arthritis listed include some type of joint discomfort and limited function. This list will try to highlight those factors that distinguish each type of arthritis. These distinctions may be important in that some forms of arthritis are treated with modalities that would exacerbate the symptoms in other types.

1. **Infectious arthritis** is the inflammatory reaction that occurs in response to a pathogen, usually bacteria, in the joint space. Antibiotics will be needed that are appropriate for the pathogen and are able to penetrate into the joint space. Antibiotics can have trouble getting to where they are needed in the joints. The cartilage within the joints does not have its own blood supply, so it's not like that tissue is going to be awash in antimicrobial. An infected joint will cause progressively worse pain, stiffness, heat, redness, swelling, chills, and fever. If not treated promptly and appropriately, the patient can get irreversible joint damage and toxemia. Examples of infectious arthritis include:

   a. Acute Lyme arthritis

   b. Chronic Lyme arthritis

   c. Other infectious etiologies causing joint inflammation

   d. Septic arthritis can be a medical emergency. Whether the infection started in the joint and moved systemically or started systemically and then localized in the joint, is immaterial. Once you have a septic patient, concentrate on targeting the correct pathogen with the appropriate antibiotic, penetrating the joint space, and treating long enough and hard enough to be effective. Remember that pathogens like Bb can be especially difficult to isolate from joint aspirate. Just because you can't easily grow them or see them under the microscope, does not mean they aren't there. If a patient with a septic joint is not responding to the first choice antibiotic, consider that you are not targeting the actual pathogen. Ineffective therapy can lead to permanent joint damage, systemic sepsis, and death.

PEARL: The arthritis associated with LD is often called migrating or traveling arthritis because the discomfort can move from joint to joint. Thomas McPherson Brown was the first to associate infection with arthritis and successfully treat with antibiotics. Critics could not tolerate his success.

2. **Rheumatoid arthritis** is an autoimmune condition that affects not just joints but also many other body systems. The joint problems in RA just happen to be the most obvious component. In RA, the joint lining and cartilage are the most damaged. RA is a symmetrical arthritis that affects fingers, wrists, knees, and elbows and can lead to severe deformity. Usually

RA affects people 20 years and older and may take weeks or months for full presentation of symptoms. The hands can provide many diagnostic clues, especially the PIP and MCP joints. There are clear signs of inflammation including swelling, fatigue, and low grade fever. Severe deformities may evolve including ulnar deviation of digits, spindle shaped joints, swan neck anomalies, and other debilitating deformities of the hand that severely limit function. On X-ray, findings include narrowed joint space, bone erosion, and multiple abnormalities. Lab tests often show anemia and a positive ESR and RF. Extra-articular features are common including fatigue, malaise, anorexia, and lymphadenopathy. RA is often treated with steroids and other immunosuppressants.

3. **Juvenile rheumatoid arthritis**: What used to be referred to as JRA, is now called **juvenile inflammatory arthritis** or JIA. There are several syndromes that are labeled JRA and some are quite different from the others. In general, JRA (JIA) presents with skin rash, fever, joint pain, and loss of joint function. JRA can be disabling and limit activities. This is a systemic disorder that affects kids less than 16 y/o. Although JRA is rare under 6 months old, the youngest child diagnosed was 6 weeks. There are two age groups where JRA diagnoses peak: between 1 and 3-years-old and between 8 and 12-years-old. More girls are diagnosed with JRA than boys. The etiology may be infectious or immunologic or a combination. One version of JRA acutely presents with a fever up to 103° and a rheumatoid rash of red macules. There can be growth disturbances in the bones at the site of the affected joints. The knee is the most commonly involved joint site. The joint pain may come and go. In some versions of JRA, only a minority have a positive RF. Some patients have dramatic organomegaly of the spleen, liver, and lymph nodes. There can be cardiac complications and eye involvement. Some have HLA-B27 antigens like many adult RA patients. There are no real X-ray changes. JRA might be hard to distinguish from Lyme disease and should keep popping in and out of the differential diagnosis as more information is gathered.

PEARL: Reading the descriptions of the possible presentations of the various forms of JRA, I have to wonder how many Lyme cases were misdiagnosed as JRA over the past 2 decades. Without targeted antibiotics, perhaps these kids had a longer clinical course than they would have had, if a diagnosis of Lyme had been made when appropriate. Just like Lyme was originally thought to be primarily an arthritic disease, JRA may be mislabeled and misunderstood on into the future.

4. **Osteoarthritis** (OA) or degenerative joint disease (DJD) is the most common arthritis affecting both large and small joints of the hands, feet, back, hip, vertebral column, and knee. OA is usually due to wear and tear of the joints but can also result from trauma. OA begins in the cartilage and leads to the two opposing bones eroding into each other so the patient ends up with bone on bone. At first there is minor pain, but then the joint pain becomes continuous and may be problematic at night. The discomfort can be debilitating and often prevents normal activities. OA affects weight bearing areas like the back, spine, and pelvis. Usually OA is most common in the older population who had prior trauma or consistent stress on the joint. Excess body weight can add to the stress on the joints. OA may take months or years to get symptomatic. There is NO evidence of inflammation, NO lab findings, and NO systemic signs. X-rays show narrowed joint space, osteophytes (spurs), osteosclerosis (thickening), and subchondral cysts. On PE, there can be numerous nodules such as boney enlargements at the PIPs and hard nodules or enlargements of the tubercles of the phalanges of the fingers. Otzi, a mummy from around 3000 BCE, that was recently found along the border between what is now Italy and Austria (where my grandfather was born), had osteoarthritis. He probably got it the old fashioned way, by walking too far over the Dolomites. Or…Otzi's joint disintegration could be associated with the Borrelia *burgdorferi* found in DNA samples taken from this "Iceman."

5. **Psoriatic arthritis**: These patients usually get skin lesions first and later arthritis. They have continuous joint pain, stiffness, and swelling. There are periods of remission and then recurrence.

6. **SLE arthritis**: Lupus is a collagen vascular disease that can present with severe arthritis, rash, extreme photosensitivity, hair loss, kidney problems, lung fibrosis, and constant joint pain. Remember lupus patients can get bitten by ticks, too.

7. **Traumatic arthritis**: A single traumatic event or repeated small traumas can result in DJD type changes in a number of joints.

8. **Gout** is prevalent in the general population. Arthritis from gout is caused by deposits of uric acid crystals in the joint space. These crystals cause inflammation. Early on in the clinical course, one joint is involved, most often the MTP joint of the great toe. Later ankles, knees, and elbows can be affected. The pain can be excruciating and crippling. Joints can become swollen and lose function. An acute attack may come on over a few hours. During a gout attack, the big toe

is the epitome of what inflammation means. Swollen, red, hot, painful! Inflammation does not present any better than this. X-rays might show punched-out bone erosions and tophi which are crystal deposits in tissue near joints.

9. **Ankylosing spondylitis** is a chronic progressive condition involving the joints of the spine, the costovertebral joints, and the sacroiliac joints. Sclerosis (fibrosis) of the SI joints is a hallmark sign. The changes here are similar to those seen in RA. Ankylosis (stiffening, immobility) may occur, giving rise to a stiff, straight, immobile back. Usually ankylosis starts in the SI joints and low back, reaching the neck only late in the clinical course. This condition is not common in young kids but depending on the underlying etiology can cause significant decrease in ROM and spastic tenderness of muscles. The patient may need to turn the whole body to look sideways and the neck thrusts forward. Ankylosing spondylitis should be part of the differential diagnosis when assessing joint involvement in Lyme disease.

10. **Systemic arthritis** or general joint inflammation, can be secondary to diseases such as hepatitis, IBD, sarcoid, and many others.

PEARL: Joints that are already injured or diseased may be more prone to additional compromise. When a joint hurts, we tend to naturally splint or guard it, thereby restricting motion, as well as fluid flow and nerve conduction. The joint can stiffen as in frozen shoulder. Stagnation may allow a burrowing spirochete a great haven, right near the cartilage buffet. When movement is subsequently attempted, additional stress can be placed on the joint, resulting in an increased potential for injury. Inflammatory changes can cause a cycle of increased responses, thereby increasing symptoms. We know that Bb likes to hit you when you're down. Treat Lyme joints with respect.

INDIVIDUAL JOINTS

Shoulders:

The shoulder is a common site for Lyme involvement, often one-sided. One of the most mobile joints in the body, the shoulder is comprised of the clavicle (collar bone), the scapula (shoulder blade), and the humerus (top arm bone), and a lot of cartilage. Bb seemingly love cartilage.

A healthy shoulder is always trying to balance between the mobility it needs to perform all its many tasks and the stability required to lift, push, pull, and throw. Quite versatile, the shoulder can abduct, adduct, flex, elevate, depress, extend, and rotate. This means you can throw a ball, shrug, and

snuggle. Because the shoulder is so mobile and so active, it is the site of many injuries including dislocation. The rotator cuff is a group of muscles and tendons that serves to stabilize the shoulder. The cuff is particularly susceptible to stress, sprains, strains, and tears. Check for inflammation including redness, swelling, and heat. Assess for fluid in the joint space, point tenderness, general achiness, full ROM, and stability.

Be careful to avoid frozen shoulder. Once the patient feels discomfort in the shoulder, she tends to subconsciously immobilize the shoulder and her HCP may contribute to that stasis with slings and wrappings. In these cases, the shoulder can stiffen almost to the point of inflexibility. Have the patient bend forward at the waist and using her hand trace the alphabet in the air above the floor using LARGE letters. This activity should take the shoulder through much of its ROM without stress. Passive ROM can be used as well. PT may be needed if the stiffness is not caught early.

Lyme can present in one or both shoulders. Often there is a general discomfort in the shoulder that may remain or move off to other joints.

PEARL: An athletic patient is going to be more at risk for shoulder injuries. Since the shoulder is a prime site for Lyme involvement, look carefully as you try to uncover the cause of the discomfort. Remember more than one pathology may be active at a time and one condition may make a patient more susceptible to another.

Elbows

The two elbow joints are the hinges between the upper arm and the forearm. These joints can flex, extend, pronate, and supinate. To examine: bend and straighten with the patient's hand touching the shoulder and then extending back out to 180 degrees. Then, with the arms at the sides and elbows flexed, turn the palms up and down. Look for signs of inflammation such as swelling, redness, or heat. Assess fluid in the joint space, and point tenderness. The bicipital reflex can be tested in the crook of the elbow.

Common abnormalities of the elbow:

• A tender lateral epicondyle of the humerus can be tennis elbow or tendonitis.

• Olecranon bursitis includes swelling and other signs of inflammation of the bursa around the elbow. This condition may result from trauma or from arthritis (Lyme, gout, RA).

• Little kids, more often than we would like, experience radial head subluxation. Also called nursemaid's elbow, the condition often follows a sudden pull up of the child's extended arm, as we all have done in trying to get a two-year-old out of the street and onto the sidewalk before she gets squished. While not especially painful, the child will sit with the arm flexed and pronated. She will not be able to supinate. The radial head needs to be repositioned back into its proper place. Orthopedic PAs are quite good at this since they do it so often. Parents should refrain from doing the reduction themselves, unless they are orthopedic PAs.

• Hitting the funny bone is not pathognomonic for anything related to Lyme but I thought you might be interested. When there is a sharp blow to the end of the ulnar bone you are actually smacking the ulnar nerve that passes close to the surface through the ulnar groove. This results in a brief pins and needles sensation that can be quite uncomfortable.

Wrists

The wrist joints connect the forearm to the hand. Look for inflammation, point tenderness, and any limits to the full ROM. The wrist can flex, extend, and rotate.

To test for carpal tunnel entrapment: Hold the wrists in full flexion (back of the hand toward the head) for 60 seconds. If numbness and tingling develop over the distribution of median nerve (palm side of the thumb, index, and middle fingers and part of the ring finger) this suggests compression of the median nerve at the wrist. Carpal tunnel is not common unless the wrist has been exposed to repetitive motion over long periods of time. However, other factors like congenital anomalies can contribute to the problem. The more you know, the more you can rule out when looking for TBI changes.

Ganglia are cystic, round, non-tender, swellings along tendon sheaths or joints. They appear commonly on the dorsum of hands and wrists. These can be confused with subcutaneous nodules found in bartonellosis and Strep or with the nodules under the skin that occasionally accompany rheumatoid arthritis or rheumatic fever. Life is a constant differential diagnosis.

Fingers

Also called digits or phalanges, the fingers can flex, extend, abduct, and adduct. They are capable of very fine movement. To examine the ROM, flex and extend the fingers. Spread the fingers wide and then adduct them back to neutral. Have the patient make a fist. Look for signs of deformities and inflammations such as swelling, redness, and heat. If there is pain, is it localized or diffuse? Many manifestations of arthritis appear in the hands. Distinguishing between the various types of arthritis can be a challenge. Remember that more than one

process may be active at a time. Steroids and immune modulators used to treat one form of arthritis may exacerbate another. Keep your wits about you as you sort through the physical findings. Look just above in the *Arthritis* section for the distinguishing features of the different types of joint inflammation found in the fingers.

PEARL: A good indicator of Lyme in the fingers is subtle arthralgia. On exam, mild tenderness is elicited on gentle palpation. Using the index finger and thumb, lightly touch the joints. Many Lyme patients will pull their fingers away as though they were pulling away from a flame, almost reflexively before the sensation could reach their awareness. With Lyme there may be slightly swollen finger joints and digits.

Also in the fingers you are going to want to look at the nails for paronychia and feel the temperature of the digits. Cold extremities are a hallmark of Bartonella infection.

Sacroiliac Joint

The sacroiliac joint is the articulation between the sacrum and the innominate bone of the pelvis. Even though this joint normally has very limited motion due to interlocking surfaces, the SI joint can be the site of much discomfort. On physical exam, palpate the SI area for tenderness and signs of inflammation. Osteopathic manipulations might relieve discomfort in the SI area.

Hips

The hip is the joint between the femur and the acetabulum of the pelvis. This joint has an extensive ROM and can flex, extend, abduct, adduct, and both internally and externally rotate. Of course, in such a busy place, much can go wrong. When examining the hip look for abnormal ROM, signs of inflammation such as heat, redness, swelling, and pain. The hip joint is a common site for arthritis, bursitis, tendonitis, fractures, strains, snapping, and referred pain from the lumbar region. Necrosis of the joint can occur when blood flow is compromised causing cells to die. When this occurs in kids, the term **Legg-Calve-Perthes** disease is used. This condition can lead to permanent damage and arthritis.

While you're in the vicinity, check bilateral femoral pulses. If there is significant discrepancy in the strength of the pulse between sides, look up the chain to see where the problem might be.

In kids **hip dysplasia** is not uncommon. Here the hip is either dislocated or out of position due to congenital, developmental, or traumatic causes. While not painful, hip dysplasia can lead to impaired walking and early arthritis.

With the infant supine and the hips and knees flexed, completely abduct the thighs until the skin hits the surface of the table. Limited abduction and a palpable clunk as the femoral head slides into the joint socket are signs of hip dislocation. Females and breech deliveries have a higher incidence of dysplasia.

> *PEARL: Hips of all infants should be examined for dislocation. With the baby supine, flex the legs to right angles at the hips and knees. Abduct until the outside of each knee touches the exam table. When the dislocated head of the femur (which is behind the acetabulum in these cases) goes back into place it will click, The click will be heard during the abduction. You will also see and feel it going back into place. Place your middle finger over the greater trochanter of the femur and the thumb over the lesser trochanter. As the child gets older the click is less and you will have to rely on the feel of the joint as it abducts.*

In older patients the hips can be examined at the same time as the knee when the patient is supine. Test rotation by rocking each leg back and forth with a rolling motion at the thigh. Any pain now cautions for a very gentle rest of exam.

> *PEARL: In checking for hip disease have the standing patient shift weight from one leg to the other. The pelvis will tilt to the bad hip when weight is borne on the affected side and will remain level when the weight is borne on the unaffected side (Trendelenberg sign).*

Knees

The knee is the mid-leg joint at the articulation of the femur and tibia. The patella, or knee cap, is a sesamoid bone that sits in the tendon of the quadriceps muscle. Along with the shoulder, the knee is the prime site for Lyme arthritis. What is it about the knees and shoulders that make Bb target them? Both are very active and both have a disproportionate amount of cartilage. Both are prone to damage from many causes, where on-going subclinical inflammation may be present. Both have deep places where a pathogen could lie dormant for extended periods and perhaps elude high concentrations of antibiotics as they float by in the blood. What do these two joints share that make the Lyme focus there so often? Why do some patients get shoulder pain and others knee pain? A few get both and some neither. What an intriguing pathogen!

Careful examination of the knee is warranted even if the patient has no current complaints. When Lyme flares it can present similarly to past episodes or in completely different ways. Document any baseline abnormalities.

Examine the knee for signs of inflammation such as redness, swelling, pain, and heat. Look for fluid in the joint and examine the patella for point tenderness and mobility. Assess stability and ROM.

There are many ways to examine the knee. First observe and compare one knee to the other. There should be normal hollows around the patella. Loss of normal hollows indicates fluid or increased synovial density. Thickening, bogginess, or tenderness suggests inflammation of the joint.

Look for knock knees or flexion contracture, which is an inability to fully extend. Look for any deformity or muscle atrophy. Palpate the area above and on both sides of the patella. Note tenderness, thickening, or bogginess. Palpate the tibiofemoral joint space for fluid. Examine the popliteal space for pulses and swellings. Popliteal cysts are not uncommon.

Rotate the hip internally by pulling the knee medially. As you move the knee place a hand over the knee to feel crepitation which suggests irregular articular surfaces. Ask the patient to bend the knee up to the chest pulling it up against the abdomen. If the opposite thigh rises when performing this maneuver, there could be a flexion problem in the original knee. Place the patient's foot on the opposite knee. Pull the bent knee laterally to rotate at the hip. Arthritis will cause pain and restricted ROM on this maneuver.

Check for effusion which is free fluid in the joint space. Use the bulge sign to check for fluid. Milk the tissue on the medial aspect of the knee upward a few times. Press the knee behind the lateral aspect of the patella. Look for a bulge of fluid going back to the medial side. A bulge indicates fluid in the knee. This test is good for detecting even small amounts. The bulge might be harder to detect if the fluid in the knee is under pressure in the joint space.

> *PEARL: Effusion is not required to make the diagnosis of a Lyme joint.*

> *PEARL: The knees can be swollen with Bartonella.*

Check the knee for stability, especially if the patient reports a sensation of "giving way" or "buckling." With the patient supine, flex the knee 90 degrees, sit on the foot, grasp the leg below the knee and attempt to move the joint forward and back. If there is laxity (easy mobility) when moving the knee forward, it could be an anterior cruciate problem. If the increased mobility is backward, consider a posterior cruciate defect.

A torn meniscus presents with local tenderness or pain on adduction or abduction of the knee. An audible click also suggests a torn meniscus. Housemaid's knee, or coal miner's knee in western PA, is **prepatellar bursitis,** a superficial swelling sharply limited to the area in FRONT of the kneecap. Boney enlargement is found in degenerative joint disease, which is not common in children.

> *PEARL: To look for loose **patellar-femoral syndrome**, examine the knee with the thigh tight. With the patient*

standing or supine and with the patella held down gently, instruct the person to contract the thigh muscle. A grinding sensation under the knee indicates the presence of patellar-femoral syndrome.

A common knee ailment in kids is the condition called Osgood-Schlatter disease. Also called **osteochondrosis,** OS is a painful inflammation of the epiphysis of the tibial tubercle on the tibial shaft. Common in active teens, OS frequently affects both legs with pain in the knees. This condition is probably due to cumulative trauma in bones before there has been a chance for complete fusion of the epiphysis to the main bone. The most commonly involved area is the site of the insertion of the patellar tendon which serves as the anchor for all the thigh muscles. Severe disease can result in permanent tubercle enlargement. The most common age for OS is between 10 and 15 y/o. Repeated knee flexion against the tight quadriceps like when riding a bike, running, or stair climbing have been associated with OS. Genetics and a locally deficient blood supply can also contribute. Symptoms include aches that continue even at rest, swelling, local heat, with pain and tenderness under the knee cap. Pain is worse during activities that move the patellar tendon on the tibial tuberosity. OS might be identified early by noting a swelling at the tibial tuberosity and eliciting pain with gentle palpation. OS could be important during the differential diagnosis phase of TBI management.

PEARL: Lyme cost me more than a quarter inch of leg length on the affected side. Seemingly the pathogen munched away at the cartilage until I had bone on bone. Shoe lifts now partially compensate. Don't let Lyme surprise you. All kinds of unexpected things have been documented.

Ankles

The ankle connects the leg to the foot and is comprised of the tibia, fibula, and talus. Examine the ankle for ROM, tender points, swelling, fluid, heat, and stability.

To examine the ankle, dorsiflex and plantar flex the foot. Stabilize with one hand and then hold the heel with the other. Invert and evert at the subtalar joint and then invert and evert the forefoot. An arthritic joint will be painful when moved in any direction, but usually a sprain will only be painful when the involved ligament is moved. Laxity is noted when the joint moves too freely when it should be snug in its ligament and tendon protected sanctuary.

The Achilles tendon is the big tendon attaching the calf muscle to the heel. This is a good place to check reflexes. Nodules along the Achilles tendon are consistent with RA, but can also be found with Bartonella infections. Achilles tendonitis and tears used to be just the bane of middle-aged men. However, the use of fluoroquinolone antibiotics and their association

with Achilles tendonitis has put this tendon back on the map for the rest of us as well.

Tinel's sign is positive when pain or tingling result after tapping on the lateral part of the lower fibula. This is the path of the superficial peroneal nerve. This discomfort on tapping suggests nerve entrapment. Swelling below the lateral malleolus suggests the synovial effusion of RA. The bursa in the ankle can also become inflamed.

Edema from an inadequately pumping heart can settle around the ankles as well as in the bases of the lungs. Fluid accumulates at the ankles because of gravity. Shoe pressure can keep fluid off the feet and pushed up into the ankle area.

Feet

In babies, feet are cute. After age 4, they can be something else indeed. Pay attention to the feet of TBI patients since you might gather much useful information. As with all the joints, look for full ROM, signs of inflammation, swelling, point tenderness, generalized pain, abnormal temperature, and skin lesions. Compare the right to the left. The calcaneus is the heel bone and it articulates with the talus, a tarsal bone that is part of the ankle.

How to examine the foot: Start with the heel. Place the foot at a right angle to the lower leg. Palpate the heel with firm pressure. If there is pain, consider a heel spur. Look at the color of the feet. If the toes are cold, pale, or blue (cyanosis), consider Raynaud's phenomenon, which can be associated with both bartonellosis and borreliosis. Edema and big veins suggest venous insufficiency. Tenderness at the small metatarsophalangeal joints could be early RA. Evert and invert the mid-sole area. Flex and extend the toes. These usually move as a unit. Look for deformities and lesions.

Common findings on the foot exam:

- **Flat feet**: A normal foot arch should have concavity. In the case of flat feet, also called fallen arches, the entire sole will be flat across the floor. This is most apparent when the patient stands, since there is no visible arch and the entire length of the sole touches the floor. Shoes will be worn more on innersoles and heels. If there is any question, wet the bottom of the patient's feet and have him stand on paper. A flattened, brown, paper shopping bag is good. The outline of a normal foot will have a curved space medially where the sole does not touch. A flat footed person will wet the whole paper since the entire sole touches the paper. There will be no curved cutout where the arch should be. Flat feet can be tender on long walks, but as a former army doctor I still don't know why having flat feet keeps people out of the service. For those of us without flat feet, the commanders didn't care if our feet were tender, blistered, raw, or had fallen off, as long as we kept going.

- **Morton's foot**: A short, hypermobile 1st metatarsal with a long second toe may cause mobility problems and discomfort throughout the foot. Morton's toe is not uncommon. If the toe is symptomatic, a pad under the 1st metatarsal may help.

PEARL: If the person has Morton's toe, with the 2nd toe longer, she may be prone to flat feet, genu valgum (knock knees), femoral anteversion, and have a tendency toward foot, shin, knee, and hip pain, as well as discomfort in the tibialis anterior muscle.

- **Morton's neuroma**: A neuroma is a mass of nerve cells tangled in vascular tissue that may be uncomfortable. In the foot these masses usually reside in the tissue between the digits, most commonly at the base of the 3rd toe. These spots can hurt, especially when pressure is applied. To assess the neuroma, apply firm pressure with the thumb at the metatarsal heads.

- Heel pain in kids can be **epiphysitis** of the calcaneus.

- **Heel spur**: A sharp or pointed spur can develop below the heel because of repeated insult to the area. Most often spurs are due to the pull of the plantar fascia on the heel. Spurs can also develop in people with unequal leg length, almost as a protective callous, as the one heel repeatedly hits harder than the other. The pain of a heel spur can mimic plantar fasciitis and the sole pain associated with Bartonella.

- **Arthritis**: Pain on manipulation of the toes is often some kind of arthritis, unless there has been recent trauma. RA can present in toes. Psoriatic arthritis will cause sausage-shaped digits. Acute gouty arthritis usually affects the 1st MTP joint of the great toe and can be very painful. Gout causes a tender, hot, dusky-red color that extends beyond the margins of the joint. Here you must also consider cellulitis.

PEARL: Lyme involvement in the toes presents as painful tenderness at the IP joints with swelling. There may be tenderness at the base of the big toe MTP joint as well.

- **Cellulitis**: A soft tissue infection, cellulitis can spread and affect the joint space. This condition can be dangerous in diabetics who have poor wound healing, poor vasculature, muted sensation, and trouble with antibiotic penetration to distal areas. Cellulitis is red, hot, and swollen. If the lesion gets bigger, the infection is spreading. Treat.

- **Plantar fasciitis**: This inflammatory process is important in TBIs. Sole pain is a frequent complaint in bartonellosis, babesiosis, and occasionally Lyme. The mechanism by which these pathogens affect the fascia is unknown. Usually the cause of plantar fasciitis is mechanical, with repeated pressure and stress causing irritation. Fasciitis may present as a stress fracture. The fascia is examined with the foot placed in dorsiflexion (at a right angle to the leg). With the thumbs on the dorsum of the foot, use the fingers to determine if there is fascial pain or tightness. Examine all along the sole in the arch area. Pain equals fasciitis. There may also be palpable nodules in the fascia.

- **Plantar warts**: Warts on the bottom of the feet are common. Usually caused by HPV, these warts can appear as a dark spot with stippling. As pressure is placed on the wart, a callus can appear. These can become tender as the callus presses into the softer underlying tissue. This viral infection can be dormant for months (or forever for all we know) before symptoms appear. HPV can present as one wart or several that form a cluster. Often these warts are self-limited. Otherwise, there are almost as many ways to treat a plantar wart in the literature as there are to remove a tick. In general home remedies from duct tape to Crazy glue don't work. Even professional interventions can be more aggressive than effective.

PEARL: Kids love to pick at plantar warts and soon they could also have palmar warts. They love to pick at those too.

- **Fractures**: Breaks usually present with point tenderness. Routine breaks are caused by all the routine reasons including falls, accidents, twists, stubs, and dropping heavy objects onto the foot. In contrast, a stress fracture is a fine hairline break in the bone that may be point tender but is hard to see on X-ray. These fractures are common in kids and are the result of repetitive microtrauma as seen with long distance running. Non-supportive and uncushioned shoes on hard surfaces can exacerbate the problem. Point tenderness is the primary finding, although there may be swelling as well. The stress fracture can recur if not enough healing time is allowed.

- **Ingrown toenail**: Common in older kids and adults, the edge of the nail digs into the flesh causing inflammation and the possibility of infection. The soft tissue around the nail becomes tender and red with the overhanging nail fold often oozing pus. Be careful with ingrown toenails in diabetics, when a podiatrist may need to manage this condition.

- **Masses**: Feet are the site of all manner of masses and growths including both benign and cancerous tumors, cysts, and nodules. Nodules, especially several in a line, can suggest TBI.

- **Hammer toe:** Uncommon in small children, the 2nd toe presents with a hyperextended MTP and a flexed PIP. Note that this kind of deformity can affect any toe and more than one toe at a time.

- **Corn**: A corn is a painful cone-shaped thickening of skin over a pressure point. Corns most often develop on the thin skin of the foot over boney prominences like the 5th toe ball and sole. These can be tender if the shoe pushes the hard cone into the soft tissue.

- **Callus**: Skin can thicken in areas of persistent pressure like the ball, heel, and sole of the foot. Usually this thick skin is painless.

- **Fungus**: Fungus like feet. The combination of shoes, socks, and sweat, provide fungus with warm, moist, dark, growing places. Fungus on the skin of the feet, often called athlete's foot, might be a different genus of fungus than the fungus found in other parts of the body. Also called tinea pedis, the condition can present with red, itchy, burning patches of dry, peeling, cracked skin. Fungus also happily grows under the toe nails, especially the nail of the great toe. Here the nail will thicken, turn yellow, and crack. The nail may split and crumble and eventually separate from the toe. These are quite unattractive and may take a LONG time to heal. A podiatrist may be needed. There is a new laser treatment available, which can be quite expensive. Toenail fungus may be worse in patients with diabetes and in those patients who have an immune system already busy with other infections.

- **Diabetic skin changes**: The foot is a primary site for diabetic skin changes. The incidence and prevalence of diabetes in kids has skyrocketed and Lyme can adversely impact blood sugar control. Diabetes is a disease that affects both the nervous system and circulation to all areas, which explains why diabetics get kidney disease, neuropathy, and blindness from their disease. In the foot, the patient is less able to feel sensations of pain, heat, and cold. That means she can be injured, burned, or frostbitten and not know. Also with circulatory compromise, wounds are very hard to heal since immune cells and antibiotics both have trouble getting to the affected area. The skin can be dry, cracked, and peeling. This further opens the foot to secondary infection. Fungus is common. Once a wound appears, healing time can be long and some wounds never heal. There can be problems with ischemia, necrosis, and gangrene. Amputations are sometimes necessary. Patients with diabetes, especially diabetes exacerbated by Lyme, should be vigilant about foot hygiene. Caution must always be taken in cutting a diabetic's nails. A podiatry consult might be prudent.

PEARL: Each episode of high blood sugar causes more damage to nerves and blood vessels, thereby resulting in more end-organ disease. Many diabetics do not understand this. Some feel they are getting away with something when they just cover a high sugar with insulin. In the meantime the kidneys, nerves, skin, eyes, and circulatory system progressively decline.

- **Bunions** are hell on metatarsophalangeal joints. A bunion is an enlargement of the bone and tissue of the 1st MTP joint, the big toe. The toes may angle laterally toward the second toe and the head of the metatarsal forms a large bump. The bursa may swell, enhancing the problem. The bunion may cause pain and make it difficult to fit shoes. Gait can be affected. The propensity for bunions is likely genetic and may be associated with flat feet and hypermobility in the foot. As far as I could glean, bunions have no association with TBIs. I wanted to have one thing in the book that wasn't exacerbated by TBIs.

Chapter 17-N   Neurologic Exam and Pertinent Differential– Detailed chapter contents

Neurologic Exam and Pertinent Differential

Pride is increased by ignorance; those who assume the most, know the least.

John Gay

NEUROLOGIC

Be careful in performing your neurologic exam lest it turn into a chaotic mess where you go through the motions and don't gather much useful information. Such were the neurologic exams I performed for many years. Then I recognized the importance of a well-executed neuropsychiatric exam in assessing TBI cases.

The nervous system is a complex communication network using specialized cells and numerous biochemicals, in this case called neurotransmitters, to perform many functions. The NS contains:

Central nervous system: The CNS is the command center in charge of coordinating overall physiologic processes and includes the brain and spinal cord.

Peripheral nervous system: The PNS is a network of paired nerves that connect the CNS to remote body parts and sends and receives messages from these locations.

Autonomic nervous system: The ANS regulates the involuntary action of internal organs. Functioning below the level of consciousness, the ANS controls the work of the viscera including HR, digestion, micturation, RR, salivation, perspiration, pupil size, and sexual arousal. A few of these operations can also be influenced to a degree by conscious control like the respiratory rate and urination. The ANS has been sliced and diced many ways including motor versus sensory, efferent versus afferent, PSNS versus SNS, and inhibitory versus excitatory.

TBIs caused by Bb, Bartonella, or M. *fermentans* seem to have a penchant for nerve tissue causing numerous neuropsychiatric signs and symptoms. The neurologic exam in TBIs can help you gauge the extent of the problem, assess the stage of the disease, and assist in the determination of treatment options. Resolution, continuation, or exacerbation of symptoms will also provide a pretty good idea of the effectiveness of your treatment plan. With Lyme, the patient is probably not better until his brain is better.

PEARL: Neuroborreliosis is the name given to Bb infection of the CNS. Here the pathogen enters the brain and CNS directly. In addition, sxs can occur from the humoral modulators sent out from the immune system in order to
eliminate the invaders. The many biochemical humors, such as cytokines, can cause a number of the neuropsychiatric symptoms associated with Lyme such as cognitive defects and "brain fog."

I will not survive if I try to detail all these possible permutations, but I will attempt to provide information pertinent to TBI patients. The purpose of the examination of the nervous system is to first see if there is something wrong. The NS is so complex that there is a wide range of normal. If a parameter is found to be "off" you can investigate further in related areas to see if you can identify a lesion. The problem may be general or specific. For example, encephalitis might cause general signs and symptoms, whereas a microscopic lesion in the temporal lobe may be responsible for a localized seizure. If you find an abnormality on PE, then you can start to look for the underlying cause and attempt to address the problem.

Let's start at the top:

Different areas of the brain control different functions. Theoretically, the brain evolved from back to front, with the back part near the neck and brainstem involved with the most primitive functions like breathing. As you move forward anatomically the functions get higher and supposedly more civilized with the frontal cortex involved in moderation and restraint. The **cerebrum**, or brain, is divided into two halves or hemispheres. The **cortex** is the thin, convoluted surface of grey matter with numerous ridges and folds. The grey matter of the brain is mostly **neurons** or nerve cells. These cells have thin projections called axons which conduct impulses AWAY from the neuron and are usually covered by a fatty layer called **myelin**. Neurons also have many branched dendrites that receive information and transmit it TOWARD the neuron. The brain is divided into lobes, each with individual and overlapping functions.

- **Frontal lobes**: The frontal cortex analyzes, plans, and problem solves. This is where our conscious "thinking" takes place. The prefrontal cortex is the CEO of the brain and this is the seat of control. Here is where the "artsy" right side of the brain is balanced with the analytical left half. The frontal lobes also control voluntary muscle movements including the motor area for speech. Usually one side of the brain controls the opposite side of the body. The frontal cortex is where most of what we would consider thinking goes on. These lobes are the seat of personality, behavior, intellect, judgment, and problem solving. They are responsible for what is termed "executive function" meaning self-control, planning, reasoning, and abstract thought. The term executive function always struck me as funny since the "executives" I know are the least likely to be strong in these areas.

PEARL: Defects in the white matter covering of the brain may be involved with slow recall and inappropriate associations, whereas problems with the grey matter more often relate to loss of previously stored information.

- **Temporal lobes**: Center for taste, hearing, smell, and interpretation of spoken language

- **Parietal lobes**: Coordinate and interpret sensory information including skin senses

- **Occipital region**: Interprets visual stimuli

- **Brainstem**: The brainstem is the base of the brain that connects the cerebral hemispheres with the spinal cord and is responsible for many processes that are independent of conscious thought such as breathing and heart rate. Input from all parts of the body goes back to the brain via the brainstem. CNs 3 through 12 originate there. The brainstem is an integrator, coordinating the heart rate, respiration, sensation, alertness, awareness, sleep cycles, and consciousness. The brainstem also has a role in proprioception, pain, itching, and temperature. On TV, people are always brain dead while they are still breathing and their hearts are still beating. This means that the frontal cortex is gone but the brainstem is still functioning.

- **Basal ganglion**: Deep in the cerebral hemispheres are the subconscious aspects of voluntary motion. While you may "volunteer" to perform a certain movement that doesn't mean you have to think about HOW to perform all aspects of that movement. If we had to consciously orchestrate every muscular aspect of getting a spoon to our mouths, we would starve to death. The BG handles all this for us and enables us to acquire motor routines and habits. The BG will select which of several motor options to perform. Lesions in this area can cause abnormal movements, which will be important later in assessing abnormal motion potentially associated with TBIs. The basal ganglion likely has some involvement in the abnormal movements found in conditions such as rheumatic fever, Parkinson's, Huntington's disease, and Lyme. The BG has some function in emotion and behavior control and is linked to some aspects of Tourette's and OCD. (In case you are wondering why you are knee deep in the basal ganglion, this all relates to TBIs eventually. I leave out most of the stuff that doesn't have an association with TBIs.)

- **Cerebellum**: Connected to the brainstem is the cerebellum which is involved with balance, posture, coordination, and the timing of movements. The frontal lobe allows all the muscles needed for running or swimming to move, but it's the cerebellum that actually coordinates and synchronizes the activity. This part of the brain controls the various characteristics of movement like speed, acceleration, and trajectory. The cerebellum allows you to go faster, if you want to, without thinking about how to do so. The cerebellum also allows for the intricate muscular interactions that permit writing, dressing, eating, playing musical instruments, and the smooth tracking by the eye muscles. Interestingly, the cerebellum is also involved in attention span and the emotions of pleasure and displeasure in ways not clearly understood. If the patient's disease is causing a lack of coordination, a change in balance, or an inability to learn a new motor skill like an unfamiliar dance step (that would have been easily mastered before), consider involvement of the cerebellum.

PEARL: With Lyme, there can be problems with attention and focus that weren't obvious before the infection. The patient might have trouble maintaining attention and present as easily distracted.

- **Limbic system**: Within the temporal lobe is the limbic system which is associated with emotions including aggression and repetitive behaviors. Memory is also housed here. The limbic system governs emotion and behavior, memory, happiness, pleasure, decision-making, reward patterns associated with addiction, sexual drive, and the overall sense of well-being.

The major parts of the limbic system include:

Hypothalamus: This very busy area maintains homeostasis where all physiologic processes are kept in balance including water, salts, sugars, and fats. The hormone leptin influences appetite through the hypothalamus and may be associated with obesity. The hypothalamus integrates the SNS and PSNS and regulates hunger, thirst, and response to pain and pleasure. This part of the limbic system is involved with sexual satisfaction, anger, and aggressiveness. The hypothalamus is involved with the EXPRESSION of emotion, not its generation. So this organ determines how a person reacts to fear or panic and may explain why some people itch for a fight. Neurosecretions are the modulators of the activity of the hypothalamus through the ANS and the pituitary.

Hippocampus: A seahorse shaped structure with an important role in memory.

Amygdala: When this small area in the temporal lobe is stimulated, aggression and rage result. When the amygdala is removed the same subject is indifferent. The amygdala is associated with mood, arousal, and emotions both positive and negative. Here the emotional parts of memories are retained. The amygdala is responsible for identifying danger. This is probably the seat of the fight or flight response. TBIs such as bartonellosis, M. *fermentans*, and Lyme can incite rage and aggression.

ASSESSMENT OF THE NERVOUS SYSTEM

MENTAL STATUS

Mental status is defined in many ways and evaluation should demonstrate the functional state of mind as judged by behavior, appearance, responses to stimuli, speech, cognition, abstract thought, memory, and judgment. In addition to the mental status, the complete neurologic exam also includes evaluation of cerebral and cerebellar function, motor activity, muscle strength, balance, gait, reflexes, CN function, coordination, and sensory perception including pain. Lyme and several of the other TBIs are known to impact the mental status and other aspects of the nervous system. The degree of involvement can range from undetectable to incapacitating. Each part of the assessment should add to the complete picture. You will need to multitask to finish the exam; otherwise the person will be elderly before you compile the results. You can gather much information on neurologic status throughout the entire patient encounter. For a full TBI neurologic exam, assess:

A. **Level of consciousness:** (LOC) The degree of awareness of the patient is an important indicator of neurologic function. The LOC can range from alert and interactive to comatose. Failure to respond even to painful stimuli can suggest significant problems. Assessment tools such as the Glasgow Coma Scale offer a quick standardized account of consciousness. A score of 15 is normal, 7 indicates coma, and brain death is 3 or lower. Comparison of results over time or after an intervention can be used to assess progress or deterioration.

B. **Affect:** The "affect" refers to general demeanor, especially the facial expression indicating mood. Is the person conveying happiness or despair? Does the body language reflect the circumstances? Does the patient adjust expression in response to the changing environment? Is the change appropriate? A blunted affect is one where there is a muted emotional response to every situation. A flat affect is the absence of emotional reaction, no matter what the circumstances.

C. **Orientation:** Depending on age the patient should have a sense of time, place, and person.

What's your name?

Who's here with you?

Where's Mommy?

Who am I?

What day is today?

When is your next birthday?

How old are you?

What grade are you in?

What is this room we're in?

Even very young kids should know if it is morning or after lunch and that they are at the doctor's office and who came with them. This conversation will need to be targeted to the age and circumstances of the individual patient. A person delirious with a 105 fever will not be well oriented.

PEARL: With Lyme treatment, the joints tend to get better before the brain gets better. If the joints improve, the brain has a good chance of improvement.

D. **Mood and interactions:** If the person is acutely ill, her mood might appropriately be dour. How is the patient interacting with others? Is the individual open, cooperative, angry, evasive, hostile, tearful, distracted, nervous, too happy, or hyper? Do her perceptions of her situation accurately reflect her current circumstances? Sometimes it is perfectly reasonable to scream bloody murder.

E. **Cognition:** The ability to think. Thoughts should be clear, realistic, and follow a logical flow. Cognition can be assessed using various methods.

Intellect is defined in a hundred ways and intelligence means different things to different people. There are many tests and screening methods, all with significant limitations. Since every parent at my son's school swore her child had an IQ of 214, I often wondered where the average IQ of around 100 came from. Do children with average intelligence exist? Not in Unionville, PA.

Intelligence quotients or IQ tests are often used as a measure of intellectual prowess. Unfortunately, they appear to have considerable bias and limits. They do not assess creativity, practical problem-solving, or flexibility of thought. They are incomparably boring and some of the smartest kids just stop in the middle of the tests and amuse themselves in other ways.

IQ tests do not account for differences in life experience. In *Guns, Germs and Steel*, Jared Diamond talks about a primitive society on a south seas island that he considered the most intelligent people on Earth. After studying many cultures, Diamond based his conclusion on their ability to arrive at creative solutions to problems and their capacity for abstract thinking. These people would have done very poorly on standard IQ tests since they cannot read and they don't have #2 pencils.

For our purposes, we are trying to establish a baseline of cognitive ability so that the patient's progress can be evaluated over time. We can see if what we're doing to help is working.

PEARL: Even with their limitations, standard IQ tests may have a place in the management of chronic Lyme disease. There are reported cases of patients whose IQ numbers dramatically improved after adequate treatment.

Means to assess cognition in the office include:

1. **Basic knowledge:** Does the 9 y/o know things that a typical 4th grader should know? Adjust the questions to the age and circumstance.

   Name a planet.

   Who is George Washington?

   What is 4 X 5?

   Name 3 colors.

2. **Vocabulary:** Another means to measure intellect is by the number of words the person uses and understands. Make sure the words are age appropriate. You can ask the patient what a word means or to make a sentence using the word. Make sure that the word would be familiar to the individual in the context of his life circumstances.

3. **Analytical ability:** Have the patient repeat a series of numbers first forward and then backwards. Start with 2 numbers and move up. For older kids and adults, you can have them start with 100 and subtract 2 or 3 or 5. (Personally, I hate this particular test.)

4. **Problem solving:** Have the patient try to solve a simple life problem. How would he get around a big puddle without getting his shoes wet? Or, ask the patient to name as many uses as she can for a common object: a spoon, a ball, a basket, a brick, a tire.

PEARL: Attention span deficits and distractibility have been associated with Lyme. How long can the person remain on task?

5. **Coherent logic:** Have the patient tell a little story. The result should be age appropriate.

PEARL: There are many ways to determine if the cognitive function is basically in the ballpark. For kids who seem to be falling below their age appropriate ability, cognitive testing may be indicated. Be familiar with the resources available to do this type of testing in your area or know how to contact the local Lyme group which might be able to make a referral.

PEARL: A patient in a manic state will have a flight of ideas. Schizophrenics will be incoherent and use neologisms or made-up words. These behaviors have nothing to do with their underlying intelligence but may make them seem less intelligent.

F. **Abstract Thinking:** Abstract concepts are those that do not have an immediate obvious meaning and require some interpretation. The following tasks will need to be made age appropriate.

1. **Proverb** interpretation is one way to assess abstract thought:

   April showers bring May flowers.

   A penny saved is a penny earned.

   Birds of a feather flock together.

   A bird in the hand is worth two in the bush.

   You can't tell a book by its cover.

   One good turn deserves another.

   Great minds think alike.

   Scratch my back and I'll scratch yours.

   Never look a gift horse in the mouth.

   Do unto others, as you would have them do unto you.

   The early bird catches the worm.

   Faith can move mountains.

   Two heads are better than one.

   Honesty is the best policy.

   Laughter is the best medicine.

   First things first.

   The best things in life are free.

   United we stand, divided we fall.

   Live and learn.

   There's no place like home.

   When the cat's away, the mice will play.

   Lions don't need to roar.

   One or two proverbs will do nicely, although some people like this game. See how rigid the answers are. Usually the more concrete the answers, the less intellect and ability for rational thought is present. (Think politicians.) If the answers are totally off base, consider conditions where the patient is out of touch with reality or delusional. (Think politicians.)

PEARL: Thinking can be quite literal and concrete in autism and in ADHD.

2. Comparisons

Ask how two items are alike or different:

A banana and an orange

A drum and a piano

A car and a bike

A dog and a bird

G. Judgment: The ability to make considered decisions, come to reasonable conclusions, and to decide between options.

Why shouldn't you play in the street?

What should you do if a stranger asks you to help look for his lost puppy?

What do you do if you get lost?

When would you call 911?

Why don't you take things that belong to someone else?

Why does your pet need fresh water every day?

Would you rather wear a black or white shirt if you are walking at night?

H. Memory: The capacity to retain and recall information. Normal memory can remember people, items, or events over both the short and long-term. Depending on age, ask:

What happened this morning? What did you have for breakfast?

What happened at your last birthday party?

Can you remember things you study for tests in school?

ADDITIONAL NEUROLOGIC ASSESSMENTS

To make a diagnosis, in addition to the history and PE, additional assessments may be needed.

A. Reflexes: Involuntary responses to stimuli. They are predictable and purposeful and adaptive. They rely on an intact neural pathway between the stimulus and the responding organ called the reflex arc. The end-organ can be a muscle or gland. Reflexes allow you to pull your hand out of fire before your brain even realized there was a fire. Otherwise, your hand would be crispy by the time you did all the thinking needed to get out of danger. When a predicable reflex is not present or that reflex is of greater or lesser intensity than expected, look for a problem in the circuit. There are abnormal reflexes that appear when certain lesions exist. When they are present, the problem is present. **Infant automatisms** are actions performed without thought in newborns and babies. These are sometimes called reflexes but there are slight differences. They are listed later in this chapter.

Reflexes can be superficial or deep tendon responses. Deep tendon reflexes can be assessed at insertions of a major tendon onto a bone. The patient should relax in a neutral position and using a reflex hammer (although many other things can also be used), the examiner should firmly strike the tendon insertion on one of the most common sites: biceps, triceps, patellar, or Achilles. Normal response is a quick extension and contraction. Reflexes should be symmetrical and compared side to side.

If the patient cannot relax, other muscles can be used to distract her attention. For testing of arm reflexes, have the patient clench her teeth or if leg reflexes are difficult to assess, ask the patient to grasp opposite wrists and pull.

Reflexes are graded:

4+ Hyperactive (suggesting an upper motor neuron lesion)

3+ Brisker than normal but not necessarily diseased

2+ Average normal

1+ Low normal

0 – No reflex elicited

Superficial reflexes can be tested using a key or the pointy side of the reflex hammer to stroke in the abdominal, plantar, or gluteal regions.

If reflexes are hyperreactive check for clonus. Clonus is a spasm between opposing muscle groups (the flexors versus the extensors, for example) caused by a hyperactive stretch reflex from an upper motor neuron lesion. To check for clonus at the ankle, support the knee in partial flexion. Sharply dorsiflex that foot. Look for rhythmic oscillations of the foot. Clonus suggests a lesion.

Another abnormal reflex finding is the Babinski response. Using a moderately sharp object like the metal point of the reflex hammer, stroke the plantar (bottom) surface of the foot from the heel, curving over to the ball. If the great toe dorsiflexes, then there is a potential upper motor neuron lesion in the area of L4, L5, S1, and S2.

B. **Cranial Nerves**: A cranial nerve is one of 12 pairs of nerves arising from the brain or brainstem. They exit through holes in the cranium. If a problem is found with a cranial nerve, try to trace it back to the etiologic lesion. Follow it home.

CRANIAL NERVES:

CN 1 Olfactory: Smell. Have the patient close her eyes. Occlude one nostril and test each nostril separately by identifying clear common odors like coffee or peppermint. In the army they used banana oil to see if our gas masks were sealed. If you could smell the banana oil, in a real gas attack you would die.

CN 2 Optic: Vision. Test visual acuity, visual fields by confrontation, and examine the fundus

CN 3 Oculomotor: Eye movement. Test pupil constriction, elevation of upper lid, and the many EOMs

CN 4 Trochlear: Downward and inward movement of the eye. Follow the finger with the eyes

CN 5 Trigeminal: Motor: Jaw clench with masseter and temporal muscles and lateral movement of the jaw. Sensory: Facial sensation. Use a Q-tip and a pin prick, "Sharp or dull?" to assess. Involvement of CN 5 in Lyme pathology can result in severe facial pain.

CN 6 Abducens: Lateral and conjugate movement of eye. Follow finger with eyes. Bb's affect on CN 6 can cause double vision.

CN 7 Facial: Motor: Muscles of the face. Check for any asymmetry: puff out cheeks, raise eyebrows, frown, smile, close eyes so tight they can't be opened, and show teeth. This is the nerve involved with the Bell's palsy that is so often associated with Lyme. Sensory: Taste on the forward 2/3 of the tongue. Use drops of sweet, salty, bitter, and sour to assess taste if indicated.

PEARL: If Bb can get at the facial nerve so easily, what stops them from affecting the other CNs? Nothing. Other CN involvement just might not be as apparent as a drooping face or an eye that can't blink.

PEARL: Another way to test for the facial paralysis of Bell's palsy is to have the person open both eyes and then close one. On the paralyzed side the eye will not be able to close and the muscles not innervated by CN 7 will try to help. The muscles of the orbit and cheek will contract in an effort to close the eye. An involuntary movement that accompanies a voluntary movement is called synkinesis and this blink synkinesis in Bell's palsy can persist for months or years after the paralysis has dissipated.

CN 8 Acoustic: Hearing and balance. Use a tuning fork to test both air and bone conduction. Balance can be assessed using all the methods listed in the balance section below.

PEARL: You might mistake a child's response to the mother's non-verbal communication for the ability to hear. The hearing-impaired and their caregivers often learn to communicate in non-verbal ways. A child may appear to be following directions when he is actually responding to his mother's subconscious hand signals or facial expressions. To rule out this possibility, turn your back to the person and speak. Ask him to repeat what you have said.

PEARL: A problem with auditory processing may be mistaken for hearing loss. The individual may be able to hear just fine but have trouble processing what she has heard.

CN 9 Glossopharyngeal: Sensory input from the pharynx and middle ear. One muscle innervation. To test, have the patient say "ah" and watch for any asymmetry in the movement of the soft tissue of the throat. Note the gag reflex upon stimulation of the back of the throat

CN 10 Vagus: Motor: Movement of palate, pharynx, and larynx. Ability to swallow. To test, have the patient say "ah" and watch for symmetrical movement of the palate and uvula which deviate away from the paralyzed side of a vagus lesion. Impairment of the vagus nerve by Bb can cause a variety of GI problems for the Lyme patient including Bell's palsy of the gut. Sensory: Pharynx and larynx. Hoarseness has many causes and one can be a lesion of the vagus.

CN 11 Spinal Accessory: Motor: sternomastoid and upper trapezius. To test, shrug against hand pressure. Turn head to each side against examiner hand resistance

CN 12 Hypoglossal: Motor: tongue. Note fasciculations (fine twitching). Stick out the tongue and note any asymmetry, deviation, or atrophy. In 12th nerve paralysis the tongue tip will deviate toward the affected side.

C. **Balance:** The ability to maintain the center of gravity over the base of support. Balance can be impacted by a number of physical conditions including muscle strength, coordination, damage to the vestibular mechanism in the inner ear, or to problems with CN 8. A patient with nystagmus should have balance checked carefully. Balance can be greatly impacted by Lyme and other TBIs. With young kids, check balance by putting their head forward, then back, and next tilting left and right. Observe their ability to maintain balance. For walking children, have them stand on one foot, then walk with one foot in front of the other. After that, ask them to stand with eyes closed and assess the degree of wobble. With eyes still closed, see how well they do on each foot alone. With each of these tasks, there will be slight instability even in healthy people. Patients with impairment will have difficulty.

Problems with balance can be due to CNS lesions, vestibular problems in the ear, structural problems like leg length discrepancies, certain medications, deconditioning, and cerebellar dysfunction. Since Lyme targets the CNS, try to seek out the root causes of any balance issues.

For older children and adults, have the patient stand with feet together without any support of the arms, first with eyes open and then with eyes closed. Assure the patient that you will protect him from falling. Normal patients have only minimal, if any, swaying. If there are cerebellar problems, the patient may have difficulty standing with feet together, whether the eyes are open or closed. If the patient is imbalanced because of poor position sense, his vision can compensate for this sensory deficit. He can stand very well with eyes open, but loses balance with eyes closed. This inability to maintain balance when the eyes are shut and the feet are close together is called a positive **Romberg sign**. If the patient lists to the left or right this may suggest which side of the brain is more affected.

D. Proprioception: Knowing where the body is in space is called proprioception or position sense. Is the patient bumping into things? To test, move the toes and fingers up and down and from side to side and see if the patient can discern their position.

PEARL: Related to abnormal proprioception (but not the same) is optic ataxia, which is more of a spatial perception distortion. Here the patient has a hard time targeting movements in space. He will bump into doorways even when trying hard not to.

E. Gait: The manner of walking is called the gait. Have the patient walk across the room at least several steps and then turn around and come back. Observe posture, balance, and arm swing. Movement should be natural with arms swinging freely at the side. When turning, the face and head should lead. Ask the patient to walk heel-to-toe in a straight line. If there are problems with this maneuver, perform the Romberg test described earlier.

There are many types of abnormal gaits, from those that are stiff and rigid with little arm movement to the staggering, unsteady gait seen with cerebellar lesions. Parkinson's patients often walk on their toes as though pushed forward and usually have short steps where their feet barely clear the floor. The trunk will lean forward when walking if the quadriceps are weak.

PEARL: Be vigilant for any gait abnormalities. In Alzheimer's, gait changes might signify the presence of disease even before cognitive problems appear.

F. Coordination: The working together of several muscles to produce a specific movement. The cerebellum and a number of high-level structures are probably involved in the timing and coordination of movements. There are several ways to assess coordination. Ask the person to walk on toes and heels. If feasible, have the individual get up from the floor from a supine position and then sit. From there, have the patient stand. The muscles have to work in complex synergy to accomplish these tasks.

Another good way to evaluate coordination is by observing rapid movement. Request that the person pat his head as fast as he can. One at a time, touch each finger with the thumb in order. Ask the patient to touch your outstretched index finger and then her nose, alternating sides several times. If these movements are awkward or inaccurate, there can be a problem with the cerebellum. If the task is only difficult when the eyes are closed, there is probably a lack of position sense

G. Motor Function: As a part of the neurologic exam we want to see how the nerves are stimulating and working with the muscles. We want to observe the action of the muscles, overlooking any structural impairment for a minute, to assess the nerves. This examination will involve tone, strength, movement, and the search for abnormalities.

Tone: The amount of tension or resistance to movement in a muscle. Tone allows us to maintain a certain position. To assess, palpate the muscle both at rest and during contraction. Observe muscle tone by holding the hand while putting the elbow and shoulder through a gentle range of motion. Tone is described as:

Flaccid: No tone, limp, weak, lax, soft. Paralyzed muscles are flaccid.

Normal: Balanced between contraction and relaxation

Spastic: Always somewhat tensed as though on the verge of spasm

PEARL: Hypotonia is a cardinal sign of gestational Lyme. Extensive discussion of hypotonia is contained in Chapter 30: Special Populations.

PEARL: Overdevelopment of muscles for age suggests a hormone problem or use of steroids or other enhancers. Assess how the muscle development correlates with the Tanner score. Overuse of steroids can cause episodes of rage.

Strength: The amount of effort a muscle can exert against resistance is strength. Muscle strength should be symmetrical. There are many ways to assess muscle strength including:

- Can the patient do a deep knee bend? Weak quadriceps make knee bends difficult.

- Muscle strength can be tested against examiner resistance in both the UE and LE.

- Ability to maintain arms held forward for 20 to 30 seconds with palms up and eyes closed. Note if one arm pronates or if there is a downward drift.

PEARL: Make sure you document your findings in a way that allows you to use the results to determine how the patient is doing on the next visit. Is she getting stronger or weaker? What other factors aside from the course of the Lyme disease could cause such change?

- With arms in front and palms down try to depress arms against resistance.

- Raise arms overhead with palms forward for 20 seconds. How long can the patient maintain this position? Check resistance to arms being forced down.

- Test flexion and extension of forearm against resistance.

- Have the patient make a fist and try to resist your pushing it down to test dorsiflexion strength.

PEARL: The wrist will be weak in radial nerve disorders.

- Assess the grip. Have the patient curl the fingers together as hard as possible. A normal grip is tight enough to make it hard for you to pull apart. Of course, little children and the elderly will not be as strong. The grip is lessened by forearm muscle weakness and hand diseases.

- Spread the fingers and try to force them back together. There will be weak abduction in ulnar nerve disorders.

- Test hip flexion strength by placing a hand on the thigh and asking the patient to raise the leg against it.

- Place hands outside knees and ask the patient to press the legs against the hands.

PEARL: If muscles are weak proximally, then you likely have a myopathy. If muscles are weak distally, then you likely have a neuropathy.

- Muscle strength in the knee is assessed for both flexion and extension. For flexion: flex the leg with the foot resting on the bed. Tell the patient to keep the foot down as you try to raise it. For extension: support the knee and ask the patient to straighten the leg while you try to stop him.

- For the muscles around the ankle, use plantar flexion and dorsiflexion of the foot against your resistance.

PEARL: Lyme can decimate muscle strength. Be careful that you are assessing muscle strength and not general weakness, fatigue, apathy, or sleepiness.

Movement: Muscles may look tough but they don't do much without some nerve telling them what to do. Movement should be symmetrical and viewed here from the perspective of the nerve. Watch for differences between sides. This examination of movement can be done at the same time as the ROM maneuvers done to examine the joints. If something isn't moving, and there isn't a problem with structure or muscle, look to the nerve to see if you can find out what's the matter.

Abnormalities in motion: There are a number of abnormalities which may look like problems with motor function that could manifest in Lyme and other TBI patients. These include tics, fasciculations, twitching, choreiform motions, tremors, and clonus/myoclonus. These are all described in the later section *Problems with the Nervous System*.

H. **Sensation:** The perception of the information picked up by the nerve dendrites and sent back to the brain for interpretation. Here we are looking at the skin sensations: pain, temperature, light touch, position, vibration, and discrimination. Sensation is usually tested on the skin of bilateral extremities. If you find an area of abnormality, try to map out the extent of the problem. This can help identify the source.

*PEARL: Patients with Lyme and other TBIs are often **hypersensitive** to sensory stimulation. Many cannot tolerate light or sound. Others cannot bear touch whether it is of human contact or the softest cloth. These people do not want to get dressed or keep clothes on. Some perceive abnormal smells or tastes. Be aware of this potential hypersensitivity as you assess the patient.*

- Light touch: Can the patient perceive a stimulus to the skin? Have the patient close his eyes. Then using a Q-tip or cotton ball on the hands and feet, ask the person to tell you when he feels the touch.

- Temperature: The sensory nerves in the skin can distinguish a whole range of temperatures. The nerve damage in diabetics can cause them to lose this ability and they can burn or freeze their skin unintentionally. To test temperature perception, use tubes filled with warm and cold water against the skin. If pain sensation is normal, there is probably no need to assess temperature.

- Position: Knowing where the body is in space is called proprioception or position sense. To test, move the toes and fingers up and down and from side to side to see if the patient can discern the position.

- Vibration: The oscillating or moving back and forth around a point in a regular, periodic fashion. A good synonym is quivering. Vibration allows sound waves to be interpreted as hearing. Using a low pitched tuning fork, place the vibrating fork over the DIP of the finger and IP of the big toe. Ask the patient if he feels the vibration. If he only feels pressure during this test there could be a problem with vibrational sense. Vibration can also be tested by placing the base of the vibrating tuning fork against any boney prominence like the elbow, knee, or ulna. If vibration sense is normal distally, there is no need to test more proximally.

- Discrimination: The ability to tell the difference between two sensory stimuli. Testing the ability to discriminate sensations quickly fatigues the patient, so do this assessment in as few attempts as possible. Stereognosis is the ability to identify an object by touch alone. Use a coin, pencil, key, or other small familiar object and see if the patient can tell what it is, using only her fingers. Older children should be able to determine what number you write in the palm of their hands with your finger. Normal discrimination should allow for the identification of common textures. Assessment of two-point discrimination uses sharp objects like pins to stimulate two places at once. How close can the pins get and the patient still tell it is two stimuli instead of one?

Abnormalities in sensation can manifest in Lyme and other TBI patients. **Hypersensation** is a huge problem in these patients. In some cases there are sensations of burning, pins and needles, and electrical currents shooting through tissue.

PEARL: Sensory deficit in muscles that control thumb abduction and opposition can cause the muscles to become weak and atrophied.

I. **Pain**: An unpleasant sensory and emotional experience caused by actual or perceived tissue damage. Pain can range from mild discomfort to excruciating and incapacitating sensations. Use a pin to detect pain alternating the blunt side of the pin with the point.

    Pain is just about universal in Lyme patients. Whether it is head pain or joint pain, or any other location, these patients hurt. Assess the person's pain threshold. Is it high or low? Many patients underestimate or overestimate the degree of discomfort. Ask the patient. Maybe there is a way to break the pain cycle. Of course, if the pain is secondary to a TBI, the best way to treat the pain is to treat the TBI.

    *PEARL: Pain has a productive role in communicating signals to the body that something should be done to stop the sensation. Usually, once the acute damage is resolved, the pain alarm goes off. Unfortunately, sometimes the pain cycle continues. The limbic system gets involved and the more the pain cycle continues, the more the pain is perceived to be increasing. The patient can overestimate the degree of pain. This is called **pain amplification syndrome**. Be aware of this possibility as you consider the pain in your patient.*

    Headache is a localized pain common to almost all infections and TBIs. Some think they can tell the pathogen by the headache location, intensity, and pattern.

J. **Speech:** The verbal expression of thoughts. There are many areas of the brain involved with speech, so there are lots of places for things to go wrong. Listen to the individual speak. Assess loudness, clarity, pace, volume, coherence, and relevance.

    If there are speech problems, try to determine how the deficit might be associated with the TBI, if at all. Some speech problems like lisps are not likely related to TBIs.

K. Developmental Milestones: Noting the developmental milestones in children may be important since active Lyme is known to potentially impact many aspects of growth and maturation. Unambiguous documentation will be useful in tracking progress.

Milestones are very individual. Unfortunately, parents often become competitive when it comes to how fast their children are moving past development landmarks. I have heard so many whoppers. Just when you think you've heard it all, some ambitious parent comes up with something new. You might be surprised at how many babies come into this world tap dancing, fencing, and quoting Shakespeare in Swahili. The good news is that most kids are average and that's just fine. In terms of assessing TBI patients, we are more concerned about the status of the individual child than who was actually the first child on the moon.

We are not only interested in what the child can do right this minute but also whether the child improves or deteriorates from visit to visit. This comparative assessment can be extremely important in determining if the treatment plan is working. Developmental and behavioral problems are often a primary concern to parents. While it may take a few minutes to assess these milestones they will be helpful as you follow the child over time.

Treatment should be continued at least until the child improves (plus a therapeutic cushion). You can't know if the child is getting better or worse unless you clearly document the status at each visit. Assess and document.

PEARL: There are many published lists of developmental milestones. One compilation is listed here. Find the version that best suits your practice.

General developmental milestones:	
GM = Gross Motor FM = Fine Motor	
2 to 4 weeks	Fixation on objects
1 month	GM: When prone holds head up (range 0 to 3 months)
6 weeks	GM: Lifts chin sometimes when prone Social: Smiles socially (range 4 to 12 weeks)
5 to 6 weeks	Coordinated eye movements when following an object
2 months	GM: Arms extend forward. When prone head steady at shoulder (range 1 to 4 months) FM: Pulls at clothes Speech: Cooing (range 1 to 4 months)

3 months	Eyes should converge. Reaches for objects. Swats at objects (range 2 to 5 months) GM: No more Moro startle reflex
4 months	GM: Rolls from front to back (range 3 to 6 months) FM: Reaches and pulls objects to mouth Speech: Responds to human voice. Laughs. Turns to voice (range 3 to 6 months)
5 months	Rolls back to front. Sits with support (range 4 to 7 months) FM: Transfers object from one hand to the other (range 4 to 7 months)
6 months	GM: Can put weight on hands when on belly. Sits independently (range 5 to 9 months) FM: Grasping at objects Speech: Responds to name. Babbling (range 5 to 9 months) Social: Begins to be nervous around strangers (range 6 to 12 months)
7 months	GM: Creeps on belly (range 5 to 10 months) FM: Eats with fingers (range 5 to 10 months)
8 months	Crawls on hands and knees (range 6 to 11 months)
9 months	GM: Pulls to stand (range 6 to 12 months) FM: Finger-thumb grasp or pincer (range 7 to 10 months) Speech: Mama Dada (range 6 to 10 months) Social: Separation anxiety begins (range 9 to 24 months)
10 months	Babinski just about gone Social: Some sharing. Understands "NO" (range 9 to 18 months) GM: Walks with support (range 9 to 18 months) FM: Pincer grasp. Throws Speech: 2 words more than Mama Dada Social: Drinks from cup. Helps to dress. Uses mom as home base
15 months	GM: Walks without support (range 9 to 18 months)

	FM: Draws line
	Speech: Jargon (range 10 to 18 months)
	Social: Points to what is needed. Uses spoon (range 12 to 18 months). Can follow one step command (range 12 to 20 months)
18 months	GM: Climbs steps without support
	FM: Scribbles
	Speech: Says name and more than 10 words. Points to body parts (range 12 to 24 months)
	Social: Good spoon use. Imitates adult work. More independence begins
2 years	GM: Kicks ball. Runs. Climbs 2 steps. Jumps on 2 feet
	FM: Undresses. Starts to show handedness (range 18 to 30 months)
	Speech: 2 word sentences. Pronouns often incorrect. "NO"
	Social: Parallel play (range 12 to 30 months). 2 step command (range 22 to 30 months)
3 years	GM: Tricycle
	FM: Copies a circle
	Speech: Prepositions. Says first name (range 30 to 40 months). Pronouns more appropriate
	Social: Dresses and undresses except buttons. Begins toilet training (range 24 to 36 months). Cooperative play (range 24 to 48 months)
4 years	GM: Hops on 1 foot
	FM: Copies an X
	Speech: Tells a story
	Social: Conservative play. Toilet trained. Can do buttons
5 years	GM: Skips. Catches ball
	FM: Copies square. Prints own name. Ties shoes
	Speech: Says alphabet. Uses future tense
	Social: Attached to opposite sex parent
6 years	GM: Rides bicycle
	FM: Copies triangle
	Speech: Starts to read
	Social: Sense of right and wrong
7 years:	FM: Printing. Writing. Tying shoes. Buttons. Scissors. R/L discrimination

After the child starts school, you can see how her development is progressing through comments from teachers and her social interactions with other kids, neighbors, pets, siblings, etc. If there appears to be a deficit in one area, do more observations and documentation. Reassess this area carefully on the next visit.

L. **Emotional maturity**: Maturation is the process of development where the individual reaches certain milestones and eventually becomes independent. Overall maturation is an integration of physical, mental, intellectual, emotional, and social components. Emotional IQ, or EQ, is the evolution of the ability to recognize and manage emotions in a way that allows for life satisfaction and stable relationships with others. Maturation is very individual and one aspect can *mature* faster than others. For example, a teen can be physically mature for his age but emotionally lagging. As they say, "Some people never grow up." Stereotypically, females mature in almost all ways before males. Certain conditions like autism can cause a person to miss emotional and social cues and thereby affect perception of his maturity by others.

Maturity can take longer than we expect, especially when it comes to organizational skills and judgment. Many mistakes that parents make in raising children are due to thinking that kids are capable of understanding and performing beyond their normal age capacities. Despite a number of Russian studies saying that babies can be toilet trained by 3-months-old, that is not a realistic expectation in other cultures. Reading these studies suggests it is the caretaker who has been trained and not the infant. So keep expectations in perspective and know what is reasonable for each age group especially before you decide a child is delayed or gifted. While all parents love to hear their child is gifted, this label has done as much harm as negative labels, especially when applied by people not qualified to make this type of assessment. That being said, few things are sadder than a child who is not living up to her potential for whatever reason. Our job here is to help patients take advantage of life opportunities despite underlying TBI.

AGE-SPECIFIC FINDINGS

Infants, especially newborns, are neurologically very different from older kids and adults. At birth, the CNS is not fully developed, so "normal" findings now do not guarantee there is no problem. For HCPs that means our target "normal" is always shifting. Since TBIs can significantly impact the nervous system, each age group must be assessed from a realistic perspective. A 2 y/o will never seem to progress if you start out evaluating him against 4 y/o parameters. You are looking to see that the child is within range and keeps progressing and not regressing. Cortical function is one of the last areas to develop, so you might not be able to get a full idea of overall potential in the neonatal period.

Babies have automatic responses to certain stimuli. These are called **infantile automatisms**. If they do not have these infantile reflexes, or if the automatisms persist after they should be dissipating, this could imply a significant problem. In general, we know that when kids are born with congenital Lyme, the Bb can have a major impact in all areas of development. We have no idea how an individual child might be affected. Manifestations are probably multi-factorial. Problems that we have been labeling idiopathic developmental delays may actually be sequelae of TBIs.

Be aware of the unique characteristics of the neonate as you examine children for evidence of a TBI:

- Infants are more flexible than any other age group and more sensitive to touch, pain, and temperature.

- If there is no withdrawal from a pain stimulus, then the child is either numb (and doesn't feel it) or paralyzed (and can't do anything about it). If the pain is felt as indicated by crying or a change in facial expression, but the child does not withdraw from the noxious stimuli, then the child could be paralyzed. In contrast, a child with a spinal cord lesion will withdraw but will not cry or change expression.

- Normal newborns lie symmetrically with semiflexed limbs and legs slightly spread at the hips. The head can be to one side or midline. Usually the neonate holds her hands in fists. Tremors of the extremities and trunk can be normal for several days and are worse with crying.

- Resting tremors lasting more than 4 days suggest there may be a problem in the CNS. Any asymmetrical movements should prompt a more extensive look for neurologic or congenital problems or birth injuries.

- Breech babies are more likely to have unusual postures with legs and head extended.

- Normal children will have spontaneous, symmetrical movements of their arms and legs.

- It is best to examine newborns and infants when they are not crying, but this may be a long wait and experienced HCPs will learn how to listen carefully between sobs.

- Hip abduction testing should be done at the end of the newborn exam since this may upset the child.

- Feet may be in odd positions immediately after birth. Make notes describing any deformities and watch them over time. If abnormalities seem significant or unresolving, refer.

- Infants almost always look flat-footed because of fat on the sole.

- Infant automatisms:

  1. Blink reflex: Eyelids close in response to sudden bright light. This reflex disappears in about a year. Absence can mean a visual defect.

  2. Acoustic blink: Eyelids close in response to a sudden loud noise. Absence can mean diminished hearing.

  3. Palmar grasp: Grasping motion that disappears in 3 to 4 months. Press a finger against the palmar surface of the baby's hand and the child should respond by making a fist. Compare both hands. Persistence beyond 4 months may signify cerebral problems. Babies normally hold their hands in fists for the first month.

  4. Rooting reflex: With the baby's head midline, put a finger on the side of the mouth. The newborn will root in the direction of the finger and the mouth will open. Absence of this reflex is a significant problem. Look for the rooting reflex in those babies thought to be infected with Babesia at birth. The reflex should return if properly treated. The rooting reflex disappears at 3 or 4 months.

  5. Trunk curve: Hold the infant horizontally and prone in one hand like a French bread. Use the other hand to stimulate one side of the back about an inch from midline from the shoulder to the butt. The trunk should curve to the stimulated side. No curve indicates a potential lesion of the spinal cord. This reflex disappears at about 2 months.

  6. If you pinch the nostril of an infant this will cause a reflex opening of the mouth and the tip of the tongue will rise. This tests CN 12.

PROBLEMS WITH THE NERVOUS SYSTEM

Some of the following terms are signs and symptoms of neurologic problems and others are diagnoses. Any or all have been associated with TBIs either as part of the pathologic presentation of the disease or as part of a co-morbidity. Consider these conditions when compiling a differential diagnosis.

A. **Pervasive Developmental Disorder** refers to delays in development of multiple basic functions such as socialization and communication. PDD can be recognized in infancy and is almost always identified prior to age 4. In retrospect, most caretakers realize there were problems earlier that they did not recognize or they rationalized away. PDD is also called the **autism spectrum of disorders** or ASD. Since it is a spectrum, not all kids show the same signs, symptoms, or clinical course. One child may not fit exactly into any one category since there is such a wide range of involvement and severity. In addition, a child may shift on the spectrum as she does better or worse over time. Most often PDD is divided into the following categories:

1. **Atypical autism**: Also called PDD not otherwise specified or PDD-NOS, atypical autism is probably the most common of the PDD diagnoses. This condition is usually considered milder than standard autism but this is often a matter of semantics. Atypical autism manifests in significant social and communication deficits. These children will act differently than other kids in their age group. They do not connect well with others and have trouble reading expressions and social cues. They don't know how to respond when others laugh or cry. Thinking is quite literal and concrete. There is no sarcasm, irony, or figurative language. These kids do not babble and have delayed or limited speech. They often repeat words and have trouble with pronouns. They have poor non-verbal communication and a very narrow set of interests. Interestingly, the difference between a diagnosis of autism and PDD-NOS may depend on which term the family finds more acceptable.

PEARL: The APA is looking to revise the diagnostic criteria for autism in the next edition of the DSM. In January 2012, the expert panel assigned this task announced their intention to curb the autism epidemic by calling certain types of autism something else. Sound familiar? While most would agree that the current diagnostic labels need clarification, changes should be made based on what makes medical sense, not simply to save money.

PEARL: The biggest issue around autism, whatever the cause, is lack of reciprocity.

2. **Autism**: Symptoms start in infancy and are usually apparent by age 2 and include withdrawal, unresponsiveness, and impaired communication. Some autistic people live chaotically with no routine while others stick rigidly to repetitive behaviors. Some have a compulsion for uniformity in their environment with everything precisely ordered. Infants may fail to react to touch or affection with a total lack of responsiveness. Some of the repeated behaviors can be self-destructive

with head banging, eye scratching, or hair pulling. Arm flapping is not uncommon.

PEARL: In common with many Lyme patients, autistic kids can have extreme sensitivity to sensory stimuli like loud noises and light.

PEARL: Age 18 months is about the time when children should be interacting. Autistic kids often miss this milestone.

Autistic kids can "look right through you" as though you aren't there. Both verbal and non-verbal language is impaired and they may repeat a word or sound over and over like an echo. In some cases, with early intervention autistics can interact socially with others by the teen years, but most are always considered odd. They range from functional to total incapacity as they get older. There remains much controversy over autism. Is it genetic or environmental or a combination? Is it due to mercury in immunizations or too many vaccines too close together? A recent report suggested that numerous spontaneous mutations were found in the genes of a subpopulation of autistic kids. These mutations were speculated to be due to environmental toxins. Could some of these toxins be due to infectious agents like Bb? Fewer of these mutations were needed to cause the disease in boys than girls, which could explain the gender disparity. As with so many of these complex and poorly understood syndromes, the cause is probably multifactorial.

PEARL: Dr. Bransfield reports success with open-ended antibiotic treatment in managing the autism-like syndrome secondary to Bb infection.

Because Lyme and autism are so often mistaken for each other, we need to spend a little more time making a distinction. While the five categories of the autism spectrum are listed here, these have little meaning to most laypeople and to many HCPs as well. Even professionals have difficulty making distinctions within the spectrum. Most of us have a vague notion of the types of signs we will encounter when someone mentions autism. The general perception of a child with autism is one who:

a. Displays social and communication deficits

b. Interacts differently than other kids the same age

c. Doesn't connect well with others

d. Has trouble reading expressions and social cues

e. Doesn't know how to respond when others laugh or cry

f. Demonstrates thinking that is quite literal and concrete. No sarcasm, irony, or figurative language

g. Engages in a very narrow set of interests, but can focus intently on those

h. Is socially withdrawn and unresponsive

i. Can live chaotically with no routine

j. May stick rigidly to repetitive behaviors

k. Will demonstrate a compulsion for uniformity in this environment with everything precisely ordered

l. May fail to react to touch or affection or may present with a total lack of interaction

m. Might engage in repeated behaviors that can be self destructive with head banging, eye scratching, or hair pulling. Arm flapping is not uncommon.

n. Can be hypersensitive to colors, light, sound, tastes, or touch

o. Can "look right through you" as though you aren't there

p. Can have impairment of both verbal and nonverbal language. May repeat a word or sound over and over like an echo. Might not be able to process what is heard. Often is not able to verbally express ideas

q. Falls on a spectrum ranging from mild social awkwardness to the need for helmets to prevent self-injury

r. If Asperger's, may be intellectually gifted, while socially inept

s. Likely to always be considered odd

How are Lyme and autism related? Some sources believe all autism is due to Bb infection, while others see no relationship at all. We do know that Lyme often presents with an **autism-like syndrome**. We have very little insight into those cases where a child with autism is subsequently infected with Bb or a child with Lyme develops the autism he would have developed whether or not he was bitten by a tick. Too early in our learning curve. How can you tell autism from autism induced by Lyme? The Lyme-related condition often improves with antibiotic treatment.

PEARL: In March, 2013, the lay media reported that more autism was being diagnosed "in older kids." I wonder if some of these cases might be autism-like syndrome?

There is considerable anecdotal evidence in the literature that suggests that appropriate antibiotics, at the correct doses, for adequate duration can improve or cure Lyme-induced autism (autism-like syndrome). In kids with autism due to Bb infection consider: amoxicillin AND azithromycin OR cefdinir (Omnicef) AND azithromycin. Many Lyme-induced autism cases need treatment for 3 to 6 years. In these cases, relapses may occur when the antibiotics are discontinued prematurely. If recurrence occurs, restarting the antibiotics usually causes the sxs to subside once again. Recurrence is less common if treated adequately.

The medical profession, along with society, is just beginning to realize that children with autism eventually become adults with autism. This will confound our assessments of Lyme and autism even further. ALWAYS when you see an autism-like presentation put Lyme on the differential diagnosis list.

3. **Asperger's syndrome:** I am not being the least bit facetious when I say that Asperger's is almost a prerequisite to study rocket science at Purdue. These are the kids who in third grade are taking college level math and my son Chris used to say were "wired funny." This is not in any way disparaging. After meeting dozens of these kids, I believe that some Asperger's personalities are perfect for engineering. Academically, the Asperger's students may have an advantage, but in groups they may struggle. There is no doubt that these kids have impaired social skills and limited interactions. But in contrast to autism, there are no significant delays in language, cognition, or developmental skills. In fact, many Asperger's patients are exceedingly intelligent. They have the advantage of being able to focus intensely for long periods within their area of interest. You're in trouble if you want them to do things they aren't passionate about. They do not have the social distractions that lure the other kids away from the goal. Yet, none seem to think they are missing anything.

At Purdue there are the engineering majors and then there are those who *were* engineering majors and now are majoring in lighter fare. Guess where the higher percentage of Asperger's might be? In my opinion, there seems to be a clear disadvantage for those kids who do not have Asperger's in studying rocket science. Chris has several TBIs, but not Asperger's and he has to study extremely hard to compensate. Some Asperger's kids do math problems for fun and text one another over the summer to see if one of them "figured it out." Many of these individuals learn to play the social game in order to function in society, though most remain on the margins. That isn't to say that some people with Asperger's do not suffer mightily, depending on the severity of the condition. Usually the parents take a while to learn what is going on and to find a learning environment that matches the child's excessive skills in some areas and deficiencies in others. One child said to me, "Another word for Asperger's is gifted," and in many cases that's true. Unfortunately, Asperger's kids are not smarter than the rest of us about tick bites and they might have concurrent TBIs.

PEARL: In November 2011, Purdue was listed near the top of US colleges with the toughest grading. I couldn't tell if they were number 3 or number 5 since I couldn't figure out the graphics in the news article. I guess there is an advantage to being "wired funny" that I do not possess.

4. **Rett's syndrome:** Rett's disorder is a multiple-deficit disorder of development that may include hand-wringing or hand-washing. Rett's almost always occurs in girls starting at around 6 months of age and can present with breath holding, hyperventilation, seizures, loss of communication skills, and a gradual decline in motor and cognitive functions. Hand skills are lost and there is less interest in social interaction. Head growth slows and retardation ensues. Rett's is uncommon and is sometimes included as part of the autism spectrum and sometimes not. You will likely never see a case and it is included here for completeness.

5. **Childhood disintegrative disorder:** CDD is relatively rare, but the most perplexing of the autism spectrum disorders. Sometimes it isn't included as part of the spectrum because unlike the other conditions, CDD has a late onset of symptoms in a *previously normal* child. Onset of first signs occurs between 3 and 10-years-old. These kids were developing normally when they regress. Attained skills are lost. The reversion can be rapid over days or weeks but can take longer. Older kids can even ask what is happening to them as they watch themselves deteriorate. (I find that very sad.) After a period of normal development, the child loses both expressive and receptive language skills, social interactions decline, and the ability for self-care is gone. There is loss of control over bladder and bowels and diminished play and motor skills. They have increasing problems with social interactions as they become progressively more retarded. Retardation can then become severe and CDD is considered a low functioning form of autism. Hallucinations and seizures may be present along with repetitive behaviors. When reviewing your differential diagnosis, consider whether an underlying infectious process could

be causing or contributing to the changes seen in these previously normal children. What a tragedy to overlook a treatable underlying condition!

*PEARL: A general understanding of autism is important for the HCP working with Lyme patients. There is an **autism-like disorder** that accompanies some cases of Lyme. When the Lyme is treated with appropriate antibiotics, the autism symptoms can regress. Whether the autism-like presentation is due solely to Bb or there was an underlying predisposition to autism is an area of much speculation. Just as the term "Lyme arthritis" is thrown about, the term "Lyme autism" is also used and appears in the literature. This may be a total misnomer since there is so much debate over the etiology. A high percentage of autistic kids are positive for Bb even in the suboptimal world of Lyme testing. If we had accurate testing methods, the percentage would likely be higher. Whether the Lyme caused the autism or the autism is a co-morbidity of the Lyme, or if they just aggravate each other, we don't know. If the kid improves on Lyme antibiotics, the Lyme probably contributed.*

PEARL: Be careful with diagnostic codes. Some insurance companies will not cover PDD but will cover PDD-NOS. Go figure.

PEARL: The presence of Mycoplasma might influence the presentation of autism in ways similar to Bb. Again, the MOA by which these pathogens could influence the clinical picture is only beginning to be recognized. In any case, if the autism is associated with an underling infectious etiology, antibiotics may help when conventional therapeutics are ineffective.

PEARL: A CDC review noted that 10 out of the top 15 states with the highest incidence of autism overlap with the states with the most Lyme disease. Of course, there could be a dozen explanations for this but one reason could be some kind of causal association. Lyme is just one of the infections with which autism has been linked. We're missing something here.

B. **Specific Developmental Disorder:** SDDs are developmental delays that are specific to one area such as motor coordination, speech, language, or learning. The ICD 10 codes and the DSM-IV categories are so confusing and conflicting about these conditions, that you will wonder how to differentiate a specific developmental disorder from an atypical autism. Splitting these hairs may not make any difference to the patient, but it may to the insurance companies.

C. **Encephalitis:** A severe inflammation of the brain, encephalitis is often caused by mosquito or tick-borne pathogens but can be due to other causes. Usually there is a sudden onset of fever, headache, vomiting, stiff neck and back, and signs of neuronal damage such as changes in consciousness, paralysis, ataxia, and psychoses. With encephalitis there can be intense leukocytic infiltration of brain tissues and the meninges, causing cerebral edema. Degeneration of ganglion cells and diffuse nerve cell destruction can occur. The infectious agent may directly damage the tissue. After an acute phase, the signs and symptoms may persist for days or weeks. Encephalitis may leave permanent damage and can be fatal. Sometimes encephalitis can be hard to distinguish from other febrile illnesses like severe gastroenteritis and meningitis. Depending on the suspected etiology, treatment with antivirals or antibiotics and intensive supportive care might be required.

PEARL: There is Lyme encephalitis.

*PEARL: Lyme **encephalopathy** is the symptom set that accompanies the encephalitis and also refers to other clusters of NP sxs that are caused by neuroborreliosis such as cognitive disorders and brain fog.*

PEARL: Bb has been implicated in acute disseminated encephalomyelitis.

D. **Meningitis:** An inflammation of the meninges, the covering of the brain and spinal cord. Most commonly the inflammation is the result of an infection, although there can be other reasons. Therefore, signs of meningitis are initially those of infection: fever, chills, and malaise. As the disease progresses, there will be signs of increased ICP such as headache, vomiting, and papilledema. Soon the signs of meningeal irritation develop including nuchal rigidity.

To check for signs of meningeal irritation:

- Brudzinski test: A positive test occurs when forward motion of the neck is impeded by pain and resistance. With the patient lying on her back, try to raise the head with your hands. Brudzinski is positive if there is pain or resistance or if the hips or knees flex when attempting the move.

- Kernig's test: With the patient supine, flex the leg at the hip, and then straighten the knee. Note pain or resistance.

Any pain or resistance during these maneuvers suggests meningeal inflammation. But there might also be inflammation from arthritis, injury, disc disease, or inflexibility. In the case of meningitis, the patient could be showing other signs of acute inflammation and infection.

The PE might show exaggerated symmetrical DTRs, vision problems, and changes in consciousness. Opisthotonos is a spasm in which the back and extremities arch backwards so that the weight rests on the head and heels. You see this once and you remember. An eye exam looking at the fundus may reveal signs of increased ICP such as papilledema. Lab tests, imaging studies, and a lumbar puncture with culture may be prudent. Although all these diagnostic methods will likely be negative for Lyme, even when it is the casual agent, other co-etiologies might be uncovered.

Meningitis can be viral, bacterial, fungal, or aseptic. Aseptic means that testing failed to uncover any pathogens. As we have learned over and over with Lyme, *not detected does not mean uninfected.* Perhaps the testing methods were not adequate to uncover the pathogen. Treat the patient, not the lab test.

Infants with meningitis may show signs of infection and be fretful and refuse to eat. Vomiting may lead to dehydration and this dryness may prevent bulging of the fontanelle which would otherwise occur. The swollen fontanelle is a sign of increased ICP. As meningitis progresses, there may be twitching, seizures, or coma. The mortality rate is especially high in infants.

PEARL: There is Lyme meningitis.

PEARL: In addition to clinical symptoms, signs of CNS involvement include CSF protein elevation or pleocytosis, altered pressure, abnormal MRI or EEG, intrathecal antibody production, positive PCR, or isolation of a pathogen from cultures. Most of these signs are NOT clearly present even though the patient may be showing obvious signs of nervous system inflammation. Pleocytosis in an increased cell count. The term is used primarily to refer to a high white cell count in CSF. Why don't they just say a high white cell count in the CSF?

PEARL: The concurrent presentation of Lyme meningitis, radiculopathy, and involvement of cranial nerves is called the triad of neurologic Lyme.

E. **Stroke:** A stroke is an infarction in the brain due to either bleeding or blockage that results in residual damage. A cerebrovascular accident or brain attack presents with sudden impairment. Diminished oxygen supply causes damage or death to brain tissue. The site where the injury occurs will dictate where the symptoms appear. A TIA (transient ischemic attack) is a CVA that clears within a day or two. In contrast, a stroke leaves residual damage. Usually a CVA causes one-sided symptoms. To assess for a CVA: Ask the patient to smile, speak, and raise the hands over the head. With a CVA, the patient might experience asymmetrical difficulty with any of these tasks. CVAs are rare in young people but the incidence goes up with DIC and with any end-stage complications. A stroke might need to be ruled out when a person presents with Bell's palsy.

F. **Cognition Deficits:** Cognition is the ability to think. Cognitive problems are some of the most common and important sxs of LD but can also be important manifestations of Bartonella, M. *fermentans*, and Babesia infections. In order to assess cognitive ability, HCPs look at basic knowledge, vocabulary, analytical ability, problem solving, and the presence of a coherent line of reasoning. Thoughts should be clear, realistic, and follow a logical flow. Tager's work showed that Lyme patients can have significantly more cognitive and psychiatric disturbances than controls. These deficits were still found after controlling for anxiety, depression, and fatigue. Cognition problems in kids can be the primary presenting sign and impaired cognitive function can make it hard to sustain attention, learn new things, and recall information. Cognitive glitches can severely impact developmental milestones. Manifestations of cognitive difficulties with Lyme might include poor processing of incoming information, plodding thoughts, slow ability to catch on, illogical reasoning, trouble with reading or writing, word searching, limited recall, difficulty in learning new concepts, impaired concentration, confused ideas, and diminished ability to express thoughts. Have a high index of suspicion especially in areas where the person had no prior problems or where there is a sudden, drastic change.

PEARL: While they do not fall neatly under the cognition label, judgment and abstract thought could also be impacted by Lyme. Further, patients may have difficulty with imagination. Imagination is the ability to create something new in the mind that had not existed before. Organizing, planning, and prioritizing can also diminish from Bb infection as well as with other TBIs. Likewise, handwriting can suffer and neat penmanship might deteriorate into illegibility. There may be an increase in spelling errors and insertion of the wrong word in both writing and speaking. There might be slow retrieval of well-known information. Data can be stored incorrectly. A patient might reverse the sequence of letters, words, or numbers, never having done so before. There can be an alarming decrease in the ability to understand spoken language,

PEARL: Logigian et al reported that neuropsychiatric testing could uncover cognitive deficits not apparent from routine mental status exams.

G. **Delayed Developmental Milestones:** Developmental milestones are a set of skills that can be used to assess where a child stands in terms of how she is developing compared to her peers. Usually aptitude in several areas is observed, such as gross motor, fine motor, language, cognition, and social interaction. These skills can be quite variable, but documenting milestones can be especially useful in TBI patients because the HCP can see how the child is doing now compared to past performance. We are not only interested in what the child can do right this minute but also whether the child improves or deteriorates from visit to visit. This comparative assessment can be extremely important in determining if the treatment plan is working. These developmental markers can be of obsessive concern to parents. They are most useful to the HCP in helping to follow the child over time.

H. **Abnormal Movements**

Tic: An involuntary spasmodic muscle contraction usually involving the brief, rapid movement of the face, mouth, head, neck, shoulder, or trunk. Tics can resolve for a while, only to return. Tics can be simple or complex and are usually stereotypical and repetitive, but NOT rhythmic. Simple tics include things like blinking, winking, shrugging, grimacing, or repeatedly clearing the throat. Tics often begin in childhood and mimic parts of normal behavior. Complex tics can include both movements and vocalizations and are disabling in some cases. Tourette's syndrome is an inherited multiple tic disorder that begins in childhood and can include both motor and vocal tics. Tics are associated with PANDAS and are common in TBIs.

Fasciculation: A muscle twitch that is a small, local, involuntary muscle contraction visible under the skin. Fasciculations are most common in the eyelid. A significant number of Lyme patients complain of fasciculations and in the presence of corroborating history or ROS, these twitches strongly suggest LD.

PEARL: Twitches or fasciculations can be transient and physiologic in rapidly growing teens.

PEARL: Abnormal activity in the PNS can cause twitching and fluttering of the triceps, calves, or thighs.

Chorea: Movements that are choreic are brief, purposeless, involuntary acts of the distal extremities. Sometimes the patient can merge these movements into a purposeful action that masks the abnormality.

Tremor: A tremor is a repetitive rhythmic movement caused by muscle contractions and relaxations that are described by: 1) pace of the rhythm slow to rapid, 2) amplitude, 3) distribution or location, and 4) whether at rest versus when performing intentional movements. Parkinson's has a resting tremor while cerebellar disease has an intention tremor. Anxiety can be associated with trembling.

Postural tremors: During a prolonged posture, tremors can occur and may be exacerbated by anxiety and hyperthyroidism.

Intention tremors: Tremors occur during intentional movements such as when reaching or pointing and are likely due to cerebellar lesions.

Resting tremors: Tremors occur when extremities are at rest.

Clonus/Myoclonus: Clonus describes spasms that alternate between antagonistic muscle groups like the flexors and extensors of a joint.

Apraxia: An inability to execute purposeful, previously-known acts despite physical ability and willingness. This is likely a nerve problem, as opposed to muscular. Speech apraxia is trouble saying words correctly and consistently. There can be a rearrangement of sounds so that potato becomes topato.

Tardive dyskinesia: Abnormal movements occur as a late complication of long-term use of certain psychotropic drugs. Most often the dyskinesia affects the tongue, lips, and face. There can be repetitive opening and closing of the mouth, grimacing, protrusion of the tongue, or deviation of the tongue and jaw.

I. **Neuropathy: A** problem with the nerves due to damage or disease. There are several types which may overlap. Peripheral neuropathy is damage to the nerves in the peripheral nervous system, while entrapment neuropathy includes the symptoms that come from compressing a nerve in an enclosed space, as in carpal tunnel syndrome. Radiculopathies can result in severe, incapacitating pain in some cases.

Neuropathies can be due to systemic illness such as diabetes, collagen vascular disease, RA, sarcoid, lupus, alcoholism, toxins, heavy metals especially lead and mercury, lightening strikes, electrocution, endocrine dysfunction, solvents, too much B6, too little B12, A, E, or B1, radiation, fluoroquinolone toxicity, or infections. Autoimmunity may play a role. One nerve may be involved or many. Direct injury can cause nerve damage as can ischemia or inflammation. Stings from sea nettles cause neuropathies. There are many ways to damage a nerve.

Depending on the nerve and location, signs and symptoms can include: weakness, loss of muscle mass, fasciculations or twitches, tremors, muscle fatigue, diminished sensation, pain, cramps, spasms, loss of balance, lack of coordination, tingling, numbness, sensation of wearing a glove or sock, burning, freezing, jabbing, electric shock sensation, extreme hypersensitivity, diminished function, sensitivity to touch, pins and needles, or feeling of the foot falling asleep.

PEARL: A burning sensation is a common complaint in Lyme.

Neuropathy involving the ANS causes problems with involuntary functions of the internal viscera such as abnormal regulation of BP, HR, RR, and sweating. There can be problems with digestion and urination including incontinence.

On PE those with peripheral neuropathies will show sensory and motor loss depending on the nerves involved. Reflexes may be diminished or absent. Neuropathy can present like myopathy and it may be hard to distinguish the two. Foot drop has been reported in Lyme patients.

If damage is not permanent, treat the underlying cause, like the TBI. In many cases of nerve damage, there may be more than one cause. Diabetics can be bitten by ticks.

Terms and conditions pertinent to neuropathies in TBI patients:

- **Sciatica**: The sciatic nerve is the largest nerve in the body and inflammation can cause extreme discomfort. This nerve passes from the pelvis down the back of the thigh and inflammation causes pain that follows its course. The pain is sharp and shooting and movement makes it worse. There can be numbness and tingling present. Sciatica can be due to compression, trauma, or inflammation. Infections such as Lyme have been associated with sciatica. While heat, PT, and NSAIDs may help, treat the underlying cause if possible.

- **Carpal tunnel syndrome** is compression of the median nerve in the wrist and can be unilateral or bilateral, presenting with paresthesias, pain, and weakness in the radial palmar aspects of the hand. Pain can be incapacitating and is often more severe at night.

- **Neuralgia** is severe sharp pain along the course of a nerve caused by pressure on nerve trunks, nerve damage, toxins, inflammation or infection. Shingles is called herpetic neuralgia.

- **Neuritis** is inflammation of a nerve and the term is used in the literature in association with Lyme. Brachial neuritis has been reported with Lyme.

- **Paresthesias** refer to the symptom described as numbness and tingling. These are definitely associated with Bb infection and appear, by most counts, in a majority of Lyme patients. The severe sole pain associated with Lyme and other TBIs could be the result of dysesthesias.

- **Formication** is a tactile hallucination described as the sensation of bugs crawling inside or outside the body.

J. Amnesia: An inability to recall past experiences and can be either recent, distant, or both

K. Delirium: An acute state of confusion common with high fevers

L. Heavy metal damage: Heavy metals can cross the BBB and get into the CSF. Mercury (Hg) can be especially neurotoxic and symptoms include burning, numbness, and electric shooting sensations. The term "mad as a hatter" refers to the poor souls who were exposed to high levels of mercury used in the manufacturing of felt hats in England in the 18th century. These workers would present with dementia, emotional lability, memory problems, and insomnia. Along with the excessive salivation that can occur with Hg poisoning, they must have made quite the spectacle as they roamed the streets of London after midnight. More information on the effects of heavy metals is found in Chapter 26: *Alternative Treatments*.

PEARL: Why does this text spend so much time on heavy metal poisoning? The signs and symptoms of metal toxicity can be very similar to those of TBIs, especially in terms of the neuropsychiatric manifestations. Further, exposure to heavy metals is thought to prolong or intensify Lyme sxs. The HCP will want to discern what might be causing the problem. Remember, two pathologies may be active at once.

M. Tic douloureux is trigeminal neuralgia which is an irritation of the trigeminal nerve causing severe lightening-like stabs of pain. The location of the pain will depend on which branch of the nerve is involved. Pain is momentary but can occur repetitively for hours. The condition can subside for months and then return.

N. Tourette's syndrome: Tourette's is an inherited multiple tic disorder that begins in childhood. Similar tics are found in association with PANDAS. Simple tics may progress to multiple and complex tics including respiratory and involuntary vocalizations. The vocal tics can begin as grunting and evolve to compulsive inappropriate utterances. Severe cases can be physically and socially disabling. Sometimes the tics can be suppressed briefly.

O. Speech problems:

Aphasia	Impairment of communication, including speech, due to some brain disorder
Mute	Inability to speak
Selective mutism	Patient speaks only in certain situations such as when alone or to friend
Apraxia	Inconsistent or rearrangement of sound so that potato becomes topato
Dysphasia	Errors or uncertainty in word choice
Dysarthria	Slurred speech due to motor problems involving lips or tongue
Dysphonia	Raspy, hoarse voice
Aphonia	Whisper
Paralysis of palate	Nasal tone
Parkinson's speech	Monotone, weak
Depression	Slow, flat, monotonous speech
Ataxia	Defective speech due to muscle incoordination, usually a cerebellar problem

*PEARL: **Stammer**ing is common in Lyme, and occasionally stuttering will be observed. While these terms are often used interchangeably there are differences. **Stutter**ing includes hesitations, repetitions, and pauses which the speaker refers to as blocks. There can be prolongation of some sounds or the repetition of the first syllable of a word in a spasmodic fashion like C - C - C- Cat. Anxiety is not associated with the onset of stuttering, but can develop in social situations after the person is known as a stutterer. The term stammering more correctly refers to tripping over words, which we all do from time to time. The monarch in the movie The King's Speech had a stutter. Will Rogers and Jimmy Stewart had stammers. Unfortunately, many of the patients for whom this book is written have no idea who these people are.*

PEARL: Some Lyme patients will use childish speech patterns or stop mid-sentence or use incomplete sentences.

P. Pain: A complex feeling reflecting real or perceived tissue damage and the affective response to this perception. Pain is an unpleasant sensory and emotional experience. Pain can range from mild discomfort to excruciating, incapacitating sensations. Pain can be acute or chronic, constant or intermittent, sharp, dull, throbbing, stabbing, pressing, vice-like, sudden, rebounding, localized, cramping, boring (as in penetrating), crushing, point tender, generalized, achy, knife-like, electric, lightning bolt, intractable, cutting, refractory, or a combination of any of these descriptors. The pattern and presentation of pain can help identify the pathogen or problem in some cases. For example, a throbbing pain is likely due to the irritation of some arterial vessel.

Pain is just about universal in Lyme patients. Whether it is head pain or joint pain, or any other location, these patients hurt. Assess the patient's pain threshold. Is it high or low? Many people underestimate or overestimate the degree of discomfort. Ask the patient. Maybe there is a way to break the pain cycle. Of course, if the pain is secondary to a TBI, the best way to treat the pain is to treat the TBI.

Headache is a localized pain common to almost all infections and TBIs. Some think they can tell the pathogen by the headache location, intensity, and pattern. Some TBI authors provide guides on making the diagnosis based on the description of head pain provided by the patient. I do not know how valid or consistent these diagnostic recommendations might be. I see no harm in taking them into consideration as long as you do not discount a diagnosis because a patient doesn't have the "right" kind of headache. Look for how the pain fits into the overall clinical picture. Pain is a complaint of most TBI patients especially pain in the head, joints, and extremities. Migrating joint pain is a hallmark of Lyme.

Try to document the nature and severity of the pain in a way that you will know what you were talking about on the next visit. Ask the patient if the pain is different from last time. Ask what makes the pain better or worse. How did your physical exam impact the pain?

Pain is subjective and hard to quantify. However a pin can be used to detect pain sensations on the skin, alternating the blunt side of the pin with the point. Many hospitals and pain clinics now use a 1 to 10 scale, where 1 is barely perceptible and 10 is intolerable. The following is a list of pain terms that might be useful in documenting the pain experienced by a TBI patient.

- **Acute:** Acute pain is associated with a recent event such as trauma or other tissue damage that remains for the short-term as the damaged sensory tissue heals. Acute pain is usually defined as lasting less than a month. At the onset of pain the SNS may be stimulated causing tachycardia, increased respirations, elevated BP, sweating, and dilated pupils.

- **Chronic:** Pain that persists beyond a month can be the result of on-going tissue damage, scarring, or abnormal pain loops within the nervous system. Long-term pain is probably multifactorial. Chronic pain can be difficult to manage and the patient may experience frustration, depression, lassitude, or sleep disturbances.

- **Tenderness:** Pain to palpation, touch, or movement is sometimes called tenderness.

- **Ache:** The term ache is used to describe persistent discomfort and often describes the joint pain or overall discomfort accompanying infection or inflammation. "I ache all over."

- **Discomfort:** This sensation is perceived to be less severe than pain and is more of an un-ease.

- **Pain amplification syndrome:** Pain is a survival mechanism signaling to the body to act in order to rectify a bad situation. Usually, once the acute painful situation has settled, the pain alarm shuts off. Unfortunately, sometimes the pain cycle continues. The limbic system gets involved and the more the pain loop persists the more the pain is perceived to be increasing.

- **Migrating pain:** Lyme disease is known to have migrating joint pain. The pain may start in one joint and then move to another with or without resolution at the original pain site.

- **Neuropathic pain:** Chronic pain can occur after an insult to any level of the NS and may be the result of aberrant communication between the sensory and motor systems.

- **Neurogenic pain syndrome:** Here the patient has so much pain that the brain is set to respond abnormally even to the smallest amount of discomfort. The pain threshold is altered.

- **Neuralgic pain:** Neuralgia is pain that follows the distribution of a nerve. The pain of shingles is herpetic neuralgia. Usually, neuralgia is severe, sharp pain along the course of a nerve that is caused by pressure on nerve trunks, nerve damage, toxins, inflammation, or infection.

- **Referred pain:** Pain that seems to be in one place but is actually originating someplace else. This is common with dental pain, and in pain in the ear, jaw, gallbladder, heart, and appendix.

- **Growing pains**: Growing pain is a nonspecific term used to refer to pain felt in the joints or limbs of growing children. There is no evidence that the pains have anything to do with growth. Of unknown etiology, growing pains are very common in the elementary school age group. I wonder if some of what we called growing pains over the years might have been associated with TBIs, especially the shin discomfort of bartonellosis. There is also a possible association with rheumatic fever.

PEARL: Unfortunately, the term growing pains is often used as a "catch-all" diagnosis for any leg pain in kids especially if the HCP doesn't feel like spending any time on the problem. My friend's 4 y/o grandson was diagnosed with growing pains twice before his bone pain was found to be associated with an underlying leukemia. Don't be cavalier with other people's pain.

To assess whether a person can even sense pain, use a pin to detect pain sensations on the skin, alternating the blunt side of the pin with the point. Remember Lyme patients can experience numbness as often as tingling with their paresthesias.

People commit suicide over pain. Do not minimize their complaints. If the pain is due to a TBI, relief may occur if the TBI is appropriately treated. In some cases, when pain persists, aggressive action may be needed to help the person live around the pain. Chapter 25: *Ancillary Treatments* talks more about how to deal with pain.

Q. **Retardation:** Below average intellectual function, is usually recognized during the developmental period. Retardation is sometimes identified early and can include impaired learning, weak cognition, and problems with social adjustment and maturation. IQ measures are often inaccurate in these cases. Retardation can be genetic or from infections early in gestation. The cause is probably multifactorial and includes metabolic disorders, syphilis, birth anoxia, injuries, toxins, and environmental exposures. The term retardation has largely been replaced with more specifically-termed "cognitive impairments." A number of Lyme patients who have been labeled retarded have experienced significant improvement in cognition with appropriate antibiotic treatment.

R. **Brain injury:** I wish I had a dime for every parent in the ER whose kid had a concussion that I brushed off with a "Just keep an eye on him." Besides, he couldn't really have a concussion since he didn't lose consciousness. Then I had my own concussion and found a new respect for this injury. Concussions are very common, especially in athletes and after accidents. Despite what we learned in med school, you do not have to lose consciousness to have a concussion.

The mechanism of injury is the brain banging around inside the very hard and very confined space of the skull. The tissue is at least bruised and swollen. While no structural lesions are apparent, the patient may be dazed or confused immediately after the injury. There may be altered consciousness for seconds or minutes. The patient may be "knocked out." Pupils and other brainstem functions should all be intact. If they are not, consider that there might be a bleed or other injury causing the problem.

Concussions are getting a lot of attention these days with athletes dropping like flies. Much to my uncle's dismay, Stanley Crosby of the Pittsburgh Penguins missed most of the 2011-2012 season due to a concussion. Just a few years ago he would have been back on the ice immediately, risking re-injury and permanent damage. Residual effects can be cumulative.

Today, athletic trainers have started to use a series of questions to assess concussions and to help determine when a player can go back on the field. Recently, these questions to decide when the person is healed enough to be re-injured have come under scrutiny. At least it's keeping some players on the sidelines a little longer, providing more recovery time.

Fallon reports that kids with Lyme resembled kids with head injuries; that is, they had short-term memory loss, difficulty finding the correct word, and problems with concentration. Performance on IQ and spatial reasoning tests were especially impaired. They could still remember and learn but they processed information slowly and needed more time for even the most basic tasks. I am a unique specimen in that I experienced mental status changes due to both Lyme and a closed brain injury. I must say that after-the-fact, the syndromes seem essentially identical to me. Add to the symptom cluster that I simply did not care, and you will have a good description of my mental status. For months…

Post-concussion syndrome can affect a patient for extended periods with headache, dizziness, a dazed feeling, difficulty concentrating, varying degrees of amnesia, depression, apathy, and anxiety. All these symptoms may be due to neuronal damage. The academics often scoff and say the person is malingering. I sat in a daze for 3 months not even reading or watching TV. I invite those academics to experience their own concussion.

No, Lyme does not cause concussions. But people with post-concussion syndrome do get Lyme or they had

Lyme before they got the concussion. A concussion can cloud the clinical picture and delay healing.

PEARL: Recently, amantadine was reported as speeding the recovery from traumatic brain injury. I wonder if it might help with the invasive and biochemical brain injury associated with Lyme. Amantadine is also used to treat Parkinson-like syndromes, which have been described in some Lyme patients.

S. **Parkinson's disease:** I am occasionally surprised with onset of Parkinson's symptoms in a young person. Nevertheless, Parkinson's is primarily a disease of older people. The TBI physician needs to be aware of Parkinson's because this condition defines many neurologic abnormalities and is often used as a reference point. Parkinson's presents as progressive muscle rigidity, akinesia or loss of muscle movement, and an involuntary, shaking, "pill-rolling" tremor. Parkinson's affects certain areas of the brain and involves abnormal levels of dopamine. The akinesia makes walking difficult and the patient has a slow, shuffling gait, where the feet barely clear the floor and the steps are small as he walks bent forward. The voice may be high-pitched and monotonous with the face mask-like (flat affect). Dysarthritis and dysphagia can be present.

PEARL: There have been Parkinson-like syndromes noted in conjunction with Bb infection. I don't know if there is any causal relationship.

T. **Alzheimer's disease:** Alzheimer's is a progressive loss of cognitive function including judgment, abstract thought, and memory. Plaques in the grey matter and cortex of the brain seem to be the focus of the pathology. Alzheimer's patients can't do many AODL and can't learn new things. This disease should appear on the differential diagnosis of Lyme in adults. Spirochetes have been isolated by a number of researchers from the brains of Alzheimer's patients. Judith Miklossy in Switzerland found spirochetes in the blood, CSF, and brain tissue of 14 Alzheimer's patients. Alan MacDonald has been making this association for some time.

U. **Multiple sclerosis:** MS is the progressive demyelination of the white matter of the brain and spinal cord. Sporadic patches of demyelination cause widely disseminated and diverse neurologic symptoms. One cause is hypothesized to be an insidious infection triggering an autoimmune response, but toxins and allergies have also been implicated. MS is probably multifactorial with both genetic and environmental contributors.

While the age of discovery is usually past the pediatric range, MS often takes a long time to diagnose and the

disease process may have started long before the patient was able to confirm anything was wrong.

Some authors think Lyme can be a direct cause of MS. Whether that is true or not, MS and Lyme should always be on both differential diagnosis lists. They have many factors in common including a nervous system target, a vague and confusing symptom set, a waxing and waning presentation, and minimal diagnostic support from testing. Both are interminably misdiagnosed. Patients in both camps are often told the condition is "all in their heads," which is absolutely true but not in the way these snide HCPs mean.

MS is characterized by exacerbations and remissions of symptoms. When in a flare, MS is a major cause of disability in young adults. Signs and symptoms depend on the extent of demyelination and flares may be brief or last for hours or weeks. The pattern is unpredictable, with symptoms hard to describe.

The first signs of MS may be vision problems including double vision. Sensory impairment includes numbness and tingling (paresthesias) in one or more extremities, trunk, or face. Then comes muscle dysfunction including weakness and clumsiness. Emotional lability, apathy, and lack of judgment are common. We used to describe an MS personality as having a flat, artificial, chronic pseudo-happiness. Often on physical exam, there is CN involvement, abnormal reflexes, optic neuritis, and impaired cutaneous sensation. The ANS can be affected as evidenced by urinary incontinence and other urinary symptoms. (Does sound a lot like some Lyme cases, doesn't it?) Both can display white matter lesions on MRI in conjunction with UMN lesions and encephalopathy.

PEARL: In mid-2012, successful treatment of MS using combination antibiotics for a minimum of one year was reported. The antibiotic suggestions were quite similar to some of those used for Lyme and Chlamydia infections.

V. **Motor neuron lesions:** The motor neuron diseases are a group of neurologic conditions that selectively affect motor neurons, which in turn control the muscle activity involved in speaking, walking, breathing, swallowing, and movement of the skeletal muscles. Skeletal muscle is innervated by a group of neurons called lower motor neurons which project out from the spinal cord to the muscle cells. The LMNs themselves are innervated by upper motor neurons (UMNs) that come from the motor area of the cortex of the brain. By careful physical examination, an HCP can determine whether the UMN or the LMN is the source of the problem. Lyme can present both kinds of lesions. The information gathered can be used as part of the overall diagnostic process.

Every muscle in the body requires both UMNs and LMNs to function and the signs described below can occur in any muscle. While thought to be impacting only the motor neurons, these conditions are often associated with emotional lability and problems with cognitive function, mood, and sensation. Perception of heat and touch can be affected.

UMN lesions: Skeletal muscle is innervated by a group of nerve cells called lower motor neurons. To repeat earlier material, these neurons project out from the spinal cord to the muscle cells. The LMNs themselves are innervated by upper motor neurons (UMNs) that come from the motor area of the cortex of the brain. Lesions in the UMN will lead to increased muscle tone (**hypertonia**) in the extensors of the legs and/or the flexors of the arms. On exam, there will be a clasp knife response where initially the patient resists the motion of the examiner, followed by total relaxation. Clonus describes spasms that alternate between antagonistic muscle groups like the flexors and extensors of a joint. The PE will show spasticity, brisk reflexes, and pathologic reflexes like a positive Babinski. Recall that the Babinski sign is where the big toe raises (extends) rather than curls down (flexes) with stimulation of the sole of the foot. Babinski is definitely abnormal in adults and those over a year old. With UMNs there is NO muscle wasting. Examples of UMN disorders include: MS, stroke, brainstem lesions, cerebral palsy, symptoms from injuries, and symptoms accompanying hydrocephalus.

*PEARL: **Cerebral palsy** is motor impairment due to brain lesions that probably arose early in fetal development. **Hydrocephalus** is the buildup of fluid in the brain either from too much being present or the inability of the fluid to drain. Hydrocephalus can cause a bulging fontanelle and papilledema and the pressure can cause damage to the motor neurons and other parts of the NS.*

LMN lesions: Lower motor neurons emerge from the spinal cord to innervate skeletal muscle cells. A problem with a LMN might affect the nerves traveling from the spinal cord to specific muscles. The signs and symptoms are OPPOSITE to those of an UMN lesion and include flaccid paralysis like that found in Bell's palsy, muscle loss, muscle atrophy, fasciculations, **hypotonia**, and hyporeflexia. There is no Babinski sign. Examples include polio, Guillain-Barré syndrome, muscular dystrophies, and peripheral neuropathies. The flaccid paralysis and fasciculations associated with Lyme would be characterized as LMNs. A characteristic finding in children with gestational Lyme is hypotonia, although the pathophysiologic mechanism is not yet understood.

*PEARL: **Charcot-Marie-Tooth** is a pediatric, progressive, neural-based atrophy of the muscles that are supplied by the peroneal nerves. The muscles atrophy, reflexes are lost, and the muscles become so weak that the foot drops. **Polio** is a viral inflammation of neurons that causes atrophy of muscles. Through vaccination, polio was nearly eradicated from the planet. Due to several paranoid dictators who felt immunization was a plot to overthrow their governments, polio is not quite gone. **Muscular dystrophies** are a group of hereditary diseases that cause progressive muscle weakness.*

PEARL: Lyme disease is known to cause Bell's palsy, a peripheral motor neuron disorder, and perhaps others that are not yet recognized as associated with Bb.

Combined UMN and LMN disorder: While there are a variety of palsies and atrophies that result from motor neuron lesions, the most familiar combined disorder is Lou Gehrig's disease (ALS). This syndrome is almost always diagnosed in middle aged males, but not always. The signs and symptoms of ALS are caused by death to both UMNs and LMNs in the cortex, brainstem, and spinal cord.

Amyotrophic Lateral Sclerosis: ALS or Lou Gehrig's disease is a motor neuron disease that causes muscle atrophy. Usually onset is later in life and the condition is often fatal within 3 to 10 years after diagnosis. Death is due to aspiration or respiratory failure. Genetics is involved in many cases and the pathophysiology is likely an autoimmune reaction. There have been associations with infectious agents. Symptoms include fasciculations, atrophy, and weakness especially in the forearms and hands. There is often impaired speech, chewing, swallowing, and breathing especially if the brainstem is affected. Choking and drooling occur and patients can become depressed or show excessive laughing or crying as other parts of the brain are sclerosed. Lyme is part of the differential diagnosis of ALS, as ALS should be on the differential diagnosis list of Lyme in older teens. There is a small population of kids diagnosed with Juvenile ALS. When examining for TBIs, keep that in mind.

PEARL: In adults, there has been speculation that Bb are a causal agent for ALS. One source noted that 4/54 ALS cases reviewed were also positive for Lyme.

W. **ADD/ADHD**: Attention deficit disorder and attention deficit hyperactivity disorder are common diagnoses in pediatric practices. I come from the generation of parents who were led to believe that half the kids in school had one of these conditions. The label was then used as the excuse for every possible untoward event the child encountered, from bad grades to armed robbery. In fact, one official definition of ADHD is that it is the disorder that prevents a child from achieving his full potential. As a practicing physician, I was often asked to assess kids with ADHD before comprehensive testing was widely available. Many of these kids were just over the line of normal behavior, while others had to be pried off the ceiling before I could start the exam. There is a wide range of behaviors under the ADD/ADHD umbrella and the clinical presentation can vary considerably between individuals. For our purposes, remember that kids with ADD/ADHD get TBIs and TBIs can cause symptoms similar to those seen in ADD/ADHD. Both of these scenarios can make the evaluation more difficult.

ADD: This syndrome is characterized by inattention, distractability, disorganization, procrastination, and forgetfulness. There is little or no hyperactivity or impulsivity. Signs and symptoms can include: anxiety, little cognitive vigor, slow thinking, daydreaming, procrastination, confusion, weak memory, short attention span, distractibility, low energy, loss of focus, wandering thoughts, restlessness due to anxiety, inability to relax, shyness, withdrawal, and immaturity. The person may appear to be not listening, but this is probably because he is not processing the information. Often he doesn't express emotions because of anxiety and fear of disapproval. ADD kids can have poor time management and are often late. While they can delay gratification, they will try too long at a task and get frustrated. They want to succeed but can get overwhelmed. Concrete thinkers, they will try until they burnout. ADD students process information slowly, but once they understand, they are able to use the material. They are poor readers and spellers and have trouble with math. Still, they want to please. They make poor criminals because they think slowly and can't get away in time or come up with a good excuse for bad behavior. They understand the consequences of their behavior, but may self-medicate with alcohol or marijuana to reduce anxiety. Just as with all these syndromes, ADD can present within a broad range of behaviors.

ADHD: Neurobehavioral condition characterized by inattention, hyperactivity, and impulsiveness, These patients can have deficits of serotonin, dopamine, and norepinephrine. ADHD causes problems with attention, impulse control, hyperactivity, and lack of awareness of the consequences of actions. ADHD patients have poor sustained effort because they cannot maintain focus. They race from task to task, are easily bored, lose things, need external motivation to stay on task, are restless due to motor activity being in overdrive, and crave excitement and stimulation. People with ADHD are often egocentric, don't care how well

they connect, can be rejected by others because of inappropriate behavior, are intolerant, often misjudge the time needed to complete a task, are frequently frustrated, need instant gratification, and are not tolerant of any obstruction, leading to irritability, anger, and aggression. They are not team players and may have learning disabilities like dyslexia. These patients miss information and don't learn from mistakes. They comprehend information but then can't use it. They impulsively lie. In contrast to ADD individuals, they make great criminals and there are a disproportionate number of ADHD people in prison. While it's hard for them to stay in school and keep a job, they don't fully grasp the repercussions of bad behavior. They may do many things to excess such as talk, spend, gamble, lose their temper, continuously move, and eat. Their drug of choice can be cocaine. They have no internal STOP signal, no guilt, and no remorse.

PEARL: The first sxs of ADHD usually appear between the ages of 3 and 6-years-old. Diagnosis can be delayed because almost every kid seems to be hyper sometimes and we all have trouble paying attention occasionally. (Perhaps in the middle of a hundred page chapter in a textbook on TBIs.) Sometimes vision and hearing problems mask ADHD. Once a kid starts talking non-stop and it's annoying, not cute, and can't follow any directions, put your antennae up. These kids get bored easily and rarely complete a task. They can't sit still even to watch a favorite TV show. Impulse control will be a problem but all kids have trouble controlling impulses sometimes. The key is how often these behaviors manifest. Is she ever able to control an impulse? Can she ever wait her turn? Does anyone ever get to finish a sentence when this child is around? Remember children with ADHD grow into adults with ADHD. Society is just beginning to realize this.

X. Reye's syndrome: Reye's is an acute childhood illness that damages many systems including the kidneys and heart and causes an incapacitating encephalopathy with increased ICP. Reye's syndrome has been associated with aspirin use in kids and has a very high mortality rate even with treatment. Death is due to cerebral edema and those who survive often have residual brain damage. Aspirin's association with Reye's syndrome is the reason it is no longer recommended in children.

Y. Guillain-Barré syndrome: An LMN deficit, GBS is an acute infectious polyneuritis that can progress rapidly to a potentially fatal muscle weakness with distal sensory loss. GBS can persist into a chronic phase. About half the patients have a history of a prior febrile illness. GBS may be a cell-mediated immune response where the immune system attacks the peripheral nerves in autoimmune fashion. GBS causes inflammation of both sensory and motor nerve roots. Usually signs of the precipitating infection are gone by the time the neurologic manifestations present. Muscle weakness starts in the legs and progresses upward. In severe cases patients have had to be placed on a ventilator because respiratory muscles were too weak to breathe. Some patients with Lyme have presented with a GBS-type picture with weakness moving up the body and increased white cells in the CSF.

Z. Myasthenia gravis: This disease manifests as a sporadic but progressive weakness with intense fatigue of the skeletal muscles that is exacerbated by exercise and repetitive movements. The pathologic mechanism is a failure to transmit nerve impulses at the neuromuscular junction involving acetylcholine. Myasthenia gravis usually affects muscles innervated by the cranial nerves such as the face, lips, and tongue and can be mistaken for Bell's palsy. MG has an unpredictable course that can wax and wane.

AA. Sensory hypersensitivity: A number of Lyme patients complain of hypersensitivity to one or more senses including light, smell, sound, or touch. Some need to be in a darkened room because even minimal light is too intense. Others want no sound and even soft music is overwhelming. Some cannot stand any clothing touching, even the softest cloth. When I had Lyme, a smell of cedar trees which was pleasant to my co-workers nauseated me. Some patients need sunglasses during the day, even indoors. Kids with Lyme often experience excessive sensitivity to any of the senses. There are several hypotheses attempting to explain why this might be so. Bb may cause direct harm to cranial nerves thereby impeding normal function or for a number of reasons may interfere with normal sensory processing.

PEARL: About 80% of all sensory input comes from the eyes.

AB. Processing difficulty: Processing is the formation of associations that enable one to interpret large amounts of information, make sense of the input, and respond in an appropriate way. Many of the neuropsychiatric complaints associated with Lyme may be processing problems. Countless amounts of information enter the NS each moment from the various senses and monitoring systems. The brain must sort and integrate all this data and then respond. If the circuits get overloaded, the person just can't effectively process or manage all the input. The response to this excess stimulation can range from numbness to hypersensitivity. The system either shuts down or tries to integrate all the input. **Sensory integration defect** (SID) is a term used to describe the situation where the individual cannot handle all the sensory data that is gathered. She might then react with either too much or too little response to the overwhelming input. Therefore, the patient can suf-

fer a range of sxs from dullness to intense perception of the involved sense. Symptoms of processing problems might include:

- Hyper-awareness of noise, light, or touch. Some patients respond with attempts to DECREASE the input by asking for dim lights, no clothes, or barely audible music. Others prefer to INCREASE the stimulation, asking for firmer and longer hugs in order to help them process the clearer, more consistent input. The person may either over or under touch.

- Abnormal perception of pain or temperature

- Avoidance of physical contact

- Aversion to certain textures

- Deflection of any stimulation of hands, face, or feet

- Strong antipathy toward grooming such as hair brushing, washing, or teeth cleaning

- Either avoidance of all clothing on skin or insistence on covering all skin. May frequently adjust clothes

- Coordination problems

- Abnormal activity levels

- Fear of heights or discomfort with personal space

- Striking out

- Additional manifestations of what appear to be processing problems include hand flapping, repetitive movements, obsessive spinning of items, or walking on tiptoe

Notice that autism, ADD, and Lyme can share several of these manifestations. We do not know enough about the involved circuitry to know which sxs might belong predominantly to which syndrome. Of course, if more than one condition is involved with disruption of sensory processing, a real diagnostic and management challenge is in the offing. In all cases, the ability to sort and integrate information will have a lot to do with how well the child is able to communicate and learn. If you can't efficiently process sensory input, you are going to be at a real disadvantage during social interactions and in learning situations. While it is too early for us to put all this in perspective, be aware that some Lyme patients may be unable to process information normally.

PEARL: Hyperacusis or hypersensitivity to sound is common in newborns with Bb.

PEARL: Hypersensitivity is one of the most common complaints of TBI patients. Many want nothing to touch their skin and can't tolerate even a light bed sheet. They can become housebound because they don't want to wear shoes and socks because they can't stand the sensation. Remember, the NS is a prime target of Lyme, Bartonella, and M. fermentans. Much of what TBI patients tell us and what we find on exam could be due to Lyme and its co-conspirators and their effects on the nervous system.

PEARL: As with all recently recognized syndromes, SID has other labels including multiple sensory disintegration and sensory processing disorder.

AC. Seizures: A seizure is a paroxysmal event associated with abnormal electrical discharges of neurons. An alteration in brain signals due to electrical instability triggers a seizure in a person once the signal goes beyond the individual's seizure threshold. The presentation of the seizure depends on the size of the stimulus and the location of the abnormal event. Isolated seizures do not necessarily mean epilepsy. A person can seize for any number of reasons including alcohol withdrawal, toxins, some drugs, tumors, infarcts, metabolic problems like hypoglycemia, trauma, hypoxia, infections, and fevers. Encephalitis, meningitis, and brain abscesses can all be associated with seizures.

Epilepsy is diagnosed when there are recurring seizures in some pattern, usually supported by an abnormal EEG. Seizures might last for seconds or hours. In some cases the patient will experience an aura, a sensation that the seizure is coming on. This premonition might be due to the beginning of the abnormal electrical discharges within the focal area of the brain. The aura can include unusual smells or tastes, visual disturbances, GI distress, a rising or sinking sensation in the stomach, or a dreamy feeling. Multiple sources say that some dogs can sense an on-coming seizure and some are being trained to perform this service. After a seizure a patient can experience a postictal state where she is confused, dazed, and tired. She will usually not recall the seizure experience at all. Status epilepticus is a continuous episode that can occur with all types of seizures. Chapter 25: *Ancillary Treatments* contains more information on seizures.

When observing a seizure you might see the following variations.

Generalized:

- Grand mal: The patient may cry out due to a rush of air out of the lungs over the vocal cords. The patient then falls and loses consciousness. The body stiffens and the tonic/clonic part of the seizure begins. Skeletal muscles spasm and relax rhyth-

mically, most obviously in the extremities. CPK might be elevated after a seizure because of all the muscle activity. A grand mal seizure may include incontinence and tongue biting. The seizure usually lasts 2 to 5 minutes. In the postictal state, the muscles can be sore and the patient complains of confusion, headache, or weakness.

PEARL: Grand mal seizures have been documented in cases of congenital Lyme but we currently don't know if there is a causal association.

- Petite mal: Absence seizures occur primarily in kids and present with a change in consciousness, blinking, an eye-roll, blank stare, or slight mouth movements. The patient retains her posture throughout the episode. A petit mal seizure only lasts a few seconds but can occur many times a day.

Localized:

- Partial: A partial seizure is a local malfunction with symptoms specific to the area with the dysfunction. A partial seizure may start locally and then move to become generalized.

- Jacksonian: This seizure begins locally and then spreads. There will be jerking and tingling in an extremity. For example, the thumb may begin the process and then the seizure activity spreads to the hand and arm.

- Complex partial: These seizures often begin with an aura or sensation that the seizure is coming on and include psychomotor and temporal lobe seizures.

PEARL: Complex partial seizures have been observed in patients with chronic Lyme. Temporal lobe seizures might be precipitated by Lyme disease.

Febrile seizures can be tonic/clonic, or partial with posturing. In fact, febrile seizures are more often associated with an abrupt *change* in temperature than the actual number on the thermometer. Febrile seizures could potentially occur in any of the TBIs, especially if the temperature cycles high and low.

PEARL: With LD, estimates of associated seizure activity vary widely. A reasonable estimate that comes from Dr. Vijay Thadani at Dartmouth is that about 10% of Lyme patients will have one seizure in their lifetime and 5% will go on to develop a pattern of epilepsy. Therefore, the incidence of seizures in the LD population is about the same as for non-epileptics, but slightly higher for epilepsy compared to the general population.

PEARL: Anecdotally, seizures have been associated with B. henselea. These seizures had not been controlled with anti-seizure medicine but responded to antibiotic therapy.

AD. Fatigue/Apathy: Should fatigue and apathy be listed as problems of the nervous system? I don't know, but I couldn't find a better fit. They are often a significant part of brain fog and other NP manifestations of Lyme and other TBIs. Fatigue can be either mental or physical and usually both systems are tired to the point of exhaustion.

The brain of a healthy person is usually isolated from the potentially caustic effects of the immune response. In contrast, patients with chronic inflammation may have immune cells infiltrating their brains. These cells, in the course of trying to do their job, release a number of powerful chemicals that have been associated with fatigue, tiredness, and a listless feeling, as well as numerous other neuropsychiatric symptoms. In the case of Lyme, the physical presence of the spirochetes and the biochemical assault from the immune humors may both contribute to what the patient experiences.

Often the fatigue associated with Lyme does not respond to rest or traditional therapies like modafinil. Apathy might be improved with bupropion (Wellbutrin), but in all cases the condition is likely to have the best outcome if the underlying infection is addressed.

AE. Sleep problems: Sleep problems are common in TBIs. Chapters 25 and 27 discuss ancillary treatments and supportive measures to address rest and sleep. With Lyme, the patient might lose his normal 24-hour sleep cycle. Here we are talking insomnia and disturbed sleep patterns and not sleep apnea, which can be a co-morbidity but is not usually associated with the TBI. Aside from a sleepy patient, you are unlikely to pick anything up on PE, and routine sleep studies, which are sometimes performed to market CPAP machines, are of little value. Despite the overwhelming fatigue, sleep for Lyme patients is often not refreshing. Poor sleep affects memory.

PEARL: Sleep is critical for recovery and healing.

AF. Memory deficits: Memory problems are a large part of "brain fog." There are many aspects to a solidly-functioning memory such as short-term, long-term, storage, processing, and retrieval. It does no good to put something into memory if it has no way to come back out. Lyme has been implicated in all manner of memory dysfunction. Short-term memory seems to be the first impacted with slow recall and poor retrieval.

AG. Brain fog: Brain fog is an almost universal complaint in Lyme, affecting more than 90%. Unless you have experienced brain fog, it is hard to describe. I experienced brain fog both with Lyme and with a concussion. Although defined as a cognitive dysfunction, to me it felt more like having a heavy, wet blanket draped over my brain. Brain fog is associated with confusion, forgetfulness, and difficulty concentrating. Brain fog has also been linked to menopause, pregnancy, post-operative confusion, fibromyalgia, mood disorders, toxins, ADHD, endocrine problems like thyroid dysfunction and diabetes, concussion, Sjorgren's syndrome, adrenal disease, mold exposure, allergies, some drugs, hypoxia, sleep dysfunction, parasites that target the brain, and heavy metals especially mercury, lead, and copper. Brain fog can also be found in babesiosis, bartonellosis, and M. *fermentans* infection.

Bransfield defines brain fog as a slowness, weakness, and inadequacy of thought processes. There is a limited ability to concentrate and to multitask and initiative can be greatly curtailed. There is little capacity for abstract thinking. Memory is significantly impaired. The person does indeed feel as though she were in a fog, perhaps missing short periods of time where she can't recall what she did. He believes that the broad-based symptom complex around brain fog may be due to toxins such as cytokines contributing to the cognitive dysfunction.

The patient with brain fog complains of mental confusion and lack of mental clarity. She often feels detached from the condition and disoriented. There may be difficulty following conversations. When I drove to the bottom of my little street, I couldn't remember which way to turn to go to the gas station. I had to pull over and think. I had lived here 25 years. I realized I shouldn't be driving and made it back home without hurting anyone.

Glutathione might help brain fog. Memantine (Namenda) may help with processing speed, decrease word misuse, improve word retrieval, and diminish fuzzy thinking, allowing for better comprehension and focus.

Usually the fog is constant and doesn't wax and wane. The fog clears with treatment**.** Brain fog is subjective and there are no physical findings. The person realizes there is something wrong with how he is thinking. Brain fog may be a type of Lyme encephalopathy and is occasionally called "Lyme fog." Bransfield recommends that the existence of brain fog be accepted so that the patient can learn to recognize its effects. Then she can use her areas of strength to compensate for those areas where she is weak.

PEARL: Dr. Bransfield has developed "The Neuropsychiatric Lyme Assessment" available online at http://www.mentalhealthandillness.com.

Chapter 17-O Psychiatric Exam and Pertinent Differential – Detailed chapter contents

Section 17-O

Psychologic Exam and Pertinent Differential

Having discovered an illness, it's not terribly useful to prescribe death as a cure.
George McGovern

PSYCHOLOGIC

TBI patients often present with significant neuropsychiatric signs and symptoms. Sometimes the distinction between neurologic and psychologic symptoms is hard to make. Even some HCPs believe neurologic symptoms are valid, while the psychiatric symptoms would go away if the patient just tried hard enough. As modern medicine gets better at measuring biochemicals and brain waves and more adept at interpreting PET and other scans, the ability to document supportive evidence for psychiatric symptoms will validate patient experience. Maybe we will finally become a society that can stop torturing sick people.

No one knows why some TBIs target nervous tissue in a way that causes so many diverse and intense symptoms. There is much speculation. Perhaps the Bb spirochete does actual physical damage to nerve tissue, just as its syphilitic cousin does. Maybe toxins are to blame. The powerful biochemicals associated with immune response may be at fault. Many individual humoral modulators have been shown to be associated with everything from aggression, to brain fog, to sleep disturbances. Autoimmune mechanisms may be at work. Patients are known to have antineuronal antibodies present with on-going Strep infections and possibly with Lyme and other TBIs as well. Researchers at the University of Oklahoma have demonstrated the association between these specific antibodies and the symptom complex called PANDAS. These antineuronal agents are known for the significant and often severe neuropsychiatric symptoms found with PANDAS. Do antineuronal antibodies have a role in TBI psychiatric presentations? There could be a combination of factors *or* none of these theorized mechanisms may be in play. The causative mechanism may be something we have not yet imagined. There does seem to be a synergistic effect when more than one co-infection is present. Of the TBIs, Lyme, Bartonella, and M. *fermentans* seem the most often implicated in neuropsychiatric presentations.

> PEARL: *In addition to Bb, Bartonella, and Mycoplasma, other co-infections can impact the neuropsychiatric body system including: Borrelia* hermsii, *Rickettsia* rickettsii, *Coxiella* burnetti, *and Francisella* tularensis.

> PEARL: *Symptoms most often associated with PANDAS include a sudden exacerbation of tics, OCD, anxiety,*

panic, hyperactivity, and emotional lability. A number of Lyme patients have been known to fit this pattern and have displayed aggressive, oppositional, and violent behavior. If antineuronal antibodies are responsible for some of this behavior, additional medical research could be life-changing for them.

> PEARL: *Tager's work documents the increased rates of anxiety, mood changes, feelings of ineffectiveness, and behavioral disorders associated with LD. Tager cautions that kids with LD may be misdiagnosed with primary psychiatric conditions when they actually have the NP sxs of an infectious disease. Addressing one without the other may lead to less positive outcomes.*

Denial is the hallmark of many psychiatric conditions. Reinforce to patients that you can best help them if you know their whole story. They will not be in trouble because of anything they tell you. A few teens might think it is clever or funny to "out smart" the HCP by providing answers that they learned on the Internet or by saying what they think the HCP wants to hear. Some minimize their psychiatric symptoms and others are melodramatic and catastrophic. Be prepared for either extreme.

> PEARL: *Hajek et al found a higher prevalence of antibodies to Bb in psychiatric patients than in healthy subjects.*

Reinforce that you have no other agenda other than to help the patient feel better. Tell the person that there is probably nothing he can say that you haven't heard before. You have no intention of judging any of his thoughts or behaviors. While you cannot allow him to continue to hurt himself or others or harm animals or property, there is always a way to come to mutual resolution on these complicated issues. Older kids and teens may want to speak to you privately without a parent present at least for part of the exam. Others are comfortable with caretakers in the room.

> PEARL: *In many cases of TBI-induced psychiatric sxs, treating only the symptoms will be insufficient. The underling infectious agent must be managed as well. Using only psychotropics will usually not resolve the problem. Think in terms of combination treatment with psychotropics PLUS antibiotics.*

This psychiatric evaluation is a subjective assessment of the patient's emotional state. Unlike a thermometer or a BP reading which give concrete numbers, with the psych exam you will need to use clinical judgment based on what you know about the various conditions and how they can be altered and exacerbated by TBIs.

Some HCPs are so uncomfortable with psych evaluations that they not only avoid the topics, but they actively steer away from any mention of psychiatric conditions. I once worked with a doctor who bragged that NONE of his patients were depressed because he was such an exceptional physician that he kept them all happy. When I came on board, ALL my patients were depressed. These were the SAME patients who had routinely seen him. The truth was that he was so uncomfortable with the topic of depression that no one had a chance to broach the subject. These were the same patients, just waiting for an opportunity.

TBI patients may have significant psychiatric manifestations of their disease. Do not skip this part of the exam because you feel uncomfortable. A friend's son with probable Lyme committed suicide and I could have intervened but didn't think it was my place. You are the HCP, it is not only your place, it is your obligation. You do not have to cure the problem; you just have to recognize it. Partner with a psychiatric professional who understands TBIs. With you managing the TBI and your colleague working on the psychiatric aspects, you have a better chance of treatment success. If the psychiatric symptoms are due to a TBI, they are less likely to get well if the TBI is not effectively addressed. As you look over the psychiatric examination parameters listed below, make sure all questions are age appropriate.

There is a large book called the Diagnostic and Statistical Manual of Mental Disorders (DSM) that contains all currently accepted psychiatric diagnoses. The most recent edition is the DSM-IV. The next edition should be the DSM-5, purported to arrive in 2013, where the traditional Roman numerals will be replaced by Arabic numbers. Apparently, you aren't really mentally ill until your diagnosis makes the DSM. The conditions below can be found in the DSM-IV complete with lists of diagnostic criteria. For the purposes of this *Compendium*, I tried to focus on those aspects that could impact the diagnosis and treatment of TBI patients. To find the DSM-details for each condition, type the name of the condition and DSM-IV into your Internet search engine and you will be rewarded. The "official" diagnosis can be important for insurance purposes. What is considered an invalid claim in 2012 might be fully covered in 2013. Most patients can't wait that long.

The next few pages cannot hope to include all possible psychiatric diagnoses that could potentially be associated with TBIs. The list tries to take into account the most common conditions that might be caused, exacerbated, or mistaken for a tick-borne disease and thereby help establish a baseline for comparison over the course of the disease.

Dr. Robert Bransfield has compiled several thousand peer-reviewed references demonstrating the association between infections and mental health sxs. I know because he gave me a stack of them to read for this book. There are more than 200 articles showing association between Lyme or other TBIs and NP sxs. (I did read every one of those. Every one.) Many of the sxs involve problems with cognition or processing, but a number discuss mood problems, anxiety, depression, and aggressive tendencies. Lyme can cause aggression in dogs and other animals. We all have seen its influence in the story of the infamous, attacking Connecticut chimp.

PEARL: Famous author, Amy Tan, for years suffered with depression, anxiety, pain, and strange hallucinations before finally being diagnosed with Lyme. After seeing 11 doctors and spending over $50,000, she was convinced she had lost her mind. She was unable to write and had lost her creativity, struggling to get from word to word. Antibiotics have allowed her to resume her creative life, although she still occasionally flares.

Many of the pertinent conditions listed below overlap and it is difficult to draw a diagnostic line between them. For example, a depressed patient can also be anxious or a person with OCD can have panic attacks. Many are associated with other disease states and are common in Lyme, bartonellosis, and M. *fermentans* infections. Certainly these TBIs, if not the initiating cause of some psychiatric conditions, can at least aggravate them. As one patient with multiple TBIs complained about his new onset panic attacks, "I feel like there is a tidal wave of biochemicals washing over me that I can't control." He's probably right.

Psychiatric conditions that have been associated with TBIs:

A. Mood disorders

A mood is the usual emotion sustained by a patient over time that affects the person's perception of the world. All non-neonatal TBI patients had an emotional baseline prior to the TBI and this baseline might be altered depending on the severity and duration of the illness. A mood disorder is a disturbance of feelings that falls outside what could be considered a normal range. While everyone has variations in mood over time, a mood disorder involves the abnormal mood becoming the predominant characteristic of the personality to the detriment of the patient. Fallon interviewed Lyme patients and found that 84% of those with a positive Lyme test had mood problems. Of those reporting depression, 90% had never experienced mood problems prior to the disease. The most familiar mood disorders include:

1. **Dysphoric disorder** (Dysthymia)

With traditional dysphoria, the depressive symptoms begin subtly in childhood and may remain low-grade for many years. There might be intense feelings of depression, discontent, apathy, and significant unhappiness. The clinical course may be punctuated with periods of major depression. Distinguishing between dysthymia, dysphoria, and depression can be tricky and not clinically helpful. Dysthymia may actually be more of a personality problem since the underlying temperament is gloomy and pessimistic, with no sense of humor or capacity for fun. The patient may be passive, lethargic, skeptical, hypercritical, complaining, self-denigrating, and preoccupied with failure and negativity. (And *then* they get bitten by a tick.)

2. **Depression**

Also called unipolar depression, this abnormal mood includes feelings of sadness, apprehension, and gloom, where the patient takes no pleasure in usually enjoyable experiences such as food, friends, hobbies, or entertainment. The sad feelings occur just about every day and can also include changes in weight or appetite, altered sleep patterns, hopelessness, low energy or motivation, feelings of worthlessness or guilt, difficulty concentrating, and recurrent thoughts of death or a wish to end it all.

Depression is one of the most common psychiatric disorders and is often coupled with anxiety. While it is normal to have occasional situational sadness when something sad happens, depression that persists and that interferes with usual activities is not normal. Unfortunately, depression is quite common in all age groups.

Depression can be episodic. An acute exacerbation of depression may present with sadness, irritability, anxiety, and hopelessness. These patients appear miserable and have poor eye contact. Some show no emotion and appear completely flat. Often they feel their lives have no purpose. Many experience sleep disorders. The majority of completed suicides had expressed feelings of depression prior to the event.

Identification of depression is occurring at younger and younger ages. Whether this is due to better recognition of the sxs or whether more young kids are getting depressed is anyone's guess. Maybe both. Some dysphoric moods are inevitable and it is appropriate for a person to feel sad under sad circumstances. However, when patients become irritable, stop eating, show little energy, have sleep problems, and take no pleasure in anything for more than a few days, something more may be going on.

Decades of epidemiological data has associated depression with a wide variety of other diseases such as endocrine conditions, thyroid problems, DM, collagen vascular diseases like lupus, heart disease, chronic pain, fibromyalgia, many infections, back pain, concussion, cancers, seizures, trauma, MS, stoke, Parkinson's, sleep apnea, malnutrition, anemias, many drugs like steroids, withdrawal from addiction, alcoholism, and dementia. Some literature sources believe that any chronic illness or chronic pain syndrome lasting longer than a few months results in clinical depression. More than a few authors felt that it would be abnormal NOT to be depressed under those circumstances.

By far the most common reason for depression is idiopathic which is the medical term for "Who knows?" In all cases, whether depression is associated with another condition or whether it stands alone, the disorder is hypothesized to be due to an imbalance of neurotransmitting chemicals like serotonin and norepinephrine. However, a 2012 hypothesis suggests that depression may not be due to such an imbalance, but rather stress-related damage to neurons.

Finally, we get back to the physical examination. There are a number of available, validated assessment tools to use in helping make the diagnosis of depression. If depression is suspected, consider the following list of questions to help determine the level of pathology. These questions may need to be adjusted for age, but most elementary school kids will understand the majority of them:

Do you feel sad?

How sad do you feel?

Do you feel sad almost all the time or just when something sad happens?

What makes you happy?

When you feel sad, what do you do to feel better?

What do you plan to do next week?

What are you looking forward to?

What do you plan to be doing next year?

Do you ever think about hurting yourself?

Have you ever cut, burned, or hurt yourself in any way?

Have you ever thought about killing yourself?

Do you ever think that death world be a relief?

Have you ever tried to kill yourself?

How did you plan to do it?

What stopped you?

What would happen if you died?

How do you think your family would feel?

IMPORTANT: If the patient is in any way inclined toward suicide, immediately refer to an appropriate mental health professional. If there is unavoidable delay, get a temporary contract with the patient to do no harm until they reach specific help. Do not allow them to leave your office alone.

If you are a front line HCP, you are probably very comfortable treating depression with a variety of modalities. Recall the new warning on many antidepressants that says that suicidal ideation may be more common in teens using antidepressants. If you are not comfortable treating younger patients with depression, please refer to a specialist. We all have areas of strengths and weaknesses. Know yours and refer when appropriate. See Chapters 25 and 27 for additional treatment guidance.

PEARL: Dr. Bransfield makes an interesting point. Based on discussions with colleagues, he wonders if perhaps the leading cause of death in Bb infections, and some of the other TBIs that so significantly impact the neuropsychiatric system, is suicide.

3. Bipolar disorder or manic depression

In contrast to unipolar depression where sadness is the primary or sole feeling, the emotions in bipolar disorder alternate between highs and lows. The mood swings from euphoria to despair with spontaneous recoveries in between. The episodes are cyclic although in most patients one extreme will dominate. The first signs usually begin in adolescence.

For the most part, the depressed periods present as they do with unipolar depression, although they may be more hypochondriacal and suicidal than the average depressed person. The manic periods are quite different. The patient may be depressed for a few days and then wake up one day excited and refreshed. They are elated and often talking non-stop about grand plans. Behavior may be inappropriate and risky. One patient I saw took her corporate credit card and bought thousands of dollars worth of Laura Ashley sheets. As in many cases, she became irritable and hostile when her manager tried to interfere with her redecorating plans. Manic people can be flamboyant and ostentatious and full of themselves. As I learned the hard way,

you cannot reason with them. They seem to have limitless energy and accelerated activity levels, as though they were in fast forward mode. They can't shut down.

Manics tend to love life when they are manic and have no desire to return to a situation where depression is a risk. They think they no longer need their medicine. People around them become exasperated. They can be exhausting to deal with. They lose their inhibitions and may become tactless and make inappropriate sexual overtures. They don't think they need sleep and truly believe they have the answer to all life's problems if only others had the sense to listen. Lyme patients have presented with such significant mood swings that it was mistaken for bipolarity.

B. Suicidal behaviors

While the majority of people with suicidal behaviors have pre-existing depression, some do not. Never lightly dismiss any suicidal ideation or behavior. Those at most risk are patients with long-term depression, chronic illnesses, or drug or alcohol problems. Red flags include previous suicide attempts, well-thought-out plans, or actions that show a determined mind-set like buying a gun or giving away possessions. The harder they have tried to conceal their plan when they are discovered, the greater the risk. Some patients seem to have no clear plan but repeatedly engage in "death wish" type behaviors like drag racing and mixing dangerous drug combinations. Recently there has been an alarming increase in suicidal behaviors in teens and even younger kids. While girls think of suicide more often, boys are more successful at committing suicide. The victim feels isolated and incorrectly believes there is no one she can turn to. Life is not worth living and problems are insurmountable. They choose a long-term solution for a short-term problem.

To repeat: If the patient is in any way inclined toward suicide, immediately refer to an appropriate mental health professional. If there is unavoidable delay, get a temporary contract with the patient to do no harm until they reach specific help. Do **NOT** allow them to leave your office alone.

Be aware of suicidal blackmail. "If you don't do what I say, I will kill myself." I have a particular antipathy for this type of manipulation and I have suggested the following response with considerable success: "I cannot give you drug money (or your own car or a tattoo or Prada shoes), but neither can I allow you to hurt yourself. I will have to call the police now to help me deal with this." (GASP! Many parents cannot even imagine calling the police on their own child. Sadly, in out-of-control situations sometimes it's the only reasonable thing to do.)

C. Anxiety/GAD/Stress

Anxiety is an excessive feeling of nervousness, apprehension, uncertainty, worry, or fear. The feeling can be mild or paralyzing. The duration can be acute, intermittent, or chronic. A patient can worry about only one thing like a particular friend or upcoming event, or she can worry about everything as is often the case with general anxiety disorder.

Initially the person may feel mild tension and nervousness. The symptoms can increase to a moderate level and then become severe to the point of panic, which can last a few minutes to an hour. Chronic anxiety persists for long periods and can impact AODL.

Repeated studies have shown that anxiety is associated with chemical changes in the body, especially in levels of cortisol and epinephrine. We don't always know which came first, the anxiety or the chemical change. A number of the immune-modulating chemicals have also been linked with increased anxiety levels. Either way, there can be considerable end-organ damage connected with persistent stress especially involving the cardiovascular system.

PEARL: Anxious patients may present with shaking or tremulousness, which is not the same as fasciculations. This is anxiety-related and can be severe.

Whether a TBI is the cause or the aggravator of the feeling of anxiety, it is likely that the persistent anxiety increases inflammatory changes and delays healing. While there are numerous articles about "good stress being motivating," in the case of TBIs it is probably prudent to keep things as calm as reasonable. We will want to modulate the effects of stress and provide coping mechanisms. This will allow the best chance for recovery.

People with anxious personalities tend to lack confidence and have a hard time making a decision. Too many options can overwhelm them. Shyness might limit social interactions. Emotions are contagious. An anxious HCP will make the caregivers nervous, making the patient nervous.

With general anxiety disorder, the patients are always anxious about everything and never relax. They are always in an unpleasant and uncomfortable state. They worry about reasonable things and unreasonable things. My mother used to worry about how the astronauts chewed their food. Not just wondered about it, she worried about it.

Although GAD can begin anytime, initial sxs often begin early on in childhood. Normally, kids will have three phases of extraordinary anxiety: 8 months, 2 years, and 5 years. These are parts of the typical milestone maturation process as they learn to get along in the world. In contrast, overly anxious kids might not be able to leave their parents because they fear for their own or their loved one's safety. They need reassurance and continuously ask, "What if this happens? What if that happens?"

GAD manifests as excessive, chronic, usually daily anxiety and is a condition that can last for months or years. General anxiety can start in young kids and be careful of the child they refer to as "the little mother." She's probably driving her siblings crazy. Some anxious patients believe that worry somehow inoculates them from harm and that sufficient worry will protect the people they are concerned about. To them, worry means you care. People with GAD worry most when they run out of things to worry about. Chronic or incapacitating worry needs to be addressed.

PEARL: The chronic stress that often accompanies TBIs can impede recovery.

PEARL: While teens often say they smoke cigarettes because it calms them down, the anxiety level of the smoker actually increases over time. The baseline anxiety level intensifies so that more and more cigarettes are needed to keep the smoker feeling normal. Addiction is part of the smoking cycle and smokers become extremely anxious if their next cigarette is delayed.

PEARL: Separation anxiety can be intense and incapacitating in some kids with TBIs.

D. PMS/ PMDD

Premenstrual syndrome consists of a wide range of symptoms that occur a few days prior to menses and usually stop at the onset of bleeding. PMS may be due to changes in hormones and we know Lyme can affect hormone balance. PMS might include physical, behavioral, and emotional signs and symptoms: bloating, cramping, breast tenderness, changes in bowels, altered eating habits with cravings, less tolerance for noise or light, mood swings, difficulty concentrating, annoyance, fatigue, anxiety, edginess, forgetfulness, irritability, hostility, anger, poor judgment, sluggishness, and lethargy.

PMDD or premenstrual dysphoric disorder can cause severe depression, irritability, and tension prior to menses. PMDD is considered more severe and potentially disabling than PMS.

E. Obsessive-Compulsive Disorder

OCD is characterized by recurrent thoughts (obsessions) and subsequent behaviors (compulsions) over which the patient gradually has less and less control. Obsessions are intrusive and repetitive thoughts, feelings, impulses, or urges. The patient may repeat unhappy thoughts or experiences over and over in his mind (ruminations) even when doing so does not make him feel better. Compulsions are irresistible actions that are usually repetitive. Once a patient acts on an obsession it becomes a compulsion. The performance of the compulsion is done to relieve the anxiety caused by the obsession. Maybe, if I check the door lock just one more time I can stop worrying that the dog will get out and get lost. Maybe, if I check just one more time.

To assess for possible OCD ask:

> Do you have thoughts that return over and over in your mind? Do you worry a lot about your brother getting lost or a pet getting hurt?

> Do you worry about germs?

> What things do you worry about?

> Do you do certain things over and over like washing your hands or checking to make sure the door is locked?

> Do you need constant reassurance that you're doing the right thing?

Usually the older OCD patient recognizes that the thoughts and actions are abnormal and unhealthy but cannot control them. They just keep coming. OCD can develop as early as middle school in both males and females. The OCD patient might try to talk himself out of the irrational thoughts but reasoning and logic do not penetrate. The underlying fears are unrealistic, but biochemistry is very powerful.

Uncertainty feeds OCDs. The harder the person tries to answer the unanswerable, the more obsessed he becomes. Nothing is ever guaranteed and yet OCD patients demand certainty. Counselors often encourage these patients to embrace uncertainty rather than continually fight against it.

PEARL: With any of the psychological conditions, sometimes it's difficult to tell what was pre-existing, what is solely caused by the TBI, and what is compounded by the presence of the infection. Probably there is some kind of genetic predisposition for some of these NP sxs. Consider

that the pathogen might be contributing in some fashion. Don't expect all things to be clear. Still it is truly unfortunate if the underlying exacerbator is an infection that is not addressed.

OCD patients often have underlying rigid and immature traits. They tend to have low stress tolerance, poor insight, and have trouble making decisions. On the other hand, they are likely to be conscientious and have high aspirations. They take responsibility seriously. With limited creativity, they can have difficulty finding alternative solutions to problems and tend to be perfectionists who can be morally judgmental. Most are nervous, tense, and apprehensive. Their thoughts and behaviors can be annoying to themselves and others and they may need constant reassurance. OCD can be a part of a continuum that includes anxiety and panic and all may interfere with normal functioning.

Usually the OCD patient will do whatever he thinks might relieve the anxiety caused by the obsessive thoughts. Most often, relief is sought through the performance of the compulsive behavior, usually over and over again. If the obsession is that the person might get sick from germs, then the compulsion might be to wash the hands every 24 minutes or exactly 12 times for 30 seconds each time. Unfortunately, the action does not relieve the anxiety caused by the obsession.

Early on in the clinical course, the patient might be able to force himself to control his preoccupations. Then a trivial incident might trigger the onset of compulsive behavior that then persists. OCD can evolve to phobias about germs and required rituals might be needed before the individual can go outside or drive a car. Some OCD patients over-analyze to the point of incapacity. They may need perpetual affirmations from others to convince themselves they are doing the right thing.

The median age of onset for OCD is around 19, but now in retrospect many patients realize that sxs began much earlier. In fact, rituals and ceremonies are common and within normal boundaries in young kids. There is a difference in being neat and tidy and being compulsive. Sometimes it's hard to draw the line, but when pathologic behaviors begin to interfere with real life, this signals a problem that needs to be explored.

Traditional OCD develops slowly. This is in distinct contrast to the OCD that is associated with PANDAS which has a sudden onset of OCD-like symptoms. I spent a disproportionate amount of time in this section on OCDs because I think there might be a common mechanism between PANDAS and some of the neuropsychiatric conditions associated with TBIs. If you don't know about the possibility, you might not make the connection when it is present. (I also spent an inordinate amount of time trying to figure out if there was a hyphen or not in manic depression and obsessive-compulsive. I became my own example.)

PEARL: OCD has been associated with a number of infections: Strep, Japanese B encephalitis, HSV-1, EBV, Mycoplasma, the virus responsible for the influenza of 1918, Coxsackie viruses, and now likely Bb, Bartonella, and M. fermentans.

PEARL: OCD, especially in the context of PANDAS, can be very hard for caretakers and other by-standers to assimilate. Even many HCPs do not understand why a child should choose to act this way. Well, it's not a choice, it's a biochemical maelstrom. Those who easily dismiss these thoughts and behaviors as controllable must never have experienced or witnessed an infection-induced, biochemical, neuropsychiatric complication. Biochemistry is extremely powerful and willpower cannot overcome chemistry. No matter how hard the patient tries and how much they want to feel better, they cannot force the chemicals to recede. This fact is especially true if an on-going infection is continuing to spur the problem along. Fortunately, treating the underlying infection can help. In the meantime, counselors can teach techniques to deal with the symptoms. The best therapeutic approach may be to concomitantly treat the persistent pathogen, along with the presenting symptoms.

F. Panic Attacks

A panic attack is a time of intense fear or apprehension that may be accompanied by palpitations, sweating, trembling or shaking, a feeling of shortness of breath, smothering, or choking, chest discomfort, flushing, GI discomfort, dizziness, numbness or tingling, unsteadiness, detachment from the feeling, loss of control, and the fear of going crazy or dying. The patient may have a sense of imminent danger or doom and an overwhelming urge to escape. The attack is sudden with a peak in about 10 minutes.

As an ER doc for many years, I know that the acute episode of panic is usually gone by the time the patient reaches the ER. If you have never experienced or witnessed a panic attack, do not be too quick to dismiss these episodes. Clearly, panic attacks are a biochemical phenomenon likely attributable to a rush of epinephrine. Epinephrine, or adrenaline, is the "fight or flight" hormone, but in panic attacks it can be hard to tell which came first, the stimulus for the attack or the biochemical flood.

Panic attacks are common and may begin in childhood or the teen years. Usually the onset is sudden and the surprise aspect of the attack can be one of its most unsettling components. Some people have triggers like flying, heights, public speaking, or a stressful event that seems to bring on the attack. Others can be minding their routine business and be accosted by a hormonal deluge. Some say they barely had time to pull off the road before they were overwhelmed. Patients can live in fear of the next attack.

Willpower will not avert an attack and most CBT therapists counsel the patient to accept that the panic is coming and that it will be all over in a few minutes and in that spirit say, "Hit me with your best shot." They teach patients how to ride out the biochemical onslaught. Other HCPs feel that taking an anxiolytic at the first hint of an attack might help avert a crisis. Many patients are exhausted after a panic attack, almost like a mild postictal state.

PEARL: The majority of Lyme patients and those infected with Bartonella and M. fermentans experience some degree of neuropsychiatric symptoms along with their TBI diagnosis. This includes episodes of panic in some cases. CBT can be life-changing for these patients. As they learn coping strategies, the TBI should be addressed concurrently. Some authors think that an anxiolytic like Xanax taken at the first inkling of a panic attack might help stem the tide. Others believe that benzodiazepines are counterproductive. It doesn't hurt to see what works for the individual patient. They may just need to know that a rescue medicine is available if needed.

G. Thought disorders

Not exactly a separate diagnosis, disorganized and irrational thought processes are usually part of other morbidities. Nevertheless, the HCP needs to be tuned into the thought processes of the TBI patient. Clearly, a person with a 104 fever might have altered consciousness and delirium and will not be especially cogent. Nevertheless, in chronic patients, pay careful attention to the logic flow. You will be able to ascertain the level of coherent thought as you talk to the patient about her history and symptoms. If something is just "not right" pursue your instincts until you get a better handle on what is going on.

With certain TBIs, the patients might complain of the sensation that they are going crazy or losing their minds. This feeling can be bad in Lyme and even worse with Bartonella or M. *fermentans.*

H. Psychosis

Psychoses are a group of diseases where the patient withdraws into herself and fails to distinguish reality from fantasy. Symptoms can start as early as age 12, but the first episode can occur anytime throughout the teen years and into early adulthood. There is a significant personality change with unusual emotional responses.

Psychoses are chronic conditions that handicap the patient in social interactions, in school, and at work. A disproportionate number of homeless people have some degree of psychosis. In these conditions, the thoughts are disorganized and the individual pursues extreme withdrawal into his own fantasy world. Behavior is often bizarre and inappropriate in ways that make sense only to that person.

The first signs of psychosis may be a strange pattern of fatigue, insomnia, and headache. In schizophrenia the person loses interest in real life. Ideas or objects may have special reference only to him. The individual is confused and agitated, with no capacity for abstract thought. They become very literal and very concrete. They may have distorted vision and auditory senses with a flat affect and low motivation. Hallucinations are common in some cases, with the patient seeing, hearing, or sensing things that aren't real. The patient may be plagued by delusions which are false beliefs that are not supported by reality. He might think the radio is talking to him or the government is trying to control him. Delusions seem to focus on sex, politics, and religion. Government and church conspiracies are common themes. Voices may tell the patient to make abrupt, life-changing decisions. There is a feeling that life has changed and no longer seems real, like watching yourself on TV. I remember a case that still haunts me from 30 years ago when I was on rotation in a psychiatric hospital. A woman came up to me heartbroken and crying. She was absolutely devastated. When asked the problem, she said, "I just killed the Virgin Mary." This was completely real to her.

Paranoid schizophrenics are extremely delusional with scattered irrational thoughts of persecution and conspiracies. They hear voices telling them what to think and do and they believe that life is outside their control. Paranoid schizophrenics believe that others are running the show and they are just watching. These are extremely sad cases.

No one knows the effect of TBIs on psychoses. Some TBI patients suffer with incapacitating delusions. Whether these delusions were somehow affected by TBIs is unknown. If there is an association, perhaps by treating the TBI, the delusions will see some improvement. No one knows.

I. Paranoia

The paranoia referred to here is not the same as the paranoid schizophrenia referred to previously. This is more of a paranoid personality type. Although these people have a distorted view of reality, they do not live in a complete fantasy world. We interact with these folks every day.

A paranoid personality believes that no one likes him or that everyone is talking about him. Usually these are cold and distant personalities who are controlling and morbidly jealous. They believe that others are working against them. They can be suspicious and resentful. They resist change and demand justice with righteous indignation. They can react with hostility and anger and rarely see their role in a bad situation. Often they overblow their own importance and influence. This personality type is not common in kids. It takes years to get this nasty.

J. Aggression/Anger/Violence/ODD/Acting out

Some TBI patients have a volatile and aggressive component to their disease. In the realm of TBI co-infections, Bb, Bartonella, and M. *fermentans* all seem to potentiate aggressive behaviors. If you see rage, think Bartonella. Whether these patients had an underlying predisposition for aggression, or the TBI started that ball rolling will not be known anytime soon.

A young man went out-of-control and killed himself and others. His family said he had become aggressive and violent after contracting Lyme disease. The young man had begged the medical community for help. Why provide help when there was nothing wrong that a short-course of doxy wouldn't clear right up? An IDSA member said that it was not possible for Lyme to cause aggressive behavior. Of course, a short time earlier, a chimp went on a rampage attacking a woman in CT in a very well-known case. The veterinary community quickly explained the chimp's behavior by saying that the animal's Lyme disease had likely contributed to his aggression.

Although some patients will deny the obvious, others are proud of their aggression. Some questions to help assess the aggression potential:

Have you ever been in a physical fight? With siblings? With others?

Has anyone ever physically abused you?

Are you a bully? Are you being bullied?

Do you have trouble controlling yourself?

Do you have trouble managing your anger?

What makes you want to hurt someone?

Have you ever mistreated an animal or pet?

In what situations do you think violence might be the best way to solve things?

Do you own any weapons?

Have you ever hit a boyfriend or girlfriend?

Have you felt more angry or violent since you got sick?

If anything sets you off, what would it be?

Do you ever feel you cannot control your temper or that you might hurt someone else?

Some terms to help clarify aggressive behavior:

- Acting out: Behaving on impulse in antisocial ways including, drinking, doing drugs, shoplifting, behaving promiscuously, and throwing tantrums. Acting out may be a way to get attention but the behaviors are damaging to the person, others, animals, or property. Acting out helps express feelings that might be better expressed in more constructive ways.

- Aggression: Ready to attack or confront, often without provocation

- Assault: Intentional physical attack

- Violence: Inflicting physical injury

- ODD: **Oppositional defiant disorder** is an ongoing pattern of disobedient, hostile, or defiant behavior, with a total disregard for authority. The individual appears stubborn and angry. The anger is excessive and persistent manifesting with temper tantrums, angry outbursts, and the desire to annoy others on purpose. Patients with ODD often blame somebody else for their problems and are easily annoyed. They are rigid, resentful, and seeking revenge. Their behavior causes distress to others and interferes with academics and social relationships. Pete Rose attributes his problems with gambling and exclusion from the Baseball Hall of Fame to ODD.

PEARL: Drugs tried as mood stabilizers include SSRIs, other kinds of antidepressants, anti-convulsants, and atypical antipsychotics. Lithium has been shown to decrease aggression and other NP sxs. However, in all these cases if the underlying cause is an on-going TBI infection, you are not likely to get far in treatment unless the infection is adequately addressed.

The term "Lyme rage" has been used to refer to the intense anger that has been associated with some cases of borreliosis. A number of patients have been surprised by episodes of road rage they had not experienced previously. Several authors have suggested that Bb can rewire the human brain causing behaviors that would normally be unknown to the patient. Dr. Bransfield has found a connection between LD and aggression in a small but significant group of patients. Antibiotic treatment decreased symptoms. Most Lyme patients are not violent but a small percentage develops a neuropsychological dysfunction that increases the risk of aggressiveness. At the same time, they may have a decreased tolerance for frustration, irritability, depression, and cognitive impairment. Sounds like a bad combination and a recipe for disaster. There are several cases when aggression and violence could be linked to the underlying infectious TBD. In most of these cases, we do not know if Lyme was the sole instigator or co-infections such as Bartonella and/or M. *fermentans* could have played a role. Aggression, when related to an underlying TBI infection, can respond to appropriate antibiotics.

K. Personality disorders

Personality disorders are difficult to handle. These people think no one likes them and they're right. When I was a medical student I was told that when you review your schedule for the day, any patient that you'd rather get mauled by Dobermans than see, had a personality disorder. People with personality disorders are inflexible, irritating, and annoying. They are outside the norm for the cultural standards and this causes distress in others who go out of their way to avoid them. I have worked in clinics where doctors would fight over who had to see the personality disorder patient. These patients may not respond to emotional stimuli and cues in the same way as other people.

There are many kinds of personality disorders. Here are the ones most likely to be seen in a TBI practice:

Borderline personality: These patients have an unstable self-image and they believe they were deprived in childhood and feel empty, angry, and entitled. They may be relentless seekers of care. This is a common disorder and can begin evolving in childhood.

Antisocial personality: These are the infamous psychopaths and sociopaths touted by the media. These people ignore the feelings of others and are callous and exploitative. Recent theories have claimed that the majority of CEOs of large companies are psychopaths. This comes as no surprise to people who have worked in large companies. The terms psychopath and sociopath are hard to differentiate. Both have a complete disregard for the welfare of others, no remorse over bad actions, a dismissive attitude around rules and morals, and a tendency toward violence and emotional outbursts. Antisocial personalities are known for messing up other people's lives while playing the victim themselves. Psychopaths are thought to be more genetically determined. They are considered better organized than sociopaths and better able to imitate normal behavior. They can be charming and manipulative and easily get others to trust them. They walk among us and are often our bosses. Sociopaths have more of a social influence on their behavior such as extreme poverty or criminals in their upbringing. Psychopaths are the sociopaths of privilege.

Impulsive and reckless, antisocial types see nothing wrong with their ruthless behavior. Rules are for the little people and do not apply to them. These patterns start in childhood and are often identified ten years later in the courtroom. About 10% are thought to be identified by the criminal justice system. (So they end up in jail, in the board room, in politics, or as the former head of the IMF.) More are identified in the courtroom than in the clinic. Most are never diagnosed. Their need for instant gratification and their ruthless disregard for the well-being of others often lead them to become quite successful. I remember my boss from the subcontinent pounding the table and spitting, "I WANT PROFITS NOW!" This guy was one of the richest people in his country at the time and quite the psychopath. Superficially charming, intelligent, and completely self-centered, he was unable to tolerate any frustration. Antisocial personalities are capable of violence. This same business wizard hired thugs to beat up his mom and brother because they questioned some trivial business deal. When this incident was all over his nation's news, he was most upset that the camera did not capture his good side. Amoral, irresponsible, bullying, and defiant, these antisocial people do not express normal emotions and are often proud of their cruelty to animals and to people beneath them on the social ladder.

Narcissistic personality: This subset thinks they are superior and attempt to exploit others because they feel entitled to do so. Impulsive and irresponsible, they do not handle frustration well and do not anticipate the consequences of bad choices.

Passive-aggressive personality: Passive-aggressive traits are very common and everyone engages in passive-aggressive behavior from time to time. To avoid normal expressions of emotion in conflict situations, these individuals will appear inert or passive. The submissive charades are designed to control, manipulate, and avoid responsibility. The individual may agree to do something she has no intention of doing. Then through procrastination, inefficiency, sabotage, or unrealistic protests of disability or ineptness, she avoids completion of the task. Much of this

behavior conceals frank hostility, which these personality types otherwise cannot handle. This is their way of coping. Passive-aggressives will avoid confrontation, yet still endeavor to get the outcome they wanted in the first place. Since they do not manage negative emotional situations well, they will cover those feeling with passivity and acquiescence. This annoys others since the actions are often fairly obvious and would be easier to accept if the passive-aggressive person would just be open about what she wanted.

L. Self-harm/cutting/self-aggression

Unfortunately, self-harm has become relatively common in the high school and college age population. Cutting, which was virtually unheard of when I was in college, is now being reported in grade school. Cutting seems to come from various motivations. In recent cases, one teen Lyme patient cut herself because she felt numb and wanted to feel something again. Another, an Asperger's male, cut himself on the arms and chest so he could display similar scars to those he saw on a character in a videogame. Some cutters believe they have no other emotional outlet, cutting to express their feelings and vent. One psychologist thinks that cutting is more common in Lyme patients than in the general population, but I found no evidence other than the I&P of cutting is increasing across all young age groups. If you have a patient who is cutting, they are saying something but the message may not always be clear.

Self-harm can occur out of a desire to punish oneself or from self-hatred. While many of the harmful behaviors are active, others are passive-aggressive in that the person will act out in ways that have a high risk of causing harm. Impulsive and reckless behaviors like drunken driving, drag racing, promiscuity, sexual asphyxiation, smoking, and substance abuse are common in these individuals. The more aggressive persons may also be antisocial and oppositional. In the two cases mentioned, both cutters were quite gentle, shy, super-intelligent, and passive personalities.

In the November 21, 2011, issue of *People* magazine, Darrell Hammond disclosed that cutting was his way of creating a crisis that was manageable. Living with Lyme can certainly feel unmanageable at times. Cutters can cause physical pain to distract themselves from their emotional pain. For them, cutting decreases anxiety.

M. Hypochondriasis

A hypochondriac may complain to get attention or he may be a narcissist who genuinely thinks his every hiccup is a stroke and each pimple is terminal cancer.

Young kids are rarely hypochondriacal. In general, what they tell you is real. As they get older, they may learn that some behaviors get more attention than others. Nevertheless, in all the TBI kids I saw in preceptorships, I did not observe one child that I thought was hypochondriacal.

Hypochondriacs are preoccupied with their bodily functions and health and fear acquiring disease. No matter how much reassurance they are given they cannot believe they are not about to succumb to a rare and deadly malady. They often misinterpret physical findings. Nevertheless, they are suffering, it just isn't for the reason they think.

In adults, hypochondriasis is somewhat common especially with the media "educating" patients hourly on what could be wrong this time. These are the patients who insist on the antibiotics for their cold and then think the diarrhea they get from the antibiotics means they have colon cancer. These patients have trouble managing anxiety and they account for a large number of visits to PCPs. In our litigious society, we prescribe the antibiotic and order the MRIs even when we think they are not indicated. God bless us, everyone.

N. Eating disorders

Eating disorders are reaching epidemic proportions. A surprising number of five-year-olds admit to having been on a diet. The majority of teen girls say they would rather be dead than be ten pounds overweight. Patients with TBIs who are restricting calories or other nutrients may have less chance of healing. Here are several eating disorders to watch for:

- **Body dysmorphic disorder**

  Body dysmorphic disorder is an obsession with appearance and the feeling that the body does not measure up to unrealistic standards. This condition is most common in teen girls who think they are fat irrespective of their actual weight. This disorder may interfere with normal interactions with others. Males may become obsessed with body building, leading to excessive weight lifting, steroids, and protein shakes that can damage the kidneys.

- **Anorexia**

  Anorexia nervosa is a disturbed sense of body image, a morbid fear of obesity, and refusal to maintain a minimum body weight. Self-imposed starvation leads to emaciation, nutritional deficits, electrolyte imbalances, muscle atrophy, hypotension, constipation, restlessness, anxiety, balding, cold extremities, disappearance of any fatty tissue, amenorrhea, dry skin, intolerance to cold, dysrhythmias, and death. While by all outward appearances this is a physical problem, anorexia is a severe mental illness that is both chronic and terminal if not aggressively treated. Mortality is estimated at 5% to 15% even with advanced medical support.

  Usually anorexics are teen females who are often meticulous, compulsive, perfectionistic, and intelligent. While they barely consume anything, these girls can be obsessed with food: its purchase, preparation, presentation, and consumption by others. They will spend hours planning and preparing a meal only to cut a pea in thirds and leave a portion on the plate. They also may expend considerable energy hiding their starvation from others. They may purge (self-induced vomiting) which can result in dental caries from the stomach acid. Rotting teeth in a girl who is otherwise obsessed by her appearance is sometimes the first sign there is a problem.

  Anorexics usually start out at a normal weight and then come to believe they have an urgent need to lose pounds. They are successful, often losing more than 20% of their body weight quickly. They will use any means necessary including starvation, excessive exercise, appetite suppressants, laxatives, amphetamines, emetics, and fat absorption blockers. They seem to have a death wish.

  Multiple websites are now on-line to encourage more drastic starvation and outlining ways to hide the problem. One offers tips on how to survive on a hundred calories a day. While still predominantly a female problem, more males are now beginning to show signs of anorexia.

  Anorexia has a high mortality rate. In my experience, this is one of the hardest conditions in all medicine to manage. Patients are in abject denial with rigid personalities and their defenses are often impenetrable. They rationalize and are frankly delusional about the reality of their situation. As an occupational and preventive medicine physician in industry, I had a number of anorexics in the workplace. Preoccupied with food, they were often ineffective employees who frustrated their co-workers. One could not attend meetings because she had to stay close to her potassium packets. (Huh? Couldn't she bring them with her?) Passive-aggressive and narcissistic, they can make themselves as unlikeable as humanly possible, almost testing people to see how outrageous the behavior could become before there were consequences. Despite the most aggressive medical care available, they would not avail themselves of help or would completely disregard medical advice. Over the years, two young anorexics that I was involved with in the workplace died, despite superhuman efforts by others to help them turn things around. Their denial was stronger than any that I have ever experienced. Often facile manipulators, the families in both cases were quite enabling. Some anorexics do get better, but both their HCPs and families have to remain strong.

- **Binge eating disorder**

Binge eating disorder is chronic, excessive eating without purging. Anorexics are usually uncomfortably thin. Bulimics are slightly overweight. Binge eaters are often obese. Binge eating may be associated with addiction to carbohydrates, compulsions, and stress relief. This makes sense since people tend to binge on "comfort foods" that have high amounts of processed carbs, fat, and salt. Bingers cannot seem to stop eating. Be careful in TBI patients, since Lyme can affect blood sugar levels and may compound the problem.

- **Bulimia**

The bulimic eating pattern consists of recurrent episodes of bingeing followed by purging. Purging is self-induced vomiting either by sticking a finger down the throat or using emetics. Many learn to vomit at will. These patients may develop dental caries from the erosion of teeth from stomach acid. They may go to great lengths to hide their behavior. Like binge eaters, they can't stop eating, but they follow their binge with purging. They are also prone to using laxatives and fat blockers. Fat blockers have exceedingly unpleasant side effects and can prevent the absorption of fat-soluble vitamins. Presumably, the oozing of unabsorbed, fetid oil from the anus has limited the OTC version of one these agents from becoming a blockbuster.

O. Munchausen Syndrome

Munchausen syndrome involves repeated fabrication of signs and symptoms of disease in order to get medical attention. While Munchausen's appears to be similar to hypochondriasis, this condition is more malevolent. While hypochondriacs worry about trivial matters, their concern is real and motivated by some valid perception. In contrast, Munchausen patients make things up, often in dramatic and convincing fashion to get attention. When one doctor tires of them, they will doctor shop and start over. They have been known to purposely harm themselves, change normal test results, and pry open healing wounds

in order to continue the ruse. Their whole life revolves around keeping the charade going. Children rarely, if ever, present with Munchausen syndrome. The syndrome is named after Baron Karl Friedrich Hieronymus Freicherr von Munchausen, who was known to tell a few tall tales back in the 1700s.

In Munchhausen by proxy, a caregiver fabricates medical problems for another, usually a child, in order to get attention. These individuals have been known to falsify the medical history, alter records, and lie about previous test results. Unfortunately, this diagnosis has become yet another political hot button. In the Lyme world, certain academics have accused parents of Munchhausen by proxy. This almost always occurs when the HCP could not make a diagnosis in a sick child and the parents kept pushing for answers. Since the brilliant physician could not be wrong, the parents must be making things up.

P. Phobias

Phobias are persistent, unrealistic and intense fears that impact behavior. Usually the anxiety is focused on a specific object, event, or other stimulus. The most familiar phobias include: agoraphobia (the fear of open space or of leaving the house), claustrophobia (the fear of enclosed spaces like an MRI tube), fear of flying, fear of germs, or fear of public speaking. Many people share these common phobias. Some phobias are bizarre like fear of cheese, fear of mustaches, or fear of clowns. There are hundreds of named phobias. Some phobias impinge on AODL. John Madden and Whoopi Goldberg will not fly. They have to find other ways to travel. Those with a fear of elevators will not make an appointment above the 4th floor. Children can be phobic of the dark, strangers, storms, animals, or any number of things.

Phobias can be affiliated with panic attacks, GAD, and OCD. These fears are real whether the threat is real or not. Reasoning and logic will not make a phobia go away. CBT can help.

A social phobia is intense anxiety in social situations and can apply to a specific event or to social situations in general. This is more than shyness where the person feels vaguely uncomfortable until he warms up. Phobias can impede social interactions and limit relationships. A social phobic will avoid the scenarios that trigger her anxiety and may become isolated.

Q. Post-Traumatic Stress Disorder

Because of an overwhelming traumatic event or series of events, a patient with PTSD mentally re-experiences the event with intense fear, anxiety, helplessness, and horror.

The person relives the experience through flashbacks or nightmares. She will go to great lengths to avoid a stimulus that will trigger these flashbacks. PTSD is common after abuse, rape, abandonment, assault, crime, torture, violence, and severe accidents. Sadly whole generations are growing up with PTSD in areas with war, upheaval, famine, and natural disasters. Assess whether the patient is in a high risk population.

Persons with PTSD might numb themselves against emotion. They can startle easily, have short tempers, suffer problems sleeping, and feel angry as though they are always on guard. They may have a heightened sense of arousal and be hypervigilant. PTSD can impact normal life functions.

R. Addiction

Addiction has many definitions and much debate over what constitutes a "real" addiction. For our purposes, an addict has a life characterized by the compulsive use of a substance or the performance of a behavior that ultimately causes harm to the addict. Addiction is often framed in terms of dependency, tolerance, and withdrawal.

When a person first starts what will become an addiction, he uses a substance for pleasure and enjoyment. The first cigarettes and the first beers are used for fun, to feel relaxed, or to fit in. As the addiction develops, the individual has to use the substance just to feel normal. That is dependency, since the person "depends" on the substance to be normal. A person can be physically dependent, psychologically dependent, or both. Tolerance means that you have to use more and more of the addictive substance to get the same high. Watch the patient who other people brag, "Boy, he can really hold his liquor." That means he has built up a tolerance to the substance and has to hold more and more to get his old buzz. That is NOT something to be proud of. More is needed to get you to the same place. Withdrawal symptoms are the physical and psychological consequences of stopping the substance that you are addicted to. Alcohol withdrawal can be fatal. In other types of withdrawal, the person just thinks he's dying.

A person can be addicted to alcohol, opioids, cocaine, amphetamines, and any number of other substances. There is also evidence that some people are addicted to certain foods, sex, gambling, shopping, excessive exercise, pornography, and other deleterious behaviors. Somehow the addictive substance affects the brain circuits, reward centers, and biochemical receptors. While cocaine and alcohol affect the physiology differently, the resulting addiction is similar. Despite repeated, severe, adverse consequences, the intense physical and psychological pull is hard to ignore.

PEARL: When I worked at Eastern Pennsylvania Psychiatric Hospital as a college intern, we studied the addiction potential of dozens of compounds. Guess which was more addicting than opioids, alcohol, amphetamines, heroin, and all the rest? Nicotine.

Unfortunately, there are TBI patients who have addictions. The road to recovery is going to be especially difficult for these individuals. Their bodies just won't have the needed energy to mount a good fight. These patients will need to be managed on a case-by-case basis. Treatments may need to be adjusted and compliance may be an issue. Don't focus so much on one condition that you forget all about the other.

S. Substance Abuse

The actress Drew Barrymore may have been an alcoholic before she was a teenager. Do not underestimate the age of first drink and the amount of drinking by kids and teens. Teens often brag to peers about how much they can drink. Or as the transportation security personnel at the local airport are heard to say EVERY time as we go through the line, "I was SOOO drunk last night." Alcohol is a solvent, like drinking paint thinner. Alcohol may kill brain cells, and at the very least adversely impact receptors. If you have a TBI, you already have Bb doing enough harm so that additional damage to the brain and nerves will be quite unnecessary. Please reinforce this concept with patients with TBIs, who otherwise may not get well.

Kids, as young as elementary school, have been known to abuse many kinds of substances from cough syrup to glue. Prescription drugs, particularly narcotic analgesics and neurologic stimulants, are all the rage today. Also frequently abused are amphetamines, cocaine in various forms, barbiturates, phenycyclidine, marijuana, and hallucinogens. Also possible are mushrooms, solvents, salvia, the hallucinogen Ecstasy, and date rape drugs such as Rohypnol, Klonopin, Xanax, GHB, and Ketamine. Just about any drug can be abused as witnessed with kids taking Viagra until they pass out or PPIs so that they can drink more beer with less stomach distress the next day. Michael Jackson taught us that even the most unlikely drugs can be abused such as the anesthetic propofol.

Know that anytime your patient is taking substances to alter her consciousness, the results of your physical exam are going be altered as well. Damage to the nervous and other body systems will delay healing. While many substances like marijuana do not seem to cause physical dependence, they can be quite emotionally addictive. I remember a physician co-worker who would crow, "The Eagle has landed," each time his marijuana supply arrived. He had other issues as well.

PEARL: Marijuana use might impact the immune system. Marijuana in any form could potentially compromise a TBI patient's immune defense.

PEARL: Some patients with long-term Lyme can no longer tolerate alcohol and will announce that they no longer drink. While I found this phenomenon reported in several different sources, I could not find any theories as to why this might be happening.

T. Conversion disorders

A conversion reaction or disorder is the involuntary loss of a body function without a good explanation. This reaction can be sensory with loss of sensation, excessive sensitivity to strong stimuli, loss of the sense of pain, or tingling or crawling sensations. Conversion disorders can involve motor function as well, with involuntary movement of the arms, legs, and vocal cords or disorganized movements such as tics, tremors, or twitches. Visceral conversion might include swallowing, burping, coughing, or vomiting. Anecdotally, infections are thought to have instigated some conversion reactions.

PEARL: If a conversion reaction is due to an infection, the symptoms will diminish if treated with appropriate antibiotics. If the reaction is situational and non-infectious, antibiotics will have no effect.

U. Dreams/Nightmares

Dreaming is conducive to good mental health. Theoretically, dreaming helps to sort through the myriad inputs of the day and sooth the rough emotional edges that the conscious mind didn't have time for earlier. Memories can be modified to be more soothing. Nightmares aren't nearly so pleasant. TBI patients often report bad dreams or more vivid dreaming. Nightmares aren't all bad. Sociopaths apparently do not have nightmares. Anyone still having nightmares probably retains some aspect of social consciousness.

V. PANDAS

Pediatric autoimmune neuropsychiatric disorders associated with Streptococcal infections are controversial, of course. In patients with a known Strep infection of the throat, scarlet fever, or impetigo, there can be a sudden onset of neuropsychiatric symptoms such as OCD, tics, or Tourette's.

The mechanism may be similar to rheumatic fever that occurs with a Strep infection except instead of the autoimmune system attacking the heart, valves, and joints, the antibodies attack the brain cells. The basal ganglion seems to be the primary target and this is the site responsible for movement and behavior. In Strep-associated rheumatic fever there can also be abnormal involuntary movements, referred to as Sydenham's chorea or St. Vitus dance.

Here is one of the most important paragraphs in the book. In RF the antibodies attack the *self* cells of the heart, valves, joints, and apparently parts of the brain. This same mechanism could also be the case for PANDAS with the brain being the focus instead of the heart. This is called molecular mimicry which means that the antigens on the cell walls of the Strep are similar enough to the antigens on the cell walls of the target tissue that antibodies mistake one for the other. In RF the target tissues are heart, joints, kidneys, valves, and brain, while in PANDAS, the target is primarily brain.

In both cases of Strep-associated disease, the abnormal movements presented as chorea in RF and tics in PANDAS, are believed to be due to the antibodies cross-reacting with neuronal brain tissue in the basal ganglia. The antigens on the brain tissue MIMIC the antigen on the Strep and the antibody ends up damaging *self* brain tissue instead of non-*self* pathogen tissue. Symptoms occur because the damage occurs in the area of the basal ganglia that controls movement and behavior.

PANDAS cause a dramatic, almost overnight onset of symptoms with motor or vocal tics, emotional lability, anxiety, OCD manifestations, enuresis, and deterioration in hand writing.

PEARL: While PANDAS were thought to be solely a Strep-associated phenomenon (hence the name), a significant percentage of PANDAS cases are positive for Bb. Lyme hits both cardiac and brain tissue just like Strep apparently does in RF. What if the concept of molecular mimicry applies to Bb as well as Strep? There is anecdotal speculation that Bartonella might be implicated in this same mimicry mechanism. But so little is known about Bartonella that this idea is currently just conjecture that hopefully will prove clinically useful in the future.

Some studies have shown that PANDAS improve with antibiotic treatments. Other studies are equivocal. I can't wait to see what Dr. Cunningham in Oklahoma finds. I hope her results are life-changing.

Chapter 18   ORDERING APPROPRIATE TESTS – Detailed chapter contents

Chapter 18

ORDERING APPROPRIATE TESTS

If you torture a number long enough, it will say anything you want.
Statistician Barbara Miller

For the purposes of this *Compendium,* a test will be one of a number of information-gathering techniques that will help HCPs, patients, and caretakers better understand and treat TBIs.

Since management of TBIs can be challenging on a good day, we should welcome any help we can get. Therefore a number of modalities will be reviewed so that we can make the best use of our time and resources. While some studies may be forced upon us, (like the use of ELISA testing for Lyme by certain insurance and medical groups), other tests certainly have their valid place in the care of TBI patients.

As long as we keep things in perspective and understand the advantages and disadvantages of the various modalities, we should be able to use the results wisely. I will try to balance the pros and cons and outline any known limitations of the pertinent exams. What is the sensitivity and specificity of the test you are about to order? Will it provide the information you need? Would an alternative give you more useful information? Are you ordering this test to keep from getting sued? While a lumbar puncture might keep you out of court, it won't help the patient much when you recognize that it is very difficult to retrieve TBI pathogens from spinal fluid. You could have a child with a dangerous meningitis presenting with a negative LP because you did not understand the limits of the test you ordered.

In fact, false negatives provide false confidence that could actually harm the patient. Some HCPs look for reasons to talk themselves out of what they clearly see before them. False negatives buy the HCP some time, but do nothing for the patient. We want positive results when they should be positive and negative results when they should be negative. Reality! What a concept. Test results NEVER absolve you from your responsibility to take care of the sick person in front of you. I don't care how often the ELISA is negative or the Western blot doesn't show the right bands. As long as you don't dismiss a diagnosis solely on the basis of a negative test result, both you and the patient should be okay.

Spreen Theorem: *Never* order a test if the result will have no impact on case management. If a test result would not make you change your diagnosis or treatment plan in any way, don't order the test. If an X-ray result will not change your thinking no matter what it shows, and you plan to do what you were going to do anyway, don't order the X-ray. I know there is something to be said for baseline results, but you know what I mean here. Do baselines if you will draw on them in the future, but use good sense when it comes to ordering tests. Some fishing may be reasonable if you are looking for clues as to what might be happening with your patient. But don't order tests just because you can. Have some rationale for your requests.

In assessing and managing TBI patients, there are many reasons why we might want to have supportive evidence beyond our own senses. Sometimes we just need the support of an unbiased observer, at least until we have the courage of our convictions. Evaluations can include lab tests such as blood, urine, sputum, spinal fluid, throat and other cultures, tissue pathology, EKGs, or imaging studies such as X-rays, MRIs, CAT or SPECT scans, and PET studies. Additional information also can come from such evaluations as nerve conduction studies or psychological testing and innumerable other modalities.

There are four basic reasons why we might request a study:

- To help support a diagnosis

- To rule out concurrent conditions and co-morbidities including co-infections

- To follow the course of the disease or the effectiveness of treatment

- To look for adverse reactions that may result from therapy, especially from medications

PLEASE remember that many of the HCPs, caregivers, and patients with whom you will be discussing these tests will have NO idea what you are talking about. When labs were first ordered on my son, I was told how much they would cost and how I had to write a check immediately because the HCP didn't intend to carry the likes of me on the books. Having never heard of Babesia until that moment, I certainly did not understand what was being ordered. When the results came back and titers were thrown around like confetti, I again had no clue. AND I had even studied before going back to the office for the results.

Have mercy. Explain exactly what is happening. In my opinion, a good teacher is one who can explain quantum theory to a 4th grader. (Dr. Schmuckler, that's you!) Prove yourself a good doctor by explaining these complex and unfamiliar ideas in a way that can be understood. If you are on the receiving end, make the HCP explain until you understand. Don't be a grinning fool like me, pretending I knew when I didn't. Just like you, I was so worried about my child that the doctors could have said anything and I would be agreeing as long as I thought it would help him. I am a physician with two specialty board certifications and two master's degrees in science. My husband is a PhD physical chemist. My son is working on his PhD in rocket science. We aren't dumb. We just didn't know. Don't be afraid to ask.

Inescapable general advice:

- Each lab has its own way of doing things so look at the normal values for the lab doing the test, not the "normals" from the hospital lab where you were an intern. (I know you still have them.)

- Don't order labs you will never use because you are compelled to do so in order to get a great "package" deal. By forcing you to pick a "panel" of tests, the lab suggests you are getting a SPECIAL offer. The cost of 24 tests will be half the cost of the three tests you actually need. You will get into more trouble from labs-you-never-wanted-in-the-first-place than you ever will from abnormal labs that you know how to handle.

- Don't order labs just to show how smart you are. I spent thousands of dollars building the ego of a TBI doctor who loved to order tests I did not understand to show superiority (whether the tests were indicated or not).

- Don't order labs when the same information is more easily obtained in other ways. Remember the H&P.

- Know that lab "normals" can be different for various ages, sexes, and races. White cell "normals" for newborns change within hours.

- If you do not understand a study: call the lab, call an expert, or call your mother before you write the order. Call all the above before you try to interpret it.

- Specimens must be handled correctly or they could be ruined. Patient specimens are precious, especially if you stuck something sharp somewhere obscure to get it. Some samples need spun, some need frozen, some need left alone. Most need a particular tube to be used for collection. Don't be the reason a good specimen goes bad.

- If you get an abnormal lab result that you do not know what to do with, document it anyway. You cannot disguise it with a fedora and a trench coat. In the chart, admit there is an abnormal result. You might want to consider why. You might not. Say you will continue to follow its progress. Then follow its progress until it no longer makes sense to do so.

- Understand the limits of your test. If a study is not designed to show something, then it cannot show it. Don't have unrealistic expectations.

- Discuss the results of any studies with the pertinent people – in a way they understand. As I learned in Swedish culture class (when I worked for a Scandinavian company), smiling and nodding does not mean comprehending.

- Know if the patient needs to be fasting or fed or if any other special provisions need to be made.

- Try not to change labs midstream, unless the initial lab quality is hideous. There is enough variation within a lab to worry about, let alone between labs.

- Do NOT order a test if the result will have no impact on patient care. If you are going to do whatever you planned on doing from the beginning, no matter what the test says, why are you getting the test?

- Do NOT order a test you never plan to look at. A friend of mine was recently diagnosed with two primary cancers. When gathering information to take to the cancer center, he noticed that a 3-year-old routine chest X-ray showed a lung lesion. This X-ray had been ordered as part of the pre-op for a minor elective surgery. The radiologist clearly said this lesion should have further work-up. The results were sent to his family doctor and both the surgeon and anesthesiologist who ordered the pre-op testing. No one looked at the result and the lesion sat there for 3 years perhaps making new cancer cells all over the place. If you're not going to pay attention to the result, don't order the test. If you order the test, you are responsible for addressing the result.

- NEVER rule out a possible diagnosis based on the result of a lab test alone. *Not detected does not mean uninfected.* If I can only get one point across in this book...

- Always treat the patient, not the test result.

While the next chapter will deal with interpretation of results, I want to share what I learned from nearly two decades in drug development. With thousands of people in hundreds of studies, I had to look at a lot of test results. At FDA meetings, I could recite the abnormal LFTs for each of the patients in each of the studies, complete with patient number and site location. The term "Within Normal Limits" or WNL can cover a number of sins. Yes, "normal" values are determined by each lab based on the composite results from hundreds, if not thousands, of test subjects. But your concern should be the one patient sitting in front of you. While her test results may say "WNL" throughout the duration of your involvement, that does not mean that nothing is going on. Our friends at the big commercial labs have even made it easy to scan a lab report with absolutely no thought required. If there is no asterisk beside the result, you can turn the page. All "normal," thank goodness.

Of course, medical practice is not as simple as that. Especially for studies looking at the liver and thyroid, the "normal" for that particular patient may be more important than the lab normal. For certain LFTs, the normal range can vary greatly. If a patient starts at the low end of normal and gradually trends upward, perhaps doubling his number with each subsequent test, something might be adversely influencing that liver function. Livers may be hurting from effects of the disease or because of adverse reactions to medication. More than a few people have been told they have a "normal" thyroid when the results are NOT normal for them. Because we usually do not have baseline numbers documenting a value that was historically normal for that individual, we are stuck with the general WNL result. In the army, we used to panic over lab results flagged as abnormal because normal was based on 18-year-old white guys. Women and various ethnic groups, along with those of us older than 18, were indeed different, but not necessarily abnormal. Figuring this out cost time and money.

In data, whether from a large population or for an individual, always look for patterns and trends. A **pattern** is the recurrence of an event again and again over time. A person takes a drug and his AST elevates. The next time he takes the same drug, his AST elevates. Patterns do not need to be perfect to suggest that you should pay attention. If you don't compare the new result to the old result, you are not going to see a pattern. Patterns can seem to occur by chance, but if the same thing keeps happening over and over, it is likely there is some causal association. I will provide you with much more guidance on determining causal association when we discuss adverse reactions to drugs later in the chapter. Always treat the patient and not the test result.

Trends are more likely to creep into the data set. To spot a trend, you have to look at a number of data points. That's why you monitor lab work over time. A trend is a general movement of findings; a drift in a certain direction. Trends can be subtle or earth-shaking. (You would be surprised by how many earth-shaking trends are still missed or ignored.) H&H can trend down suggesting bleeding or other causes of anemia. (My hemoglobin dropped from 16 to 9 after my knee replacement. Those values were all WNL, but not for me. I

am normally between 15 and 16. I was so weak I could barely walk.) Creatinine can trend up indicating a possible kidney problem. LFTs can creep up, doubling or tripling the patient's normal. However, because the values are still WNL, they are ignored or even celebrated. Trends are gently leading you to discover something. If you don't look, you won't see. It is much easier to just say "All is WNL," but that shortchanges your patient. Look at the last test results and the ones before that. Pretend you are a detective like Sherlock Holmes. Make decisions based on what you learn.

The rest of Chapter 18 will consider the four primary reasons to order studies in TBI patients and which tests will best serve these purposes. The information in this chapter provides insight on selecting which tests might provide useful information for your individual patient. Next, Chapter 19: *Scientific Foundation and Interpretation of Study Results* will describe the study procedures and will tell you what to do with the results once you get them. So, the remainder of this chapter will be a list of possible options and the next chapter will detail the underlying science to enable the most comprehensive interpretation of the results. For tests of immune parameters, much of this same material was introduced in the *Gentle Immunology* chapter.

I.   STUDIES TO PROVIDE SUPPORT FOR DIAGNOSIS

Diagnosis of a TBI must be a clinical decision. Almost always, case management and treatment must begin long before you get back any test results. Essentially, no test for TBIs screams the name of the pathogen. The methods listed are fraught with unreliability, inaccuracy, insensitivity, and non-specificity. And that's when things are going well. While a veteran TBI practitioner will be able to work around the flaws in diagnostic testing, most of us are too inexperienced and insecure to pull that off. Use this text for support. False positives are rare in TBI assessments. False negatives abound. Always take in the whole clinical picture when making a diagnosis. While study results can provide support, they cannot make the diagnosis. That takes clinical judgment; putting together the results of history, physical, and clinical course, in addition to any supportive test results. NEVER rule out a possible diagnosis on the basis of a lab test alone. That makes you foolish and potentially dangerous. Proceed with caution and don't let a lab result keep you from making the best decisions for your patient.

A.   Routine lab tests that may provide support for a TBI diagnosis:

1.   **Complete blood count** (CBC) including white cell differential and platelets. This test can provide clues regarding the etiology of symptoms including differentiating between bacterial, viral, parasitic, and

allergic causes. Anemia with a low H&H may be a sign of Babesia infection. A high eosinophil count may indicate allergies rather than infection, or suggest parasites.

2. **Clotting panels** may demonstrate a tendency toward hypercoagulation consistent with Babesia or Bartonella. Lyme can also impact clotting.

3. **Blood smears** involve looking at a thin layer of peripheral blood under a microscope. Technicians can look at either white or red cells for diagnostic purposes in TBIs. The most diagnostic smears include:

   • **Morulae** in white cells in ehrlichiosis

   • **Maltese cross** formations in red cells infected with Babesia

Smears are relatively quick and inexpensive tests. Many smears today are automated, making them less useful for our purposes. While smears can be done at any local lab, use caution. Write "manual exam" on the lab request since automated readings tend to be less sensitive. The more experienced the tech is in reading peripheral blood smears, the more accurate the results. How long will the novice tech look for the rare parasite? The manual exam takes patience; otherwise, a false negative will result. In babies born with babesiosis, a high pathogen load can make detection of the Maltese crosses easier. However, do not rule out a diagnosis on the basis of a negative peripheral blood smear.

4. A routine **urinalysis** showing red cells or bilirubin can be consistent with babesiosis. If UA results suggest an infection, a culture with sensitivity test can be requested. Here you would be looking for the usual suspects that cause UTIs such as E. *coli.* TBI pathogens rarely are uncovered on urine cultures. In Lyme-induced interstitial cystitis, the signs and symptoms might say infection but the routine cultures consistently come up "clean." Here Bb may be the infectious agent and the usual testing methods do not allow for its recognition. The HCP will need to be aware of the possibility of a Bb etiology and make the diagnosis based on clinical suspicion.

5. **Cultures** are sometimes collected in TBI patients looking for infectious etiologies. TBI pathogens are notoriously difficult to grow from any body fluid. Routine cultures looking for the pathogens that traditionally grow in urine or blood or any number of other body fluids just aren't going to grow TBI pathogens. With the exception of tularemia, which are aerobic

bacteria that love to be out in the air infecting lab techs, there is little value in ordering *routine* cultures in this population, solely for the purpose of ruling out a TBI. Even cultures that are designed to grow Bb and other TBIs often do not grow the etiologic organism. Methods just aren't that reliable as yet. *Not detected does not mean uninfected.* Negative or no results can only be used to conclude that the selected technique did not grow organisms.

Is there any usefulness in ordering routine blood cultures or urine cultures in a TBI patient? Probably not, if you are looking for help in diagnosing the TBI. You are more likely to grow other pathogens that are part of a concurrent infectious process – or are the sole etiology of the infectious condition. With a UTI, the culture might identify E. *coli,* which is good since you would want to know about the presence of this pathogen so you could treat appropriately. That doesn't mean there might not be other pathogens contributing to the clinical condition. If proper treatment does not resolve symptoms, consider that more than one infectious agent might be operating.

Whenever you have a patient with a persistent fever of unknown origin or a sepsis, a blood culture may be prudent. These samples are usually a series of blood draws, most often three, separated by several hours and drawn from different body sites. These methods attempt to take into account the peaks and troughs that may occur in pathogen cycles and, therefore, allow for the best chance of capturing the organism. Routine blood cultures will not be looking to culture TBI pathogens, common or otherwise. Cultures for those organisms would need to be ordered for the specific organism of interest.

The same holds true for cultures and analysis of CSF and joint aspirate. Aspirate or collagen from an involved joint is sometimes used for analysis. Here you might be able to look for actual spirochetes under a scope. But, don't get your hopes up. Bb seem to know we're coming and manage to make themselves scarce. You WILL need to make your diagnosis based on clinical judgment, so warm up to that idea.

While we would all love to culture live spirochetes from a culture specimen, it's not going to happen in most health care facilities. Of course, if you have a septic or otherwise symptomatic patient, order the routine culture. People sick with TBIs can also be sick for other reasons as well. You may find another etiology contributing to the problem but it won't likely be a TBI pathogen. Cultures for the individual TBIs usually require special collection, handling, and media use.

You pretty much need to have an idea of what you are looking for before you order the culture. Even then the chance of growing pathogens like Bb are slim. If you are determined to make a diagnosis based on culture results, call the lab and ask for guidance on what to order and how to collect.

PEARL: Despite their limitations, cultures for Lyme, especially when taken from biopsy or other tissue samples, can provide a better chance of identifying the Bb pathogen than many other tests. Results of a retrospective study recognized the sensitivity of cultures in comparison to other testing. A more definitive blood culture for Lyme is being refined at Advanced Laboratory Services in Pennsylvania (1-855-238-4949). Perhaps this culture will prove more helpful than those used in the past and will become the gold standard in supporting the diagnosis of Lyme. I can dream.

Tissue from biopsy, surgical remnants, or birth products can provide test samples that allow for more accurate testing. Assessments of Ag/Ab complexes as well as DNA and RNA testing through PCR and FISH are more likely to uncover true positives if the sample is tissue rather than the various body fluids. If a culture is going to grow out a pathogen, tissue samples will likely serve you better than body fluids.

Biopsies can be taken during scopes, birth, or surgery. Do not let these rare opportunities to collect a specimen pass you by. When you hear your patient is having a procedure, discuss the possibility of tissue sample collection. In intractable cases consider muscle or skin biopsy.

6. **Lumbar punctures** (spinal taps) are often ordered in symptomatic patients with possible TBIs. While they may show signs of inflammation and even infection, their yield for TBI pathogens is notoriously low. Nevertheless, if a patient presents with a meningitis-like syndrome, you would be remiss in not looking for white cells or other signs of pathology including pathogens (both TBI and non-TBI), and measuring opening pressure. Remember, all diagnoses are not TBI-based and you may find other causal agents. TBI microbes are frustratingly difficult to culture from CSF. Nevertheless if an LP was done and CSF is in hand, depending on the clinical presentation, take full advantage of this available specimen. Consider sending the CSF for a TBI panel looking for antibodies for those TBIs in your differential. Cultures, WB, Lyme DOT assay, and PCR, can all be done on CSF. Please use a lab familiar with TBI testing. A negative result for TBIs on the LP does not prove anything. Never dismiss a TBI diagnosis based on a negative LP.

7. **Imaging studies** tend to not be especially helpful in making the diagnoses of TBIs. While Lyme may present with brain lesions similar to those seen with MS, these findings are nonspecific and tend to manifest later in the clinical course when you should have already figured out what's happening by other means. In some Lyme cases, SPECT scans are thought to show hypoperfusion of the brain which may improve with treatment. Here areas associated with slow thought processes have been correlated with decreased perfusion on the SPECT scan. X-rays will show what X-rays show: joint effusions and consolidations in the lung and gas in the GI tract, all of which provide data on the patient's condition but do not help make TBI diagnoses. By the way, effusion does not need to be present for a joint to be infected with Lyme. We need to stop finding excuses to disregard TBIs. Ultrasounds will be important later when we are monitoring for untoward drug effects, but they usually do not add to the diagnostic evidence. Despite the limits on imaging techniques as a means to diagnose TBIs, these test results will cross your desk. Here is a quick synopsis regarding the most common imaging studies that may be part of a TBI work-up:

a. **X-ray:** A plain X-ray is an image produced on photographic film made by passing radiation through a body part. X-rays are best at distinguishing gas from liquid and liquid from solid, especially bone. Plain films are good at identifying fractures and other bone abnormalities and seeing if there is a solid where air should be, or air where liquid or solid should be. CXRs can identify pneumonias, pulmonary edema, and some masses. Abdominal X-rays can see free air, obstructions, and stones. Recently, there has been media concern over how much radiation exposure from X-rays is safe. Unfortunately, many X-rays are ordered for the wrong reasons such as reassuring the patient or parent or to give the perception that the HCP is doing something about the complaint. Many times the HCP knows the X-ray will show nothing that will alter the pre-determined diagnosis or treatment plan. Ironically, many patients feel much better after an X-ray has been taken, even without knowing the result. So the act of taking an X-ray can have a placebo-effect in some people. X-rays are relatively inexpensive, readily available, and generally not harmful if ordered in moderation. They are best reserved for high contrast situations when not trying to parse out fine distinctions between types of soft tissue.

b. **CAT scan**: CT or computed axial tomography allows the formation of a 3-D image from pictures taken around a single axis of rotation. Images are taken in slices and then reconstructed in multiple dimensions. Although more expensive and less available than plain X-rays, CAT scans can focus on the area of interest and can distinguish different soft tissues, one from the other. Still there is exposure to ionizing radiation. Initially CAT scans took a long time and kids needed to be sedated to get usable images. But, technology is improving all the time making the procedure shorter and less confining. CTs can be done with or without contrast, but contrast allows for better resolution and better distinctions between tissues. Nonetheless, contrast is not without risks and is best avoided in patients with any kidney compromise. Paradoxically, contrast can be used in patients who are on kidney dialysis since the kidneys are already shot and no more damage can be done. With IV contrast, some patients feel a warm sensation near the injection site along with nausea and discomfort. Allergies are possible. CTs of the head can help detect infarcts, tumors, calcifications, bleeding, and bone injuries. In the lungs CAT scans can look at the parenchyma in ways that a 2-D X-ray cannot do. These scans can show emphysema, fibrosis, and signs of pulmonary emboli. CT scans are very sensitive in assessing the abdomen and pelvis showing tumors and organomegaly. They can be especially useful in examining an acute abdomen. Virtual colonoscopy is now possible through CAT scanning. CT scans can be used to assess bones and can detect fractures, especially around joints because the image is gleaned from multiple perspectives. CAT scans are more expensive than X-rays and less accessible but they are becoming almost as common and provide resolution advantages.

PEARL: A 2013 study from Brigham and Women's Hospital in Boston showed that 83% of radiologists failed to see the image of a dancing gorilla in a CT scan of the chest even though they knew they were being evaluated and the average radiologist looked at the scan four times.

    c. MRI: Magnetic resonance imaging used to be called more accurately nuclear magnetic resonance. The label nuclear was removed because laypersons were concerned about radioactivity. In fact, the term had nothing to do with radioactivity but instead refers to the nuclei of atoms and how they align in a magnetic field. By using radio waves, some of the nuclei can be temporarily realigned and when they relax back to their natural state they emit a signal that can be processed to create an image. Different tissues can be clearly distinguished. MRI uses no ionizing radiation but still provides good soft tissue resolution making it especially useful for assessing the brain, heart, muscles, and connective tissue. Cancers are often delineated. In some cases, contrast agents can

help better identify vessels, tumors, or inflammation sites especially in joints. Many times cancers can be recognized. The large magnet may pose a risk to persons with indwelling metal such as pacemakers and cochlear implants, as well as some artificial joints and stents. Always review the possibility of internal metal prior to moving forward with an MRI. This includes bullets and shrapnel since the magnet can potentially heat or move the metal object which has been reported to be decidedly uncomfortable.

PEARL: To compare CAT scans and MRIs consider: MRIs are best for soft tissue imaging while CTs are better for bones and calcifications. With MRIs multiple plane imaging is possible while with CTs the image is limited to the transverse plane. CTs involve ionizing radiation whereas MRIs do not. Different contrast agents are employed, with CTs using iodine or barium most often, and MRIs using gadolinium and manganese. MRIs are better for identifying tumors in the brain, whereas CT scans might be better for solid tumors of the abdomen and chest. CAT scans are less susceptible to subject motion than MRIs. MRIs may be more confining and noisy. CAT scans are usually more available, faster, and cheaper than MRIs. Still, MRIs are a better choice if the patient will need repeat exams over a short time because there is no ionizing radiation involved.

    d. PET scan: Unlike X-rays, CT scans, and MRIs, positron emission tomography looks at function not just structure. By measuring accumulation of radioactivity in areas of more intense metabolism, the PET scan highlights those locations with more activity than the surrounding tissue. These places are often the sites of dysfunction or disease and show up brighter on the scan. PETs show blood flow and chemical activity. The images have good resolutions and fast results. The tracer decays fast so PETs are limited to assessing activity of only short-term tasks. These studies are especially useful for examining neurologic, cardiac, and cancer problems. Cancer cells show up brighter because they have a higher metabolism than surrounding tissue. Still, not all cancers are caught by PET scans and some other lesions can resemble cancer. For heart disease, PET scans are used to detect sections of decreased blood flow and potentially help identify patients that could benefit from intervention. In the brain, PET can highlight parts of the brain that are most active when the patient is performing various tasks and so PETs have been used in many research projects. These scans can be helpful in the work-up of tumors, memory disorders, and seizures. PET scans do use a radioactive substance that is instilled through injection, inhalation, or ingestion but the radioactivity is low level. Still, caution must be used when scans are performed in pregnant or nursing women since the radioactive tracer may reach the fetus or breast milk. Here too the subject must lie still or images may blur and some patients feel claustrophobic.

Using PET scans, Moeller found hypometabolism and decreased activity in the temporal lobes of Lyme patients, which may correlate with memory problems. Regional blood flow studies in patients with Lyme encephalopathy suggest disruption of the cerebral white matter and interference with the neural tracts between regions. Sensory hyperacusis may be associated with increased activity in the thalamus as well as additional action in the auditory and visual regions of the cortex.

e. **SPECT scan**: Single-photon emission computerized tomography provides information regarding the function of organs. A radioactive substance is used to create 3-D pictures illustrating how blood flows and what tissue areas are more or less active. SPECT can be used to help diagnose or monitor conditions. In Lyme, SPECT has been employed to assess affected tissue before and after treatment. The results show a light color where activity is low and a darker or brighter color where activity is high. In examining heart function, SPECT can show clogged vessels and diminished pump efficiency. With bone studies, SPECT is good for uncovering hidden fractures and the progression of healing. Likewise SPECT is sometimes used to highlight bone cancer progression and treatment effects. Most useful in studies of the brain, these scans can tell which parts of the brain are affected by dementia, clogged vessels, seizures, injuries, and for our purposes, encephalitis. The tracer is radioactive, albeit in very low amounts and some patients experience allergies. The radioactive material is not recommended in pregnant or breast-feeding women since the tracer may cross the placenta and get into the milk. In LD, SPECT has demonstrated a global hypoperfusion.

PEARL: In comparing SPECT and PET: SPECT is usually more restricted in the type of activity it can monitor over time but the SPECT tracers persist so this modality can be used to monitor longer-term brain functions. This, in turn, means the study will take longer to complete than a PET scan. PET tends to have better resolution, while SPECT is cheaper, using less equipment and personnel for each test. In both modalities new techniques are improving the testing all the time. SPECT used to be done more often to assess Lyme and the effect of treatment. But since baselines were rarely available and the test is not highly specific, this use has diminished and we are back to relying most often on clinical judgment.

PEARL: Fallon has used SPECT scans in Lyme patients. After Lyme patients received antibiotic treatment the hypoperfusion seen on SPECT improved along with the clinical presentation. Bransfield has also reported similar results. Before treatment the Lyme patient had extensive hypoperfusion primarily in the frontal and temporal lobes. The parietal and occipital areas were also involved. After treatment considerable improvement was observed.

f. **Ultrasound:** US uses high frequency (ultrasonic) sound waves to measure the energy as the sound moves through tissue. (I have never asked how dogs react to ultrasound machines, since these sounds are at a frequency higher than those audible by humans.) If anything impedes the flow of the sound, the energy will be reflected back in what is called an echo. The echo signal can be received and recorded and thereby tell the location, size, and other features of the entity that interrupted the path of the wave. US allows for good visualization of subcutaneous tissues such as tendons, muscles, joints, and internal organs. Probably the most familiar application of ultrasound is to look at the fetus in the womb. While this use provides critical information about the size and status of the baby, US units in malls have a thriving business selling pre-birth photos. With lower frequency sound waves, there is less resolution but the assessment can penetrate deeper. With higher frequencies you can see the small stuff but can't go as deep. Since US is good for soft tissue it is commonly used in examinations of the liver, kidney, and heart (here called echocardiogram). After trauma, US can be used as a rapid way to assess the abdomen and pelvis for blood. An especially important application of US in Lyme patients is to assess for gallstone formation in those patients on Rocephin. US is not as good at looking at organs in the abdomen because fat and gas can impede resolution. The carotids are a good target, as is the bladder, where US can look for retained fluid. Often US is used to assess tissue and fluid in the scrotum. Since US cannot penetrate bone it is not a good choice for looking at the brain since it does not readily pass through the skull. There is use for US in assessing musculature, especially when looking for cysts, and in the CVS looking for obstruction. As with most diagnostic methods, the better the technician, the better the image. US is sometimes used as a therapeutic agent in OT and PT, but this modality is not as popular as it was a few years ago. Sometimes US is used to break up stones in the kidney or gallbladder and is occasionally used to treat cysts and tumors.

PEARL: US is excellent in distinguishing fluid from solid and, unlike many other techniques, provides "live" images allowing the technician to focus on the prime areas of interest (Most people are thrilled to see their baby's heart beat.) There seem to be no adverse events due to US, either short-term or long-term, even with repeat studies. US is painless, easily accessible, and equipment is essentially portable. Even though it is relatively cheap, the results provide good spatial resolution. In contrast, US cannot penetrate bone and is significantly impeded by gas, making it a poor option for imaging of the lung or the pancreas where gas in the GI tract diminishes resolution. US is also not a good choice in those who have fat deposits over the targeted areas.

8. Other tests might provide diagnostic clues. CPK muscle component may be high in babesiosis due to savage rigors and in RMSF for reasons not entirely clear. A triad of abnormal lab results is sometimes seen in ehrlichiosis including low WBCs, low platelets, and elevated LFTs. Otherwise, with high LFTs, think Q fever. While these findings may all support a diagnosis, they are nonspecific and I wouldn't trust their diagnostic reliability. Psychological testing may be helpful in differentiating M. *fermentans* from the many other causes of neuropsychiatric symptoms. Or not, since these diagnosis are difficult under the best circumstances. Nerve conduction studies, blood gases, pulmonary function tests, endoscopies, EKGs, and a number of other modalities might provide useful information on the patient's status, but will not generally help with TBI diagnoses.

B. Specialized Diagnostic Testing

The specialized testing available to support the various TBI diagnoses are often useful when positive and meaningless when negative. A positive test usually suggests that AT SOME POINT there was antigen present from the organism in question. Otherwise, there would be no circulating antibody against that particular antigen or no DNA or RNA particles specific to that pathogen. Since antibodies and nucleic acids can persist after active infection is gone, most tests show that antigen WAS present at some time. The pathogen can still be present and active but it can also be dead and gone. This means the patient was exposed but may not be actively infected now. Some compensation for this time lag can be made by testing for both IgM and IgG. IgM is usually the initial antibody to respond, and its detection supports the idea that infection might be early in the clinical course. In contrast, IgG comes in later and some forms take years to develop. IgG suggests either current infection or infection in the not-so-distant past. With Lyme, the immune system may be so altered that these usual patterns can't always be relied upon to help define the clinical status.

Even the most sensitive tests are fraught with problems. Tests that measure protein or nucleic acids from the ACTUAL pathogen are likely to be the most reliable. However, almost all current methods are still prone to insensitivity, nonspecificity, cross-reactivity, bad timing, and unrefined technology where all the glitches are yet to be worked out. Add to this, blatant political, financial, and personal agendas. In some cases, test strains are used that could not possibly match the strain in the sick patient, or bands are selected that do not correspond to an accurate representation of the pathogen, and limits are placed on whose samples can qualify for more definitive testing. Now, you have a real mess.

Bottom line advice before you order any testing:

• Know the limits of the tests you are selecting.

• NEVER rule out a diagnosis based on a negative lab test.

• Correlate all lab findings with the clinical picture.

• Use all the supportive test results as just another piece in the diagnostic puzzle.

• Ultimately, diagnosis is a clinical decision.

1. **Searching for antigens, antibodies, and Ag/Ab comple**xes:

Many supportive diagnostic tests are based on the fundamental binding of antigens to antibodies. These chemical reactions involve the attachment of Ag to Ab in complexes. They bind, and they bind very specifically like a key fits into a lock. Although there is minimal cross-reactivity between some pathogens, in general, the Ag/Ab relationship is a marriage between one antigen and one antibody.

When testing to determine if a patient made antibodies against a specific antigen, make sure that the antigen used as the standard against which the antibody is being tested has a chance of being the antigen that inspired the antibody in the sample. Antigen from Germany is less likely to match with antibody produced by a patient in Pocopson, Pennsylvania, resulting in a false negative test. Putting in a reference strain that could never have induced the antibodies in the test sample puts the patient in a Catch-22 situation. They can't be positive, but they would be positive, if they were given a realistic chance to be positive. Amazing how many HCPs are willing to believe the test result before they would believe the sick patient in front of them.

When ordering a supportive diagnostic test you will likely never write the words "agglutination study." More often you will check a box in front of the pathogen you are investigating. The lab will then determine the method. Each lab has its own menu and deciding which tests to order can be daunting. Instead of just checking off items that you think might be useful, consider which studies might be most beneficial to diagnosing a particular patient.

PLEASE CALL THE LAB if you have any questions. In all cases of potentially supportive diagnostic laboratory tests, if you or your staff are not VERY familiar with how to order, collect, pack, and ship the sample, CALL the lab. Find a lab you trust and establish a relationship. Tell them what you suspect clinically and ASK which tests to order and how to collect and ship the samples. These tests can be extremely expensive and insurance does not always cover them. You do not want to be the reason a specimen is useless.

Some of the antibody detection methods listed below are based on agglutination and include tests of precipitation, electrophoresis, radioimmunoassay, and cytometry. Various other modalities are available, all with strengths and weaknesses. Not all the possible techniques are included here, only the most commonly encountered in the literature and in practice. Don't assume that if you understand how to interpret one method, you will automatically be able to interpret other techniques. There is no shame in not knowing, only in not asking.

Even with all the stars aligned, you can usually only tell if the patient was EVER exposed, not if there is now active disease. You might be able to get some chronology by testing both IgG and IgM but this is hit or miss depending on when the samples are drawn. Of course, it is better to order both IgG and IgM in an attempt to catch one, rather than missing both. That great HCP Wayne Gretsky said, "You miss 100% of the shots you don't take."

The following Chapter 19: *Scientific Basis and Interpretation of Study Results* will help you decipher test findings as you try to reconcile the results with the clinical picture. The remainder of the *Specialized Diagnostic Testing* section below should help you better understand what you are ordering before you check the box.

Most of the antibody or antigen testing methods listed below can be used in attempts to identify the presence of the various TBI pathogens. Just remember, there is almost NO WAY an antibody can be around today if

its corresponding antigen wasn't originally there to induce its formation.

The biochemistry supporting the science of antibody detection is outlined in both the *Gentle Immunology* chapter and in *Scientific Basis and Interpretation of Study Results*. In case you are not reading this text word-for-word (and I would be shocked if you weren't), here is a recap pearl.

PEARL: Antigens are proteins, and these proteins cover essentially all living cells. When the immune system finds a protein that is foreign, or non-self, it constructs a MATCHING antibody that can bind with that antigen in a specific lock and key fashion. One antigen, one antibody. Because of the nature of RNA and DNA, the system cannot make any other kind. Based on this premise, a number of testing methods have been developed that recognize and measure either antigen and its corresponding antibody, or antibody and its matching antigen. Antibody tests are indirect in that they are the response to an antigen that must have been around at some point. Usually you can't prove that an organism is present NOW, only that it had been present.

One or more of the following tests might be used by a lab in looking for the specific antigens and antibodies of a particular TBI. The scientific foundation and guide to interpretation for all these modalities are in Chapter 19:

- Agglutination methods

- Electrophoresis

- Immunofluorescence assay **(IFA)**

- Radioimmunoassay (RIA)

- ELISA

- Western blot (WB)

- Complement fixation techniques

- Lyme DOT blot

2. **Looking for nucleic acids**

There are a number of advantages in testing for RNA and DNA when looking for support in diagnosing TBIs. Most importantly, you cannot have nucleic acids from a pathogen present if the pathogen itself was not present at some point. The primary nucleic acid based tests, which are defined in the next chapter include:

a. **PCR** – The polymerase chain reaction looks for **DNA** of pathogens that are in the differential diagnosis.

b. **FISH** – In contrast to PCR, the fluorescent in-situ hybridization assay looks for **RNA** from the pathogens of interest.

II. STUDIES TO RULE OUT CONCURRENT CONDITIONS AND CO-MORBIDITIES

A. Tests for co-infections

Testing for any of the listed co-infections is reasonable **IF** the tests are clinically indicated, that is, 1) if a TBI patient is not getting better despite seemingly reasonable treatment, 2) if the patient is getting worse, 3) if this seems to be the worst case of Lyme you've ever seen, 4) if the signs and symptoms do not show any recognizable pattern, or 5) if the clinical course seems otherwise confounding. If one or more of these conditions exist, now may be the time to look for co-infections. Remember that under current conditions, a tick is likely to transmit more than one pathogen. If you live in an area endemic for some of the co-infections, where, say babesiosis may be as common as Lyme, you may want to look empirically at some of these conditions. Look at the specific recommendations under each potential co-infection listed below for advice on diagnostic testing.

PEARL: Diagnostic support for essentially all the following infectious diseases can be sought by attempting to measure Ag/Ab binding. Depending on the methodology and knowledge of appropriate test strains, there are varying degrees of success. One pathogen might be identified with a high degree of sensitivity and specificity while others are very unlikely to be uncovered using current technology. But still we look and order and search. Sometimes we get lucky and other times we just spend the patient's money. I guess it's only natural to pursue the positive test results that support our initial impressions. It's satisfying to have evidence that our clinical judgment was correct. But, don't go overboard. Order what actually might help identify the causative agent. Call the lab and ask, "If I am thinking about tick relapsing fever, what tests do you have that might help support my preliminary diagnosis?" (You don't have to sound as stiff as that sentence.)

Remember, diagnosis of TBIs is based on clinical judgment. Positive results from diagnostic testing can only support a diagnosis. Negative results, for many reasons, do not rule out anything. Negative just means "not detected," but it doesn't mean "not infected." Most of the TBIs can be assessed by using some form of antigen or antibody detection system to help support diagnosis in addition to the suggestions listed below. In every single case, if you don't know what you are doing, call the lab.

1. **Lyme disease:** Some insurers and medical groups require that ELISA testing be positive before a Western blot can be performed. There is no valid reason to use ELISA as a screening test for Lyme diagnosis. Start with a Western blot and know how to interpret the results beyond what the lab slip says. Specifically order both an IgM and IgG Western blot. Recall that ordering antibody tests too soon in the clinical course will result in a false negative. Antibodies, even IgM, take time to form. In especially hard cases, consider a Lyme DOT blot test which looks for bits of the Bb in the urine. NEVER rule out Lyme solely on the basis of a negative ELISA or Western blot. Use the history, physical, and your clinical judgment to make the diagnosis. Treat the patient, not the test result. Bb are notoriously difficult to confirm using any diagnostic method. Because of the pathogen's tendency to hide, alter, encyst, and go dormant, you may NEVER come up with that positive confirmation you so desperately crave. If the history and physical corroborate the suspicion, the patient likely has Lyme. Samples can be sent for PCR and FISH, and you might consider that new blood culture under development at Advanced Laboratory Services. But always remember, for now, Lyme is a clinical diagnosis.

2. **Babesiosis**: Order and follow the H&H. Look in the urine for RBCs or bilirubin. The muscle component of CPK may be high from the savage rigors. Hypercoagulation may be a sign of Babesia. Some authors recommend 30 days of at-home urine dipsticks for blood. Again, the basis for a diagnosis of babesiosis is clinical. After I learned more, I realized my son was a textbook case of Babesia infection: tick-bitten and 4 days later presenting with rigors and fevers near 106° with drenching sweats and air hunger. His diagnosis could have been made without any diagnostic lab testing. Fortunately, treatment was started long before the lab tests were back. Nonetheless, the testing did show the existence of several co-infections and later helped decide the best combination of medicines and how long to treat. Diagnostic testing for Babesia can include blood smears looking for Maltese cross formations in the red cells, IFA, PCR, and FISH. Clongen will test for several different Babesia species. Screen for at least 2 strains if possible: B. *microti* and B. *duncani* (which may also include the strain formerly named WA-1), since these two respond to different treatment regimes. If you cannot assess for both, then treat as though both are present. If FISH is positive, that is very strong support for a Babesia diagnosis.

3. **Ehrlichiosis/Anaplasmosis:** Morulae can sometimes be seen in WBCs by experienced observers. There may be a triad of lab results that support the diagnosis including low WBCs, low platelets, and elevated LFTs.

However these findings can occur in a number of other conditions. Diagnostic testing can include HME and HGA titers (either IgM or IgG) or PCR. For these diseases, treat fast based on clinical judgment.

4. **Bartonellosis**: Diagnostic testing can include IFA and PCR. Efforts to identify common strains of Bartonella such as B. *quintana* and B. *henselea* are often first attempted using antibody tests. Remember, there is much taxonomic confusion around Bartonella and we may think we want to test for B. *henselea* when we are actually looking for BLOs. PCR is sometimes used to screen, but positive yield may be low. Antibody tests may fail to detect Bartonella even when it is present by PCR testing. Since Bartonella stimulates vascular development, the measurement of vascular endothelial growth factor (VEGF) can suggest the presence of this pathogen. Elevated levels <u>might</u> mean that the person is infected with Bartonella since the pathogen may use this factor to enter into the cells making up the blood vessels. VEGF is performed at many commercial laboratories and cancer hospitals. Note that Bartonella is not the only reason VEGF can be elevated, and high levels could mean many things including cancer, so don't miss other important reasons for an elevation.

5. **Mycoplasma** *fermentans*: This pathogen presents challenges in all respects. Diagnostic testing can include IFA and PCR which may help uncover active cases. If the H&P supports the diagnosis of M. *fermentans*, consider addressing this difficult pathogen without confirmatory lab data since you might NEVER get it. In the meantime, the patient gets sicker and sicker. Note that professional psychological testing may help in the long-run with diagnosis and treatment in these patients.

6. **Colorado tick fever**: Diagnostic testing can include IFA for the tick pathogen and complement fixation techniques.

7. **Powassan viral encephalitis**: Standard serological tests have been reported successful in supporting the diagnosis of POW. I have never ordered a test for Powassan encephalitis. Most physicians have not, including most TBI experts. Call your most trusted lab and see what they recommend.

8. **Q fever**: Here you are looking for evidence of Coxiella *burnetii*. IFA, PCR, complement fixation, and agglutination antibodies have all been used to identify this pathogen. If LFTs are especially high, think Q fever.

9. **RMSF**: Since RMSF rarely if ever becomes chronic and since it so readily responds to antibiotic, there is usually no need to do a routine screen. Generally, it's all over before the results get back. If you think of RMSF, treat it before you test it. Treat on first suspicion and don't wait for confirmation by antibody or other testing. If testing is needed, IFA is the standard choice with a sensitivity over 90%. RMSF can increase CPK. Identification of Rickettsia has been made from biopsies of skin lesions. RMSF antibodies in asymptomatic patients probably represent past exposure and not current disease.

10. **Tularemia:** This pathogen is one of the few of the TBIs that grows well in cultures. In labs, personnel must be protected since it is highly contagious and lab workers are at risk. This bacterium loves air and stays viable in blood and tissues. In tularemia, most show a leukocytosis, but total WBCs may be normal with a disproportionate amount of PMNs. Diagnostic testing can include the usual suspects: antibody detection, IFA, or PCR.

B. Tests for concurrent infections

In addition to tick-borne co-infections, patients can be suffering from a number of concurrent conditions. Since even sick people get sick, we must be vigilant so that we are not overlooking something that can impede recovery. Concurrent illnesses can be infectious or result from any manner of other etiologies. We may never know which came first: the TBI or the co-morbidity. Did the patient's abnormal blood sugars predispose to a more intense manifestation of Lyme, or did Lyme cause a disruption of normal glucose metabolism? We can only play the hand that is dealt us in trying to help these patients. Take action, rather than place blame.

Infections – With Lyme there is an alteration of the host's immune system, potentially resulting in a greater susceptibility to other infections or to an increase in the intensity of these diseases. The most common infections you might be looking for in a TBI population are listed below. Order testing for these pathogens when clinically indicated. The following possible diagnoses marked by an * are of particular interest in TBI patients.

1. **Hepatitis A, B, C**

   A: HAV antibodies – IgM for current infection and IgG for past infection

   B: HBV assessments:

   > HbsAg - current infection, acute or chronic
   >
   > HbsAb - previous infection or past vaccination
   >
   > HbeAb - current infection, assesses infectivity

   C: HCV-Ab: current or previous infection (80% chronic) HCV-RNA

2. **Streptococcus:*** We don't pay as much serious attention to Strep as we did in the past. Today, if a child gets a sore throat, the parents want the instant test and the antibiotics. Be aware of the importance of monitoring TBI patients for Strep. In some patients, Strep can have significant sequelae such as rheumatic fever, forms of toxic shock, glomerulonephritis, and PANDAS. Strep can also complicate the diagnosis and delay the recovery in TBI patients. So think about Strep and look for it, if clinically appropriate. Cultures are first-line testing. If you remain suspicious after a negative culture, consider antibody testing against Group A β-hemolytic Streptococci. Testing usually involves agglutination with antigen from the throat mixed with known Strep antibody. Specificity is good, but sensitivity is only moderate. In TBIs, look for Strep when the patient experiences tics, OCD, or signs of PANDAS.

PEARL: The role of antineuronal antibodies is just beginning to be explored primarily as they relate to the symptoms of PANDAS. Initially, pediatric autoimmune neuropsychiatric disorders were only thought to follow the body's mismanagement of a Strep infection. Now the possibility of some TBI pathogens causing the body to make antibodies against its own neurons is appearing more likely. If you have a patient presenting with symptoms of PANDAS, look for both unresolved Strep and the presence of TBIs, especially Lyme and Bartonella.

Strep antibodies mimic those of Bartonella. This biological resemblance could possibly explain the similarity of post-acute neuropsychiatric symptoms. Consider antibody tests looking for antistreptolysin-O antibody as well as others including streptozyme DNAase B. If these come back positive in a person presenting with a PANDAS-like syndrome, then consider treatment: appropriate antibiotics including those for Strep and any involved TBIs *and* IV γ-globulin. Plasmapheresis is then used to clean up the debris from all the deceased pathogens.

3. **Herpes viruses**: Human herpes viruses (HHVs) are everywhere. Some are self-limiting, but others can result in long-term and disabling problems. In TBI patients who are difficult to diagnose, look especially for CMV and EBV. Herpes simplex viruses notoriously evade the immune system by messing with presenting antigens on the cell surface and in many other ways. Chicken pox now may mean shingles years from now. The majority of children have either HHV-1 or HHV-2 or both.

   a. <u>HHV-1</u> – Also called herpes simplex virus 1 or HSV-1. This virus causes cold sores and is ubiquitous and contagious. In some populations, essentially everyone has been infected. The effect HSV-1 has on the immune system is demonstrated each time a "run down" person develops a cold sore. If the immune system is healthy, cold sores are rare. If the immune system is compromised, cold sores will manifest. They often appear when a person is battling a cold, hence the name. There is a questionable link between HSV-1 and Alzheimer's disease.

   b. <u>HHV-2</u> – Also called herpes simplex virus 2 or HSV-2. This virus is the etiologic agent for genital herpes and is common and contagious.

   c. <u>HHV-3</u> – Represents a group of common, contagious viruses that result in a number of well-known diseases. HHV-3 is the varicella zoster responsible for chickenpox, shingles, and herpetic neuralgia. Again, the effect of these viruses on the immune system is sometimes obvious and other times obscure. Although individuals rarely get chicken pox twice, that does not mean the virus leaves the body. Hiding inactive in the dorsal root ganglia along the spine, the virus will emerge again when the individual is especially debilitated for other reasons. The skin lesions of shingles and the intense pain of herpetic neuralgia are the evidence. The virus lies dormant in the ganglia (clumps of nerves forming small centers of activity positioned on both sides of the spinal cord) until conditions become favorable for their reappearance. The symptoms surface years later distinctly on one side of the body. The skin lesions usually look like a strip of concentrated chicken pox. The connection between chicken pox and shingles took years to make and even longer for herpetic neuralgia.

   d. <u>HHV-4</u>* – Epstein-Barr virus is thought to be the cause of infectious mononucleosis and generally provides adaptive immunity. (Nonetheless, I have a positive EBV test in my hand from when my son was sick in middle school and another positive from last summer. Both clinical presentations were identical, with huge lymphadenopathy, severe sore throat, fever, and incapacitating fatigue. When Chris was symptomatic last summer his HCP said he couldn't possibly have mono twice. I later learned that EBV can reactivate in people with some defect in their immune system.) Early in the disease course, antivirals such as Valtrex or Acyclovir might be considered to attenuate the severity of symptoms.

   e. <u>HHV-5</u>* – Cytomegalovirus often goes unnoticed and remains an asymptomatic infection indefinitely. However, CMV can be a life-threatening condition in the immunocompromised. As with many of the HHVs, CMV can remain latent in the body for long periods. CMV can be transmitted to the fetus and congenital CMV can cause problems in the newborn. About 1 in 150 neonates are born with CMV. This infection can be especially problematic in babies also at risk for a congenital TBI, where it can compromise diagnosis and recovery. Once present, the virus stays for life. CMV can be tested in urine, eye fluid, serum, breast milk, respiratory lavage, CSF, birth tissues, and biopsy specimens.

   f. <u>HHV-6</u> –This herpetic virus can cause roseola, also called exanthum subitum. While usually self-limiting, this infection can cause seizures and encephalitis. Over the years, inconclusive association has been made between HHV-6 and autism and various chronic fatigue-type syndromes. Look for evidence of HHV-6 in TBI patients who do not respond to conventional treatments or who are difficult to diagnose.

   g. <u>HHV-7</u> – No attributable disease but may cause a roseola-like syndrome

   h. <u>HHV-8</u> – Responsible for Kaposi's sarcoma in the immunocompromised

4. Mycoplasma *pneumoniae** - This pathogen is NOT the Mycoplasma *fermentans* listed with the potential TBI co-infections. M. *pneumoniae* is the causative agent for atypical pneumonia also called "walking pneumonia." Many signs of M. *pneumoniae* mimic those found in TBI patients, especially fever and respiratory symptoms including dry and frequent cough. Antibody testing can be used to identify M. *pneumoniae*. This pathogen has been found in ticks from drags in Connecticut by a team from the University of New Haven led by Eva Sapi. Whether this pathogen should be *promoted* to co-infection is yet to be determined.

5. Candida* overgrowth can complicate the presentation and management of TBI cases. Fungus commonly overgrows in people on antibiotics or in those who have depressed immune systems. Antibiotics can eliminate the "good" flora in the GI tract allowing for a fungal surge. A repressed immune system, like that common to the TBI infections, enhances the imbalance. Since Candida is a normal flora, it is sometimes hard to tell when the line has been crossed. Symptoms that have been attributed to Candida overgrowth mimic those of many TBIs and include: allergy-like symptoms, anxiety, hyperactivity, ADD, signs of inflammation, GI complaints, lethargy, eye problems, fatigue, rashes, urinary tract problems, yeast infections, dandruff, lactose intolerance, OCD, muscle and bone pain, weakness, dermatitis, itching, swelling, and white tongue. Of course, Candida might confound

the clinical picture in TBIs. Testing can be done to look for Candida proteins, but antibody levels such as IgA, IgM, and IgG are probably a more sensitive screen. A high sugar diet, antacids, and steroids can all contribute to the problem. Adding probiotics to a course of antibiotics might help keep the flora in the gut in balance and the fungus in check. An entire section is devoted to Candida overgrowth in Chapter 21: *Differential Diagnosis and Concurrent Disease* with additional information in *Ancillary Treatments*.

6. Parasites: Consider Chlamydia and the parasites that result in filariasis, amebiasis, and giardiasis.

7. Chlamydia *pneumoniae* has been found in tick drags in CT. At this point, we have no idea whether C. *pneumoniae* causes disease in these populations and, if so, whether it is a co-infection or a concurrent infection. Split those hairs. What is important is to think of C. *pneumonia* in recalcitrant patients when the clinical picture suggests it as a possibility.

PEARL: Recall that Dr. Sapi from the University of New Haven has identified Chlamydia pneumoniae, *Mycoplasma* pneumoniae, *EBV, and CMV in her Connecticut tick drags. She has found these potential pathogens with and without Bb present.*

C. Assessment for co-morbid conditions

In addition to their TBI, patients can have an unrelated pre-existing condition OR be more susceptible to other conditions because of the TBI. For example, Bb can so impact hormonal balance that a patient might have first-time thyroid problems. In others, unrecognized problems with sugar metabolism may be pushed over the edge of diabetes with a Bb infection. Either way, concurrent medical conditions can mask or overshadow TBI signs and symptoms, complicating diagnosis and treatment and delaying recovery.

Too often we find a scapegoat diagnosis and stop there. Do NOT get trapped in an evidence-based medicine algorithm that restricts your thinking and ability to be flexible. An individual can have two or more pathologic processes active at one time. Do not presume that the tick is the sole culprit.

In each case, especially where a major body system is significantly impacted, such as the heart or the nervous system, presume that there may be more than one etiology supporting the pathology. What would you do for this patient if TBIs were not a factor? Always consider the problem through TBI lenses and then take them off. Do the work-up you would do with a TBI and without. Remember, people die from TBIs. They need all their cylinders firing. All body systems must be allowed to perform optimally.

Conditions like heart problems, diabetes, congenital problems, autism, autoimmune disorders, underlying respiratory problems, thyroid dysfunction, and neuropsychiatric diagnoses all need to be put on the table for review. Some of these issues may have been subclinical for years, and now the presence of a TBI brings them to light. For example, neuropsychiatric problems are common in TBIs. Is the problem only the TBI? Rule out other medical reasons for the symptoms such as thyroid defects, parathyroid imbalance, hypercalcemia, deficiencies of Vitamins B12 or D, porphyria, SLE, syphilis, or Wilson's disease. The almost limitless number of autoimmune and immune-influenced conditions should be considered here. The list of these conditions is contained in the *Differential Diagnosis* chapter as well as in the *Patient History* form.

In some cases, heavy metal poisoning might be responsible for at least some of the symptoms attributed to TBIs. Screening for heavy metals can be performed by most commercial labs. Usually a urine sample is collected. The metals most commonly tested include: antimony, arsenic, bismuth, boron, cadmium, cobalt, copper, lead, mercury, selenium, tellurium, thallium, and zinc. If you have a sick person who is not getting better, think of what else might be contributing to their distress. Don't dismiss the contribution that might be made by fungal overload, heavy metals, allergies, and other less common etiologies.

III. STUDIES TO FOLLOW CLINICAL COURSE OR EFFECTIVENESS OF TREATMENT

Once the diagnosis is made, or you are as close as you are going to get for the time being, it's time to manage the case. This might be a matter of logic and common-sense. Parameters that measure as "bad" when the patient is actively ill, should get better as the person recovers. For example a low H&H in babesiosis should improve as the patient gets better. If the patient is deteriorating, one would expect a deterioration in her lab work as well. Do recognize that the picture painted by lab results might lag behind the actual clinical picture. Of course, the premise of this entire text is to manage the patient, not the test result. If the patient is not feeling better, your efforts are not successful, no matter what the lab numbers say. Remember the best way to tell how a patient is doing is by asking the patient.

A. Testing to Follow Specific TBIs

In all cases, TBI treatment strategy should be based mostly on how the patient feels. Nonetheless, here are a few disease-specific tests that might help with your case management.

1. **Lyme:** CD57 NK cells are thought to be suppressed ONLY in Lyme disease. Measurement of CD57 looks at this specific subpopulation of NK (natural killer) cells. Low counts are seen in active Lyme disease. Theoretically, the lower the count, the sicker the patient. This measure is less useful in kids than adults since children tend to make fewer NK cells overall. While this test may provide guidance, always treat the patient not the test. LabCorp performs CD57 testing. Interpretation advice is provided in Chapter 19.

PEARL: There is some hint in the literature that NK cells may also be suppressed in some cases of autism. Fascinating!

2. **Babesiosis:** Hemoglobin and hematocrit can be followed to assess anemia status. Blood and bilirubin in urine should decrease as the patient improves. One author recommends daily urine dipsticks for red cells. Since urinary changes are not subtle when present in babesiosis, just visually checking the color should probably suffice. In recovery, CPK should normalize, as should evidence of hypercoagulation. Maltese crosses should be harder to observe in the red cells as the patient improves, but they aren't always the easiest marker to spot to begin with. Haptoglobin is a protein to which Hb released from lysed red cells is bound. Measurement of haptoglobin can be used as a screen for hemolytic anemia. If the patient has sxs of anemia but haptoglobin is normal the anemia is not likely due to hemolysis. If haptoglobin is low, then hemolysis could be the underlying etiology. Haptoglobin can be measured serially in babesiosis to track anemia status.

3. **Ehrlichiosis/Anaplasmosis:** The lab triad of low WBCs, low platelets, and elevated LFTs is not specific enough to be a reliable way to follow the clinical course of the disease. Similarly, while morulae should lessen in the white cells as the patient improves, they may not have been caught early on, so following treatment effect by counting morulae is not reliable.

4. **Bartonellosis:** While Bartonella may increase coagulability more than any other TBI, a return to more normal clotting is not specific enough to use as a measure. A few authors mention the use of VEGF levels to assess clinical status. Since *Bartonella* stimulates vascular development, the measurement of vascular endothelial growth factor could potentially suggest the presence of this pathogen. Elevated levels <u>might</u> mean that the person is infected with Bartonella since the pathogen may use this factor to enter into the

cells making up the blood vessels. Changes in levels of VEGF could allow monitoring of an individual's progress. If VEGF declines or returns to normal then, the antibiotics may be doing their job. These results could help with decisions regarding length of therapy. VEGF is performed at many commercial laboratories and cancer hospitals. Note that Bartonella is not the only reason VEGF can be elevated. While decreasing VEGF may provide support regarding the effectiveness of treatment of bartonellosis, count on the patient more than the test. Comparing sequential changes in neuropsychiatric testing might help monitor treatment effect.

5. **RMSF:** Recovery from RMSF should return CPK to normal but we don't know if or why CPK might be raised with RMSF in the first place.

Alas, you are essentially left to rely on your clinical judgment to assess how well your patient is doing and if your treatment plan is effective. Ask the patient.

PEARL: Rely on your patients to tell you how they are doing. They are much more reliable than any lab result. Even very young children can tell if they are "all better," "better," or "not better." They can make impressive, fine distinctions that can match the sensitivity and specificity of just about any test. If they say they're not better, believe them and pursue a management course that will help them improve. Don't provide their answers for them: "You're feeling all better now, aren't you, little Boris?" That approach might make you feel better, but it doesn't do anything for the underlying condition of the patient. Let them tell you their reality in their words. In fact, simply ask, "What would make you feel better?" This might steer you to a more targeted treatment plan.

B. Assessment of Immune Function

The presentation and intensity of TBIs are closely related to the function of the immune system. Some of these studies can be ordered at the initial visit, like HLA-DR2 and DR4 to see how much of the clinical presentation of Lyme might be an autoimmune tendency. These patients might need a different treatment approach than those who do not present these specific antigens. Further, if the disease is not responding as well as hoped, a more comprehensive examination of immune function may be indicated. Both Lyme and the presence of co-infections can impact immune response, often in unexpected ways. A number of the following assessments might also help with the differential diagnosis. Much of the material below is explained in Chapter 19: *Scientific Basis and Interpretation of Study Results.* To better understand what is happening with your patient from an immune perspective, consider:

1. **RF** (rheumatoid factor) is an immunoglobulin (antibody) present in the serum of 50% to 95% of patients with rheumatoid arthritis. Although not specific for RA, RF is helpful in diagnosing that condition. Testing for RF is useful in the differential diagnosis of rheumatoid arthritis and other connective tissue diseases. Without either great sensitivity or specificity, IgM of RF is present in the serum of patients with a variety of infectious processes such as leprosy, TB, syphilis, bacterial endocarditis, hepatitis, influenza, and numerous collagen vascular diseases such as lupus and scleroderma. While it will not give you a diagnosis, RF might steer you in parsing out what is happening with your case. Order RF if you want to have more insight into which mechanism might be operating in a Lyme patient with predominate joint complaints. Patients with pre-existing RA, get bitten by ticks, too. More than one thing can be happening at a time.

2. **ANA** (antinuclear antibody) is a group of antibodies that react against normal cell protein. Found in a number of immune disorders such as lupus and other connective tissue diseases, ANA is likely present in many autoimmune conditions. Order an ANA if your differential includes Lyme, SLE, RA, CREST, Raynaud's, mixed connective tissue disorders, or other conditions with a possible autoimmune component.

PEARL: Do not get antinuclear antibodies and antineuronal antibodies mixed up.

3. **Complement** is a group of proteins that play an important role in immune response through a complex cascade of reactions. Complement is known to be consumed when antigen/antibody complexes are formed. Antibodies can't do all the work themselves so their efforts are *complemented* by these biomolecules. If complement levels are low it might be inferred that complement is being used in the formation of antigen/antibody complexes, which in terms of TBIs might be a good thing. But, if complement consumption goes too far and there is not enough complement around for the antibody to use in latching onto its antigen, the whole defense system is at risk. The measurement of complement in immune complexes is starting to be used in the search for understanding and ultimately in diagnosing inflammatory, autoimmune, rheumatologic, and infectious diseases. Individual complement levels are sometimes measured in the management of TBI patients. Their role in TBIs is just beginning to be explored. Levels of circulating immune complexes can be measured serially to determine the effect of treatment or help assess clinical status. Tissue from biopsies can be used to look for Ag/Ab complexes.

a. **Complement C1Q** is measured using a binding assay to find sites on immune complexes and the amount of those complexes in the circulation. C1Q complex levels may shed some light in puzzling cases. If levels are low, the result suggests an autoimmune mechanism in play; if high, a persistent, on-going infection is suggested.

b. **Complement C3** is used in the diagnosis and management of diseases such as kidney problems and lupus and in many inflammatory conditions. When antibodies bind to a foreign protein, C3 attaches to the complex and signals for help from other parts of the immune cascade. C3d is a fragment of C3 that serves as a sign to certain B cells. Likewise, immune complex C3d may suggest that a persistent infection is driving an autoimmune clinical presentation.

REDUNDANT PEARL: C3d levels might provide information in Lyme cases. These molecules reflect the prevalence of toxins and infectious agents and may prove to be a good monitor of overall pathogen burden and indicator of an on-going inflammatory process. A result > 40 is an index of persistent inflammation. If the person seems to be improving, but C3d levels are still at 40 or above, something pathological is probably still going on inside this patient, either a simmering infection or an autoimmune process.

c. **Complement CH50** levels can be used to monitor complement deficiencies and to assess disease progression in patients with lupus, nephritis, or a variety of infections. CH50 is a measure of the overall health of the complement system and indicates how much complement is available to mount an attack. CH50 can be used to follow autoimmune conditions.

d. **Complement individual immunoglobulin profiles:** Quantitative measures can be done for each of the distinct immunoglobulin (antibody) proteins. In many specialized diagnostic tests, both IgM and IgG should be ordered to help with the chronology in each individual's case and to avoid missing the presence of antibodies due to fluctuating levels in the blood. Each result could have potential clinical significance.

PEARL: When concerned about adequate immune response, consider ordering total complement, C1Q, CH50, and C3d.

PEARL: One hypothesis as to why so many serologic tests are false negatives is that most antibody is tied up with complement and antigen and therefore not available in sufficient quantities to bind with the test reagents.

PEARL: More detail regarding the role of complement is provided in Chapter 3: Gentle Immunology *and in Chapter 19:* Scientific Basis and Interpretation of Study Results.

4. **ESR** or erythrocyte sedimentation rate is a nonspecific measure of the speed at which erythrocytes (red blood cells) settle out of unclotted blood. ESR suggests the presence of inflammation and generally monitors the onset and progress of inflammatory disorders. In TBI patients, ESR is used to detect the presence of inflammation and to help rule out autoimmune disorders. Rarely does the ESR tell you anything you don't already know: that a patient is inflamed or infected. Serial readings might suggest therapeutic response.

5. **CRP** (C-reactive protein) is an abnormal protein detectable in blood only during active phases of certain illnesses. CRP is therefore associated with the presence of inflammation and is used to help rule out autoimmune disorders. In TBI patients, CRP is used as a nonspecific marker of inflammation and is occasionally useful for discriminating between diagnoses and for monitoring clinical course. CRP can increase a thousand fold in inflammatory conditions and will respond to inflammation in 6 to 10 hours. The protein has a short half-life of about 6 hours and is most useful in the first 24 hours of the disease process when ESR is still normal.

PEARL: Chapter 3: Gentle Immunology *has a detailed section discussing MHCs (HLAs) and CDs that are referred to below.*

6. **HLA markers**: As part of the MHC system, human leukocyte antigens are protein markers primarily on white cells that distinguish between *self* and non-*self.* HLA-DR2 and HLA-DR4 markers are especially pertinent to Lyme patients. These markers are found in a subpopulation of the general populace who will tend to respond to Bb infection with an autoimmune reaction. Think about ordering HLA-DR2 and HLA-DR4 in Lyme as early in the work-up as possible. Since these markers are known to suggest the potential for an autoimmune presentation, their presence can significantly impact treatment decisions. Consider HLA-DR2 and HLA-DR4 levels in those patients who have on-going, intractable, intense, or atypical presentations of Lyme. Since it is hard to predict early on who will develop these autoimmune type manifestations, ordering HLA-DR2 and HLA-DR4 at initial work-up may be prudent.

PEARL: The presence of HLA-B27 indicates that the person is predisposed to the spondyloarthropathies, other rheumatoid problems, and IBS.

7. **CDs**: Clusters of differentiation are groups of protein markers on the surface of white blood cells that serve to identify and classify the cell types. Each marker has a specific function within the system like passing along biochemical signals. CD subsets that may be important for the TBI patient include:

    a. **CD4** is a marker found on essentially all T helper cells, some macrophages (monocytes), and even a few B cells. CD4 is responsible for sending signals from the T cell receptor. CD4 is sometimes ordered as a part of an immune evaluation in TBI patients.

    b. **CD8** is found on T suppressor and T cytotoxic cells which are important in the defense against viruses.

    c. **CD57** marks a subpopulation of NK (natural killer) T lymphocytes. These are thought to be suppressed ONLY in Lyme disease (and perhaps select autism cases). In theory, the lower the CD57, the more suppression of these Lyme-specific NK cells and the more active the Lyme disease. So, the lower the count, the sicker the patient. Suggestions on interpretation of CD57 levels are outlined in Chapter 19. Note that kids and teens do not make NK cells in the same proportion as adults, so measurement of CD57 may not be as useful in the pediatric population. As always, treat the patient and not the lab report. LabCorp performs CD57 testing.

8. **Interleukins**: ILs are cytokines (biomolecules) that help regulate the immune system, inflammation, and the formation of blood cells. Various IL families are made by different cells and have unique roles. ILs appear critical to normal function of the CNS in ways not clearly understood but seem to impact the hippocampus and its role in memory, learning, and nerve signal potentiation. ILs currently play a role in assessment and treatment of certain cancers such as melanoma and kidney carcinoma. ILs have been measured in conjunction with TBIs, but the specifics of their possible role(s) has yet to be clearly defined. Some researchers and HCPs use measures of ILs such as IL-6 and IL-IB in TBI management. Future work may reveal a less ambiguous function for these molecules.

PEARL: Smith et al have shown that IL-6 may mediate the immune reactions in pregnant rodents that lead to changes in gene expression, cell histology, and abnormal behaviors such as those seen in autism and schizophrenia. Interesting...

9. **TNF-α:** Tumor necrosis factor-α is a cytokine that is sometimes measured to assess the degree of chronic inflammation. This molecule is a growth factor for both immune cells and the osteoclasts that break down bone. Sometimes TNF is part of a broader cytokine panel. Since TBIs can be associated with significant chronic inflammation and on-going infections, elevated TNF-α may be measured in these patients (...if we indeed know what defines a normal level). As mentioned earlier, do not order tests if you already know the answer or the result would not alter anything in your management plan.

10. **ECP:** Eosinophil cationic protein is a biomolecule that is released during degranulation of eosinophils and is related to inflammation, asthma, and parasitic infections. ECP testing is sometimes used to assess level of inflammation, disease progression, and response to treatment. Will the test result tell you anything you don't already know? ECP is toxic to neurons so in patients with neuropsychiatric symptoms, ECP may provide additional information.

11. **Antineuronal antibodies:** As outlined in Chapters 2 and 19, work with antineuronal antibodies is an up-and-coming development in neurologic and immunologic sciences. In some patients association with Strep, Bb, or Bartonella seems to result in an autoimmune-type reaction where neurons in the nervous system are mistakenly targeted for elimination. These conditions can present with OCD, tics, anxiety, panic, aggression, and other intense neuropsychiatric problems. Currently, specific testing to identify antineuronal antibodies are not readily available. Yet if you have a TBI patient with neuropsychiatric manifestations, consider somewhat less specific testing from Quest called the anti-ganglioside antibody panel 3. These studies measure anti-lyso-ganglioside, anti-tubulin, and anti-dopamine 1 and anti-dopamine 2. This testing can be useful in uncovering what might be happening with TBI patients with severe, intractable neuropsychiatric manifestations. Call the lab for guidance. These patients may respond to a different treatment regimen than traditionally used, therefore the possibility of antineuronal antibodies should be considered when a patient presents with intense neuropsychiatric symptoms. More detailed information is provided in Chapter 19.

PEARL: As you order the testing in the work-up for antineuronal antibodies, make sure you are also working to uncover the underlying infectious agent so an appropriate antibiotic regimen can be targeted to that pathogen. Treatment with IV IgG has NOT always been shown to be effective in these cases UNLESS proper and adequate antibiotic therapy is included. Here, look for Strep, Bb, and Bartonella. You may need to treat empirically.

C. Therapeutic Drug Levels

Some HCPs swear by drug levels. I have not had the best luck. Drug levels were hard enough to do in the rigid confines of clinical trial work for commercial drug development. There we had all the resources imaginable at our disposal. I consider them a colossal pain in the neck with little return on investment. After you mess with fasting and non-fasting, timing-after-dose, peaks and troughs, slow versus fast metabolizers, all the possible confounders from hydration level to whether or not the subject drank grapefruit juice and ate kale, plus the myriad lab variations, the juice just ain't worth the squeeze. Before drawing routine therapeutic levels, I would first make sure the drug is being taken as directed and adjust the dose as needed. Next, I'd consider a different medicine. Therapeutic drug levels give you numbers but they may have little relationship to the patient's reality. If you feel better ordering drug levels, ask the lab the best way to order such testing in terms of peaks and troughs and reference ranges for that particular drug. Always correlate lab results with the clinical presentation. After that diatribe, I do order drug levels in a number of cases such as on-going use of vancomycin and digoxin. Further, in those patients where you believe everything is being done correctly, and still the patient is not responding as expected, drug levels may provide a clue that the person is not achieving the levels needed for optimal effect.

Okay, I surrender. If you decide to draw drug levels, the trough should be drawn just before the next dose is due. The peak draw will vary depending on the particular drug you are assessing. Take the medicine and then wait the time specified when the level should peak for that particular drug. Perhaps two to four hours or longer. Do not use the approach my husband experienced in the local hospital where they continued to draw his blood *before* they gave him *any* of the medicine.

IV. STUDIES TO LOOK FOR ADVERSE REACTIONS TO TREATMENT

If you are planning an aggressive or long-term course of antibiotics consider baseline CBC, LFTs, as well as BUN and creatinine. This will at least give you a ball park from where you can monitor for AEs. Now, this baseline will not necessarily be "normal" for the patient since they are already sick or you wouldn't be planning a treatment program for them. This is just a place to start your vigil.

Just because an adverse event occurs in *association* with the use of a drug does NOT mean that the drug *caused* the event. Drug companies like to find every excuse to explain why the drug did not cause the problem. In contrast, government regulators try to blame the drug for everything wrong in the west end of the galaxy. The truth, as always, lies somewhere in between. Your obligation is to parse out this truth. You do that by drawing baselines and following appropriate lab work for patterns and trends. Based on your best information gathering and common-sense, you must decide if it looks like *this* drug is hurting *this* patient at *this* time. Your job is not to decide if this drug is the worst drug ever to be found in the cosmos, nor should you feel compelled to defend the drug from all detractors. Focus on this patient, this time.

If you suspect that the medicine is causing a problem, weigh the risks and benefits. You may need to consider a dose adjustment or a change in drugs. Unfortunately, depending on the severity of the illness, types of co-infections, allergies, or drug intolerance, treatment options may be limited. In discussion with patients and caretakers, try to make the best decisions regarding the course of action.

Just because an adverse event is listed in the product label does not mean all or any of your patients will experience this event. In contrast, just because it has never been seen before does not mean your patient will not be the first to experience this new event. (You could finally make it into *The New England Journal of Medicine*!)

Forgive the redundancy, but I am fanatical about not getting stuck in the false security of the WNL test result. Recall that a pattern is the recurrence of an event again and again. A person takes a drug and her creatinine elevates. The next time she takes the same drug, her creatinine elevates. Patterns do not need to be rigid to suggest that you should pay attention. If you don't compare the new result to the old result, you are not going to see a pattern. Patterns can seem to occur by chance, but if the same thing keeps happening, it is more likely that there is some causal association.

Trends are more likely to slink into the data set. To spot a trend you have to look at a number of data points. That's why you monitor lab work over time. A trend is a general movement of findings with a drift in a certain direction. Trends can be obvious or subtle. Hematocrit can trend down, suggesting bleeding or other causes of anemia. Creatinine can trend up, indicating a possible kidney problem. Trends are leading you to discover something. If you don't look, you won't see. It is much easier to just say all is WNL, but that shortchanges your patient. Look at the last test results and the ones before that.

I spent nearly 20 delightful years checking to see if association meant causation. Association means something occurs concurrently with something else. A exists alongside B. Causality means A *caused* B. That is a BIG difference that people mix up all the time, especially the media. After years spent in occupational medicine looking to see why the workers at the fibers plant in Mexico City had high red cells counts (it was the altitude and the smoking, not the benzene), I developed a system of analyzing data that helps determine if one event causes another. I do not take credit for this logic process. I picked it up and put it together from many mentors and long-forgotten sources over the years.

A. Logic Steps Used in Causal Assessment

1. **Timing** – If Event A occurs AFTER Event B, then Event A could not have caused Event B. So if a patient has low potassium before taking a drug, then the drug did not cause the low potassium. If your thumb is red and swollen BEFORE it is hit by a hammer, the hammer did not cause the initial symptoms. That is not to say that the drug can't later contribute to the low potassium or that the hammer hit did not increase the pain in the thumb. To cause something to happen, the causal agent must be in place before the impact. For A to cause B, A has to be in place before B, not after. You can't have an allergic reaction to PCN before you take it. Blood thinner cannot thin blood before it has been administered, even in Lilith's[1] hospital.

2. **Bioplausibility** – Could this event even happen or does it defy the laws of science? An antibody against antigen A will not bind with antigen B except in some cases of cross-reactivity. Just won't happen. Can't. Implausible. But don't be fooled. Just because you don't understand a scientific concept does not mean it is outside the realm of possibility. Make sure it is actually implausible before you discredit the idea. The problem could be you.

3. **Challenge/Rechallenge** – This is the best way to assess causality. If A causes B and you take A away and then B goes away, that's strong support for causality. If you reintroduce A, and then B reappears, you nailed it. It's pretty hard to talk your way out of that one.

4. **Confounders** – What could be confusing this picture? In the workers I studied in Mexico City, three things confounded the theory that benzene caused them to have high RBC counts: 1) high altitude causes an increase in red cells; 2) smoking causes an increase in red cells; and 3) benzene should lower the red cell count, not raise it. These three facts were all confounders to the hypothesis that benzene raised red cell counts in these workers.

5. **Consistency with what's expected for drug and class** – Every person who has gone to medical school has heard the adage, "If it walks like a duck and quacks like a duck, it's probably a duck." Drugs in the same class tend to act similarly. Further, if the drug has done it before, it could do it again. The best predictor of

future behavior is past behavior. If Rocephin has been known to cause gallstones in some patients, and your patient on Rocephin develops gallstones, consider that it might be the Rocephin.

6. **No better explanation** – If you've looked and looked and thought and thought and brainstormed all kinds of alternatives and still can't find another explanation for an adverse event, it very well could be the drug, darn it.

B. Known Drug Reactions

Some medications commonly used in treating TBIs merit special mention. All long-term use of antibiotics should be followed for potential problems. Drugs have to be metabolized and eliminated from the body in some fashion. In most cases, the liver and kidney take care of these jobs. So if the drug is going to cause harm, it is most likely to do so in the places where it is most concentrated or spends the most time. If you know how a drug is metabolized and excreted you will know the best places to look for problems.

In general, a minimum screen for adverse drug events includes a CBC, basic LFTs such as ALT, and a BUN and creatinine to assess kidney damage. Try to establish baseline values before the medicine is started. These are not true baselines because the illness may also be skewing the results, but this is as good as it's going to get for now. Then follow these parameters at regular intervals. To start, about every 2 weeks is prudent. Of course, any adverse drug events that the patient notices should be reported to you immediately so you can determine if the plan needs to change (like stopping, adjusting, or changing the medicine). When you receive the follow-up results, don't just look at them, *interpret them*. Are there any patterns or trends suggesting damage? Compare the entire string of results available to you.

Some antimicrobials in our TBI arsenal have documented adverse consequences. That does not mean that every patient at every dose will have a problem. After months of Ketek, my son's LFTs remained fine. Most patients will NOT have any untoward consequences. Just so you can be prepared for anything, here is a list of suggested lab tests that will give you the best chance of catching potential problems. This list just mentions the potential lab abnormalities, not all possible AEs associated with these drugs. Check the *Antimicrobials* chapter for more information. For the following drugs, consider monitoring the listed parameters in addition to the CBC, ALT, BUN, and creatinine.

1. **Vancomycin:** Consider kidney function and therapeutic drug levels. (This doesn't mean that all of a

sudden, I am a big advocate of therapeutic drug levels, but if you have a patient on long-term, high-dose vanco, here might be a place to think about drug levels.) If levels are high, regroup.

2. **Fluoroquinolones:** (Such as ciprofloxin) Baseline EKG to watch for QTc prolongation. (If I did an EKG on every patient I ever started on Cipro, the entire medical system would be bankrupt...Oh, it is.) Look for liver and kidney problems, cardiotoxicity, pancreatic damage, and assess muscle wasting with CPKs. Baseline kidney function is useful.

3. **Macrolides:** With Biaxin (clarithromycin), Zithromax (azithromycin), and Ketek (telithromycin, actually a ketolide), monitor the QT and compare to a baseline EKG. Follow electrolytes, K, Ca, Mg, along with kidney and liver function. With long-term use, every 2 weeks is prudent. If macrolides are used with statins there may be myopathy. (CPK alert!) There have been deaths reported in conjunction with Ketek use. Because of allergies, my son had few options and had to remain on Ketek for months. He was monitored closely and had no known adverse effects. When using Ketek, order an EKG before starting treatment, as well as baseline LFTs. Another EKG can be performed 24 to 48 hours after the first dose. Then repeat the EKG and LFTs monthly. Most TBI-focused clinicians have not seen significant untoward effects with Ketek.

4. **Sulfa/trimethoprim:** (Bactrim, Septra) Follow liver, kidney, urine, and blood

5. **Rocephin:** (ceftriaxone) Here the big problem can be GALLSTONES. Rocephin is eliminated from the body through the bile, and stones can form from the high concentration of salts. Before you start a course of Rocephin, ask if there is a personal or family history of gallstones. Get a baseline US of the gallbladder and then follow regularly throughout the course of treatment. The stones usually diminish once the antibiotic is discontinued. Rocephin should not be used in premature babies with bilirubin problems. Keep an eye on that liver.

6. **Flagyl:** (metronidazole) Consider CBC with differential, WBCs, and electrolytes

7. **Rifampin:** (rifamycin) This drug stains the urine and other body fluids orange-red, so don't think you have red water fever when you are just being dyed by the drug. Draw CBC and LFTs at baseline and throughout the treatment course.

8. **TCNs:** Consider CBC with differential. Watch the hemoglobin, LFTs, and kidney functions. Monitor over the long-term. Note that doxycycline is often used in patients with renal impairment since it does not seem to accumulate in the kidney or increase the BUN. Still keep watch. Minocycline has rarely been associated with a lupus-like syndrome, including positive test results for SLE. Some of the literature cites this syndrome as irreversible, while others say the patient returns to normal after the minocycline is stopped. Rarely, minocycline has been associated with a thyroiditis and an autoimmune hepatitis requiring long-term treatment with azathioprine and prednisone. Most of these patients were on long-term minocycline for dermatologic conditions. Order liver and thyroid functions if clinically indicated and compare to baseline. Drugs past expiration usually just lose potency, but TCNs can become toxic when old.

9. **Quinine:** This product can cause hemolysis in patients with G6PD deficiency. Get a CBC with differential looking for thrombocytopenia. Watch for hematuria. Get a baseline EKG and follow for abnormal heart rhythms. Monitor the kidney, liver, and urine

10. **Lariam:** (mefloquine) Watch for QT prolongation. Monitor calcium levels and LFTs

11. **Aralen:** (chloroquine) Watch the liver and check CBC for porphyria. Use with caution in G6PD deficiency

12. **Plaquenil:** (hydroxychloroquine) Monitor liver, CBC, and muscle CPK. Use with caution in G6PD deficiency

13. **Mepron:** (atovaquone) Monitor liver. May diminish CoQ 10 levels

14. **Malarone**: A combination of atovaquone and proguanil. Watch liver and kidney

15. **Clindamycin:** (Cleocin) Consider liver, renal, CBC with differential, stool for C. *difficile* if symptomatic, kidney functions, and lytes for hydration

The above list is just for selected antimicrobials known to cause certain abnormal findings on lab testing. This is not a comprehensive list of all possible adverse events observed with these drugs. For a more inclusive catalog of AEs see the *Antimicrobials* chapter. If you want even more, read the product label.

With all antibiotic use, the occurrence of prolonged, frequent, loose stool should prompt the search for C. *difficile*. The biggest culprit is clindamycin, but any antibiotic can be responsible.

PEARL: Actually LOOK at the test results. Don't just scan down the page looking for the checkmarks in the normal range. Especially when looking at AEs that could be caused by a certain drug regimen, be vigilant. A patient can be within normal range in sequential tests and yet consistently trending to the abnormal. There could be something happening with this patient even though she remains WNL. If a patient has doubled or tripled her value and went from low WNL to high WNL, pay attention. Watch throughout the treatment course and take the time to assess the overall situation. Monitor the individual, not just the normal boxes. Look for patterns and trends. A pattern is something repeating over and over and a trend is a creeping up or down. Be especially vigilant with thyroid function and LFTs.

Possible Testing on Your First Visit with a TBI Patient

This patient may be new to you but not new to the TBI world. Many TBI patients have seen more than a dozen HCPs in their quest to get well. The person comes in with reams of paper and files. As part of their history, see what work-up they've already had done. You may find some valid reports that will save time and money now. Just as likely, you may have to start from scratch. If possible, have them send in copies of their records and results for your review prior to their first visit. Then spend time poring over these old reports.

Old negatives are no more valid than new negatives. While a positive test result may support a diagnosis, a negative test result merely says there was no evidence of the pathogen in this sample, using the testing methods of a certain lab on a particular day.

Based on what you already have in hand and the presentation of the patient, consider:

1. For Lyme: IgM & IgG Western blot, order ELISA only if required by insurers. (Recognizing that if the result is negative, the insurer will likely resist paying for anything else.) Consider Bb blood culture. The new methodology used by Advanced Laboratory Services appears to be highly sensitive. This test is best done BEFORE the patient is started on antibiotics or herbals or after the antibiotic has been discontinued for at least a month. In some cases, the HCP might be reluctant to discontinue treatment in order to draw the culture sample. Try to think of this option prior to the first dose of antibiotics if possible. Currently the lab requests 4 tubes of blood that may be too large a volume to extract from the smallest patients.

2. For ehrlichiosis/anaplasmosis: HME and HGA titers, white cell smears for morulae

3. For babesiosis: Red cell smear for Maltese crosses, cultures, IFA, PCR, and FISH. Maltese crosses are usually only seen in acute cases. Looking for RNA using FISH has been most useful in identifying the *microti* species.

4. For bartonellosis: IFA and PCR, although BLOs are likely the etiologic agent

5. For Mycoplasma *fermentans:* IFA and PCR

6. Depending on clinical presentation and history: Chronic fatigue panel, Chlamydia, HHV-6, HHV-8, Strep culture, Strep antibodies, M. *pneumoniae* antibodies, CMV IgG and IgM, and EBV. (Patients with Lyme can have a false positive heterophile mono screen without having EBV infection.)

7. Routine studies for baseline and diagnostic clues: CBC with differential, selected metabolic panel, kidney function tests such as BUN and creatinine, liver function tests such as alkaline phosphatase, ALT, AST, bilirubin. Some do initial thyroid functions with anti-thyroid antibodies as well as cortisol baselines.

8. Some HCPs do immune/autoimmune panels that could include ANA, RF, ESR, total complement, C3d, C4, CH50, IgA, IgM, IgG and subclasses, IgE, IL-6, TNF-α, anti-thyroid antibodies, antithyroglobulin, and HLA-DR2 and 4. This last test would be ordered to help determine if a Lyme patient is predisposed to an autoimmune type presentation that would require a different treatment approach. Consider HLA-DR2 and HLA-DR4 on potential Lyme patients early in the work-up cycle. Presence of these markers can change treatment strategy.

9. Make sure you order a baseline and follow-up EKG and other tests if the drugs you plan to use may cause problems in specific organs or you anticipate a pathogen like Lyme that may significantly impact the heart or other systems over time. Likewise, vision and hearing baselines are often prudent.

Do not order a test to which you already know the answer. Remember these people are already selling their car to pay for this work-up. Some docs order tests just because they can. Some order the test to show they know more than you.

Some authors recommended tests whose purpose I could not fathom even after I looked them up and searched and searched. Ask yourself, "Do I really need this test result? What will I do with it when I get it? Can I get my answer another way?"

Testing Considerations for the Intractable, Recalcitrant, Confounding Patient

Patients with complicated, prolonged TBIs can be challenging. Even the most experienced TBI specialist gets stumped, puzzled, and perplexed sometimes. Treating TBIs is HARD. Never give up. Never, not ever. Not once.

For the especially prolonged or complex cases consider: Immune/autoimmune panel if not already done, serial PCRs for suspected TBIs, a mycology panel, Lyme urine/blood /tissue PCR, Lyme DOT blot, reverse Western blot, look for RMSF, Brucella, Q-fever, tularemia, West Nile Virus, or Borrelia *lonestari*. Your checklist might include a repeat ANA, DS DNA, C3, complement C1Q, CMV and other HHVs, and Candida IgA, IgM, IgG. Look for more species-specific Babesia antibodies. Dig deeper for Bartonella. Really dig deep for the Mycoplasmas, not just M. *fermentans* but also M. *pneumonia*. Look for antibodies. Call your trusted lab and see what other more definitive testing might be possible. Try FISH.

If they just won't get better, or if they are getting worse, consider the possibility of any co-infections, an entirely wrong diagnosis, or the need for a totally new treatment plan. After you also consider that you never should have gone into medicine in the first place, TRY AGAIN. NEVER GIVE UP. Try again . . . and again. Imagine Winston Churchill crusading against TBIs, "We shall not flag or fail. We shall go to the end. We shall fight in France. We shall fight on the seas and the oceans. We shall fight with growing confidence and growing strength in the air. We shall defend our island, whatever the cost may be. We shall fight on the beaches, we shall fight on the landing grounds, we shall fight in the fields and in the streets, we shall fight in the hills. We shall never surrender."

Laboratory Information

TBD specialists often use Specialty Laboratories, Imugen, Clongen, IGeneX, and LabCorp. Routine lab tests and smears can be done at a TRUSTED local lab or hospital. Just because a lab is affiliated with your local hospital does not mean it is a good lab. If there was a national award for most false negative test results, I know a local lab that would qualify. You have to know enough to uncover what they don't know.

Please realize that even the most experienced TBI docs call the lab with some frequency. Occasionally, a lab will introduce a new procedure or discontinue an old test. More often than not, more than one laboratory will be needed to accommodate all the tests ordered for a single patient. No one can keep up with all the changes. If you do not KNOW the answer for sure, CALL THE LAB.

Just because a lab is listed below does not mean that these are the only good labs. I include the labs below because I know they do the kind of specialty work needed by TBI patients and because I am trying to make life easier for you by providing contact information and a pertinent menu. There may be many other fine labs out there that also do high quality work. Most labs will provide you with an order form that can serve as a checklist for your requests. Many will give you pages or pamphlets on ways to interpret the results and how to explain the findings to patients. Many do not mind being called for guidance and some are available for questions over the Internet. One way I choose my labs is by ease of contact, in addition to their technical acumen. As of mid-2013, here is a list of lab options. Some may no longer be available and the numbers may have changed, but I had good intentions:

1. **Medical Diagnostic Laboratory (MDL)** does ELISA and PCR among other tests. Phone: 1-609-570-1000 or 1-877-269-0090, www.mdlab.com. This lab has recently become entirely automated, which means that with some testing you might have to ask if human review is possible. They will evaluate ticks and their contents.

2. **Clongen** has a broad menu of organisms usually with the capacity to test for multiple strains. For example, they can test for several strains of Borrelia. They will provide test kits so that you can be sure your samples are properly collected and handled. Phone 1-301-916-0173. Fax 1-301-916-0175, www.clongen.com.

3. **Imugen** in Norwood, MA, has a good reputation for serologic testing. Phone 1-781-255-0770 or 1-800-246-8436

4. **IGeneX** provides testing for a number of TBIs as well as strains of the different pathogens using IFA, PCR, FISH, Lyme DOT blot, and antibody testing for the majority of the TBIs. Phone: 1-800-832-3200, www.igenex.com.

5. **Fry Clinical Laboratories** will use blood smears to attempt direct visualization of Babesia even when antibody testing is negative. Phone: 1-480-991-4555

6. **Specialty Laboratories** has had success in identifying Bartonella *henselae* IgG and IgM. Phone: 1-800-421-7110. This lab is now an independent sub-unit of Quest. In most cases you can have blood samples drawn at a local Quest site and then properly shipped to the Specialty Laboratories division.

7. **Advanced Laboratory Services** in Pennsylvania has developed what appears to be a more definitive blood

culture for Bb than previously available. I have talked to these people at length and found them very helpful. They have an excellent tool but also recognize its limitations. Phone: 1-855-238-4949.

Unfortunately, as with all serious illnesses, there are unscrupulous vendors out there waiting to take advantage of the vulnerable and naive. In the TBI community we often hear of a new lab or a new test that will revolutionize the diagnosis of a certain TBI. Rarely do these promises come to fruition. More likely is the follow-up rumor a few months later saying the lab was closed or the test didn't pan out. I wince when I witness how readily those who should know better buy the marketing spin. *Caveat emptor.* Your best defense is knowledge.

Testing the Tick

Despite how often we have been told to save the tick and show it to your HCP, no one really seems to care when you do. Occasionally a veteran TBI doctor will have the tick tested to see what pathogens may be lurking. Nonetheless, a layperson can commission her own analysis of the tick if she is so inclined, no doctor's order needed. Clongen will do this testing if you use their special form. They will test for Lyme (Bb), Babesia *microti,* and Bartonella *henselea*. This test can be ordered by a layperson AND if the specimen is not a tick you will not be charged. (Of course, they don't send your bug back either.)

Some state health or agriculture departments will identify ticks for you. Usually, they will tell you the species and the degree of engorgement as a way to tell how long the tick may have been present. One specimen was turned away because the tick was not sufficiently engorged. Today, we know that absence of engorgement does not guarantee absence of transmission. In fact, Willy Burgdorfer found that Bb in the salivary duct can be transmitted effectively, if not efficiently. Still Connecticut will not test a tick unless it is engorged. In New Jersey (if funding is still available), the state may test a tick for you. Inquire at 1-877-Tick-Test. Check state laboratories and veterinary schools.

PEARL: Until you find out exactly how the lab wants the tick shipped, save the tick, preferably alive, in a jar with moist paper towels.

The result may help convince an HCP that a patient actually has a TBI. Or, at least inspire him to look for a TBI in the person bitten by said tick. Or, as is often the case, he might ignore you. NEVER delay evaluation or treatment while waiting for test results on the tick (or the patient, for that matter).

Chapter 19 SCIENTIFIC BASIS & INTERPRETATION OF STUDY RESULTS - Detailed chapter contents

Chapter 19

SCIENTIFIC BASIS AND INTERPRETATION OF STUDY RESULTS

*Not detected does **NOT** mean **un**infected*

K. Spreen

Absence of evidence is not evidence of absence.

Some guy on Criminal Minds

Everyman takes the limits of his own field of vision for the limits of the world.

Arthur Schopenhauer

Now that I told you dozens of possible tests to order, the least I can do is suggest ways to interpret the results when they appear on your desk. Most results need to be compared to lab normals or previous results from the individual patient. Remember each bit of information is just one part of the overall clinical picture. Do not let test results override your judgment.

Don't obsess over units. Units are what they are and will be recorded based on the methods used by the reporting lab. With that said, units should make sense. When my son was little we were called by a near-by renowned children's hospital saying to bring Chris in IMMEDIATELY. He had no thyroid hormone. One parent was to rush in with the child while the other picked up his records from the pediatrician. When we arrived in Philadelphia with a happy, healthy kid, the doctor sheepishly informed us that the lab had misplaced a decimal and there was actually no problem. Focus on the nuances involved in the interpretation of the results. Since TBIs can do strange things to lab results, always keep your TBI filter on, but don't be blinded by it.

If possible, get a baseline for those parameters you intend to follow over time. Then look at the previous results when the new ones come in. Do not look just to confirm something is WNL, but also look for any patterns or trends working in the patient. The last chapter explained patterns and trends in lab data. Please keep that discussion in mind as you follow patients over time.

While I perpetually preach to order only those lab tests that you can use and that you understand, the existence of "metabolic panels" will provide you with many results that you not only don't need but that you wouldn't understand if your dog's life depended on it. There are dozens of packages or panels to choose from. Each commercial lab has a menu of panels that include 8, 18, 24, 36 or more tests. These are a "great deal" since the 24 tests are often cheaper than running the three studies that you actually want. I do not need a random glucose or a chloride or a CO_2 level on a wiggly 3-year-old, but here they come. This is all well and good until you get an abnormal that you have no idea what to do with and are stuck following it into eternity just because it's there.

For routine purposes, I prefer a "light" panel that includes basic LFTs and kidney function tests. After you establish some parameters on your patient, you can always come back and order testing targeted to the individual case.

The following list provides basic information on a variety of tests that may be pertinent to the management of TBI patients. The items include a minimal description of the test and what the result might mean to your patient. Any known confounders to interpretation are mentioned.

I. BLOOD COUNTS

Complete blood counts or **CBC**s usually include hemoglobin, hematocrit (H&H), red cell count with indices, reticulocytes, total WBCs, and a differential count that provides the proportion of each of the different type of white cell present.

Hemoglobin (Hb) is the iron-containing pigment of red blood cells that carries oxygen. Hb gauges the O_2-carrying ability of the blood and is measured in g/dL. In TBI patients, Hb can be useful in the diagnosis, monitoring of clinical course, and treatment success, especially in cases of babesiosis. Also, Hb can help when looking for AEs from medications used to treat TBIs. Hb levels vary considerably with age, gender, and race: highest at birth (15 to 24 g/dL) and lowering throughout childhood. In those over 15 y/o, Hb normals vary with gender with male levels between 14 to 18 g/dL and females 12 to 16 g/dL. Hemoglobin will be low in anemia, blood loss, and fluid overload.

PEARL: Haptoglobin is a protein that binds with free Hb released from lysed red cells and thereby decreases the oxidative capacity of the bound Hb. The haptoglobin-Hb complex is then removed, usually by the spleen. Measurement of haptoglobin can be used as a screen for hemolytic anemia and can be ordered in cases where babesiosis is suspected. If the patient has sxs of anemia but haptoglobin is normal the anemia is not likely due to hemolysis. If haptoglobin is low, then hemolysis could be the underlying etiology. Haptoglobin can be measured serially in babesiosis to track anemia status. This protein can also be increased in some inflammatory conditions and decreased in hemolytic disorders.

Hematocrit (Hct) is the percentage of the total blood volume that is made up of red cells. Hct varies with age, gender, and altitude. Menstruating females tend to have a lower level. The normal adult ranges from 42% to 54%, with kids slightly lower at 35% to 49%. Newborns are around 50%. Hct will be low in blood loss, anemia, over-hydration, and in cases where there is volume dilution such as pregnancy, edema, and long-term bed rest. Hct is high in polycythemias, dehydration, posttransfusion, and long-term exposure to high altitudes.

Reticulocyte count: Reticulocytes are immature RBCs that usually constitute between 0.5% and 1.5% of the total circulating red cells. More than 1.5% reticulocytes usually means that the body has pumped up the manufacture of red cells in order to compensate for some kind of loss. Here the body needs more oxygen-carrying capacity as is the case with many anemias, after severe bleeding, or when the individual is getting acclimated to high altitudes. Fewer than 0.5% reticulocytes can mean bone marrow suppression such as might be seen with the use of chloramphenicol.

Total WBCs: White blood cells are counted and then a "differential" count is completed where each individual type of white cell is reported as a percentage of the total. This differential can help determine if an infection is bacterial or viral. (Bacterial infections tend to have more overall WBCs and more PMNs than viral infections.) Remember that TBIs, especially Lyme, can mess with the immune system and therefore not show typical patterns. The presence of co-infections can muddy the waters even more. From my son's experience, I know it does no good to yell at a Lyme patient because their differential does not show them to be mounting the proper defense.

Total WBC counts are measured in amount per cc and decrease from birth to adulthood. A neonate will have about 20 x 10³ cells/cc and a child will range around 10 x 10³ cells/cc. Total normal WBCs in an adult range from 4 to 11. Check the normals for your lab. Look at the *Gentle Immunology* chapter if you would like a review of each of these different white cells.

- **Neutrophils** (often referred to with the broader abbreviation of **PMNs**): The life span of a neutrophil is less than 24 hours so rapid changes can be observed in the immune response by measuring neutrophils. Neutrophils are the most common of the granulocytic white cells. Technically, the term PMN includes all the granulocytes, but neutrophils are in such a majority that the term PMN is often used just to refer to them. Depending on age, neutrophils comprise 35% to 70% of the total white cell population.

  High neutrophils: Acute bacterial infection, inflammation, stress, tissue damage from necrosis or burns, vomiting, strenuous exercise, spirochetes, Rickettsia, and parasites have all been known to increase neutrophils.

PEARL: Mature neutrophils have a segmented nucleus. Less mature neutrophils are called <u>bands</u> *or stabs because instead of the mature poly-lobed nuclei they have band-like nuclei. If there is something really bad going on (like acute appendicitis), all the PMNs will be called into action and the system will start cranking out more. Some will have to serve before they are mature and these bands will comprise a higher percentage of the overall population. The term "shift to the left" comes from the days when white cell differentials were done by hand and the bands were recorded on the left side of the page. Today the term "left shift" means that a lot of young PMNs are in play. Something is going on that needs to be addressed by you as well as by the immune system. Bands can be quite high postoperatively.*

  Low neutrophils: Low levels can be found in viral infections such as hepatitis, influenza, any of the HHVs, Colorado tick fever, collagen vascular diseases, drugs that suppress the bone marrow, and with use of a few antibiotics. Any overwhelming infection can make it hard for the immune system to keep up. Malaria lowers the neutrophil count and Babesia may as well.

- **Eosinophils** are quite the interesting granulocyte, most closely associated with allergies, asthma, and the response to parasitic infections. Although nonspecific, eosinophilia is associated with collagen vascular diseases, and Bb appear to have an affinity for collagen. In newborns, eosinophil levels range from 20 to 850/cc; by 1 year, the range is 0 to 450/cc. A zero eosinophil count is not uncommon in a healthy adult. Eosinophils are involved with antigen/antibody reactions and are useful in recognizing parasites, allergies, hay fever, asthma, skin disorders, and drug hypersensitivity. Steroids can lower eosinophil counts.

- **Basophils** are the least common of the granulocytes and are involved with heparin, histamines, and serotonin. They are also the least understood of white cells. If you start seeing basophils on a patient's differential count think allergy or inflammation. They are involved with IL-4 and joints and chondroitin metabolism. Probably the more basophils counted on the differential, the more inflammation inside the body. Basophils normally are only 0.01% to 0.3% of the total white cell population. Basophils might be the circulating form of mast cells but there are slight differences in composition.

- **Lymphocytes** comprise about 20% to 44% of the circulating white cells and include the B and T cells. Here we are concerned only with absolute numbers. Later, in the *Immune Marker* section of the chapter, we will discuss measuring individual components of the lymphocyte pool. In children less than 8-years-old, there may be as many lymphocytes as neutrophils.

  High lymphocytes: Viral infections such as hepatitis, CMV, EBV, and most of the HHVs can increase the number of lymphocytes. Some bacteria increase total lymphocyte counts. Syphilis is known to increase lymphocytes, but the pattern is not yet clear for Bb. Lymphocytes increase in ulcerative colitis and other chronic inflammatory conditions. Very high lymphocyte counts may mean leukemia.

  Low lymphocytes: Immunodeficient conditions including AIDS, lupus, renal disease, and terminal cancers can lower the lymphocyte count. HIV is a virus that targets T cells and significantly lowers the T cell count. Low T cell levels place the patient at risk for all manner of opportunistic infections. Absolute lymphocyte count can be used as a surrogate marker for CD4 counts in emergencies. Less than 1000 cells/cc predicts a CD4 of less than 200 cells/cc. Steroid use decreases lymphocyte levels.

- **Monocytes** circulate in the blood for about a day and then settle into the tissue where they are called **macrophages**. RMSF can increase monocyte counts but this is a tidbit you can't do much with. At birth 1000/cc is normal and it goes down from there. `

PEARL: Since Bb may cause a significant, even predominant, monocytic response, we may need to focus more on monocytes as we attempt to understand the complex pathophysiology of Lyme. This concept was introduced in Chapter 3.

Blood smears involve looking at a thin layer of peripheral blood under a microscope. They are relatively quick and inexpensive tests. Technicians can look at either white or red cells for diagnostic purposes in TBIs. The more experienced the tech is in reading peripheral blood smears, the more accurate the results. Many smears today are automated, making them less useful for our purposes. When the smear reveals findings consistent with a known pathogen, there is relatively high sensitivity and specificity. If you see morulae or Maltese crosses in TBI patients with historical and clinical corroboration, these findings strongly support their respective diagnoses. Note that these observations are very much dependent on when in the clinical course the sample is taken. A positive is essentially pathognomonic, while a negative means nothing. *Not detected does NOT mean uninfected.* Never discount a diagnosis on the basis of a negative test. In conditions like DIC, the smear will show a minefield of broken erythrocytes and a scramble of other cells making more subtle distinctions difficult.

- Specifics regarding the Maltese crosses found in babesiosis: With Babesia infection, crosses can sometimes be seen in the RBCs, often with a pale center. Since Babesia reproduce in the RBCs, they often form a tetrad composed of four sex buds that look like Maltese crosses. When you see these crosses, you are probably looking at B. *microti*. One RBC can hold about eight parasites. Since intracellular Maltese cross formations are not usually seen in malaria, they can be useful in the differential diagnosis. Finding the parasite inside the RBCs under the microscope is usually possible only in the first few weeks of infection. A thin blood smear is preferred over a thick one since the parasites are easier to see in a thin display. Most often a Giemsa stain is used.

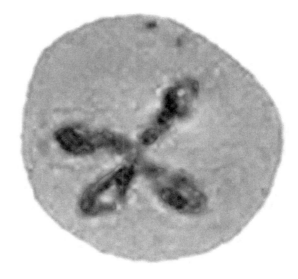

Maltese cross
Source: CDC. Accessed March 2013

- Specifics regarding the morulae found in ehrlichiosis: Pathogens can also be observed in white cells. Ehrlichia like to live in the white cell vacuole. Here they form clusters called morulae which are mulberry-shaped clumps of bacteria. Since the vacuole floats in the cell's cytoplasm, these morulae can sometimes be seen in blood smears under a microscope. Positive Wright-stained smears of monocytes containing morulae are diagnostic for E. *chaffeensis.* Finding morulae on the blood smear is helpful in diagnosing both ehrlichiosis and anaplasmosis.

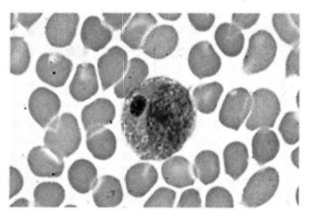

Morulae
Source: CCD. Accessed March 2013

Platelet count – Platelets are sticky cell fragments critical to the clotting process. Although they are often counted as part of a CBC they will be further discussed in the *Coagulation Panel* section just below.

II. COAGULATION PANEL

Coagulation is the complex cascade of reactions that result in clot formation. Many pathogens associated with TBIs adversely impact coagulation. Here we worry about the following:

- Bleeding and anemia associated with pathogens like Babesia

- Hypercoagulation found with Bartonella, Babesia, and Lyme

- Hypercoagulation-associated excess inflammation where the blood is thicker and stickier

- DIC, which is an overconsumption of clotting materials often observed in the end-stages of many of the TBIs, is detailed below.

Bleeding can lead to anemia which can have significant sequelae including weakness, dizziness, and hypotension. In most cases of bleeding or hemorrhage, we prefer for the bleeding to stop. In general, this involves clotting using the complex coagulation system. When clotting does not know when to stop, the condition is referred to as hypercoagulation. Risks of hypercoagulation include thrombus (a stationary clot within the vascular system which can impede blood flow), or emboli (a travelling clot with the potential to snag or occlude anywhere in the vasculature). Either of these conditions can result in tissue ischemia especially of the heart, lungs, or brain.

Disseminated intravascular coagulation or consumptive coagulopathy (**DIC**) is not so much a sign of TBI as a sign of severe end-stage disease. DIC is often fatal. Once you start seeing signs of DIC, you can stop worrying about the tick and concentrate on keeping your patient alive. Of course, the best treatment for DIC is to eliminate the underlying etiology. That means you must go back to worrying about the tick as well as everything else you need to worry about with DIC.

DIC is a pathologic activation of coagulation that often happens in the terminal stages of many TBIs. DIC leads to the formation of small clots inside the blood vessels throughout the body. These multiple small clots use up the coagulation proteins and platelets and disrupt all aspects of normal coagulation. Abnormal bleeding occurs with seeping into the skin, GI tract, and pulmonary tree. Wounds won't stop oozing and small clots disrupt kidney function and normal blood flow to organs, which can quickly malfunction.

Once you have a patient with DIC, you know fear. DIC contributes to multiple organ failure, which can lead to death. DIC patients are severely ill and going into shock, often bleeding from the mouth, nose, and blood draw sites. They may exhibit massive bruising. Both PT and PTT are prolonged and fibrinogen is reduced with considerable clot and fibrin debris due to all the concurrent fibrinolytic activity. Severe thrombocytopenia ensues, and blood smears show a wasteland of broken RBCs and debris. Early on, there may actually be an increase of clotting factors with a normal PT and PTT. Do not allow these normal results to lull you into a false sense of security. If your patient is severely ill, all hell can break loose quickly in terms of coagulation. The prognosis for DIC is grim. If there is evidence of DIC, regroup fast. Treatment is to reverse the underlying cause, but with TBIs that might be wishful thinking. Provide all manner of supportive care and aggressively treat for the likely TBIs. DIC work-up can include PT, PTT, platelet count, fibrinogen levels, bleeding time, and peripheral smear.

While there are MANY tests for clotting and coagulation, here are the studies you will most frequently encounter with TBIs:

Platelet count – Platelets are sticky cell fragments critical to the clotting process. Platelet counts vary considerably with age:

Premature	100,000	to	300,000/cc
Newborn	140,000	to	300,000/cc

Infant	200,000	to	475,000/cc
Adults	150,000	to	400,000/cc

Order a platelet count in patients with frank or suspected bleeding, purpura, petechiae, or long bleeding times. If the patient is severely ill, begin to monitor for impending DIC, as you work frenetically to avoid that outcome.

> Low platelets can be seen with bone marrow depression, some drugs, RBC transfusion, DIC, coagulopathies, sepsis, severe hemorrhage. Platelets can be transfused to make up for deficits.

> High platelets might be observed with infection, platelet transfusion, splenectomy, tissue damage, hypothermia, iron deficiency, surgery, and burns.

International normalized ratio (INR) – The liver is responsible for production of coagulation factors. The INR measures a patient's speed of coagulation and compares it to a control. If the INR is higher than the control, it means the person is taking longer than usual to clot. If lower, she is taking less time than usual to clot. The INR becomes your life when you are taking certain anticoagulants. For TBI patients, the INR would likely show up in a clotting panel if you are assessing suspected problems with coagulation. INR can also serve as an insensitive measure of liver function. The higher the INR above the lab standard the more likely there will be unwanted bleeding.

Prothrombin time (PT) – Prothrombin time is the clotting time of plasma. The PT is quite insensitive and does not become abnormal until more than 80% of the liver's capacity for synthesizing clotting factors is lost. As a result, PT is a poor marker of liver function, but it is sensitive to rapid changes in the ability to form clot. PT is almost always a part of a coagulation screen, especially if DIC is suspected. The usual PT ranges from 10 to 13 seconds and is compared to the lab's reference range. Order PT in cases of severe illness, advanced liver disease, Vitamin K deficiency, or when low fibrinogen is suspected. PT results are often used to manage the effect of anticoagulants. Prolonged PT may mean liver damage.

Partial thromboplastin time (PTT) – This measurement is used as a screen for coagulation problems and takes into account all clotting factors except Factor VII. The normal PTT varies by lab, but the range is about 20 to 34 seconds. PTT is prolonged when there are deficits of clotting factors, liver problems, and DIC.

Bleeding time – This measurement is used to assess platelet function. A standard cut is made in the patient's skin and the time until the cut stops bleeding is recorded and compared to a reference time.

Fibrinogen – Also called clotting factor I, fibrinogen is used to assess the tendency to bleed abnormally and the risk of thrombosis. The results depend on the method used and should be evaluated based on the lab normal. Usually normal ranges of fibrinogen are between 1.5 and 2.8.

> High fibrinogen is sometimes seen with acute inflammation and tissue damage, pregnancy, OCPs, malignancy, smoking, older age, periodontal disease, and high cardiac risk. Vets sometimes use fibrinogen levels to assess inflammation in horses.

> Low fibrinogen levels can mean the clotting factors are being consumed faster than they can be replaced (like in DIC), liver disease, or bleeding.

III. URINALYSIS

Ah, the lowly UA. If you've never peed in a cup, you haven't been living in the USA in the 21st century. Entire books have been written about what can be done with a few mls of urine.

For office or home use, a variety of dipsticks are available that allow quick testing of urine for several parameters such as sugar, ketones, blood, white cells, or nitrates. Not especially sensitive, they provide a mostly qualitative quick check. In almost all cases a microscopic exam is the better choice, since a dipstick misses about a quarter of the positives it is looking for. Nonetheless, dipsticks can provide an inexpensive way to follow a factor of interest over time. One author recommends 30 days of urine dipsticks to follow babesiosis patients for urinary blood. This is probably overkill since some strains are more prone to hematuria than others and simple visualization might provide almost as much information.

Here we will focus on UA results as they pertain to TBI patients.

Inspection – Dark or red urine suggests the presence of red cells or bilirubin, which is a breakdown product of erythrocytes. Since babesiosis in cattle is called red water fever, red or dark urine can be used to support that diagnosis or to follow the progress of the disease. Cloudy urine suggests infection, which may be totally separate from the TBI. Some food metabolites and drugs, such as rifamycin, can also discolor the urine.

RBCs – Normal is 0 to 2 cells. Any more red cells than that indicates bleeding. Red cells are usually present in the urine of menstruating females. RBCs can also suggest infection or stones in the system.

WBCs – Normal is 0 to 2 cells but this depends on how clean the sample was on collection. "Clean catch" or midstream urine is hard to collect in adults and nearly impossible in kids.

Catheter collection can be unpleasant at any age and should be avoided unless there's no other way to get the information you need. If white cells are found in a urine specimen, try again to do a clean collection. More than 5 WBCs is considered a marker of infection. Correlate the results with clinical presentation. If signs of infection are present and are consistent with UTI symptoms, a urine culture may be indicated.

Protein – A trace of protein is normal, but more than that suggests problems with kidney filtration, infection, febrile illness, pregnancy, or bleeding.

Glucose – If the kidney is working properly, all the glucose that passes through should be reabsorbed. Sugar in the urine suggests problems with glucose metabolism, steroid use, thyroid dysfunction, infection, OCPs, or inadequate kidney function.

Ketones – Acetone in the urine suggests a problem with glucose metabolism, extended fasting, or acute febrile illness. Normal urine should test negative for ketones.

Bilirubin – Bilirubin is a breakdown product of red cells and gives urine its normal yellow color. Too much bilirubin can spill into the urine and make it orange or brown. High levels are often due to excessive destruction of red cells which can also yellow the whites of the eyes and the skin. In these cases, you will want to find the source of the surplus. Bilirubin in the urine also suggests liver disease or obstruction of the biliary tree.

Nitrites – The presence of nitrites in the urine suggests bacterial infection, especially by E. *coli*, the most common etiologic agent of UTI.

Casts – A variety of casts can be seen in urine using high powered microscopes. They form in the shape of the duct or tube where they were made. They are constructed from red or white cell debris, bacteria fragments, or crystals.

hCG – Usually absent, hCG is a hormone that appears in the urine of pregnant women.

PEARL: Interstitial cystitis is a common problem with Lyme disease. By all indications, the patient appears to have a routine UTI with dysuria, hesitancy, nocturia, and suprapubic pressure as the bladder fills. While mostly a diagnosis of middle-aged females, interstitial cystitis can occur in kids and can be hard on them and their parents. The UA can show signs of irritation since the bladder presents as chronically inflamed and irritated with pain, discomfort, and the constant need to void. The condition is poorly understood. The symptoms drive the patient crazy. Repeated UAs and cultures turn up negative over and over again. Frustrated HCPs don't know what else to do, so they keep ordering UAs and cultures. Patients are repeatedly treated for traditional UTIs without relief. This disconnect between clinical complaints and negative testing should alert the HCP to the possibility of a TBI as the potential underlying cause. Symptoms seem worse at menses. Occasionally, the Lyme spirochete has been picked up with cystoscopy, and biopsy of the bladder trigone has revealed Bb by PCR.

IV. CULTURES

With rare exceptions, TBI pathogens do not culture well. Nonetheless, cultures are ordered on TBI patients by HCPs who are looking for both tick-borne pathogens as well as other more common infectious agents. When positive, Lyme cultures are essentially 100% sensitive, but yield is disappointedly LOW.

PEARL: If you just write for a culture and sensitivity, you will get a test that looks for the usual suspects. Of course, this can be useful for several reasons. First, they aren't called the usual suspects for nothing. These pathogens are the most common causes of infection in most cases. One of the critical premises of this book is that more than one thing can be happening at a time and more than one pathogen can be infecting the patient concurrently. Routine cultures are unlikely to grow most TBI pathogens. Since routine culture media and standard conditions are designed to facilitate growth of the most common etiologic agents, the environs are unlikely to be favorable to most of the TBIs. You rarely find what you aren't looking for. Just because a culture comes back without evidence of a TBI does not rule out TBI.

You can try to culture just about anything: urine, blood, mucus, lavage fluids, stool, throats, eyes, nares, urethra, joint aspirate, CSF, wounds, and biopsy tissue. Usually, the "deeper" the source of the sample, the more likely you are to get the obscure germ you are looking for. Successful culturing of pathogens depends on adequate sample collection, storage, media selection, and appropriate growing conditions that include correct oxygen levels, temperature, humidity, nutrients, etc. A wound culture, for example, can grow out any number of pathogens. Conditions can be selected that predispose for the growth of particular organisms. Once cultured, the growth can be tested for its sensitivity to various antimicrobials. This sensitivity information can be invaluable in selecting proper antibiotic treatments.

Sometimes cultures are collected in TBI patients by HCPs looking for a specific tick-borne pathogen. Unfortunately, the TBI agents are notoriously difficult to grow in culture. Being able to culture spirochetes from body fluids or tissues would be great but current methodology does not make that easy. Of course, if a culture is positive, the sensitivity is 100%. (Hard to contaminate a sample with a spirochete that was just ambling by. The Bb would have had to come from the patient sample.) The problem with cultures is that the yields are so low. Even if all conditions are right and the stars are aligned, it's hard to get Bb to grow in culture. Some of the other agents like Bartonella and M. *fermentans* can also be notoriously recalcitrant.

The routine cultures looking for the pathogens that traditionally grow in urine or blood just aren't going to grow TBI pathogens. Occasionally, attempts are made to culture Bartonella. Since B. *henselea* only circulates in the blood intermittently, a number of consecutive specimens would need to be collected. These attempts, although heroic, are often futile. In these cases, a positive culture would be considered confirmatory. However, a negative culture could just mean that the specimen was collected at a time when no organisms were circulating, so none could be collected. Further, we may be trying to grow B. *henselea* when the actual infectious agent is a BLO.

Nevertheless, there is a role for cultures in TBI patients. Multiple case reviews have shown positive results on cultures in patients who were negative on antibody testing. So if you have a decent sample, attempt cultures for appropriate TBI pathogens. As we know from the abundance of co-infections, more than one pathogen can be active in an individual at a time. These concurrent infections can be tick-borne or not. While a culture may not turn up a TBD pathogen, you might find another culprit contributing to the problem. If your head is spinning over which cultures to order or how to correctly collect samples, call your trusted lab.

Listed below are several cultures that may be pertinent in TBI patients.

Urine cultures – UTIs are common in all age groups. The most common cause is E. *coli*. A "clean catch" or clean catheter specimen should show no growth if there is no infection. Growth of 10^5 or more per ml is a sign of infection. A lower amount of growth would be considered significant in symptomatic patients or for those with nitrites present. If a urine culture is to be repeated, keep 4 hours between samples. Please refer to the *Urinalysis* section above describing interstitial cystitis. When the bladder is perpetually irritated but repeat cultures are negative, consider a TBI as the underlying cause of symptoms.

Streptococci culture – The most common cause of bacterial pharyngitis is Group A β-hemolytic Streptococci. A Strep infection places the patient at increased risk of rheumatic fever, toxic shock Strep syndrome, glomerulonephritis, and PANDAS. A number of rapid Strep detection methods have been developed including ELISA and various agglutination techniques involving antigen from the throat mixed with known Strep antibody. Specificity is good but sensitivity is only moderate. If clinically indicated, look for Strep in your TBI patients. Be especially vigilant in TBI patients who present with OCD, tics, or PANDAS. In these cases, tests for Strep antibodies might also be warranted.

Joint aspirate for culture – While a "hot" joint may inspire a culture of the aspirate, do not rule out Lyme on the basis of the lab not seeing or growing spirochetes. *Not detected does NOT mean uninfected.*

Blood cultures – Routine blood culture results rarely produce TBI pathogens, especially if the culture conditions are designed to grow the most common causes of sepsis. Any positive result should be addressed. If the patient does not improve consider that an undetected pathogen may be contributing to the problem.

PEARL: A more definitive blood culture for Bb shows promise. New methodology used by Advanced Laboratory Services appears to be highly sensitive. This test is best done BEFORE the patient is started on antibiotics or herbals or after the antibiotic has been discontinued for at least a month. Experienced clinicians might be reluctant to discontinue treatment in order to draw the culture sample. Think of this option prior to the first dose of antibiotics if possible. Currently the lab requests 4 tubes of blood that may be too large a volume to extract from the smallest patients. Call for additional advice (855-238-4949).

Cultures for C. *difficile* – Clostridium *difficile* (or C. *diff*) are bacteria that cause severe diarrhea in those patients whose normal gut flora has been eliminated either by strong broad spectrum antimicrobials or use of certain specific antibiotics. Once the normal gut bacteria is gone, the C. *diff* has no competition for local resources and it overgrows and takes over the gut, releasing a potent toxin. C. *difficile* can lead to serious complications, not the least of which is savage, incapacitating diarrhea with dehydration. The signs and symptoms can progress to pseudomembranous colitis and toxic megacolon, which can be life threatening. Suspect C. *difficile* infection in any patient with diarrhea who has been treated with antibiotics within the past 2 months or whose frequent, loose stools began within about 3 days after hospitalization. When suspected, send a stool specimen for culture and for analysis of toxins. If these first tests are negative, send one or two more specimens ordering the same tests to be repeated or ordering different methods. PCR testing is available, but culture of the organism remains the gold standard since it is the most sensitive and specific. ELISA is used for the analysis of toxins. Note that many hospitals test for only one of the strains of C. *difficile,* so there are a high number of false negatives. Some say that a CT scan of the colon showing wall thickening of greater than 4 mm has as good a PPV as the ELISA for detecting C. *diff*. Currently, testing requires stool (not swab) for toxin studies, but a rectal swab is okay for cultures. Symptoms usually improve when the causative antibiotic regimen is stopped or changed. C. *difficile* usually responds well to metronidazole (Flagyl) or vancomycin.

PEARL: In all cases, make sure that the sample collection, storage, and shipping are appropriate.

V. GLUCOSE

Almost all metabolic panels include a random glucose level whether you want it or not. By all accounts, this is worthless unless the result comes back at 644. Even fasting blood sugars have little value. Parents say their child is fasting and then you see the empty juice box in the purse. That does not mean glucose should be ignored in TBI patients. Lyme can significantly affect sugar metabolism. If you are concerned about blood glucose levels, order HbA1c to assess sugar control over time or a 2 hour post prandial sugar. In addition to abnormal sugar metabolism, glucose levels can be high due to liver disease, stress, steroids, and inflammation like that found with infection.

VI. LIVER FUNCTION TESTS

Liver function tests (LFTs) provide basic information about the liver's performance. The liver has the primary responsibility for metabolizing drugs using innumerable enzyme pathways. If the liver is not healthy, drug levels could become toxic. Baseline levels should be obtained to determine whether the liver can function adequately to process these chemicals. LFTs can then be monitored to see if the liver is being adversely affected by the disease or harmed by the treatment.

Patients with TBIs that are treated with medications that can cause liver damage should have regular LFTs. Note that a test result that is WNL does not mean that nothing is happening in the individual liver. Results that are markedly changed from previous testing can provide important information. A patient whose LFTs go from the low end of normal to the high end should be monitored. Compare results and look for trends. Do not allow a liver to fry on your watch.

The following are some frequently used LFTs.

Transaminases are enzymes that catalyze reactions in the liver. Damage to liver cells causes these enzymes to leak into the blood circulation where they can be measured. Higher than normal levels may mean there is a problem with full hepatic function. Normal levels vary with gender, race, and body fat.

- **AST**- Aspartate transaminase (formerly SGOT) is used as a biomarker of liver injury and the overall integrity of the liver cells. If the hepatic cell is injured, AST will increase in the blood as it spills out of the broken cell. AST is not as specific to the liver as is ALT. Because it has other sources as well as the liver, AST is sometimes used to measure red cell damage as well as injury to the heart. The usual reference range is 10 to 35 IU/L, but this varies with lab, gender, and race.

- **ALT** - Alanine transaminase (formerly SGPT) can be correlated with liver function. When there is an elevated ALT, damage to liver cells should be suspected. Causes of the liver damage that can increase ALT include: infections such as hepatitis, α 1-antitrypsin deficiency, certain kidney and muscle conditions, medications (synthetic penicillins, ciprofloxacin [Cipro], nitrofuratoin [Macrobid,] isoniazid, antifungals such as ketaconazole and fluconazole [Diflucan], and certain Chinese herbs. ALT rises fast in acute liver damage such as acute hepatitis or acetaminophen overdose. The normal reference range is 9 to 40 IU/L depending on age and lab methods. ALT is a more specific indicator of liver problems than is AST. If you had no other parameter to monitor in assessing affects of the disease or treatment on the liver, you could do worse than follow ALT. Get a baseline if possible.

Bilirubin (BR) is a breakdown product of heme which is part of the hemoglobin in RBCs. The liver is in charge of clearing the blood of bilirubin. Bilirubin is taken up into the liver cells (hepatocytes), conjugated (modified to make it water soluble), and then secreted into the bile. Bile is then excreted into the intestine where the bilirubin helps give stool its brown color. An increase in total bilirubin can cause jaundice and dark urine. Bilirubin gives urine its yellow color, but excessive BR will make it darker. Likewise, bilirubin is responsible for the yellow color of bruises. Conjugated bilirubin is also called direct bilirubin, and comparing levels of conjugated and unconjugated bilirubin may help tell the source location of a liver problem. Note that many neonates have excessive bilirubin which can be entirely separate from any consideration with TBIs. The normal reference range is 0.2-1.2 mg/dL depending on the lab.

PEARL: Patients with Gilbert's syndrome have normal AST and ALT but the direct and total bilirubin levels are high. Rarely are they jaundiced. These patients have a decreased capacity to metabolize bilirubin which is thought to be a genetic variant and not pathologic.

Gamma glutamyl transpeptidase (GGT) is reasonably liver-specific and will go very high for even minor subclinical liver problems. GGT can be helpful in identifying a one-time elevation in LFTs. In the ER, we found GGT useful in identifying recent drinking binges. In TBI patients, we are more worried about long-term liver damage, especially those that might result from on-going use of medications. Nonetheless, GGT may show up on a metabolic profile.

Albumin is a protein test of liver functionality and detailed separately in the *Protein* section below.

Alkaline phosphatase (ALP or **AP)** is an enzyme found in the cells of the biliary ducts of the liver. AP is elevated in bile duct obstruction, cholestasis, or infiltrative liver disease. Also found in bone and placenta, AP is higher in kids since they have growing bones. AP can be used as a marker of liver or bone disease and the reference range is 30 to 120 IU/L. Normals vary with age and pregnancy.

Lactate dehydrogenase (LDH) is sometimes included on a broad metabolic panel. LDH is an enzyme found in many body tissues including the liver. If elevated, investigate liver damage.

VII. KIDNEY STUDIES

TBIs, especially Lyme, are known to impact the kidneys. Medications used to treat TBIs impact the kidneys as well. BUN and creatinine are good measures of kidney function. Levels should be drawn at baseline and then followed at regular intervals both to assess the progression of disease as well as to monitor for untoward treatment effects. Baseline levels may be skewed since the patient is sick to start with and may have an altered "normal." Nonetheless, the results should demonstrate that the patient's kidneys are strong enough to handle the treatment regimen proposed.

BUN or blood urea nitrogen is a useful measure of kidney function, hydration, and nutritional status. Only BUN will suggest the patient's hydration level and readings can change quickly in response to fluids. BUN measures the amount of nitrogen in the blood in the form of urea. Urea is a by-product of protein metabolism in the liver that is then removed from the blood in the kidney. BUN can be used to help determine if the kidney is healthy enough to handle the proposed treatment regime. Since many drugs are excreted by the kidney, the organ must be able to handle their filtering and subsequent removal. Otherwise, a drug could back up to dangerous levels. The reference range for BUN is 8 to 18 mg/dL. BUN is considered more of a "quick" look at kidney function since it changes rapidly as the patient's condition and hydration level adjusts. In contrast, creatinine gives a better long-term look at how the kidney is functioning.

High BUN: In general, BUN will go up if:

- You have too much nitrogen as in a high protein diet
- You have low blood volume like in dehydration, hemorrhage, or shock
- There is an increased absorption of nitrogen in the kidney like in malnutrition and kidney disease
- TCNs can raise BUN levels.

Low BUN: Over-hydration, pregnancy, and steroid use can all lower BUN.

Creatinine is a breakdown product of muscle metabolism and, depending on muscle mass, is produced at a fairly con-

stant rate by the body. Creatinine levels in the blood compared to the urine can be used to calculate creatinine clearance which reflects how fast the kidney is filtering and is one of the best measures of kidney function. A rise in creatinine suggests damage to kidney cells.

Males tend to have higher levels of creatinine than females because they usually have more muscle mass. The usual reference ranges are 0.7 to 1.2 mg/dL in males and 0.5 to 1.0 mg/dL in females. Age also affects the level. More important than the absolute value is the trend over time.

Creatinine is an important baseline test to make sure the kidney is healthy enough to handle proposed treatment. Since most medicines are excreted by the kidney, if kidney function is suboptimal, drug levels can accumulate to dangerous levels. After baseline, creatinine levels should be assessed regularly throughout the course of the disease and treatment. Look for patterns and trends. I said, "LOOK FOR PATTERNS AND TRENDS." Is the creatinine creeping up? Medications may be starting to hurt the kidney. Consider a dose or drug change.

High creatinine might mean something is impacting kidney function such as damage to kidney vessels, infection, autoimmune disorders, drugs or toxins, stones, reduced blood flow due to shock or heart failure, heart disease, diabetes, or muscle injury.

Low creatinine levels are rare and usually of no concern. Vegetarians have lower creatinines.

As a drug safety physician, I was constantly looking for adverse drug effects. If I had only a limited number of tests to run they would be CBC, ALT, BUN, and creatinine. Even slight alterations in any of these assessments suggest that a drug might be doing harm. An example of a pattern would be an increase in creatinine after a drug pulse and a decrease after a drug break. Even if all results are WNL, patterns and trends can provide pertinent information. Just looking at the WNL checkbox, you can miss what is actually happening with the patient. We can all be busy, trying to get through the day, but kidney function is too important to leave to cursory lab reviews. Compare the current level to the last level and to the one before that and to baseline, if available. Watch out for that kidney, or it will come back to bite you. Make any appropriate adjustments to treatment to spare the kidney function.

BUN and creatinine determine how well the kidney is filtering waste from the blood. Decreased blood flow to the kidney can result in a high BUN-to-creatinine ratio. This can occur in conditions where the heart pumping is inadequate, there is an increase of protein in the blood, excessive bleeding occurs, or in cases of dehydration. Malnutrition and low urea levels due to liver problems can cause a low BUN-to-creatinine ratio. If you start seeing worrisome signals of kidney malfunction, look at potential causes in more depth. You may want to look at ratios, urinary creatinine, and creatinine clearance.

VIII.   METABOLIC PANEL REMNANTS

Extensive metabolic panels often leave us with lab results we may not want or know how to handle. Nevertheless, they will appear on our desks. I do not mean to minimize their importance, but they tend to be nonspecific, and gross abnormalities in asymptomatic TBI patients are uncommon. The most common tests that could impact TBI patients include:

Electrolytes

Electrolytes are charged ions. Since they can conduct electricity in solution they are called *electro*lytes. Most body processes at the cellular level rely on electrolytes. Too much or too little can cause cellular and system malfunction. Usually the "electrolytes" on a lab request form include sodium (Na), potassium (K), chloride (Cl), and CO_2 (carbon dioxide, sometimes measured as bicarbonate or HCO_3^-). Primarily these ions help regulate the balance between salts and water and the acid/base equilibrium. "Lytes" are essential for heart rhythms, muscle contraction, nerve conduction, and kidney function.

A.   **Sodium (Na)** – Sodium is important for salt and water balance and electrical conduction. Na is critical for brain, nerve, and muscle function. Sodium allows electricity to flow and thereby enables communication between cells. Sodium "obligates" water, so wherever there is too much sodium, the ion will be pulling water toward it. If there is too much sodium inside a cell, water will flow in and expand (or explode) the cell. If there is too much sodium outside the cell, water will flow out, shriveling the cell.

> Range: 135 to 145 mEq/L depending on age with slight variations by lab

> High sodium (hypernatremia): Kidney disease, low water intake, loss of water due to diarrhea or vomiting

> Low sodium (hyponatremia): Liver disease, kidney dysfunction, heart failure, burns, excessive sweating

PEARL: The use of high sodium sports drinks to replace the sodium lost through sweating during exercise is largely overkill and marketing. Only under extreme conditions does low sodium become an issue in these cases.

B.   **Potassium (K)** – Potassium is necessary for cell function, especially the regulation of heartbeat, nerve conduction, and muscle operation. My memories of the ICU as an intern include perpetually trying to keep K levels normal. Low potassium can be quickly fatal.

> Range: Adult   3.5   to   5.0   mmol/L
>
> Newborn   3.2   to   5.5   mmol/L
>
> Infant   3.4   to   6.0   mmol/L
>
> Child   3.3   to   4.6   mmol/L

(mmol/L converts to mEq/L in this context)

High K (hyperkalemia): High potassium can be due to decreased kidney function, medicines such as steroids, muscle necrosis, IV or other K supplements, or acidosis. Hemolyzed blood or repeated fist clenching during a lab draw can artificially increase K.

Low K (hypokalemia): Low potassium can be due to urinary loss, GI loss, or redistribution of K from the extracellular space to inside the cells. The most common causes include medications such as diuretics and penicillins, kidney disease, excessive loss due to heavy sweating associated with high fevers or other causes, vomiting, diarrhea, eating disorders, abnormal aldosterone, increased Na, hypercalcemia, malabsorption, cancers, DKA, or severe B12 anemia.

C.   **Chloride (Cl)** – Chloride is needed to maintain a normal fluid balance.

> Range in serum: 98 to 108 mmol/L

> High chloride: Diarrhea, kidney disease, overactive parathyroid, acid/base imbalance

> Low chloride: Loss in urine, excessive sweating, vomiting, stomach secretions, kidney or adrenal disease, acid/base imbalance

D.   **Carbon dioxide, bicarbonate,** or HCO_3^- – Inside the body most of the carbon dioxide is in the form of bicarbonate, so a measure of CO_2 is really a measure of HCO_3^-. Bicarbonate acts as a buffer to maintain normal acid/base balance. The body pH can be affected by foods, medicines, and the function of both the kidneys and lungs. When you start seeing significant changes in CO_2, you might be dealing with either metabolic or respiratory acid/base imbalances. This would be more common in TBI patients who are severely ill. Steroid use tends to increase CO_2 levels, while some antibiotics like the TCNs can decrease bicarbonate levels.

Calcium

This mineral is essential for the formation and preservation of bones and teeth. Calcium is also required for the proper operation of nerves, muscles, and heart tissue. Calcium allows for the chemical reactions necessary for clotting, enzyme function, and the work of hormones. Most calcium resides in bone, and the amount in blood is very carefully regulated. If blood calcium becomes low (hypocalcemia), bones release more to bring the levels back to normal. If blood calcium is too high (hypercalcemia), some will be stored in bone and the rest excreted into the urine and stool. Abnormal calcium levels can suggest problems with bones, kidneys, pancreas, parathyroid, Vitamin D metabolism, or magnesium deficiency. Patients who are immobilized for long periods and those with rhabdomyolysis may have high calcium levels.

Magnesium

Finally, we have a remnant of the metabolic profile that can have an important role in TBI patients! Magnesium plays a critical role in normal muscle, nerve, and enzyme action. This mineral is involved in reactions involving energy use. Many symptoms associated with Lyme such as fatigue, twitches, weakness, and speech problems are also associated with low magnesium levels. A magnesium level should be considered in TBI patients presenting with these problems. Normal magnesium levels range from 1.5 to 2.5 mg/dL, depending on the lab.

Phosphorus

Often there is a relatively elevated phosphorus with a normal calcium. The clinical significance of this is unknown and just one of those things that comes with a "great deal" metabolic panel.

> *PEARL: I know an antihypertension drug that was not approved because of an incidental lab finding that came from a "great deal" metabolic panel. Saved a few thousand dollars and lost millions. The abnormal labs in this case were not clinically significant but the pattern could not be ignored.*

Protein

Albumin is a protein made specifically by the liver and is the primary protein found in blood plasma. The level of albumin suggests how well the liver is working to make proteins. If something is inhibiting the manufacture of protein in the liver, albumin levels will be low. From the perspective of TBI management, albumin can be affected by acute or chronic inflammation. While not an especially sensitive test, albumin provides a heads up that all is not well. If the liver is so preoccupied or damaged that it cannot synthesize its main protein, then the patient is not going to be able to heal and recover optimally. The lower the albumin level, the worse the prognosis. In fact, albumin levels can be inversely related to risk of death.

> Range: 3.5 to 5.5 g/dL depending on the lab and other factors such as age and nutritional status. Normal ranges can be very different for newborns, children, and adults.

High albumin: Usually the only clinically significant cause of an elevated albumin is dehydration.

Low albumin: Albumin can be decreased in debilitating diseases and in either acute or chronic inflammation. Low levels can be seen with liver disease, malabsorption, malnutrition, starvation, renal dysfunction, significant loss of skin or GI tissue, loss of protein from the gut, diarrhea, fever, chronic illness, burns, edema, or hypocalcemia.

IX. STUDIES OF IMMUNE FUNCTION

There are many reasons you might have ordered an assessment of the various immune parameters. You might want to know how hard the immune system is fighting, how specifically, or if it is railing against it*self* as well as foreign invaders. You might have ordered some of these tests on your first visit with the TBI patient or you might be ordering them later if the patient is not responding as you had hoped. The results of some of this testing can help with the differential diagnosis. Most of these tests are nonspecific, but each can provide information that in some cases may be just the clue you need to help turn the tide for the individual patient.

We know that both Lyme and the presence of co-infections can impact immune response, often in unexpected ways. Use each piece of information as yet another piece of the puzzle. You have seen some of the material below in the last chapter. More detail is provided here to help with interpretation.

Rheumatoid factor (RF): Without either great sensitivity or specificity, the IgM of RF is present in the serum of patients with a variety of infectious processes. The presence of RF might support the presence of an inflammatory process but will not give you a TBI diagnosis.

Antinuclear antibody: ANA is found in a number of immune and autoimmune disorders such as lupus and other connective tissue diseases. Some medicines, such as PCNs and TCNs, increase the ANA. ANA is usually measured by ELISA or immunofluorescent microscopy (IFA). ELISA results are reported as titers. Dilutions of 1:320 usually indicate an elevated ANA. Different patterns on immunofluorescent testing suggest different diseases like SLE, mixed connective tissue disease, Sjogren's syndrome, RA, CREST, Raynaud's phenomenon, and others. ANA is present in lupus. If there is no elevation in ANA, the diagnosis is probably not lupus. ANA tests are best used to determine if there is more going on than meets the eye, such as multiple etiologies or an underlying immune problem.

There is no need to repeat a negative ANA immediately. Because immune compromise can be episodic, repeat the ANA at a later date to follow changes. Chronic hepatitis and other conditions can cause falsely positive ANAs. About 4% of

Caucasians may be positive for ANA without any known underlying pathology. This number increases in healthy people over 65.

A number of medications including minocycline are known to rarely cause a drug-induced lupus. ANA results can be followed over time to assess clinical progression, treatment response, or adverse drug events. In TBI patients, ANA might be examined to see if there is an autoimmune component to the clinical presentation. Patients with an autoimmune reaction to borreliosis (Lyme) respond to a different treatment approach compared with those who are not autoimmune. Those with autoimmune disorders have a variety of symptoms such as low grade fever, joint pain, fatigue, or unexplained rashes. High ANAs may explain why these symptoms predominate or persist in some patients.

PEARL: If the ANA is elevated consider ordering an anti-DS DNA test. If anti-DS DNA is correspondingly NOT elevated, then the increased ANA is probably of no clinical significance.

Complement levels: Complement are proteins in the serum that act to destroy foreign invaders. For example in the **classical** complement pathway, antibody-binding initiates the immune cascade calling in other immune molecules to help. An **alternative** complement pathway works without needing antibodies to start the process. Repeated activation of the complement process uses up the available complement proteins. When complement levels are low, complement is probably being used in the formation of antigen/antibody complexes. This result can be deemed good in that the complement is being consumed in mounting a defense. But complement consumption can go too far and when too much is consumed before it can be replenished, there is not enough complement around to help form the Ag/Ab complexes.

Once complement is activated it will begin to work with or without the antibodies to punch holes in the cells of the pathogen eventually destroying the invaders. You have seen much of the following information on complement in the preceding chapter. Here is additional detail on interpretation. Remember, only order tests that will provide information that you don't already know and that have the potential to impact case management.

Complement C1Q results should reflect the amount of circulating immune complexes. If the amount is low, suspect that something is broken higher in the immune cascade. This complex attaches to the complement fixation sites of antibodies. C1Q inhibits immune complex-induced interferon production and is linked to SLE and other immune diseases. Lack of C1Q is the biggest indicator for SLE. Almost everyone with deficiency of C1Q gets lupus, and low levels will correspond with flares. C1Q

has a role in the cytokine production process, regulates production of IFN-α, impacts overall complement activity, and is involved with the process of making immune complexes. If levels are low, an autoimmune mechanism might be in play; if high, a persistent, on-going infection is suggested.

Complement C3 is used in the diagnosis and management of diseases such as kidney problems and lupus and in many inflammatory conditions. When antibodies bind to a foreign protein, C3 attaches to the complex and beckons for aid from other parts of the immune cascade. C3d is a fragment of C3 that serves as a signal to certain B cells. Likewise, immune complex C3d may suggest that a persistent infection is driving an autoimmune clinical presentation. C3 is the component of complement found in the highest concentrations in plasma and is elevated with a number of inflammatory problems. C3 is low in lupus, bacterial endocarditis, some kidney diseases, bacterial septicemia, end-stage liver disease, and some fungal infections, presumably because the complement is being used in the formation of Ag/Ab complexes. Low levels means C3 is doing its job. Too low might mean there is not enough available to do everything that needs to be done.

PEARL: C3a and C4a are inflammatory markers that some HCPs monitor to determine disease status. C3d levels may provide information on the clinical condition. These molecules reflect the prevalence of toxins and infectious agents and may prove to be a good monitor of overall pathogen burden and indicator of an on-going inflammatory process. A result > 40 is an index of persistent inflammation. If the person seems to be improving, but C3d levels are still at 40 or above, something pathological is probably still going on inside this patient, either a simmering infection or an autoimmune process.

Complement CH50 levels can be used to monitor complement deficiencies and to follow disease progression in patients with lupus, nephritis, or a variety of infections. One normal reference range in serum is 35 to 55 CH50 units/ml. CH50 is a measure of the overall health of the complement system and it helps us monitor how much complement is available to mount an attack. CH50 can be used to follow autoimmune diseases.

Complement individual immunoglobulin profiles: Quantitative measures can be done for each of the distinct immunoglobulin (antibody) proteins. Presence of IgM and IgG can help with the chronology of the infectious process and provide information about the underlying pathology.

IgM – High in early infectious states especially viral, parasitic, and autoimmune diseases. In Lyme, some patients never convert from IgM to IgG. Here

IgM may be the predominant responder throughout the clinical course. Drawing blood too soon after the bite will show a negative result since the antibodies will not have had a chance to form. A positive reaction would then be due to "left-overs" from earlier bites.

IgG – Comes in later in the immune reaction after IgM and remains after the infection is gone. Indicative of past, on-going, or chronic infections. Also present when there is an autoimmune component to the immune response.

IgA – Infections of respiratory, GI, or renal systems. Low IgA is the most commonly recognized deficiency of antibodies but the significance of this finding in TBI patients is not clear.

IgD – No one seems to care about IgD but that's probably because we don't currently know enough to worry. IgD may be an immature antibody.

IgE – This antibody can be elevated in allergies, asthma, and parasitic infections.

Erythrocyte sedimentation rate: The **ESR** is a nonspecific measure of the speed at which erythrocytes (red blood cells) settle out of unclotted blood. Blood to which an anticoagulant has been added is placed in a tube, and the distance the cells fall in one hour is the ESR. Normally the rate is less than 10 mm/hr for males and slightly higher in females. The clumping of the cells depends on proteins released during inflammation. Therefore, the ESR suggests the presence of inflammation and is used to monitor the onset and progress of inflammatory disorders. For example, ESR can help tell the difference between acute MI and angina, since no inflammation is present with angina.

In TBI patients, ESR is used to detect the presence of inflammation and to help rule out autoimmune disorders. The rate varies with age and gender. This measurement is used less now than in the past since more specific tests have become available. ESRs are still used in the diagnosis of temporal arteritis, RA, multiple myeloma, and monitoring of these conditions as well as lupus. ESR is not especially good for screening asymptomatic people to see if they have a disease because of its low sensitivity and specificity, although it is routinely ordered in such cases. ESR is high in many infections and systemic diseases. Rarely does the ESR tell you anything you don't already know: that a patient is inflamed or infected. Serial readings might suggest therapeutic response. Those with ESRs over 100 should be sick enough to have an identifiable disease. Very low ESRs can mean steroid use.

PEARL: If a patient has low IgG levels, he should also have a low ESR because ESR depends on the presence of IgG.

C-reactive protein: CRP is an abnormal protein detectable in blood only during active phases of certain illnesses. One hypothesis suggests that IL-6 and TNF-α produced through inflammatory processes induce CRP production. Elevated CRP is therefore associated with the presence of inflammation and can be used to help rule out autoimmune disorders. In TBI patients, CRP is used as a nonspecific marker of inflammation and is seldom useful for discriminating among diagnoses or for monitoring clinical course. CRP can increase a thousand fold in inflammatory conditions and will respond to inflammation in 6 to 10 hours. The protein has a short half-life of about 6 hours and is most useful in the first 24 hours of the disease process when ESR is still normal. Recently the literature has been aflutter with the revelation that inflammation in cardiac patients can be a bad sign and that elevated CRP shows a high risk for bad outcomes in heart disease. In TBI patients, CRP might help recognize the existence of concomitant diseases such as RA, Reiter's syndrome, rheumatic fever, vasculitis, and IBD. CRP could also help to uncover the presence of co-infections and might be used as a tool to monitor for treatment response and as a nonspecific aid in differential diagnoses. CRP is lower in viral infections than in bacterial infections and lower in asthma than in bacterial infections.

HLA markers: These protein markers, as part of the MHC system, are found primarily on white cells and help the immune system to distinguish between *self* and non-*self*. HLAs are some of the thousands of markers on the surface of our cells that identify us as "us." HLAs are located on the surface of leukocytes and help determine what molecules our immune system will confront and to what degree. We have thousands of HLA identifiers (proteins/antigens) on our cells to prevent us from eating ourselves up. The basic science underlying these markers is explained in Chapter 3: *Gentle Immunology*.

HLA-DR2 and HLA-DR4 are markers found in a subpopulation of the general populace. They are just two of the thousands of antigen markers present in humans. Their presence suggests which patients will tend to respond to Bb infection with an autoimmune-type reaction.

About 15% of individuals in the general population have specific HLA markers that identify them as a singular group that will not react predictably to the B. *burgdorferi* infection. About 15% of us have HLA-DR2 markers, and about 15% have HLA-DR4. Some have both. Recently, scientists have learned that individuals with high levels of these two specific markers are at an increased risk of presenting an autoimmune-type picture when infected with Bb. This autoimmune presentation may be more severe and may include increased joint involvement and muscle pain, along with a more aggressive inflammatory response, since, in addition to attacking the foreign Bb, they are also assaulting the *self.*

Their genetics predispose these patients to a more difficult clinical course, and they do not seem to respond to traditional therapies. Adding hydroxychloroquine (Plaquenil) to the treatment regimen appears to help this subpopulation by alleviating symptoms and decreasing the autoimmune reaction. If HLA testing can recognize those at risk for this atypical presentation, they may be helped sooner and more efficiently.

Not all individuals with HLA-DR4 and HLA-DR2 markers trigger this type of immune reaction. For those who do react with autoimmune manifestations, there appears to be a correlation with the antibody bands 31 or 34 on Western blot that makes them more inclined to present in this way. Antibodies 31 and 34 may take a year to evolve after initial tick exposure. Knowing the patient's proclivities could help in their case management. They can be treated, just not solely in the traditional way. An individual's HLA markers should not change over time, so once these have been ordered, there is no need to repeat, unless you feel the test was not valid for some reason.

HLA-B27 is another one of the identifying markers found on cells. This particular antigen on the cell surface is associated with ankylosing spondylitis. About 6% of the Caucasian population has the HLA-B27 marker which is associated with back pain including ankylosing spondylitis and IBS. These people tend to have more general achiness and arthralgias. Not everyone with HLA-B27 has ankylosing spondylitis but essentially everyone with AS has the B27 marker.

Clusters of Differentiation: CDs form a group of protein markers on the surface of white blood cells. They are used to classify immune cell types and establish international nomenclature standards. Each marker has a specific function within the system such as passing along biochemical signals. CD levels are measured as a percent of total lymphocytes. T cells are mostly labeled CD1 through CD8, while B cells are categorized generally from CD19 to CD24. CD subsets that may be important for the TBI patient include:

> **CD4** is a marker found on essentially all T helper cells, some macrophages (monocytes), and even a few B cells. CD4 is responsible for sending signals from the T cell receptors. HIV binds to these CD4 receptors on T lymphocytes. HIV prefers to infect

the cells that are CD4+. As the HIV progresses, the number of CD4+ cells decreases. When they get low enough, the symptoms of AIDS manifest. Measuring CD4+ levels can help us gauge where the AIDS patient is clinically. Watching these trends can enable us to see how the patient is progressing. CD4 levels less than 200 are a prerequisite for the diagnosis of AIDS. The lower the CD4 the more severe the illness, so CD4 is used as a marker of clinical status. CD4 is sometimes ordered as a part of an immune panel in TBI patients.

CD8 is found on T suppressor and T cytotoxic cells which are important in the defense against viruses.

CD57 is used as a marker by some practitioners to determine when treatment of Lyme can be discontinued. CD57 marks a subpopulation of NK (natural killer) T lymphocytes. These are thought to be suppressed ONLY in Lyme disease (and perhaps some autism cases). Measurement of CD57 looks at this specific subpopulation of NK cells. Low counts are seen in *active* Lyme disease. So, in theory, the lower the CD57 level is, the more suppression of these Lyme-specific NK cells and the more active the Lyme disease. Overall, the lower the count, the sicker the patient.

CD57 less than 20	Advanced or highly active Lyme
CD57 20 to 60	Active Lyme
CD57 over 60	Less active or recovering
CD57 greater than 200	Normal

Some believe that treatment for Lyme is needed until CD57 is greater than 150. During treatment there may be only small changes observed until late in the course, when values increase dramatically. Possibly, the lower the number when treatment is stopped, the more likely a relapse. As with all testing, the CD57 should be correlated with the *clinical condition* of the patient. High CD57 levels have been documented in very sick people and low levels in some who feel great. Nonetheless, the CD57 is used as one tool for tracking disease progression, treatment response, and likelihood of relapse. As always, treat the patient and not the lab report. While this test may provide guidance, it does not absolve the HCP from looking at the whole clinical picture.

PEARL: Children do not make NK cells in the same quantity as adults; therefore, CD57 may not be as useful in monitoring Borrelia activity in kids as it may be in older patients.

Interleukins: ILs are cytokines (biomolecules) that help regulate the immune system, inflammation, and the formation of blood cells. Various IL families are made by different cells and have unique roles. ILs appear critical to normal function of the CNS in ways not clearly understood but seem to impact the hippocampus and its role in memory, learning, and nerve signal potentiation. ILs currently play a role in assessment and treatment of certain cancers such as melanoma and kidney carcinoma. ILs have been measured in conjunction with TBIs, but the specifics of their possible role(s) have yet to be clearly defined. IL-6 and IL-IB are sometimes measured in TBI patients to get clues about immune response and inflammation.

TNF-α: Tumor necrosis factor-α is a cytokine that is sometimes measured to assess the degree of chronic inflammation. TNF can be part of a broader cytokine panel. Since TBIs can be associated with significant chronic inflammation and on-going infections, elevated TNF-α may be measured in these patients although the definition of a normal level remains somewhat ambiguous.

ECP: Eosinophil cationic protein is a biomolecule that is released during degranulation of eosinophils and is related to inflammation, asthma, and parasitic infections. In these cases, the level of ECP will be elevated. ECP testing is sometimes used to assess level of inflammation, disease progression, and response to treatment. Be careful. Levels of circulating ECP can vary greatly between individuals and even within the same patient. ECP is toxic to neurons so an elevation may help explain what is happening in patients with neuropsychiatric symptoms. You may need to discuss the results of ECP testing with the reference lab to garner the most benefit from the study.

Antineuronal antibodies: The human genome is about 90% identical to that of bacteria. Because of this molecular mimicry, when the immune system is assaulted and is in combat mode, it is understandable that some of the less specific components of the response may mistake *self* antigens for bacterial antigens. An autoimmune reaction may result where neurons in the nervous system are mistakenly targeted for elimination. This phenomenon has been well-described in some children with a Strep infection. Termed pediatric autoimmune neuropsychiatric disorders associated with Streptococcal infections (PANDAS), these conditions present with sudden onset or change in intensity of OCD, tics, anxiety, panic, aggression, and other intense neuropsychiatric problems.

PEARL: PANDAS-like presentations have been associated with infectious processes involving Bb and Bartonella infections. Dr. Madeleine Cunningham at the University of Oklahoma is working to quantify some of these clinical

impressions. Currently, the specific testing methods used by Dr. Cunningham to identify antineuronal antibodies are not commercially available. Yet if you have a TBI patient with PANDAS-like manifestations, don't just hope they will go away. This type of autoimmune presentation can be life-altering. Quest has an anti-ganglioside antibody panel that includes anti-lyso-ganglioside, anti-tubulin, and anti-dopamine 1 and anti-dopamine 2. If <u>even one</u> of these parameters is found to be present, then there can be interference with nerve transmission in the patient. Some insurance plans cover this testing. These results can be the key to deciphering what is happening to your patient. Since there is an aggressive treatment regimen including <u>antibiotics</u>, IV γ-globulin, and plasmapheresis, that has been found to be useful in patients with antineuronal antibodies, consider the possibility and do what you need to do to determine how autoimmunity might be involved.

X.   SUPPORTIVE DIAGNOSTIC TESTS

The basic premise of this section is that negative diagnostic tests don't mean much in TBIs. Negative tests just mean not detected, NOT that the patient was never infected with the pathogen of interest. There are many reasons why a diagnostic test can be negative. Remember, NEVER rule out a diagnosis based on a negative test for a TBI. To date, the tests are just too insensitive and nonspecific. Use positive results as just one more piece of the bigger picture. A positive result doesn't mean you can stop thinking. There could be more than one thing going on concurrently in your patient. Diagnosis of a TBI is a clinical decision. We must get over our 20th century inclination to treat the test instead of the patient.

A.   Searching for antigens, antibodies, and complexes:

An antigen is a protein. This protein can be foreign if it comes from a pathogen, allergen, or toxin **OR** a *self* protein if the immune system is cleaning up cellular debris or there is an autoimmune malfunction. An antibody is interchangeably called an immunoglobulin, which is formed through the stimulation of T cells and the maturation of B cells in response to a specific antigen. As you interpret test results, here are some basic concepts to help you understand what you are seeing.

A **titer** is the concentration of a substance in solution. For example, the titer of antibodies present in a sample can be calculated by determining the *lowest* concentration where those antibodies are still able to combine with a known amount of antigen. The lowest concentration is also referred to as the *highest* dilution. If the concentration of antibody is too low (the dilution is too high), there will not be enough antibody present in the solution to react with the antigen; therefore, there will not be sufficient amounts of reaction product to measure.

Titration is the process by which we measure titers. A measured amount of one solution is added to a known quantity of another solution until a reaction between them is complete (as defined by some preset parameters). By measuring a quantity, such as a specific reaction product that forms between the known and unknown substances, the concentration of the unknown entity can be calculated. This is the premise on which many of the tests used to determine the presence of an antibody or antigen is based.

Serology is the study of the components of serum. You will read and hear terms like sero-negative and sero-positive, which are slightly misleading. While much diagnostic testing is done on serum, it is also performed on many other fluids and tissues. Many HCPs throw these terms around without having any idea of what they actually mean. In general, the term serologic testing refers to the process of dilutions and titer measurements looking for Ag/Ab complexes. Any number of methods might be used to obtain these results. Take the term serology as a general moniker for a wide variety of methodologies looking for evidence to support diagnosis.

Essentially, the more "intimate" the specimen source, the higher the yield of useable results for all the listed tests. Tissue samples are usually the most reliable. One group of patients tested negative for Babesia using blood samples. When tissue from biopsies taken during endoscopy and surgery were used instead, the same patients all tested positive. While most testing can be done using blood, serum, or urine, any sample that can be collected during biopsy, surgery, or at birth can be invaluable. Sensitivity and specificity in most of these tests is marginal under the best conditions, so collecting a sample that gives the greatest chance for pathogen detection is important.

Qualitative methods are useful when all you need is a yes or no answer. Is an entity present or not? The most familiar example is testing patients for blood donor compatibility. The patient's antigen-containing red cells are mixed with known antibodies to a particular blood group. If they clump inside the test tube, they are likely to clump inside the person, and that would be bad. But here all you need is a YES or NO qualitative result.

Quantitative testing measures the *amount* of antibody present in correspondence to a particular antigen. This measurement is usually accomplished using a series of dilutions. The MOST dilute combination that shows agglutination is identified. The *least* concentrated dilution that still shows agglutination is given as the test result. Details of the interpretation of these techniques are provided below so that you can better understand what you are ordering.

With general serology or Ag/Ab testing, results are provided as titers or dilutions. A starting dilution of 1:8 means one part component-of-interest in 8 parts of total test solution. An assay starting with a dilution of 1:8 could then have results with values such as 1:16, 1:32, 1:64, 1:128, 1:256, 1:512, 1:1024, etc. A test result of 1:16 shows minimal interaction between the antigen and the specimen. In that case, there must be little, if any, antibody specific for that antigen in the test sample. In contrast, a finding of 1:1024 suggests a whopping reaction and indicates that there is a large amount of the antibody in the sample able to react with the antigen. In other words, even at very high dilutions making the concentration of the test agent proportionately LOW, there is STILL enough antigen present to react. For example, a titer of 1:160 or higher is suggestive of Babesia infection.

Each pathogen will have a titer level associated with a particular test that is considered positive, others that suggest there is no reaction, and many that are considered equivocal, borderline, or uninterpretable. If 1:16 is little or no reaction and 1:64 is thought to be positive, what does 1:32 mean? These are the cases that are most difficult to interpret. My thought is that if there is enough antibody present to cause any reaction, you should consider that finding suggestive of the diagnosis. Something triggered that reaction, no matter how mild.

In almost all cases where we talk about antigen testing against sample antibodies, we could just as easily be talking about antibody testing against antigen. Usually the antigen is the KNOWN, since the proteins can be extracted from the recognized pathogen and used as the test strain. The antibodies from the patient have been made in response to some antigen stimulus. Let's see if they were made in response to the pathogen we suspect as the cause of the illness. The patient sample is washed over the known, affixed antigen. Any number of methods (dyes, bands, fluorescence, radiation, complement consumption, etc.), are then used to determine if there are now measurable Ag/Ab complexes. Reverse methods check antigen against known antibody. If there is no binding, then NO (or not enough) antibody was present that could have been inspired by the known antigen used as the reference marker. This doesn't mean the antigen was never present, just that no antibody was recovered in the test sample.

PEARL: NEVER discount a TBI diagnosis on the basis of a negative test result. A lab finding is just one piece of a BIG puzzle. The tests are just not reliable enough under the best of circumstances to rule anything out on the basis of one finding. Look at your patients. They will tell you what you need to know. In our litigious society, courage is needed to go against a lab result. Knowledge can provide the courage.

Many of the pathogens causing TBIs have isolated antigens that can be used in such testing. Positive results can vary between labs. A positive result must be statistically different from a negative one and has meaning only if correlated with the clinical picture. Further, a negative result just means "not detected." The patient could still have been infected. If the lab where the sample is being tested is using antigen from pathogen strains from Bartleby, Maine, and your patient was infected in Pocopson, Pennsylvania, it is possible that you will get negative results even though you have a very sick patient. Please check with the lab, especially if you don't do this every day or are testing for a pathogen that is not in your usual repertoire.

PEARL: The biggest concern with TBI testing is false negatives not false positives. Is the person sitting in front of you sick? If the answer is yes, you might have a false negative OR you could be looking for the wrong pathogen. Your focus might have been in the wrong ball park looking for TBIs when you should be looking at some other condition in the differential diagnosis or concurrent disorder list. Okay, just regroup. False positives very rarely occur in testing for TBIs, although the IDSA appears deathly afraid of that possibility. The worst that could happen if you act on a false positive has far less meaningful consequences than if you don't act because of a false negative.

PEARL: Yesterday I was told of an interesting twist to the complexity around testing for Lyme. In one case where the patient tested positive repeatedly for Lyme at different labs, the HCP was determined to keep trying still more labs until he got a negative result. Since false positives are rare (to say the least), I have no idea what this HCP was after. He had a patient with a positive test with all the corroborating history and clinical presentation and he was treating her appropriately. A positive test was a miracle, a gift, considering the testing environment. Did he think that a negative test would make the Lyme go away? Would it mean the disease was no longer present or was never there? Would a negative test signify cure? Just when you think you've heard it all….

PEARL: Western blot, ELISA, and numerous other serological and agglutination techniques depend on the ability of an antigen to bind with its specifically-designed antibody. Most of these test methods involve the adherence of a known antigen to a surface and then washing a sample of unknown antibodies over the antigen. If the antigen and antibody can bind, they will. Then, depending on the method – dyes, radioactivity, florescence, or location on a test strip – the antigen/antibody complex is recognized and documented. Serologic tests use the smallest amount of antigen (or the largest amount of dilution) to determine if binding occurs. The presence of antibodies that could only have been manufactured after exposure to a specific antigen, provides

supportive evidence that the antigen had been around either now or in the past. Today, thousands of antigens, corresponding to hundreds of pathogens, have been isolated and are available for supportive diagnostic testing. Somewhere, your target pathogen probably has some antigen stored waiting for you to check the right box (and send the right check). Essentially all pathogens can be sought – with different degrees of success – through Ag/Ab binding.

While there may be some cross-reactivity, where one type of antibody binds with two or more antigens making test interpretation more difficult, for the most part we can assume that one antibody was made in response to a specific antigen.

PEARL: In any of these Ag/Ab detection methods, some mild cross-reactivity may occur, complicating the interpretation. Set aside what I said about only one lock, only one key, and marriage between one antigen and one antibody. Sometimes, there is a little fraternization. Yes, occasionally, the key can semi-fit into another lock. This is usually a partial fit, just enough to confound us. Usually, cross-reactivity causes a weaker binding than does the "made-for-each-other" Ag/Ab complex binding. The key prefers its own lock. For diseases like Lyme, we have already identified the patterns that are likely to indicate cross-reactivity. We know how to watch out for them and work around them.

Now, let's track down a few antibodies. …

You probably won't have much choice as to which tests are performed in looking for the antigens or antibodies of interest in your patient. Still the more you know, the more you will understand as you interpret test results. Test interpretation depends on the technique used. If there is a method that you have found to be more reliable than another, discuss that possibility with the lab.

1. **Agglutination methods** – In some cases, the binding of an antigen to its antibody causes a clumping of antigen/antibody complexes in a process called agglutination. The amount of clumping can be measured. Different labs may employ an assortment of techniques and the definition of a positive test may vary. Agglutination studies can be qualitative where a positive outcome is said to occur if any clumping is detected. Qualitative methods are useful when testing patients for blood donor compatibility and the patient's antigen-containing red cells are mixed with antibodies to a particular blood group and all you need is a yes or no answer. Quantitative testing measures the amount of antibody present in correspondence to a particular antigen. This measurement is usually accomplished using a series of dilutions. The MOST dilute combination that shows agglutination is given as the test result. Note that in the

interpretation of these tests the terms "most dilute" and "least concentrated" mean the same thing. It's enough to make your head spin.

2. **Electrophoresis** – A separation technique that uses an electrical field to move molecules based on their size and charge. A complex mix of antigens is placed on a plate coated with an agar gel where an electric field is then used to separate the various components. Wherever there is an antigen/antibody reaction, a precipitate will form on that section of the gel. The more reaction, the more precipitation. Depending on the specifics of the technique the precipitate can be visualized using dyes, radioactivity, or fluorescence. This testing is used as a qualitative analysis when looking at a mixture of antigens. Rough quantities can also be estimated by looking at the amount of precipitate present with each antigen. Electrophoresis is often tacked onto other techniques such as PCR.

3. **Immunofluorescence assay** - IFA can be used to detect antibodies in a sample. The specific antibodies are labeled with a compound that causes them to glow bright green when viewed under UV light. Most simply, IFA uses a single antibody that is chemically linked to a fluorescent molecule. The antibody recognizes the target antigen and binds to it causing the fluorescence. The glow can be detected under a microscope using a UV light. Usually a known antigen is fixed to a test plate and test samples are added at various dilutions. When antibody in the sample binds to the antigen on the plate, the complex fluoresces. IFA counts on the specificity of the antibodies to their antigen in association with specialized dyes to allow visualization.

Different methods can be used to enhance specificity and IFA can be used on tissue sections and cultures under a microscope. The problem with IFA is with timing. The older the sample the more potential for cross-reactivity and therefore less specificity. Time also results in loss of activity of the fluorescent molecule.

PEARL: If there is a lot of fluorescence, the test may be hard to interpret. The reader can't understand the test because she can't tell if the findings are specific or nonspecific because the system is overwhelmed.

4. **Radioimmunoassay** – RIA can be used to identify either antigen or antibody. This technique is sensitive and specific and can be used to measure the concentration of antigen by use of its corresponding antibody. The converse can also be done where the antibody can be quantified by use of its matching antigen, called radiobinding technique.

RIA is less expensive than many other analytic techniques. However with a number of pathogens, RIA has been replaced by ELISA. We will examine the catastrophic improper use of ELISA in detecting Lyme disease below. Although there are a number of variations, usually with RIA, a radioactive label is placed on the protein and then the amount of radioactivity in the Ag/Ab reaction product is measured. Rosalyn Yalow received the Nobel Prize for her work developing RIA.

5. **ELISA** – Enzyme-linked immunosorbent assay can be used to detect the presence of an antibody or antigen in a sample. ELISA testing has gotten a bad rap because of the controversy surrounding its inappropriate use in testing for Lyme disease. There is nothing inherently flawed about the ELISA test. There are a number of valid uses for this methodology in testing for a variety of infectious diseases. The ELISA test is an inanimate entity and cannot be held responsible for its unscientific and unethical use by humans. ELISA results can support diagnoses for other TBIs or other pathogens and should be reviewed just like any other test results: Who did the test? How did they do it? With the methods and pathogen strains used to make the antigens or antibodies, does this test have a reasonable chance of providing pertinent information for a particular patient?

ELISA tests simply detect the presence of an antigen or antibody. Usually an unknown amount of antigen is fixed on a surface. Then a specific antibody is washed over that surface giving it the opportunity to bind with the antigen. A dye is added so that a visual demonstration of the formation of antigen/antibody complexes can be observed. Antigens will bind only with their matching antibody (and vice versa). One kind of antigen binds only with its specific antibody. If they don't match, they do not bind.

PEARL: You can't use an antigen that has no chance of binding with the antibody and expect detection of Ag/Ab complexes and valid results. Biochemistry does not work that way.

ELISA can be effective in detecting the presence of a number of pathogens. Unfortunately, its history in detection of Lyme disease has been dismal, not because of inherent flaws in the methodology of the ELISA, but because of choices made regarding how the test should be interpreted that do not have a solid scientific foundation. If proteins from strains of pathogen are used that cannot match the antibody made by the patient, you will not get a positive test result. This causes a very high number of false negative tests. When the panel determined that only those ELISA tests that were deemed positive would be sent on for confirmatory WB testing, many sick people were left without options. Based on faulty methodology, very ill patients were told that they did not have Lyme, and there was no recourse. Estimates using the current test strains for Bb will miss between 30% and 50% of positive cases.

PEARL: Estimates of missed cases vary in the published literature but AT LEAST 30% are thought to be missed and this is a conservative estimate.

With all that being said, ELISA results cannot be ethically used to rule out Lyme disease. Most knowledgeable HCPs do NOT order ELISA testing in support of a Lyme diagnosis unless they are forced to do so by insurance companies. The surveillance criteria require that the ELISA be positive before the sample can be sent for more diagnostic testing such as the contrived WB test. Remember the goal has been to decrease the incidence of Lyme. By not recognizing clear cases, the numbers will decline. Numbers should not become more important than sick people. One author proposed that if your HCP orders ELISA screening to support a diagnosis of Lyme, then perhaps that HCP does not know much about Lyme and you should find another doctor.

PEARL: In defense of the CDC, they have admitted that it is inappropriate to use their **surveillance** *case definitions "for establishing* **clinical** *diagnoses, determining the standard of care necessary for a particular patient, setting guidelines for quality assurance, or providing standards for reimbursement." Still, the CDC surveillance criteria are used daily in clinical practice and this shortchanges many sick patients.*

For further details about the problems inherent with the ELISA and Lyme, see Chapter 11: *Controversies around Lyme*. Also, Pam Weintraub in *Cure Unknown* provides a comprehensive overview.

PEARL: In January, 2012, I came across a similar situation where the "authorities" decided to decrease the incidence of a condition by changing the diagnostic parameters. The autism spectrum of disorders has overlapping and confusing descriptions and most practitioners would welcome clarity in this regard. A panel from the APA was formed and their mission was to adjust the diagnostic requirements that would define autism in the next edition of the DSM. Unfortunately, the panel decided that there was an autism epidemic that they planned to "nip in the bud."(Their words not mine.) Panel members admitted to trying to decrease the number of insurance claims and to save money on special programs for autistic children. Writer William Rostler said, "You won't find a cure by

saying there is no problem." Just as when the "authorities" sought to decrease the Lyme epidemic by making it nearly impossible for the majority of true cases to get an "official" diagnosis, renaming the problem will not change the number of sick people. The true incidence of the condition will stay the same and we can only pretend that it is different, but that won't change the facts. Personally, I would prefer that the panel just admit that they are trying to make it harder for kids to qualify for resources so they are going to develop different funding criteria. But a condition by any other name is still going to be that condition. The same number of people will still be sick, but there will be fewer called sick. The child will wake up tomorrow with the same signs and symptoms as he had yesterday but a name change will have miraculously affected a cure. Similarly, local officials at a Chester County, Pennsylvania, hospital brag that they have greatly reduced the incidence of Lyme, when they have only reduced the identification of true positives. How sad that these autism regulators have not learned lessons from previous mistakes. The media war over re-categorizing autism has now begun.

6. **Western blot (WB)** – The Western blot method uses the principles of electrophoresis to separate out proteins by length and structure. The proteins are then identified using antibodies specific to the target antigen. WB looks at both the type and amount of antibodies present. This test is more sensitive and specific than ELISA since it shows more positive results when the results are actually positive.

WB is recognized by the NIAID (National Institute of Allergy and Infectious Diseases, a division of the National Institutes of Health) as the most useful method for detecting Bb *antibodies* currently available. WB can be used to measure both IgG and IgM. In most infectious diseases the IgM tend to appear first and wane after the first few weeks and *usually* do not recur. These are followed by IgG which are regarded as the major enduring Ab response in chronic infections. However in LD, IgM may persist for years suggesting persistent infection or reactivation of latent infection. This type of IgM endurance is also known to occur in toxoplasmosis, leishmaniasis, and CMV. A number of studies point to the importance of IgM in recurrent or persistent LD. As with all things Lyme, keep an open and flexible mind.

Many companies now provide antibodies against thousands of proteins to be used in Western blot testing. Here again we have a problem. The key to sensitive and specific WB testing (getting positives when the reality is positive and negatives when the reality is negative) is in selecting antigens that have a chance of connecting with the antibodies present in the sample. If you put in antibodies to one strain of pathogen, and only another strain of the pathogen is present, you will most likely get a result that will be interpreted as negative.

Your goal is to select an antigen that is close enough to the antigen that first inspired the antibody so that there is the possibility of reacting with the antibody present in the patient sample. WB results are influenced both by the strain used as the testing standard as well as the timing of sample collection. Sometimes the endemic region is known and the antigen selection can be based on this information. If the antigens chosen as the test standard are from a similar strain as the one that caused the patient's disease then the test can be expected to show good sensitivity and specificity. If no, then not so much.

If you will be working with a number of TBI patients, you will be ordering WBs and looking at WB results. The literature is full of WB references. Unfortunately, politics, hubris, greed, and what-can-only-be-described-as-lunacy, have tainted this test for the diagnosis of Lyme disease. NEVER rule out the diagnosis of Lyme based on arbitrary band criteria on a Western blot test. The good news is that if you understand the science behind the test, you can circumvent the bad criteria choices made by those with secondary agendas and actually use Western blot results to help Lyme patients.

Just to complicate your life, a **reverse** Western blot is an **antigen** detecting test where the urine is exposed to known Bb **antibodies**. A full discourse on the history of the WB controversy as well as the insight and knowledge needed to interpret WB testing in 2013 is provided in the adjacent box. Fasten your seat belt, it's going to be a bumpy ride.

PEARL: Remember that antibodies take time to develop. Taking a blood sample immediately after a tick bite is not likely to produce a positive result due to that particular tick. An instantly positive test is likely due to exposure in the past or on-going, active infection from a prior bite.

THE WESTERN BLOT SAGA

Western blot (WB) – First, let me apologize for the length of this section. There is so much history and controversy around the use of WB testing in support of the diagnosis of Lyme disease that I felt the need to explain in detail. For those of you who interpret WBs daily, this may seem to be much ado about nothing. But for those of us who do not read these bands often, the interpretation can be confusing. The science itself is quite comprehensible, but when politics deliberately confounds the science, we mere mortals need a little extra time. There were hundreds of articles on this topic. In some, I even had trouble corroborating the bands that the CDC would accept, let alone the dozens of other so-called "better" approaches. I had stacks of articles sorted by which bands were approved by various sources. In some of the literature, the CDC did not appear to agree with themselves.

Description: The Western blot measures the antibodies your body makes against an infection—nothing more, nothing less. The WB looks at both the type and amount of antibodies. This test is more sensitive and specific than ELISA since it shows more positive results when the results are actually positive. The Western blot can detect specific antigens using gel electrophoresis to separate the proteins; then these proteins are transferred to a membrane where specific antibodies from a patient source are used to determine what antigens are present.

Known pathogen proteins (antigens) are separated by weight and spread on a surface. The lighter proteins move more readily than the heavier ones. A sample from the patient is washed over this stripe of known antigens. If antibodies against the pathogen are present in the specimen, a vertical line will form where the antigen and antibody react. This band forms wherever an antigen and corresponding antibody meet along the way. The band is a line of antibody/antigen complexes, a fingerprint that can ONLY be made if an antibody meets up with its matching antigen. With few exceptions, an antibody can bind only with its exact antigen so there will be a band formed only at that precise spot on the WB, *IF* that specific antigen is present. Biochemically, it doesn't work any other way.

There are a number of valid methods used to gather WB test results. Most common is the reading of the bands that form on the substrate material when antigen binds with antibody. Stained bands then indicate the presence of the antigens to which the patient's serum contains antibody. Because the antigens should be selected specifically for their ability to react with the antibodies against the pathogen of interest, we know the bands that *should* form if their corresponding antibodies are present. The patterns that form in the test result are compared to the patterns that are known to form when the matching antibodies are present. By comparing what is known with what appears after the patient's antibody is added, interpretations can be made.

Sounds reasonable and direct and valid. Of course, things aren't that simple. We are not yet so advanced that we have access to test antigens for all the various strains of pathogens of interest. With TBIs, there can be dozens or even hundreds of strains. We might suspect a certain pathogen based on history and clinical course, but we're lucky if we know we're picking between spirochetes and Rickettsia, let alone the hundreds of variants. Usually, we don't know what we don't know. We check the box for Babesia and the lab throws in the antigens it has available. Occasionally, *IF* we know the geographic location where the patient was infected, an enlightened lab can target the test to organisms known to be endemic to the area. But they work off checklists, too. Sometimes the strains used are closely related to those present in the patient, causing equivocal results.

Timing is critical for sensitive WB testing. In most infections, IgM is the first antibody present, and amounts produced are large. IgM decreases over time as the immune system has time to make IgG. As the infection decreases, IgM decreases. IgG is produced once an infection has been going on for a while and levels may remain high even after the active infection is gone. Looking for both IgM and IgG bands on the Western blot gives a better idea of where an infection might be in the clinical course. If you order only one or the other, you might miss the whole thing. IgG testing too early in the infectious process will give a false negative since it hasn't had time to become established yet. IgM testing too late in the process may be negative because the IgM has been mostly replaced by IgG. For most pathogens, IgM shows a current infection and IgG shows either active or past infection or previous exposure. Paradoxically, Lyme may not follow this traditional pattern. Usually about a week is needed to be able to detect antibodies to an infectious agent. Serologic testing done before this time can be too early, and patients may be told they don't have the disease when testing a short time later would be positive. Certain IgGs may take years to manifest.

In Lyme, Western blot may not be positive early in the course of the disease. In fact, some researchers believe that Lyme may actually cycle IgG and IgM as symptoms wax and wane. There may be more reasons than you know for a Lyme WB to be negative. Order both IgG and IgM antibodies tested so you mitigate the risk of missing one if they cycle. Cycling antibodies might help explain the fluctuating symptoms found in Lyme. Some researchers believe that IgM may persist in LD, while IgG might never establish a substantial presence.

Many companies now provide antibodies against thousands of proteins to be used in Western blot testing. Always use caution in interpreting any WB test. Again, the key to sensitive and specific WB testing (getting positives when the reality is positive and negatives when the reality is negative) is in selecting antigens that have a chance of connecting with the antibody present in the sample. If you put in antibodies to one strain of pathogen and only another strain of the pathogen is present, you will get a result that will most likely be interpreted as negative. Remember, the test antigen selected should be as close as possible to the antigen that could have originally stimulated the antibody formation in the patient in the first place. Western blot techniques are commonly used with HIV, hepatitis B, and mad cow disease. There is Western blot testing for everything else, and then there is WB testing for Lyme. This brings us to the…

Controversy: In 1994, on what I can only imagine was a dark and stormy day, representatives from the CDC and public health agencies met in Michigan to decide what constituted grounds for a diagnosis of Lyme disease in patients with symptoms lasting longer than 4 weeks. They came up with the Dearborn criteria, also called the CDC surveillance guidelines. Pam Weintraub provides a comprehensive review of the process in her book *Cure Unknown*.

Today we know that many of the participants at the Dearborn conference had various secondary agendas. A number were on the payroll of the vaccine industry, and others belonged to the insurance companies. Even real estate speculation came into play. Let's consider the possible motivations:

- Certain WB bands were left off the list of positive results even though they were the most specific for Lyme because of the impact on vaccine clinical trials and interference in the development of vaccines between competitors.

- The fewer "valid" cases of Lyme, the less insurance companies would have to pay in terms of expensive long-term treatments, IV regimens, or more sensitive (and expensive) supportive lab tests. A claims adjustor could more easily say, "The tests are negative. She doesn't have Lyme. We're not paying for anything else."

- If there is less Lyme around, realtors do not have to worry about clients avoiding endemic areas. Lyme, Connecticut, anyone?

- The CDC had been promising to decrease the I&P of Lyme, and a great way to do that is to not recognize the diagnosis. Just ask all of us in West Chester, Pennsylvania, who have negative tests and bad disease. Congratulations, you've almost wiped it out (and us along with it.)

While it's easy to lob criticism from the cheap seats, there is no excuse for the irrational and unscientific restrictions imposed in Dearborn that have hurt thousands of TBI patients. Here are a few of the scientific flaws in the Dearborn conclusions that impede the diagnosis of Lyme disease:

- Only some forms of the Lyme pathogen can be detected by Western blot. Antigens selected as the standards for positive tests were based on a single European strain of the spirochete, while there are a number of variants in the US that we know of. Many HCPs felt that it was absurd to rely on a European isolate as the reference strain when that was not likely to reflect the disease in the US. Since the protein on the spirochete's coat could be different in the various strains, the antigens would also be different. Therefore, there would be little likelihood that antibodies formed in the patient would be able to react with the antigens on the test strip. Another false negative.

- Antigens were selected from a patient population who no longer fits the current profile. Back then, Lyme was thought to be mostly a rheumatoid disease with occasional CNS complications, hence the name Lyme arthritis. Antigens selected were from patients who had swollen knees and measurably damaged nerves. This definition is much more restrictive than the multisystem disease that we now know Lyme to be. By the nature of the WB, the diagnosis could only be made in patients who were similar to this small subpopulation, greatly cutting the number of true positives.

- Of the many possible antigens, just 10 were anointed worthy of making the diagnosis and none were allowed to stand alone, although some, like band 18, certainly could. The most specific antigens of Bb were eliminated: Outer surface proteins A and B, or OspA and OspB, were eliminated from the test. Antibodies to OspA and OspB are so specific for Borrelia *burgdorferi* that they could come from NOTHING but exposure to Bb. They were so specific for the Lyme pathogen that they were chosen to make the first vaccines. There is NO WAY that antibodies could be made against OspA and OspB UNLESS Bb antigen had been present. How else would it get there? Unfortunately, these antigens were not included as part of the criteria to appease vaccine business interests. (The vaccines that these OSPs were eliminated to protect, either never made it to market or were pulled from commercial use. Therefore this bad decision was all for naught.)

The following CDC criteria were included for the identification of Lyme:

- Patients had to be positive by ELISA screening before WB testing was allowed to be performed. Since ELISA has been shown to miss between 30% and 50% of true positives, many Lyme sufferers did not even get a chance to be deemed positive by Western blot. (In fact, 30% is lower than the usual estimate. Most estimates of potential misses of true positives are much higher.)

- Serologic diagnosis of early Lyme required presence of antibodies associated with early infection. Three IgMs were selected and patients who had 2 of these 3 bands within a month of tick bite were considered positive. IgM bands "approved" by the CDC are OspC 23-25, 39, and 41.

- At least 5 of the 10 selected bands of IgG must be present for a positive diagnosis: 18, 23-25, 28, 30, 39, 41, 45, 58, 66, and 93 (83 to 93).

These decisions worked against the sickest patients and those infected longest before being diagnosed. Long-term patients are more likely to show antibodies to OspA and OspB. If these antigens were not available to be tested, then all the specific antibody on the planet cannot react with them. The sickest patients would be less likely to show positive bands on the test.

Cases positive by Dearborn are positive, indeed, but these aren't the ones we are concerned about here. We are worried about all the false negatives. Once you are tossed from the system for being negative, there is no recourse. The system does not have a built-in place for this error to be rectified. In contrast, false positives will be identified one way or another: 1) more definitive testing is done, 2) the patient gets better, or 3) the patient gets worse and is investigated for other etiologies. Essentially the worst thing about a false positive is that a patient is treated for a condition that he does not have. If there is no response, the error will soon be recognized.

Different HCPs, labs, and agencies use different patterns of bands to affirm a positive. You will want to choose a lab that provides band numbers and not just a positive or negative result based on the Dearborn criteria. That way you will be able to decide if the band patterns you see support the diagnosis of Lyme or not. Unfortunately, a number of labs still use the antigens recommended as standards by the CDC. You may be stuck with their bands, but you are not prohibited from thinking. Analyze the results on your own, and make the best decision for your patient. NEVER rule out the diagnosis of Lyme based on arbitrary band criteria on a Western blot test.

> PEARL: In summary, the CDC recommends that 1 of 3 reference strains be used. Several commercial labs use two or more reference strains and therefore are more likely to have a match between the antibody in the patient sample and the various strain antigens used as reference. Some "authorities" have criticized these labs for getting too many positives. I don't know what too many positives means. The antibody won't react unless it finds its corresponding antigen. We want positive results when they should be positive. We don't want to eliminate any chance of a positive result, and then gloat that the sick person isn't sick. Other labs use various numbers and sources of reference strains but some come from Germany, and the local hospital here must have an interplanetary source. Before you make any decisions about Lyme based on a negative WB, make sure you know the origin of the strains against which your patient was tested. It also helps to know where geographically the patient was bitten. If she just got back from a trip to Germany where she was bitten by a tick, then a German strain might be entirely appropriate. That scenario would be exceedingly rare.

Thank goodness that – except for insurance adjusters trying to avoid a claim or medical boards ripe for a kill – we are free to interpret WB results scientifically and logically.

Interpretation: In general for WB tests, most of us just check the box in front of the pathogen of interest and let the lab worry about how to do the test. Nonetheless, it is prudent to know what you are looking for in comparison to what you are requesting, because they might not be the same. If you don't know, CALL THE LAB. If the lab can explain what strain options are available along with the test methods, you have a better chance of getting information you can use.

That approach should work well for just about everything. However, because of the artificial Dearborn criteria, interpretation of WB looking for evidence of Bb is not so straightforward. Here we go:

WB results can be reported several ways:

1. A positive or negative (yes-or-no reaction between antigen and antibody)

2. By band number, which identifies a specific location on the test strip

For each antigen available for study, there is a known pattern or fingerprint of bands that should display if its corresponding antibodies are present. By comparing what you know to what you tested, some determination should be able to be made if there is a match.

Look at IgG **18, 23, 30, 31, 34, 39, 83**, and **93**. If 18 alone is present, that band is specific enough to support a diagnosis of Lyme. Any of these other bands, alone or in combination, indicates sero-evidence of exposure to the Bb spirochete. For IgM look at the same bands since the IgG started out originally as IgM. WB alone is not diagnostic for active disease, it just shows that exposure likely occurred at some point. You must take this data point and put it into the overall picture to make the diagnosis.

Many of the CDC-selected bands are quite nonspecific. In fact, you can have a positive Lyme test by CDC criteria based only on nonspecific bands with no evidence of Bb in sight. For example, band 41 suggests an antibody reaction to a pathogen that has a flagellum that might be a spirochete. The CDC surveillance criteria do not correlate with clinical reality and should not be used to make or break a diagnosis of Lyme.

In Lyme, IgM is thought to be generated first, and then in about 2 months IgG takes over, unless a persistent, active infection continues to drive IgM production. IgM band 23 is thought to be the same as IgG band 18. Most chronic patients have been infected for a long time potentially confounding their band presentation. Band 31 may take a year or longer to appear.

There are five cross-reacting bands that are shared by Bb and several other pathogens. These bands might appear, but they lack specificity and include 28, 41, 45, 58, and 66. Their appearance should not have any bearing on a decision in support of the clinical diagnosis of Lyme disease. All five are part of the CDC 5/10-required-to-be-present-to-diagnose-Lyme panel.

> *PEARL: Bands 31 and 34 may take a year to appear after the tick attachment that transmitted the Bb. These bands are associated with the increased tendency to have a Lyme-induced autoimmune presentation – especially in those who have shown the presence of HLA-DR2 and HLA-DR4 markers. The exclusion of bands 31 and 34 by the panel was prompted by secondary agendas having to do with vaccine patents and conflicts of interest. Including these bands would have allowed the WB to be significantly more diagnostic than currently seen.*

When documenting bands, the lab generally reports each of the bands with the following intensities:

–	Not present
+	Low
++	Medium
+++	High
+/–	Equivocal (indeterminate, which is not as intense as low)

As an old biochemist, I don't get too excited about intensity. To some people +++ might mean more than +. But Lyme messes with the immune system, so magnitude is not as significant as sheer presence. The body doesn't just make antibodies at random. The immune system makes antibodies against specific antigens, and it makes antibody against Bb when Bb is present. If there is a detectable band, there is antigen binding to antibody and "God's in his Heaven/All's right with the world." (Robert Browning)

There are thousands of articles in the literature touting the best band pattern to be used to identify Bb. I have read hundreds of these articles, and I'm done now. As of this moment, I will never read another article about Western blot testing in Lyme disease. I'll stick with my current approach.

Uses: The website www.mentalhealthandillness.com lists 27 reasons why someone could have a false negative Lyme Western blot. I can think of even more. That just means that most HCPs don't understand how to use this test, not that the science underlying the test is flawed. While the WB has strengths and weaknesses, just like any other analytic method, if we understand these limits and work around them, we can gather useful information from the WB.

There is inherent value in the WB, but *only* if the antigens that are used have a chance of matching up with the antibodies in the sample. This is true for Lyme and any other pathogen of interest. You can't test for something that is not there. Well, you can, but don't expect anything useful. Different labs use different antigens. A sample that produces a negative result in one lab might be positive in another. The second lab might use antigens obtained in the area where the individual was infected. If you know the geographic location where the patient was infected, the lab can attempt to select antigens with the potential of giving a sensitive result. One area hospital that shall remain nameless seems to make a special effort to use antigen that can't possibly react with sample from anyone in Chester County.

Use a lab that provides band numbers in the results. This way, you decide what is meaningful. If you do not know what you are ordering, CALL THE LAB. Never rule out Lyme on the basis of a Western blot. Even if you are testing the right strains at the perfect time and all the stars are aligned, the test is simply not sensitive enough to place all your faith there. For WB testing of any other pathogens, know what you are ordering and the strains that will be used in testing. The lab can help with both requests and interpretation. These tests are so expensive that you should expect a little customer service with your order.

Some authors swear that WB is more likely to be positive BEFORE treatment, and others are just as adamant that WB is more likely to be positive AFTER treatment. This may depend on the pathogen or the timing of the sample. If you get a negative band pattern and still believe the patient has Lyme, you can consider a retest but wait about 4 to 6 weeks for the antibodies to reestablish. Otherwise, try different diagnostic technologies such as PCR or cultures.

At best, WB is about 50% sensitive. The problem comes mostly when the false negative gives an HCP absolute confidence that the diagnosis is NOT Lyme. That's where the stories emerge of an HCP screaming at a 5-year-old, "You do NOT have Lyme!"

One review article claimed that using history alone to make the Lyme diagnosis is 76% accurate. Even if this percentage is overblown, most diagnostic tests don't even come close. Fortunately, we do not have to rely on diagnostic testing to make a diagnosis. Lyme is a clinical diagnosis.

7. **Complement fixation techniques** – Antigen/antibody complexes can be quantified by their ability to fix complement. The formation of Ag/Ab complexes will consume complement like a ravenous tick if complement is present. In contrast, free antigen or free antibody will not deplete complement. Complement fixing techniques are often used to see how much antibody is present in a sample, but the methodology can be tweaked to assess antigen as well. These methods are used primarily for pathogens that are hard to culture. Today, complement fixing has been mostly superseded by methods like PCR and FISH. Nevertheless, there are a number of references to this modality in the literature.

8. **Lyme DOT blot** – This assay for the direct detection of Lyme antigen in the urine looks for actual pieces of the bacteria. DOT is used in those who show clinical symptoms and a history consistent with Lyme but continue to test negative on antibody tests. Here, the molecules to be detected are not separated first but rather a mixture is applied directly on the test surface. One of the editors asked me what "DOT" stood for. Well, here is your answer, Doug. The specimen is applied to the test surface as a "dot." Why the letters in DOT are capitalized in much of the literature, I have no idea. This technique is one of the fastest analytical methods but provides no information about the size or nature of the molecules. Sometimes if two molecules are similar they will appear as a single result in the findings. All you get is a present or absent outcome; but, sometimes that is all you need. Lyme DOT can also be done on CSF.

PEARL: The Lyme DOT blot is a variation of the northern blot, the southern blot, and eastern blot all named by various researchers in the spirit of whimsy and competition. The reverse Western blot can be used to confirm the Lyme DOT blot. (Let me get this straight: The WB is used to correct for the insensitivity of the ELISA. The Lyme DOT blot is used to correct for the insensitivity of the WB. The reverse Western blot is used to correct for the insensitivity of the Lyme DOT blot. Thank goodness that Lyme is a clinical diagnosis!)

B. Searching for nucleic acids

There are a number of advantages in testing for RNA and DNA when looking for support in diagnosing TBIs. The primary nucleic acid based tests include:

1. **PCR** – The **polymerase chain reaction** looks for **DNA**. A positive result on PCR means that the actual DNA of the organism was found. A negative result only means that no DNA from the pathogen of interest was found in this sample – NOT that there was no pathogen in this patient now or ever. As always, a negative test does not exclude the diagnosis. Repeated (serial) PCR tests may be needed to finally show a positive. Although PCR results are more sensitive than many other tests, low sensitivity remains a problem because the test relies on such minute amounts of DNA. In 2013, PCRs are ordered like fries at the drive-through. Despite low specificity, the term PCR is on every list of diagnostic modalities for essentially all TBIs and other pathogens. PCR yield may be as low as 5% to 10% but when it is present it is clear that the pathogen was around prior to testing. References to PCR are common in the literature since a positive is highly likely to be a true positive. As always, it's great to get a positive PCR result for the organism you suspected. This proves you were a genius to think of it in the first place. It's probably safe to assume that the pathogen is still present if its DNA is found. Some of the literature says that the DNA can persist after the organism is dead but with Bb you're never quite sure if they're actually dead or just dormant. Assume live spirochetes are present if their DNA is present and treat accordingly. As always, a negative result does not exclude that pathogen from the differential diagnosis. *Not detected does not mean uninfected.* You WILL need to make your diagnosis based on clinical judgment. Yes, you will.

PEARL: In general, there is a poor recovery using fluids for PCR testing. Lyme PCR is used to try to detect Bb DNA in blood, CSF, urine, synovial fluid, or tissue. While PCR results are highly specific, yield is <u>painfully</u> low especially in fluids compared to tissue. Better to submit a tissue sample from biopsy or postsurgical procedure. Usually, the "deeper" the tissue the more likely a positive result. For example, a positive PCR is more likely from synovium than from synovial fluid. If such samples are not likely to become available, try blood or other fluids and you may get lucky and get a supportive result. Again DNA might survive for weeks after the causative organism is gone. If the information is critical, consider a diagnostic biopsy.

PEARL: One reason why it is so difficult to get a positive Bb PCR test in humans is that we may only have low levels of free floating spirochetes in the blood at a given time.

2. **FISH** – In contrast to PCR, the **fluorescent in-situ hybridization** assay looks for **RNA**. FISH is often said to be more sensitive than PCR, but in many cases this is conjecture. Finding ribosomal RNA from a pathogen might indicate an active infection. If the result is positive, FISH provides very strong supportive evidence for the suspected etiologic agent. This technique may be able to detect more species than traditional testing but this has yet to be fully demonstrated. If positive, FISH gives considerable diagnostic support. How else would specific pathogen RNA get in the sample? If negative, you are no worse off than when you started. *Not detected does not mean uninfected.*

XI. LUMBAR PUNCTURE (LP)

A spinal tap is a diagnostic (and sometimes therapeutic) procedure performed in order to collect cerebrospinal fluid (CSF) for analysis. During the procedure the pressure is checked and samples are taken for analysis. Usually the tap is done looking for confirmation of meningitis.

PEARL: Always record opening and closing pressures. Consider resting the patient on his stomach after the procedure. Most texts will say to have the patient lie on his back after an LP. This can lead to extravasation from the puncture site. If they are on their stomachs, they are less likely to "spring a leak." You should not do your first LP all by yourself. An LP done improperly in the presence of high intracranial pressure can result in herniation.

The key to interpreting LPs in TBI patients is not to expect too much. You are NOT going to see wiggly spirochetes under the microscope. You probably aren't going to grow any Lyme pathogens from the CSF either. Spirochetes are found in less than 10% of spinal fluid aspirates even in the most classic of Lyme meningitis cases. In Lyme patients with characteristic CNS manifestations and other supportive findings, only about 7% show any Bb antibodies in the CSF. That doesn't mean you shouldn't try to catch what you can. In these cases, something appears to be causing meningeal irritation whether it's due to a TBI or not. If CSF is available, depending on clinical presentation, you may want to send the sample for a TBI panel looking for antibodies or nucleic acids. WB, Lyme DOT Assay, and PCR can all be done on CSF. Yield for antibodies in these tests is low. In any case, look for signs of inflammation and infection: white cells, red cells, pathogens, proteins, and pressure. Red cells might be more indicative of trauma than infection.

PEARL: Intracranial pressure (ICP) can increase because of Lyme.

PEARL: If the patient is presenting with a meningitis-like syndrome, the CSF can be examined for white cells, and routine cultures will likely be done. TBIs are notoriously hard to culture from CSF. In Lyme patients with CNS symptoms or meningeal signs, only about 7% show any Bb antibodies in the CSF. The culture of live spirochetes is extremely difficult. In fact, spirochetes were found in only about 10% of spinal fluid samples even in the most classic cases of Lyme meningitis.

Recall that I overheard Lilith[1] in the ER say that the LP results in the child in the next bed "proved" he did not have Lyme meningitis. That is not true. Never rule out the possibility of a TBI, especially in the case of possible meningitis, on the basis of a negative lab test. Use your clinical judgment. You may want to treat empirically.

XII. BIOPSIES

Sometimes the only positive test for a TBI will come from biopsy tissue. So, if your TBI patient is having any procedure, make sure a sample is taken for diagnostic evaluation. The procedure can be anything from surgery to endoscopy. Many HCPs have had good results from biopsies of the gut. Never waste a golden opportunity to examine internal tissue. Make sure you call your trusted lab so that you can ensure that the sample is gathered and preserved properly and that you order the tests that you actually need to have run. Patients do not have endoscopies or surgery every day, especially kids, so you want to make the most of this rare gift.

While blood and serum can be used for a number of tests, tissue samples will offer a better chance of a positive yield. One group of patients tested negative for Babesia with blood samples, but when tissue from biopsies taken during endoscopy and gall bladder surgery were used, they all tested positive. Except in extreme circumstances, avoid invasive procedures for the sole purpose of diagnosis. However, if tissue becomes available during other procedures take advantage of the opportunity to obtain more sensitive test results. If you are aware of a procedure your patient will be undergoing, don't let tissue be tossed without considering if useful information could be gathered.

Urine, blood, serum, and synovial fluid can all be used to look for DNA using PCR. But even with the best methodology, it is hard to get a positive. The best yield comes from biopsy tissue, surgical remnants, placenta, or foreskin. To check a newborn for exposure, look for DNA in the placenta, umbilical cord, cord blood, and foreskin remnant. DNA can persist after the organism is gone with some sources saying the DNA lingers for 6 weeks and others saying up to 3 to 4 months.

PEARL: Chapter 10 reviews the difficulties inherent in visualizing Bb under the microscope even with the best samples.

If you are really struggling to make a diagnosis and all your instincts are pointing to a TBI but you haven't been able to confirm the diagnosis, consider a muscle biopsy. If you are going to do an invasive procedure to get tissue, order the works: cultures, Lyme DNA PCR, and tests for M. *fermentans*, B. *henselea*, and Babesia as suggested by the clinical presentation. Have the lab preserve that part of the tissue sample that is not consumed in the testing in case further examinations are indicated in the future.

PEARL: Consider asking the lab to retain all biopsy specimen in paraffin blocks that can be saved for years and recalled for future testing. As new methodologies become available, a request for a specimen can be sent. The lab holding the block will not release its block to anyone, anywhere, anytime. But they might release several microtomal cuts of the block and ship these to another lab as needed. They usually appreciate hearing the results of a test that came from their block. Pathologists, like the author of this Compendium, *need live human contact once in a while.*

PEARL: The expertise and awareness of the person assessing the tissue sample will dictate the results. Is the pathologist board certified? Has she seen spirochetes in tissue before? Does she know to look for them? After my second knee procedure I asked if anyone looked for spirochetes in the biopsy sample. I was told they had found nothing and asked why they would look for spirochetes. Why did they send tissue? If you don't look, you won't see. Unfortunately, with Lyme even if you do look, the pathogen can be obscure.

PEARL: Taking everything into consideration, nothing beats a positive culture from a biopsy for confirming the diagnosis of Lyme. In the future, perhaps the new blood culture will have this distinction. Still, I'm sure some would deny even the isolation of Bb in culture.

XIII. ENDOCRINE STUDIES

There is clear evidence that Lyme impacts the endocrine system and the endocrine system impacts Lyme. There is a higher incidence of thyroid, adrenocortical, and other endocrine problems in TBIs. This knowledge may provide a good indication for endocrine studies in correlation with the clinical presentation, including:

A. Thyroid function tests

The most common thyroid evaluations pertinent to TBI

---

1 See Glossary or Introduction for name origin

patients are T3, T4, thyroid binding globulin, TSH, and anti-thyroid antibodies. Probably more than in any other circumstance, do not be fooled by the WNL designation. Many people are told their thyroid is normal when the function is not normal for them. There is often a big range of normal and patients starting near the upper limit of normal and trending toward the lower limit of normal may have impeded thyroid function, which can be clinically important. The converse may also be true, where a patient may trend toward the high range. Even if these results stay within the normal limits they may not be normal for that particular person. Try to compare lab results from a time before the patient got sick. If thyroid function is suspect, consider checking iodine levels as well.

*PEARL: A reverse T3 test can show if the T3 is not formed adequately. Anecdotally this is not uncommon in Lyme patients. In addition to treating the underlying thyroid condition, selenium 100 to 200 **mcg** per day may be useful, although recommendations range from 70 mcg to 400 mcg daily.*

PEARL: Perhaps 10% of Lyme patients have an autoimmune-like thyroiditis.

B. Cortisol

Now called the stress hormone, cortisol has been found to be associated with the normal function of many organ systems. Imbalance of this hormone may result in a number of the symptoms associated with Lyme. Levels vary with time of day! Measurement of cortisol is done to assess function of the adrenal cortex. High cortisol levels are found in chronic inflammation, on-going anxiety, and obesity.

Bb might impact the adrenals and thereby cortisol levels. This hormone can affect stress response, weight control, and fatigue.

PEARL: Adequate adrenal function is essential for healing. Sxs of abnormal cortisol include fatigue, depression, anxiety, sleep disturbances, frequent infections, muscle weakness, burn-out, lack of motivation, feeling overloaded or overwhelmed, emotional numbness, no social interest, low tolerance to stress, and hypersensitivity to smells and noise. When adrenals are weak recovery is compromised. Cortisol levels can be checked but be careful since these levels have daily cycles. Abnormal cortisol has been shown to slow improvement in Lyme. Perhaps the Lyme is altering the cortisol levels. It's hard to say which came first but both can adversely influence the other. Licorice, ginseng, the B vitamins, and EFAs are all theorized to promote adrenal health.

C. Sugar

Sugar metabolism is imbalanced by Lyme. This does not mean that a diagnosis of diabetes is warranted, but that glucose can be unpredictably high or low. HbA1c measures sugar balance over time. High sugars, no matter how they are labeled, can cause damage to small blood vessels and nerves and, overtime, can create a myriad of symptoms that confound the management of and recovery from Lyme. Don't miss an underlying diabetes because Lyme is also presenting with fluctuating blood sugar levels. Remember that high sugar levels aren't just numbers that can easily be controlled with an insulin shot. Each high number means real damage to nerves and small vessels in the patient.

PEARL: Most infectious processes will raise the blood sugar levels temporarily due to inflammation. Lyme seems to do a better job at this than most infections. Be vigilant.

D. Vitamin D

Vitamin D is an intrinsically-made hormone. Additional sources come from food and sun exposure. Most Americans, especially children, are woefully lacking in Vitamin D. Deficiencies in this vitamin can lead to symptoms that may mimic Lyme symptoms including difficulty concentrating and balance problems. Vitamin levels – especially for D, B12, and B6 – might be helpful. Too much Vitamin D has been associated with kidney stones.

E. Human Chorionic Gonadotropin (hCG)

This hormone is present in the urine when a woman is pregnant. Consider treating pregnant women infected with Bb with combination antibiotics that hit both the free-floating spirochetes as well as the intracellular forms of Bb for the duration of the pregnancy.

XIV. IMAGING STUDIES

For the most part, imaging studies such as X-rays, MRIs, CT and SPECT scans, and PET studies are used in TBI patients the same way that they are used in everyone else. There do not seem to be consistent findings to suggest that they provide additional information in either the specific diagnosis or management of TBIs. MRIs of the brain in chronic Lyme occasionally show a similar pattern to that found in MS, but this finding cannot be relied upon. Some HCPs use SPECT scans of the brain since Lyme seems to show hypoperfusion. Since there is usually no SPECT scan from before the TBI infection for comparison, the results are not always easy to interpret. Nonetheless, there are reports of considerable improvement in brain perfusion in Lyme patients with adequate treatment. Most HCPs do not routinely order imaging studies in case management of TBIs.

With one exception, of course. Ultrasound of the gallbladder is often needed to follow patients on Rocephin therapy. Rocephin is eliminated from the body through the bile. Stones can form from the high concentration of salts. Before you start a patient on a course of Rocephin, ask if there is a personal or family history of gallstones. Get a baseline ultrasound (US) of the gallbladder and then follow regularly throughout the course of treatment. The stones usually diminish once the antibiotic is discontinued. Consider US of the GB on Rocephin patients every month and then for 3 consecutive months after cessation of the treatment. This process is detailed in the Rocephin section of Chapter 24: *Antimicrobials* and in Chapter 25: *Ancillary Treatments*.

PEARL: The risk of gallstones might be lessened by the use of Actigall.

XV. MISCELLANEOUS EVALUATIONS

Any number of tests such as EKGs and EMGs can be used to gather useful information in making the differential diagnosis and in following the clinical course. Serial EKGs may be appropriate when the treatment regimen includes antibiotics that can prolong the QT interval or induce dysrhythmias. Various neuropsychiatric testing, done by a professional, can provide information pertinent to differential diagnosis, especially in M. *fermentans* and bartonellosis.

PEARL: I talk here about getting EKGs to monitor for prolongation of QTc as though that were the easiest thing in the world. I have looked at hundreds of EKGs for this purpose, and I can tell you it's hard as hell. Many cardiologists, who say they know how to do it, do not. I had to consult with a rare QT expert to review my work before I was comfortable submitting to the FDA. If you are dealing with a drug known to prolong the QT or a patient who might be predisposed to prolongation, find an expert you trust to walk this path with you.

Tests for heavy metals, toxins, and molds can be useful, especially in intractable patients. Allergy testing may be indicated in those who appear more allergic than infected. These assessments are described in Chapter 25: *Ancillary Treatments*.

Synovial fluid analysis is sometimes done on patients with a "hot knee." Many TBIs are hard on the joints, especially Lyme disease. Yet, analysis of the synovial fluid is of limited value if looking specifically for Bb. Even when pathologists are looking explicitly for spirochetes, they are rarely observed even in cases where all indications point to a Borrelia infection. Further, there is a low yield of positive results for PCR. Analysis of the fluid may show signs of inflammation or infection much the same way a urine specimen might with white cells and nitrites. A total WBC count greater than 2000 in synovial fluid suggests bacterial etiology.

Consider an **antiphospholipid panel** on those patients presenting with a TBI and Raynaud's or otherwise cold extremities. Phospholipids are necessary for normal blood clotting. Abnormal results might uncover antiphospholipid antibody syndrome, which is a disorder of coagulation often involving abnormal clot formation. This syndrome has been associated with autoimmunity and pregnancy complications including miscarriage. Antibodies are formed against the phospholipid component of the cell membrane. This symptom complex is sometimes seen with other autoimmune conditions such as SLE. Rapid organ failure can ensue and the condition can be fatal. DVTs or stroke may be the first indication of a problem.

XVI.   THE "WHY WOULD ANYONE ORDER THESE TESTS IN TBI PATIENTS?" SECTION

A.   Creatine phosphokinase (CPK)

I have reconciled myself to the idea that CPK can provide useful information in some TBI patients. After being badly burned by the CPK results from a "great deal" metabolic panel during a clinical trial, I have run away from this measurement as I would run from a blood-thirsty tick. Creatine phosphokinase (some vehemently believe that the proper term is creatine kinase) is an enzyme found in muscle (both skeletal and cardiac), and brain. Damage to these areas will cause the enzyme to leak into the blood, where it can be measured. By measuring the specific CPK isoenzymes, the site of injury might be determined. Muscle-derived CPK might be high in babesiosis, where this finding could be due to the intense muscle activity associated with rigors. Muscle CPK can also be elevated in seizures, vigorous exercise, RMSF, trauma, viral infections, muscular dystrophies and other muscle disorders, long-term immobility, and rhabdomyolysis. Perhaps pertinent to TBI patients is the potential increase in CPK in metabolic disorders, sepsis, and inflammatory myopathies. Some drugs and toxins will elevate CPK. The most pertinent to TBI patients is streptococcal toxin. CPK tends to be nonspecific and usually there are better ways to get the information. Nevertheless, I apologize for not showing CPK the respect it deserved.

B.   Angiotensin-1-Converting Enzyme (ACE)

ACE was traditionally used to recognize sarcoidosis and to monitor the stage of that disease, but it is rarely used even for that purpose today because of lack of specificity. I don't know why some TBI docs order ACE levels, but it is mentioned in the literature with great enthusiasm by a few authors. I don't know what to do with the result. I offer no apologies here.

Chapter 20

MAKING THE DIAGNOSIS

"I'm in a phone booth at the corner of Walk & Don't Walk"
Unknown

A patient presents with fever, headache, fatigue, and general discomfort. What could this be? Well, off the top of my head, just about any infectious or inflammatory process known to humankind. Fortunately, patients do not visit HCPs for our sparkling wit and lively conversation. They want answers and that means we must attempt to make a diagnosis.

To diagnose, start with the similarities and then look at the differences. Consider the patient's presenting signs and symptoms and see how they are similar to the signs and symptoms of various known diagnoses. As in the case above, there are hundreds of reasons why a patient might present with fever, headache, fatigue, and general discomfort. What we need is a distinctive feature that will distinguish this particular symptom-set from all the others. So what is there about this patient's fever, headache, fatigue, and general discomfort that is distinctive? Maybe the fever is especially high, or the headache has a defining intensity or location. Maybe the onset of distinguishing symptoms or the subsequent clinical course will provide clues. Perhaps additional signs become evident over time that will set this syndrome apart from all others.

In establishing a diagnosis, the HCP attempts to answer the question, "What could this be?" A diagnosis is: 1) the method used to determine the cause of an illness, or 2) that illness. Making a diagnosis involves gathering information such as patient history, findings from the physical examination, ROS, and results from any diagnostic testing. Diagnoses are essential if we hope to effectively treat disease and offer a prognosis. An accurate diagnosis also helps standardize communication so when one person says "Q-fever" everyone knows what is being referenced.

In diagnosing we try to use logic, analysis, and experience to determine cause and effect. Old habits die hard and when making a diagnosis I revert to my days in preventive medicine and the causality logic I used then, which is further detailed in Chapter 23: *Understanding Medicines*. There I apply the following six steps as a way to assess whether one event caused another. Similar logic can be used to examine what might be causing a particular set of signs and symptoms:

A. Timing: If Event A occurs AFTER Event B, then Event A could not have caused Event B. With some exceptions such as gestational Lyme, one cannot have a tick-borne illness without having a tick bite. Unfortunately, with TBIs we don't always have the tick in-hand when the patient presents with symptoms. Still if there is any chance that a bite could have occurred, then proceed with additional evaluation.

B. Bioplausibility: Could a particular disease reasonably explain the clinical presentation? You must make sure it is actually implausible before you discredit an idea. I was initially fooled during the Phen-Fen debacle, since I couldn't imagine the mechanism by which these weight loss drugs could damage heart valves. I soon learned that just because I don't understand something doesn't make it scientifically impossible. When trying to determine plausibility, supportive lab testing can be helpful. Nevertheless, a negative test result alone should never be used to eliminate a diagnosis.

C. Challenge/Rechallenge: If the symptoms lessen or resolve with targeted treatment and then recur when treatment stops, this finding suggests a diagnosis. Further, if the symptoms then respond to re-treatment, the pattern supports a diagnosis. For example, if antibiotics are discontinued and Lyme symptoms flare, this flare supports a diagnosis of persistent Lyme. Resolution with re-treatment would be a positive rechallenge.

D. Confounders: What could be complicating the diagnostic process? With TBIs, confounders can include co-infections, concurrent diseases, immune abnormalities, underlying genetic predispositions, and any number of other factors. Determine what might be standing in the way of making a diagnosis.

E. Consistency: Does the observed pattern fit with the usual presentation of the condition under consideration. "If it walks like a duck and quacks like a duck, it's probably a duck." Unfortunately, diseases like Lyme are great imitators and can look like any number of other conditions. Further, true Lyme cases can present in a mind-boggling array of signs and symptoms. Lyme manifestations can change during the course of the disease and can vary from case to case and even in the same patient at different times. If you have any hint of Lyme, pursue the possibility even if the EM lesion is not round enough or the patient doesn't remember the tick. If there is a possibility, then give the diagnosis a chance. Don't be too quick to toss a Lyme diagnosis just because one sign or symptom doesn't fit a preconceived idea of what Lyme should be. I was told that to be a "Lyme knee," an effusion had to be present. That's not true. And, never eliminate Lyme from your differential based solely on negative lab testing.

F. No better explanation: If you've looked and looked and thought and thought and brainstormed all kinds of alternatives and still can't find another explanation for a clinical presentation, you might have to consider a diagnosis of exclusion. Here you have identified a *possible* explanation for a symptom set but you cannot say this is the diagnosis with complete confidence. Still you think you have eliminated all other reasonable possibilities. This is where I write in the note's diagnosis line "qualifiers" like: Cannot r/o babesiosis, Consider Lyme, Likely Bb infection, Inflamed L knee, possible Lyme etiology, etc.

Without a working diagnosis (hypothesis), it's difficult to make any progress with the case. Without a destination it's hard to set a course. A diagnosis is based on all those old fashioned things you learned in training like the chief complaint, history, signs and symptoms, physical exam, and supportive test findings. Then by using the type of logic listed above, judgments can be made that progress you toward a diagnosis.

Of course, computer software and practice guidelines can be used to help diagnose but these should be used as a safeguard to ensure you're not missing something not as a rigid formula that leads to an irreversible decision. Beware of algorithms that are too simple because once a patient falls outside the preordained algorithm it's hard to get back in. Algorithms can take on a life of their own and end up taking away HCP discretion. They can lead you astray. Remember, medicine is a combination of science and art. A patient is more than the sum total of his algorithm checklist.

When algorithms and practice guidelines are used to make a diagnosis, proceed with caution. While these guidelines can provide a useful and quick refresher for harried HCPs, they are often of questionable quality and their development can be tainted with bias. Chapter 11: *Controversies around Lyme* discusses the caveats around relying solely on guidelines to make diagnoses.

Use pattern recognition to better allow you to diagnose efficiently and accurately. A quick diagnosis does little good if you're fast but not accurate. Take all available information and use it to assess how likely this symptom-set fits in with what might be found with a known diagnosis. In emergency situations, some accuracy will need to be sacrificed in exchange for the need for rapid action. Still the diagnosis can be continuously revised as more information is gathered during your response.

Where you stand depends on where you sit. You cannot diagnose a condition you do not know exists. Further, you might be less likely to diagnose a problem if you have been conditioned to find every excuse not to diagnosis it. Don't be too quick to shout: "YOU DO NOT HAVE LYME!" Proving a negative is hard and you will look foolish when it becomes clear over time that, in many cases, they do indeed have Lyme.

Remember the story of the blind men and the elephant. A group of blind men approached an elephant and each was interested in knowing what an elephant was like. Each touched the elephant in only one place. The man who touched the trunk thought the elephant was like a hose. The man who touched the side thought the elephant was like a wall. The one who touched the tusk believed the elephant was like a plow. The one who touched the tip of the tail thought the elephant was like a brush. Each was correct but all missed the totality of the elephant. Your diagnostic ability will be severely limited if you take only one perspective and then become entrenched in the idea that this is the only true or correct view. We all take the limits of our own experience as the totality of everyone's experience but we will be much better practitioners if we open up to the possibilities.

Even if the probability of a condition being the underlying etiology is *near* zero that does not mean the probability *is* zero. There is always the possibility of outliers in the stats. There is always the first case to be identified. Somebody's got to do it. Diagnosis is simply a way of hypothesis testing. As such, we need to keep an open mind and a high index of suspicion.

The more common a symptom the more difficult it will be to assign a definitive diagnosis. For example, a headache can be associated with 100s of conditions. (Sometimes I wonder if it's possible to have any illness without having a headache. I have a headache right now.) If you have no more specifics, in this case, your initial diagnosis might be: Headache of unknown etiology. As you learn more you can refine the diagnosis: Muscle tension headache.

Where there are few or insensitive tests available, the harder a diagnosis might be to deduce. One source suggested moving as quickly as possible into diagnostic testing mode. Perhaps you have read the lab chapters already, but maybe not. I am not a big believer in over-testing with labs or other modalities. First, give the history, physical, and ROS a chance. As an HCP, you have been led to believe that you NEED all this ancillary confirmation and that you can't make a diagnosis using your medical skills, experience, and judgment. Many sages from

Hippocrates to William Osler have remarked that if you listen to the patient, he will tell you what you need to know. You might be surprised at your diagnostic skills if you are brave enough to use them. Too much testing can result in a bunch of equivocal results that just tangle the logic process and can be quite costly. Today there is much commentary about unnecessary testing doing more harm than good such as PSA tests, which have been the gold standard for diagnosing prostate cancer for years. Use common-sense and order what you need to help you make a diagnosis but don't order everything you can "just in case." Do what makes medical sense.

Diagnosing Lyme is a clinical judgment. There is no lab test that will bail you out here. Yes, if you find DNA bits from Bb you very likely dealing with Lyme. Nonetheless, even the most sensitive tests for Lyme have an extremely low yield of positives, even in cases that are clearly clinically real and later supported by other testing. Often you will need to have taken action before you get the test results back. There are high rates of false negatives in most current Lyme testing methods. YOU MUST MAKE THE DIAGNOSIS THE OLD FASHIONED WAY!

With that being said, diagnosing Lyme can be hard. Lyme itself has a number of aliases such as relapsing fever, Master's disease, and STARI, which may or may not be LD. So when you read the literature, you aren't always sure what you're dealing with. Like its syphilitic cousin, Lyme is a great imitator so you may go down a number of wrong paths before you find your way. Since 2013-era-ticks rarely carry just one pathogen, co-infections can cloud the diagnostic picture. The differential diagnosis and the possibility of concurrent conditions are discussed it the next chapter.

Several point systems for diagnosing Lyme have been introduced which may be useful to some HCPs. For example, an EM rash observed by the HCP would score a number of points. Disease affecting one organ system would not result in as many points as disease affecting multiple systems, etc. Based on the total number of points a Lyme diagnosis is thought to be highly likely, possible, or unlikely. Personally, I do better with a more qualitative approach, but use what tools work best for you.

Anything is possible, but as the attending HCP your job is to see what is likely. Do you need a working diagnosis now or do you have time to gather more information? Always consider the risk/benefit of action versus continuing to collect more facts.

Even in Chester County, Pennsylvania, not everything is Lyme. People occasionally do have other maladies. If you don't think it's Lyme (or whatever the patient is concerned about) say, "I don't think we're dealing with Lyme here but I'll keep an open mind as we try to figure out what's going on with you. In the meantime, let's consider…"

Sometimes you just can't come to a diagnosis either because you made a logic error, don't have enough information, the signs and symptoms are not sufficiently discernible, you waste time going down the wrong path, or the condition is too similar to others so that distinctions can't be made. OR… the diagnosis is not yet known, so it can't even be considered. You try and try to find a pattern but the presentation just doesn't fit anywhere. Consider how many things have been misdiagnosed over the years. My husband's great, great grandfather Cassius Marcellus Clay, buried in Hampton Virginia, has apoplexy listed as his cause of death. Apoplexy is often thought to refer to a stroke but the term was also used for people with cardiac arrest and any number of other things. Since there was (and is) stigma associated with some diseases, apoplexy was preferred to diagnoses like seizures or syphilis. Apoplexy, grippe, Bright's disease, and consumption were all common causes of death in the past and we don't know exactly what those terms mean. Was the bloody sputum due to TB, cancer, pneumonia, CHF, or some other cause? Just as "cardiopulmonary arrest" covers many modern bases, we might not know the real etiology. I doubt that the first diagnosed case of Lyme was the first case of Lyme. What were we calling Lyme before we knew about Lyme?

Just because symptoms are unexplained does not mean there is no disease present. Be wary of the HCP who tells a patient that she just needs to buck-up and learn to live with it, even though he might not know what "it" is. The HCPs inability to make a diagnosis does not cure the patient. Just because a diagnosis is difficult to make does not mean there isn't a diagnosis to make.

DIAGNOSTIC PEARLS:

A. When doing the H&P, remember that a patient can have two or more different disease processes going on at once. Just because they have acute otitis media does not mean that they can't also have hearing sensitivity due to a TBI. Just because they have one kind of arthritis does not mean they cannot have two. This is especially true with neuropsychiatric manifestations.

B. Do not be too quick to dismiss signs and symptoms by saying "Oh, that's just part of his Lyme." More than one thing can be happening. Concurrent conditions can occur before, during, or after diagnosis of TBI. Maybe a symptom or sign is part of the TBI and maybe it's independent.

C. Have an open mind and a high index of suspicion and see how all the pieces fit into the puzzle. Do not cherry-pick where you focus only on those findings that support a preconceived diagnosis and dismiss those that could lead you down a different path.

D. A syndrome is a group of symptoms, often found together, that loosely defines a condition. A diagnosis can be a sign and symptom package such as CHF which can occur for a number of reasons that might not be initially clear.

E. Pathognomonic refers to a sign that only occurs in one condition. When something is pathognomonic, like a primary EM rash with a scab from a tick bite in its center in a symptomatic patient, you have been given a diagnostic gift. Remember that if you choose to ignore that gift, a patient could suffer. Some argue that an EM rash with corroborating history is not pathognomonic of Lyme. Quick! Name one other condition that causes an EM rash including the scab from the tick bite in the center and the deer tick in the jar. Lilith? Lilith[1]?

F. The term rule out means using scientific methods to exclude certain diagnoses from consideration in a process of elimination. Here, the HCP gathers all available information and creates a mental sign and symptom list. Then possible candidates that could account for those signs and symptoms are reviewed and subsequently removed from consideration as it becomes clear that they do not fit the clinical presentation. Some may be thrown farther off the list than others in a priority-type elimination. Possible diagnoses are ruled out, one after the other, as the HCP works down the list of contenders.

G. Algorithms provide a step-by-step approach to problem solving. Here, sets of questions with Yes or No answers lead the user down a path to a conclusion. This is risky since anyone who does not present EXACTLY as the algorithm requires will fall off the algorithm path. Despite all the arrows suggesting otherwise, there is little recourse. While algorithms use a process of Yes or No questions to lead to a decision, questions in medicine are rarely absolute or 100% yes or no. Especially in TBIs where some acknowledged signs are found in a relatively small percentage of patients, the person can be disqualified before they have a chance.

H. Do not get obsessed with meeting all the diagnostic criteria in a guideline. If a fibromyalgia patient has only 10 points of tenderness instead of 11, use good medical judgment. Allow each patient to have his disease his way.

I. Be careful when diagnosing from practice guidelines. That approach allowed hundreds of women to die in ERs by telling them they weren't having a heart attack because they did not fit into the pattern displayed by men. And we used that when we told patients they didn't have CFS and fibromyalgia and epilepsy and autism and diabetes and hepatitis and MS and depression and the list

goes on and on *ad infinitum*. Why do we fight so hard against making a diagnosis as though it were a personal affront?

J. Probably, you will not be able to consider all possible diagnostic options that might correspond to a given symptom set. Usually in making a diagnosis the HCP is counseled to consider the most common diagnosis first. This approach could get you in trouble in the TBI world. You can't see what you don't look for. We're taught that if we hear hoof beats to think of horses not zebras. With Lyme you might want to consider zebras earlier in the process, before you realize you were hearing giraffes all along.

K. If you're just too nervous to write the word Lyme in the diagnosis box, ponder these synonyms: "Infectious process: consider Lyme, r/o Lyme, probable Lyme, possible Lyme, likely borreliosis, on-going infection with unconfirmed etiology." Note that different insurance companies will pay for some diagnoses but not others when referring to the same condition. This is true for many illnesses. I am not asking you to fabricate a diagnosis, but when you are calling a rose by any other name, you might as well use the name that is pre-approved, if it's just as accurate. For example, some third party payers will NOT cover pervasive developmental disorder but will cover pervasive developmental disorder-not otherwise specified.

L. Since many TBIs have overlapping symptoms, don't just grab the first diagnosis that makes a modicum of sense and latch on. That way you wouldn't even be able to consider other infections that could be along for the ride.

M. Very rarely is someone told they have Lyme when they don't. In contrast, false negatives are quite common. Patients are too often told they do not have Lyme when they do. If a patient remains sick, try again to answer the question: "What could this be?"

N. Be careful not to over-diagnose or the patient may get an inaccurate label. Be careful not to under-diagnose or the disease can progress because of delayed treatment.

O. If a TBI patient has a family member who is now being worked-up for MS, ALS, ADD, ADHD, CFS, Alzheimer's, or fibromyalgia, think that maybe Lyme or another TBI could be confounding their diagnosis.

P. Worst misdiagnoses of Lyme found in the literature: Allergic tension, fatigue syndrome, broken thumb, clubbed foot, dog bite, globulin binding problem, cortisol excess, pre-seizure, punctured ear drum, Qui blockage, sleeping brain, female anxiety troubles

---

1 See Glossary or Introduction for name origin

Q. Don't force a diagnosis. If it doesn't fit, it doesn't fit. Look elsewhere but don't slam any doors shut. You may want to come back. No matter how clearly defined one syndrome may be, each individual has her own clinical presentation.

A good diagnostician uses a logical process. Draw on your experience and common sense to systematically and OBJECTIVELY narrow down the field. Diagnosing is one of the fun parts of medicine – like being a detective. Do not allow flawed and restrictive guidelines or inflexible algorithms take away your clinical discretion. The experience and the knowledge of the HCP should be the key to good diagnosing.

Chapter 21

DIFFERENTIAL DIAGNOSIS AND CONCURRENT DISEASE

Imagine what you could learn if you didn't already know it all.
Famous coach and former Purdue player John Wooden

While the diagnostic process answers the question, "What could this be?" the process of differential diagnosis answers the question: "What ELSE could this be?" Much of the logic is the same but now we look at all the other potential causes for a symptom-set. In diagnosing, we are comparing a clinical presentation to the list of potential explanations. Now we are taking all those possible explanations and comparing them to one another. Actually the processes of diagnosing and establishing a differential diagnosis usually occur simultaneously, but that was too hard to organize into one chapter.

Again we will be using the causality logic described in both Chapters 20 and 23, but we will arrive at a list of candidates by comparing similarities and differences between the contenders and the actual case. A differential diagnosis (DD) helps the HCP determine which of several conditions might be producing the symptoms. Also called differentiation or "the **differential**," I will use sentences like "In your differential, you might include, A, B, and C." In distinguishing one likely etiology from another, the HCP will try to find as many possible answers as reasonable to the question: "Could this diagnosis explain this patient's clinical presentation?"

Once in a while, you will be gifted with a **pathognomonic** sign that will make your journey into the DD process short and sweet. However, to take advantage of these signs that are associated with only one diagnosis, you must know they exist and be willing to accept them as pathognomonic. I believe that an EM rash with a scab from the tick bite in the center, with the deer tick in a jar, and an appropriately symptomatic patient is pathognomonic for Lyme. Lilith[1] disagreed. Usually we aren't so lucky as to have a clear indicating sign and we are stuck with a vague and overlapping symptom-set with a dozen possible explanations.

DD involves a process of elimination where we render the probability of each candidate down to negligible levels. Lyme is the great imitator. (Actually syphilis, Lyme's spirochetal cousin had this moniker first, but the nickname fits both nicely.) There are so many confounders in the diagnosis of TBIs

that you will often be shaking your head and wondering why you filled out those med school applications. Look at the DD in TBDs as a personal and professional challenge, where if you get the answer right, you have the potential to do much good for some sick little kid.

Don't be intractable. Your working diagnosis could be wrong and your DD totally off-base. If the patient is getting worse or new sxs are appearing, regroup. You may have to pick up your logic and start over. Many diagnoses are not initially correct and I hear stories daily, from all therapeutic areas, about missed diagnoses. The patients never seem angry that a diagnosis was missed because they understand that physicians are human. Rather, many are furious when the doctor will not accept that the first try was wrong and are then unwilling to reevaluate. If the patient is not getting well, she is not still sick merely to annoy you, she may need a fresh appraisal.

Always remember, there can be more than one thing going on at a time. Some of the signs and symptoms you are trying to cover with your diagnosis may have been pre-existing. Alternatively, the patient may have had a genetic predisposition to that symptom, which was triggered or exacerbated by the current problem. Don't force things to be related when they may or may not be. Remember the term "red herring" refers to items that serve to distract you from the truth. Don't let the pungent red herrings take you down the wrong paths.

Today, DD can be done by a person or a computer using algorithms and checklists. For me and mine, I prefer the human. With all our foibles, nothing beats the "gut" feel from a master diagnostician. As always, do not be tempted to treat the computer result from an algorithm, which may or may not be clinically valid, while you ignore the patient in front of you. (I think I have told you the story of the ophthalmologist at Hopkins who did not look at me once except through a machine and then sat with her back to me as she dictated my note that had NOTHING to do with me or my chief complaint.)

In some cases you might have an almost immediate diagnosis of something like an acute abdomen, which you will then

---

1 See Glossary or Introduction for name origin

follow up with a more detailed DD to determine the source of the emergency. You can start treatment with a working diagnosis, but you will need more information as you then decide how to proceed. Other times, you will struggle with the DD over time. In cases of chronic Lyme, you might have to assess treatment response and continue to work the DD as you determine if co-infections, concurrent infections, or co-morbid conditions are complicating the picture. You might just be dealing with the variable clinical presentations that can accompany persistent Lyme disease.

There are books and computer programs that will take a sign or symptom and list all the possible conditions that could result in such a manifestation. These can be helpful especially if you are stuck, or blank, or unfamiliar with a particular symptom. These manuals are not always all-inclusive, especially for diseases that have recently been identified. There are software packages that will take a symptom set and provide a diagnosis. These can be helpful guides, but the HCP retains the final responsibility to match the diagnosis to the actual human. Do not allow expediency, or the number of patients waiting, or the call from the ER, tempt you into abdicating your responsibility to the patient sitting on your exam table.

In dealing with the DD of TBIs, always have a high index of suspicion for co-infections and possible concurrent infections. Always consider how a pre-existing condition (perhaps previously subclinical) might be affecting the TBI and how the TBI might be affecting it. With TBIs you must keep a wide prospective field. Expect the unexpected. You will never find what you are not looking for. Likewise, don't be so TBI-focused that you fall prey to thinking everything is Lyme. Balance. Zen.

There are many ways to do a DD. Here, you will take all the pieces of the puzzle that you have been able to gather and see where they lead. Take all the possibilities and hone down the likely candidates. "What ELSE could this be?" If condition A fits except for one parameter, then consider if condition B fits the clinical profile better. If B has a disqualifier, consider C. No matter how clearly defined one syndrome may be, each individual has her own clinical presentation. Just because a person does not fit a proscribed diagnosis perfectly, does not mean she does not have the disease.

Unfortunately, diagnoses become fashionable and then go out of favor. Among these are mold and heavy metals and ADD and GAD. For a while everyone seemed to be having panic attacks and then all kids had learning disabilities. Moms would compete over which child had the most impairing ADD. Overuse of certain diagnoses makes it hard for the patients who really do suffer from these diseases. In contrast, if people are sick, something is causing the problem. Dr. Sherr was told by the state health department not to worry

about babesiosis because it was just a "trendy" diagnosis. A few years later, splashed across the media is the presence of babesiosis in the blood supply, putting everyone at risk. Maybe someone should have paid attention to Dr. Sherr.

One diagnosis should eventually explain a clinical presentation better than the other possible diagnoses. This may take minutes or years. Careful. You can only recognize something you admit exists. A proponent of the IDSA Lyme guidelines is unlikely to ever diagnose chronic Lyme even if he admits that some patients may have persistent symptoms. That is why some docs see Lyme when others scream, "It's not Lyme!" when looking at the same patient.

Med students often use the mnemonic VINDICATE to make sure they don't miss any possible diagnostic considerations. This acronym comes from the Vascular, Inflammatory, Neoplastic, Degenerative/Deficiency, Idiopathic/Intoxication, Congenital, Autoimmune/Allergic, Traumatic, Endocrine processes. Here, the HCP looks at each category and determines which diagnoses under that grouping could be the best explanation for the clinical picture. Although desperate to avoid going through the DD process for Lyme, I could not morally shirk my responsibility.

The VINDICATE model is useful in many cases, just not so much for Lyme. I have developed what I hope is a more applicable version that might be better at meeting our needs. I refer to this as the:

SPREEN TBI DIFFERENTIAL DIAGNOSIS CHECKLIST

Note that this list is not all-inclusive. Some items are given more attention based on my biases as I tried to create a list that might be most helpful to your practice. Many of the terms listed in the DD checklist are signs or symptoms and not specific diagnosis. My intention is that when you see the manifestations listed you think of the diagnoses that could possibly explain their presence. These would be diagnoses to be considered in your TBI differential. Unfortunately, this checklist does not lend itself to a clever mnemonic. I tried.

Just know that DD is a process and you should consider even those items that you might think are highly *unlikely,* at least initially. You can disregard them when you have reason to believe they are no longer plausible candidates. Bring them back onto the table if your other diagnoses do not pan out, especially if the patient is not responding to early treatment efforts that were based on your initial diagnosis. Some components of the TBI differential below are in more than one category. Each could be responsible for the signs and symptoms you are observing. Always remember multiple diagnoses may be active simultaneously. Kids with JIA get bitten by ticks and tick-bitten kids may develop JIA unrelated to the tick. Here goes...

SPREEN TBI DIFFERENTIAL DIAGNOSIS CHECKLIST

Infections: Infections on the TBI differential include both those that may have traveled on the same tick and those that arrived by any other means of transmission. Here you are answering "What else could this be?" not simply "What is this?"

A.   TBIs including all known (and unknown) co-infections: Lyme, STARI, babesiosis, bartonellosis, various Mycoplasma, ehrlichiosis, anaplasmosis, RMSF, tularemia, Q fever, tick paralysis. A single tick can carry many pathogens, including those we have not yet recognized as tick-borne pathogens. Especially in endemic areas, TBIs should be a part of the DD in more cases presenting with signs of infection than they currently are.

B.   Viruses: EBV, CMV, West Nile, HHV, HIV, hepatitis, etc. When Bb are present, the impact on the immune system allows for many pathogens such as the HHV viruses to manifest including EBV, CMV, and the herpes genus responsible for chicken pox and shingles. For example, since EBV stays in the body forever, you may get manifestations of this virus along with whatever else is going on. If signs and symptoms of encephalitis appear, consider viral etiologies such as St. Louis encephalitis as well as those TBI co-infections well-known to show neurologic inflammation such as Lyme, Bartonella, and M. *fermentans*.

C.   Bacteria: Strep, (rheumatic fever, glomerulonephritis), bacterial co-infections, or other concurrent infections

D.   Parasites: Babesia, Chlamydia, and those causing filariasis, amebiasis, giardiasis

E.   Fungi including Candida and molds

Inflammation/Immune dysfunction: So many things cause the sxs of general inflammatory response that sorting through the possibilities can be tedious. Keep parsing. Try to find the distinctive piece that distinguishes your case, then see how it fits the list of contenders. One by one. A red, pinpoint rash with a characteristic progression might lead you to RMSF instead of Lyme. That doesn't mean Bb aren't there concurrently, just that they are not the primary presenter at this time. Making one diagnosis does not cure another. That's such a good point, I'll say it again. Making one diagnosis does not cure another.

Autoimmune: We know that Lyme affects the immune system and that the immune system affects Lyme. We also strongly suspect that Bb, and perhaps other TBIs, may induce antineuronal antibodies, causing the body to work against its own cells. To date, we have no idea how common this might

be or if it happens at all. Certainly, this hypothesis would explain many mysteries around TBIs. Regardless, depending on the clinical presentation, autoimmune conditions should be included in your differential as possibly induced, exacerbated, or concurrent with Lyme. Note that in those cases where Lyme is a factor, a number of these conditions will not respond as well to traditional therapies unless the Lyme is concomitantly treated. Consider the following conditions that are thought to be autoimmune: DM type I, RA, SLE, pemphigus, ALS, Addison's disease, hepatitis, aplastic anemia, atopic dermatitis, asthma, celiac disease, cardiomyopathy, Cogan's syndrome, Cushing's disease, glomerulonephritis, Crohn's disease, autism, CREST, arteritis, Dressler's syndrome, Evans syndrome, Hughes disease, eczema, infertility, encephalitis, purpura, meningitis, adrenal problems, Kawasaki's disease, Meniere's disease, connective tissue diseases, multiple myeloma, myasthenia gravis (thymus disorder), multiple sclerosis, myositis, Hashimoto's thyroiditis and other types of thyroid inflammation, ulcerative colitis, uveitis, vitiligo, Wegener's granulomatosis, Alzheimer's, polymyalgia rheumatica, polymyositis, Goodpasture's disease, cirrhosis, Wilson's syndrome, psoriasis, Raynaud's, Reiter's syndrome, sarcoid, scleroderma, Still's disease, Sjogren's syndrome, vasculitis, PANDAS, Behcet's disease, chronic fatigue, antiphospholysis, some seizures, certain blood disorders, Guillain-Barré, irritable bowel, autoimmune inner ear disease, chronic otitis media, rheumatic fever, etc.

Neoplastic: While mistaking Lyme for cancer is rare, there are times that presentations may overlap. If you are hot on the trail of a TBI, don't discount cancer if you see abnormal blood work, growing pains, large nodes or organs, masses, nodules, or bone tenderness.

Skin: I misdiagnosed my first case of Lyme as ringworm. In my defense, this was in the ER at Fort Dix in 1985 and Mr. Plummer, the PA, brought his toddler in to see what this bizarre round rash inside a concentric circle could possibly be. We all got it wrong until the dermatologist remembered reading about a strange disease coming out of Lyme, Connecticut. Lyme has been associated with a number of other rashes and skin conditions in addition to EM. Subcutaneous skin nodules and violaceous striae suggest bartonellosis. Erythematous, pinpoint rashes are associated with RMSF, etc. Look at what the skin is showing you and think about which diagnoses might explain what you see.

Arthritis: If you have a painful, non-traumatic joint, a working diagnosis of arthritis may be indicated. Then, the HCP will need to determine the cause of that arthritis. With TBIs, Lyme is the first diagnostic consideration but all other explanatory conditions from gout to JIA should be methodically excluded.

Respiratory: Air hunger can be present with babesiosis and pneumonia in tularemia. With few exceptions, most other pulmonary problems associated with TBIs are secondary to progressive or end-stage disease.

Deficiency: Vitamin deficiency such as low D or Bs, deficiencies in calcium or magnesium, and inadequate amounts of other nutrients can all be part of the differential. Mitochondrial dysfunction has been documented in chronically ill patients who appear to lose mitochondrial utility. Here the membranes can't maintain adequate potential. Lipids in the membranes oxidize so that the mitochondria are limited in producing energy. This might be contributing to the profound fatigue found with some TBIs.

Congenital: Babies can be born with active Lyme, babesiosis, or bartonellosis. You must have a high index of suspicion. Aggressively evaluate a hypotonic baby for gestational Lyme. Sometimes symptoms of gestational Lyme are not apparent at birth. Ask if the mother had active Lyme during pregnancy or ever. Babies are also born with innumerable other types of congenital issues. These problems can impact Lyme and vice versa.

Allergic: Since allergies often present with components of inflammatory response, various allergic presentations can get tangled in a Lyme differential. Allergies to foods, drugs, and environmental factors can influence the diagnostic process.

Endocrine: Vitamin D deficiency, diabetes or fluctuating sugars, metabolic syndrome, hyper or hypoactive thyroid, adrenal dysfunction, and pituitary abnormalities are considerations.

Neurologic: Lyme, Bartonella, and M. *fermentans* are especially known to cause neurologic problems including neuropathies, palsies, tics, tremors, fasciculations, hypersensitivity, headaches, seizures, various dementias, autonomic dysfunction, MS-like patterns, vertigo, pain, hypotonia, sensory dysfunction, sleep disorders, autonomic anomalies, and balance disorders. Diagnoses associated with any of these manifestations may appropriately be part of the differential. Bell's palsy can come from non-Lyme sources but in a patient with a corroborating history and clinical course, when you see Bell's palsy, think Lyme. I have witnessed physicians just patch an eye and tell the patient the symptoms would probably resolve in a few months and never even consider the underlying etiology. Lyme can cause an autism-like syndrome OR autistic kids can get Lyme disease OR there may be a mechanism whereby these two conditions exacerbate each other. Perhaps a child who would have presented at a later date with autism is bitten by a tick and then presents with sxs consistent with autism. Here, whether the infection or the autism came first may be hard to tell. Many patients with neurodegenerative disease show evidence of chronic infection. For example, there appears to be an excess of H. *pylori* and Chlamydial pneumonia in Parkinson's patients. Neurologic manifestations are some of the most important signs associated with

Lyme. You may need to spend additional time in this arena when formulating your differential.

Psychiatric: In the DD look at the possible cause of anxiety, GAD, depression, OCD, bipolar disorder, schizophrenia, PANDAS, ADD, ADHD, OCD, and panic attacks. Psychiatric disorders that do not respond to conventional treatment should have Lyme as part of their differential. Do not easily dismiss Bartonella and M. *fermentans* in these cases just because you are less familiar with them. Discovering that one of these TBIs may be contributing to the problem may explain why a patient is not improving on conventional therapies.

Cardiac: Atrial fibrillation, valve problems, dysrhythmias, or indications for a pacer could all be due to a TBI or exist as a separate diagnosis. If you have a patient who is in need of a pacer, make sure Bb are not the underlying contributor. Do not dismiss a Lyme diagnosis here based on a negative lab test. The presence of Bb in these cases is too important to rely on flawed lab studies.

Sensory: The underlying etiology of tinnitus, Meniere's, vision or eye conditions, hyperacusis or any other hypersensitivity such as those to light, touch, taste, smell, pressure, or temperature should be part of the work-up and DD.

Gastrointestinal: GI problems are often associated with Lyme and leaky gut, UC, IBS, GERD, malabsorption, elevated LFTs, and hepatitis can be evaluated as part of the TBI or as independent entities.

Musculoskeletal: A number of the TBIs cause muscle pain, nodules, and changes in tone. Depending on the presentation, other explanations for these signs and symptoms should be considered.

Genitourinary: Investigate the cause of bladder spasms, nocturia, incontinence, pelvic discomfort, and interstitial cystitis. If recurrent UTIs do not respond to traditional therapy or there are repeat negative cultures in patients with sxs of UTI, think Bb.

Toxins: Heavy metals, molds, bacterial or environmental toxins, medication, multiple chemical sensitivity, and environmental illness can all be reasonably considered in the DD if the history corroborates that possibility.

CO-MORBID OR CONCURRENT DISEASE

The terminology here can be confusing so don't get hung up on terms. Co-morbid or concurrent diseases are simply conditions occurring at the same time. Even sick people get sick. In fact, sick people may get even sicker than previously well people since they are already compromised. A person debilitated with a TBI can get sick with other things *before, during, or after* the TBI infection. Further, the TBI may increase, decrease, or not affect the other condition.

Pre-existing conditions can be present. These can be apparent or subclinical. Genetic predispositions may be known or unknown. Likewise, TBI patients can catch cold, develop high cholesterol, or suffer trauma during the course of their disease. Some TBIs result in permanent adverse sequelae.

Co-morbidities can be co-infections that arrived on the same tick as another TBI or they can be infections transmitted through totally autonomous sources. Concurrent diseases may have nothing to do with infections such as heart problems or diabetes. Still, since Lyme affects so many organ systems, either directly or through the vascular and nervous systems, every co-morbidity can be assumed to affect the Lyme, just as the Lyme should be assumed to affect the other conditions.

People can have one, two, three, or a dozen diagnoses, all related or all independent. The presence of one condition does not eliminate the concurrent presence of another. When my mom died, she had at least a dozen *active* disease processes and many others that had been pushed to the wayside by more pressing conditions. Some were related to the others, others were not. Still, they impacted each upon the other. What a mess. The only thing she didn't have was a TBI. Really.

Concurrent diseases can involve any body system. People with psoriasis get bitten by ticks as do people with Parkinson's. People with bunions and dandruff can still make it to the tall grass by the side of the woods.

While some conditions are likely either caused by the Lyme or impacted by it, others you might never consider can be influencing the clinical course of Lyme. When there is a new onset of endocrine problems or diabetes in a Lyme patient, suspect that the Lyme had something to do with it. To try to tease out which came first, the abnormal sugars or the Lyme, try to find evidence of a pre-existing condition. If no information is available, then look to see if the patient responds to traditional therapies. If there is a poor response, then consider Bb as a contributor to the problem. In these cases, you usually have to address the Lyme pathogen as well as end-organ symptoms to get resolution. Here, standard treatment without antibiotics often does not work well.

But *expect* endocrine problems to confound our Lyme cases. With TBIs you must expect the unexpected. For example, gingivitis (yes, I said gingivitis) may be impeding recovery and confounding your attempts to figure out what is going on. Gingivitis can cause a low grade inflammation that may interfere with the body's immune response to infection. Gingivitis can even change lab parameters so that you can't quite tell what is happening. Although I use gingivitis as an example here, any number of conditions can be confusing your dif-

ferential diagnosis. The more aware you are, the more able to circumvent the confounders.

Patients with co-infections or other concurrent problems are often sicker and take longer to recover than a person with a sole infectious agent or single pathology. This makes sense. Just because you are adequately treating one co-infection, does not mean you are hitting them all. Standard Lyme treatment does not hit Babesia or Bartonella so the patient can remain sick because you have missed part of the diagnosis. Keep going back to your differential and revise it as appropriate.

DISTINGUISHING FEATURES OF THE BEST KNOWN TBIs

A portion of the following chart appears on the back inside cover of the book. Each recognized TBD is listed with the following attributes included: Pathognomonic, Distinctive, Common, and Frequently observed. The most usual treatment choices are added as well. This approach is just another way to look at this complicated field of medicine.

DISTINGUISHING FEATURES OF THE BEST KNOWN TBIs

Lyme (Borreliosis)

Pathognomonic

  EM rash

Distinctive

  Migrating joint pain

  Paresthesias (numbness/tingling/pins)

  Fasciculations/twitch (especially of eye)

  Bell's palsy

  Hypersensitivity

Common

  Flu-like syndrome

  Intractable fatigue

  Brain fog

  Headache

  Pain

  Irritability

  Arthralgia

  Anxiety

  Neck crepitus

  Waxing & waning course

Frequently observed

  GERD

  Eye problems (smeared vision)

  Neuropsychiatric signs

  Cognitive deficits

  Memory issues

  Processing problems

  Difficulty with sensory integration

  Endocrine problems (sugars/thyroid/cortisol)

  Tinnitus

  Interstitial cystitis

  Cold extremities

  Cracking or popping joints

  Achiness

Primary treatment choices

  Combination TX important

  Amoxicillin or Doxycycline

  With macrolide such as azithromycin (or Ketek)

  Add cyst-buster (azole)

  Plaquenil for autoimmune sxs

Gestational Lyme (Borreliosis)

Common

  Hypotonia

  Hypersensitivity

  Irritability

Frequently observed

  GERD

  Wilting/deflating

  Poor stamina

  Fatigue

  Cognitive problems

  Developmental delays

  Behavior issues

  Congenital anomalies

  Pallor/ dark circles under eyes

Primary treatment choices

  PCN or CS with macrolide

  May need cyst-buster

Babesiosis

Pathognomonic

  Maltese crosses *inside* RBCs

Common

  Rigors

  Sweats

  High fevers @105-6

Frequently observed

  Anemia

  Blood in urine

  Air hunger

  Headache

Primary treatment choices

  TX for both primary species

  Atovaquone PLUS azithromycin

  PLUS artemesia

Ehrlichiosis/Anaplasmosis

Pathognomonic

  Morulae in WBCs

Common

  Flu-like syndrome

Frequently observed

  Fever

  Chills

  Severe headache

  Muscle pain

  GI complaints

  Fatigue

Primary treatment choices

  Doxycycline or rifamycin

Bartonellosis

Distinctive

  Pain in tibia or sole

  Violaceous striae

  Subcutaneous nodules

  Microangiomas

  Neuropsychiatric problems

Common

  Disproportionate rage

  Behavioral issues

  Fever

  Chills

  Headache

Frequently observed
> ODD
> Gastritis
> Cold extremities
> Lymphadenopathy
> Skin lesions
> Circulation/coagulation issues

Primary treatment choices
> Combination of macrolides, TCNs, rifamycin (also possible Bactrim or fluoroquinolones)

M. *fermentans*

Distinctive
> Worst NP manifestations of any TBI

Common
> Intractable fatigue
> Headache

Frequently observed
> Cognitive problems
> Severe behavior issues
> Depression
> GI complaints
> Joint discomfort
> Immune impact
> Muscle pain
> Somnolence

Primary treatment choices
> Most challenging TBI to treat
> Combination of doxycycline & macrolide. Add rifamycin, Plaquenil, Cipro, Bactrim, and/or chloramphenicol prn

Colorado Tick Fever

Common
> Recurrent fever

Frequently observed
> Headache
> Chills
> GI problems
> Muscle and back pain
> Pain behind eyes
> Light sensitivity

Primary treatment choices
> Antiviral if caught early

Powassan Encephalitis

Common
> Encephalitis

Frequently observed
> Pain behind eyes
> Fever
> Headache
> Light sensitivity

Primary treatment choices
> Antiviral if caught early

Q fever

Common
> Fever
> Chills
> Sweats

Frequently observed
> Pneumonia
> Abnormal LFTs

Primary treatment choices
> Doxycycline or Plaquenil or fluoroquinolones

RMSF

Distinctive
> Pinpoint rash 1st on soles and palms

Common
> Headache
> Pain behind eyes

Frequently observed
> Bleeding
> Rash may not be immediate

Primary treatment choices
> Doxycycline or chloramphenicol

Tick Paralysis

Common
> Flaccid paralysis begins in legs and spreads

Frequently observed
> Paralysis can affect tongue and facial muscles
> Seizures

Primary treatment choices
> Remove tick

Tick Relapsing Fever (Borreliosis)

Common
> Cycles of high fevers and chills / Herx

Frequently observed
> Eye inflammation

Primary treatment choices
> Treat as for Lyme

Tularemia

Distinctive
> Ulcers at infection sites

Common
> Eye ulcers
> Skin ulcers
> Mouth ulcers

Frequently observed
> Large painful nodes
> Pneumonia
> Fever
> Chills
> Sore throat
> GI complaints

Primary treatment choices
> Doxycycline or CSs or chloramphenicol or aminoglycosides

Chapter 22

TREATMENT OPTIONS

The problem may be with the archer, not the arrow.

John Martin

Once you decide that you have a TBI patient sitting in front of you, how might you help him? The key to predominantly favorable results may be a core belief in success. These patients can and do get better with diligent management. Never give up. If Plan A doesn't work, regroup, and move on to Plan B. Don't be so hard on yourself. This field is new, controversial, and no one knows it all. If you're reading this text, you already know more than most.

Patients, along with their caregivers, often need reassurance. They want to know there are options available. Frequently, they want to be a part of the decision-making around their treatment. You don't need to force anyone to do anything, although encouragement might be offered when the pill is expected to be bitter.

Please explain everything to the caretakers and patients in a way that they understand. When my son first got sick, he was given a long list of medicines, many of which his mom, the physician, was quite unfamiliar. We had no idea what had been prescribed. The pharmacist couldn't read the writing and had to call the office. Even after she was told the spelling, she had never heard of these medicines either and had to order them from her central office.

Multiple medicines may be prescribed at the same time. Make sure all the instructions are in writing somewhere, so the caregiver can look and see what they are supposed to do. And, NO, the caregiver does NOT know what you mean when you say, "Atovaquone 10 cc bid with a fatty meal concurrent with telithromycin 800 mg po qd at hs….." not even if the mom is a doctor who studied before she came to your office.

If the patient is being prescribed more than two medicines, especially if they are to be given before, after, or during food intake, before bed, upon wake-up, etcetera, you might want to consider making a medicine tracking chart. Especially when you might be alternating acetaminophen and NSAIDs along with probiotics and vitamins, no one can be expected to keep all this in his head.

PEARL: Sample forms XIII and XIV, displayed in Chapter 24, show different ways to track treatment regimens. These forms will work best when targeted to the individual patient's schedule.

I was in drug development for many years (decades even). There is much to learn. Knowing that the drug label is a regulatory document rather than a way to convey medical information might help you better understand the medicine your child will be taking. When the TV announcer says, "Ask your doctor if Cialis is right for you," they say that only because the government MADE them say that. Drug companies know (and rely on) the fact that your doctor probably has no idea what the advertised drug is all about either. Nonetheless, she is likely to write for it just because you asked, whether you need it or not. (There are 17 more patients to be seen before that doctor can leave for the day and she wants you to be on your way. If writing for Cialis will get you out the door, she will probably write for Cialis. I have been there myself. I say this with apologies to all those doctors who try to do the right thing.) Remember, the words on these ads are the result of hundreds of hours of in-house meetings and discussions with DDMAC[1] at the FDA designed to say things in a certain way. I participated in these meetings for 20 years. Because I know you don't know, I have included a chapter that will explain in plain language how to decipher "drug speak." That is where I explain how we used to track sales based on the number of TV ads telling the patient to ask for a certain color pill (not my favorite color, but each to his own taste). Patients would come into offices demanding the pill and not even knowing what it was for. And not caring …they just had to have it. Drug companies LOVE direct-to-consumer advertising.

Remember that treatment of TBIs is controversial. Use your best judgment in selecting what you think will help the individual patient. Case-by-case. One at a time. Know that the controversy all but disappears in those HCPs whose own child gets sick after a tick bite.

There are so many treatment options and combinations of options for TBI patients that I had to split things into six chapters. Don't get overwhelmed. Look until you find what your patient needs.

---

1 Division of Drug Marketing, Advertising and Communication, now called OPDP

The treatment chapters are divided as follows:

As you might guess, Chapter 22: *Treatment Options* introduces you to the various approaches used in trying to help TBI patients. This chapter is short; the other chapters are interminable. They are not designed to be read word-for-word as you would a novel. Rather they are intended for you to be able to look up what you need and move on.

Chapter 23: *Understanding Medicines* outlines basic pharmacology and the foundation of drug regulation. This information will help you prescribe, use, and understand the medicines most commonly ordered in response to a TBI. Here I review how to read a drug label, including all the terms and acronyms that are thrown around as though you talk like that at your dinner table: MOA, AE, and CIs. Black box warnings are introduced, including how I once inherited a drug that got a black box warning because my predecessor was rude to the regulators. The warning had nothing to do with the safety of the drug in question and made no medical sense. (In defense of the FDA, the company guy was rude and quite passive-aggressive.) I will describe how to calculate a dose and how many ccs are in a teaspoon. The pros and cons of various modalities such as IV, po, and IM are reviewed.

Chapter 24 introduces essentially all the current antimicrobials known to be helpful in treating the array of TBIs. Remember, we are dealing with bacteria, spirochetes, protozoa, rickettsia, viruses, fungi, and probably a few critters we don't even recognize yet. Each antibiotic (or antiviral, or antimalarial, or antiprotozoal) includes a description of the drug, its mechanism of action, indications, use, dosing information, common adverse events, and recommendations for monitoring during the course of therapy. Of course, this book cannot include everything. Around me now I have dozens of texts with 1000 to 2000 pages outlining in painful detail everything there is to know about each of these drugs. One 1700 page text talks *only* about the adverse effects of antibiotics. Chapter 24 focuses on those aspects of each drug that are pertinent to TBI patients. Also included are drug combinations that might be useful in the cases of two or more co-infections.

Ancillary Treatments are the focus of Chapter 25. This includes everything from antipyretics to mittens for cold hands to psychological counseling. Just about everything that is usually accepted in traditional medicine, and has been shown to help the TBI patient, has a chance of appearing in this chapter. I am even so radical as to recommend a blanket for those patients who dare to shiver pathetically in the ER waiting room. I also discuss treatments for conditions that might come from aggressive therapy for TBIs such as fungal overgrowth and C. *difficile*.

Chapter 26 is titled *Alternative Treatments*. These modalities can be anything from herbal remedies (some of which I recommend consistently) to those that are somewhat "out there." A few I vehemently caution against. Look at this chapter to see if you have overlooked something that has the potential to help in a specific case.

Supportive Measures are the topics reviewed in Chapter 27. While these are not treatments *per se*, they include those modalities that are the foundation for the TBI patient getting well such as diet, exercise, stress reduction, and sleep hygiene.

Each patient needs an individual treatment strategy that addresses his specific case and depends on:

- TBI(s)
- Underlying health (concurrent disease, nutrition, fitness)
- Age
- Gender
- Available support and finances.

Elizabeth Maloney, MD, provides insight on the decision to treat or to extend treatment in Lyme patients. Paraphrasing her suggestions, when making treatment decisions consider:

- Time between onset of illness and diagnosis
- Severity of presenting symptoms
- Neuropsychiatric or cardiac sxs
- Is the disease progressing or holding steady?
- QOL
- Co-infections
- Ability to function and productivity
- Status of individual immune system
- Signs of on-going infection
- Ability to tolerate treatment regime
- Current or previous response to treatment
- History of relapse when treatment discontinued
- Risk/benefit of proposed plan
- Options available

Interestingly, Maloney also discusses the benefit to society in treating chronic Lyme disease, including the increased productivity from people who were previously too ill to contribute and the enhanced health of the community. By not treating, the cost to society increases through maintaining the patient in a chronically ill state, time and money devoted to intense supportive care, and loss of constructive input at work and school.

Repeatedly, delay in treatment or premature discontinuation of treatment has resulted in a Lyme syndrome that is much more recalcitrant and harder to treat and therefore much more costly over time. Had treatment been started earlier, permanent and expensive sequelae might have been averted. Bransfield asks whether some of the neuropsychiatric diagnoses that we pour so much time and resource into managing actually have an underlying infectious etiology. Think of the money spent without positive outcomes. In these cases, treating the on-going infection might allow for relief of some of the symptoms that were unresponsive to conventional therapies. The cost and labor-savings there would be tremendous. Not to mention, the relief of unnecessary suffering.

These perspectives underscore the idea that the best treatments for TBIs are those that are targeted for each individual patient. If this were strictly "algorithm medicine" there would be no need for HCPs at all. Some people would get better with no treatment. Others, like many treated in the past with inadequate therapies, would never get well. As an HCP, you must decide *how* to manage your patients. As a parent or guardian, you must decide *who* will manage your child's care. Let's hope we all make wise decisions.

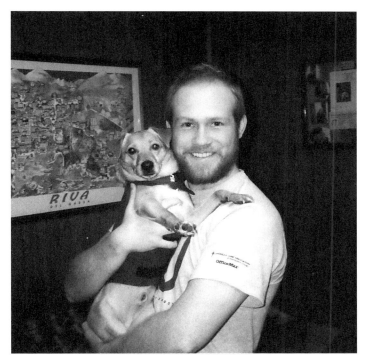

After three years of hell, "Chris Spreen, YOU are fixable."

Chapter 23 UNDERSTANDING MEDICINES – Detailed chapter contents

Chapter 23

UNDERSTANDING MEDICINES

Nobody loves me but my mother, and she could be jiving too.

B.B. King

In medical school we had a pharmacology course that went through the various drug classes and we memorized lists of drugs and their uses. As we marched through our clinical rotations, we learned from practical experience and, in general, picked a few drugs from each class and stuck to them come hell or high water. We had a first choice for otitis and a first choice for hypertension and a first choice for high blood sugars. If Choice 1 didn't pan out or if the patient dared to be allergic to the first choice, we had a second choice. If Choice 2 also proved faulty, we would dip into our *Washington Manual* or *Harriet Lane* and come up with something else. Drug selection had more to do with which sales rep was bringing sandwiches and what drug required the least effort on our part, than it did with targeting individual patient needs.

Although some things have changed (drug reps aren't supposed to bribe you anymore to use their drug) many things have stayed the same. When my knee was replaced and I tried to tell the resident that I was allergic to the codeines, he first tried to talk me out of the allergy. Was I really allergic or was it just a non-allergic bad reaction? "Codeine nearly killed me twice and I don't use it, okay?" He really wanted me to accept his Choice 1 or Choice 2. Further, I had been the physician for these specific drugs at their original drug company so I knew all about their paradoxical reactions in a small population of patients. Even further, I knew exactly which drugs I could take safely. Unfortunately, he didn't know if one came in an oral form and he didn't want me to get addicted to the dissolving formulation. (Just thinking of me, doncha know?) He had no intention of looking anything up. He wrote for his Choice 3, which the pharmacist wouldn't fill since I am allergic to the drugs in that class. My husband had to drive 40 miles to get another prescription for the drug I told the resident I *could* take in the first place.

My point is: Many HCPs do not know as much as we might hope about medicines and many don't seem especially inclined to learn. Hopefully, if you are reading this text, you are trying to get as much knowledge as possible so you can actually help people. The following chapter provides some of the basics as they pertain to TBI patients. Scan down and linger in the spots where you might need a refresher.

I. Treatment Guidance

Here is a tip that has helped me many times over the years. Unless you know the drugs in this field inside and out, you should know the phone number of a trusted local pharmacist or pharmacy school. Often times, the local pharmacist can help you immensely with routine questions. For more obscure, complicated queries I have called the library at the University of the Sciences in Philadelphia. (I apologize to the various superlative librarians there because now I know that they will be inundated with calls. Nonetheless, they have been exceptional in finding the most bizarre tidbits of information. After they were nice to me and found information I could not find anywhere else, I was their friend for life. My advice to them is to set up a fee-for-service computer hot-line. They will never lack for work.) If in doubt, ask.

The information provided in these chapters is a general overview and you must decide how best to treat each individual. Watch the specific patient. Target the therapy to the person. Each may respond differently. Even that one specific, unique, singular, peerless, particular individual patient may respond differently from one time to the next, depending on a number of factors. These determinants include their overall health, severity of illness, co-infections, underlying illnesses, ability to metabolize medicines, genetics, the capacity of their immune system, level of nutrition and hydration, concomitant medicines, concurrent illnesses..... You get the idea. The key is to pay attention to your patient. And don't be afraid to rethink a past decision and adjust your treatment plan. If the patient is not getting better on the regimen you have selected, ask yourself why. Then, regroup.

You are about to enter one of the most complex fields of medicine. There are numerous contributing factors to both health and illness. Much is unknown. Science is on the edge of important discoveries about the immune system, but we have a long way to go to find the best management course for TBIs. Unfortunately, we're stuck in the time before we have resolution on many issues. Still, if you focus on one case, keep an open mind, and *act in good faith* with no other agenda but to help your patient, you will be okay. We all make many decisions every day that we later second guess. Gather as much information as you can and move forward to help the person in front of you.

II. Drug Speak

I have spent 20 years in drug development and I know that you do not come out of medical school knowing much about how medicines work and why. You don't know beans about how to interpret clinical trial data and you certainly are unaware of how drug companies and others with secondary agendas can skew data to their own ends. You have no idea how the FDA or the CDC or NIH works. After many years and many scars from the school of hard knocks, I have a better, but still incomplete, understanding. I present some basic information here that hopefully will allow you to make the best treatment decisions for your patients.

What makes a medicine work? Who knows? Drug companies have been trying to figure this out for years. Most effective drugs are found through serendipity. Valium started out as a muscle relaxant and became one of the most commonly used anxiolytics. I remember being an intern in the 80s when a drug called minoxidil was given for high blood pressure. Minoxidil was the new "big thing." However, we noticed that our patients were getting hairy. I don't know anyone who uses minoxidil for blood pressure anymore, but I sure know that many doctors use Rogaine (minoxidil) to treat baldness. All serendipity. By the way, Rogaine is extremely toxic to cats, who presumably die hairy.

A drug that does what you want it to do is called **effective**. Anything a drug does that is outside what you want it to do is called a **side effect** or **adverse event**. The entire scope of knowledge about a drug's side effects is called its **safety profile**. Before making treatment choices for any specific condition or individual patient, the HCP should do a **risk/benefit** analysis to determine if the benefits outweigh the risks of treatment.

I was a drug safety doctor at various pharmaceutical companies for what seems like a million years and I wrote many SOPs for **pharmacovigilance** programs. These programs were all the rage a few years ago when the FDA seemed hot on them and companies were trying to earn Brownie points. As the FDA became grossly understaffed and had to focus on their highest priorities, they seemed to have bigger fish to fry. Pharmacovigilance is a process by which professionals gather safety data on medicines and then watch this data over time to see if there are identifiable patterns or trends. The idea was to gather clues that might identify potential safety issues before they happened.

Personally, I think pharmacovigilance is a great idea. Too bad no one really does it anymore. Trust me when I say that companies go to great lengths not to reveal any information that they do not have to uncover. Just call a corporate drug safety hotline sometime and see if you can get any information aside from pre-written, pre-approved, canned, standard statements.

They will grill you mercilessly regarding whether or not you might have had an adverse reaction related to their drug and then spend thousands of dollars proving you did not. (And you wonder why grandma's medicine costs so much…)

Today, what used to be called pharmacovigilance is now referred to as **REMS** or Risk Evaluation and Mitigation strategy. Again, this is an acronym referring to techniques used to identify, evaluate, understand, and prevent safety problems that could arise from the use of certain drugs. Taking what is known about a compound, a plan is written to try to anticipate and circumvent any problems that might appear in an individual patient. Unfortunately, the individual is unpredictable and does not always act like the population. For every AE, there is a first time. Currently the FDA, often requests a REMS plan be written before a drug is approved and that a Patient Information Sheet be compiled that is supposedly more user-friendly than the label. Just as with pharmacovigilance, REMS has become a way for unscrupulous vendors to sell safety and risk management programs to companies too inept or too lackadaisical to write them themselves. Be careful with what you read and always check the source and consider any secondary agendas the author may have had.

PEARL: There are now "Patient Information Sheets" which are designed to make the material contained in the package insert more comprehensible to the lay user. In some cases, they do.

I cannot imagine any drug company on the planet spending a nickel specifically developing TBI drugs in the next decade. They will only go for the blockbusters or those smaller indications that will allow them to capitalize on off-label usage. Since TBIs are currently treated with old drugs that have long become generic (and therefore barely profitable for the manufacturer) it is not worth their time. Therefore, with few exceptions only a handful of drugs have TBIs listed in their labels. This means when an HCP writes a prescription to treat a TBI, they are said to be treating **off-label**. Further, a drug is usually only approved for one or a few **indications**, based on the clinical studies conducted by the company that wants to sell the drug. That does not mean it cannot do other things very well. Most initial indications for which the drug is **approved** are based on studies that will get the company's foot into the market, are the easiest to obtain, or will allow the company the best competitive edge over a market challenger. While many companies have as their slogan "Patients First" it is really another word that starts with a "**P**" that comes first.

Any use of a drug other than what is written in the label is therefore off-label usage and that includes what the drug is used for and how it is used. IMPORTANT: Providers are allowed to use medicines off-label essentially any way they like, but drug companies are NOT allowed to promote a drug for off-label use. Do not kid yourself. Drug companies bet their economic lives on off-label usage. Pharmaceutical giants know that it is worth the free publicity they get by marketing off-label. Over and over they have paid huge fines for telling doctors about uses that are not in the label. Once they plant the seed, the doctor just might keep on writing those scripts. Why follow the rules, when it is more profitable to pay the fines? Drug companies often have more lawyers than doctors working for them. They probably have more lawyers than the FDA, as well.

Why do I tell you all this? Because you are writing off-label all day every day in your practice, and not just for TBI patients. If scripts were written only by the letter of the label, few patients would ever fill a prescription. Let me give one example, although I could give a hundred. For a diaper rash treatment that is currently on the market, the label took more than a year to negotiate. This delay occurred despite the fact that the active ingredient in this drug had been available for decades and was now available OTC in a cheaper and superior formulation. The FDA required a microscopic exam proving that fungus was present under the diaper. Let me kindly say that none of the doctors on the FDA panel had ever seen a patient for diaper rash in the US. Nonetheless, they felt obligated to insist on this. If I was taking my kid to a doctor who would NEED to read the label on a diaper rash cream, with an ingredient that was likely older than she was, and couldn't diagnose fungus *in situ*, I would find a new doctor. I know of no HCP worth her salt who would spend the time or money to scrape a kid's poor bottom to look for fungus under the scope before prescribing a more expensive medicine than what is available from the shelf at the drug store. Sure, we put the microscopic exam in the label. It wasn't wrong, it just wasn't real. Your tax dollars at work.

For TBI treatment, make sure you detail your rationale in the chart. If someone is going to come after you for prescribing a particular drug they will usually *not* do so for writing off-label. Rather they will probably try to get you for not following a certain "Guideline" or some imagined "Standard of Care." If they are determined to come after you, they will find a reason whether it is legitimate or not.

The **label** or **package insert** must accompany the product when it is sold and must appear on any promotional material. That's why you have to turn several pages after a drug ad in a magazine. The label must be reprinted (even if it is printed in a font so small as to be indecipherable, in language specifically designed to be incomprehensible). The label contains a number of standard sections that are usually of no help whatsoever to the prescriber. I once worked at a company that had a blood thinner label that was nearly 50 pages long at one point. Adverse events included bleeding from upper right gum, bleeding from lower right gum, bleeding under right little toenail, etc. We would spend hours arguing if bleeding under the left little toenail was expected or unexpected based on what was already in the label. Some of us wanted to condense this to something like: "Since this product is an anticoagulant, bleeding can occur in any tissue or organ internally or externally. This bleeding can be severe and difficult to stop and may become life-threatening." So don't always count on the label to provide you with handy information when you need it, especially in an emergency.

III. Reading a Drug Label

Whatever my feelings regarding the medical validity of a drug label, they are a part of my life and yours. Below are descriptions of standard label sections and what they mean, since a number of these terms will be included in the information in subsequent chapters.

Remember that package inserts (labels) are the result of long fights between drug companies and the FDA. (I have been in label negotiations for years.) They are regulatory documents that may not be especially useful to the practitioner. Depending on the personalities of the combatants at the different companies and divisions of the FDA, sometimes you have a ludicrous amount of information and sometimes not enough. It's all a dance. Gather the information that you can and make balanced decisions by considering the risk/benefit of any treatment plan.

A. **Drug name** (Brand and generic): In general, the brand name is capitalized and the generic name is small. The PDR only includes drugs from companies that pay money for their inclusion. Usually the PDR reproduces the label just as it appears in the package. Many generic drugs are not included since no one is going to pay for these old dogs to go to Westminster. Since many of the treatments for TBIs are primarily dispensed as generics (amoxicillin and doxycycline, for example), they can be hard to find in the PDR. In the old days, this was a big problem. Fortunately, with the web there are numerous other sources of information. The *Monthly Prescribing Reference* (www.PrescribingReference.com) is much more helpful than the PDR, providing a synopsis of the most important information for each drug. With the Internet, the problem is too much information, some of which is contradictory and some just plain wrong. If you search amoxicillin, you will get ten pages of individual sites, many of which are ads for cheap versions from India.

B. **Description:** This section includes drug class and basic chemistry. In the *Description* sections compiled below for the individual drugs, I include more drug development history than usually found in the PI, not only because I find it interesting, but also to help you remember the drug under discussion. You're more likely to remember that cephalosporins were first isolated from a sewer in Sardinia than you are to recall their precise mechanism of action.

C. **Mechanism of Action:** The MOA is a description of how the drug works. Unfortunately, most drug labels say, "Mechanism of action unknown." Information on MOA may help when combining drugs to get better efficacy. Usually you do not need two drugs doing the exact same thing. Rather, select the second drug because it comes at the pathogen from a different angle and you may have a better chance of treatment success. If one antibiotic inhibits cell wall synthesis and another works by penetrating the cystic capsule, that might be useful information to know when making your decision. There are hundreds of ways that drugs work, but the most common MOA is probably through some kind of receptor binding.

D. **Clinical Pharmacology:** Clinical pharmacology describes the interactions between a drug and a body. In assessing these complicated parameters, always remember that the goal is simply to relieve symptoms, or to cure, in a way that results in the least number of adverse side effects. Always aim for the most favorable risk/benefit ratio. Pharmacology is greatly affected by genetics, age, weight, gender, the current degree of pathology, concurrent medical conditions, compliance, and physiologic factors (such as the patient's hydration and nutrition). Individuals vary greatly in their response to an identical drug regime. Even the same patient can respond differently at different times. The label may contain the following Pharmacology sections:

Pharmacodynamics (PD) are all the things the drug does *to the body*, while **pharmacokinetics** (PK) is all the stuff the body does *to the drug*. Although there are numerous textbooks written on each of these clinical pharmacology topics, I will include here only those terms that might be useful in selecting between treatment options. Many details have been generalized and summarized below in order to remain practical.

First, a drug is **administered** to the patient. At this point, the body begins to act on the drug (PK) and soon thereafter, the drug begins to act on the body (PD). All these processes can be occurring at the same time.

A drug can be introduced in many ways, which are detailed later. The drug comes into the body either orally or parentally, which is any entry aside from swallowing. At this point, the drug gains access to the patient's system where it can do its work.

Absorption is the process by which the drug gets into the circulation. This can occur when the drug crosses any number of barriers such as the skin, the mucous membranes, the GI tract, or muscle capillaries. If the drug is given IV, it goes directly into the vein, by-passing many absorption issues.

Rarely is a drug applied directly to the tissue we want it to affect, although this is sometimes the case for dermatology drugs. After absorption, the drug begins to be **distributed** through the body, usually traveling with fluids such as blood or lymph. The drug starts to find its way into the tissue cells and the space between cells (intracellular, extracellular, and interstitial areas). Depending on the chemical nature of the drug, some can cross the BBB and the placenta and others get into the CSF and breast milk. These drug characteristics may be important in drug selection.

PEARL: TBI drugs that cross the BBB include: Rocephin (ceftriaxone), rifamycin, Bicillin, minocycline to some degree, IV doxycycline, Claforan (cefotaxime), Ceftin (cefuroxime), chloramphenicol, and Lariam.

Once present in the tissues, the drug starts to achieve **steady state**. At this point we assume that there is some therapeutic **target level** that provides the drug with the optimal chance to work. In developing drugs, researchers study a number of parameters to determine the best **dose** to do a specific job. For antibiotics this includes the **concentration** that kills a certain number of bacteria in a given time. The information gathered helps determine the "best" target concentration at which the drug will be most effective. Measuring the concentration levels over time helps decide the dosing schedule needed and the form in which the drug should be administered. For some drugs a **therapeutic window** can be defined, which is the level of drug that is effective without causing unacceptable bad effects. This window can be broad or narrow.

Some drugs have a **dose response** where more drug causes more effect. Other drugs achieve a certain response level and after that more drug does not increase positive response. As Americans, we almost always think more is better. This is not always the case and more can just mean more side effects and not more efficacy. Therapeutic window is the amount of medicine between the amount that gives an effective concentration and the amount that does more harm than good.

Almost as soon as the drug hits the blood stream, it starts to reach the liver, which is the prime site of metabolism for most drugs. So even before the drug has had a chance to do any good, some of it is already being cleared away. That's just how chemistry works. The next paragraphs will be extremely important in understanding possible drug interactions, which is a section in most drug labels.

Drugs can influence one another in many ways: changing pH, binding inactivation (that's what antidotes sometimes do in overdoses), and for our purposes they can compete for enzymes that break them down.

Drugs are eliminated from the body in two ways: **excretion** and **metabolism** (also called transformation or degradation). While the liver is the prime site for metabolism, the kidney is the main route of excretion. After urine, drugs are excreted most commonly in the feces (by way of bile or other avenues), sweat, saliva, tears, mucus, and a few may directly evaporate from the skin.

Most drugs are metabolized in the liver, although a few are broken down in the kidney, bone, or elsewhere. The primary route of metabolism is through oxidative reactions catalyzed by enzymes of the hepatic cytochrome P450 system. There are many subsystems in this network but the concept is the same. Molecules come into the liver and travel down a specific biochemical pathway where they undergo metabolic reactions, either activating, deactivating, or otherwise metabolizing them.

When you read about drug interactions, you need to think about the enzyme systems in the liver. Many drugs can affect the P450 system in a variety of ways:

- So many biomolecules might be competing for the same metabolic pathways that one or more of the competitors can back up into the circulation thus INCREASING blood levels

- The drug can inhibit the P450 enzymes and so the metabolic pathway is no longer available for chemical reactions, thus INCREASING levels of any compounds that depend on that pathway. Sometimes this action is termed down-regulation.

- The medicine can up-regulate the pathway thus metabolizing the drug faster than anticipated thereby DECREASING blood levels of the active compound.

- Other physiologic processes may also be in play.

The key point is: If the label says that this drug has interactions with other drugs, or is metabolized by the P450 system, EXPECT that blood levels of ANY medicine might be different from expected. In some cases the levels may be so impacted that the medicine will be either ineffective or toxic. On the one hand, there is *more* drug available to do the intended job. But at the same time, there is *more* drug present to cause adverse effects and toxicity. Or there is *less* drug available so that you are not getting the therapeutic levels you anticipated. Either way, you might find yourself wondering why your regime in not working. Be careful.

Be ready to think of alternative therapies or to adjust doses to levels that will likely be more effective. Be vigilant for side effects that might occur from having higher than therapeutic levels in the body. Also, as if this complicated mess were not enough, drugs aren't the only molecules competing for space in the liver's processing plant. Grapefruit juice and a number of other compounds also want access to these same metabolic pathways.

Some of the drug that is metabolized in the liver will come out inactive and get eliminated from the body in one of the ways mentioned above. Others form metabolites that are even more active than the original molecule in doing the intended job. A number of drugs are metabolized into molecules without more positive effects, but with the capacity to cause additional side effects. The various metabolites may make several passes through the liver before their mission is complete.

Once the drug is in the body, many active and passive processes occur concurrently. The drug and its metabolites are in the circulation, liver, and in various excretory locations. Pharmacokinetic parameters determine how fast the drug gets where it needs to go, how long it stays at the target, and then how long it remains in the body. These times can last for minutes or months. By now the drug should be in the vicinity of where the action is desired. For example, if there is an infection in the digestive tract and the medicine is taken orally, it will be present at the affected site as soon as it dissolves. In contrast, if the infected site is the brain, then the drug or its metabolites will need to cross the blood brain barrier. This can take a while, even longer if the drug needs to penetrate a cystic capsule or needs to infiltrate areas that are notoriously difficult to access (small toes in a brittle diabetic or deep in an infected bone).

Hopefully, all this information is considered by some brilliant pharmacologist as the medicine is being developed. While you may want a certain minimum drug level to remain at the infected site (or at the pertinent receptor sites in other conditions), other pathways are moving drug out at a consistent rate. In the kidney, each molecule has a specific **clearance** or elimination rate, almost like an identifying fingerprint. Here's where things get very complicated with differential equations and exponents. Fortunately, you do not need to do any math, just understand a few more terms.

Clearance is the measurement of a RATE of **elimination**. This **rate** refers to how fast plasma is moving through the kidney and is usually measured per minute. Each molecule has a specific clearance or elimination rate, almost like an identifying fingerprint. Clearance can occur at different rates for different drugs in different people. After a single dose, only a fraction of the drug remains in the body. To maintain a therapeutic level another dose is needed before the clearance rate overtakes the bioavailability rate.

Clearance measures the efficiency of drug removal and may involve a number of "passes" through the liver and eventually the kidney before the drug and its metabolites are all gone.

The **half-life** ($t_{1/2}$) is the time it takes for 50% of the drug to be eliminated. In other words, the time it takes for the drug concentration to fall to half its previous level. Knowing how long the drug remains in the body impacts many aspects of dose determination. Usually it takes about 4 or 5 half-lives after starting a drug to get to a steady state level and then about 4 or 5 half-lives to eliminate a drug after the last dose. The dose you use to get the target concentration you want is determined by clearance rate, half-life, volume of distribution, and blood concentration over time. Volume of distribution is the amount of drug in the tissues. Clearance is the PK parameter most impacted by all these factors in addition to disease state, enzyme levels, concomitant drugs, GFR, age, gender, severity of illness, and underlying health.

Bioavailability is the fraction of the dose that reaches the systemic circulation and is used to quantify absorption. After the drug is in the circulation it almost immediately begins to clear and the plasma concentration decreases steadily after it reaches its peak. Clearance, usually through the kidney, is part of elimination and occurs at different rates for different drugs in different people. After one dose, the body starts to process the molecule. To maintain effective blood levels, another dose is needed before the clearance rate surpasses the bioavailability.

The concept of clearance is important in determining the therapeutic range of a drug. This range is the concentration at which the drug is effective while not causing unacceptable toxic effects and is the difference between the maximum and minimum concentrations needed to get positive results without negative effect (sort of like the TV show *The Price is Right* where you guess the price without going over). As always, when selecting treatment, the goal is to end up with a favorable risk/benefit ratio. The clearance is important to decisions around dose, dosing regimen, and route of administration.

Since a certain amount of drug is being cleared each minute, if you want to keep an effective drug level in the tissue, more drug will need to be administered in plenty of time to keep the blood levels within the therapeutic range. So, you have to replace both the drug that has been cleared and the drug that will soon be cleared. The only way to get the levels you need is by adjusting the dose, the regimen, or the route of administration.

Depending on the PD/PK parameters, some drugs do better with lower doses more often (PCNs), while others like to have a bolus level resulting in a peak concentration to be most effective (TCNs). Giving drugs at shorter intervals (q 6 instead of q 8 or q 12) gives more level blood concentrations whereas longer intervals (q 12 or q 24) tends to give more obvious peaks and troughs.

IV administration provides therapeutic blood levels almost immediately, while oral administration may take an extended time to reach those same levels. IM may result in the most consistent levels. The reason you need to understand these basics is to be able to consider many options if the initial treatment strategy does not work. Do you need to give the same drug in a higher dose, in a more frequent regimen, or by a different route? Do you need to change drugs or add others? The more you know, the more options may present themselves.

E. **Indications**: Drugs do many things, some good and some bad. How you define good and bad may depend on the circumstances. Just as beauty is in the eye of the beholder, good and bad is all relative. The drug, Megace, almost always causes patients to gain weight. Most see this as an unacceptable side effect. But for those patients who have terminal breast cancer, the weight gain is a blessing. So how do you classify the weight gain? Good or evil? Early in the Megace story, weight gain was considered a side effect. Now, it's perceived as an indication.

The first thing to understand about the *Indication* section of a label is that it is a regulatory sentence which lists only those uses that have been studied in two randomized, well-(often placebo)-controlled clinical trials that prove the point. The FDA reviews the results of the studies and then approves the drug for that indication alone, only at the doses used *in the study*, specifically for the type of patients enrolled *in the study*, with the exact disease defined *by the study*, etc. Drug companies only pay for these clinical trials if they are going to make a bazillion dollars by selling the drug to the patients with the condition being tested **or** if the study will get their foot in other doors. Then they pray that doctors will use it off-label for other things until they can support those indications – **or** they make people believe they have the disease that was studied. (YOU could have Gastro-Esophageal-Reflux-Disease! Say it isn't so! I thought I just had heartburn.)

By no means does the "Indication" section hold the complete information regarding what a drug might be able to do. As previously mentioned, many drugs are used off-label each day either in terms of dose adjustments, regimen changes, or indications. See what your patient needs and match it to what the drug does. You might not know everything a drug does based on what is mentioned in the label. Keep your antennae up for new uses for every drug. Especially if a drug is old and there is little profit margin, the drug company will never spend money going after new indications even if EVERYONE at the drug company knows it is the best treatment for a specific condition. They might do a little marketing study to flatter one "expert" in the field and to publish a paper regarding this new indication. Since they cannot promote off-label, they can only publish and plant seeds that they then surreptitiously water.

Just after I finished the above paragraph at 4:32 p.m. on April 27, 2010, I checked my e-mail. I was informed by a number of former colleagues that this very day a local pharmaceutical company was fined $520 million for off-label promotion. Note that the illegal promotion brought in almost $5 billion, so did the end justify the means? I had dinner last night with two people who worked on the drug in question. These two people did everything right and above board. The criminal decisions were made at higher levels. So why isn't anyone going to jail or even losing their jobs? Oh I forgot, this company just let thousands of researchers go because they really don't need to do that much science anymore. Sorry, I digress. This might be the subject of another book. Back to the parts of a drug label.

F. **Clinical Studies:** Depending on the personalities in the specific division of the FDA, sometimes there will be detailed clinical trial results and sometimes not a word. This disparity also has to do with the years when the drugs were approved and the clinical conditions under study. Even though I have written a number of these sections for drug labels, I rarely have found an HCP who has read these sections and received any information that helped the patient in his office. If you suffer from insomnia, The *Clinical Studies* section of any drug label should clear that right up.

G. **Special Populations:** Often a drug label will have additional information regarding what is known about use of the drug in children, pregnant or nursing mothers, people with kidney or liver problems, or other pre-existing conditions. Often the label will give the cop-out phrase: "No specific studies have been done to determine the effect of this drug on pregnant women." Or "Insufficient information is available regarding use in children." (These are similar phrases to those that were recently used to explain why certain professional organizations do not believe *THEIR* guidelines need to be changed. They say there are no well-controlled, prospective clinical trials to *PROVE* that the guidelines need changed. Well, there are no studies to prove the opposite either and there never will be. Who would pay for the studies? Again, I digress.)

Pregnancy Categories:

The FDA has a system to rate drugs with respect to their safe use during pregnancy. Risk of damage to the fetus is usually the greatest in the first weeks or months of the pregnancy when the major organ systems are developing, often when many women don't even realize they're pregnant. But damage can occur at any time. A higher-risk rating of C or D may not cause any problems in a particular pregnancy. In contrast, a drug with a low rating, which suggests that the drug should be safe, may result in fetal damage. There are no guarantees. Just as each individual can respond differently to a particular drug, each fetus might be affected differently. There are no 100% assurances and many other factors will impact a drug's effect on the fetus.

The FDA categories serve as a guide. Some drugs are placed in a particular category during one part of pregnancy and then are in another category during another part of gestation. Many drugs that are CI in the first trimester become a category B or C in the 2nd or 3rd trimesters. For example, ibuprofen is considered category B in the 1st and 2nd trimesters, but is completely CI in the 3rd trimester.

PEARL: For whatever reasons, the average age at onset of menses seems to be getting younger. Consider the possibility of pregnancy even with pre-teens. Your discomfort will not protect the fetus.

The categories are supposed to take into account the risk to both the mom and the fetus. OTC drugs are usually rated for risk, but naturals, herbals, and dietary supplements usually are not. In almost every case, promotional material will tell you to "Ask your health care provider." Trust me, they don't know any more than you do about these things. Where would that information come from?

In each case, the patient, guardian, and HCP should gather the available information and then make an informed decision together, always assessing the risk/benefit in making treatment choices. Unfortunately, sometimes you have to decide between a baby being born with babesiosis and the risk of antiprotozoal drugs. A number of drugs used in TBI patients have high pregnancy category ratings, possibly introducing more risk.

PEARL: Denial of pregnancy does not mean there is no pregnancy. In the ER, I delivered a number of babies who were conceived by immaculate conception. If you are planning on using a drug with potential risk, assess the possibility of pregnancy.

Categories:

A Tested for safety in pregnancy and found to be safe. Examples: folate and Vitamin B6

B Used often in pregnancy with no evidence of major birth defects or other serious problems. Examples: many antibiotics, acetaminophen, insulin

C More likely to cause problems for the fetus or mother. Also includes drugs where the safety studies are not done or are not planned. Most of the time these drugs come with the warning that the benefits should outweigh the risks of treatment. For these drugs you must discuss and decide. Examples include Compazine, used for nausea; the antifungal, Diflucan; and the antibiotic Cipro. A number of antidepressants are category C.

D Clear risk to the fetus. Examples: alcohol, some seizure medicines, and many chemotherapeutic agents.

X Cause birth defects. Never use in pregnancy. Examples include Accutane and its imitators, some medicines for psoriasis, thalidomide, and DES.

PEARL: With pregnancy, consider the potential of having two TBI patients instead of one: the mom and the fetus. TBI patients do get pregnant and have babies. HCPs need to take this contingency into account.

H. Usage: The package insert (label) usually contains information on dose, frequency, and route of administration. Again, HCPs are able to decide how to use the medicine in a particular patient. Various studies show that the majority of medications are prescribed differently than the instructions provided in the label. Whether this is from ignorance or intent I don't know. I do know that once I learned that every patient I prescribed a Z-Pak always needed another, I soon learned to write for a refill. I had my own little Diflucan regimen for fungal infections. Their way, no cure. My way 100%. You adjust based on what you learn from experience with these drugs. Why rigidly follow rules that don't work for your patients?

PEARL: Anecdotally, some HCPs have found when treating select cases of Lyme, improvement occurred only with very high doses of antibiotics. If the patient is tolerating the dose and getting better, the risk/benefit for the off-label dose just might be favorable.

Useful usage acronyms:

IV   Intravenous

IM   Intramuscular

PO   Per os, taken by mouth

Stat   Immediately, highest priority, Latin for statim or urgent

HS   At bedtime, hs

QD   Once a day, Latin: quaque die, qd

Bid   Twice a day, 2 x/day, Latin: bis in die, bid

Tid   Three times a day, 3 x/day, Latin: ter in die, tid

Qid   Four times a day, 4 x/day Latin: quarter in die, qid

Q   Every, q, q 4 h is every 4 hours

D   day, d

/   Per. So, 1 mg/kg/day is one milligram per kilogram per day

d/c   Discontinue

Gtt(s) Drop(s)

Hr   Hour, h, hr, q 4 h is every 4 hours

KVO   Keep vein open. Just enough fluid in the IV or line to keep the vein from collapsing or clotting

PICC   Peripherally inserted central catheter, a central line. If any problems, remove until the line can be safely re-inserted. AEs: infection, pain

<u>Various modes of administration</u>: Different modes of administration can provide useful options. Drugs come in immediate release, slow release, extended release, pulsed regimens, IV, po, IM, SL, SQ or SC, suppositories, sprays, powders, patches, topicals, depots, etc. By selecting among the various options, the HCP can help control the blood concentration and thereby best maintain the levels within the therapeutic range. All modes of administration have pros and cons to be considered before making a decision.

1. Intravenous (IV): Medicine is infused directly into a vein either in a single dose **injection** (bolus) or more slowly in a dilute **infusion** over time (that is, a syringe and needle or a hanging IV bag). IV dispensing goes right into the circulation and thereby circumvents any potential absorption problems. IV allows for the best plasma concentrations and the most rapid onset of action (aside from certain unique cases such as intracardiac and intrathecal, which we won't concern ourselves with here).

Pros: The medicine goes directly into the circulation with easy access to the tissues including across the BBB and CSF, assuming the molecule can cross. IV is probably the most effective treatment modality because it gets drug where you need it in a hurry in the sickest patients. No messing around.

Cons: Even after IV administration there can be other barriers to tissue penetration that will depend on drug solubility, size, etcetera, which may affect passage into areas like the placenta and milk ducts. A prime disadvantage to IV use is that it can be very expensive and can be difficult to provide at home. Today, home IVs are more common especially with the current quality of home health nursing. Some insurance plans will cover in-home IV usage. Because IV administration can be quite effective, you must anticipate a significant Herx reaction. Depending on the antibiotic, IV dispensing may not absolve you from fungal overgrowth. Like IM injections, an IV **bolus** is irreversible. But unlike IM injections, IV **infusion** can be shut off.

The IV drug may go places you do not want the medicine to go such as across the placenta or into breast milk but this can be an issue with other modes of administration as well.

TBI implications: IV can be through a bolus (doxy) or constant infusion (amoxicillin) depending on how you want the level in the blood. Rocephin is commonly given IV in TBI patients. Other familiar IV choices include: Claforan, doxycycline, Zithromax, vancomycin, Flagyl, Diflucan, tigecycline, and immunoglobulin.

Consider IV antibiotic administration in those TBI patients who are:

Very sick

Chronically ill

Presenting with significant neuropsychiatric symptoms

Having GI or other problems which limit oral options

PEARL: IV administration can be more effective than other treatment modalities. Each HCP has his own way to determine when to use IV medicine. One prefers to start all significantly ill patients on IV antibiotics if they can handle the cost and inconvenience. Others prefer to use orals for a few months to assess patient response and then try IM or IV routes. Another camp advocates hitting very sick patients hard with a blast of IV antibiotics before the pathogens have a chance to hide or encyst. By flooding them with as much of an IV dose as they can tolerate, these HCPs believe the patient has the best chance for recovery. With this method, you must be wary of an incapacitating Herx reaction. So in the severely ill, there is the IV, then IM, then oral school and the oral, then IM, then IV school. Target the treatment modalities to the individual case. Take into consideration both the clinical and social factors and make your decision based on what would help that particular patient. Your opinion may change as circumstances change.

2. **Intramuscular (IM):** Medicine is inserted into the skeletal muscle either through a needle attached to a syringe or through a pellet embedded in the muscle.

Pros: IM tends to be a more effective modality than oral administration. IM probably allows for the most constant **steady state** levels since drug is essentially held in a depot in the muscle and effuses out into the circulation from muscle at a fairly consistent rate. IM also eliminates most compliance issues that come from taking multiple doses each day. For drugs like the PCNs that work best at consistent blood levels, frequent dosing throughout the day is recommended. A skipped dose can have significant implications. IM eliminates this potential problem.

IM may be a good choice in patients who have been sick a long time, where you are looking for a steady blood level to penetrate the hard to reach tissues. IM injections can be given at home by caretakers, home health nurses, in the HCP's office, or by self-administration. Bicillin is a common IM drug for Lyme patients. Patients tend to adapt to the IM schedule and experienced patients know there is a good risk/benefit ratio in many cases. Rocephin and B vitamins are also familiar IM candidates.

There may be less yeast and diarrhea since you are not washing the GI tract with antibiotic in the same way as you would with oral preps.

IM dosing can be cost effective, especially if the family or patient learns to administer the drug themselves.

Cons: IM injections can hurt – a lot. Patients tend to perceive the needle as huge. Once injected, the site can have a firm drug repository area and remain sore. Diffusion of the medicine is limited by the area of absorbing capillaries and drug solubility. You can try a topical anesthetic, but the needle stick for local Lidocaine would be about the same as the needle stick for the IM injection since the Lidocaine will not likely be all the places the medicine will eventually penetrate. Although the needle is perceived as the problem, the pain actually comes from the physical distribution of the medicine into the tissue. In the case of IM injections, EMLA would only mute the surface discomfort and not the residual muscle pain.

PEARL: Chapter 24: Antimicrobials contains detailed advice on ways to minimize the discomfort of IM injections.

When giving an IM injection, aspirate before injection to avoid inadvertent IV administration. If blood appears in the syringe, you could be in a vein, so reposition.

IM injections are NOT reversible. Once you put it in, you can't suck it back out. Make sure the patient is not allergic to the prep before injecting.

TBI implications: IM Bicillin is a common treatment method used in Lyme patients. Some HCPs introduce IM dosing early in the treatment strategy since it has the advantage of consistent blood and tissue levels and superb compliance. With other antibiotics, dosing may need to occur 3 or 4 times a day to achieve the same steady blood levels. In those cases, a missed dose could have significant clinical implications. IM injections are often considered in chronic patients who have been sick a long time or those who are severely ill. Since so many TBIs have GI symptoms, injections into the muscle might also be considered for those who cannot tolerate oral administration.

PEARL: When antibiotics or other medications need to be delivered by continuous infusion either IM, IV, or SQ, consider an elastomeric infusion system. This collapsible elastic-bag technology allows for more precise drug administration and enables the patient to be mobile and not bound by at-home delivery systems. Administration rates can be adjusted. Anecdotally, many patients speak highly of their experience with this device.

3. **Oral (po)**: Tablets, capsules, chewables, pills, sprinkles, suspensions, drops, fizzies, syrups, nectars, gummies, troches (pronounced tr-OH-key and NOT tr-OH-shay), lollipops, edible gels, and foams are all going into our mouths in the hope of getting medicine into our blood.

Oral administration is the most common order on drug prescriptions and we usually expect to "take a pill" when we come out of the doctor's office. The term **parenteral** refers to any means of drug administration that is NOT oral.

The PDR is filled with oral drugs that have the initials XR, ER, DR, or CR (proclaiming extended release, delayed release, or continuous release formulations). Usually these are just marketing gimmicks to extend patent life or to allow the companies to use the word "new" in their ads for another 6 months. Know that they are there and that they have something to do with

how the drug is released into the body and make prudent decisions based on this knowledge.

Pros: Orals are easy, convenient, reasonable to store, and they don't come with any sharp edges. When taken as directed, effective blood levels can be achieved and maintained. If something bad happens, like an allergic reaction, the medicine can be stopped and you only need to deal with the amount already present in the system. In emergencies, a nasogastric tube can remove the stomach contents precluding all but the most immediate absorption.

Cons: Have you ever tasted clarithromycin suspension? Never order for a child what you would not take yourself even if two caring adults held you down and begged you to swallow. You might get the first dose in, but I have yet to see a kid take the second dose. Of course, some of the liquid preps taste great and kids will ask specifically for the pink stuff or the one that tastes like bubble gum.

Absorption after oral administration is variable and often incomplete and differs from individual to individual. If not taken as directed (and sometimes even if directions are obsessively followed), blood levels can fluctuate in ways that may not be conducive to maintaining the tissue levels that you want. Levels can even be unpredictable within the same individual from dose to dose depending on many factors such as proximity to food, hydration, and underlying health. Remember that passing through the gut adds many complications to the simple premise of getting a drug from outside to inside. Keep an eye on the patient and notice how s/he is responding. You may have to adjust the dose to target the needs of the individual.

The good flora in the digestive tract can be wiped out by passing a strong, broad-spectrum antibiotic through the system. This allows for the imbalanced overgrowth of fungus, which can be difficult to handle thereafter. Discussions around the management of yeast infections are presented in Chapter 27: *Supportive Measures*.

Further, Clostridium *difficile* bacteria can cause severe diarrhea in those patients whose normal gut flora has been eliminated either by strong broad spectrum antimicrobials or by use of certain specific antibiotics such as clindamycin. Once the normal gut bacteria are gone, the C. *difficile* has no competition for local resources and it overgrows and takes over the gut, releasing a potent toxin. C. *diff* can lead to serious complications. Additional information on the identification and management of C. *difficile* is provided in subsequent chapters.

Oral medications can also directly cause GI upset. The most common symptoms include nausea, burning, poor appetite, vomiting, reflux, and burping. There may be residual metallic or other bad tastes. Some medicines are partially inactivated by stomach acid or are better absorbed with or without food.

To change the subject completely, patients tend to get quite unnerved when they notice undissolved capsules in their stool or the stool of their children. In these cases, I have been told that the medicine has leached out and it is just the capsule skin that remains, but I don't know if this is correct in all cases. I don't know if anyone knows if this is correct. If capsules appear in the stool:

a. If you are the caregiver, tell the prescribing HCP, (who probably won't know what to do either).

b. If you are the prescribing HCP, check the product label to see if there is any reference to this situation. If not, then you can try calling the company and asking for their recommendation. Unfortunately, most brand companies will waste your time trying to convince you that your patient did not have an ADR, and in many cases you will not be able to reach anyone at the generic companies. Your trusted, local pharmacist may have additional information.

c. If you have concerns that the formulation you have prescribed is not actually delivering the medicine to the patient, switch modalities.

What should you do if the patient vomits after taking a dose of medicine? If you actually see the medicine in the vomit, you can wait until the stomach settles and try to re-administer. Of course, here I am assuming that they are vomiting because of their underlying illness and not from a bad reaction to the medicine itself. If the patient vomits very soon after taking the drug, they can be assumed to not have absorbed much of the dose. Re-dose. However, if the vomiting occurs an hour or more after ingestion, assume that some of the dose was absorbed and wait until the next designated time to take the regularly scheduled dose.

Some oral preps need special storage such as refrigeration for many suspensions. This can be inconvenient when dealing with day care and school. We all manage somehow.

TBI implications: Oral medications are the most commonly prescribed formulations in TBI patients. Unless the targeted site of effect is in the GI tract, the oral preparations may take a while to get where it is needed. Several doses may be required. Remember that TBIs can significantly impact the GI tract. The drug must move though the walls of the alimentary canal to the sites where it is needed. During its travels, the molecule can encounter many barriers in the GI wall, nervous system, and capillaries, precisely the places where TBIs such as Lyme wreck havoc.

PEARL: Tid is NOT the same as every 8 hours, qid is not the same as every 6 hours, and bid is not the same as every 12 hours, although they can be. Make sure you understand this distinction. Usually when you take a drug 2, 3, or 4 times a day you take the medicine only while awake. That means a drug prescribed as tid would likely be taken when you got up and then at midday and then in the evening – for kids after school or before bed. This might mean taking one tablet in the morning, then 5 hours later another, and then 7 hours later the third. Or the medicine could be taken tid by taking it at each meal, which would be a separation of about 4 or 5 hours between doses. In contrast, every 8 hours means every 8 hours. This might mean waking the person up to give medicine. This concept is important when you are dosing say amoxicillin versus doxycycline. Amoxicillin should be given every 8 hours to maintain steady blood levels. In contrast, doxycycline works better with a higher blood level intermittently so it usually given bid or once a day. As a drug developer for many years, I know that many HCPs do not understand this concept, so follow the dosing instructions carefully.

4. **Subcutaneous (SC, sq, sub-Q)**: The drug is placed under the skin usually by a (hypodermic) needle where a small deposit of medicine is left for later dissolution. Sub-Q administration is rare in the drugs used to treat TBIs, but this section is supposed to be teaching you how to read a drug label and this modality appears in labels.

5. **Topicals**: Topical administration involves placing the medicine either on the site where we hope to see action or on the skin or mucous membranes in the hopes of absorption. I will over-generalize a bit here so that I can fit essentially every drug administration technique into this one last category. Topicals can range from the swish and spits used for oral fungus to the suppositories placed in the vagina or rectum to introduce any number of drug compounds from antipyretics, to hormones, to steroids, to antifungals. Drops that we plink into eyes and ears are topicals. I guess we can include inhalants here such as vapors. They go onto the mucus membranes carrying a medicine in hopes of local or systemic effects. Patches can be considered a topical (I am the author and I will call it a topical if I choose.) Patches are a colossal pain to develop. Absorption is unbelievably inconsistent and often the

patches are huge. No one ever remembers when they were put on or when they need to be changed. Even writing the change date on the patch isn't fool proof. They don't stick to hair and the fact that they can macerate the underlying skin is especially problematic in young children and the elderly. Usually, the younger or older the skin, the more delicate and easily damaged the tissue. Either way you will be slathering a variety of topicals onto your wards and yourself for the rest of your natural life.

TBI implications: One of the primary target organs of TBIs is the skin. Onto the skin we smear all kinds of stuff. In the PDR there are innumerable references to creams, lotions, gels, and ointments. Many of these distinctions are frankly bogus but supported by reams of fine print as to which qualifies as what. I have wasted years of my life arguing over subtle grades of petroleum jelly. (By the way, many high-priced goos in the pharmacy are just fluffy Vaseline. Read the ingredient list.)

In general, the oilier the formulation the more moisture will be kept on either side of the barrier. If the skin was already moist the water will stay put. If already dry, no water will be coming into the skin until the oil dissipates. Decide what you want your vehicle to do and then select a preparation that does just that. Also, note that whenever the skin is inflamed or compromised in any way, absorption of any active ingredient into the systemic blood supply is enhanced. The different formulations are just a variety of vehicles used either for their own therapeutic properties or as a carrier for **active pharmaceutical ingredients** (API or drug). Here is a little refresher to help you split those hairs:

Lotion – Lotion has a light, flowing consistency and is less thick than a cream. With a low to medium viscosity (thickness), lotion can spread more thinly than other formulations. This allows more surface area to be covered with the topical medication. The patient may be able to cover more area with the same amount of lotion, which might be more economical. Lotions are mixtures of oil and water and are good for scalp and skin folds and getting into crevices. Most medicated shampoos are lotions. If the instructions say shake before use, then shake before use. Otherwise, you will get one layer of the preparation and not the other and what you want may be in the part you don't get.

Cream – Creams absorb faster than an ointment but slower than a lotion. About half oil and half water, creams don't flow. They are appreciated for not being as greasy as an ointment, but are usually more protective than a lotion.

Ointment – Made of about 80% oil and 20% water, ointments stay on the skin longer than a cream or lotion. If there are active ingredients in the ointment, they often take longer to be absorbed. Ointments are viscous, semi-solids that are often referred to as greasy. They can be used by themselves as a treatment for dry skin, since they effectively keep moisture in contact with skin, or as an occlusive dressing. However, they can also be used to deliver API, either as a treatment or as a prophylactic. Many runners and surfers use ointments to keep their skin from chaffing. They are considered a good choice to moisturize dry skin. Note that moisture has to be present on the skin BEFORE the ointment is used so that the moisture is kept in place. Otherwise the ointment will just be sitting on dry surface. By itself this vehicle has very low risk of inducing hypersensitivity since it is an inert oil. Personally, I know of no one allergic to petroleum jelly. (For the six of you out there who are, no need to contact me. I surrender. I know you exist.) Many don't like the greasy feel of ointments. I recall a business development meeting with a company putting a hormone into an ointment and telling us how user friendly the formulation was. In the meantime, the stuff was so greasy it was like putting testosterone in salad dressing. By the end of the meeting the small samples we tried on our hands had ruined one guy's shirt and I messed up three pens trying to take notes. The grease was everywhere and the cleaning crews spent days removing it from the wooden table, pushing it around and around like a never-ending dose of Pledge. That product's development didn't make it out of the meeting room. But sometimes, ointment is exactly what you need when the skin needs a barricade, such as when its own barrier has been compromised.

Gel – Unlike most of the previous examples, gels are usually a mixture of oil and **alcohol.** With a high viscosity, they often melt at normal body temperatures. These vehicles tend to be *drying* because of the alcohol component and they can sting if they contact broken skin. Because of the alcohol and other additives, they may predispose to hypersensitivity reactions. Gels may be a good choice when you are treating fungus since they can be drying and fungi like it nice and moist.

Foam – Air pushed through any of the above vehicles creates a foam. Currently, prescription foams are used to deliver steroids and a few other compounds but most are runny, with high alcohol contents. Medline makes a superlative, mild, skin cleanser foam.

Powder – Powder is a carrier that can be sprinkled on skin or hair or that can be inhaled (as in cocaine). Often used as a drying agent, powder is a good vehicle for antifungals since fungus does not like dry environments.

Paste – A paste is a combination of oil, water, and powder; essentially an ointment with powder added. The compounding pharmacists at A.I. DuPont Children's Hospital in Wilmington, where I had privileges before I became consumed by this book, made the best "Butt Paste" on the planet.

PEARL: Steroids in any of these vehicles can readily be absorbed into the general circulation. You can get a nice dose before you realize what is happening. Skin that has had steroid pass through is often shiny and thin and the vessels are readily apparent beneath the surface.

I. **Duration:** How long should the medicine be taken? With TBIs, duration of treatment is often a point of contention. Remember, the drug label includes the duration specified in the clinical trials used to get approval for a specific indication. That indication is probably *not* the same as the one you are currently addressing. In most cases, you will need to determine the appropriate length of treatment based on the patient response and what you know about the probable underlying pathogen. When discussing the treatment options in the following chapters, I often do not specify a time course. One reference will say treat for 16 days and I will have no idea where they got that number. Another source will counter by saying to treat for 5 to 7 days, again with no substantiation. The product label will be useful in giving a ball park duration for the indication listed. You will have to use clinical judgment in a way that makes sense for the patient. Chapter 11: *Controversies around Lyme* reviews at length the options around the duration of Lyme treatment.

PEARL: The medical literature is all over the place. One common-sense rule is to stop treating infections when the patient stops being sick <u>plus</u> a cushion. The cushion often suggested for Lyme is at least 2 months, preferably 3, after all sxs subside. If symptoms recur, restart treatment.

J. **Contraindications:** Simply put, contraindications are all the reasons an individual should not use the specific drug. In other words, use of this medicine under certain listed conditions or circumstances may pose a particular risk. In all cases, the drug should not be used if the patient is allergic to any of the ingredients. Immunosuppressants should not be used in people with sepsis. Alcohol should not be consumed while taking certain drugs such as some cephalosporins and tetracyclines. Saccharomyces probiotics are contraindicated if you are taking Nystatin.

Aspirin is contraindicated in small kids because of the risk of Reye's syndrome. Many drugs are contraindicated in pregnancy, etc. If a drug is contraindicated in your patient, try to think of alternatives. If you decide to use the drug despite a contraindication, document your rationale. Sometimes there are few choices for a hard-to-treat patient. Analyze the risk/benefit.

K. **Warnings**: A black box warning, named after the black border that appears around the words, is the strongest message that the FDA sends in a label. The intention is to alert consumers that something very bad, even life threatening, can occur while taking this medicine. Examples include the black box warning on antidepressants alerting about the possibility of increased suicidal tendencies in children and teens. Or the possibility of tendon rupture in patients taking fluoroquinolones. Some of these warnings may be useful. Others are silly like the warning on antifungal diaper rash cream against drug resistance when there is no evidence to support such a claim and the active ingredient is available OTC. One specific case I inherited was a black box warning on an anti-alcoholism drug that was issued because the company missed a deadline in turning in some documents (before I got there). While I admit that the company was playing passive-aggressive with the FDA and deserved some disciplinary action, the black box warning made no medical sense. The warning involved the potential for liver damage in intractable alcoholics using the treatment. All the patients had pre-existing liver damage that only improved when they stopped drinking. Yet one more case where politics and juvenile behavior, on both sides, may have contributed to a warning that did more harm than good to patients. These types of overblown caveats just diminish the effect of valid black box warnings.

L. **Precautions/Cautions:** This section involves forewarnings regarding what you should know before you put a patient on the drug. Typical "cautions" include: the need for good liver and kidney function prior to drug use, or no significant mental health issues present before starting therapy, or a negative pregnancy test documented prior to initiating the first dose, or the need to avoid the sun after starting the medicine. Precautions are more a recommendation regarding vigilance than a desire to keep the drug from being used.

M. **Overdosage:** Sometimes the company will provide advice on how to handle an overdose, including antidotes, but usually they advise you to call Poison Control. Poor Poison Control! The staff is supposed to know things that the manufacturer professes not to know. Actually Poison Control knows a lot and they may have access to information from the MSDS for the active ingredient or know more about the type of molecule that was ingested.

Poison Control almost always gives helpful advice. You may want to keep the local number handy and not rely on the product label in case there is an accidental or intentional over-usage. Check your area, but 1-800-222-1222 usually gets you a knowledgeable person.

N. **How supplied:** The ways the product is available to the consumer are listed such as 250 and 500 mg tablets or gel in 4 and 12 gram tubes.

O. **Adverse events**: (AEs, side effects, adverse drug reactions, ADRs) Adverse events are (bad) experiences that happen after taking a drug. Taking any medicine will in some way alter the body chemistry. This change will result in multiple effects. I know of no drug in any class that is capable of doing just one thing. Usually the good things we call efficacy and the bad things (or surprises) we call side effects. For regulatory and legal reasons, these terms have been changed, redefined, reformulated, parsed, dissected, and debated for years.

In my humble opinion, the AE section of the label is the most misunderstood. There are armies of people at drug companies working daily to determine if something bad happened or not and if it did, was the drug at fault? Since one man's poison is another's pleasure, the splitting of hairs here is phenomenal (as is the number of clichés I can incorporate into one sentence).

There are volumes of government guidelines on how to make these decisions. The process changes frequently and not always for the better. Regulations do not have to make medical sense. That is why essentially every drug known to humankind has as its top AEs headaches, URIs, and GI complaints. The way the information is gathered, forcing clinical study participants to report every hiccup throughout the course of the trial, skews the data collection. Humans do get headaches, colds, and GI symptoms with some regularity in everyday life. When they occur during a drug study they are "collected" and if the numbers go over a certain percentage of patients they are included in the label as though they are "caused" by the drug. There are huge data bases and dictionaries that have been developed just for these purposes.

AE data can be influenced by the time of year when the study was done. If conducted during cold and flu season, essentially every patient will complain of a URI during the course of the study. If conducted in allergy season, a high percentage of study subjects will complain of allergies and the event will get "labeled." Do I believe that the eye drops I saw advertised on TV today really caused the sinusitis mentioned in the AE statement? Or is it more likely that some patients had sinus problems when they happened to be in a drug study.

While I am all in favor of not missing real problems caused by drugs, I get frustrated when the AE section in the label will not allow you to see the forest for the trees. You are so busy sorting through colds and hay fever and heartburn that you can't see that the liver is getting fried in the background. Usually the true safety profile for a drug does not emerge until it has been on the market for a while and used by the general population under real world conditions.

Just because a label says an AE occurs in a percentage of patients taking the drug does not mean that your patient will experience that event. Likewise, just because no one *ever* reported a certain event in association with a particular drug does not mean it cannot be associated with that drug in a particular patient. Anything is possible. Look at what is happening in the patient and weigh the good against the bad in terms of side effects. Look at the risk/ benefit before starting, changing, or stopping a drug.

When discussing each TBI-pertinent medication below, I will be selective in the AEs I mention. Almost every drug has listed as its most common adverse events: headache, nausea, upper respiratory infection, vomiting, and dizziness. That is how the data collection system on side effects works. That does not mean that every drug *causes* these five adverse events. Almost every antibiotic has diarrhea and overgrowth of fungus listed. That is because most antibiotics at therapeutic doses will cause some diarrhea and fungal overgrowth. I will only mention these types of events again IF that particular medication is especially noted for an association with this common occurrence.

The most important point for us is capturing the unique problems that are frequently seen with some drug classes or individual products. For example, the tetracyclines (TCNs) are known to cause photosensitivity and discoloration of kids' teeth. But sometimes you might REALLY need a TCN, so then you will want to pick one of that class that is less likely to cause those problems.

Note that just because a side effect or adverse event is *not* listed in the label does *not* mean it isn't happening right now in your patient. There is a first time for everything. I love it when an HCP looks in the label to see if the drug can cause a certain effect, as though its listing grants special permission for the drug to be the reason for an event. Does that mean if it is not listed, the event could not have been caused by the drug? I think not. I have had patients almost brag, "My doctor says my bunion is from the medicine I'm taking." What happened there, I bet, is that the clinical studies were run over a long time in a patient population that is prone to bunions. The bunions were "captured" in the data base. The drug may not have had a thing to do with this person's bunions. A little knowledge can be a dangerous thing.

The bottom line is that any drug can probably be *associated* with any event if given to enough people over a long enough time, whether it is the *"cause"* of the event or not. The AE list is not magic, authorizing some events and disregarding others. Unfortunately, some people think that if a symptom is not listed there, you can't possibly be experiencing it. The AE portion of the label is just a record compiled under numerous artificial premises where the manufacturer is trying everything imaginable to keep items off the list and the FDA is trying to include every tidbit possible.

I get scared when people who should know better read the label on their medicine and say things like "It says here I'm going to get high blood pressure from taking this." Yes, and I could become a Dallas Cowboy cheerleader. Anything is possible, just not necessarily probable. Even if 90% of the patients taking a certain drug turn green from its effects, that doesn't mean the patient in front of you will automatically turn green. Could happen. Prepare them, just don't scare them unduly. Is the potential benefit of this medication worth turning green over? Just might be. This is part of the risk/benefit analysis conducted in collaboration with the HCPs, patient, and caretakers.

When trying to determine whether your patient is experiencing an adverse drug reaction, use common-sense. The information in the label is population data, based on what was collected from a very select group. Your patient may or may not fit. Use the information as a framework, not as a holy writ. When a doctor pulls out a great big book like the PDR, everyone including the doctor seems to think that conveys some kind of extra wisdom. Remember the PDR is a commercial enterprise and companies pay to have their drugs listed.

Just because an event was found in association with the use of a drug, does not mean that the drug caused the event. When assessing a patient to determine if an event is related to taking a particular medicine, use the following analytic path:

Logic steps used in causal assessment:

1. Timing – If Event A occurs AFTER Event B, then Event A could not have caused Event B. So if a patient has low potassium before taking a drug, then the drug did not cause the low potassium. If your thumb is red and swollen BEFORE it is hit by a hammer, the hammer did not cause the initial symptoms. That is not to say that the drug can't later contribute to the low potassium or that the hammer hit did not increase the pain in the thumb. To cause something to happen, the causal agent must be in place before the impact. For A to cause B, A has to be in place before B, not after.

You can't have an allergic reaction to PCN before you take it.

2. Bioplausibility – Could this event even happen or does it defy the laws of science? An antibody against antigen A will not bind with antigen B. Just won't happen. Can't. Implausible. But don't be fooled. Just because you don't understand a scientific concept does not mean it is outside the realm of possibility. Make sure it is actually implausible before you discredit the idea. The problem could be your lack of insight.

3. Challenge/Rechallenge – This is the best way to assess causality. If A causes B and you take A away and then B goes away, that's strong support for causality. If you reintroduce A and then B reappears, you nailed it. It's pretty hard to talk your way out of that one.

4. Confounders – What could be confusing this picture? Remember the workers I studied in Mexico City with the high RBC counts. There were many confounders clouding that clinical picture.

5. Consistency with what's expected for drug and class or population – Every person who has gone to medical school has heard the adage, "If it walks like a duck and quacks like a duck, it's probably a duck." Drugs in the same class tend to act similarly. Further, if it's done it before, it could do it again. The best predictor of future behavior is past behavior. If Rocephin has been known to cause gallstones in some patients, and your patient on Rocephin develops gallstones, consider that it might be the Rocephin. Further, when looking at population data, consider looking at what you observed versus what you would expect to happen in a matching population. If the two people out of 100 in a defined population who experience high blood sugars are compared to a matching group taking a specific medicine, where 12 people out of a 100 have high blood sugars, maybe something is going on. Now you'd need some fancy statistical testing to tell if this finding is significant or coincidental, but you get the idea.

6. No better explanation – If you've looked and looked and thought and thought and brainstormed all kinds of alternatives and still can't find another explanation for an adverse event, it just might be the drug.

If after careful consideration, you believe that your patient is experiencing a side effect from a drug, what should you do?

1. Has the patient been taking the medicine as directed? If they haven't been taking the drug at all, it's going to be hard to pin an AE on drug use. Unfortunately,

patients fib mightily when it comes to compliance questions. They don't want you to get mad at them so they say they take their medicine when they most certainly do not, at least not regularly. Emphasize that this time they really must tell you the truth so that you can help make the right decision about their treatment.

2. Have they been doing better, worse, or the same on treatment?

3. Is the AE tolerable or intolerable? There is a big difference between a mild dry mouth and Stevens-Johnson syndrome.

4. Weigh the risk/benefit of continuing the drug versus stopping or adjusting the regimen.

5. Is the effect an allergic reaction or some other kind of AE?

6. Consider challenge/rechallenge. This means taking the patient off the drug to see if the problem resolves. Then, if reasonable, consider trying the drug again. Do not rechallenge if that would put the patient at serious risk.

7. Consider alternatives. Be careful when switching antibiotics since some have overlapping allergies like PCNs and cephalosporins. Be careful not to jump from the frying pan into the fire.

8. Make a decision in the best interest of the patient.

Some adverse event concepts come up again and again in labels. I will review these here and then only list the exceptional concerns when reviewing the individual drugs in the next chapters.

- Allergies: An allergic reaction is possible after taking ANY medicine. The most common signs and symptoms of an allergic reaction include: swelling of the face or throat, shortness of breath, problems swallowing, itching, anxiety, and rashes including redness, flushing, splotches, and hives. Allergic reactions can be fatal. If an allergic reaction is suspected, seek medical advice immediately.

- Prolonged QT intervals: A number of drugs have the potential of prolonging the QT interval on the EKG. If the interval gets longer and longer, this situation can translate into problems with heart rhythm. I talk often in the individual drug sections about getting EKGs to monitor for prolongation of QTc as though interpretation were so simple. From experience with 100s of QT measurements, I know this is extremely difficult

with variations between readers and even within the readings of one reader. If you are dealing with a drug known to prolong the QT or a patient predisposed to prolongation, find an EXPERIENCED expert for consultation. A few points on interpretation:

i. QTc is the QT corrected for heart rate

ii. Measure the lead that has the best T wave (V2 or V5)

iii. Measure from the start of the Q to the end of the T

iv. The slower the pulse the longer the QT

v. QTc equals the QT/the square root of the RR interval

vi. Normals: female adults less than 450 ms and male adults less that 470 ms

vii. To mitigate the risk of prolonged QT keep the potassium above 4 and the magnesium above 2 and avoid low calcium

- Impact of cytochrome P450: Often there is a section in the label that talks about drug interactions. HCPs are cautioned that one drug should not be used with another class of drug because of potential "interactions." The majority of drugs are metabolized in the liver, mostly by a series of enzymes in the cytochrome P450 system. There are many sub-categories of these enzymes and a person can spend an entire career just sorting these reactions. The bottom line is that if every drug is competing for the same enzyme path in order to get metabolized, someone is going to get left behind, at least for a while. Those that have to wait can accumulate in the blood and have higher than desired blood levels. Sometimes this can be meaningless, but in other cases high levels can lead to AEs or even toxicity. Grapefruit juice can do the same thing, competing for the same metabolic pathways as some drugs. Do you know how many hours people at drug companies and the FDA spend arguing over grapefruit juice? I recently saw a TV ad where one company says their drug is better than another drug because theirs can be taken with juice. My first reaction is that it's a sad day when the only thing better about your drug is that it can be taken with juice. (The only reason your drug doesn't have that restriction in its label is that you probably failed to make the connection in your PD study and no one caught it.) Be careful and look for signs that you may have more drug circulating than you intended. Be ready to adjust doses or change drugs.

- C. *difficile* and pseudomembranous colitis: Just about every antibiotic can cause a disruption of the normal balance of flora in the gut. Antibiotics cannot tell a good bacteria from a bad bacteria and they tend to wipe out the whole lot of them indiscriminately. Normal flora is essential to good digestion and once things become imbalanced there will begin to be absorption problems and diarrhea. Except for Clostridium *difficile,* which resists most antibiotics. As its neighbors are getting wiped out, C. *diff* is taking over the world. The problem with that scenario is that C. *difficile* produces a powerful toxin that can cause severe symptoms including: diarrhea, abdominal pain, fever, and mucus and blood in the stool. This can progress to pseudomembranous colitis where there is a false membrane on the lining of the intestine and symptoms can become severe and even fatal. Problems with C. *difficile* may start during treatment or not for weeks after the medicine has been discontinued. If symptoms appear, consider cultures and assaying the stool for toxin. Discontinue the suspect antibiotic immediately and treat with metronidazole (Flagyl) or with vancomycin po 125 to 500 q 6 for 10 days. Do NOT give drugs such as Lomotil that slow down the motion of the GI tract in order to stop the diarrhea. This type of diarrhea is caused by a toxin made by the C. *difficile.* You want that toxin OUT of you. If you give Lomotil, you will usually find that Lomotil works. It will stop the diarrhea but that means the toxin is now trapped inside. As soon as the Lomotil wears off you will learn a whole new meaning of the word diarrhea. The best course of action is to stop the causative antibiotic and treat with antimicrobials that will obliterate the C. *difficile.* Once the C. *diff* is gone, it won't be producing toxins that are responsible for the symptoms anymore. Don't forget that there was a reason that the patient was on the antibiotic in the first place. Don't let the underlying TBI run wild now. Reassess and consider alternative treatments.

- Stevens-Johnson syndrome (SJS) and toxic epidermal necrolysis (TEN): Allergic reactions to drugs can occur along a continuum from mild itching and hives to anaphylaxis. Two manifestations along this spectrum are SJS and TEN. Stevens-Johnson syndrome is a medical emergency even though the insurance company will tell you that it is not and that you are perfectly capable of handling it in your office. Trust me, these patients will try to die while you are on the phone spelling the word to the insurance reviewer. Call the ambulance before you call the insurance company. Symptoms include rashes and lesions on the mucous membranes and conjunctiva. There may be swelling. Skin loss can be severe leading to secondary infection and dehydration. They can look like severe burn patients. My last patient with SJS had sheets of skin sloughing off as though he had been flayed. And TEN is considered the more severe form of SJS. Both of these conditions have been called severe forms of erythema multiforme which in SJS appears to be every skin lesion imaginable appearing at the same moment. Some lesions are transient and others hang around a little longer: macules, papules, wheals, vesicles, bulla, appearing on extremities, trunk, face, and even the palms and soles. Some display in targets and rings. About 95% of the patients diagnosed with SJS or TEN have been taking medications. Who are the other 5%?

PEARL: In every large clinical study I worked on there were a few SJS and TEN patients. Not a lot, only a few and always about the same proportion. I never knew if this was the number of people that would have developed these syndromes anyway or if it was drug-related. I always investigated these cases thoroughly. In my experience these were a subpopulation who often had a long list of drug allergies on their chart and other allergies as well. Was it the drug or the patient? Who knows?

- Fungal overgrowth: Just as the intestinal flora can become imbalanced with use of antibiotics, yeast can overgrow as well. As bacteria are removed from the competitive environment, yeast are happy to take more than their share of the space. Overgrowth of yeast in a patient on antibiotics is most often due to Candida *albicans,* but other species can be involved. These can then cause signs and symptoms in the mouth (thrush), skin folds (intertrigo), genitals (vaginitis), and GI tract. Yeast are opportunistic, especially if the organisms that usually balance them are no longer there. If they find themselves in a warm, dark, moist place, with no competition, they will take advantage. They do enjoy themselves inside a wet diaper. They LOVE simple sugars and starches and are a chronic problem in many diabetic and overweight patients. In general, fungal overgrowth causes thick white discharge or curd-like specks in the affected area with circumscribed red patches. Often the affected areas ITCH. Once the area becomes inflamed then other symptoms of inflammation can occur such as swelling, heat, redness, and discomfort. These conditions are treated in a variety of ways. Chapter 25 includes these *Ancillary Treatments.*

- Interactions with OCPs: This is more of a precaution common to many antimicrobials than an actual AE. (I guess if you get pregnant, you might consider that an AE. In every drug company where I have worked, there would be colossal fights over whether a pregnancy during treatment was an adverse event or a blessed event. This example illustrates the difficulty surrounding AE classification.) The possibility of antibiotics interfering with birth control used to be considered a major problem. These days it does not seem to be as much of a concern. In cases where "Attention must be paid,"[1] the possibility of interaction is noted in the individual drug sections.

- Drug resistance: Resistance is the variety of mechanisms used by pathogens to avoid destruction. The pathogen wants to invade, multiply, and metabolize which may include making products toxic to the host. They want to ensure their own survival and that of their progeny. Further, they want to be left alone while they do this. In contrast, the body wants to get rid of them and will use a number of ways to do this. Antibiotics are one means to help the body get rid of pathogens and the method we are concerned with here.

For their part, the pathogens have evolved many ways to minimize the effect of antibiotics. These include rapid mutation so that the antibiotic no longer has the same target. They can change surface proteins and encyst and hide in tissue that is less penetrable to antibiotics. Sometimes the pathogens take quite a while to develop resistance to antibiotics like PCNs and TCNs. Other antimicrobials like Rifampin can have resistance develop within days or even hours. For those antibiotics that are likely to have a pathogen become quickly resistant to them, always combine these drugs with a back-up antibiotic. For example, never use rifamycin alone. Within a few doses you will have a drug on board that can't do anything. If a second antibiotic is present, it can hit the pathogen and allow the first antibiotic on-going access where it might have been completely shut out without help. That is one of the beauties of combination therapy.

PEARL: Most pathogens develop resistance to rifamycin within days or even hours. But we humans have a few tricks up our sleeves as well. NEVER pulse or interrupt a course of rifamycin. Pulsing increases the chance of mutant organisms starting a resistant population. And ALWAYS use rifamycin in combination with other antimicrobials. This way those microbes resistant to the rifamycin will be picked off by the back-up antibiotic. Many pathogens have developed a resistance to TCN, but doxycycline isn't so vulnerable and there is not so much resistance against that drug. The reason for using doxycycline in combination is not resistance but the desire to hit the multiple life forms of Bb, which doxy cannot do alone.

There are two kinds of resistance around antibiotics. The kind that develops in an individual due to the action of the infecting microbe and the kind that develops

in the population over time. For example, exposing cattle to large doses of broad spectrum antibiotics for commercial purposes allows for many pathogens to develop resistance to entire classes of drugs. This happened to TCN. This is also likely one contributor to the current MRSA pandemic in the US.

In hospitals, gorilla-cillins were used to treat everything, until the pathogens got wise. If there are millions of pathogens, most will be wiped out by an appropriate antibiotic or by the host's immune system. A few may be able to mutate in time to save themselves. Others may have already had the random mutation in place that was needed for their survival. Only a few surviving microbes are needed to quickly make a whole new generation of pathogens. These organisms were already selected to survive because they resisted the antibiotic that killed all their kin. They and their progeny are not susceptible to the antibiotic that wiped out everyone else. So, if you treat the surviving Staph with the drug methicillin again, the microbes scoff. You will have to use something else to hit them. Unfortunately, the list of "something else" becomes shorter and shorter. And the gorilla in the gorilla-cillin needs to get bigger and broader all the time to hit the pathogens that were naturally selected to survive. (One local Delaware politician said she would only believe in evolution if she saw it with her own eyes. Antimicrobial resistance through genetic mutation is happening every day right before our eyes.) When my mom got MRSA during her many hospital stays, she then passed it along. As more and more people get infected with this strain, the *population* now has what was originally an *individual* problem.

PEARL: How do you decide whether to protect the population at the expense of the individual or to protect the individual at the expense of the population? Most of us chose to protect the individual when our kid is sick and the population when someone else's kid is sick.

PEARL: Rhen suggests that H. pylori *and Mycobacterium* tuberculosis *establish persistent infections despite active immune defenses because they have evolved strategies to overcome the host defenses. While defenses can vary with anatomical location, these pathogens appear to have found ways to manipulate the host's response. These and other pathogens likely use multiple strategies to establish persistence. Persistence may be a phase in the natural history of some microbes. Therefore, effective resistance can result in persistence. Chapter 10:* Borreliosis *reviews the survival techniques used by Bb that allow it to persist causing relapses and chronic illness. Once you see how much medical sense this makes, you will understand the on-going infection explanation for LD.*

---

1 *Willie Loman's wife in Death of a Salesman by Arthur Miller*

The more exposure a pathogen gets to an antibiotic, the more chance it has to mutate and build resistance. Very recently, I worked on the development of a drug for otitis media in kids. The "authorities" came out with new guidelines, saying their old recommendations were wrong. (Wouldn't it be nice to have other incorrect authorities follow in their footsteps?) One of the reasons so much resistance grew in the pathogens that cause otitis media in kids was that we were using the right drug at the wrong dose. We were using doses way too low to matter. All low-dose Amoxil was doing was giving the natural selection process described above plenty of time to work. When parents came in saying that the pink stuff didn't work, being caring physicians we pulled out a bigger gun, which over time also allowed resistance to develop against its efforts.

We created our own problem. If we had used the appropriate dose in the first place we might not be in this current resistance nightmare with antibiotics in general. We must be careful we don't do the same thing with antibiotics in Lyme disease. "Authorities" have HCPs so scared of using appropriate doses that match the pharmacokinetics of the drug, that they give doses that are so low they are almost guaranteed to be ineffective and prompt resistant strains. Low doses will not allow the drug to be successful and will just provide the Bb time to hide and mutate. "Authorities" will then say that no treatment is needed in these patients because they had their chance to get well and they elected not to take it. Simply put, treatment with incorrect antibiotics, at inadequate doses, for too short a time is more likely to cause resistance than doing things properly in the first place.

PEARL: Ways to minimize the effects of antimicrobial resistance:

- *Don't use antibiotics. (This would only resolve the problem of mutated resistant strains, but not all the other mechanisms of resistance that would still enable pathogens to evade the immune response. Besides, this is not an especially realistic scenario in contemporary western medicine.)*

- *Don't treat at subtherapeutic doses. Some HCPs are afraid and they think they will get in less trouble if they treat at doses too low to do anything. Low doses are thought to cause more resistance than appropriate therapeutic doses.*

- *Antibiotics used for too short a duration may just cause the targeted bug to burrow until the offending antibiotic is gone and then resurge.*

- *Stop giving antibiotics for colds and URI viruses. (We all have done it.) This just allows the coexisting bacteria to evolve resistant forms.*

- *Stop the wholesale use of broad spectrum antibiotics in cattle, swine, and fowl, which then become resistance factories. Most of us have no control over this phenomenon. Be aware.*

- *Use combination drug regimens so that when one antibiotic is ineffective the pathogen will be hit by the back-up antibiotics.*

- *A continuous antibiotic regimen against Lyme is probably the most effective. This doesn't mean that the antimicrobials can't be changed and adjusted, as long as there is continuous antimicrobial coverage.*

PEARL: There are numerous mechanisms that pathogens use to resist both the immune system and the antimicrobials coming their way, including:

- *Decreased membrane permeability (so antibiotics can't penetrate)*

- *Mutation of ribosomal active sites*

- *Increase in metabolic enzymes (so that the body gets rid of antibiotics faster)*

- *Enzyme inactivation (so pro-drugs can't metabolize to active moieties)*

- *Mutations of surface proteins (so antibodies cannot recognize pathogens as non-self)*

- *Mutations at the key binding sites (this decreases the ability of the drug to bind and so decreases efficacy)*

- *Changing life forms to encysted, encapsulated, dormant, etcetera, (making it harder for the antibiotic to access)*

- *Hiding in tissues where blood flow and therefore antibiotic levels are low such as joints and extremities*

- *Lurking in tissues protected by barriers such as the BBB or placenta*

- *Changing non-self proteins to look like self proteins*

- *Transduction: A virus infecting a bacteria transfers DNA within its protein coat to the bacteria thereby protecting the bacteria by making it unrecognizable. Since the bacterial cell serves as the viral home, this mechanism protects the virus as well.*

- *Transformation: Incorporation of DNA from other sources into the bacteria that then serves to protect the pathogen*

- *Conjugation: Passing of genes from one cell to another for mutual benefit*

- *Efflux pumps which decease intracellular drug concentrations*

- *Plasma-mediated resistance genes producing proteins than bind certain enzymes (thereby protecting against the action of antibiotics)*

- *Likely many, as yet unrecognized, mechanisms*

Anyone so species-centric as to think that Homo *sapiens* are vastly superior to all other life forms, might want to ask why the microbes win so many battles. George Carlin,[2] famous scientist, said something to the effect that if our species is the best in the universe then the universe aimed rather low and settled for very little.

---

2 *George Carlin is not a famous scientist, but rather a recently deceased, irreverent comedian.*

Chapter 24

ANTIMICROBIALS

"...come celebrate with me that everyday something has tried to kill me and has failed."
Lucille Clifton

This text is called *Compendium of Tick-Borne-Disease*. Therefore, the treatments outlined will be those that the top TBI-focused practitioners have found useful in treating patients with tick-borne conditions. These methods are generally consistent with the ILADS Guidelines.

I. BACKGROUND

Antimicrobials are considered the foundation of TBI treatment and the key to success. I wish this part were as simple as one fly, one swatter. Unfortunately, selection of the appropriate antibiotic(s) will depend on a number of factors both obvious and obscure:

- The pathogen and any number of possible strains
- Potential co-infections
- Co-morbidities
- Allergies
- Tolerance of treatment regimen
- General health
- Stage of disease
- Previous treatment response
- Herx potential
- Age, gender, ethnicity.

All these confounders could play a part in treatment strategy. As with life, always be ready to regroup and move on with Plan B. In this chapter, the various antimicrobials pertinent to TBI patients will be described including their MOA, indications, usage, doses, distinctive AEs, caveats for use, and monitoring recommendations over the therapeutic course. Of course before we can move into that level of detail we will need to review several concepts.

The old fashioned **Gram stain** is still used to classify bacteria. Organisms are said to be either Gram positive or Gram negative depending on the color they retain after being exposed to an iodine solution. Why would you care? Because...antimicrobials are often selected for use based on their ability to affect either Gram positive or Gram negative organisms. In cases where the pathogen's reaction to Gram stain is known, you might want to choose an antibiotic able to hit that type of organism. The Bb that cause Lyme are, of course, equivocal on Gram stain.

A **bacteriostatic** antibiotic is one that inhibits the growth or reproduction of bacteria without killing them. They work by interfering with protein production, by impeding DNA or RNA replication, or by impairing some other metabolic process. To be effective these antibiotics must work with the immune system in order to decrease the bacterial load. The number of bacteria lessens over time because they cannot grow or reproduce. **Bacteriocidal** antibiotics actually kill the bacteria. These terms are not etched in granite and in some cases bacteriostatics will kill organisms and bacteriocidals will just muffle the population. Sometimes an antibiotic is –static at one dose and –cidal at a higher dose. These distinctions might be helpful in selecting drug combinations.

If humanly possible, get any blood tests for diagnostic purposes and cultures BEFORE you start the antibiotic. This can save you from tearing your hair out later when trying to figure out what is going on with the results. Further, baseline values will help determine if any abnormalities were pre-existing, due to the disease, or the result of an ADR. I know this is often not possible. With TBI patients, they may have been on several courses of treatment before they see you, so you may not have a choice but to draw labs after treatment has been initiated.

Some sources recommend taking peak and trough drug levels repeatedly to make sure the patient is getting appropriate blood concentrations to achieve maximum effect. As I mentioned in earlier chapters, except in special circumstances, I am not a fan. The results are too unreliable. Therapeutic drug levels are almost impossible to draw and interpret unless the patient is in a controlled setting. If you have had a patient hospitalized recently you will know it is even tricky to get useable drug levels in there.

My husband was recently an in-patient. They wanted to measure his coagulation parameters regularly after cardioversion as a baseline and then after doses of anticoagulant. However, they continued to take his blood before they gave him ANY anticoagulant. It is especially difficult to assess the blood level or the overall effect of a medicine you did not take. No amount of prompting to the staff changed this sad state of affairs. Even telling the attending, who promised to fix the oversight, did not help. The phlebotomist showed up again before the medicine nurse. Before the 4th worthless blood-letting, my husband signed himself out. (Lilith[1] works at this hospital.)

Nonetheless, if there are situations where you really believe the treatment regimen should have worked and it did not, you might want to draw blood levels to get a ball park estimate of whether you have an effective amount of medicine in the patient. Also if you are using a drug with the potential for severe toxicity, making sure you do not have dangerous levels may be prudent.

Some drugs work better at a steady state blood level, whereas others, like TCNs, work better with intermittent high peaks. Before you draw blood levels make sure you know if your therapeutic goal is an even, steady state level or a high peak/low trough blood level. You can better ensure steady levels by dosing more frequently. Of course, more frequent dosing raises the risks of more missed doses. To get higher peaks, give higher doses less frequently. Here there is a greater risk for AEs such as GI upset. Antimicrobial treatment for TBIs is often a balancing act. Where appropriate, recommendations for therapeutic blood levels are outlined in the individual drug sections below.

II. HOW TO CALCULATE THE DOSE

Dose calculation:

For those of you who calculate doses all day, I apologize. Caretakers or HCPs who do not use many antibiotics in their practice are often confused by these unfamiliar concepts. First of all, while we sometimes base dose on age, most often dosage is calculated by weight. Sometimes the manufacturers use both metric and English units in their dose recommendations, so you end up trying to figure out how many mgs to give a 20 pound child. Conversions may be necessary. Pay close attention to the instructions and be meticulous with the units. Remember when your college chemistry TA would mark your answer wrong if you forgot the units. Well, there was a reason for that.

When I first started work in the ER in 1984, I would calculate the dose so closely that I would have parents giving 5.4 cc of the pink stuff, which is just a tad more than a teaspoon. I later learned that no one would expire if I had ordered a simple teaspoon. Get close but don't be obsessive.

Make sure that when you read the dosing recommendations you are paying close attention to detail. Do not mix up grams with milligrams. Double check. The dose you get should

make sense. A 44 pound 6-year-old should not be getting 814 mg of Amoxil every 8 hours. Watch the decimal point. If a value is less than one it often has a zero in front of the decimal (0.1 or 0.44)

Let me provide an example from a call I received this morning.

"What would be the dose of amoxicillin for a 7-year-old child?"

"How much does the child weigh?"

"45 pounds"

(Thank you Dr. Schmuckler for teaching me "If..., then" math.)

If 2.2 pounds is 1 kg,

Then 45 pounds is (x) kg

Set up the equation to solve for (x). X will need to be bigger than 1 since the 45 pounds is bigger than the 2.2 pounds, so set the equation up so that it turns out that way.

X kg /1 kg x 45 lbs /2.2 lbs

This child weighs 20 kg

Since amoxicillin is dosed at 30 to 50 mg/kg/day, this child's dose would be calculated by setting up the proportion below.

If 40 mg is given for each 1 kg that the child weighs,

Then (x) mg would be given to a 20 kg child

(I picked 40 mg/kg/day because it is in the middle of the range.)

40 mg x 20 is 800 mg per day

So in a day this child gets 800 mg

Since amoxicillin is scheduled every 8 hours, we divide the 800 by 3.

800/3 is 266 mg at each of the three doses.

Amoxicillin suspension comes in several strengths. I think the 250 mg/5 ml would be well within the range for this child. So she would get 1 teaspoon (5 ml or 5 cc) every 8 hours. If you want to be a stickler for the 266 mg or if you want to go to 50 mg/kg/day then you could give 5.5 cc in the first case and 6.5 cc in the second. Here is where a medicine syringe comes in handy. But I think that life might be too short to split hairs that finely. Of course, if you select the 125 mg/5 ml formulation, then the child would get 2 teaspoons (10 ml or 10 cc) q 8 h.

---

1 See Glossary or Introduction for name origin

Underdosing poses the risk of the medicine not working, while overdosing might cause more GI problems and fungal overgrowth.

<u>Helpful conversion list:</u>

1 kilogram is 2.2 pounds

1 pound is 0.45 kg

One cc (cubic centimeter) equals 1 ml (milliliter)

One teaspoon equals 5 ml or 5 cc

One and a half teaspoon is 7.5 ml or 7.5 cc

Two teaspoons equals 10 ml or 10 cc

One milligram (mg) is .001 grams

1000 grams equals 1 kilogram (1 kg)

1000 mg equals 1 gram

III. HOW TO TAKE THE MEDICINE

A. Compliance – I am now shifting my focus and speaking to the patients reading this text. There are good reasons why you should take the full course of antibiotics as prescribed. If the prescription says 10 days, take it for 10 days. With that being said, I bet even Mother Teresa had a few bottles of half-taken antibiotics in her medicine cabinet at the ashram. The truth is, if you were given the antibiotic for a real bacterial infection, the symptoms might reappear if you stop too soon. If the medicine was ordered for what was actually a viral infection, that infection was going to run its course unaffected by the antibiotic either way. In this case, the antibiotic didn't do anything to help remove the pathogen, but probably did give you yeast and loose stool.

With TBIs, things are a little different. You might be taking antibiotics for weeks, months, or years. The important thing here is to tell your HCP the truth. I learned from studies at Tufts that patients do not want to disappoint their HCPs and so they say they take their medicine when they do not. Researchers have filmed clinical trial patients dumping their meds in a planter outside the doctor's office on their way from the parking lot. (In clinical trials, each pill is counted so the staff knows if you've been naughty or nice.) You have reasons for not taking the medicine. Maybe you couldn't tolerate the side effects. Maybe you didn't think the medicine was doing any good. Maybe you are just sick of taking medicine. That's all okay with me. We can work around all those issues. The important thing is to let the prescriber know. Some medicines should not be stopped abruptly and need to be weaned off instead. In other cases, you risk a whopping relapse. Please be honest about how you have been taking your medicine so that you and your HCP can make the best treatment decisions.

PEARL: My favorite uncle and I were visiting our small town neighbor in rehab for pneumonia. His name is Boo. He was doing a lot better and was happy to have visitors. His nurse came in while we were there and handed Boo his medicine cup and water to take his two pills. She smiled and left the room. As soon as she turned the corner, Boo tossed the medicine in the trash. He signaled us to keep quiet and we did.

B. Follow the directions – If the instructions say take with food, please take it with food. Some drugs are miserably absorbed in the first place, so give the medicine its best shot. Do not stop or restart any TBI medicine without checking with your HCP. Make sure your doctor knows all the meds you are on including OTCs, vitamins, herbals, and supplements. These are all chemicals going into the same body system and they can interact unfavorably. Teens may be especially reluctant to admit they are on birth control, antidepressants, or steroids. This information is critical to making good treatment decisions. Steroids, especially, can impede recovery in TBI patients.

PEARL: Tid means three times a day. That is not necessarily the same as every 8 hours. Every 8 hours means you take a pill and 8 hours later your take another pill (not 7, not 9, just 8). That means someone might have to set an alarm clock. Tid means that you take the drug 3 times during the day while you are awake. This can be done any number of ways. Depending on whether you need to take the drug with food or not: you can take a dose when you get up, midday, and evening. Conversely, you could take a dose at each meal. Here is where your friendly neighborhood pharmacist will know best. He will actually know why you are supposed to take the medicine in a specific way. When you pick up the medicine, ask.

Do not share medicine.

Do not stop or change medications without discussing with the prescribing HCP. The HCP may know more about what is going on with the medicines than you think. You never have to continue a medicine that you do not want, BUT some medicines cannot be safely stopped cold turkey and need to be weaned off. PLEASE give the HCP a chance to find an alternative.

C. Keep track - My mother took dozens of pills a day for her myriad problems. We would spend hours sorting them into those morning, noon, and night pill boxes. Interrupting someone while they were sorting was reason to incite violence. Heaven forbid that you mess up and have to start over. Even though she had several caretakers working on this and we had all been doing this for years, we still got confused. She was 80 and her medicine list was overwhelming.

Now, imagine being 8-years-old and not used to taking one medicine let alone several. Imagine feeling sick while adults tell you to eat, don't eat, sit up, lie down, drink more water, wait until we get you a fatty food, hold off ten more minutes before you swallow, no you can't have a snack until you have your medicine, wake up, take it all. …

Don't get medicine burn-out. Make a list, make a chart, get pill sorters, do whatever you need to make life as simple as possible. My son, a very compliant sort, after about 4 months got quite tired of counting drops and remembering to take one pill before he ate and one after and one during. Once he started feeling better he didn't see the point, but he did it and now he seems mostly recovered. He even had the best medicine list on the planet to help him. (I am so modest.) Don't let anyone kid you, keeping track can be tiresome, especially if one thing changes and that dominoes your entire schedule. So be creative and devise a system that works best for you. You may have to experiment with several tracking tools. Examples are provided below.

Make sure the day care staff and school nurse understand exactly when and how any medications need to be given. Write this down, legibly, and go over it verbally.

One HCP I know has patients on dozens of supplements in addition to prescription meds. To follow this regimen correctly is literally impossible. Personally, I take almost no medicines myself and prefer to be a minimalist. Give them what they need, in a dose that is safe and effective, and adjust as needed. While some people really are lacking Vitamin D, calcium, etcetera, do not overwhelm either their psyche or their lives with dozens of pills, drops, sprays, and lotions.

D. Sample medicine tracking sheet

Sample tracking forms follow. The first is a blank and the other is an adjusted version from a real case. Sometimes, my son's treatment regimen would change and we would have to adjust the entire tracking method. We experimented with multiple approaches before we found the approach that worked for us. Sometimes the tracking method that was perfect for one flare no longer fit with the treatment regimen of the next bout. At first we "jotted" the tracking sheets up by hand and later used the computer. Experiment until you find an organizing system that works for you. There is no one correct way.

In the blank form opposite, the medicine name and dose go at the top. Then note the time the dose is *due*. After the dose is administered, the *taken* box is checked. You will need to adjust this for the individual patient. For example, my mother ate dinner at 4 p.m. and then went to bed immediately afterward, so charts made for normal people did not work well for her. We adapted the chart for her particular case. A chart or checklist of some kind should be made to suit your patient's unique situation. There were times when we needed to tape together page extensions to account for short-term meds to be added to on-going treatments. Be flexible.

Caretakers may need help getting organized. One of the office staff might be an expert in this area and might have devised methods superior to the samples provided here.

Adopt whichever tracking method best suits you and your treatment regimen.

IV. GETTING THE MEDICINE IN

Most sick patients want to get well. They understand that the medicine is supposed to help them feel better. But some medicine really is like drinking metal. Do whatever possible to make the experience better. The drug store usually has flavor additives for about $2.99, but in some cases you'd have to buy their entire stock to improve the taste. Sometimes a medicine syringe can squirt the medicine in quick before a little kid has a chance to protest. (Most kids do learn how to spit pretty early.) You can try ice chips or popsicles to numb the taste buds. With some drugs, the aftertaste is worse than the actual taste, and can persist for days.

I know that I hate to be forced to eat something I don't like. I find it positively nauseating. Yet we still want the medicine inside rather than out. If the situation is truly intolerable, call the HCP. No person, especially a sick one, should be tortured to get the medicine in. There have got to be alternatives. In the case of Mepron, I recommend the patient learn to love it at @ $1000 a bottle. (Fortunately, Mepron is not bad. Weird, but not bad.)

SAMPLE FORM XIII: Blank Medication Tracking Sheet

For each day, list all drugs with dose. Then using the initial or name of each drug, set up the dosing schedule by placing the identifier in each cell when the drug is *due*. After the medicine is taken, check the corresponding *taken* box. Be vigilant about checking the *taken* cell, since these small details can be forgotten within seconds. Remove any categories that are not pertinent to the case.

Medication Tracking Sheet

	Day/date Drug/dose		Day/date Drug/dose		Day/date Drug/dose	
	Due	Taken	Due	Taken	Due	Taken
Wake Up						
Before food						
Breakfast						
After food						
Between food						
Before food						
Lunch						
After food						
Between food						
Before food						
Dinner						
After food						
Bedtime						
Overnight						

SAMPLE FORM XIV: Sample Medication Tracking Sheet

Here is a variation of the above form, adapted from a real case showing treatment of a draining gland infection. This example ends on Tuesday morning.

Medication Tracking Sheet

Name: _H. Spreen*_____ Date initiated: <u>December 25, 2011</u>

	Day	S	M	T	W	Th	F	S	S	M
Time	Drug or tx due	done	done	done	done	done	done	done	done	done
1 hr pre food	Probiotic	x	x	x						
a.m. with food	Antibiotic	x	x	x						
a.m.	Antimicrobial wipe	x	x	x						
a.m.	Topical cortisone	x	x	x						
midday	Probiotic	x	x							
p.m. with food	Antibiotic	x	x							
p.m.	Regular arthritis meds	x	x							
p.m.	Antimicrobial wipe	x	x							
p.m.	Topical cortisone	x	x							

*Hoagie Spreen is a dachshund.

V. PROS AND CONS OF OPEN-ENDED ANTIBIOTIC THERAPY

With TBIs, a patient may be on a long-term treatment regimen. By looking at the advantages and disadvantages of such therapy, a patient may be able to better assess her options.

Potential advantages of long-term or open-ended antibiotics:

- They work. With many TBIs, symptoms return if the antibiotic is stopped. Restarting the medicine makes the patient feel better again.

- They allow many patients, who would otherwise be incapacitated, to function despite the disease.

- Often they result in a cure, where symptoms resolve and do not return after the drug is discontinued.

- Remember that long-term antibiotics are used in many conditions without the blink of an eye: chronic OM, rheumatic fever, acne, rosacea, chronic skin infections, gum disease, cystitis, COPD, etc.

Possible disadvantages of long-term antibiotics:

- Yeast overgrowth such as Candida in the mouth, gut, and vagina

- Resistance and the potential evolution of superbugs

- Diarrhea due to toxins from resistant, opportunistic microbes such as C. *difficile* after the beneficial bacteria have been killed by the antimicrobial

- GI upset including nausea, cramps, and vomiting

- IV line irritation or infection

- Sore muscles from IM injections

- In some cases the longer an antibiotic is taken, the more likely significant and sometimes permanent AEs can result.

- In TBIs, especially at too low a dose or too short a treatment duration, the pathogen may burrow deeper into tissue where the antibiotic cannot penetrate. Similarly, the infecting microbe may encyst only to re-emerge after the antibiotic is stopped requiring additional courses of therapy. This may be the best argument for treating with adequate doses, in combination regimens, for sufficient time, to begin with.

The IDSA says that long-term antibiotics can be dangerous because they worry about C. *difficile*, infections in IV catheter lines, and superbugs. Yet, these issues can arise with short-term therapy as well. Further, creative approaches can help manage or resolve these risks. The differing opinions around antibiotic use are vetted in Chapter 11: *Controversies around Lyme.*

VI. WHY ANTIBIOTIC TREATMENTS SOMETIMES FAIL

The list of reasons why even some of the best thought-out treatment plans fail is long and varied:

- The diagnosis is wrong.

- Unrecognized co-infections may be preventing recovery.

- Antibiotic may be inappropriate for strain

- The patient may not be taking the medicine properly or at all. (A study published May, 2011, says that 50% of prescribed medicines are taken improperly. I think the number might be much higher than 50%.)

- Antibiotic is not correct for the pathogen

- Treatment duration was too short

- Dose is too low or administered in a way that does not allow the antimicrobial to be effective

- Pathogen became resistant to the antibiotic and there was no back-up

- Pathogen develops evasive techniques: burrowing, encysting, antigen shifting, etc.

- Poor health habits such as alcohol, inadequate nutrition, lack of sleep, etc.

- Concurrent conditions such as other infections, additional diseases, or outside agents such as allergies, toxins, or molds

- Herx causes interruption of treatment

- Drugs are interacting or counteracting

- Patient does not have enough immune capacity to collaborate with the antibiotic regimen

- Additional antibiotics need to be added to complement the action of the initial drug choices

- Need different route of administration

- Patient was reinfected with different strain

- Unrecognized immune defect

- Genetic predisposition to a poor response

- Too much delay between initial infection and eventual treatment. The stage when first diagnosed and treated can impact results. The longer the delay, the more treatment might be required to get a positive outcome.

- Disease had progressed to a stage where some complications are permanent

- Combination of any or all of the above

VII. MEASURING TREATMENT SUCCESS

The patient will tell you when it is probably safe to stop treatment. When the patient feels better, they are usually better. Even very young children get to know their disease pretty well after living with it for a while. They will know if something is still not completely right or if the disease is pretty much all gone.

Some kids who were infected very young or who were born with a congenital TBI don't really know what it feels like to be disease-free. Still they can provide some pretty solid information about how they are doing.

Many TBI patients are cured. By cure I mean a resolution of symptoms that do not recur when treatment is stopped. This does not necessarily happen overnight. Sometimes a number of courses of therapy are needed. Chronically ill patients are often those who have seen many doctors and tried many treatments before without success. They usually only get to a veteran TBI doc if they have been repeatedly unsuccessful in getting well. Hopefully, you will have a few "easier" cases in your mix, at least to start.

PEARL: A reasonable approach seems to be to treat until they're better. The signs and symptoms should be gone and there should be at least a short period of treatment after symptom resolution to ensure no pathogen is lurking in the shadows waiting to pounce. Consider treating until sxs are gone plus a therapeutic cushion of 2 to 3 months. We know from too much experience that pathogens like Bb can morph into various life forms allowing them to remain dormant while they wait for a more hospitable (antibiotic-free) environment. We accept the fact that TBI cousins like syphilis and malaria can resurface after periods of quiescence, so why not Bb and Babesia? If symptoms return, the logical response would be to re-treat.

Success is not just cure rates. Many of these people have been so sick for so long that incremental improvement is very welcome. Improvement is the first step. Cure is the goal.

A few "specialists" believe that their TBI patients get better with minimum or no treatment. But I could find no numbers to support this contention. From what I have experienced in preceptorships, many chronically ill TBI patients get frustrated with being told there is nothing more that can be done or there is really nothing wrong with them. They KNOW they are still sick, so they move on to another HCP. Many patients tell stories of having seen 12, 15, or 20 HCPs before finding an HCP that will listen. These specialists are mistaking run-away patients for success stories. The IDSA contends that only about 5% of Lyme patients don't get well after 10 to 28 days of treatment. Where would they get that number? No one asked me. I got well three times, maybe more, and I can still tell when Bb are resurfacing. Did they count me three times as cured or as one of the 5%? I suspect they don't know that I exist.

PEARL: If symptoms recur after treatment has been stopped for a while, there are several possible explanations including: the pathogen was dormant and is once again active OR the patient has been reinfected. If new, the infection could be an entirely different strain of the same pathogen or additional co-infections may have been introduced. With TBIs, be on the lookout for anything and everything.

VIII. DURATION OF ANTIBIOTIC TREATMENT

In general with TBIs such as Lyme, the later in the course of the disease that treatment is initiated, the longer treatment will be needed for the patient to improve.

In each specific drug section, I am usually vague about the duration of treatment for the TBIs. I might note the length of treatment recommended for some of the "official" indications just to give you a ballpark for the specific drugs. TBIs are different. As you read the Lyme chapter, you will notice that some patients recover completely with a short-course of antibiotics and some with no treatment whatsoever. Others are sick for years. With babesiosis, you will learn that the majority of cases are subclinical with the infected person never knowing they were infected at all. I am happy for those folks. Nevertheless, many of us must deal with those patients who have been sick for a long time and some are critically ill. For these cases, treatment may need to continue for months or years.

PEARL: Consider a simple approach to length of treatment in TBI patients. Treat them until they're better, plus a cushion. Once they are feeling well enough to come off antibiotics, watch. If symptoms reappear, resume treatment.

If the treatment is helping and not hurting, treat them. If the person is feeling better and is more functional on treatment than off treatment, continue treating. Consider a treatment cushion after symptoms resolve.

Some authors recommend treatment duration for the various TBIs, but these vary considerably. Because of the controversy around Lyme treatment, some local HCPs act like they are being chased by Lilith[2] when it comes to dose and duration of treatment. They treat with as low a dose, for as short a time as possible. This does not make pharmacologic sense. If you're going to treat, treat. If not, please move out of the way.

PEARL: Treating with subtherapeutic doses of antibiotics is more likely to cause resistance.

IX. WHEN TO CHANGE DIRECTION

With very ill patients who may have been sick for a long time with complicated syndromes, sometimes you feel like you are taking two steps forward and one step back. Know that if you keep trying you just might find the right combination to help the individual. How can you tell if the patient is making any progress? When should you regroup and reconsider?

- Always consider that you could have made incorrect decisions about diagnosis or treatment. See the list of reasons why treatments fail a few sections back. Consider all possible angles.

- There is no shame in being wrong, only in not thinking you could be wrong.

- Ask for another opinion from someone who understands TBIs. Patients aren't the only ones who can seek additional opinions. Consult. (I saw a poster in a medical office building that said, "If you really cared about the patients, you'd send them to someone better than you.") In the case of TBIs, I don't believe in sending the patient off because you've given up. I do believe in consultations where you gather information while you continue to be the case manager. These poor patients have already been to a dozen docs. They came to you because they heard you might be somewhat more knowledgeable about TBIs than the average HCP. That doesn't mean you need to know everything. You should have an idea of who to call in the various therapeutic areas.

- With every treatment whether short-term or long-term, medicinal or otherwise, or deciding among various combinations, you should always be doing risk/benefit analyses. Is the juice worth the squeeze?

- If the patient has reached a plateau or is going backward, regroup.

---

2 See Glossary or Introduction for name origin

- Would increasing the dose or changing the mode of administration help?

- Ask the patient if they think the current approach is working or if they might like to try something else. Ask the caregivers.

- Insist that the patient not try to please you by saying they are doing better when they are not. If the person seems wishy-washy, ask more specifically, "What is better since the last time I saw you? What is worse?"

- Would ancillary treatments or supportive measures help?

- You do not have to change everything. Keep what's working and discard what's not. Add and subtract from the core program.

- Assess whether the patient could benefit from ancillary treatments: PT, counseling, tutoring, dietary advice, vitamins, yoga, heat, etc.

- Consider the idea of challenge/rechallenge. When a treatment stops, does the patient get better or worse? If the same treatment is restarted does the patient get better or worse?

X. ANTIBIOTIC OPTIONS FOR EACH TBI

In each case, check the specific chapter or section for treatment details. The lists below include antimicrobials that should hit the named infection.

IMPORTANT CAVEAT: In all cases, the doses below were gleaned from multiple sources. Most of the doses listed are NOT from the "official" drug label, since TBIs are almost never the intended indication. The following doses are either those that some TBI experts found effective or were compiled from various references. While every effort was made to check and recheck, errors could have been made. In EVERY case check the drug label and adjust the dose as appropriate for the individual case.

- **Babesiosis**

Different species of Babesia respond to different treatments. Since we cannot definitively rule out the various strains, treat as though *both* of the primary causal pathogens are present.

Initial combination: Atovaquone (Mepron) AND azithromycin (Zithromax) AND artemesia

Biaxin (clarithromycin) or the ketolide Ketek can replace the azithromycin (Zithromax)

Malarone (atovaquone and proguanil) or other antimalarial can replace atovaquone (Mepron)

Enula might be used in place of artemesia. If for some reason artemesia is not available, consider enula as part of the combination therapy.

PEARL: Enula is considered by some to be a good antiprotozoal that can be administered starting with one drop per day up to 20 drops daily. Since enula can cause a headache, dose should not be increased until the patient can tolerate the previous level without pain. Consider enula in combination with either Mepron or Malarone PLUS azithromycin. Nutramedix has a formulation available on the Internet.

Other agents that should hit the protozoa: trimethoprim/sulfa (Bactrim or Septra), clindamycin, Flagyl (metronidazole), quinine

PEARL: Since lab testing is not reliable, always treat as though both B. microti and B. duncani are present. This means that artemesia is part of all Babesia treatment regimens.

The immunocompromised are at greater risk of treatment failure or a severe presentation of babesiosis and higher doses may be needed.

IDSA Babesia dosing:

Clindamycin: Use in severe cases requiring IV

Adults: 300 to 600 mg q 6 IV or 600 q 8 orally

Kids: 7 to 10 mg/kg IV or orally q 6 to 8, max of 600 mg/dose

Quinine: I found the doses listed by the IDSA confusing so I chose not to reproduce them here. PLEASE base dose on salt available and age of recipient. Your trusted local pharmacist should be able to assist in selecting the dose based on the accessible formulation.

Mepron:

Adults: 750 mg q 12

Kids: 20 mg/kg q 12, max 750 mg/dose

Azithromycin:

Adults: 500 to 1000 mg on day 1 and 250 daily thereafter

Kids: 10 mg/kg on day 1 up to 500 mg/dose and then 5 mg/kg daily up to 250 mg/dose.

IDSA says to use exchange transfusions if indicated: if parasitemia greater than 10%, significant hemolysis, or renal, hepatic, or pulmonary compromise.

PEARL: IDSA Guidelines for dosing can be inconsistent with the dosing recommendations in the package insert and not for approved indications.

- **Ehrlichiosis/Anaplasmosis**

Doxycycline is the DOC.

Rifamycin is effective but should never be used as a solo agent because of rapid resistance.

If doxycycline is not feasible, consider other TCNs like minocycline.

- **Bartonellosis**

Start with a foundation macrolide such as azithromycin (Zithromax) or clarithromycin (Biaxin), then add trimethoprim/sulfa (Bactrim or Septra), rifamycin, a fluoroquinolone like Cipro, or a TCN such as doxycycline or minocycline.

Treat for at least 3 months and longer if the patient is immunocompromised. For Bartonella with primarily CNS manifestations, use doxycycline WITH rifamycin AND a macrolide. Anecdotally, in recalcitrant cases rifamycin has been a key to treatment success.

In pregnant women with Bartonella, consider azithromycin and Bactrim. Since Bactrim is pregnancy category C, always do a risk/benefit analysis.

Note that one source specifically says NOT to use PCNs, cephalosporins, Bactrim, or quinolones. They don't say why. Be aware. Target your treatment to the specifics of the individual case.

- **Mycoplasma *fermentans***

Start with a foundation macrolide such as azithromycin (Zithromax) or clarithromycin (Biaxin) together with a TCN like doxycycline or minocycline. Add as needed agents such as: trimethoprim-sulfa (Bactrim or Septra), rifamycin, chloramphenicol, Cipro (ciprofloxin) or other fluoroquinolone, or Plaquenil (hydroxychloroquine).

- **Lyme Disease**

There are dozens of proposed treatment regimes for Lyme that are detailed in Chapter 10: *Borreliosis*. Entire books have been written on this topic as well as two conflicting treatment guidelines. The goals of therapy include: improvement in signs and symptoms, normalization of function, prevention of long-term sequelae, and cure. To achieve these goals, many possible approaches have been suggested including but not limited to:

1. Treating by disease stage: acute, localized, disseminated, persistent, chronic, relapsing, reinfected, etc.

2. Deciding to treat based on time from original infection: early versus late in clinical course

3. Selecting antimicrobials based on the primary organ system affected such as cardiac, musculoskeletal, or neuropsychiatric

4. Attempting to choose antimicrobials that hit various forms of Bb: cell walled spirochete, intracellular, and cystic

5. Balancing a potentially resistant drug with a back-up

6. Endeavoring to hit both Bb and likely co-infections

7. Hitting the cell wall of the spirochete

8. Determining which method of administration to use: po, IM, IV

9. Deciding whether to use the big guns first or save them for later

10. Establishing which regimen will give the desired blood levels such as steady state versus clear peaks and troughs

11. Recognizing the impact of a Herx reaction

12. Assessing the benefits and risks of pulsing regimens or drug holidays

13. Taking into account the restrictions in use of some of these antibiotics in kids as well as the safety profiles of each drug

14. Collaborating with patients and caretakers to review the risk/benefit of alternative treatments

15. Using the clinical response to determine the duration of treatment

In general, choose a cell wall antibiotic in combination with an intracellular antibiotic. Using solo agents might cause the pathogen to go intracellular or to encyst and there will be no back-up. ALWAYS consider a COMBINATION approach. For example in kids under 8 y/o consider starting with amoxicillin PLUS azithromycin. Over 8 y/o, consider doxycycline PLUS azithromycin. Chapter 10: *Borreliosis* weighs all these factors in choosing the best regimen to target the disease in the individual patient.

Cell wall antibiotics: Suitable for use against the spirochetal, free-floating form of Bb: PCNs (Amoxil, Augmentin, Bicillin), CSs (Omnicef, Ceftin, Rocephin, Claforan, Cedax, Suprax), Primaxin, vancomycin, TCNs (doxycycline, Doryx, Minocin), Tindamax. Both Plaquenil and rifamycin are likely to hit the free spirochetes but the mechanism is unclear. L-forms have no cell wall so they are not hurt by cell wall antibiotics.

Intracellular antibiotics include macrolides/ketolides (Zithromax, Biaxin, Ketek), Tindamax, and rifamycin. Once the pathogen gets inside the cell, doxycycline has less effect, but minocycline may do a little better. Tigecycline can go intracellular.

Cyst-busters: Tindamax, Flagyl. Plaquenil is thought to penetrate some cysts.

PEARL: Tindamax likely hits all three life forms of Bb.

The best drugs for crossing the **BBB** in an attempt to hit the TBI pathogens causing neuropsychiatric symptoms include Rocephin (ceftriaxone), rifamycin, Bicillin, minocycline to some degree, IV doxycycline, Claforan (cefotaxime), chloramphenicol, Ceftin (cefuroxime), and Lariam. Drugs that do **not** cross the BBB include macrolides, oral doxycycline, vancomycin, clindamycin, and Mepron.

The best drugs for musculoskeletal and joint complaints include the penicillins and Plaquenil. Consider adding Plaquenil when the patient shows sxs of autoimmune response to a Bb infection or tests positive for HLA-DR2 or HLA-DR4.

- **Colorado Tick Fever**

  Antibiotics do not work with viruses. Consider antiviral if early in clinical course.

- **Powassan Viral Encephalitis**

  Antibiotics do not work with viruses. Consider antiviral if early in clinical course.

- **Q Fever**

  Consider doxycycline (or minocycline or other TCNs). Chloramphenicol and quinolones have been reported to be effective. For Q endocarditis consider doxycycline PLUS hydroxychloroquine (Plaquenil).

- **Rocky Mountain Spotted Fever**

  Doxycycline (TCN) and chloramphenicol have both been effectively used.

- **Tick Relapsing Fever**

  Doxycycline is the DOC but success has also been shown with chloramphenicol.

- **Tularemia**

  The following antimicrobials have been effective in treating tularemia: streptomycin[3] (or gentamicin), chloramphenicol, TCNs, or Rocephin (ceftriaxone).

XI. ANTIBIOTIC OPTIONS FOR COMMON CO-INFECTION COMBINATIONS

As might have been mentioned a few times in this text, diagnoses of TBIs are based on clinical judgment. Waiting for confirmatory lab results can be time consuming. A negative result does NOT rule out the disease. If you suspect co-infections, try to select a treatment regimen that covers the possible etiologies. When my son had Lyme, babesiosis, and Ehrlichia, and was only treated for Lyme (the treatment of which should have also hit the Ehrlichia), he did get better after a few doses only to crash after two days. The Babesia was untouched by the Lyme treatment and the pathogens had a field day and nearly killed him. You must manage the case. Do not let the case manage you. Do not force a patient into an artificial treatment algorithm just because that is the easiest approach for you. Do not say as our Lilith[4] did, "He's already on doxy, what more do you want?"

> *PEARL: Make sure the patient and caregivers understand the concept of co-infections. This understanding might help them realize why the treatment plan includes multiple drugs. Don't just prescribe and run. Make sure there is some type of follow-up contact in the not too distant future such as a phone appointment in one or two weeks. The sicker the patient the sooner the contact. Make sure the patient and caretakers know to call if symptoms get worse, there is no improvement, or if a significant side effect occurs. If the patient or caregiver thinks a side effect is significant then that meets the definition of significant. They should be prepared for a Herx reaction. They should call if the Herx is unbearable. Counsel them to never stop or change medicines without contacting you. If signs of an allergic reaction appear such as trouble breathing, they should seek help immediately, and then call you to discuss next steps.*

The following chart shows the most recognized co-infections along with their DOCs and alternative antimicrobials. Those infections that should be treated with combination therapy are marked with an *. DOCs or foundation antimicrobials are marked with a +. Effective substitutions or appropriate components for a combination regime are marked with a √. This same graphic appears as an insert on the book cover.

---

3 *Aminoglycosides are a class of antibiotics rarely indicated for treatment of TBIs aside from tularemia. However, if given for other reasons in TBI patients they might increase the risk of kidney damage. They include: gentamicin, tobramycin, amikacin, kanamycin, streptomycin, and neomycin.*

4 *See Glossary or Introduction for name origin*

ANTIMICROBIAL OPTIONS FOR SELECT CO-INFECTIONS

	PCNs: Amoxil, Augmentin, Bicillin	Doxycycline (Doryx), Minocycline	CSs: Omnicef, Rocephin, Ceftin	Macrolides: Azithromycin, Clarithromycin, Ketek	Azoles: Metronidazole, Tinidazole	Rifamycin*	Mepron (Atovaquone) (or quinine derivative)	Artemesia*	Plaquenil* (hydroxychloroquine)	Fluoroquinolones (Cipro, Levaquin)	Bactrim (sulfa/trimethoprim)	Chloramphenicol	Aminoglycosides (Streptomycin, Gentamicin)	Clindamycin	Antivirals
Lyme Adult*		+	√	√	√	√			√	√					
Lyme Child*	+		√	√	√	√			√	√					
Babesia* B. microti				√	√		+		√		√			√	
Babesia B. duncani								+							
Ehrl/Ana		+				√									
Bartonella* BLOs		√		+		√				√	√				
RMSF (Rickettsia)		+										√			
Other Borrelia* (STARI,TRF)		+	√	√	√	√			√			√			
Viral: CTF, POW															√
Q fever Coxiella		+							+	√		√			
Tularemia (Francisella)		√	√									√	+		
M. *fermentans*		+		+		√			√	√	√	√	√		

* = Always consider combination therapy

+ = First DOC or foundation for combination

√ = May be effective choice or use as part of combination regimen

XII. FINALLY: THE DRUGS

Drug classes are somewhat artificial, but we have to organize somehow. Many of the categories overlap. Drug listings in this chapter are as up-to-date as possible. Drugs do change labels and the available body of knowledge shifts. Much on-line and published information is incorrect, unreliable, or misleading. New drugs are coming on board all the time and others are falling by the wayside. We can only do our best with the information at-hand. Use the listings below to help you make reasonable treatment decisions.

Antimicrobials are any agents that diminish the pathogen load or otherwise enhance the body's capacity to fight infection including antibiotics, antimalarials, antivirals, and antifungals.

- Antibiotics: Drugs that are effective in treating bacterial infections and include the penicillins (PCNs), tetracyclines (TCNs), cephalosporins (CSs), sulfas, and several other classes. Many more exist and some are not quite classifiable. I will focus only on those pertinent in the treatment of TBIs.

- Antimalarials: For the treatment of TBIs, the term anti-malarial is limiting. While these agents certainly address malaria, for our purposes they are better termed **antiprotozoals**, since they also handle Babesia.

- Antivirals: Agents that diminish the effects of viral infections. These agents are given only a mention in this text.

- Antifungals: Drugs that target fungal infections. These medicines are detailed in Chapter 25: *Ancillary Treatments*.

Each class will be described along with the most commonly used agents within each grouping. In general, the brand name of a medicine is capitalized while the generic name is not. Not all brand names are included in these sections. I have included those that are most commonly used or seem to be preferred by TBD specialists.

More than a PDR, I find the *Monthly Prescribing Reference* to be a useful asset in day-to-day practice. While you can subscribe monthly, you can also order occasional issues and get the practical information you need.

PEARL: All dosing information listed below is to provide you with a foundation from which to work, NOT to define the exact dose to be used in an individual patient. This information has been gathered from product labels, literature reports, and the experience of experts. There is great variability in what different sources find to be effective and safe. Every effort was made to provide the most up-to-date

and accurate information, but things change in medicine. In all cases, check the package insert and target your prescribing to the specific case.

A. ANTIBIOTICS

General Penicillins (PCNs)

Description: Alexander Fleming, a Scottish scientist, first discovered penicillin in the late 1920s. Originally derived from fungi, PCN was the first drug effective against such serious diseases as syphilis and the various manifestations of Streptococcus. Anyone over 70-years-old today is probably alive because PCN saved them at some point. PCN is still the most commonly used antibiotic worldwide. Many pathogens are now resistant to the original PCNs.

MOA: PCNs work by inhibiting cell wall synthesis. If certain bacteria cannot make a cell wall, they cannot reproduce and grow. After PCN administration, the pathogen cannot form cross-links in the cell wall. As the wall weakens, it eventually breaks and often the pathogen underneath dies. Therefore, penicillins are considered bacteriocidal. PCNs are more effective against the cells that are rapidly dividing than against mature, resting cells that aren't making new cell walls at the moment. This may explain variations in their effectiveness against spirochetes. Because of the MOA, PCNs work well with other antibiotics that can go inside the cell and cause damage there such as tinidazole or the macrolides.

Usage: Sustained "cidal" levels are needed for at least 3 days to be effective, so try for sustained blood and tissue levels. If you miss a dose of PCN, take it as soon as you remember and take the next dose 3 to 5 hours later. Then go back to your usual schedule. Usually PCNs can be taken with or without food but food often helps with GI upset. Give one hour before other antibiotics if possible.

Indications: PCNs are well-known for their effectiveness against Staph, Strep, syphilis, and gonorrhea. In terms of TBIs, PCNs are used in children with Lyme in combination with other agents. Since they are effective against spirochete-induced syphilis, one would expect activity against the spirochete Bb as well.

Use in TBDs: Since TCNs have restricted use in pediatrics, PCNs are often selected, especially in combination with other agents, to treat Bb. Amoxicillin is the DOC for borreliosis in kids under 8 y/o. This is the drug that the combination regimen should be built around. Combining this cell wall antibiotic with a good intracellular agent like azithromycin might be a prudent first choice. PCNs should appear higher on the option list if the patient's symptoms are primarily musculoskeletal. IM Bicillin has a number of advantages over oral agents and is considered a good foundation drug for combination therapy in Lyme disease.

Cautions: Just as PCNs are the most commonly used antibiotics worldwide, PCN allergy is the most commonly reported drug allergy. Allergies to PCN are widespread and can be fatal. Also, because of structural similarities, there is cross-reactivity with cephalosporins. So an allergy to any of the PCNs makes a patient more at risk for an allergic reaction to cephalosporins and vice versa.

PCNs may interfere with OCPs, so use caution in females of child bearing age. Potassium levels can be altered by penicillins.

AEs: Allergies are the most common problem with PCNs. Any sign of an allergic reaction, contact the HCP so that a decision can be made about continuation of treatment. Most common allergic manifestations include rash, hives, and breathing difficulties. If the person is starting to struggle in any way, call 911 or get them to the nearest ER.

As with almost all antibiotics, PCN use can result in fungal overgrowth, diarrhea, or pseudomembranous colitis.

Monitor: In long-term use monitor blood, liver, and kidney function. Watch potassium

Specific PCN Options:

There are many PCN options. Here are the most commonly used in TBI patients.

1. **Amoxicillin** (Amoxil)

   Description: Broad spectrum PCN antibiotic considered more effective than oral PCN. Amoxicillin has been combined with probenecid to increase efficacy.

   Indications: Well-known to all parents who have ever been up all night with a child with an ear infection. Often called "the pink stuff." Multiple uses including OM and other infections of the ears, nose, throat, respiratory, and GU tracts. Used in combination against H. *pylori*, the organism implicated in many GI ulcers

   Use in TBDs: Common adjunct in combination with other agents to treat Lyme, especially in patients who present predominantly with musculoskeletal complaints. Since TCNs have restricted use in pediatrics, amoxicillin has a larger role in the treatment of Lyme in kids than in adults. Amoxicillin is the DOC for borreliosis in kids under 8 y/o. This is the drug that the

combination regimen should be built around. Combining this cell wall antibiotic with a good intracellular agent like azithromycin might be a prudent first choice.

Usage: Use higher doses in severe infections and lower doses if the kidney is impaired. PCNs can be taken with or without food, but food might help decrease GI upset.

PEARL: Amoxicillin is effective only if the affected tissue is saturated with the medicine at all times, so you need to give adequate FREQUENT doses. Ideally, you would give the drug tid or qid, but the more frequent the dosing, the greater the likelihood of missed doses.

Cautions: Allergy may manifest as Stevens-Johnson syndrome or anaphylaxis. This is a medical emergency. Call the ambulance.

Cross allergies with cephalosporins are possible.

A number of bacterial species have developed resistance to plain amoxicillin.

Dosing: Amoxicillin comes in capsules, tablets, chewables, drops (50 mg/ml), and suspension (either 200 or 250 or 400 per 5 ml).

<u>Adults:</u>	500 -2000 mg q 8 up to 6 grams/day
<u>Children:</u>	
Neonates and infants < 3 months:	Maximum 30 mg/kg in divided doses q 12
Over 3 months:	25 to 45 mg/kg in 2 divided doses q 12 OR
	20 to 40 mg/kg in 3 divided doses q 8
Older kids:	50 mg/kg/day divided into 3 divided doses q 8
Kids > 40 kg:	500 - 875 mg q 12 or 250 q 8

PEARL: One regimen in pregnant women suggests a combination of amoxicillin 1 gram q 6 with azithromycin for the duration of the pregnancy.

Probenecid has been added to amoxicillin in adults at 250 to 500 mg q 8 to enhance efficacy but this is not usually considered necessary today since Augmentin comes with its own efficacy enhancer.

Amoxicillin is used in pregnancy with doses adjusted to severity of illness and presumed pathogen at doses up to 1 gram q 6.

AEs: Can cause falsely high sugars in blood and urine testing, blood dyscrasias, GI upset, diarrhea, overgrowth of fungus, and all manifestations of allergic reactions including anaphylaxis.

Monitor: In long-term use monitor blood, kidney, and liver function.

2. Amoxicillin plus clavulanate (Augmentin)

Description: Combination of the PCN based antibiotic amoxicillin and the enzyme inhibitor clavulanate. The blending of these two components results in a greater range of action against organisms that are resistant to plain amoxicillin.

MOA: A number of bacteria produce an enzyme called β-lactamase that is able to inactivate amoxicillin and allow resistant forms of the pathogens to overgrow. By inhibiting this enzyme, the clavulanate enables the amoxicillin to do its job.

Indications: Sinusitis, OM, lower respiratory infections, skin infections, and UTIs

Use in TBDs: Frankly, if you are looking for an amoxicillin based product, basic amoxicillin should do the job, especially if you make sure the dosing is frequent enough to allow for steady blood levels. Usually, amoxicillin doesn't rip apart the GI tract the way this combination product can.

Usage: Take with meals

Cautions: Augmentin can cause savage diarrhea that can contain blood and lead to dehydration. Often this settles down in about 3 days, but be cautious. In children in diapers, this can be especially uncomfortable since it can exacerbate the overgrowth of fungus and cause very painful rashes. If the side effects seem to be more than the patient can tolerate discuss the risk/benefit and possible alternatives.

May interfere with action of OCPs.

Dosing: Comes in tablets, suspension, and chewables in many strengths. Base the dose on the amoxicillin component.

Adults:	250 to 500 mg q 8 or 500 to 875 mg q 12

Children:

Less than 3 months:	30 mg/kg/day divided into 2 doses q 12
Greater than 3 months:	25 to 45 mg/kg/day in 2 doses q 12 OR
	20 to 40 mg/kg/day in 3 doses q 8

Dosing differs for the immediate release formulations versus the extended release so make sure you know which one you are prescribing. Check the label if there are any questions.

PEARL: The more frequent the dosing regimen, the more potential for missed doses. The less frequent the dosing regimen, the more ups and downs in the blood levels. In general, with PCNs you want the steady levels that come from frequent dosing. With TCNs you want intermittent high blasts that come from higher doses less frequently. Remember to reinforce the need to take the medicine as prescribed.

AEs: Diarrhea, allergies, pseudomembranous colitis, nausea, vomiting, cramps, and thrush

Monitor: In long-term use monitor blood, kidney, and liver function.

3. Benzathine PCN (Bicillin-LA)

Description: This PCN is given by IM injection, allowing for all the advantages provided by using an IM repository of drug, including steadier blood levels compared with those found after oral administration. Of course, disadvantages come along with that as well, such as pain at the injection site. Bicillin is a long-acting penicillin G with an efficacy close to that of IV agents. There are essentially no GI AEs and minimal yeast.

MOA: While Bicillin injections into the muscle aren't EXACTLY a depot as an injected pellet would be, they do provide for a drug repository from where the medicine can consistently dispense over time. For a PCN to be effective, blood levels must be sustained for at least 72 hours. Bicillin IM allows for these continuous levels.

Indications: IM Bicillin is a common treatment method used in Lyme patients. Some HCPs introduce IM dosing early in the treatment strategy since it has the advantage of consistent blood and tissue levels and superb compliance. With other PCNs dosing may need to occur 3 or 4 times a *day* to achieve the same steady blood levels. A missed oral dose can have significant clinical implications. IM injections are often considered in chronic patients who have been sick a long time or those who are severely ill. Injections into the muscle should also be considered for those who cannot tolerate GI administration. There is more than 20 years experience using IM Bicillin in Bb. In many cases, Bicillin IM has shown to be more effective than oral preparations and blood levels are close to those found after IV treatment, if the dose is adequate.

Use in TBDs: Many Lyme patients seem to do quite well on IM Bicillin. Often, Bicillin is not considered until the patient has been sick for a long time or is severely ill. Actually, Bicillin is a good foundation drug for combination therapy in TBIs. If the patient is very sick, weigh the pros and cons of IV versus IM. There may be advantages to considering Bicillin earlier in the course of treatment. From experience, Bicillin therapy seems to offer some indication of appropriate length of treatment. In a number of cases, symptoms will resurface when the Bicillin is stopped and remit when the Bicillin is restarted. Over time in many cases, Bicillin can be totally discontinued when symptoms do not recur. Dosing a few times a week instead of 3 or 4 times a day can provide a compliance advantage. Some sources recommend that Bicillin be given with a cystbuster since that is likely to improve efficacy. Consider Bicillin as one part of a combination regimen.

Usage: Bicillin is usually administered *3 to 4 times a week*. This intermittent dosing allows for about 72 hours of continuous blood levels prior to the next dose. IM Bicillin is comparatively cheap. GI AEs are rare and there is less yeast overgrowth. In general, IM Bicillin has a good safety profile. The family can inject at home or the Bicillin can be self-administered. Nevertheless, kids, especially teens, can get tired of getting stuck all the time.

PEARL: While Bicillin can be self-administered, everyone that I know who tried it themselves said, "Never again!"

A typical course of IM Bicillin in a Lyme patient can last 6 to 12 months. If, after discontinuation, symptoms recur, consider resuming Bicillin or re-assessing the overall treatment strategy.

When giving an IM injection, aspirate first to avoid an inadvertent IV administration. If blood appears in syringe upon aspiration, you could be in a vein. Reposition.

May be used in pregnancy

AEs: Minimal GI side effects and rare yeast overgrowth since the antibiotic is not washing over the entire GI tract. Strong safety profile. May cause a significant and prolonged Herx reaction requiring a dose adjustment. Injection site reactions including redness, swelling, palpable bump where the medicine deposited, and rarely infection. IM injections hurt. They can leave a firm, palpable bump of medicine under the skin. The injection site can become infected, but this usually can be avoided by using good injection technique.

PEARL: IM Bicillin can hurt. Doug Fearn, President of the LDASEPA, offers the following insight on administering the IM Bicillin injections:

"Learning how to do Bicillin injections can seem intimidating, but it is actually quite simple and a caregiver is likely to have more compassion for the patient than the HCP in a busy office. At-home administration is also much more convenient for the patient and saves the expense of an office visit.

The injection can be painful. The needle is a large gauge and Bicillin is a thick cream-like liquid that is more difficult to inject than a typical light liquid injection. The medication must be kept refrigerated to maintain its potency and the Bicillin thickens further in the cold. It is best to remove the dose from the refrigerator at least thirty minutes before injection. Alternatively, you can place it in a shirt pocket where your body heat will warm it up more quickly.

Bicillin is injected in what is euphemistically called the "hip," but it is really into the large muscle of the buttocks. A doctor or nurse can help you locate the proper location. The area is swabbed with an alcohol prep pad first to disinfect the skin. If you administer the injection while the alcohol is still wet, it will sting, so let it dry before injecting.

Some patients prefer standing for the shot and others find lying down is more comfortable. In either case, the shot will be significantly less painful if the muscle is completely relaxed. It will be easier to insert the needle into a relaxed muscle, too. If the patient is standing, have them put most of the weight on the foot opposite the injection side, and ask them to consciously relax the muscle as much as they can. It's worth waiting a few extra seconds for them to accomplish this before the needle is inserted.

Exercising the muscle immediately before the injection can help, too. If the patient is able, a brisk walk, or a trip up and down a flight of stairs, can help get the muscle ready for a pain-free injection.

It may seem less painful to slowly push the needle through the skin and into the muscle, but actually a quick insertion is far more comfortable. Hold the skin taut between two fingers and rapidly insert the needle (almost like throwing a dart). Your nurse-instructor can show you how deeply to insert the needle. Once in place, it is necessary to pull back on the plunger a bit to make sure no blood appears in the syringe. Blood would indicate that the needle is in a blood vessel, which is not good. Reposition the needle and aspirate again, looking for blood. How common is blood? I never had that happen in over 150 injections I administered.

There are two schools of thought on how quickly to inject the medication. Some patients find that a slow injection, over a period of several minutes, is less painful. Other patients would rather have the procedure over with as quickly as possible. In any event, the time spent injecting the medicine should be at least thirty seconds.

Sometimes you and the patient will feel a sudden "pop" as a large amount of the Bicillin suddenly enters the tissue. The plunger on the syringe will quickly jump more deeply, and the patient will feel a jolt of extra pain. When this happens, it is usually best to relax pressure on the plunger and wait a few seconds. If the patient tenses up, remind them to relax.

Once the plunger hits the bottom, the injection is done and the needle can be removed. Be sure to pull the needle out in a straight line, perpendicular to the skin, to minimize pain. Some patients find that withdrawing the needle is more painful than the insertion, so perform this step carefully, but quickly.

As soon as the needle is removed, place a sterile gauze pad over the injection site and hold firmly for a minute or so. Gently massaging the area with the pad can help the medicine disperse and often helps mitigate the pain. It is normal for the injection site to bleed a little, although sometimes it does not bleed at all. Cover the site with a Band-Aid.

Have the patient get up and walk around if they are able. More strenuous exercise is even better for many people, so encourage them to walk for a few minutes. For most patients, the pain quickly subsides, although the area may have a dull ache for hours, especially if the injection process was less than perfect or the patient was tense during the injection.

The next time the injection is due, it should be done on the opposite side.

Sometimes a hard knot will form at the injection site. This usually disappears in a day or two, but may persist longer in some cases."

Cautions: The injection must be deep enough to reach the muscle. This can be a problem with novice administrators who can barely get through the skin without weeping. Self-injectors usually learn quickly to get down to business. Since IM Bicillin can be quite effective, the dose may need to start low since a strong, prolonged Herx can occur. Some Herx reactions have lasted for weeks. Chapter 28 is called *Understanding the Herxheimer Reaction*. One significant disadvantage of IM injection is its irreversibility. Once you push that plunger, the medicine is in and you cannot suck it back out (and it's there for days leeching into the system). Make sure the patient is not allergic to the drug before you administer an IM injection.

Dosing:

For Teens and Adults: 1.2 to 3.6 million units divided into 2 to 4 doses per week (Some argue that 1 time per week is sufficient but this does not seem to jibe with the 72 hour sustained blood levels needed for maximum efficacy.)

The muscles of the butt are usually the preferred injection site since there is considerable muscle mass. Xylocaine topical ointment at 5% or EMLA cream can be applied to the targeted area 30 to 60 minutes prior to injection. Icing the area prior to the needle stick is also sometimes recommended. Unfortunately, the surface skin and subcutaneous tissue are not the sites of the most pain anyway, so superficial treatments aren't going to help much. IM should go deep in the tissue and that is where the most pain will be felt. I would not use a deep local anesthetic with vasoconstrictors since this could alter the physiology of the underlying tissue and impact absorption for several hours. After injection, the site can be gently massaged or dressed with warm, wet compresses or soaks. Ice will slow absorption and warmth might enhance blood flow and distribution.

PEARL: One regimen in pregnant women with Lyme suggests Bicillin 1.2 million units IM one to three times per week plus azithromycin.

Monitor: If treatment is long-term consider basic routine screens of CBC, LFTs, BUN, and creatinine.

4. **Primaxin** (combination of imipenem and cilastatin)

Description: The antibiotic component is imipenem, an antimicrobial closely related to the PCNs and CSs, but usually classified separately as a carbapenem. With a broad spectrum, Primaxin is usually reserved for serious, susceptible infections.

MOA: Impedes the ability of the pathogen to make cell walls so eventually they die

Indications: Sepsis, LRIs, UTIs, and infections of skin, bone, and joints. Also used for endocarditis, gynecologic infections, and infections due to multiple pathogens.

Use in TBIs: Primaxin has been used as an alternative treatment for Lyme.

Usage: Dosage is based on the imipenem component. Can be given IM or IV

Cautions: Kidney dysfunction. May increase risk of seizures so use caution in patients with underlying seizure disorders. May have less reported allergies than other PCNs but still need to be aware of potential allergic cross-reactivity in those allergic to PCNs or CSs.

Dosing:

Adults: IM: 500 to 750 mg q 12

IV: 250 to 500 mg q 6

Children:

IM: Not recommended in small children

IV: Less than 30 kg, not recommended.

Less than 1 week:	25 mg/kg q 12
1 to 4 weeks:	25 mg/kg q 8
4 weeks to 3 months:	25 mg/kg q 6
Greater than 3 months:	15 to 25 mg/kg q 6
Maximum 2 to 4 gram/day	

AEs: Confusion, seizures, electrolyte imbalances, dizziness, sleepiness, and abnormal LFTs

Monitor: Make sure creatinine clearance is sufficient to handle elimination of the drug. Monitor LFTs and electrolytes.

General Fluoroquinolones

Description: Scientists were trying to synthesize chloroquinone to treat malaria in World War II. They accidentally came across another class of antibiotics, which are now called quinolones. When these drugs were later modified by substituting a fluorine atom for a hydrogen, the class came to be called fluoroquinolones. These are very powerful broad-spectrum antibiotics that are prone to high resistance and great risk of overgrowth of fungus

and *C. difficile* possibly resulting in pseudomembranous colitis. After their financial potential was recognized, many formulations were developed and more than 10,000 compounds have been synthesized.

MOA: Fluoroquinolones work by preventing bacterial DNA from unwinding and duplicating. So, no baby bacteria. These drugs are bacteriostatic.

Fluoroquinolones inhibit the cytochrome P450 enzyme system in the liver. As a result, the blood concentrations of certain other drugs taken concomitantly could increase. Use caution with other medications such as antidepressants, antipsychotics, caffeine, and theophylline.

These drugs rapidly cross the blood-placental barrier and appear in breast milk and thereafter are extensively distributed in the tissues of the fetus and newborn. If you do not want to expose the fetus or neonate, consider alternatives.

Indications: Fluoroquinolones have many uses from STDs, anthrax, severe lower respiratory infections, genitourinary infections, PID, pyelonephritis, prostatitis, skin infections, bone and joint infections, and traveler's diarrhea.

Most experts recommend not using these agents as first-line unless there are no other options. Don't throw a fluoroquinolone at every sick patient just because you think it will kill the pathogen. It most likely will, but no need to use an elephant gun to kill a butterfly.

Fluoroquinolones are not recommended in kids under 18 although this class is prescribed frequently in kids. Always consider the risk/benefit before you prescribe and justify your decision in the patient's chart.

Use in TBDs: Quinolones enter cells easily and so may be considered for use against intracellular pathogens like Mycoplasma and are often considered when M. *fermentans* is suspected. Mycoplasma is not a butterfly and you want to select agents that have the best chance of eradicating this harmful pathogen. Fluoroquinolones may also hit Bartonella and the Coxiella that cause Q fever. With M. *fermentans* and Bartonella, the diagnosis may be hard to make. If the patient is not getting well and the clinical picture is compatible with these pathogens, antimicrobials that hit these organisms might be considered. Do a risk/benefit assessment.

Usage: In general, pick something else as first-line treatment in order to avoid the myriad possible side effects. Do as I say, not as I do. When I go to Mexico to work with the native people on the Guatemala border, I pop Levaquin like candy to prevent tourista. Those of us who do, don't get diarrhea. Those of us who do not; well, it gets ugly. Of course, we are a bunch of HCPs who can keep an eye on one another.

If you choose a fluoroquinolone, be vigilant. Sometimes a fluoroquinolone is what a patient needs. Consider the risk/benefit.

Fluoroquinolones can be taken irrespective of food with plenty of water. These drugs are best not taken with mineral supplements or multivitamins with minerals especially iron, calcium, aluminum, or magnesium. Do not take within two hours of antacids.

Cautions: Fluoroquinolones have black box warnings. Black box warnings are the highest level of warning required by the FDA. These warnings can be valid but, as with all things that involve the government and corporate interests, they can be political. Many HCPs do not know a black box warning from a shoebox. Read them and consider what the warnings might mean for each individual patient. Many generic forms of the drug do NOT contain the black box warning on the label, (although they're supposed to) so you might not be aware of their existence from the package insert.

Do not take fluoroquinolones with steroids or Rifampin. Make sure the patient has adequate renal function prior to prescribing. If a fluoroquinolone is necessary and renal function is compromised adjust the dose appropriately. Taking with antacids or products containing calcium, iron, or zinc may decrease absorption. Resistance to fluoroquinolones can occur very fast, even within one course of treatment. Use in combination with other agents is prudent. Since quinolones can make the patient jittery, try to avoid caffeine during treatment.

Some consider the fluoroquinolones the most dangerous drugs on the market. (At least they are effective. Working in drug safety for a long time, I have a list of drugs that I think are much less safe than fluoroquinolones.)

Here is a list of problems that *might* be associated with use of fluoroquinolones. As noted in the previous chapter, just because an event is listed as having occurred in a blue-eyed, Tasmanian coal miner in 1984, does not mean it will absolutely happen to your patient. Just be aware of the possibilities:

- Very high risk of colonizing MRSA and C. *difficile* (Some think the risk of C. *difficile* overgrowth exceeds that of clindamycin.)

- High rates of resistance

- Pseudomembranous colitis

- QTc prolongation, torsades de pointes,

- Nephritis, renal failure, seizures, CNS toxicity, hyperthyroidism, liver problems, rheumatic disease, cardiotoxicity, pancreatitis

- Rhabdomyolysis (muscle wasting)

- Stevens-Johnson syndrome (SJS), toxic epidermal necrolysis (TEN)

- Children and elderly are at greater risk of AEs.

- Tendonitis and tendon rupture (black box warning) with a higher risk in those over 60-years-old, steroids users, and transplant patients

- Musculoskeletal disorders

- Photosensitivity and phototoxicity

- Contraindicated in: epilepsy, QT prolongation, CNS lesions or inflammation, pregnancy (unless no options), and in nursing mothers

- Use in children only if severe infections where there are no other options. (Make sure rationale is documented in patient chart.)

- Theophylline, NSAIDs, and steroids increase toxicity

- Significant changes in blood sugars

- Peripheral neuropathy (irreversible nerve damage)

- When used in pregnant females, there is risk of spontaneous abortion and tissue levels in the fetus

- Found in breast milk

- Higher numbers of adverse events in patients with panic disorder or depression

This list is not intended to be exhaustive, just informative.

Dosing: Duration of treatment depends on severity of illness and patient response. Some recommend serum drug levels during extended therapy to avoid an overdose but use common-sense and ask the patient to call with any problems.

AEs: One controversial theory on the mechanism by which the fluoroquinolones cause so many adverse events is the damage they cause to healthy mitochondrial DNA in the patient. In addition to the items listed in the "Cautions" section above, fluoroquinolones have been associated with phototoxicity, confusion, erythema multiforme, anemia, visual changes, loss of vision, involuntary muscle movements, double vision, diminished color vision, fever, eosinophilia, pseudotumor cerebri (intracranial hypertension), fungal overgrowth, allergic reactions, and GI disturbances. As mentioned in the previous chapter, association does not necessarily mean causation. Did the fluoroquinolone CAUSE the observed erythema multiforme or was this manifestation part of the underlying pathology that the fluoroquinolone was selected to treat? Blaming the wrong agent for causality leaves the real culprit free to harm again.

With several anthrax scares in the past decade, many unexposed persons took fluoroquinolones prophylactically and a number of AEs were reported. Again, here it is hard to separate the frenzy from actual ADRs.

The mechanism by which the fluoroquinolones cause CNS problems is hypothesized to be a neurotoxin inhibition of GABA (γ-aminobutyric acid). The rate of CNS toxic events is estimated to be between 0.2% and 2%. Risk factors for neurotoxicity include: old age, renal insufficiency, prior CNS disorders, use of CNS medications, and drug interactions such as those with NSAIDs or theophylline. Almost all fluoroquinolones need dose adjustment in the case of renal compromise, a history of seizures, acute psychosis, manic episodes, concomitant CNS medicines, and visual or auditory hallucinations. Monitor closely in case of the need for dose adjustment or discontinuation.

Monitor: EKGs, ROS, PE, blood, liver, kidney function, concomitant medication list

Specific Fluoroquinolone Options:

1. **Ciprofloxacin (Cipro** and over 300 brand names worldwide)

   Description: All information in the *General Fluoroquinolones* section may apply to ciprofloxacin.

   Indications: Infections of the lower respiratory tract, skin, bone, joints, sinuses, UTIs, infectious diarrhea, typhoid, GC, and with metronidazole for complicated abdominal infections. Used both post-exposure and as prophylaxis against anthrax

   Use in TBDs: Cipro has been reported to have efficacy in the treatment of Bartonella and M. *fermentans.* Also used against the Coxiella that causes Q fever

   Cautions: Cipro inhibits cytochrome P450 enzymes interfering with the metabolism of certain other drugs, increasing their blood concentration. Use caution with

other medications such as antidepressants, antipsychotics, caffeine, and theophylline. Ciprofloxacin also might interact with many supplements, herbal treatments, and thyroid medications.

Dosing: Available in tablets 100 mg, 250 mg, 500 mg, 750 mg, suspension 250 mg/5 ml and 500 mg/5 ml, and IV solution.

   Adults: 500 to 750 mg q 12 hours

   Children: Not recommended in under 18 unless severely ill and no other options and only for susceptible pathogens: 10 to 20 mg/kg q 12 hours with a maximum of 750 mg/day

AEs: Increased side effects in patients with pre-existing mental health complaints and cases of suicidal ideation and attempts. Panic, anxiety, and psychosis have been reported during or after Cipro treatment.

Monitor: Elimination of ciprofloxin is primarily through the kidney so establish adequate kidney function prior to starting Cipro and throughout treatment. Monitor as for any fluoroquinolone.

2. **Ofloxacin (Floxin)**

   Description: All information in the *General Fluoroquinolones* section may apply to ofloxacin.

   Indications: Chronic bronchitis, PID, community acquired pneumonias, GC, UTIs, skin infections, prostatitis, and abdominal infections. Floxin is not recommended in kids under 18, but you do see kids on this medicine. Be careful, especially in monitoring patients you get referred from other HCPs.

   Use in TBDs: Anecdotally, Floxin has been reported to have efficacy in the treatment of Bartonella and M. *fermentans.*

   Usage: Take on an empty stomach with plenty of water. Maintain adequate hydration

   Cautions: Be careful in patients with conditions that may increase seizure risk. Discontinue in patients with CNS effects, photosensitization, or tendon problems. Ofloxacin is category C for pregnancy and not recommended in nursing mothers.

   AEs: CNS stimulation, nervousness, anxiety, seizures, phototoxicity, GI complaints, insomnia, headache, dizziness, tendon problems

Dosing: Available in 200, 300, and 400 mg tablets

Over 18: 200 to 400 mg q 12 hours

Monitor: CBC, LFTs, kidney function. Monitor as for any fluoroquinolone.

3. Levofloxacin (Levaquin)

Description: All information in the *General Fluoroquinolones* section may apply to levofloxacin. Levofloxacin is a commonly used antibiotic and probably the most potent fluoroquinolone.

Indications: Serious or life-threatening bacterial infections due to susceptible bacteria

Use in TBDs: Has been used against infections due to M. *fermentans* and Bartonella. Some HCPs choose Levaquin as the DOC for BLOs using 500 mg daily for one to three months. Do a risk/benefit assessment and document your rationale for use in the patient chart.

Usage: Ensure that the patient has adequate renal function prior to prescribing and adequate hydration throughout therapy. Take solution on empty stomach. Generally well tolerated with almost no stomach upset. Some sources say that use of magnesium and Vitamin C lessens the risk of tendonitis.

Mepron or Malarone may lessen efficacy.

Dosing: Available in tablets (250 mg, 500 mg, 750 mg), injectable (5 mg/ml), and solution (125 mg/5 ml or 250 mg/10 ml). There should be a dosage guide in the label.

Children:	Under 18 not recommended
Adult:	250 to 750 once daily. If infusing, administer slowly over 60 to 90 minutes.

AEs: May cause confusion

Monitor: As listed for previous fluoroquinolones. Stop if any sxs of tendonitis.

General Macrolides

Description: Macrolides are mostly antibiotic drugs but also include a class of macrolide immunomodulators.

MOA: These molecules inhibit protein synthesis by impacting tRNA. Usually macrolides are bacteriostatic but they can become -cidal in higher doses. They may also decrease inflammation.

Indications: Wider range of effectiveness than PCNs and can be effective with more difficult pathogens including Mycoplasmas

Use in TBDs: Erythromycins do concentrate well in tissues and penetrate cells so they should be good agents for Lyme and certain other TBIs. But they have not performed as well as might be expected. Bb often resides inside a cell vacuole with low fluid pH. The acid may inactivate the azithromycin or clarithromycin, so consider using these agents in combination with hydroxychloroquine (Plaquenil) to raise the vacuolar pH.

Usage: In general, do not use two macrolides together and this includes clindamycin, which is technically NOT a macrolide but is similar enough to overload the metabolic enzyme systems. Also, since these agents use similar MOAs, you don't need to hit the pathogen the same way twice.

Cautions: Use with statin drugs can cause significant myopathy because of inhibition of the P450 enzyme system. Macrolides have been associated with QT prolongation that has led to torsades de pointes.

AEs: With macrolides, enterohepatic recycling occurs. These drugs are absorbed from the gut and then sent to the liver and eventually excreted into the duodenum via bile. The drugs and their metabolites can build up and often cause nausea.

Monitor: CBC and LFTs. If there is new muscle pain, consider CPK testing.

Specific Macrolide Options:

1. Erythromycin (EES, ERYC, E-Mycin)

Description: Antimicrobial spectrum similar to PCNs but broader and often used for patients with an allergy to PCNs or CSs. Not used as much in TBI patients as clarithromycin or azithromycin and is included here because it is the standard name in this class. Essentially all the information in the *General Macrolides* section applies here. This is your grandma's macrolide.

All erythromycins are easily inactivated by gastric acids so all oral formulations must be protected by enteric coating or attached to stable salts or esters. Erythromycin inhibits P450 enzymes so use can increase the blood concentration of other drugs that are metabolized by this same enzyme system, especially statins.

Use in TBDs: Erythromycin is not an adequate mono-therapy in Lyme or other TBDs.

2. Clarithromycin (Biaxin)

Description: Unlike erythromycin, clarithromycin is acid-stable and so can be taken orally without being protected from stomach acids. This drug works in many cases, it is just hard to tolerate due to bad tasting suspension, metallic aftertaste, and GI upset.

MOA: Readily absorbed and penetrates most tissues and white cells. Due to high concentrations in phagocytes, clarithromycin is transported to the site of infection. During phagocytosis, clarithromycin is released and can be present at high levels, especially in liver and lung tissue. Concentration at the infected site can be much higher than in the plasma and infected tissue is where you want the drug to be localized.

Indications: Used in sinusitis, bacterial bronchitis, and pneumonias

Use in TBDs: Clinically clarithromycin is thought to be more effective in Lyme than azithromycin but is less often selected because it is not as well tolerated.

Usage: When I was in active practice, I used a lot of Biaxin in adults. When the suspension became available, I was thrilled. Almost exactly 12 hours after I wrote my first prescription I got a call from the parents. They were able to get the first dose in the kid, but the second was impossible. While one parent was talking to me on the phone, I could hear the other parent chasing the poor child. That was not my last call about that product. Clarithromycin, in suspension, is probably the worst tasting stuff you can imagine (like fruit flavored liquid metal). Maybe they've improved it since I last tried, but the aftertaste seems to last for decades.

Take with food. If the kidney is compromised, either half the dose or double the dosing interval.

Cautions: Watch out for QT prolongation and use with caution in patients with a slow heart rate. Many pathogens develop resistance to clarithromycin. This drug may decrease the effectiveness of OCPs. Clarithromycin may also interact with HIV drugs. If there are liver or kidney problems, low potassium or magnesium, be wary and monitor carefully. Biaxin is not recommended in pregnancy or for young children.

Dosing: Available in 250 mg and 500 mg tablets and suspension 125 mg/5 ml and 250 mg/5 ml.

Adults: 250 to 1 gram q 12. Most common dose is 500 bid.

Children:

Less than 6 months not recommended

Greater than 6 months: 7.5 mg/kg q 12

Not recommended in pregnant women or very young children.

Hydroxychloroquine 200 to 400 mg/day can be added. The combination appears to enhance efficacy. Amantadine has also been used to increase the efficacy of clarithromycin at 100 to 200 mg/day, but I could not find the supportive mechanism for this combination.

AEs: Diarrhea, nausea, abdominal pain, vomiting, facial swelling, irritability, headaches, dizziness, motion sickness, rashes, altered senses of smell and taste, metallic taste that lasts after the drug is stopped, dry mouth, anxiety, hallucinations, nightmares, jaundice, liver disorders, kidney problems including failure, increased BUN, irregular heartbeats, chest pain, shortness of breath, false positives on cocaine drug testing, ototoxicity, delirium, mania, muscle pain when taken with statins, and fungal overgrowth. Allergic reactions have been reported from mild rashes to Stevens-Johnson syndrome and TEN. Leaves a bad metallic taste in the mouth. May cause excessive yeast. Poor GI tolerability in the doses needed to be effective.

Monitor: If long-term use, order regular EKGs looking for QT prolongation, CBC, LFTs, kidney function, and electrolytes

3. Azithromycin (Zithromax)

Description: Zithromax is readily absorbed and penetrates most tissues and white cells. Due to high concentrations in phagocytes, azithromycin is transported to the site of infection. During phagocytosis, it is released and can be especially high in the tissues. Concentration at the infected site can be much higher than in the plasma.

Azithromycin may be more effective against Hemophilus *influenza* than other macrolides. Some pathogens have developed resistance.

Indications: Bacterial infections of the sinuses, ears, throat, tonsils, lungs, skin, and urethra

Use in TBDs: In TBI patients, azithromycin is commonly used against Lyme in combination with other agents. Often selected as part of the regimen if M. *fermentans* is suspected. Azithromycin is effective against malaria when used in combination with artemesia and so is presumed to work against Babesia. With Lyme, expect a rapid and severe Herx, which may be a sign of efficacy. Appears quite effective when used IV in Lyme patients. In pregnant women with Bartonella, consider azithromycin with Bactrim. Used as part of combination regimen in pregnant and nursing mothers with Lyme.

Usage: Azithromycin is not destroyed by stomach acid so there is no need for enteric coating to protect the tablet and is therefore good for oral administration. Better absorbed on an empty stomach

PEARL: Azithromycin comes in prepackaged "packs" with 3 or 5 days of medicine inside. Patients love them because they validate the fact they are "really sick." In my experience, the patient gets better within the 3 to 5 days covered by the "pack" if they have a virus and didn't need an antibiotic in the first place – OR the 3 to 5 days is not long enough and they call asking for a refill because they are still sick. If I think they really have a bacterial infection that will benefit from this package, I write the refill on the original script.

Azithromycin is pregnancy category B which means it is not expected to be harmful to the unborn baby. May pass into the breast milk

A loading dose is often recommended, but a number of HCPs do not load when treating Bb. To load in adults start with 500 to 1000 mg on the first day and then 250 to 500 mg daily thereafter. In kids, 10 mg/kg on the first day up to 500 mg and then 5 mg/kg daily thereafter up to 250 mg/dose.

Dosing: Available as 250, 500, and 600 mg tablets and oral suspension 100 mg/5 ml and 200 mg/5 ml

Adults: 250 to 500 mg daily (higher doses up to 1200 mg/day may be considered in certain cases) given twice a day

Children:

Less than 6 months   Not recommended
Greater than 6 months   5 to 10 mg/kg/day up to 500 mg/day

PEARL: Azithromycin is often recommended as part of the combination regimen used in pregnant women with Lyme, usually 500 mg bid.

PEARL: IDSA recommends using a loading dose when treating babesiosis.

Azithromycin seems to be more effective in TBI patients when given IV but must be given through a

central line due to the caustic nature of the formulation. IV doses range from 500 to 1000 mg daily in both children and adults.

Hydroxychloroquine 200 to 400 mg/day can be added to enhance efficacy. Amantadine has also been mentioned in the literature as an enhancer but the MOA has not been divulged that I could find. (Makes me wonder if the patient actually had a primary viral infection and the antibiotic was just along for the ride.)

PEARL: If azithromycin is given parenterally (any way but the alimentary canal) results can be excellent but expect a rapid and severe Herx.

PEARL: In a March 12, 2013 report, azithromycin was associated with dysrhythmias likely associated with QT prolongation.

Monitor: Baseline and intermittent EKGs for QT prolongation and dysrhythmia

4. **Telithromycin (Ketek)**

Description: Telithromycin is thought to be the most effective drug in the class. Ketek is not strictly a macrolide but rather a ketolide, which is structurally related. Ketek is stable in the intracellular acid environment and is probably the most effective of the class for Bb. The bottom line is that this drug works but is despised by the FDA because of its safety profile. Whether their impression is valid or a little over-reactive is yet to be determined. Do not discount this drug. As with my son, who was allergic to a number of the medicines that might have been a first choice for his combination of co-infections, sometimes options are limited. His long course of Ketek was carefully monitored and there was no hint of ADRs. Ketek is said to build less drug resistance than many other antibiotics. Organisms are less likely to become resistant to the ketolides because they have a double-binding site. (I don't know what that means either.)

MOA: Ketolides interfere with protein synthesis and are much stronger than the original erythromycins. Ketek distributes throughout the body and has a high concentration at the site of infection due to release from phagocytes.

Indications: Susceptible bacterial infections of the lungs and sinuses. Especially useful in respiratory infections resistant to other macrolides

Use in TBDs: Effective against Bb. In fact, some HCPs speculate that Ketek may be the best oral agent for Lyme. This drug can be hard for some patients to tolerate, so use may be limited for that reason. Ketek has also been used anecdotally against Bartonella, Mycoplasma, and other Borrelia species.

Usage: Ketek is a CYP3A-4 inhibitor and interacts with Rifampin, statins, Diflucan, and numerous other drugs through competition for the same metabolic cytochrome enzymes.

Ketek is pregnancy category C which means there could be harm to the fetus and the drug should be used with caution in nursing mothers. Ketek should be avoided in pregnancy. Always conduct a risk/benefit assessment and document your rationale.

Ketek has little impact on the E. *coli* in the GI tract, so there is less diarrhea than with many other agents. The molecule is acid stable so it can be taken orally and not be inactivated in the stomach. Ketek can be taken with or without food which can be an advantage when on a multi-drug regimen.

Cautions: Do not use in cases of QT prolongation, slow heart rate, hypokalemia, renal impairment, myasthenia gravis, or liver dysfunction. Pregnancy category C. Use with caution in nursing mothers. Ketek can cause a strong and long Herx. Numerous drug interactions

Dosing: Not recommended for kids under 18

Adults: 800 mg daily. Available as 400 mg tablets

AEs: GI upset, headache, dysgeusia (distorted taste), dizziness, transient visual disturbances such as delayed accommodation, trouble focusing, and blurred or double vision. Ringing in the ears has been discussed in the literature. False positive results for cocaine and amphetamines on drug tests have been associated with Ketek. As a certified Medical Review Officer for drug testing, I admit that I do not know what the mechanism of this reaction would be but I'm sure somewhere somebody has a reasonable explanation, (especially the guy who passed the drug test by blaming the result on Ketek.)

Liver abnormalities have been noted but generally are thought to be reversible. Nonetheless, liver failure and subsequent death have been associated with the use of Ketek. The potential for liver damage is one reason the FDA is so uncomfortable.

Strong and prolonged Herxheimer reactions may occur.

PEARL: The FDA removed previously approved indications for Ketek and instituted a black box warning that Ketek should not be used in patients with myasthenia gravis, a disease that causes muscle weakness. Dr. Graham, a drug safety physician with the FDA, was especially resistant to the approval of this drug and one clinical investigator is currently in prison for falsifying safety data on this product. Graham, often controversial, makes points that should not be lightly discounted.

Monitor: Measure the QT interval before starting this drug, but this is not always possible. If on baseline EKG, or patient history, the QT is prolonged or the heart rate is slow, reconsider your options. If you are not comfortable assessing QT prolongation, make sure you have a back-up who can read these EKGs for you. Monitor the EKGs regularly throughout the course of treatment. After Ketek is stopped, do another EKG to document a normal interval.

Try to establish a baseline LFT and kidney function to ensure the patient is stable enough to handle this drug and then religiously monitor these systems.

Watch for eye problems such as blurring, changes in accommodation, and double vision. These disturbances are thought to be transient but be vigilant.

PEARL: Because of limited options, this drug was used in my son. Of course, at the time it was prescribed I had never heard of it or the disease that it was supposed to eradicate. Knowing what I know now, I would use the Ketek and continue to monitor carefully.

Consider blood work every two weeks and at a minimum monthly. Measure CBC, electrolytes, LFTs, BUN, and creatinine.

Be cognizant of the possibility of drug interactions because Ketek is a CYP3A-4 inhibitor. Check QTc and LFTs. Since the use of Ketek can be a hot button issue, protect yourself and the patient when you use this drug by monitoring appropriately AND documenting in the patient's chart your rationale for selecting this medicine.

PEARL: Do not get all these "T" antibiotics mixed up: telithromycin (Ketek), tinidazole (Tindamax), tigecycline (Tygacil). You think you won't, but you will. Be careful.

5. Pediazole (macrolide and sulfa)

Pediazole is a combination of 200 mg erythromycin with 600 mg sulfisoxazole in 5 ml suspension. Used for H. *influenzae* otitis in children but in TBI patients may be applicable where you would consider a macrolide or a sulfa. If you are allergic to sulfa, you will be allergic to Pediazole, but otherwise the drug appears to be well tolerated. Pediazole has been used long-term in many children as a preventive measure against recurrent AOM. Pleasant tasting in oral suspension.

General Lincosamides

Description: Lincosamides are very similar in structure and function to the macrolides but tend to be effective against more species. Clindamycin (Cleocin), a lincosamide antibiotic, is most often used to treat very serious anaerobic bacterial infections but is also effective in protozoal diseases like malaria and babesiosis. See "Antimalarial" section below.

General Sulfonamides

Description: Sulfas were among the first commercial antibiotic drugs, starting in the 1930s, and they prompted a sulfa craze with hundreds of manufacturers. Tons of sulfa drugs were sold with no regulatory oversight. In 1937, hundreds of people were poisoned after taking a sulfa elixir. This tragedy helped lead to the passage of the Federal Food, Drug and Cosmetic Act of 1938. Sulfa was used throughout World War II and was credited with saving countless lives including FDR's son and Churchill himself. Soldiers were given first aid kits containing sulfa powder to sprinkle on open wounds and this saved tens of thousands.

Specific Sulfa Options:

1. **Sulfonamide and folic acid inhibitor** (Sulfamethoxazole 400 mg and trimethoprim 80 mg in brands like **Bactrim** and **Septra**. The doses are double in Bactrim DS and Septra DS, that is, 800 mg and 160 mg). These are "sulfa" drugs so if you are allergic to sulfas, you are allergic to this.

   MOA: The synergy between trimethoprim and sulfamethoxazole is well documented. Because they inhibit successive steps in the folate synthesis pathway, they have greater efficacy when given together than they do separately. Bacteria are unable to take up folic acid from the host due to enzyme inhibition so the bacteria are deprived of two essential nucleoside bases needed for DNA replication. Folic acid (folate) is an essential precursor to synthesize DNA nucleosides. These agents are bacteriostatic.

Indications: Sulfas are often the DOC for UTIs and have been used successfully in many bacterial, protozoal, and fungal infections including OM, Pneumocystis pneumonia, travelers' diarrhea, shigellosis, bacterial bronchitis, and MRSA.

Use in TBDs: Thought to be effective against malaria and likely some activity against Babesia as well. Bactrim can be considered as a part of combination therapy in bartonellosis. In pregnant women with Bartonella, consider azithromycin and Bactrim. As always, do a risk/benefit analysis since Bactrim is pregnancy category C. There is speculation that Bactrim may also hit M. *fermentans*. There is considerable controversy around whether or not Bactrim hits Bb. If Bactrim does hit Bb it doesn't seem to do so very well. The consensus appears to be to choose other alternatives first. I do not understand why an HCP would select Bactrim for Lyme with so many other options, but stranger things have happened.

Usage: Do not take with Vitamin C. Take with large quantities of water to prevent crystalluria. Best absorption if taken without food: 1 hour before or 2 hours after meals. Bactrim is pregnancy category C.

Cautions: ALLERGIES! While PCNs may have the most frequent reports of allergies, the sulfas may have the most severe. Contraindicated in porphyria. Use with caution when liver or kidney impaired. Do not use in patients with folate deficiency or G6PD deficiency. Sulfa drugs may acidify urine, causing precipitation of various crystals. Any sign of allergic manifestations, call the prescriber immediately before taking the next dose. If breathing difficulties or swelling occurs, seek emergency help.

Dosing: Available in tablets: Sulfamethoxazole 400 mg and trimethoprim 80 mg in brands such as Bactrim and Septra. The doses are double in Bactrim DS and Septra DS, that is, 800 mg and 160 mg. Also in suspension: sulfa 200 mg and trimethoprim 40 mg in 5 ml. Can be given IV in slow 60 to 90 minute infusions

Adults: One DS or two regular tablets q 12

Children: Over 2 months: 8 mg/kg trimethoprim and 40 mg/kg sulfa in two doses q 12.

For routine UTIs, 14 days of treatment is recommended.

AEs: Allergies, blood dyscrasias, agranulocytosis, aplastic anemia, hemolytic anemia, low platelets, low white cell counts, porphyria, headache, depression, seizures, hallucinations, nausea, vomiting, diarrhea, abdominal pain, anorexia, drug fever, mydriasis, liver failure, hepatic necrosis, nephrosis, oliguria, anuria, hematuria, crystalluria, jaundice, erythema multiforme, Stevens-Johnson syndrome, general rashes, TEN, photosensitivity, urticaria, pruritis, hypersensitivity reactions, and anaphylaxis. Patients with HIV report a higher incidence of AEs on sulfa drugs. Elderly and pregnant women, especially if the drug is taken in the last 6 weeks of pregnancy, could have higher rates of side effects. Sulfa can displace the bilirubin from albumin and there could be an increased risk of kernicterus in the newborn.

Monitor: Urine, blood (CBC), liver (LFTs), and kidney function. Since sulfas are metabolized in the liver and excreted by the kidney, you will want to ensure the on-going health of these systems in long-term treatment.

2. **Pediazole** (macrolide and sulfa)

Pediazole is a combination of 200 mg erythromycin with 600 mg sulfisoxazole in 5 ml of suspension. This combination product is used for H. *influenzae* otitis in children. In TBI patients, Pediazole may be applicable whenever you would consider a macrolide or a sulfa. Those allergic to sulfa will be allergic to Pediazole, but otherwise the drug appears to be well tolerated. Pediazole has been used long-term in many children as a preventive measure against recurrent AOM. This medicine is pleasant tasting in oral suspension.

General Cephalosporins (CSs)

Description: Cephalosporins were first isolated from a sewer in Sardinia in 1948. (I once had a business associate with an identical pedigree.) These drugs are organized into different generations largely in chronological order. The later generations are said to have better efficacy and safety. But remember, a first generation in Japan might be a second generation in Spain. The early generations aren't used much anymore. The later generations get better blood concentrations and have a longer half-life so they don't need to be taken as often. Cephalosporins can be effective when PCNs and TCNs fail. While there are dozens of cephalosporins in each generation, TBI patients are most likely to come across the few described in more detail below.

MOA: Cephalosporins are bacteriocidal. They have the same MOA as other β-lactams such as PCNs but are not as vulnerable to the penicillinases. They disrupt the pathogens' cell walls, so that proper structural cross-links cannot form and the integrity of the cell wall is lost and breaks. Most bacteria have cell walls that protect them and once the cell wall is broken the bacteria die.

Cautions: Because of similar chemical structures, cephalosporins have cross-reactive allergies to PCNs. If you are allergic to one class, you are at increased risk of allergies to the other. Some cephalosporins have been associated with clotting problems and some cause a disulfiram-like reaction after drinking alcohol.

AEs: Generally cephalosporins have few side effects compared to other antibiotics. Here diarrhea, nausea, rash, electrolyte abnormalities, allergies, vomiting, headache, dizziness, overgrowth of Candida, pseudomembranous colitis, superinfection, eosinophilia, and fever have all been reported.

Specific Cephalosporin Options:

1. **Cefuroxime (Ceftin)**

Description: A 2nd generation cephalosporin and the most common oral cephalosporin used in TBI patients

Indications: Infections of the throat, tonsils, sinuses, lungs, middle ear, skin, urinary tract, and "early" Lyme. Unlike most other 2nd generation cephalosporins, cefuroxime can cross the blood brain barrier.

Use in TBDs: Unlike essentially every other antibiotic mentioned in these pages, Ceftin is actually indicated for the treatment of "early" Lyme. The Ceftin package insert, in fact, uses the term "Spirochetes" under which it simply says, "Borrelia *burgdorferi*." The final instruction under Ceftin Tablets (number 8 to be precise) says that these tablets can be used in "Early Lyme Disease (erythema migrans) caused by Borrelia *burgdorferi*." With all empathy to the drug developers at the company, they were just trying to get the indication on the books and get a good performance review. They felt no compunction to understand the disease. Although incidence rates vary, Lyme presents with an EM rash in less than half the cases.

Beyond the label, some authors believe Ceftin kills Bb only when the pathogens are active. Once threatened by an antibiotic, the Bb may hide deep in the tissue or encyst in a hard shell. When the treatment stops, the pathogen perceives that it is safe to re-emerge and they reappear along with the symptoms of the infection. Higher doses and repeated courses may be needed to eradicate the organism, which can be quite resilient. Consider an aggressive combination regimen, adding intracellular and cyst-busting agents, as appropriate.

Ceftin may be good in Amoxil and doxy failures. Some HCPs chose Ceftin when the patient has an EM rash, especially if concurrent infection with common skin pathogens is suspected (although that concept does not make medical sense to me).

Usage: Give with food. Can be used during pregnancy

Cautions: PCNs and CSs are structurally similar, so if the patient is allergic to one they have a higher risk of allergy to the other. Antacids may decrease absorption.

Dosing: Available in 250 and 500 mg tablets and in 125 mg/5 ml and 250 mg/5 ml suspension

Adults: For Lyme 500 mg to 1 gram bid

Children:

> Greater than 3 months: 20 to 30 mg/kg per day in two divided doses. This translates to 125 to 500 mg bid depending on the patient's weight with a maximum of 1 gram/day
>
> Over 13: 250 mg to 500 mg bid

PEARL: Ceftin has been suggested as part of a combination regimen for pregnant women with Lyme, usually 1 gram q 12 plus azithromycin.

PEARL: Other common 2nd generation cephalosporins include cefaclor (Ceclor) and loracarbef (Lorabid).

PEARL: I do not know any experienced TBI doctor who uses Ceftin as a solo agent against Lyme despite the "official" indication.

2. Ceftriaxone (Rocephin)

Description: A 3rd generation –cidal antibiotic, Rocephin is the most common IV treatment for Lyme. Ceftriaxone can be administered po, IM, or IV.

MOA: Rocephin blasts the spirochetes by stimulating a gene that limits the amount of the biomolecule, glutamate. Excessive glutamate at the nerve endings has been tied to ALS and suppression of this molecule may eventually become a treatment for ALS.

Indications: Gonorrhea, susceptible septicemia, PID, meningitis

Use in TBDs: Rocephin is commonly used intravenously in Lyme disease especially in those patients who are severely or chronically ill and is considered a good foundation drug on which to build a combination drug strategy.

Rocephin started to be used for Lyme in the 1980s. In some cases, it seems like nothing else will work but long-term IV Rocephin. Rocephin appears to kill Bb but may take longer to get the overall –cidal effect than a drug like tigecycline, which may kill *in vitro* within 24 hours. Still, Rocephin is the tried and true IV therapy for Lyme. Since the medicine can be given in a split bid dose instead of a continuous infusion, this regimen is convenient for at-home use.

Rocephin may cause spirochetes to go into cystic form. Some controversial sources say this is reason enough NOT to treat Lyme with IV Rocephin. Nonetheless, there is a subpopulation of Lyme patients who do not do well off their Rocephin and relapse when the medicine is discontinued. To be functional, they prefer the treatment. Always consider combining the Rocephin with an intracellular agent. A cyst-buster can be added to the Rocephin regimen to mitigate the possibility of relapse.

Fallon showed that with Rocephin therapy, the patients with the most symptoms when the drug was started showed the most improvement. Their pain decreased more and they had better cognition. The mechanism that Fallon described had to do with glutamate transport. This may partially explain how Rocephin helps resolve neurologic symptoms. Unfortunately, Rocephin itself may cause neurological problems over time. Some practitioners report that a number of their Lyme patients did not achieve the success with IV ceftriaxone that they had expected. Treatment in TBIs is always a balancing act.

IV therapy is postulated to be many times more potent than oral dosing in killing Bb so consider IV Rocephin when you find a patient with severe, intractable, chronic, or later-stage symptoms.

PEARL: Some practitioners prefer to use Rocephin early in the clinical course of Lyme rather than wait. Try to target the plan to the individual case.

PEARL: Glutamate is a neurotransmitter. Do not get this mixed up with the antioxidant glutathione.

Usage: IM or IV Rocephin comes in vials of 250 mg, 500 mg, 1 gram, and 2 grams. Often given 4 days in a row each week. Rocephin can be infused in the HCP office, by home health personnel, or by caretakers. Pulsing the IV regimen may decrease the likelihood of gallstones, i.e., **4 days on and 3 days off**.

Rocephin also comes in 300 mg capsules but this drug's primary advantage seems to lie in the ease of its IV administration.

Rocephin may alter the absorption of other drugs and should not be taken near other medications. Give one hour before or 4 hours after any other medicines. Rocephin may also interfere with absorption of fat-soluble vitamins.

One common regimen in older, larger children: 2 to 4 grams daily either as 1 or 2 grams IV bid or the entire dose slowly infused, four days in a row each week for 14 or more weeks. Regular three day breaks seem to lessen complications like biliary stones and colitis and is less costly with a better QOL. So as to reduce the number of needle sticks, consider a capped IV with a heparin lock.

PEARL: Most Rocephin patients have a PICC line with the medicine going directly into a central vessel. About 30% have midline access. Others are successful with peripheral veins.

Rocephin can be used in pregnant females.

Cautions: Gallstones can form in patients on ceftriaxone. Rocephin is a unique antibiotic in that it is eliminated from the body in the bile in high concentrations. In the gallbladder, the ceftriaxone combines with calcium and becomes insoluble, forming particles that can grow into stones. Most of these stones dissolve once the antibiotic is discontinued, but until they are gone, they can cause problems. Since Rocephin has a 95% biliary excretion and can form sludge and crystallize in the biliary tree causing stones and colic, patients tend to do better if pulsed 4 days in a row out of the week, with a 3 day break. (I know I have repeated that point too often, but it's important.)

Most people who take Rocephin do NOT get gallstones. About 2% of kids on long-term Rocephin did have GB problems and about 1% had to have their GBs removed.

Before starting Rocephin ask the patient if they have ever had gallbladder problems. Is there a family history? Order a baseline GB ultrasound and then follow the patient with regular ultrasounds of the gallbladder throughout the course of therapy. Make sure the patient knows to contact you if there is any RUQ discomfort after starting the Rocephin treatment. Other common symptoms of gallstones are epigastric pain, vague nausea, occasional vomiting, bloating, and gassiness. Pain can radiate into the back or shoulder. Usually the pain increases after food but otherwise remains fairly constant. Often, Actigall is ordered to dissolve current stones and to try to prevent more from forming. Actigall at 1 to 3 tabs per day is co-administered.

More information on Actigall is found in Chapter 25: *Ancillary Treatments.*

PEARL: Order a baseline US of the GB and then another every month throughout the treatment course. For those who are at a higher risk of stone formation (past personal history or family history), USs may need to be done weekly. After discontinuation of the Rocephin therapy, consider US of the GB for three consecutive months after the cessation of treatment.

If the patient develops gallstones, stop the Rocephin and find an alternative antibiotic for the patient's TBI. Continue the Actigall until resolution. Of course, more aggressive treatment for the stones may be needed if there is obstruction or other complications. Don't forget about the underlying TBI while you are dealing with the gallstones.

PEARL: Make sure the patient and parents understand the risk of Rocephin therapy. Together weigh the risk/benefit of this IV treatment.

Rocephin should not be used in premature babies with bilirubin problems. Do not give to hyperbilirubinemic neonates especially if premature. Use a lower dose if known hepatic or renal dysfunction. Never mix ceftriaxone with calcium containing solutions. There have been cases reported of calcium-ceftriaxone precipitates in lung and kidney.

PCNs and CSs are structurally similar, so if the patient is allergic to one s/he has a higher risk of allergy to the other.

Dosing: Recommended doses vary in the literature.

Adults: 1 to 2 grams IM or IV once daily or in 2 divided doses. Max 4 grams/day

Children: 50 to 75 mg/kg per day in 2 equally divided doses q 12 up to 2 grams/day

PEARL: Rocephin has been used in pregnant women with Lyme. One suggested course is 2 grams IV four days on and three days off per week.

The sicker the patient, usually the higher the dose. *Pulse* the regimen four days on and three days off to reduce the risk of gallstones. A peripheral IV line with cap can minimize needle sticks.

Concomitant Actigall can be used to prevent gallstones. The Actigall can be given orally.

AEs: in addition to stone formation, Rocephin has been associated with abdominal pain, constipation, dyspepsia, diarrhea, nausea, vomiting, headache, and dizziness. High blood sugars and IV site reactions have also been reported.

Monitor: Gallbladder ultrasounds at baseline and regularly throughout treatment. Keep an eye on the liver functions. Monitor CBC and LFTs q two weeks and increase to weekly if any abnormalities are uncovered.

PEARL: Other common 3ʳᵈ generation cephalosporins: cefdinir (Omnicef) and cefixime (Suprax)

3. Cefotaxime (Claforan)

Description: A 3ʳᵈ generation –cidal antibiotic, Claforan can be given IM or IV. Considered by some to be equivalent to Rocephin in safety and efficacy. Claforan may be less susceptible to resistance than many other PCNs and CSs.

MOA: Inhibits cell wall synthesis in the pathogen. The cell wall assembly is arrested. The organism can't make new walls or stop the old walls from breaking. The cells eventually die through lysis.

Indications: A broad spectrum antibiotic used in moderate to severe illness when caused by a susceptible organism. Often selected in life-threatening situations. Used in sensitive pneumonias, UTIs, GU and gyn infections, PID, sepsis, bone, joint, or skin infections. Claforan is used in CNS infections including meningitis.

Use in TBDs: Seems to penetrate the BBB and can be considered if there are neurologic symptoms. Considered by some to be equivalent to Rocephin in safety and efficacy in Lyme patients, seemingly without the gallstone complications. There may be transient changes in LFTs. Once IV administration is decided upon, begin the infusions as soon as feasible to try to decrease the chance of progression to the point where full recovery is less likely. Claforan may be less susceptible to resistance than many other PCNs and CSs. Further, there seems to be less impact on the gut flora than with a number of other antibiotics.

Usage: Make sure that an IM injection hits deep into the muscle. Aspirate before injection to avoid inadvertent IV injection. For IV infusions of Claforan, ensure that the injection is slow (at least 3 minutes).

Can be used in pregnancy

Cautions: Claforan does not seem to have the same problem with gallstones and biliary complications as does Rocephin.

Dosing:

For mild infections, Claforan can be given in single IM doses of 0.5 grams. While this drug can be administered q 12, the more frequent the dosing, the better the efficacy. Every 6 to 8 hours is often selected, but continuous infusion is probably most efficacious. If the plan is to give greater than 6 grams/day, consider a pulsing regimen of 4 days on and 3 days off.

Adults:

Mild infection:	1 to 2 grams IM or IV q 8
Moderate:	6 to 8 grams/day giving 2 grams per dose q 6 to 8 hours
Life-threatening:	2 grams IV q 4 h up to 12 grams/day

Children:

0 to 1 week:	50 mg/kg/dose q 12 h IV
1 to 4 weeks:	50 mg/kg/dose q 8 h IV

1 month to 12 yrs:

Less than 50 kg: 50 to 180 mg/kg IM or IV divided into 4 or 6 equal doses

Greater than 50 kg: Adult doses up to a maximum of 12 gram/day

PEARL: One regimen suggested for pregnant women with Lyme is 6 grams daily either through continuous infusion or as 2 grams IV q 8 plus azithromycin.

Use IV at higher doses if the patient is really sick. Continue treatment until symptoms resolve and do not relapse upon discontinuation. This may be several months in TBI patients.

Claforan must be given **at least** q 8 or more frequently to keep up the blood levels. This is less convenient than the bid dosing of Rocephin. If giving more than 3 or 4 doses a day, continuous infusion may be more prudent, as well as more efficacious.

A pulsed dose schedule is often selected. Four or five days on with a 2 or 3 day interim break

AEs: Injection site reactions. Seems to have less impact on intestinal flora and the subsequent sequelae than other cephalosporins

Monitor: Kidney function

4. Cefdinir (Omnicef)

Description: Oral cephalosporin

Indications: Pneumonias, bronchitis, sinusitis, pharyngitis, tonsillitis, skin infections, AOM

Use in TBDs: Omnicef is often a good choice when selecting an oral cephalosporin. Omnicef in combination with Zithromax can be used when treating a child with a first bout of Lyme.

Usage: Pregnancy category B. Do not take with Mg or Al antacids or iron supplements. Separate by 2 hours

Dosing: Available as 300 mg capsules or 125 mg/5 ml or 250 mg/5 ml suspension

Adults :	> 13 y/o:	300 mg q 12
Kids:	6 months to 12 years:	7 mg/kg q 12 with 600 mg/day max

PEARL: One regimen suggested in pregnant women with Lyme is 300 to 600 mg bid plus Azithromycin.

AEs: GI upset, headache, rash, allergies

<u>**General Azoles**</u>

Description: Azole antimicrobials have far-reaching uses against a wide variety of pathogens from fungus to anaerobic bacteria to protozoas like Entamoebas, Giardia, and Trichomonas and all their corresponding manifestations. Often these drugs are included in the list of antimalarials since the causative agent of malaria is a protozoan as is that of the TBI babesiosis. These agents are considered to be cyst-busters and may be effective in those pathogens that are thought to encyst when challenged by antibiotics. For this reason azoles are often useful as part of **combination** therapy in TBIs. Metronidazole and tinidazole are the most commonly used of this class in TBI patients. Grapefruit seed extract may also have a similar mechanism.

MOA: Although the mechanism by which azoles operate is complicated, they seem to interfere with the energy making apparatus inside the pathogen through diversion of electrons. Most of these drugs form cytotoxic metabolites that eventually destroy the cell. Some may cause the unwinding of the DNA helix in the genetic material of the microbe.

Cautions: With azoles, the patient should avoid alcohol during treatment and for 3 days afterward. These drugs should not be used within weeks of disulfiram. Azoles do have a number of drug interactions. They can inspire significant Candida overgrowth. Probiotics might help with fungus and GI upset. Watch for neurologic adverse events.

PEARL: There are anecdotal reports of tolerability problems with generic azoles compared to branded products. Given my experience with generic companies, I recommend using caution in all cases. If you wouldn't drink the water...

Specific Azole Options:

1. Metronidazole (Flagyl)

Description: One of the first azoles to be developed, metronidazole was found to have very high activity against Amoebas and Trichomona.

MOA: A -cidal agent, metronidazole likely interferes with energy production and DNA replication inside the pathogen cell. Metronidazole is taken up by diffusion into the cell of select anaerobic bacteria and sensitive protozoa. Inside the microbe, the drug is metabolized in a way that results in products toxic to the pathogenic cells. These toxins accumulate in anaerobes and form unstable molecules. These reactions usually happen only in anaerobic microbes and protozoal cells so there is relatively little effect upon healthy human cells or aerobic bacteria.

Indications: Extremely broad spectrum, metronidazole is used to treat all manner of protozoal infections including Entamoebas, Giardia, and Trichomonas species. Flagyl is classified as an antimalarial by many sources and is quite effective against the Plasmodium protozoan that causes malaria. Babesia is a protozoa as well.

Used against anaerobic infections of the abdomen, skin, bone, joints, CNS, lower respiratory tract, endocardium, and for a number of gyn infections including sexually transmitted vaginitis. Flagyl is also indicated prior to abdominal surgery and dental procedures. Flagyl can also be used to treat Helicobacter *pylori*, the bacteria implicated in peptic ulcer disease, and is thought to be effective in many cases of MRSA.

While many antibiotics have the potential to cause C. *difficile* overgrowth with its savage diarrhea and potential for pseudomembranous colitis, Flagyl is that rare antibiotic that does NOT cause overgrowth of C. *difficile*. In fact, metronidazole is the DOC in treating this condition.

Use in TBIs: Flagyl is a common agent used to treat TBIs in combination with other antimicrobials. In Lyme, Flagyl is often considered when the presentation is predominantly neurologic. Bb are thought to encyst, especially in and around CNS tissue. Flagyl is thought to penetrate these cysts, leaving the pathogen vulnerable. With some pathogens, the Flagyl may make a direct kill.

PEARL: When Bb are present in a hostile environment like when exposed to antibiotics, the organisms can go into a cystic form. Here they can remain dormant until conditions are more favorable, like when the antibiotic is stopped. Then the Bb can revert back into the spirochete form. Conventional treatments for Bb like PCNs, CSs, and TCNs do not usually penetrate the cystic form. However, metronidazole seems able to enter these cysts. Then the Bb can be damaged either by the Flagyl itself or by the concomitant antibiotics that are able to get to the Bb after Flagyl breaks down the door. If the patient is chronically infected, consider metronidazole with one or two other antibiotics. This ensures that all Bb forms are targeted. Caution: TCNs, such as doxycycline, may inhibit the effect of Flagyl so watch using metronidazole with TCN combinations.

For Lyme, Flagyl is effectively combined with Bicillin or with Ketek or Zithromax. The combination of Biaxin and Flagyl should hit both Bb and Babesia. In patients who are experiencing a Herx from other antibiotics, an added cyst-buster may be what is needed to break through to some of the pathogens not reachable by cell wall or intracellular antibiotics.

Flagyl is commonly part of the **combination** strategy used in the treatment of Babesia *microti*. Since Bb and Babesia are so often found together, Flagyl might be considered when you are trying to hit these two TBIs at once.

Usage: Some providers prefer to pulse Flagyl 2 weeks on and 2 weeks off. For novice users, Flagyl is sometimes hard to tolerate. Pulsing may help. Usually the therapy is started with oral Flagyl, but this can be hard to endure. Give with food to decrease GI distress. Since metronidazole has a unique MOA, it is often selected to complement other drugs in combination therapy.

Metronidazole may be a carcinogen and mutagen that might cause birth defects and pre-term births. Contraindicated in the first trimester of pregnancy, it is considered category B in the 2nd and 3rd trimesters. Not recommended in young children unless other options are limited. If you decide to use this drug in a young child, be sure to document your rationale in the medical record and note that the caretakers and patient understand the risk/benefit.

Flagyl can be administered IV and this may attenuate some of the GI distress associated with the oral preps. While on metronidazole, avoid all alcohol including cough medicines or mouthwashes with alcohol. Some sources recommend that the patient take a daily multivitamin with B complex when taking Flagyl, presumably to moderate neurologic effects. Probiotics may help with the likely fungal overgrowth and GI upset.

A **loading dose** is often used to prime the blood level.

Cautions: Make sure the patient is tolerating the oral formulation. Dosing with food and using a pulsed regimen may make the medicine more endurable.

If taken with alcohol, Flagyl may cause a disulfiram-like reaction of nausea, vomiting, confusion, cramps, headache, flushing, tachycardia, and SOB. Do not use with disulfiram. Do not use with hepatotoxins. Use with caution in patients with a history of blood dyscrasias, CNS problems, or retinal or visual field disorders.

Flagyl may result in a strong Herx reaction in TBI patients.

There may be additional adverse events associated with taking metronidazole with antidepressants in the SSRI and SNRI categories. Flagyl can be irritating to the nervous system causing irritability and spaciness. In the long-term, Flagyl can affect peripheral nerves causing tingling and numbness. If symptoms are mild, lowering the dose may eliminate the problem. Who decides what is mild? With neurologic symptoms, consider discontinuation. Always consider the risk/benefit relationship. B vitamins might help diminish these symptoms.

Metronidazole is not recommended in pregnancy.

Dosing: Available in 250 and 500 mg tablets and 375 capsules. Injectable formulation for IV use is 500 mg/100 ml. Infuse over at least one hour

Adults: 250 to 750 mg po tid translated to 15 mg/kg (loading dose) and then 7.5 mg/kg q 6 hours with a maximum of 4 grams/day

Children: Use in children only if options are limited. Otherwise, not recommended

    Less than 120 pounds: 250 mg tid

    120 to 150 pounds: 500 mg tid

AEs: Use of metronidazole may cause reddish-brown urine. Yeast overgrowth is common. Depending on the pathogen, there may be a strong Herx reaction.

Overall, Flagyl is thought to have a good safety profile but it is not always well tolerated by some patients. There is a difference between **safety** and **tolerability**. To put this another way: The drug won't kill you, but you might wish it had. Some patients have no AEs at all and others must stop the drug.

AEs reported with use of Flagyl include: leukopenia, neutropenia, vertigo, headache, ataxia, incoordination, confusion, irritability, depression, restlessness, weakness, fatigue, drowsiness, insomnia, neuropathy, paresthesias, stimulation, seizures, myopathy, flattened T wave on EKG, blurred vision, diminished visual fields, nasal congestion, abdominal cramping, stomatitis, nausea, vomiting, anorexia, diarrhea, constipation, proctitis, dry mouth, dark urine, polyuria, dysuria, pyuria, incontinence, cystitis, itch, flushing, overgrowth of non-susceptible organisms, glossitis, metallic taste, fever, abnormal blood chemistries, allergic reactions including rare Stevens-Johnson syndrome, and thrombophlebitis. Injection site irritation has been associated with IV use.

Monitor: Consider at least monthly blood work: CBC with WBC differential, LFTs, and blood chemistries including electrolytes, BUN, and creatinine. Watch for new or increased tingling, numbness, and neurologic signs indicating a need for dose adjustment or discontinuation. Regularly assess vision and visual fields.

2. Tinidazole (Tindamax)

Description: Tinidazole is a second generation nitro-imidazole useful against both sexually transmitted and water-borne protozoa such as Amoebas and Giardia.

PEARL: Do not get tinidazole mixed up with tigacycline or telithromycin. One is an azole, one is a tetracycline, and one is a macrolide. Make sure the one you are writing for is the one you want.

MOA: The MOA likely interferes with the pathogen's cell wall, energy production, and DNA replication.

Indications: Protozoas such as Trichomona, Giardia, and Amoebas

Use in TBIs: Tindamax gets the cystic form as well as the spirochetal form of Bb and may be even better at penetrating the cyst than metronidazole. Tindamax hits all three of the Bb life forms: spirochetal, intracellular, and encysted. (In comparison, Flagyl hits primarily the cystic form.) Tindamax may be better tolerated than Flagyl. In TBIs it is often pulsed either in alternate weeks or two weeks on and two weeks off. The regimen varied in the literature. Tindamax is used in combination therapy for Lyme and may be effective against the protozoal agent of Babesia as well. Unlike Flagyl, Tindamax can be used in kids.

PEARL: Pulse Tindamax in a way that best suits the individual case.

Usage: Take with food. Tindamax is probably better tolerated than Flagyl.

This drug was designed to be effective with short treatment courses from one dose to a few days, but may be needed longer-term with some of the TBIs.

Tindamax is CI in the 1st trimester of pregnancy and is considered category C for the 2nd and 3rd trimesters. Not recommended during nursing and no breastfeeding for three days after the last dose.

Available in 250 mg and 500 mg tablets.

Fungal overgrowth is common and probiotics might help.

Cautions: Tindamax interacts with alcohol and disulfiram, potentiates anticoagulants, and is antagonized by CYP450 inducers and potentiated by CYP inhibitors. Since no one but a world-renown azole pharmacologist knows what that means in real life, be aware that azoles can mess with just about any other medicine the patient is taking. Check the label and keep an eye on the patient. Adjust doses as needed to accommodate the necessary medications. Here is a good place to NOT tax the system with non-essential supplements.

Tindamax boasts a LONG list of potential drug interactions including herbals, grapefruit juice, vitamins, anticoagulants, antifungals, numerous antibiotics, anti-convulsants, and immunosuppressants. The list is so long that it even includes zafirlukast, a drug I worked on a million years ago that may no longer be available. I guess they didn't want to leave anything out. If you are planning to put a patient on Tindamax, check the medications that the individual is taking against the list in the package insert. This doesn't mean you can't use Tindamax, it just means that you should be vigilant for altered blood levels of either Tindamax or the concomitant drug.

Do not take with cholestyramine (Questran) which is sometimes given to prevent gallstones. Use with caution with pre-existing CNS disorders, liver dysfunction, or blood dyscrasias. Consider discontinuing the drug if neurologic effects occur. A Herx reaction may take place. Similar drugs have caused cancer in lab animals.

PEARL: Anecdotally, Tindamax has been associated with severe neurologic events such as problems standing and walking. Be vigilant.

Dosing:

Adults:

> Depending on what you are treating: 2 gram single doses for 3 to 5 days or longer in a pulsed regimen

Children:

> While Flagyl is not recommended in children, Tindamax can be given in kids three and older.

Less than 3-years-old:	Not recommended
Greater than 3-years-old:	50 mg/kg with a maximum 2 g per day in a pulsed regimen

PEARL: Although both are considered cyst-busters, Tindamax might be better at entering the cyst than Flagyl. Tindamax is probably as effective as metronidazole, but better tolerated, although Tindamax has its own tolerability issues.

AEs: With Tindamax neurologic side effects are the most significant, although not common. Fungal overgrowth is common. Other AEs include: GI complaints such as abdominal pain, dyspepsia, cramps, constipation, anorexia, metallic taste, headache, tiredness, weakness, dizziness, transient leukopenia or neutropenia, and abnormal serum chemistries. Rarely seizures, numbness, and peripheral neuropathy have been reported.

Monitor: Watch for the onset or exacerbation of neurologic signs and symptoms. Adjust dose or d/c if neu-

rologic effects occur. Document your rationale. Watch the liver and blood parameters. Measure WBCs before, during, and after treatment. Serum chemistries such as electrolytes, BUN, and creatinine may be abnormal.

General Rifamycins

Rifamycin (Rifampin, Rifabutin, Rifampicin, Rifadin, Mycobutin)

Description: Rifampin is bacteriocidal. In 1957, a soil sample was taken from a pine forest in France and transported to a lab in Milan. There, Professor Piero Sensi discovered a new bacterium that produced antibiotic activity. Piero Sensi's favorite French crime story was called *Rififi* about rival gangs and a jewel heist. Hence, the name rifamycin.

MOA: Inhibits DNA-dependent RNA polymerase thus impairing RNA synthesis. Therefore the pathogen cannot make the RNA chains it needs to survive. Rifampin can also inhibit RNA synthesis in the host cells but the doses needed to hurt the host are much higher than the doses used to impede the pathogen. Rifampin is -cidal for both intracellular and extracellular organisms and does hit the cell wall.

Indications: Primarily used to treat Mycobacterium like those that cause tuberculosis and leprosy. The distribution of rifamycin is high throughout the body and so it should be effective for those susceptible conditions where multiple body systems are affected such as TB, leprosy, and some TBIs. Rifampin helped many patients in the 1960s suffering from drug resistant TB. Also used in combination to treat MRSA and gonococcal meningitis

Use in TBDs: Rifampin has good penetration across the BBB and into the CSF. Its lipophilic nature allows it to penetrate the BBB and it works well in a number of the etiologies of meningitis, encephalitis, and other infections involving nerve tissue. Rifampin may be effective for Bartonella, Ehrlichia, and Bb. Rifamycin may be a good option in those patients where doxy or other first-line choices are contraindicated. Rifampin has been used as the foundation drug in TBI combination therapy, where the rifamycin remains constant and other drugs are changed around it. In TBIs, Rifampin readily penetrates into the meninges and brain making its way into the cells. This medicine has the potential to act fast against both intracellular and extracellular organisms and reaching dormant organisms lurking in macrophages.

PEARL: Anecdotally, rifamycin has been successful in treating Bartonella infections where other regimens have failed.

Usage: Do not take with food or milk. Take one hour before or 2 hours after a meal since food decreases blood concentrations.

In treating diseases like tuberculosis, rifamycin is used daily for months without any break to minimize resistance. *Always* use Rifampin in combination with other antimicrobials to decrease the impact of resistance, so if one agent doesn't get the bug, the other will.

This antibiotic is considered a big gun. Some HCPs like to pull this agent out early and try to subdue the pathogen with shock and awe. Others prefer to reserve this type of antimicrobial for the sickest patients and for those showing signs of meningitis or CNS effects. This is a judgment call based on the individual case. I prefer to use the most effective treatment available when it is determined that it might be useful.

Rifampin has many potential drug interactions especially with steroids, ketaconazole, and anticoagulants. Best not used concomitantly with fluoroquinolones

*PEARL: Most knowledgeable practitioners suggest that Rifampin **NOT** be pulsed in order to minimize resistance and AEs. So while other antimicrobials may be pulsing, Rifampin would be given with no "drug holidays" or breaks.*

Rifamycin is pregnancy category C and can cross the placenta and be excreted in breast milk. This drug is not recommended during pregnancy or nursing.

Pre-existing liver problems may predispose a patient to drug-related jaundice and hepatitis which can be fatal. Hepatitis associated with Rifampin rarely occurs in patients with normal liver function at baseline. Rifampin may decrease Vitamin D levels and a supplement may be prudent during treatment.

Cautions: The big problem with Rifampin is resistance. Susceptible bacteria can become resistant in a one-step process sometimes in a matter of hours after the first dose and often in as little as one to two days. Here, resistance is due to a change in the target of the drug, specifically DNA-dependent RNA polymerase.

PEARL: ALWAYS use Rifampin in combination with other antibiotics to counteract the high level of resistance mounted by many of its susceptible pathogens.

Rifamycin is a VERY red solid compound which can cause body fluids to turn red-orange (urine, sweat, tears). Contact lenses can be permanently discolored and there may be an orange-red ring around the toilet bowl. Tell the patient (and the parents) that the urine, tears, and other body fluids may be orange-red. (Otherwise, they may call the Vatican.) This coloration can be frightening if not expected. In contrast, if there is no color in the urine, the dose or frequency of administration may need adjustment. In these cases, make sure the medicine is taken farther away from food and milk.

Rifampin up-regulates the cytochrome P450 system in the liver and so increases the rate of metabolism of many other drugs that use this enzyme system. Drugs like warfarin, chloramphenicol, and OCPs may be less effective. In the early 1970s, women taking rifamycin reported high rates of irregular bleeding and unwanted pregnancies. While with many antibiotics the warnings about decreased efficacy of birth control might be overstated, with rifamycin err on the side of the conservative. Suggest back-up measures in females of reproductive age, especially if they are on prolonged treatment. Use supplemental birth control until at least one cycle after the rifamycin is stopped. Also consider possible interactions with statins, digoxin, other cardiac medicines, protease inhibitors (antivirals like those used to treat HIV and hepatitis C), steroids, and oral hypoglycemics. Rifamycin interacts with antifungals and may decrease serum concentrations of both drugs.

Dosing: Available as 150 mg and 300 mg capsules and for IV injection in 600 mg vials

Adults: 300 to 600 mg two times a day
Children:

Less than one month:	5 mg/kg q 12
Greater than 1 month:	10 mg/kg q 12 with a maximum of 600 mg/day

AEs: Liver problems are the most significant AEs. Pre-existing liver problems may predispose a patient to drug-related jaundice, hepatitis, and liver failure which can be fatal. Hepatitis associated with Rifampin rarely occurs in patients with normal liver function at baseline.

The most common AEs are rash, nausea, vomiting, and a flu-like syndrome. GI problems such as stomach upset, nausea and vomiting, cramps, and diarrhea have resulted in the need to discontinue treatment. CNS complaints include fatigue, drowsiness, headache, dizziness, ataxia, confusion, poor concentration, numbness, pain in the extremities, and muscle weakness. Other reported AEs include breathlessness, flushing, dysphoria, confusion, visual problems, watery eyes, fever, hives, blood dyscrasias, allergies, and itch. Urine may be pink.

Monitor: Get a baseline LFT and continue to follow the liver throughout therapy, at least monthly.

General Tetracyclines (TCNs)

Description: TCNs are considered bacteriostatic antibiotics, originally developed after the screening of soil samples yielded antibiotic-producing microbes, the Streptomyces. Tetracyclines have a broad spectrum of action against both Gram negative and Gram positive organisms and do especially well against those pathogens that are good at resisting cell wall antibiotics like Mycoplasma, Chlamydia, and Rickettsia.

Use has been limited by resistance that occurs through various mechanisms, especially when used as the sole antibiotic against such diseases as gonorrhea. TCNs are widely distributed in most body fluids including bile, mucus, synovial fluid, and pleural fluids but NOT in cerebral spinal fluid. TCNs can accumulate in bones, liver, spleen, and teeth.

While the individual TCNs have their own idiosyncrasies, most can be discussed in general as a member of the class.

MOA: TCNs inhibit cell growth by interfering with the translation of mRNA into protein. They work at the level of the ribosome, which just might be my favorite organelle.

Indications: TCNs are usually effective for Chlamydia, Mycoplasma, Rickettsia (the causal agents of RMSF and Q fever), spirochetes (the etiology of borreliosis and syphilis), and tularemia. TCNs are commonly prescribed for long-term dermatological use in acne and rosacea. Here they are hypothesized to have both anti-inflammatory and antimicrobial properties.

Use in TBDs: Doxycycline is the gold standard therapy for Lyme disease. Unfortunately, use is restricted in children. TCNs are usually effective for Chlamydia, Rickettsii, spirochetes (borreliosis and syphilis), and tularemia. Doxycycline, or another TCN, is also the first choice for treatment of ehrlichiosis/anaplasmosis.

For the most part, as detailed below, the risk posed to kids is greatly diminished by the time they are 8. In emergencies, consider TCNs in pediatric TBI patients if the drug would only be needed for a short one or two week

course. While this short-term usage will not eliminate all potential hazards, it will minimize damage that might be incurred in a longer course of treatment. In the meantime, the child can be stabilized. As always, with each decision, weigh the risk/benefit ratio. Make sure both the patient and parent understand any risks and are part of the decision-making process. Document your rationale.

PEARL: Use caution if used as a single agent against Borrelia. While the TCNs are excellent at hitting the spirochetal form, they also might inspire the microbes to go intracellular or to form cysts. Think combination therapy for best results.

Usage: TCNs can be given po or IV. With oral use, the intestinal flora will change within two days. Since TCNs are incompletely absorbed, a lot of the product reaches the lower parts of the GI tract. E. *coli* and other normal flora can be obliterated. GI complaints can result and the stools often become soft and yellowish. There can be a significant overgrowth of yeast. If diarrhea appears, ensure that the cause is not C. *difficile*. Rarely, these symptoms will evolve into pseudomembranous colitis. Be vigilant.

Oral TCNs can be hard to tolerate. Usually TCNs are not recommended taken with food. TCNs should be taken two hours before or after food to ensure the best chance for absorption. While food may decrease the GI irritation from TCNs, it's not worth the impact on absorption. Yet, some patients absolutely cannot bear these drugs without something in their stomachs. Occasionally, tolerance improves with time.

Take TCNs with a full glass of water. Do not take TCNs near the ingestion of magnesium, aluminum, iron, or calcium, or foods high in these minerals like beef or dairy. Review the ingredients in multivitamins, supplements, antacids, and laxatives.

IV administration allows for higher doses of TCNs to be administered that could not be tolerated orally. Unfortunately, thrombophlebitis is not uncommon when TCNs are given by vein especially when one vein is used over and over. Just as the oral formulations can irritate the GI tract, the IV preps are very irritating to the veins and patients often complain that the infusion hurts – A LOT. If you need an IV preparation, take this into consideration as you make your selection. IV administration may eventually allow a slow passage of TCN across the BBB, but usually the juice ain't worth the squeeze. There are other medicines that accomplish that task much more readily.

PEARL: With TCNs, we like to have good peaks and troughs. We're not as interested in steady state levels here as in the big boluses of drug beating on those spirochetes.

That is why you can dose TCNs once or twice a day in contrast to many other antimicrobials that work best at steady state and must be given frequently to maintain constant blood levels. In general, TCNs are given in higher amounts less frequently to get good intermittent blasts of drug into the blood. This approach is in contrast to other antimicrobials like the PCNs that are administered at lower doses more frequently to keep the levels at a consistent steady state.

Cautions: Although thousands of prescriptions are written each day for the TCNs, there are a number of things to keep in mind about this drug class. Each of the bullets below could also be included as part of the potential AE section. Be cognizant of these potential hazards when using TCNs.

- Microbes can develop a slow step-wise resistance to TCNs similar to that of PCNs. A combination regimen is one way to combat resistance. Because TCNs have been routinely used in animal feeds there is currently considerable microbial resistance to this drug class.

- Use with caution in patients with renal and liver impairment. TCNs may worsen renal failure and is more likely in those with pre-existing conditions. Of the TCNs, doxycycline seems to have less significant problems than the other TCN formulations, with less effect on the BUN. Hepatic toxicity is usually only associated with higher doses of 2 grams or more per day.

- If taken with alcohol, some TCNs can cause an adverse reaction much like the drug disulfiram (Antabuse). Symptoms include nausea, vomiting, headache, flushing, cramps, and confusion.

- TCNs can mitigate the effect of Flagyl (metronidazole) which is often selected to attack cystic forms of Bb as part of combination therapy.

- Conventional wisdom was that TCNs lessened the effect of OCPs but now the evidence is not clear. A number of patients are on OCPs, so be careful.

- Phototoxicity is a problem with some TCNs like doxycycline. A small but significant number of patients will experience a mild to severe burn reaction when exposed to sunlight. The important thing to remember is this reaction is OUT OF PROPORTION to what might be expected under normal circumstances. Some people really fry in a very short time. This is called a **phototoxic reaction.** Not all patients experience this phototoxicity but all should be prepared for it. While high SPF sunscreen should always be recommended, these screens may not be protective enough. Even sunscreens over SPF 35 and those with Helioplex may be insufficient. Preach hats and long sleeves and sun avoidance. Along with this reaction there may be pigmentation of nails after sun exposure and even a separation of the nail from the nail bed (onycholysis). Goodness knows why that might happen. Warn the patient. Teenagers especially believe this won't happen to them. "I never burn. I'm a really good tanner." There will be tears when they look like a painful lobster. Re-enforce that the problem can occur after minimal sun exposure, with only one or a few doses of TCN on board, and with tanning lights as well as the real sun.

- If given during pregnancy, the TCN can deposit in the fetal bone and teeth, where it chelates with the available calcium. TCNs are discouraged in women greater than 18 weeks pregnant because that is the time when the fetal calcified tissues are developing. Discoloration of the teeth of the child can be permanent.

When given to babies the greatest risk of a problem is in those who are treated with a TCN before their first teeth are fully developed. Discoloration can also occur in the permanent teeth if given to kids between 2 months and 5 years. As the teeth are being calcified the TCN binds with the calcium. At first, the teeth will become yellowish, but then a permanent brown-grey color is evident. Horizontal dark bands on the teeth have also been observed.

Discoloration can develop whether the TCN regimen is short-term or long-term. The dose seems to be more critical than the length of treatment. The higher the dose to body weight ratio, the more discoloration. Kids up to 8-years-old are susceptible.

TCNs can cause depression of bone growth as measured by fibula length. This decline is reversible if the treatment period is SHORT. Extended TCN treatment in children can lead to permanent length loss and bone weakness.

- Many types of hypersensitivity reactions are associated with TCNs such as rashes, itching, eye irritation, hives, and exfoliative dermatitis. These symptoms can persist after the drug is discontinued. Angioedema and anaphylaxis are rare.

- Yeast overgrowth and bacterial superinfections have been associated with TCNs. If a patient on TCNs experiences diarrhea this could be due to irritation or to overgrowth of opportunistic organisms. Make sure you are not dealing with C. *difficile*.

- A strong Herxheimer reaction may occur in TBI patients treated with TCNs.

- Long-term TCN use can change blood chemistries and CBC results including: atypical lymphocytes, abnormal granules in granulocytes, and low platelets consistent with thrombocytopenic purpura. In lab testing TCNs can decrease hemoglobin, platelets, blood ammonia, and cause abnormalities in urine and blood glucose. Diabetic testing may be falsely high.

- TCNs can be irritating both orally and intravenously. The bigger the dose, the greater the irritation. GI complaints such as nausea, vomiting, burning, and distress are usually worse at the onset of treatment and diminish over time. The "usual" things we do to minimize GI side effects are not tenable with TCNs. We cannot take TCNs with food because that decreases absorption, which is not the greatest to start with. We are reluctant to lower the dose because that would lower the peak blood concentration that makes the TCNs most effective. IV administration allows for doses at higher levels than could be tolerated po. But the veins get ragged pretty fast since the formulations are so irritating. Rotate infusion sites, if possible. Believe the patient when they say it hurts.

PEARL: Be very careful using a tetracycline alone against Bb. While the TCNs are great at eliminating the spirochetal form of Bb, they are much less effective against intracellular or cystic spirochetes. Used alone, these drugs can cause the microbes to burrow or encyst. Think in terms of combination regimens, not solo agents.

AEs: Certain side effects are common in the TCNs because of their MOA, metabolism, and distribution. Some of these events can be quite formidable. Read the caution list above and change the syntax and you will have a fairly complete AE list. Not all patients will experience all these events or even a few.

The common AEs are GI upset, headache, allergies, rashes, and urticaria (hives). Uncommon but potentially significant AEs include thrombocytopenic purpura, pancreatitis, and aseptic increased ICP. When the TCN is discontinued the ICP generally returns to normal. Both pseudotumor cerebri and vestibular toxicity with dizziness has been associated with TCN use. (Is the increased ICP due to the TCN or the underlying infection?)

Vestibular toxicity manifests with dizziness, ataxia, nausea, and vomiting and has been reported with minocycline. The symptoms start soon after the initial dose and stop after the drug is discontinued. This appears to be a dose-related reaction.

Monitor: Keep a careful eye on patients treated long-term with TCNs. The younger the patient the more vigilance should be expected. Since TCNs are excreted primarily in the kidney, watch the kidney function with a BUN and creatinine at baseline and throughout treatment. Watch the liver. Check CBC with differential and platelet count. Compare the levels over time not just to see if the results are WNL, but to look for patterns and trends that might be happening within the individual patient.

Specific TCN options:

1. **Tetracycline (Sumycin)**

   If you write for TCN these days you are likely to get a generic product. Few write for plain TCN anymore because of possible resistance and because the semi-synthetic products have fewer side effects and better efficacy. TCN is included here for completeness.

2. **Doxycycline (Vibramycin, Doryx, which is enteric-coated doxycycline)**

   Description: Semi-synthetic TCN that is the most commonly used TCN in TBI patients. Doxycycline appears to have fewer side effects than other TCNs and is at least as effective, so it may be the most appropriate when a TCN is needed in TBIs. The information above in the *General Tetracyclines* applies to doxycycline as well. In conversation, the drug is often called doxy.

PEARL: Do not get vancomycin and Vibramycin confused.

PEARL: I opted for the $4 generic instead of the $900 Doryx for my son (even though I know from professional experience that a number of imported generics do not contain the listed quantity or quality of API), I knew the benefits that Doryx might have in terms of absorption and tolerability over the generic doxycycline. I bought the generic and then had to go back and buy the Doryx. Even I revert to the dark side from time to time, even when I know better.

   MOA: Doxy kills spirochetes directly whether they are dividing or not. If the dose of doxy can be spiked once a day, even if trough levels are low, the drug can be very effective. The spike level is what counts with this drug. Doryx is an enteric-coated form of doxycycline. The coating minimizes dissolution in the stomach and allows more of the active drug to get to the SI where it is then absorbed. This delayed release usually makes Doryx better tolerated than traditional formulations since there may be less stomach upset.

Use in TBDs: Used for RMSF, Lyme, and ehrlichiosis/anaplasmosis. Doxycycline is sometimes used in the prophylaxis of malaria and hypothetically might also be effective, at least in combination, against babesiosis. I know that doxy didn't work out so well for my son's babesiosis. Doxy is the gold standard treatment for adult Lyme. Consider doxy early in TBI treatment because it covers several prominent co-infections.

Unfortunately, in some quarters, doxy is relied on too heavily to treat Lyme. Uneducated practitioners often feel that single agent, low dose, short duration doxy for 10 to 28 days will cure ALL Lyme, ALL the time. This is most definitely not the case. Controversy has made them cautious. They think that if they just give a little bit they won't get into trouble. They give less medicine to a very sick patient than they would give to someone with mild acne. While they would treat the acne for years without batting an eye, some will only treat the Lyme for two weeks or a month.

First, low doses of doxy do not give the bolus (high peak) levels needed to hit the spirochetal form of Bb. Many doctors do not understand that some drugs work best at steady state, while others work best with intermittent high peak levels. Doxy is one that works best with the high peak levels. Second, short duration therapy with doxy alone can cause the Bb to go into survival mode, hiding in a number of ways until it is safe to come back out. Frequent dosing is unnecessary. You are not going for consistent levels here, but rather the blast and relax approach. Further the more frequent the dose, the more chance for a missed dose. With frequent low doses you do not achieve the desired high peak level. You end up only with the false confidence that the patient has been cured under your watchful eye. Solo antibiotics can do more harm than good. They induce the pathogen to go intracellular or to encyst. When no back-up antibiotic is then available to go after the cyst or follow inside the cells, the hidden spirochetes become a repository for future infection. When the patient returns still sick, the Liliths[5] of the world ask, "What more do you want? He's already on doxy."

For Lyme, doxy needs to be given in doses high enough to impact the circulating spirochetes and long enough to get those spirochetes that later emerge from inside tissues or cysts. Inadequate dose and duration will likely make matters worse and may set up a chronic disease state. Treatment should be stopped when symptoms completely resolve along with a cushion to allow for any re-emergence of Bb in various life forms. If symptoms recur, then restart treatment. And this time, for goodness' sake, blast 'em when they are out in the open. Consider a loading dose and then *high, infrequent* dosing, once or twice a day. Make sure a back-up antibiotic that better hits the intracellular and cystic forms is part of the combination package. Chapter 10: *Borreliosis* goes into detail on how the life cycle and various forms of Bb should impact treatment decisions.

Doxycycline can be given in TBI patients either po or IV with all the inherent advantages and disadvantages of those respective modalities listed above.

Doxy does not penetrate well inside cells but it is the preferred drug used to target the free spirochetal forms of Bb.

Try to find different treatment options in kids under eight. Use with caution in kids eight and above since bones can still be growing. Discoloration can develop in teeth if given to kids up to five-years-old whether the TCN regimen is short-term or long-term. Here, the dose seems to be more critical than the length of treatment. The higher the dose to body weight ratio, the more discoloration. Herein lies the doxy conundrum: You need the high concentrations to be effective but higher concentrations can be associated with more problems.

Doxycycline can cause depression of bone growth as measured by fibula length. This decline is reversible if the treatment period is SHORT. Extended TCN treatment in children can lead to permanent length loss and bone weakness. In general, the risk posed to kids is reduced by the time the child is about eight. Only consider TCNs in pediatric patients if options are limited and if the drug would only be needed for a limited one or two week course. While this short-term usage will not eliminate all potential hazards, it will minimize damage that might be incurred in a longer course of treatment. In the meantime, the child can be effectively treated while suitable alternatives are identified.

PEARL: Some TBI experts select minocycline over doxycycline in pediatric patients who need a TCN. Doxy has become so much a part of the Lyme community lexicon that we forget there are other TCN choices that may offer advantages.

---

5 See Glossary or Introduction for name origin

Usage: Take with a lot of water. There may be decreased absorption with antacids or laxatives containing calcium or high iron supplements or foods.

If you need a TCN in a patient with renal compromise, consider doxycycline since it does not seem to accumulate in the kidney or cause a significant rise in BUN.

PEARL: Doxy can be hard on the stomach. Consider Doryx, the enteric-coated formulation of doxycycline, since more of this is absorbed in the small intestine.

IV doxy often requires a central line since the formulation is so caustic. Nonetheless, this form of administration can be very effective because the blood levels can be higher than with oral preps. A single *large* daily dose optimizes the kinetics of pathogen-killing with this drug. Often a PICC (peripherally inserted central catheter) is used to deliver doxycycline directly into the blood stream.

GI complaints seem to diminish over time. Do not increase an oral dose if the patient is having trouble tolerating the lower dose. If the patient is tolerating the current dose, you can try an increase, if clinically appropriate.

Cautions: Doxycycline can be used carefully in patients with renal impairment. Watch for changes in red and white cells. Look for retinal or visual field problems. Don't use with known hepatotoxins, disulfiram, or alcohol. May antagonize atovaquone

If taken with alcohol, doxycycline can cause an adverse reaction much like the drug disulfiram (Antabuse) including nausea, vomiting, headache, flushing, cramps, and confusion.

Not recommended in pregnancy or nursing

Dosing:

Dose recommendations vary with reference. Base doses of TCN on parameters specific to the individual case.

Adults or children over 100 **lb**s: Can start with a 200 mg loading dose and then 100 to 200 mg q 12 hours either po or IV. Switch to the other modality (oral or IV) as appropriate. Up to 600 mg/day. Note that some load with a higher dose such as 400 mg over a 24 hour period, followed by 200 bid. I found no source that dosed at greater than 600 mg/day.

Children: There is both syrup and suspension available (25 mg/5 ml and 50 mg/5 ml).

For kids under 100 **lb**s: 2 mg/**lb** in 2 divided doses for the first day and thereafter 1 to 2 mg/**lb** daily. Maximum dose in small children is considered 200 mg per day.

For kids over 100 **lb**s: Start with a 200 mg loading dose and then 100 to 200 mg q 12 hours either po or IV. Switch to oral or IV as appropriate. Up to 600 mg/day

In children less than 8-years-old, consider other first-line therapy.

PEARL: Notice that this dosing source mixes metric and English measuring traditions. I don't know why. Be careful.

PEARL: For ehrlichiosis/anaplasmosis and RMSF in adults consider 100 mg bid. For children 4 mg/kg/day in two divided doses. In children less than 8 years old, use of doxycycline in these cases is usually short-term which decreases the risk.

PEARL: Although I am not a fan of therapeutic drug levels, they may provide information in cases where treatment is not working when all indications suggest that it should. If the levels are low at tolerated oral doses, try an IV formulation or change drugs. Therapeutic levels vary in the literature but one suggestion is that the level should peak above 10 and trough above 3 to get levels that allow for maximum efficacy.

PEARL: Doxy is only effective with intermittent high blood levels.

AEs: Of the TCNs, doxycycline seems to have less significant safety problems than the other TCN formulations, with less effect on the BUN. However, minocycline may be better tolerated. Remember, safety and tolerability are not synonymous.

Photosensitivity is possible, as well as GI upset, rash, blood dyscrasias, leukopenia, neutropenia, vertigo, headache, ataxia, lack of coordination, confusion, irritability, depression, restlessness, weakness, fatigue, drowsiness, insomnia, neuropathy, paresthesias, mental stimulation, flattened T waves on EKG, blurred vision, difficulty with visual focusing, nasal congestion, GI cramps, nausea, vomiting, anorexia, diarrhea, constipation, dry mouth, proctitis, dark urine, polyuria, incontinence, cystitis, decreased libido, dyspareunia, dry vagina, sense of pelvic pressure, itch, flushing, overgrowth of Candida, coated tongue, and metallic taste. Doryx makes the cheeks and hands hot in some patients.

Monitor: As with the monitoring recommendations listed above for the TCN class, watch blood counts especially RBCs, WBC differential, and platelets, along with liver and kidney functions.

REDUNDANT PEARL: For doxy a high spike blood level is more effective than sustained blood levels. That is why an initial bolus is recommended. It is better to give higher doses less frequently than lower doses more frequently. So 200 bid is more effective than 100 qid. Likewise, an IV dose of 200 mg once a day may be more effective than dosing 100 bid. I wouldn't tell you twice if it wasn't important.

PEARL: Why do some HCPs dislike doxycycline for Lyme? When doxycycline is used ALONE, some patients (perhaps 10% to 15%) appear to develop a syndrome that is hard to treat. Using doxy as part of a COMBINATION approach is prudent. So be careful when following certain guidelines and using doxy as a solo agent. For whatever genetic or otherwise predisposing reason, you may be putting a sub-population at greater risk for a recalcitrant clinical course.

3. **Minocycline (Minocin)**

   Description: A semi-synthetic TCN

   Use in TBDs: Many TBI-competent physicians choose minocycline over doxycycline when they need a TCN in the pediatric population. Doxy has become so much a part of the Lyme community lexicon that we forget there are other TCN choices that may offer advantages. Consider minocycline for sensitive pathogens

   Usage: Do not take with antacids, laxatives containing calcium, or high iron supplements or foods. Minocin is somewhat better absorbed than the other TCNs when taken with food, but it's still better to take on an empty stomach with water.

   Cautions: All cautions and usage suggestions for the general TCNs and doxy listed above also apply to minocycline.

   Minocycline is not recommended in pregnant or nursing mothers because of potential adverse effects on bones and teeth and minocycline may interfere with OCPs.

   If the patient complains of dizziness, consider vestibular toxicity and determine how the symptom needs to be addressed. You may need to consider an alternative drug since lowering the dose is not usually the best option in TCNs. Minocycline has been associated with a lupus-like syndrome.

   Dosing:

Adults:	Loading dose: 200 mg po or IV then 100 mg q 12	
Children:		
	Over 8:	4 mg/kg/day po or IV initially then 4 mg/kg daily divided q 12. Give IV in 500 to 1000 ml solution without calcium over 6 hours
	Under 8:	Consider other antibiotics first

   PEARL: Not all practitioners choose to load first. Some HCPs begin with 50 mg bid. If there is no headache after about a week, try 100 mg q 12.

   See doxycycline section above for a discussion on use in pediatric emergency situations.

   AEs: In addition to the usual TCN AEs, minocycline may be associated with neutropenia, eosinophilia, light headedness, dizziness (if dizzy check for vestibular toxicity), pericarditis, dysphagia, glossitis, anorexia, GI distress, nausea, vomiting, diarrhea, enterocolitis, lesions in the anogenital region, increased BUN, maculopapular and erythematous rashes, photosensitivity, increased pigmentation, urticaria, thrombophlebitis, hypersensitivity, and fungal overgrowth.

   Minocycline may be more associated with **vestibular toxicity** than other TCNs. Symptoms include dizziness, ataxia, nausea, and vomiting. If this condition is going to occur it most commonly starts soon after the initial dose and then resolves quickly after the drug is discontinued. This appears to be a dose-related reaction in susceptible individuals.

   Minocycline has been associated with pseudotumor cerebri that may be hard to resolve.

   PEARL: Minocycline is listed as standard therapy for both RA and Lyme by the Arthritis Foundation.

   PEARL: Minocycline may cause more dizziness than doxycycline. If the patient gets dizzy on Minocin, consider doxycycline (Doryx).

   Monitor: Papilledema, signs of vestibular impairment

4. Tigecycline (Tygacil)

Description: Tigecycline is a **glycylcycline.** Look at that word! Is there any reason on earth to have a word like that? Whatever happened to phonics? I dare you to sound that word out. I get stuck after the first "cy." There is an entire website explaining the pronunciation of that word, which purports it to be: gli-sil-si-klen with the third i and only e long.)

PEARL: Do not get all these "T" antibiotics mixed up: telithromycin (Ketek), tinidazole, (Tindamax), tigecycline (Tygacil). You think you won't, but you will. Be careful.

Classified as both –cidal and –static, depending on dose, pathogen, and literature source.

MOA: Inhibits protein synthesis on the ribosome. Tigecycline is not always classified as a TCN. Of course not, it's a glycylcycline. During development, care was taken to introduce structure that would help circumvent resistance mechanisms. Tygacil seems to bind to the ribosome in a unique way. The MOA is similar to doxy and the TCNs but its chemical structure is such that it does NOT allow itself to be pumped out of Bb cells like a number of other antibiotics. Tigecycline is 100 times more effective against Bb than doxy. Instead of just inhibiting the spirochetes, tigecycline kills them. Rocephin kills them too but it takes much longer to do so. Tigecycline kills them within a day.

Indications: Gram positive, negative, and anaerobic pathogens. Used often in infections of the abdominal organs, skin, and in community acquired pneumonias.

Use in TBDs: The mechanism of tigecycline is similar to that of doxycycline. However, its chemical structure is such that it gets inside the Bb cell and then it cannot get back out, which is good news in terms of efficacy. Tigecycline appears to be many times more effective against Bb than doxycycline. Instead of just inhibiting the spirochetes like doxy, tigecycline kills them in their proverbial tracks. Tigecycline kills the Bb within 24 hours *in vitro* and appears to work rapidly *in vivo* as well. Tigecycline has been used in the treatment of patients with both Bb and babesiosis, with positive results. Tygacil seems to have less problems with resistance than other TCNs.

Usage: Tygacil is an IV product given by a slow infusion. No dosage adjustment appears necessary for patients with renal impairment.

Anecdotally, patients who eat DURING the infusion may have much less nausea and vomiting than those who do not. The mechanism by which this might occur is unknown.

If the same IV line is to be used to administer other drugs, flush the line thoroughly between dosings. Do not give Tygacil in the same line as IV omeprazole or esomeprazole. That last sentence means nothing to you but I worked on the development of these two drugs and to type their names made me wax nostalgic.

Cautions: Tigecycline is not recommended in patients under 18-years-old. This seems more restrictive than the limits placed on the other TCNs. I could not find any rationale for this except that it has not yet been tested in these populations. (And it may never be. The drug company will likely be happy with any off-label use rather than spend the money on an expensive clinical trial, where they are not likely to get much return on investment.)

Use in children would have at least the same caveats as listed with the other TCNs above. Use only when no other options are available in line with the severity of the child's illness. If pancreatitis develops consider alternative therapy. Be cognizant of the possibility of C. *difficile.* Be cautious using this product in patients with liver impairment.

May cause fetal harm if given during pregnancy. Unsure of the consequences of use during nursing. Pregnancy category D

Dosing: Over 18: Initial dose of 100 mg followed by 50 mg q 12

Duration of therapy should correspond to the severity of infection and the patient's progress.

AEs: Most common AEs are nausea and vomiting. Seems to be better tolerated than other IV TCN formulations, but can still be hard to endure. Hepatic dysfunction has been reported. This antibiotic has similar AEs to other TCNs.

Monitor: LFTs looking for patterns and trends, not just that the results are WNLs. Elevated SGPTs have been reported.

Miscellaneous Antibiotics

1. Vancomycin (Vancocin)

Description: Vancomycin was first isolated from a soil sample collected from the jungles of Borneo by a missionary. (Wouldn't a missionary in the wilds of

Borneo have other things to do besides collecting soil samples?) The compound was so effective against PCN-resistant Staphylococcus *aureus* that it was given the name vancomycin from the word vanquished. Nonetheless, vancomycin never became first-line treatment because, except for its use in the GI tract for C. *difficile,* it is not absorbed when taken orally and must be given IV. Drugs that were even better against resistant bugs were soon developed. Early trials used such impure forms of vancomycin that it was called Mississippi mud. Unfortunately, these early formulations caused severe and permanent side effects and the drug never regained its reputation. Actually, vancomycin is an excellent drug and it is unfortunate that the bad rap from early formulations limits its use today.

PEARL: Do not get vancomycin and Vibramycin, a tetracycline, mixed up.

MOA: Glycopeptides inhibit the synthesis of cell walls in susceptible microbes by impeding peptidoglycan synthesis. The antibiotic binds to the amino acids in the cell wall, which prevents addition of new amino acid units to the peptide chains.

Indications: Vancomycin is used against MRSA, C. *difficile,* and is used liberally pre-op in orthopedic surgery. Very good against Gram positive organisms. Less effective on Gram negative since the large drug molecule cannot penetrate their outer membrane. Indicated only for life-threatening infections by susceptible pathogens that are unresponsive to less toxic treatments. Consider all other options first. The CDC has "guidelines" on the appropriate use of vancomycin. Vancomycin is commonly used as a preoperative medication for orthopedic and other surgeries, but this is usually only a few doses.

Use in TBDs: IV vancomycin is one of the best drugs for treating Bb but the perceived toxicity limits its use. Vancomycin does NOT penetrate the CSF or cross the BBB. Consider combination therapy if there are neuropsychiatric symptoms.

Usage: Currently vancomycin is considered the treatment of "last resort." Certainly consider using vancomycin before you lose a patient. People die of TBIs every day. Mortality is grossly underreported because death certificates use euphemistic causes like cardiopulmonary arrest. If vancomycin can turn the case around, consider its use before it's too late.

Use oral vancomycin to treat C. *difficile* in the GI tract when Flagyl is not effective. Oral vancomycin is a particularly good choice. Since the oral formulation does not cross the intestinal lining the drug is exactly where it needs to be to do its job. Since pseudomembranous colitis can be an untoward side effect of many antibiotics, including those used to treat TBIs, you may encounter vancomycin one way or the other.

For indications other than C. *difficile,* vancomycin is given IV. Here, vancomycin is a good candidate for pulse therapy to minimize toxicity. The IV formulation is extremely caustic and is usually delivered using a PICC line to decrease the risk of injection site irritation and thrombophlebitis. The drug must be administered in a dilute solution at a maximum rate of 10 mg/minute because of pain and inflammation at the injection site and the possibility of **red man syndrome**. This reaction usually occurs within a few minutes after the start of a too-rapid infusion. This mast cell reaction releases histamine and causes flushing and a red rash on the face, neck, and upper torso. Hypotension, swelling, and shock have been observed. Slow infusion prevents this reaction and antihistamines may help decrease the signs and symptoms.

Cautions: To protect yourself, make sure you CLEARLY document your rationale for using this drug in the chart. Some HCPs even use a type of "Informed Consent" document or patient treatment waiver. That seems somewhat over-reactive to me but you can't be too careful in this litigious environment. Make sure the patient and caretakers understand the risk/benefit ratio and are part of the decision-making process.

The two most significant AEs associated with use of vancomycin are ototoxicity and nephrotoxicity. Ototoxicity has been associated with use of vancomycin. Ototoxicity is any situation that causes an adverse effect on the 8th cranial nerve or the sense of hearing. No one knows the exact mechanism by which vancomycin might be responsible for this presentation. Some patients, like those with pre-existing hearing problems may be at more risk. Of course, there is considerable debate over whether hearing damage is dose-related or not. Some sources strongly believe that the higher the dose of vancomycin, the more likely there are to be hearing problems. Others feel that the dose has no relationship to the occurrence of ototoxicity. There is even debate regarding whether the hearing loss is temporary or permanent. The reality probably involves a combination of factors, as is usually the case.

With nephrotoxicity, association has been established but causality is still indeterminant. In the first cases of nephrotoxicity, the patients had also received other drugs known to harm the kidney. Early formulations were notoriously impure and these impurities might have been responsible for the kidney damage. Today, the reality is hard to discern. The incidence of vancomycin related nephrotoxicity is thought to be about 5% which is similar to some of the PCNs and cephalosporins.

With all that being said, use vancomycin with caution in renal insufficiency and in those with pre-existing hearing loss. Assess the hearing and kidney function at baseline and throughout treatment.

Vancomycin is pregnancy category B.

Dosing:

Oral: Oral preps of vancomycin are available as 125 mg and 250 mg capsules. These are used only for enterocolitis and pseudomembranous colitis associated with C. *difficile.*

Adults: 0.5 to 2.0 g daily in 3 to 4 divided doses for 7 to 10 days

Children: 40 mg/kg per day in 3 to 4 divided doses for 7 to 10 days. Maximum 2 g/day

Intravenous:

Use: 15 mg/kg q 12. (This dose is recommended for patients with endocarditis and should handle cases where patients are just as sick in other organ systems.)

PEARL: *One regimen suggested for the treatment of C. difficile is 125 to 500 mg po q 6 h for 10 days.*

In renal impairment, start with this dose and then base further dosing on renal function results.

AEs may increase if doses exceed 4 g/day.

AEs: Early formulations caused kidney damage and hearing loss but with current vancomycin preps these events are rare. However, nephrotoxicity may be more likely in patients with pre-existing kidney problems and in those taking aminoglycoside antibiotics, which are rarely used in treatment of TBIs.

Common AEs include: nausea, rash, blood dyscrasias such as eosinophilia, fever, and superinfections.

Red neck or **red man syndrome** occurs occasionally when IV infusion of vancomycin is too fast. This reaction usually starts within a few minutes after the initiation of a too-rapid infusion. This mast cell

reaction releases histamine and causes flushing and a red rash on the face, neck, and upper torso. Hypotension, swelling, and shock may occur. Slow infusion prevents this reaction and antihistamines may help decrease the signs and symptoms.

Other AEs include: anaphylaxis, TEN, erythema multiforme, neutropenia, leukopenia, tinnitus, dizziness, ototoxicity, thrombocytopenia, bleeding, florid petechial hemorrhages, bruising, and purpura.

AEs associated with IV injection include: pain at the IV site, necrosis, phlebitis especially if injected too fast, and red man syndrome which is thought to be a histamine reaction to a rapid bolus.

Monitor:

- Hearing: If possible obtain a baseline hearing test and then monitor hearing throughout the course of treatment. Since by the time you decide vancomycin is the only remaining option, baseline testing may no longer be feasible. Do the best you can to keep track of any hearing deficits.

- Kidney function: Baseline BUN and creatinine. Consider twice a month follow-ups

- CBC with differential and platelets. Baseline and throughout treatment course. Consider twice a month testing

- There is considerable debate in the literature around the value of therapeutic blood levels. Some authors feel they are essential to ensure that blood levels are not in the toxic range. Others feel these tests add very little to the mix because they tend to be so unreliable and influenced by so many extraneous factors. What do you do if the patient's hearing is diminished but the blood levels are low? What do you do if this person is getting sicker? This is the treatment of last resort, remember? What do you do if the levels are too high but the patient is getting better? Before you order the test make sure you know how you will answer these questions.

Talk to the lab that will be running the test to ensure samples are collected properly and that you know how to interpret the results. Here, toxic levels are best assessed by looking at the trough (that's as low as it goes) and if that is high you might have a problem. With vancomycin, antimicrobial activity depends on how long the drug stays at therapeutic blood levels.

Appropriate levels vary by source but here is a ballpark: Peak between 18 and 26 **mg/liter** and trough 5 to 20 **mg/liter**. The recommendation is to wait at least until after the third dose to start measuring levels.

Some believe that peak levels have NOT been correlated with either efficacy or side effects so serum concentrations are not necessary. Others think this information is critical in making future treatment decisions. You decide how you might use this data to help your patient.

Consider blood levels if the patient is also 1) on an aminoglycoside[6] 2) taking other drugs affecting the kidney 3) experiencing inability to metabolize drugs properly 4) a hemodialysis patient 5) on a very high dose 6) on an extended treatment course, or 7) acknowledging a pre-existing abnormal kidney function or hearing deficit. Some think that there is an increase in nephrotoxicity when trough levels are above 10 **micrograms/ml** but others disagree. There are documented cases of nephrotoxicity when blood levels were in the "therapeutic" range.

Unfortunately monitoring vancomycin levels to ensure they are not toxic can be false security. Ototoxicity, like nephrotoxicity, is rare and may have little relationship to blood levels. So while monitoring blood levels may make the HCP feel vigilant, it does NOT guarantee protection from either of these potential AEs. Watch the patient.

2. **Chloramphenicol** (Numerous brand and generic formulations, many of which may be unavailable)

Description: A broad spectrum bacteriostatic produced by a Streptomyces organism and first isolated from soil samples in Venezuela. Late in 1947, chloramphenicol was used in a typhus outbreak in Bolivia with good results. The drug went out of favor later in the 50s because of its association with serious and fatal blood dyscrasias. Use is again picking up because of its excellent activity against anaerobic pathogens and because of the significant resistance now building against newer drugs. Chloramphenicol is widely used in low income countries because it is cheap and available there. Chloramphenicol seems to be effective against the pathogen, probably a fungus, which has wiped out many frog species in the last two decades.

MOA: Inhibits protein synthesis near the same ribosomal active site as macrolides and clindamycin and competes with them. Chloramphenicol has one of the best penetrations of the BBB of any antimicrobial.

Indications: Used mostly for serious susceptible infections such as typhoid, typhus, and RMSF, and in potentially sensitive meningitis when safer options are not feasible. Employed against rickettsial typhus and the three primary causes of bacterial meningitis: H. *influenza*, N. *meningitides*, and Strep. *pneumoniae*. Effective against almost all anaerobes such as Bacteroides. Chloramphenicol may hit MRSA. Used in combination with PCNs for brain abscesses.

PEARL: Do not get typhus and typhoid fever mixed up. Typhus is caused by a Rickettsia. Typhoid fever, also called typhoid, is a form of salmonellosis. Chloramphenicol is able to hit both pathogens. Apparently, many authors, like this one, often get these terms confused.

Use in TBDs: Often considered first-line against RMSF. While TCNs are often considered the DOC for rickettsial diseases, chloramphenicol is preferable in pregnancy, renal compromise, the severely ill who need IV treatment, and for those in whom TCNs are contraindicated, not tolerated, or cause allergic reactions. Chloramphenicol may be effective against Mycoplasma species and the Coxiella species that causes Q fever, but is not indicated for Lyme. This drug has been used anecdotally for tularemia and TRF. Chloramphenicol crosses the BBB.

Usage: In some parts of the world, chloramphenicol is available as capsules, suspension, and in IV, IM, and ophthalmic formulations. Currently IM might not be available in the US and Europe. These things change by the minute. I can find ten sources that tell me how much an IM dose costs in the US (less than a $5 foot-long) and just as many other sites that lament that oily chloramphenicol is no longer available in the US and Europe. WHO considers chloramphenicol an essential drug and, at least for a time, recommended that field doctors carry IM doses in their bags for emergency use in meningitis cases.

Remember, the affable, trusted, neighborhood pharmacist I told you to befriend? Well, if you have a hankering for oily chloramphenicol for IM injection, she might know if it is currently available. Intermittently, oral formulations may be hard, or even impossible, to come by at your standard pharmacy. Then you have no choice but to select another drug or route of administration.

---

6 *Aminoglycosides are a class of antibiotics rarely indicated for treatment of TBIs although they are sometimes used to treat tularemia. However, if given for other reasons in TBI patients they might increase the risk of kidney damage. They include: gentamicin, tobramycin, amikacin, kanamycin, streptomycin, and neomycin.*

Chloramphenicol is metabolized by the liver and excreted by the kidney, so keep an eye on these body systems before and during use. Baseline evaluation should ensure adequate function to withstand the rigors of therapy.

The oral formulation can cause nausea, vomiting, or a bad, lingering taste.

Cautions:

Dose should be reduced in those with known liver impairment. They just don't have the guns to handle this drug.

The risk of aplastic anemia does not preclude use of chloramphenicol in severely ill patients where there are limited options. Do a careful risk/benefit assessment and ensure that both the patient and caregiver understand the potential risk. Involve all parties in the treatment decision. Document your rationale for selecting this drug. Never use the drug blindly without having some idea of what you are treating just because you think it will probably hit the pathogen.

PEARL: Here is one example of how I might document this choice: "6 y/o w/ hx of tick bite 5 days ago now presents w/ fevers >104 not well modulated by alternating acetaminophen & ibuprofen. Petechial, red, pinpoint rash started on palms & soles & now on face, back, & trunk. Severe ha & some confusion & delirium associated w/ fever spikes. Child rapidly getting worse & less responsive. Doxycycline is not recommended in this age group & this child is so ill as to likely benefit from IV drug administration. No other antimicrobials likely to hit this probable Rickettsia as well as chloramphenicol. Mortality if untreated about 30%. Confirmatory blood work for RMSF pending. Discussed risk/benefit with parents & they understand the potential threat. Need to balance possible risk for significant blood abnormalities w/ the risk of inadequately treated disease. Baseline lab work drawn. Will monitor frequently for signs of abnormal blood cells & adequate liver & kidney function. Will draw therapeutic drug levels if clinically indicated." Yes, that is how I actually write my chart notes, although I use a lot more abbreviations in my real charts than I did here. I was drilled by armies of lawyers in the pharmaceutical industry. As you can imagine, I am really a fun date. Will this type of note prevent you from getting sued? Of course not. Lawsuits rarely have anything to do with the practice of good or bad medicine. This comprehensive note, however, makes you look like you have thought out the course of action and know the underlying medicine. This note will give you something to say on the stand and is within the standard of care in most places.

Resistance to chloramphenical is likely due to an enzyme inactivation of the drug by certain pathogens. But as has been recently observed, resistance to chloramphenical may be less than the resistance now building against some of the newer antimicrobials.

Patients treated with chloramphenical can experience a significant Herx reaction. See Chapter 28: *Understanding the Herxheimer Reaction.* Prepare all parties.

Chloramphenicol uses the P450 enzyme system so its use may increase the half-life of other drugs that use this same metabolic system. Rifampin decreases the half-life of chloramphenicol. Chloramphenicol impedes the body's production of Vitamin D and other hormones such as testosterone and DHEA. Also, chloramphenicol may lower resistance to viral infections and be associated with motor neuron disease. This drug is likely a carcinogen. Chloramphenicol can pass into breast milk and so use caution during breast feeding.

Dosing: Available (sometimes, in some places) as capsules 250 mg, suspension 125 mg/5 ml, and IV, IM, and ophthalmologic formulations. Dozens of brands. Oral is preferred but there may be circumstances where IV or IM is indicated.

Because of the way the IV needs to be formulated, *less active drug is ultimately available in the system.* IV levels are only about 70% of those achieved orally, so the daily IV dose needs to be *higher.*

Give in equally divided doses q 6 to 8 hrs. Continue until the patient is well and the symptoms are completely resolved for at least 2 days.

Adults: The same dose is recommended for all the rickettsial diseases. Some recommend a loading dose to start and thereafter the same daily dose for maintenance only divided q 6 to 8 hours.

Oral: 50 mg/kg/day in divided
doses q 6 to 8 h

IV: 75 mg/kg/day

Children: In kids with a fever and petechial rash the differential would include N. *meningitides* and RMSF, both covered by chloramphenical.

Oral: 50 mg/kg/day in divided
doses q 6 to 8 h

IV: 75 mg/kg/day

Kids less than 2 weeks:
Maximum daily dose is 25 mg/kg

Older infants:
Up to 50 mg/kg/day

In adults, oily chloramphenicol is given as a single IM injection of 100 mg/kg (with a maximum dose of 3 grams) and then repeated if no clinical response in two days. WHO recommends oily chloramphenicol as first-line in low income regions for meningitis since it tends to be cheap and available. At times, chloramphenicol appears on the WHO essential drug list.

PEARL: I worked a great deal with physicians from WHO when developing western medicines in Asia. Just because a doctor is from WHO or CDC or NIH or IDSA or the FDA does not mean they are more knowledgeable or insightful than the rest of us.

AEs: Adverse drug reactions have limited the use of chloramphenicol. Those with pre-existing liver disease seem to have the most problems especially with inadequate erythropoiesis.

Chloramphenicol can cause bone marrow toxicity in two ways:

Suppression is a direct drug effect on the human cell mitochondria that first manifests as a falling Hb. The body cannot uptake iron and incorporate it into heme to make hemoglobin. Look for reticulocytopenia (low number of immature red cells) which occurs 5 to 7 days after the start of treatment. If there are not enough baby cells, there aren't going to be sufficient fully functional mature cells.

Some reports suggest that suppression is more often noted after a cumulative dose of about 20 grams. Suppression of the bone marrow appears to be fully reversible once the drug is discontinued and is not a predictor of long-term untoward effects such as cancer.

Aplastic anemia is due to defective red blood cell production secondary to problems with the bone marrow. With the use of chloramphenicol, the aplastic anemia is idiosyncratic, which means the condition is likely due to a predisposition in the individual. These tendencies may be genetic as suggested by pancytopenia in twins taking the drug. Aplastic anemia is rare, unpredictable, and seemingly unrelated to dose, but may be associated with length of treatment. The condition is often fatal. Incidence is low, but the mortality rate is high. Those that recover may be at higher risk of later leukemias. Aplastic anemia may be less likely if the drug is given IV rather than oral, but cases have been reported after both routes of administration.

In line with the suppression of bone marrow, all manner of blood cell abnormalities have been reported with the use of chloramphenicol including leukopenia and thrombocytopenia. If you have a baseline before you start treatment, you will be able to track the status. Here is one place where you will want to look at reticulocytes. Remember the importance of not getting stuck in the false security of the WNL paradigm. Look at patterns and trends and compare the patient's last result to the current result. Refer to Chapter 19: *Scientific Basis and Interpretation of Study Results.*

IV chloramphenicol has been associated with **gray baby syndrome**. Some newborns, especially the premature, do not yet have the fully functioning enzyme systems needed to metabolize and excrete chloramphenicol. As a result, the medicine can build up in the system. This toxicity can be fatal. The child may vomit and not suckle. Respirations can become irregular and rapid and cyanosis can result. The baby becomes flaccid and ashen gray. Intermittent loose green stool and abdominal distension have been noted. Heart problems can occur and there is a significant mortality. Those who recover seem to recover entirely. Although only a little chloramphenicol is removed by dialysis, this treatment has been used in children with grey baby syndrome and in cases of overdose with some success.

Chloramphenicol can be irritating causing nausea, vomiting, and bad taste. Also reported are blurred vision, paresthesias, and an optic neuritis with loss of nerve cells and fibers. A number of allergic manifestations including various rashes and swelling are known.

Herx reactions have been documented.

Monitor: CBC with differential, reticulocyte counts, and platelets, along with LFTs, BUN, and creatinine at baseline and frequently thereafter. Some recommend twice a week while on therapy. No one knows if early detection helps stop progression of blood dyscrasias, but you may be dealing with someone with a genetic predisposition toward problems. Err on the side of the conservative. Vitamin D levels may be clinically indicated, as might prophylactic treatment with supplements. The baseline liver and kidney functions should be used to determine if these organs are healthy enough to withstand the treatment regimen and then followed to assess damage.

Some sources recommend blood levels of chloramphenicol especially in neonates, patients with abnormal LFTs, children under 4, the elderly, and patients with renal failure. One reference suggests that peak levels one hour after dose should range between 15 and 25 mg/L and the trough, taken immediately before the next dose, should be less than 15 mg/L.

No one seems to know if high levels predict any untoward consequences or not and if there is any predictive value to this testing. Unfortunately, if the child is critically ill and other treatment options have been ruled out, you then have an unbearable decision to make. Should you continue the chloramphenicol and take your chances with the AEs or d/c the drug and take your chances with the underlying disease? Weigh the options carefully, discuss the risk/benefit with the patient and caretakers, and document your rationale.

PEARL: I learned something in the school of hard knocks doing clinical research: Patients, especially small patients, do not have an unlimited blood supply. In cases where you might be running out of RBCs, do not order endless blood tests if not truly indicated. An anemia may result caused by your zeal, and that complicates the clinical picture.

B. ANTIMALARIALS

Description: I refer to these drugs in this text as antimalarials since that is how they are usually referred to in the literature. For our purposes, they would be better labeled antiprotozoals. Note that the azoles described above could have just as appropriately been included in this section. Don't get distracted by the categories. These are just ways to help sort through too much information.

PEARL: Do not mix up proguanil and Plaquenil and Primaquine.

You might not need all the medicines listed below in your practice repertoire. But they are good to have if your original plan of attack does not seem to be working out.

Selected antiprotozoals:

1. Quinine (Qualaquin)

Description: Quinine is a bitter alkaloid obtained from the bark of the cinchona tree. Medicinal properties were first found by the Quechua (Inca) Indians of Peru and Bolivia. The Indians used the bark to halt shivering from fevers. Peruvians would mix the ground bark of the cinchona tree with sweet water to offset the bitter taste thus producing what we now call tonic water.

After the Jesuits came to South America, they quickly learned the benefits of cinchona bark. Malaria had caused the death of many popes, cardinals, and countless parishioners. Most priests trained in Rome had seen malaria and its effects. Brother Salumbrio was an apothecary Jesuit stationed in Lima, Peru. He saw the Quechua using the cinchona bark and the curative effect on malaria patients. He sent the bark back to Rome to be tested as a malaria treatment. The bark became known as Jesuit's bark and evolved into one of the most profitable products ever sent back to Europe.

The name quinine came from the Inca word "quina-quina" which means bark of bark or holy bark. In Europe, the bark was ground to a fine powder and mixed with fluids (usually wine). Quinine began to be used for the prophylaxis of malaria in the mid-1850s.

Whatever you think of the philosophy of the Jesuits, they were often astute businessmen. The Peruvian government and the church became desperate to keep their monopoly on cinchona bark. They outlawed the exportation of seeds and samplings. But the Dutch (also quite entrepreneurial and non-Catholic to boot) were able to smuggle the seeds out of South America. By the 1930s, the Dutch were producing 97% of the world's quinine in Java. In WWII, when the Germans controlled Holland and the Japanese had the Philippines and Indonesia, the Allies were cut off from their quinine supply. The US quickly started cinchona plantations in Costa Rica. This was too late and thousands of Allied soldiers died from malaria.

Quinine was one factor responsible for the colonization of Africa by Europeans. Prior to its use the continent was known as the "white man's grave." Quinine's efficacy allowed colonists to swarm in and take over.

Today, there are many derivatives and synthetic versions of quinine. While many of these are more tolerable and safer, the natural bark quinine is still probably the most effective against malaria.

MOA: The mechanism of action is unknown but quinine is considered a general protozoal poison. Further, quinine demonstrates a variety of physiologic effects which are not clearly connected. In addition to antiprotozoal effects, quinine has antipyretic actions (fever-reducing), analgesic effects (pain-killing), and anti-inflammatory properties. Quinine reduces shivering through at least two mechanisms: killing the protozoal pathogen directly and somehow addressing temperature regulation. Quinine's isomer, quinidine, is used as an anti-dysrhythmic drug and so it's expected that quinine would have some impact on heart function as well. With these diverse actions, quinine appears to be the perfect treatment for malaria, since this molecule seems to address both the pathogen and many of the most troubling symptoms.

Indications: For malaria, quinine was the standard of care for hundreds of years. Today quinine is mostly reserved for severe chloroquine-resistant malaria. Given IV in these cases, quinine can be life-saving.

Quinine is no longer considered the DOC for malaria and should be used only when other options are not available. Quinine is still the WHO first-line drug for pregnant patients with malaria.

Quinine preparations are also used to treat lupus, leg cramps, and arthritis with varying degrees of anecdotal success. In 2011, quinine in tonic water was touted as the best cure for nocturnal muscle cramps.

Use in TBDs: Quinine is no longer recommended by the WHO as first-line treatment for malaria. Currently, quinine is used only when artemesia is not available or when the patient is severely ill. IV quinine is then used to address incapacitating cerebral malaria. In these cases, quinine is considered life-saving. While Mepron and artemesia are excellent antiprotozoals in their own right, they are not necessarily easy to pull off the shelf in an acute emergency. You might want to treat the patient while you are tracking down the artemesia and taking a second mortgage on the house to buy the Mepron. Don't discount a treatment because it has been around a long time. In these cases, the medicine has survived because it works. Similarly, Mepron and artemesia have supplanted quinine as the treatment of babesiosis. Nevertheless, keep these tried and true remedies in your repertoire. You never know when your babesiosis patient might need them.

Usage: Oral quinine is VERY bitter and may cause vomiting. If a dose is vomited soon after ingestion, wait until the stomach settles and try again. Giving quinine during or after food might help tolerability. Once ingested, the quinine is readily and almost completely absorbed.

Derivatives such as chloroquine (Aralen) and hydroxychloroquine (Plaquenil) provide viable options if the patient cannot tolerate quinine. Take with food.

IV administration is currently reserved for severe, life-threatening cerebral malaria. Since safer and better tolerated treatments are now available, consider alternatives if the patient is stable. There are po, IV, IM, and rectal formulations available in some countries.

Quinine is very sensitive to UV light and will fluoresce in direct sun.

Quinine is pregnancy category D. Nonetheless, the WHO still endorses quinine as the first-line treatment for uncomplicated malaria in pregnancy.

PEARL: Quinine is the flavor in tonic water, bitter lemon, gin and tonic, and many other beverages around the world. Because of its fluorescence it is often selected as a lab standard. When available, quinine is sometimes used as a cutting agent in street drugs like heroin and cocaine.

Cautions: Quinine has a complex and poorly understood MOA, but appears to affect many body systems. Even at therapeutic doses the patient can develop **cinchonism**: ringing in the ears, headache, disturbed vision, and nausea. Cinchonism is a cluster of symptoms which can occur after repeated doses with quinine. With on-going or higher doses, cinchonism can progress. Respiration can be stimulated at first and then become depressed. Body temperature and blood pressure can fall and the patient will become extremely weak. As the pulse slows, the patient lapses into a coma, with pulmonary edema and death from respiratory arrest.

PEARL: Mild cinchonism doesn't mean you must d/c quinine immediately. If the patient needs the drug and there are no viable alternatives, monitor them like a hawk.

Both auditory and visual problems can occur either as part of the cinchonism syndrome or separately. Drug is recommended to be stopped if hemolysis occurs. With the information I had, I could not tell if the hemolysis they are referring to in the literature was due to the drug or the condition the drug was trying to treat (namely malaria and babesiosis). If the hemolysis is due to the disease it will continue, and perhaps increase, if the suspected drug is stopped. If the drug is the cause, the hemolysis should stop or decrease when the drug is discontinued.

PEARL: Quinine and derivatives such as chloroquine and hydroxychloroquine can cause retinal and visual field changes.

If there is an accidental overdose, call Poison Control on the way to the ER. Then have the ER staff call Poison Control. Quinine is extremely toxic in overdose. Be careful in patients with myasthenia gravis and those with difficulty swallowing. Quinine's effects on muscle may cause respiratory problems and dysphagia. Quinine is CI in those patients with pre-existing tinnitus and optic neuritis. Use caution in patients with a history of atrial fibrillation, heart block, and conduction defects. Quinine can cause bleeding in G6PD deficiency but this hemolysis is usually rare and mild.

Dosing: Quinine dosing can be complicated because you have to know what formulation you have. Quinine is always dosed as a salt and there are at least a half dozen kinds of salt preparations. All can be administered po or IV and the gluconate salt can also be given IM and rectally. Different formulations are available at different times and in different countries and dosing recommendations differ for all. If your heart is set on using quinine, call your trusted local pharmacist and see what is available. Consider the alternatives listed below as well.

One published IV regimen of quinine is:

Loading: 20 mg/kg of quinine base
Maintenance: 8 mg/kg of quinine base q 8 h

PEARL: IV quinine is only intermittently available in the US. When not available and IV quinine is desired, quinidine is substituted.

Load with 20 mg/kg in 400 ml NSS and infuse over 4 hours then follow with 8 to 10 mg/kg in a 4 hour infusion q 8 h. The maximum dose of the salt is 1500 mg daily.

Oral quinine sulfate is available in the US as 324 mg tablets under the brand name Qualaquin. The oral adult dose is two tablets q 8 h.

AEs: In addition to cinchonism described above, the most important quinine AEs include those listed below. Quinine derivatives can also cause these events.

- Ototoxicity: The mechanism here may be direct damage to the 8th cranial nerve. Manifestations include tinnitus, decreased auditory acuity, ringing, and vertigo. Auditory problems can remain after treatment is discontinued.

- Visual changes: The mechanism is probably direct neurotoxicity against the optic nerve or vascular changes. Reports include spastic constriction of the retinal vessels, pale discs, edema, blurred vision, optic atrophy, distorted color perception, diplopia, night blindness, restricted fields, and scotoma. Blindness has rarely been documented. Residual problems can remain after quinine is stopped.

- GI: Multiple GI complaints are likely from local irritation including nausea, vomiting, pain, dysphagia, and diarrhea.

- Skeletal muscle: Respiratory distress involving the accessory respiratory muscles has been reported.

- Kidney: Renal damage and failure

- Liver: Quinine is primarily metabolized in the liver, so the liver is a potential site of problems.

- Pancreas: Lower blood glucose levels have been observed.

- Cardiac: Since quinine is an isomer of quinidine, a cardiac drug, AEs around cardiac rhythm and function have been reported. Use with caution in patients with pre-existing atrial fibrillation.

- Skin: Often hot, flushed, or sweating (Is this the drug or the underlying disease?) With cinchonism, the skin can feel cold. Many types of rashes and skin conditions have been reported including angioedema.

- CNS: Headache, apprehension, central vomiting, excitement, confusion, delirium, and syncope

Monitor: Some say you do not need to monitor quinine patients if the dose is given orally. Err on the side of the conservative. Try to get baseline hearing and visual testing (including fields, acuity, and color). Some recommend cardiac monitoring at the first dose and then regular observation. Check CBC for hemolysis and LFTs and kidney function tests including BUN and creatinine. Blood glucose readings may be low.

APOLOGY: I spent a lot of words on a drug that you will likely never use and will never be used in your TBI population. I did this for several reasons. First quinine was the foundation therapy for protozoal infections for centuries. Knowing the background may help you understand the state of antiprotozoal medicine today. Secondly, many of the common, viable antiprotozoals today are derivatives of quinine.

2. Mefloquine (Lariam, Mefaquin)

Description: Developed in the 1970s at the Walter Reed Army Institute of Research as a synthetic quinine. I worked there for a summer once with a crazy researcher with a long beard who was into heavy metal music. In its day, Walter Reed was a fabulous hospital.

MOA: Disrupts calcium metabolism in pathogen cells which can lead to cell injury and death. Lariam readily crosses the BBB, accumulates, and appears to be able to get at the pathogens inside neurons.

Indications: Prophylaxis and treatment of certain kinds of acute malaria

Use in TBDs: Alternative treatment for Babesia. There is speculation that mefloquine may have efficacy against Bb.

PEARL: Mepron does not always get Babesia infection out of the brain so sometimes the patient will need Lariam since it is much better at passing the BBB.

Usage: Take with food and plenty of water. Because of the significant side effect profile, consider all options. Assess the risk/benefit ratio and make sure the patient and parents understand the potential risks of therapy. Ensure that they are part of the decision-making process. Document your rationale.

Cautions: Discontinue if there are CNS disturbances, heart problems, psychiatric symptoms, seizures, or hepatic impairment

Caution when used with drugs that cause QT prolongation. Do not use with quinine, quinidine, or chloroquine since concomitant use may result in EKG changes. Do not use with β-blockers since this combination could prolong QT intervals.

Complete all live oral bacterial vaccinations before starting Lariam.

Caution in pregnancy and nursing. May interact with anti-epileptics.

A strong Herx reaction may occur, depending on dose and pathogen. Make sure the patient understands the Herx reaction prior to initiating therapy. See Chapter 28: *Understanding the Herxheimer Reaction.*

Caution in using in patients with a history of psychiatric problems, depression, or anxiety.

Dosage: Available in 250 mg tablets which can be crushed and added to food or water. "Official" dosing recommendations are for prophylaxis and weekly administration. For TBIs, doses would need to be determined on a case-by-case basis.

AEs: Nausea, vomiting, diarrhea, dizziness, syncope, abnormal heart rate, myalgia, fever, headache, chills, rash, abdominal pain, fatigue, anorexia, tinnitus, seizures, cardiac arrest, encephalopathy, emotional disturbances, depression, anxiety, paranoia, aggression, nightmares, insomnia, birth defects, neuropathy, hallucinations, vestibular damage (balance), CNS signs, eye problems, vivid dreams, brainstem signs, pneumonitis, and eosinophilic pneumonia.

Some of these events result in permanent sequelae. Because of the significant side effect profile, consider all options. Based on the individual case, Lariam might be the best choice.

Monitor: Follow liver, cardiac, and visual function in long-term use. Monitor EKG regularly throughout the course of therapy.

3. **Chloroquine (Aralen)**

Description: Derivative of quinine

MOA: Binds to and alters the properties of both microbial and mammalian DNA. Chloroquine only hits the intracellular pathogens.

Indications: Suppression and treatment of certain malarias

Use in TBDs: Antiprotozoal for babesiosis

Usage: Give right before or after meals. Use IM when oral therapy not possible

Do not take near cimetidine, penicillins, antacids, or kaolin

Dosing: Available as 500 mg tablets and injectable 50 mg/ml. Dose amounts vary by source.

For malaria:

Oral:

Adults:	For malaria treatment: 1 gram loading and then 500 mg 6 hours later, then 500 daily for 2 days
Children:	For malaria treatment: 16.7 mg/kg then 8.35 mg/kg (max 500 mg) then may repeat at 6, 24, and 36 hours. Maximum 1 gram in 24 hours

IM:

Adults:	For malaria treatment: Load with 200 to 250 mg IM. May repeat in 6 hrs. Maximum 1 g in 24 hours and then may administer again up to 1.875 g after 3 days
Children:	For malaria treatment: 6.25 mg/kg IM, may repeat in 6 hrs. Maximum 12.5 mg/kg/day and maximum 5 mg/kg/dose

Cautions: Do not use if patient has underlying retinal or visual field changes, hepatic or auditory dysfunction, alcoholism, psoriasis, porphyria, seizure disorders, or G6PD deficiency.

Consider stopping if blood, vision, or hearing problems occur. If blood dyscrasias occur, consider alternative treatments. Caution in elderly and children and with concomitant hepatotoxic drugs. Avoid excess sun exposure. Overdosage can lead quickly to toxicity.

Not recommended in pregnancy or nursing. Ensure that adequate birth control is in place if the drug is going to be used in females of child bearing potential.

There is currently considerable resistance to chloroquine from some malarial strains.

AEs:

General: Headache, pruritis, photosensitivity, GI upset, skin lesions, mucosal pigment changes, cardiomyopathy, myopathy, anorexia, abdominal cramps, diarrhea, nausea, vomiting, hepatitis

Blood: Dyscrasias: agranulocytosis, leukopenia, pancytopenia

Vision: Retinopathy, blurred vision, difficulty in focusing, corneal changes, retinal problems such as narrowing arterioles, macular lesions, pallor of optic disc, optic atrophy, and patchy pigmentation. These changes may be irreversible and occasionally lead to blindness.

Ototoxicity: Nerve deafness, vertigo, tinnitus

CNS: Stimulation, fatigue, nightmares, seizures, psychosis, irritability, neuromyopathy

Monitor: CBC with differential, platelets, reflexes, vision, hearing, LFTs. Baseline and periodic eye and hearing checks in long-term use

4. Plaquenil (hydroxychloroquine)

PEARL: Do not mix up proguanil (component of Malarone), Plaquenil (hydroxychloroquine), and Primaquine (another antimicrobial).

Description: Derivative of quinine

MOA: Binds to and alters the properties of both microbial and mammalian DNA and increases the pH in antigen-presenting cells. In terms of decreasing inflammation, there is a complex MOA. Hydroxychloroquine blocks toll-like receptors which recognize DNA-containing immune complexes leading to interferon production. Interferon causes dendritic cells to mature and present antigens to T cells. By decreasing the signals from the toll receptors the drug reduces the activation of the dendritic cells and thereby lessens the inflammation. If you understand all that, you don't need this book. Don't bother looking in the *Gentle Immunology* chapter because that won't help. Fortunately, here's a sentence even I can understand: With parasites, hydroxychloroquine may stop the parasite from metabolizing the hemoglobin inside the RBC, thereby impacting the cell's survival.

Indications: Susceptible malaria, inflammation in RA, SLE, Sjogren's syndrome, and other rheumatic disorders. Lyme arthritis. May have antifungal properties

Use in TBDs: Antiprotozoal also used in Lyme to potentiate the effect of other antibiotics (macrolides). In Lyme arthritis, hydroxychloroquine may have both an anti-spirochetal and anti-inflammatory MOA. This dual effect is reason to consider Plaquenil when a Lyme patient has predominately joint or autoimmune-type presentations. May be useful in patients who test positive for HLA-DR2 or HLA-DR4 which indicate a tendency for an autoimmune reaction to Lyme. In the TBI literature, there is considerable reference to the use of hydroxychloroquine. Consider in Lyme especially when arthritis is a major presenting component. Often co-administered with clarithromycin or with azithromycin to enhance their efficacy. In TBIs, almost always used in combination in order to come at the pathogens from multiple angles. Consider with Bb, M. *fermentans*, and Babesia co-infections. Used against Q fever endocarditis

PEARL: A potentially important use of Plaquenil (hydroxychloroquine) is in those Lyme patients who test positive for HLA-DR2 and HLA-DR4 markers. The presence of these markers suggests which patients might respond to Bb infection with an autoimmune-type presentation. These patients do not respond well to traditional antibiotic regimens alone, but Plaquenil seems to be a useful addition in these cases.

Usage: Give right before or after meals. Some say to take with food or milk.

Dosing: Available in 200 mg tablets

For malaria:

Adults: Initially 800 mg, then 400 mg at hours 6, 24, and 48 hrs after 1ˢᵗ dose

Children: Dose is calculated based on body weight and should not exceed adult dose

For rheumatic disorder such as SLE or RA:

Adults: Initial: 400 to 600 mg daily. After stabilized in about 4 to 12 weeks, go to:

. Maintenance: 200 to 400 mg daily (in divided doses) with food or milk

Children: Not established. Base dose on weight and do not exceed adult dose

For long-term use, calculate the best dose to avoid eye toxicity. This dose can be calculated using patient height and weight. The manufacturer can provide the formula. A trusted pharmacist may be able to help.

Cautions: Be careful and monitor closely, especially any long-term use in children. Watch for retinal or visual field changes, hepatic dysfunction and auditory problems. Long-term use in a small children is not recommended.

Use with care in alcoholism, psoriasis, porphyria, seizure disorders, and G6PD deficiency. Those with G6PD can develop significant anemia and children taking hydroxychloroquine are most vulnerable. Avoid other hepatotoxic drugs.

Most serious problems associated with the eye are usually with long-term use. Toxicity from hydroxychloroquine is seen in two areas of the eye: the cornea and the macula. The cornea can develop keratopathy with epithelial deposits. These are NOT dose-related and are usually reversible. In contrast, problems in the macula can be related to dose and length of treatment. Reduction in visual acuity, a clear bull's eye lesion on the macula, and atrophy of the retinal pigmented epithelium have all been documented.

Caution in pregnancy and nursing. Hydroxychloroquine is secreted in breast milk.

AEs:

General: Headache, dizziness, GI upset, weight loss, abdominal cramps, diarrhea, heart problems, decreased appetite, nausea, vomiting, acne, anemia, blood disorders, pigmentation of skin, hives, itch, diminished reflexes, emotional changes, hearing loss, liver problems including failure, loss of hair, muscle

paralysis, weakness, muscle atrophy, nightmares, tinnitus, skin inflammation, scaling, vertigo, leukopenia, and thrombocytopenia. Hydroxychloroquine might worsen psoriasis and porphyria.

Eye problems: Hydroxychloroquine can affect both the cornea and the macula. The cornea can develop keratopathy with epithelial deposits. These are not dose-related and are usually reversible. In contrast, problems in the macula can be related to dose and length of treatment. Signs include reduction in visual acuity, a clear bull's eye lesion on the macula, atrophy of the retinal pigmented epithelium, and color blindness. Altered eye pigmentation has also been reported.

Monitor: Try to get a baseline comprehensive eye exam. Also, do a baseline hearing test and blood work including CBC with differential and platelets and LFTs. Document reflexes and muscle strength on baseline PE and then assess regularly over time. Follow vision and hearing regularly if hydroxychloroquine is used long-term, at least several times each year. Better to err on the side of the conservative. Check eyes, even if there are no signs or symptoms.

5. Atovaquone (Mepron)

Description: An antiprotozoal of the naphthalene class that is almost insoluble in water. Atovaquone is claimed to be a primary component of henna used to color hair in India. Who knew?

MOA: The specific MOA is unknown but atovaquone is thought to impact the cytochrome complex III mitochondrial electron transport system of the protozoa. By doing so, critical enzymes cannot be synthesized and therefore nucleic acid and ATP synthesis is suspended and the pathogen dies. (Wouldn't it just be easier to smother it with a pillow?)

Indications: Atovaquone is indicated to treat and prevent PCP (Pneumocystis *carinii* pneumonia) in those patients who cannot tolerate Bactrim. PCP is common in AIDS patients and in some transplant patients. Atovaquone may have an advantage in these patients since it does not seem to cause myelosuppression. Also, commonly used to treat toxoplasmosis and malaria.

Use in TBDs: Atovaquone is used to treat the protozoal causes of malaria. In fact, the antimalarial Malarone is a combination atovaquone and proguanil specifically indicated for that purpose. Since Babesia is a similar protozoal pathogen, atovaquone has also been used to treat babesiosis with considerable anecdotal success. Often used in combination with Zithromax (azithromycin), atovaquone would be expected to handle the Babesia and help with co-infections such as Bb. Remember that Mepron probably only hits the B. *microti* species and other agents will need to be added to handle the B. *duncani*. Mepron does not always get infection out of the brain so sometimes you need to consider an alternative antiprotozoal like Lariam since it is much better at passing the BBB. The combination of Mepron, Zithromax, and artemesia is probably best in going after Babesia. Case reports suggest that Mepron may have efficacy in hitting Bb, so Mepron might be a good choice when Bb and Babesia are co-infections.

Usage: Pathogens have not yet demonstrated strong resistance to atovaquone.

Must take with *fatty foods* for best absorption. Mepron should be taken with balanced meals that include *fats*. Take about the same time every day. *Shake* the bottle. Atovaquone is practically insoluble so the suspended particles must be well mixed for appropriate dosing.

Measure carefully. Even though a teaspoon equals 5 ml or 5 cc, that does NOT mean a kitchen teaspoon. Kitchen teaspoons can vary considerably. The spoon must be a measuring or medicine teaspoon. Drug stores have them or you can use a 5 cc syringe. If the medicine is prescribed to be dosed at more than a teaspoon, you can use a larger syringe. If you use a kitchen teaspoon, which I used for many years, you will likely overdose or underdose.

Mortgage the house. Atovaquone is expensive. Comparison shop.

Safety and efficacy have not officially been established in kids. No problems specific to the elderly have been documented but the elderly may have liver, kidney, or heart problems that might put them at greater risk of side effects. Lower doses may be prudent.

A common dietary supplement, enzyme CoQ 10, may interfere with the efficacy of Mepron so check the ingredient list on any multivitamins or supplements to make sure they do not include this enzyme.

Atovaquone works best when the blood levels are steady. Try not to miss a dose and if you do, take the missing dose as soon as you remember. However, if it is almost time for your next dose just skip the missed dose and go back to your usual schedule. Do not take a double dose to make up for the one you missed. Plasma levels have been correlated with treatment efficacy, so take the medicine as directed.

Some patients do not like the taste and some do not like the texture and thickness. There are far worse. I find Mepron pleasant. My son found "the feel of it" strange.

Atovaquone is highly bound to the plasma proteins so be careful using this medicine with other drugs highly bound to plasma proteins since they may compete for binding sites. Use with Rifampin will cause lower systemic levels of both drugs. Be cautious when used concomitantly with tetracyclines and some seizure medicines. Dosage may need to be adjusted.

Mepron is pregnancy category C. The doses used for testing in the pregnant animals were proportionately much higher than are used in routine human treatment protocols.

Cautions: Always weigh the risks/benefits before deciding on a treatment regimen.

Be careful in patients with pre-existing GI or liver problems. Be careful in patients who cannot take the medicine with fatty foods. They may have poor absorption.

Monitor patients with pre-existing liver disease or GI disorders (stomach or intestinal problems). Watch for limited efficacy as well as safety and tolerability issues. They may not be absorbing the product adequately. Mepron may decrease CoQ 10 levels.

Effects on the fetus or nursing baby are not known. Assess pregnancy status prior to embarking on a long-term course.

PEARL: Anecdotally, Mepron has been used in a number of pregnant women without adverse consequences.

Dosing: Available in a bright *yellow* suspension (like drinking a daffodil) at 750 mg/5 ml. Also 250 mg tablets. No specific dosing information has been established for the treatment of malaria or babesiosis.

Adults and over 13 years: 750 mg (1 teaspoon or 5 ml) bid with food or 1500 mg (2 teaspoons or 10 ml) once daily with food. Measure accurately.

For PCP: 750 mg bid for 21 days

For babesiosis: Treatment may need to be continued for months.

PEARL: In children with babesiosis, IDSA recommends 20 mg/kg q 12 with a maximum of 750 mg/dose.

AEs: Despite comments about taste and texture, Mepron seems to be well tolerated. Since the patients prescribed this medicine are often quite sick, deciding which treatment emergent AEs are due to the Mepron versus the underlying disease or concomitant therapy can be difficult. About ¼ of the subjects in clinical trials discontinued due to an AE. Remember these patients had PCP and probably AIDS during the studies. Always consider the risk/benefit of every treatment. If options are limited, the ratio may shift. Use the causality checklist presented earlier to help you determine the etiology of an AE.

Reported AEs include: Cough, hoarseness, trouble breathing, fever, chills, back or flank pain, chest tightness, wheezing, anxiety, depression, sleep disturbances, hoarseness, black or tarry stools, bleeding gums, various skin lesions, bruising, white patches in mouth, skin peeling, pinpoint rash, tiredness, weakness, vomiting, yellow eyes or skin, sweating, loss of strength, stuffy or runny nose, allergic reactions including severe symptoms, itching, joint or muscle pain, bloating, blood in urine or stool, thrombocytopenia, neutropenia, hyponatremia, anemia, blue lips, nails or palms, diarrhea, constipation, dark urine, bruising, dizziness, rapid heartbeat, headache, indigestion, hives, swelling, light-colored stools, poor appetite, nausea, and pain in the stomach, abdomen, or side. To an old drug developer like me, this is the usual list of suspects. Everything and nothing. Mepron might make the urine orange-tinged.

Monitor: Watch CBC with differential, platelets, and liver function

6. **Malarone** (combination of atovaquone 250 mg and proguanil 100 mg)

Description: Malarone is a combination of atovaquone 250 mg and proguanil 100 mg. The information provided in the previous section regarding atovaquone also applies here as well. Proguanil is effective against some protozoans, in specific stages, and is sometimes used alone as a prophylactic antimalarial. Since these two agents work by different mechanisms the combination is thought to provide better efficacy against protozoas.

MOA: Proguanil works by stopping the protozoa from reproducing once they get inside the RBC. This drug inhibits the enzyme dihydrofolatereductase that is involved in the reproduction of the pathogen and known to be quotessperescent.

Indications: Prophylaxis and treatment of malaria

Use in TBDs: Consider in babesiosis since both components appear to be effective antiprotozoals

Usage: Take at the same time each day with fatty food or milk. Repeat dose if vomiting occurs within one hour. Can take with folate

Do not take with enzyme CoQ 10 or Rifampin. Be cautious when used concomitantly with tetracyclines and some seizure medicines

If the patient is severely ill or not responding, consider other treatment.

Malarone is pregnancy category C. Use with caution during nursing

The good news about this drug combination is that there is actually a pediatric formulation. Instead of reading over and over about no data being available regarding use in kids for many of the other drugs, this combo actually has information!

Cautions: Be vigilant in monitoring patients with pre-existing depression, anxiety, or psychiatric conditions. Consider alternative therapies when symptoms that appear out of the ordinary occur during treatment.

Dosing: Available in tablets containing atovaquone 250 mg and 100 mg proguanil. Malarone pediatric tablets have 62.5 mg atovaquone and 25 mg proguanil. These tablets can be crushed and taken with something nice and fatty like pudding.

For malaria:

Adults: Daily po dose for malaria treatment: 1 gram:400 mg (4 tablets) to start for three days and then one tablet a day thereafter

Children: Daily po dose of the pediatric formulation for malaria treatment:

Less than 5 kg:	Not recommended
5 to 8 kg:	125 mg:50 mg (2 pediatric tablets)
9 to 10 kg:	187.5 mg:75 mg (3 pediatric tablets)
11 to 20 kg:	250 mg:100 mg (4 pediatric tablets)
21 to 30 kg:	500 mg:200 mg (can use 8 pediatric or 2 adult tablets)
31 to 40 kg:	750 mg:300 mg
Greater than 40 kg:	1 gram:400 mg

Cautions: Caution in renal impairment with creatinine clearance less than 30 ml/minute, hepatic dysfunction, the elderly, pregnant, or nursing. Malarone interacts with Rifampin and the atovaquone component is antagonized by TCNs.

With use of proguanil watch for signs of depression and anxiety when taken long-term. These symptoms may come on gradually and may be beyond the ordinary in terms of the variations in mood in everyday life. Always consider the risk/benefit ratio when deciding on whether to stop or change a treatment.

AEs: GI upset or pain, headache, anaphylaxis, asthenia, anorexia, vomiting, pruritis, sullenness, anxiety

Monitor: Make sure the kidney is healthy enough to handle the drug. Draw a baseline BUN and creatinine and then follow the kidney function throughout the treatment course. Draw baseline LFTs and CBC. Monitor periodically. Watch for mood changes and anxiety.

PEARL: Notice that 25% of the patients in clinical trials using Mepron discontinued use due to AEs. That is A LOT! At the same time, less than 1% of those using Malarone discontinued their study participation due to AEs. That's hardly any. Why? They were using the same drug. It is highly unlikely that combination with proguanil altered the safety profile of atovaquone so much as to wipe out essentially all AEs. Consider the study populations. In one case, the patients had PCP and AIDS. In the other they had malaria. Look at the AE list for Mepron. Many of the AEs for Mepron are the signs and symptoms of PCP and AIDS. Took me 20 years to see what might be real in a data set.

7. Clindamycin (Cleocin)

Description: Clindamycin is a bacteriostatic lincosamide.

MOA: Works by inhibiting protein synthesis in the pathogen via interference with translation on the ribosome. Clindamycin is thought to use this MOA in impeding the synthesis of toxins from a number of pathogens such as Strep.

PEARL: Clindamycin, erythromycins, and chloramphenicol all bind to the same area on the ribosome and when used together may cause significant interactions. There should not be much reason to use these agents together since there are alternatives.

Indications: Serious susceptible infections where less toxic antibiotics won't help. While most often considered a strong antibiotic for anaerobic bacteria, clindamycin is also quite effective against protozoal diseases like malaria and babesiosis. Often used in infections of the respiratory tract, skin, soft tissue, intra-abdominal cavity, pelvis, genital region, bones, joints, and for sepsis. Clindamycin does NOT penetrate into the CNS and is NOT for the treatment of meningitis. Clindamycin is often used as a topical acne prep and for antibacterial prophylaxis before dental procedures.

Use in TBDs: Clindamycin is effective against protozoal diseases like babesiosis. Because of slow action, clindamycin cannot stand alone against these protozoa but is considered an effective ancillary treatment. The combination of clindamycin and another antimalarial is considered a standard therapy for babesiosis. Clindamycin may not be a good choice if penetration is needed across the BBB or for meningitis.

Usage: Clindamycin can cause considerable GI irritation. Initially the patient can try taking the medicine while sitting up since lying down seems to cause more irritation. If the patient has no problem after several doses, then the patient can lie down after taking the medicine. This is often good news since these people are often quite sick.

In terms of absorption, clindamycin can be taken with or without food. Take with a full glass of water. To be most effective, blood levels should remain steady and so the medicine needs to be taken at regular intervals. For example, take every six hours instead of qid.

Clindamycin is pregnancy category B.

Cautions: Use only for serious infections since clindamycin can have potentially fatal side effects. The bacteria Clostridium *difficile* is completely resistant to clindamycin. Because the strong clindamycin is wiping out most other bacteria, C. *difficile* is overgrowing and producing a toxin that can cause severe diarrhea, dehydration, pseudomembranous colitis, and toxic megacolon: all potentially fatal. While just about every antibiotic can cause these problems, clindamycin is known for **C. *difficile* overgrowth**. Pseudomembranous colitis associated with the C. *difficile* toxin was first identified in association with clindamycin. Now, forever more, clindamycin will be considered the drug that causes C. *diff*.

Clindamycin may antagonize macrolides. Use caution in nursing.

Dosing: Adjust the dose to the severity of the illness. Cleocin comes in capsules (75 mg, 150 mg, and 300 mg) and solution 75 mg/5 ml made from granules.

Oral:

Adults: 150 mg to 450 mg every 6 hours

Children: 8 to 25 mg/kg/day in 3 or 4 divided doses

In kids less than 10 kg, make sure they get at least 37.5 mg tid

Injectable for IM or IV

Adults: 0.6 to 2.7 **gram** daily in 2 to 4 equally divided doses. Maximum IM injection is 600 mg with no more than 4.8 **gram**/day

Children:

Neonates: 15 to 20 mg/kg/day in 3 to 4 divided doses

Greater than one month: 20 to 40 mg/kg/day IV or IM in 3 to 4 divided doses

PEARL: For severe Babesia, IDSA recommends that clindamycin be used only as an IV.

For neonates and severely ill children, professionals experienced in using clindamycin should do the dose calculations. If you are not comfortable, consult.

AEs: Poor clindamycin. You'd think all the C. *diff* in the world was its fault. Actually, just about any antibiotic can cause *difficile* overgrowth, but clindamycin was the first and will likely always be the primary drug associated with this syndrome.

Let's put this in perspective. About 2% to 20% of clindamycin patients get diarrhea. Depending on the source, between 0.01% and 10% of those taking clindamycin develop pseudomembranous colitis characterized by diarrhea, abdominal pain, fever, and mucus and blood in the stool due to the C. *difficile* toxin.

Chapter 23: *Understanding Medicines* has more details on the diagnosis and treatment of C. *difficile* overgrowth. Problems with C. *difficile* may start during treatment or not for weeks after the medicine has been discontinued. We are FINALLY remembering to think back in the patient history to see what they might have been taking previously that could be causing the current problem. If symptoms appear, consider cultures and assaying the stool for toxin. Discontinue the clindamycin immediately and treat with metronidazole (Flagyl) or with vancomycin po 125 to 500 q 6 for 10 days.

Do NOT give drugs, such as Lomotil, that slow down the motion of the GI tract in order to stop the diarrhea.

This type of diarrhea is caused by a toxin made by the C. *difficile*. You want that toxin OUT of you. If you give Lomotil, you will usually find that Lomotil works. It will stop the diarrhea but that means the toxin is now trapped inside you. As soon as the Lomotil wears off you will learn a whole new meaning of the word diarrhea. The best course of action is to stop the antibiotic that is causing the problem and treat with antimicrobials that will obliterate the C. *difficile*. Once the C. *diff* is gone, it won't be producing toxins that are responsible for the symptoms any more. I know, you just want it to STOP!

But clindamycin is not all diarrhea all the time. There are other reported AEs: rashes in about 10%, itching, GI upset, nausea, vomiting, jaundice, renal problems, blood dyscrasias, arteritis, anaphylaxis, arthritis, jaundice, increased LFTs, hepatotoxicity, thrush, and metallic taste.

Monitor: Assess blood, renal, and hepatic function. Keep track of loose stools and hydration status. Watch *neonates* closely. They are very susceptible to dehydration and if they are on an aggressive antibiotic like Cleocin, they already have enough troubles.

8. **Azoles**

Description: Azole antimicrobials are detailed in the *Antibiotic* section above and include metronidazole (Flagyl) and tinidazole (Tindamax). They have shown efficacy against all kinds of microbes from fungus to anaerobic bacteria to protozoas like Entamoebas, Giardia, and Trichomonas and all their corresponding manifestations. Often these drugs are included in the list of antimalarials since the causative agent of malaria is a protozoa, as is that of the TBI babesiosis.

9. **Artemesia** (arteminisin, artemisinine, artemisian, artesunate, quinghaosu, artemether, artemisinin)

Description: This is my least favorite drug. Not because I don't think it works or because I think it has a hideous safety profile. I don't like this drug because it is so hard to pin down. For the last 3 years I have had a list taped to my monitor with various spellings of artemesia. I stopped at 26 because my sticky-note got full. But to say there are hundreds of variations is not an exaggeration.

One Internet reference said there were more than 3,000,000 registered importers and exporters of artemesia. "REGISTERED." Imagine how many unregistered traffickers there are. Even if the Internet source misplaced a decimal or two, that would be 300,000 or 30,000 or 3,000. That's a lot of entrepreneurs out there pushing artemesia. Not bad for a medicine I never heard of a few years ago.

How did I choose "Artemisinin" as the name I would mostly use as opposed to all the other variations? I had to select one or go daft. I learned that if you pick the wrong formulation, or a manufacturer who makes an impure product, you could be recommending a toxin. I had to be careful. I needed to find a product that was fairly reliable and stick with it. My husband had found Artemisinin on the Internet after we were told our son needed it. We had no idea what we were buying, especially since we could not read the physician's hand-writing. We were lucky to come close. We ordered Artemisinin. Our son got better and nothing bad happened so I figured this was as good a place as any to start. I had a hard time remembering the name so I decided, "There is both **art** and **sin in** medicine." Not great, I know, but it helps. I still have to look at the sticky-note on my monitor each time I want to spell it.

*PEARL: I use the term **artemisia** to refer to the plant source or active ingredient. I use the term **artemesia** to refer to the medicinal herbal used to treat protozoa. I use the term **Artemisinin** to refer to the combination product we used at our house.*

Artemisia is derived from an herbal plant native to many Asian countries, not regulated by the FDA, and not available by prescription. There are no requirements on how it is made, purified, or packaged. The HCP must tell the patient to take it, usually in combination with several other medicines. Often, they jot the name on a scrap paper. Our HCP just said. "Look on the Internet." Where, if you have the money, you get the goods.

Artemesia has been used medicinally for more than 2000 years. There are extant curing recipes from the 1st century BCE. Respected in TCM for millennia, artemesia has been used to treat skin problems and malaria. The earliest mention is from 200 BCE in a work called: "Fifty-two Prescriptions." The first reference as a malaria remedy was from 4th century CE writings found in Han dynasty tombs.

Artemisia is most often extracted from the herb Artemisia *annua*, a staple in traditional Chinese medicine. Usually, this herb is modified by some type of processing and mixed with any number of other herbs to form a therapeutic compound. Artemisia is also found in shrubs like wormwood. Artemisia *annua* and variations of the wormwood are found around the world,

even near the Potomac River in Washington, DC. Nevertheless, there is now a shortage of wormwood leaves. To extract the active compounds the peaceful wormwood must be extremely stressed (much like the author of a textbook on TBIs).

In the 1960s, the Chinese army set about finding a good treatment for malaria. By 1972, they had found artemisia in wormwood. Locally, the herb was called quinghaosu. This herb was tested against 200 others from TCM and was the only one effective against malaria. The quinghaosu (artemisia) cleared the malaria parasites from the human body faster than any other drug in history. The findings were finally published but largely ignored. Some of this disregard had to do with politics, since the government did not want outside interests exploiting the local market. Some of the snub was intentional due to greed, since drug companies with competing antimalarials were interested in keeping the effectiveness of artemesia under wraps. (Imagine politics and greed influencing medicine. Unheard of!) Despite being used medicinally for millennia, the active ingredient in artemesia was not isolated until the 1970s.

Published in the Chinese Medical Journal in 2006, the results of the army testing were still met with skepticism, since artemesia seemed too chemically unstable to be used in a large population. This doubt was soon dispelled and WHO recognized the benefits of artemesia as the most effective antimalarial and now recommends it as first-line combination treatment against malaria.

UC Berkeley may have engineered a way to synthesize artemisia from yeast. (I feel more names coming.) Other researchers say they can get artemisia from a plant closely related to tobacco. Doctors without Borders (with whom I will volunteer if I ever finish this book) are working with farmers in Mozambique to grow a shrub from cuttings so the locals can make an artemisia tea.

PEARL: Coartem is a combination brand of artemether and lumefantrine, two antimalarials that may be commercially available in the US by the time this Compendium *is published.*

MOA: You'd think that with 3,000,000 people out there selling the stuff, someone would have figured out how artemesia works. Many theories regarding the MOA have been discredited. One proposed MOA that is still standing involves the parasite inside the RBC. When the pathogen is exposed to artemesia, it consumes excessive hemoglobin, releasing free heme.

This heme is then involved in a complex cascade of reactions that leads to the formation of free radicals. These free radicals eventually destroy the parasite cell. As with many humans, the parasite's gluttony becomes its undoing.

Artemesia appears to be most effective against the pathogen when it is inside the RBC, also called the intraerythrocytic state of infection. Still, this herb likely hits both the sequestered and circulating parasites. The therapy works quickly and the cell of the parasite is impacted soon after exposure to the medicine. Hypothetically, artemesia is effective at certain points of the parasite life cycle when other drugs aren't nearly as useful. This has something to do with the digestive vacuole of the parasite, the electron transport chain, the generation of local reactive oxygen species, and the depolarization of the mitochondrial membrane. You can't ask a drug for more than that.

Artemesia may have anti-cancer effects using a similar mechanism. Working best in areas like the liver, where there is a high concentration of iron, artemesia comes in contact with the iron and becomes unstable. The subsequent chemical reactions release highly reactive oxygen species which reduce angiogenesis and VEGF. Since cancer tissue seems to have a disproportionate concentration of iron, some believe that artemesia may have potential as an oncology treatment.

When using artemesia as a long-term treatment, care must be taken not to stress the liver. If used continuously without a break, the liver goes into overdrive in order to metabolize the compound. In this case the liver does its job too well. Artemesia has a very short half-life of only a few hours. The liver is metabolizing it rapidly. There is a significant drop in blood levels over a five day treatment course. After about 3 or 4 days the blood levels will be very low and you will not have an effective treatment. Then, the liver needs a break. Therefore, the best way to dose artemesia is by **pulsing**. One regimen pulses 4 days on and 3 days off because that matches the natural physiology of the liver. While some practitioners pulse 2 weeks on and 2 weeks off, 3 weeks on and one week off, 12 days on and 2 days off, or even pulse monthly, these regimens do not correspond with what is happening in the liver. The drug will be over-metabolized in a few days and the patient will be left with ineffective treatment for the rest of the course. The 4 days on and 3 days off schedule makes physiologic sense.

Indications: WHO recommends artemesia in combination with other antimicrobials as first-line treatment for malaria. The medicine should not be used alone because of increasing resistance. The artemesia hits the protozoa hard and fast and then the secondary drug, presumably with a longer half-life, is there to mosey along and clean up the stragglers or the ones who were resistant to the artemesia. Artemesia seems to be effective against both the fulciparum and vivax forms of malaria.

Artemesia has also been found to be useful in treating schistosomiasis and is being actively investigated for its anticancer potential.

Use in TBDs: Artemesia is the DOC for malaria. Babesia is a similar protozoal infection. The traditional antimalarials and macrolides that hit B. *microti* do not hit B. *duncani*. For this you need artemesia. The distinction between the two Babesia strains is hard to make. The patient is lucky if the HCP even considered Babesia, let alone which kind. So, if Babesia is suspected assume both strains are present. (You can't prove a negative.) Always treat both strains. Artemesia should probably be part of every Babesia treatment regime. Just as in the treatment of malaria, artemesia should not be used alone in case resistance is building. Always use artemesia as a part of a combination treatment strategy.

Usage: Take 15 to 30 minutes before meals. Use for longer than 3 months may result in additional AEs.

There are dozens of formulations all with different names and dosing instructions. Know what you have in hand prior to consumption. Artemesia is available over the Internet in just about every conceivable form – *IF* you can find a reliable source. Sometimes I have no trouble pulling up Dr. Zhang's Artemisinin at hepapro. com and other times it seems to have evaporated into the ether. Holley Pharmaceuticals provides 50 to 100 mg capsules. Some health food stores have variations of the core product. Know the source. Be careful.

Formulations include oral, rectal, IM, and IV. The oral preps are tablets, capsules, and teas. There continues to be debate over whether the water needs to be warm or boiling to make a therapeutically effective tea. (Welcome to my world.) Artemisia is not especially water soluble.

One promoter boasted that their production process *might* soon be up to GMP standards. Try to find a reliable source. Your HCP might have a supplier that has provided consistent product over time. If you are the HCP, some patients will be able to provide insight to you. In this arena, the game changes all the time.

Do not use as a monotherapy. In general, follow the dosing instructions for the formulation you have in hand. Artemesia in NOT good for malarial prevention. Because of its extremely short half-life, doses would need to be given too often to make the prophylaxis worthwhile. Patients can relapse after treatment is stopped.

Artem**esia** may be the least effective of the myriad formulations and probably has the most side effects. Artem**isinin** may be better with fewer adverse events. Many of the other versions are mixtures of various herbs and components from TCM. Art**esunate** is a more recent version. Both the IV and IM forms of artesunate were found to be superior to quinine in treating malaria in adults and kids with fewer severe AEs. Without standardization, comparing the various forms is tricky.

You may want to comparison shop. While there is a considerable range in prices, I have little advice to offer here. I would like to say that you get what you pay for, but I don't know if that is the case. Blogs are confusing and make you scream out for an exorcist. Either the writer is rapturous in praise of a product or a particular brand nearly killed him. You never know who is actually doing the writing. Could be the brother-in-law of the competitor. If you know someone who had a good experience, see what they used. Consider Dr. Zhang.

Cautions: Let the liver recover by using a pulsing dose regimen roughly 4 days on and 3 days off. When you restart the drug after the "holiday," the liver will not be so hyper and you will get decent levels again for several days.

Dosing: The doses found in the literature generally refer to the WHO recommendations for the treatment of malaria. Further suggestions are all over the place. In general, artemesia has a very short half-life and needs to be dosed frequently.

WHO recommendation for malaria: 1200 mg on day one and 600 mg per day thereafter (in divided doses.)

Another regimen in adults is 4 tabs at hours 0, 8, 24, 36, 48, and 60. Others give the second dose at hour 4 instead of hour 8. I don't know why this type of distinction is made or if there is any scientific support for one approach over the other.

PEARL: One approach uses 250 mg of artemesia tid to treat kids with babesiosis, 4 days on and 3 days off.

The directions for Dr. Zhang's Arteminisin are 1 pill tid. Start with the 100 mg tabs tid and then go to 250 tid. Some authors prefer the higher dose first. This Arteminisin formula can then go to 1200 mg daily in divided doses.

Treatment should be pulsed and may be needed in babesiosis for months. Reassess in 30 to 60 days. Babesiosis patients may relapse when treatment is stopped and a new course might need to be started. Pulsing is likely the most effective approach with 4 days on medicine and 3 days off.

AEs: Artemesia is well tolerated in the doses used against malaria. Most common AEs include: nausea, vomiting, dizziness, blood abnormalities, and liver dysfunction. Usually it's hard to tell which events are due to artemesia and which are from other drugs in the combination therapy or the underlying disease.

The MOA of artemesia is closely linked to iron metabolism. Iron levels may be impacted with long-term use of this product.

Monitor: Chris's first HCP never mentioned the need to pulse so Chris probably wasn't getting effective levels for quite a while. Also not mentioned was the need to stay on the artemesia as long as you are treating the protozoa. Since artemesia is not a prescription and doesn't need to be "officially" renewed, this treatment can fall by the wayside. The "Patient Instructions" sample form should help minimize that omission.

10. Enula

Description: Herbal that may be effective against babesiosis and Lyme. Not regulated by FDA so standard information is not available. The herb in one formulation gets its Latin name Inula *hellenium* because Helen of Troy was supposed to have carried a bouquet of these plants with her as she was abducted from Sparta. Ancient Greeks and Romans used this herb to treat indigestion, sciatica, asthma, and bronchitis.

Indications: Various promotional materials list indications as: antiparasitic, antiprotozoal, antibacterial, Lyme disease, digestive health, asthma, bronchitis, and microbial defense.

Use in TBDs: Recently discussed as a possible treatment for babesiosis and borreliosis. Enula might be used in place of artemesia. If for some reason artemesia is not available, consider enula as part of the combination therapy for babesiosis. Enula can be combined with either Mepron or Malarone PLUS azithromycin.

Usage: Usually 20 drops is listed as the maximum daily dose and the most recognized regimen uses twice a day dosing. Since enula can cause a headache, the dose should not be increased until the patient can tolerate the previous level without pain. Nutramedix has a formulation available on the Internet.

Dosing: Start with one drop in water bid and slowly increase to 20 drops a day. Twice a day dosing is often mentioned in the literature.

AEs: Headache. Perhaps mild nausea. AE profile still being established

C. ANTIVIRALS

Description: There are medications that are used to treat viral infections. Traditional antibiotics do NOT treat viruses. Unfortunately, antivirals usually must be initiated as close to the onset of infection as possible to be effective. This is often not possible with tick-borne viruses. Nevertheless, certain viral TBIs and some co-morbidities, like HSV and EBV, might benefit from early antiviral intervention. By inhibiting the ability of a virus to reproduce, antivirals can prevent the disease from progressing, diminish the severity of symptoms, or shorten the duration of the illness. Other times, they just give the patient bad dreams. In general, these agents must be used early in the clinical course before there is mass replication of the virus. Too late and the damage is done. If you have a patient who you think has a viral infection that might benefit from an antiviral, you might consider:

1. Acyclovir (Zovirax) is used primarily for HSV but is active against most of the herpes viruses in varying degrees including: HSV-1, HSV-2, varicella (chicken pox, etc.), EBV (one possible cause of mononucleosis), and CMV. Acyclovir is not active against dormant viruses lurking in nerve ganglia. Can give with food. Use caution in renal impairment

    Doses:

    Adult:

Acute treatment:	200 mg q 4 hrs (5 times a day) for 10 days
Chronic treatment:	400 mg bid or 200 mg 3 to 5 times per day for up to 12 months

    Children:

Not recommended in kids less than 2	
Older children:	20 mg/kg qid for 5 days. Check insert for maximum dose.

2. Tamiflu is indicated for the prophylaxis of influenza in those over 13 y/o and for influenza treatment in those over 1 y/o but not sick for more than 2 days.

    Doses:

    Adults and kids over 13:   75 mg bid for 5 days

    Children: Tutti-frutti flavored suspension. Treat for 5 days and longer for prophylaxis

<15 kg:	30 mg bid
15 to 23 kg:	45 mg bid
23 to 40 kg:	60 mg bid
> 40 kg:	75 mg bid

3. Relenza is indicated to treat influenza in patients sick for less than 2 days. Not recommended in kids less than 7 y/o and CI in airway disease. Relenza is sold in blister packs to be used in an inhalation device. Discontinue if bronchospasm occurs or if there is decreasing respiratory function. Use 2 inhalations (10 mg total) bid at least 2 hours apart on 1ˢᵗ day and then 2 inhalations q 12 hrs for 4 more days.

    All three may cause GI upset. None are indicated for TBIs. All are frequently used off-label. Most people treated for influenza have a virus but NOT influenza.

D. ANTIFUNGALS

Description: This class is described in Chapter 25: *Ancillary Treatments.*

Chapter 25   ANCILLARY TREATMENTS – Detailed chapter contents

ANCILLARY TREATMENTS

One word that brings me joy is dungarees.

Nick Flynn

While the foundation of treatment for Lyme and most other TBIs is antimicrobials, many other things are going on in these patients that need to be addressed. The diseases all have a myriad of symptoms, from pain to fever to anxiety to nausea, which the patient will want you to modulate. Patients don't want to split hairs over semantics; they just want to feel better. Some of the antibiotics will cause side effects like diarrhea and fungal overgrowth that will need to be managed. As always, we need to strike a balance. While we want to decrease the misery, we don't want to dampen the immune system so much that the patient can't mount a good defense. Remember that many of the symptoms we are minimizing are the evidence of immune response. Fever can be our friend. This chapter provides treatment suggestions for the most common signs, symptoms, and conditions associated with TBIs. As usual, I have no logical classification scheme. Just the problems as they raised themselves in my mind.

I.   CONCURRENT CONDITIONS IN TBI PATIENTS

A.   Pain

Along with fatigue, pain is an almost universal complaint of Lyme patients. From headaches to joint pain to muscle soreness to generalized achiness, just about every patient complains of some kind of discomfort.

1.   In TBIs, try Tylenol (acetaminophen) first. Although acetaminophen works by inhibiting cyclooxygenase in much the same way as the current class of COX 2 inhibitors (Celebrex), it does not seem to mute the immune response to the same degree as most of the traditional NSAIDs might.

Acetaminophen has the advantage of also helping to normalize temperature and helps mute the discomfort of fever. Unlike a number of other pain medicines, acetaminophen is not known to cause GI distress and is not associated with GI bleeding. Acetaminophen is a liver toxin so use caution in patients with underlying liver dysfunction or those concomitantly using other drugs that also affect the liver. Be aware of potential liver damage with long-term use. So do not give "extra" to help the patient feel better faster, since the liver may pay the price. Follow dosing recommendations carefully.

2.   NSAIDs (nonsteroidal anti-inflammatory drugs) are commonly used to treat pain. There are numerous brand names but the most commonly used are the ibuprofens, Motrin and Advil. These agents work well in modulating pain and fever but may suppress the immune response more than acetaminophen. NSAIDs are known to cause GI irritation and should be taken with food.

PEARL: Personally, I have often alternated acetaminophen with ibuprofen since these two agents have different MOAs and a different dosing schedule. I have had considerable success here in controlling symptoms without risking overdose.

3.   Aspirin is no longer indicated for children because of its association with an acute type of encephalitis called Reye's syndrome.

4.   A number of patients have long-term, incapacitating musculoskeletal pain associated with Lyme or other TBIs. In these cases, opioids have been used to ameliorate the symptoms. Percocet is a combination of oxycodone and acetaminophen and Vicodin is a combination of hydrocodone and acetaminophen. These are big guns and many HCPs are not comfortable prescribing these medications because of abuse and addiction potential. Nevertheless, if you are treating TBIs, you will have patients genuinely suffering from severe chronic pain. If you are uncomfortable prescribing these medicines, know a reputable pain clinic that can manage the pain portion of these cases. Do not let your case get away from you. You still need to manage the TBI. A long time ago, I was a physician at the drug company that sold Percocet and this drug was my responsibility. My rule of thumb was that if the patient was taking more than a dozen a day, he might be feeding an addiction as well as treating his pain. You will need to strike a balance between helping a patient in agony and not feeding an addiction. Sometimes the pain is so savage that you have to get the patient

functional again and then worry about the addiction. Under those circumstances, you need to talk to the pain specialist to see what other options might be possible.

5. Medical marijuana has been used to modulate pain in TBI patients. While the pain might be mitigated with its use, be careful because marijuana may suppress the immune system and the sxs of Lyme might be exacerbated. In addition to immune suppression, studies have shown that marijuana might cause genetic aberrations with gene dislocation and disassociation. We know that Bb adversely impacts immune response and may alter genetic material. We certainly do not need additional ways to impact the immune system and genetic material in Lyme patients, since Bb already can do that on its own. Further, the paranoia sometimes associated with use of marijuana does not seem conducive to healing in the Lyme population. These patients may already be dealing with multiple NP sxs. Further, dementia associated with marijuana use has been reported. Medical marijuana users might begin to think everything is great and thereafter underestimate the complexity of their disease. An almost blind euphoria might ensue with the patient unaware of the true nature of their underlying condition. Ask if the benefits outweigh the risks, especially when alternatives are available. With that being said, you may decide that your patient is in dire need of this treatment. In those states where medical marijuana is legal, there has been very loose oversight of its use. The patients who could genuinely benefit have often been shut out while others take advantage of the system. If you are amenable to trying this type of treatment, know the law in your state and how to order and dose appropriately.

PEARL: Synthetic marijuana is a mixture of herbs thought to be responsible for numerous ER visits.

6. Neurontin (gabapentin) has been mentioned in the literature for pain relief in TBI patients. Others have tried pregabalin for the widespread muscle pain in fibromyalgia thought to be due to hyperactive nerves. Anecdotally, a number of Lyme patients have found relief with the use of gabapentin. Others have reported no effect. One source said, "When it works, it works, but when it doesn't, it doesn't." You won't know unless you try.

7. Various ancillary treatments have been used in attempts to ease the pain including heat, ice, massage, acupuncture, and biofeedback.

B. Fever

Fever is an almost universal sign of systemic infection. Remember that fever is a manifestation of the inflammatory process and a sign of the immune system defending its body. Some pathogens cannot tolerate high temperatures and the fever itself is contributing to the demise of the infectious agent. Nevertheless, fever can be miserable and most patients appreciate some relief. Many parents panic when their child gets a high fever and all grandparents blame the parents for any reading over 101. There is no need for alarm. Some associated signs of high fever like delirium, hallucinations, lassitude, and lapsing consciousness are not easy for caretakers to witness. Remember, you want to moderate the response, not obliterate it. In fact, febrile seizures are more often associated with a rapid temperature *change* than the actual number on the thermometer.

As with pain, try acetaminophen first and then NSAIDs. Again, alteration of these two agents can be tried. Since Tylenol is given every 4 hours and ibuprofen every 6 to 8 hours, you can make sure the patient is well covered. With many of the TBIs you can set your clock by when the antipyretic is wearing off and when the fever again climbs. If the fever cannot be regulated by alternating acetaminophen and ibuprofen, perhaps an antibiotic or antiviral should be considered. While an excellent antipyretic, aspirin is contraindicated in kids because of its association with Reye's syndrome.

A record of temperature readings along with the times that antipyretics were given may be useful to the HCP. Different pathogens may present with distinct fever patterns. Remember that any use of antipyretics changes the usual fever course of the disease and so your record becomes more documentation of your diligent nursing, than a distinctive fingerprint that might help identify a pathogen. That's okay, these patterns are often not that characteristic anyway.

PEARL: Sample Form XV is called the Symptom Tracking Sheet and, although it can be used to follow any number of signs and symptoms, fever is one of the most commonly recorded.

Keep patients comfortable. If they are hot, help cool them. If they are cold, help warm them. No, Lilith[1], giving a patient with rigors a blanket will not cause a fever. You don't need to place people in tubs of ice. All things in moderation. An abrupt change in temperature is more associated with febrile seizures than a high number on the thermometer.

PEARL: Fever does not have to be treated. There is no inherent prohibition against fever. If the patient is tolerating a low grade fever you do not have to bring out the entire armamentarium to combat a temperature reading of 99.8. If the patient is uncomfortable or unable to rest, treat.

---

1 See Glossary or Introduction for name origin

Ways to help cool someone down gently: cool compresses, cool sponge baths, cool packs in groin and axilla (bags of frozen peas wrapped in a towel work nicely), if conscious try ice chips or popsicles, and fans.

Ways to warm someone up: blankets, electric blankets, warm compresses, mittens, hats, socks, warm drinks, and warm packs in the groin and axilla. There are reusable microwaveable hot packs. Careful. These can get VERY hot. Diabetics cannot always tell if they are being burned.

Don't obsess about getting the temperature back to "normal." If the person is acutely infected, you can give her all the acetaminophen and ibuprofen she can tolerate, all the cool baths on the planet, and that temperature is not going to be "normal" until it is good and ready (often with the help of antibiotics). If you can get the person comfortable enough so she can sleep, that is the most conducive path to healing.

If the child has a **febrile seizure**, the seizure will be much more frightening for the parent than the child. First, don't panic. Allow the child to seize. The seizure in itself will not cause the child harm, but it will scare the hell out of you. Kids don't die from febrile seizures. Gently place him on the floor ON HIS SIDE. No matter how many times you've seen the TV detectives place a tongue depressor inside someone's mouth so that they "don't swallow their tongue" you don't need to do that. That is a good way for the person to splinter the stick in half along with your finger. If he is on his side with his mouth tilted down he cannot aspirate vomit and gravity will not be pulling the tongue back to occlude the airway. Keep them away from sharp corners where they could hit their heads or hurt themselves. Most seizing patients will be incontinent and once the seizure is over will be dazed and tired for a while. I like to check all kids after a febrile seizure, if only to reassure the parents. I've seen many febrile seizures in the ER. It's different when it's your kid. A febrile seizure does not mean your child is epileptic.

PEARL: Antipyretics can mute the highs and lows of the fever cycles, but will not usually put the numbers back into the normal range. By alternating ibuprofen and acetaminophen, Chris's temperature peaks would come down to 102° or 103°, which was much better than 104° and 106°. Until the antibiotic kicked in, the temperature did not come back within the normal range. Nevertheless, you feel better at 102 than you do at 105. Chris's delirium diminished with antipyretics and he was conscious for longer periods. When he was late taking the next antipyretic dose (we didn't want to wake him when he was sleeping), the temperature would spike again.

C. Nausea

Nausea is a common symptom in most of the TBIs as well as a common adverse effect of many medicines used to treat these conditions.

There are many prescription medications and OTC treatments available:

1. Phenergan (promethazine) comes as tablet, syrup, injection, or suppository. When you're nauseated, an injection or suppository can be a blessing. Phenergan has been around so long that I was once the product physician. This drug was approved back when not much data was needed to show efficacy. Now the FDA says they have no evidence that it works. Well, no one is going to do efficacy trials on an old generic. I think Phenergan just might help some with nausea and help calm the queasy patient. There seem to be few side effects aside from a little drowsiness and dizziness, so if it helps swell, if not, then no harm done.

Adults:	25 mg to start and then 12.5 to 25 mg q 4 to 6 hrs
Children:	Not recommended in under 2
	0.5 mg/**lb** with maximum of 12.5 mg q 4 to 6 hrs

    Contraindicated in dehydrated patients, Reye's syndrome, and the very ill

2. Tigan (trimethobenzamide) is available in capsules, injection, or suppositories.

    Contraindicated in dehydrated patients, Reye's syndrome, or the very ill

Adults:	200 mg rectally 3 or 4 times a day
Children:	Not recommended in preemies or neonates
	Less than 30 **lbs**: 100 mg 3 or 4 times a day
	30 to 90 **lbs**: 100 to 200 mg 3 or 4 times a day

3. Zofran (ondansetron) is a serotonin blocker available as a tablet, liquid, dissolving tablet, or injection. Given 1 to 3 times per day. Use caution in those susceptible to dysrhythmia or QT prolongation

4. Medical marijuana has been used to treat nausea. This option is likely to be considered when the nausea is intractable despite other remedies and causing problems with hydration and nutrition over the long-term. As stated in the *Pain* section above, be careful with

marijuana use in Lyme patients for many reasons, especially when there are viable alternatives. Different states have different rules.

5. OTC medications that may help nausea include Mylanta, Maalox, and Pepto-Bismol. Alka-Seltzer contains aspirin and would be contraindicated in kids.

6. There are innumerable home remedies for nausea including: peppermints, ginger ale, flat cola, Coke syrup, 7Up, acupressure, wrist pressure, ear lobe pressure, eating light or not eating at all, crackers, ginger tea, ginger candies (eaten like gummies), various other teas, broths, avoidance of milk and dairy, no alcohol or caffeine, and avoidance of spicy and greasy foods. A mixture of a half teaspoon of baking soda (bicarbonate) in warm water is an old-time remedy featured prominently in *Three Stooges* shorts.

D. GI Imbalance

The GI tract is filled with millions of bacteria performing numerous functions critical to the survival of the host. More than 400 different kinds of bacteria live in the human gut. These symbiotic relationships can become imbalanced by the effects of antibiotics on the intestinal tract.

Probiotics generally contain either "good" bacteria or "good" yeasts. By "good" here we mean strains that we would like to reproduce and colonize in lieu of those that have been destroyed. The most commonly found bacterial genuses used for this purpose are variations of Lactobacillus, Acidophilus, or Bifidobacterium. Saccharomyces yeast is also commonly used as a probiotic. Speculation is that the new colony will start to stabilize in about two days after starting the probiotic. These genuses do well in the human GI tract and fit right in the neighborhood.

Of course, the live or dehydrated microbes must first pass through a gauntlet of hazards in the GI tract including the acid in the stomach, the base in the SI, and the antibiotic that already wiped out everyone else. The idea is to overcome these obstacles with sheer numbers. Commercial probiotic formulations contain millions and billions of organisms. (They use scientific notation to count them on the bottles at Walmart.) Hopefully, at least some of this mass quantity will survive to colonize the gut. Like bunnies, it should only take a few to create a whole new generation.

Unfortunately, as with so many good ideas originally designed to help people, unscrupulous marketers enter the fray. I have found a bazillion probiotics on-line. Since both my son and mother were on probiotics for extended periods, I learned a thing or two. The most expensive is not necessarily the best. Although not a guarantee of quality, try to find brand name products with stable suppliers and availability. Just as I advised when discussing generic drugs (maybe you didn't get to that chapter yet), if you wouldn't drink the water in the place where it was made, maybe you should think twice about using that product. Aside from promotional claims, I couldn't find a reason to pick one species over another.

Probiotics do seem to reduce side effects from antibiotics. Generally, encourage patients who are on any antibiotic regimen to also consider probiotics. The side effects appear benign and include gas, rumbling, and bloating, but not much else. These side effects usually diminish after a few weeks of use. If the probiotics are discontinued, the intestinal flora seem to revert back to the way they were in about a week. Depending on the prior status, that can be good or bad news.

Probiotics are best taken an hour or two before food or antibiotics. If the patient is taking more than one kind of probiotic at a time, they can be taken together. A few recognized brands include:

1. UltraFlora: Combination of Acidophilus and Bifidobacteria. Take at least 10 billion organisms tid.

2. Culturelle: A formulation of Lactobacillus GG

3. Various Acidophilus brands are indicated to help with digestion and detoxification. Take an hour or two before or after antibiotics, at least 10 billion organisms per dose.

4. Florastor (a Saccharomyces yeast): This formulation contains live yeast cells and is suitable for all ages 2 months to adults and is meant to be taken by people on antibiotics. This product is sometimes sold from behind the counter in pharmacies so you have to ask for it, even though it does not require a prescription. (I don't know why Florastor is often sold behind the counter. Do drug dealers sell yeast on street corners? I must have missed something.) Usual dose is one twice a day. Florastor is probably not a good choice for those on yeast free diets or those taking antifungals. Saccharomyces yeasts are often available in health food stores.

5. Theralac is a mix of five different bacterial species. The promotional material says this product is the #1 probiotic for Lyme patients because it strengthens the immune system. I could not find confirmation that this product was #1 for Lyme patients or how the product actually strengthened the immune system and how

this was measured. Unsupported claims make me nervous. Because probiotics are food supplements, their promotional material does not need to go through DDMAC. Maybe I'm crabby because I spent the best years of my life trying to get promotional pieces through DDMAC review. Dosing directions for Theralac: One capsule daily but if loose stools develop, can increase to two times a day. Theralac may not be affected by time of dose or whether taken with or without food, as are other brands.

PEARL: Sometimes you will see the term prebiotic and wonder if that is the same as a probiotic. Probiotics are potentially living organisms given to people (or animals) to enhance the growth of the helpful flora in the gut. Prebiotics are foods (usually fibers) that provide nourishment for the good flora. Much of this distinction is a way to market various products. In general, the natural intestinal flora are pretty happy eating whatever is around and seem to flourish on the same thing that the mean character ate in the book The Help, *except they know what they're eating and she didn't.*

E. Diarrhea

Diarrhea can be part of the clinical presentation of a TBI or can be a side effect of many medicines. Antibiotics can cause loose stool by way of several mechanisms: direct irritation of the GI tract, the imbalance of normal flora, and the overgrowth of non-susceptible, opportunistic microbes such as C. *difficile*. The distinction between these mechanisms is critical, since what treats one etiology, exacerbates another.

First, one loose stool does not constitute diarrhea. Frequency is the determining factor. Often diet can temporarily loosen stool. Once the diet adjusts, the consistency of the stool should return to normal. Watery, bloody, or explosive diarrhea is a problem. Diarrhea can be a serious and even fatal condition in children and the elderly. The smaller the person, the greater the risk. Be obsessively vigilant about hydration. If a patient has a few loose stools, but is drinking, you have less reason for concern than if she is reluctant to take anything by mouth.

Treatments:

1. Identify and eliminate the likely underlying cause.

2. Probiotics: As noted in the *GI Imbalance* section above, the earlier in the course of antibiotic treatment that probiotics can be initiated, usually the better for the normal flora in the gut. Ideally, start the probiotics before the antibiotic and continue throughout the course of treatment, even during bouts of diarrhea.

Probiotics may help prevent diarrhea or lessen its severity but they are not a panacea and diarrhea can still occur.

3. Anti-motility drugs: DANGER! DANGER! WILL ROBINSON! These medicines work!

Only consider slowing the motility of the GI tract IF you are certain that the underlying cause of the diarrhea is not an endotoxin like that made by C. *difficile* AND the patient is at risk of imminent dehydration or demise. With diarrhea caused by endotoxins, you want that poison OUT of the system, not trapped in the GI tract indefinitely. In those cases, you want the diarrhea to continue within reason.

Imodium (loperamide): Sold OTC, Imodium slows the motion in the GI tract. Do not use if you are trying to avoid constipation. Use caution in cases of ulcerative colitis or in cases where the diarrhea might be caused by an endotoxin.

Adults:

Acute:	Start with 4 mg then 2 mg after each loose stool with maximum of 16 mg/day. Stop if no improvement after 48 hours.
Chronic:	4 to 8 mg/day

Children:

Do not use in kids less than 2-years-old. (Here's where the manufacturer mixes pounds and years with metric and English and, heaven forbid, that your child does not fit into the same age and weight category! Just gives you something else to worry about.)

24 to 47 **lbs** (or 2 - 5 years)	1 mg up to tid for 2 days
48 to 59 **lbs** (or 6 - 8 years):	2 g then 1 mg after each loose stool with a maximum of 4 mg/day for 2 days
60 to 95 **lbs** (or 9 -11 years)	2 mg then 1 mg after each loose stool with a maximum of 6 mg/day for 2 days

*PEARL: Do not mix up loperamide with **Lomotil**. Imodium is a much less aggressive treatment than Lomotil. Giving too much Lomotil can be damaging. While you should not be paralyzed with fear over using Lomotil when indicated, you should maintain a very healthy respect for what this drug can do. I have prescribed both of these agents many times over the years. I never give the full recommended dose to start. Once the medicine goes in, you can't get it back out. You could have trouble getting the GI tract moving again. I wait to see the response before I give more.*

Most diarrhea does not stop instantly after the first dose. Do not over-treat. If the patient is starting to decline, ensure that you have eliminated the underlying cause of the diarrhea and that you are adequately hydrating.

Lomotil (opioid and anticholinergic, that is: diphenoxylate and atropine) This prescription drug comes in a tablet or as a liquid. Lomotil will slow or stop the movement of the GI tract. Use only if you are sure that no endotoxin is causing the underlying diarrhea and that the patient is not at risk for ileus or toxic megacolon. We used atropine at Aberdeen Proving Ground as an antidote to nerve agents. DO NOT OVER-TREAT.

Adults:

Acute:	2 tabs or 10 ml qid
Maintenance:	2 tabs or 10 ml daily

Children:

Not recommended in kids less than 2 y/o

2 to 12 years: 0.3 to 0.4 mg/kg in 4 divided doses until diarrhea controlled

4. Hydration is critical in the treatment of diarrhea. Dehydration is the biggest risk for any person with diarrhea and can be accompanied by electrolyte imbalances. Water is the best hydration agent. Broths are good, as are teas and ice pops. Both alcohol and caffeine can be dehydrating so avoid those in all ages.

PEARL: Despite heavy advertising, sports drinks and liquid nutritional supplements are not usually necessary. Rarely does a kid with diarrhea get sodium depleted in a way that is not compensated by the next food that he ingests. The kids in the ads are way too healthy-looking to be dependent on a sports drink or liquid nutritional aid. They're actors, not patients. If your child likes Gatorade, by all means let her drink it within reason, but don't feel obligated to buy expensive drinks when, in most cases, water is best.

What about milk? Yet another controversy. Milk contains lactose which is not always easily digested by older people, especially blacks and Asians. If the GI tract is already macerated because of savage diarrhea, the enzymes usually present might not be readily available even in those who usually have no trouble digesting milk sugar. On the other hand, milk has great protein, which is always a good idea for a healing patient. If the individual had trouble digesting milk before, diarrhea is not going to help. If the person wants milk, serve low fat varieties in small amounts, especially when diarrhea is active, and see how well it is tolerated.

Sometimes patients just don't feel like drinking. Games can help. If a child's favorite number is three, then he can take three sips every three minutes. If the patient's skin starts to look wilted, if pinched skin does not spring back into place immediately upon release, the eyes and mouth are dry, or the person is barely peeing, she could be on her way to dehydration. Evaluate this patient further. The younger or older the person, the sooner the evaluation. If you can't get an appointment with your regular HCP, go to the ER. Intravenous fluids may be needed.

5. **Pepto-Bismol** can be tried in diarrhea from any underlying cause. Pepto sooths the GI tract and supposedly binds endotoxins. GI motility is not impeded. Because Pepto contains aspirin-like salicylates, use with caution in kids with viral syndromes because of the possible association with Reye's syndrome. The bismuth in the product (the pink part) can darken the tongue and make the stool black.

Pepto-Bismol is sold over the counter as liquid, chewables, and caplets. I think that part of the therapeutic value of Pepto is the coating the liquid gives the GI tract. But some people don't like the taste or texture of the liquid. To actually bind toxin, however, you must take lots of Pepto.

Adults:

Take 2 caplets or chewables or 30 ml of the liquid. Only chew the chewables, not the caplets. Take q 30 to 60 minutes with a maximum of 8 doses/day.

Kids:

Take the caplets with water and do not chew them

Less than 3 years (14 to 18 lbs): 2.5 ml (half teaspoon) every 4 hrs if needed with maximum of 6 doses/day

18 to 28 lbs:	5 ml, repeat q 4 with maximum 6 doses/day
3 to 6 years:	1/3 tab or 5 ml*
6 to 9 years:	2/3 tab or 10 ml*
9 to 12 years:	1 tab or 15 ml*

*Repeat q 30 to 60 minutes if needed with a maximum 8 doses per day.

6. Identify and treat C. *difficile* as outlined in the next section.

7. Diet: Often people with diarrhea don't feel like eating. For short periods, eating is optional, drinking is not. For the past several decades the BRAT diet was universally recommended for patients with diarrhea. Bland and low in fiber, this diet consisted of bananas,

rice, applesauce, and toast. While that might be okay for a few days, the BRAT diet is nutritionally weak and has largely fallen out of favor.

Some authors recommend no solid food for 24 to 48 hours with diarrhea, but that approach seems to be unnecessary. Of course, the literature contains hundreds of dietary options, most attached to a small fee, that are designed to calm the diarrhea once and for all.

Again, a sensible approach is probably the most conducive to healing. The body will give strong clues regarding what it can tolerate. Nutritional supplements are rarely needed. Infrequently do routine cases become salt depleted. Initially, start with broths, rice or light noodle soup, crackers and things that are not too spicy, sugary, or greasy. The first real meal after significant diarrhea probably should NOT be a carnivore's delight onion pizza and a beer. Don't worry about a "balanced" diet in the short-term. Some people can handle dairy but for others, dairy seems to exacerbate the problem. Some do well with eggs, which are an excellent source of protein. Since these are TBI patients, protein will be needed to make antibodies and other components of the immune response.

PEARL: Each family seems to have its own menu of "feel better" foods. Some like chicken noodle soup, others popsicles, and still others have the smiley face print on the toast. Short-term, kids love to have these "special" foods. They'll let you know when they can handle a hot dog. Remember that when you're a sick kid there's no better place to be than on grandma's lap.

Lactose (milk sugar) can exacerbate loose stools in those people who are lactose intolerant.

8. Chapped bottom: Diarrhea can make small (and large) bottoms raw. Because the antibiotic that caused the diarrhea might also cause a fungal overgrowth, consider that a diaper rash might be fungal in these kids. (See the section on treating fungal overgrowth below.) In other cases, apply barrier creams or ointments to the area as soon as you realize that there may be trouble ahead. Many children's hospitals compound their own "butt pastes" that act as a barrier between the skin and the irritating diarrhea. Otherwise, there are many choices OTC. (*NOTE: The white ones, usually with zinc oxide, will take the color out of fabric.*) Keep the area meticulously clean and dry. After each loose stool, clean with warm water and mild soap and rinse well. Gentle cleaning wipes can also be used. Dab dry, don't rub. In some cases when skin is macerated, the diaper or underwear may need to stay off so the skin can air dry. This is unappealing in kids with diarrhea

but some bottoms are just too sore to be immediately re-covered. Get the newspapers out of recycle or sit on the grass outside. (Just watch for ticks.)

F. Clostridium *difficile*

Humans cannot survive without the "good" bacteria that live all over us, inside and out. The digestive tract is filled with millions of symbiotic bacteria that help with digestion, aid in the absorption of vitamins and other nutrients, maintain normal pH levels, enhance the immune response, and synthesize important molecules that we cannot make for ourselves. To survive, we need them and they need us. Just as we do with snakes and sharks, humans seem to feel an overwhelming compulsion to obliterate every bacteria that comes across our paths. This is not necessary. We simply don't need all the Lysol and Clorox the marketers say we need.

On a normal day, all this natural flora is nicely balanced in and on the body. But when an antibiotic is introduced to fight an infection, the equilibrium can shift. This antibiotic, usually given orally, washes over the GI tract. Antibiotics cannot tell a good bacteria from a bad bacteria from the host's perspective. The drug goes after whatever organism happens to be vulnerable to its chemistry. Most of the common intestinal bacteria, like E. *coli,* can be susceptible to many of the antibiotics used to treat TBIs. Depending on the bacteria and the antibiotic, entire populations can be wiped out. For example, clindamycin and the fluoroquinolones do a pretty effective job at cleaning out susceptible bacteria in the gut.

Alas, a few bacteria are not susceptible to the common antibiotics. Microbes like Clostridium *difficile* are not depleted by the usual antibiotics. As the neighbors are wiped out, there is more room and resource for the C. *difficile* to reproduce. PARTY! This organism, which was just another member of the normal flora days before, now overgrows and becomes an **opportunistic i**nfection. The big problem comes when the C. *difficile* makes an endotoxin. The more C. *difficile*, the more toxin is made and released. This toxin can lead to a condition called pseudomembranous colitis with severe diarrhea, dehydration, electrolyte imbalances, toxic megacolon, and, in some cases, death. This diarrhea is frequent, often explosive, watery, and may contain blood or mucus. Further, diarrhea from C. *diff* can be accompanied by cramps, urgency, abdominal pain, and fever. A pseudo or false membrane forms over the intestinal lining.

While just about every antibiotic can cause these problems, clindamycin is known for C. *difficile* overgrowth because C. *difficile* is totally resistant to clindamycin. When this particular antibiotic is in the vicinity, C. *diff* is completely unaffected, while other bacterial species are eradicated *en masse*. The elimination of most of the normal flora can be due to either a strong broad-spectrum antibiotic or from the long-term use of most antibiotics. And here the definition of long-term is well within the IDSA's 30 day maximum allocated to treat Lyme disease. Not all patients in these circumstances develop C. *difficile* overgrowth, but the HCP must be vigilant.

Problems with C. *difficile* may start during treatment or not for weeks after the medicine has been discontinued. If symptoms appear, consider cultures and assaying the stool for toxin. Diagnostic tests used to help identify C. *difficile* are described in Chapters 19: *Scientific Basis and Interpretation of Study Results.*

Suspect C. *difficile* infection in any patient with diarrhea who has been treated with antibiotics within the past two months or whose frequent, loose stools began within about three days after hospitalization. When suspected, send a stool specimen for culture and for analysis of toxins. If these first tests are negative, send one or two more specimens, using the same tests to be repeated or ordering different methods. PCR testing is available, but culture of the organism remains the gold standard since it is the most sensitive and specific. ELISA is used for the analysis of toxins. Note that many hospitals test for only one of the strains of C. *difficile,* so there are a high number of false negatives.

Treatments:

1. Immediately discontinue the causative antibiotic. Symptoms usually improve when the causative antibiotic regimen is stopped or changed.

2. Don't forget that you were treating a TBI with that antibiotic you just stopped. Find an alternative treatment for the TBI. Recall that continuous antibiotic coverage for Lyme, within reason, is probably preferred.

3. Aside from the possible consideration of anti-motility drugs, most of the treatments recommended in the *Diarrhea* section above apply to the treatment of the diarrhea associated with C. *difficile*.

4. With C. *difficile*, you do not want to stop the diarrhea (unless it is incapacitating or life-threatening). You want the endotoxin OUT of the system and that is what the body is trying to accomplish with the diarrhea.

5. To stop the diarrhea in these cases, you must stop the production of endotoxin and to stop the endotoxin

factory, you must eliminate the C. *difficile*. Most antibiotics do not hit C. *difficile* and that's how we got in this mess in the first place. Fortunately, we have two antimicrobials that do.

a. Flagyl (metronidazole): 7.5 mg/kg po q 6 h for 7 to 10 days with a maximum dose of 4 **g**/day

b. Vancomycin: 125 to 500 mg po q 6 for 10 days. In this case, the oral route is preferred because the site of action is the GI tract. (Those snotty C. *difficile* sure are going to be surprised.)

G. Fungal overgrowth

Just as antibiotics can wreck havoc on the balance of intestinal flora, they can also affect the equilibrium between bacterial species and fungi. Like the symbiotic bacteria, fungi live in a mutually advantageous relationship on the host's skin and in the moist, mucus membrane-lined areas of the body such as the mouth, nose, sinuses, throat, groin, GI tract, and vagina. When broad-spectrum antibiotics come on board or when antimicrobials are used for extended periods, the balance can be upset and yeast can overgrow. In these cases, a number of fungal species can become opportunists and invade the host where they previously lived in balanced coexistence.

Primer on fungi, yeast, and molds

First let's clear up the terms fungus, yeast, and mold. Often they are used interchangeably, but that is not entirely correct. Yeasts and molds are types of **fungi**. In the five Kingdom taxonomy scheme, fungi are one of the five, the others being Plants, Animals, Monera (Bacteria), and Protists (Protozoa and Algae). Fungi comprise over 25% of the earth's biomass with over 200,000 species. They can include yeasts, molds, mushrooms, lichens, rusts, truffles, and smuts. Fungi are everywhere.

Many fungi are edible including mushrooms, the blue in blue cheese, and truffles (which are only slightly more expensive than TBI treatment). They are used to raise breads and to ferment wines, beer, and soy sauce. Alexander Fleming discovered penicillin from mold and today a number of drugs and enzymes are extracted from fungi. Several cholesterol-lowering drugs such as lovastatin are made from the Aspergillus mold. The immunosuppressant drug cyclosporine is also mold-derived.

Yeast are budding, single-celled organisms. **Mold** grow filaments called hyphae and they use spores to reproduce. Molds are multicellular and their connected network of branching hyphae tubules are considered all one organism, which is called a colony. Fungi tend to grow in circles, like ringworm, which causes a round skin lesion that can be mistaken for the EM rash of Lyme.

PEARL: Not only is Southern Chester County, Pennsylvania, where I am now sitting, the deer tick capital of the world, it is also the mushroom capital. We know our fungi.

PEARL: Lyme patients continuously exposed to mold may be less likely to improve. They may experience brain fog, fatigue, and myalgias and it can be hard to tell what symptoms might be from Bb and what might be from mold. Both Bb and mold can overwhelm the immune system and make it hard to get well. Mold reactions in TBI patients can be important for two reasons: Symptoms can be similar to those of TBIs and thereby confuse the diagnosis. Also, the impact of hypersensitivity on the immune system can lessen the TBI patient's chance of recovery.

In general, fungi LOVE warm, dark, moist places like the forest floor or the inside of a diaper or skin fold. That being said, many fungi can survive freezing and boiling, which accounts for moldy countertops in Antarctica and fungi floating unscathed in hot springs.

Fungi can cause multiple medical problems. I will focus on those that most impact TBI patients. While people can get a yeast infection or fungal overgrowth, they are not often said to be moldy. Mold does its damage to humans in other ways. Yeast infections and mold sensitivity in TBI patients are not the same beast. They must be managed differently because one is an infection and the other is a sensitivity reaction. The next section in this chapter will deal with mold allergies, but right now we are focusing on fungal overgrowth.

Unlike plants, fungi cannot make their own food. Once they acquire food, they must digest their lunch using enzymes. Chemicals that are just home-grown digestive juices to the fungi can be toxic to the host. These **mycotoxins** can ultimately cause a number of health problems in a body. The fungi are not intentionally making poison specifically to get you. Their normal physiologic processes can result in chemicals that cause problems in the host such as: inactivation of enzymes, release of free radicals, and interference with WBCs and other parts of the immune system. While toxic to the host, the fungi don't even know what a WBC is, let alone have a focused desire to target a wayward lymphocyte. Elton John would simply say it's the circle of life.

Although many fungi can become opportunistic, especially in the immunocompromised, those infections are beyond the scope of this text. We are already familiar with common fungal infections such as jock itch, ringworm, dandruff, athlete's foot, and that creepy yellow fungus that grows under finger and toe nails. These can be caused by different species and so are treated in different ways. Some can be quite stubborn. Here we will focus on those fungi that overgrow as a result of antibiotic therapy in TBI patients.

Overgrowth of yeast in a patient on antibiotics is most often due to Candida *albicans*. This mass escalation in numbers can then cause signs and symptoms in the mouth (**thrush**), skin folds (**intertrigo**), genitals (**vaginitis**), and GI tract. Yeast are opportunistic, especially if the organisms that usually balance them are no longer there. If they find themselves in a warm, dark, moist place, with no competition, they will take advantage. They do enjoy themselves inside a wet diaper. They LOVE simple sugars and starches, and overgrowth can be a chronic problem in many diabetic and overweight patients.

Sxs of systemic fungus include general allergic manifestations, anxiety, eye irritation, diarrhea, gas, cramps, lethargy, eye fatigue, rashes, increased urination, white tongue, itch, problems with hair follicles, weakness, and NP sxs including nervousness, OCD, panic, and dementias. Mold allergies are discussed in the next section.

PEARL: Broad spectrum antibiotics aren't the only reason for fungal overgrowth. Other contributing factors include: high sugar diet, OCPs, steroids, antacids or other anti-ulcer medicines such as PPIs, DM, chemotherapy, immunocompromise, and pregnancy.

PEARL: Since Candida are normal flora, it is sometimes difficult to tell when there is systemic overgrowth. Symptoms can be similar to much other pathology. Antigen testing can be done looking for Candida proteins, but searching for antibodies: IgA, IgM, and IgG, is likely more sensitive.

Fungal overgrowth might cause thick white discharge or curd-like specks in the affected area or circumscribed red patches. Often the overgrowth areas ITCH. Once the area becomes inflamed then other symptoms of inflammation can occur such as swelling, heat, redness, and discomfort. These conditions are treated in a variety of ways.

Treatments:

1. To the degree possible, keep the affected area clean and DRY.

2. At least during the time of active fungal infection, try to minimize the amount of processed sugars and white flours consumed. There are low glycemic and anti-yeast diets available that may serve this purpose. Even high sugar fruits and juices can make a fungus feel like it is in fungal heaven, since these foods tend to cause a spike in blood sugar. The strict anti-yeast, anti-mold diets usually recommend no fermented products like wine, beer, vinegar, or yeast breads. Others also limit caffeine, cheese, chocolate, high fructose fruits, mushrooms, and nuts.

3. Antifungals come in troches to dissolve in the mouth, formulations for swish and spit or swish and swallow, topicals for skin manifestations, all manner of vaginal preparations, and various oral preps to treat systemic infection. Some common antifungals include:

   a. **Diflucan** (fluconazole): Comes in tablets and suspension

      Adults: Depending on the level of fungal infection: 200 to 300 mg on day 1 and then 100 mg daily. Treat systemic infection for 2 weeks or longer if needed. Some suggest continuing treatment for 2 weeks after symptoms have disappeared in systemic infections or meningitis.

      Kids: Individualize the treatment to the child and degree of infection. Systemic infections are treated longer at higher doses than localized infections. All doses are once a day.

      Neonate: Seek advice from a neonatologist.

      Over 2 wks: 6 mg/kg/day on day one, then 3 mg/kg/day for at least 3 weeks for systemic infection, then treat at least 2 weeks after symptoms resolve. Higher doses have been used in systemic Candida. The maximum dose is 12 mg/kg/day. Higher amounts have been used in meningitis. The maximum for all children is 600 mg/day.

   Fluconazole is pregnancy category C. Check LFTs if used long-term. For example, if the patient is treated weekly for more than 3 weeks, consider LFTs. If

treatment is on-going, monthly LFTs are prudent. Diflucan might involve CYP450 enzymes. AEs include nausea, headache, rash, and vomiting.

   b. **Ketoconazole** (Nizoral) comes in many formulations and is a very common antifungal. This drug is the poster child of drug interactions. I don't know if it actually has more drug-drug interactions than any other drug, or because it is a standard test drug for pharmaceutical companies, it just SEEMS to have more interactions. Just remember if you are using this drug long-term there could be higher blood levels or other effects on concomitant products. There are too many formulations to address all dosing recommendations. You will need to assess which area needs treatment and read the package insert. Usually duration of therapy is at least two weeks.

   c. **Miconazole** can be used orally in troches 4 times per day for 7 days. Let one troche dissolve slowly in the mouth. You do not want to chew or swallow the troches whole because you want the medicine to bathe the affected area. Vaginal preparations of miconazole are also common to treat yeast infections. The miconazole molecule is also used in photographic film development. (That tidbit woke you up.)

   d. **Nystatin** (Mycostatin) comes in many formulations with various brand names. You can drop it on, swish and spit, swish and swallow, and dab this stuff just about anywhere. Nystatin can be taken orally, although it's not well absorbed, and in some countries it is injectable.

   e. **Clotrimazole** (Mycelex): In kids over 3, dissolve one troche slowly in the mouth 5 times a day for prevention or treatment of oropharyngeal candidiasis. These local preps do not treat systemic fungus. Note that these troches are indicated for prophylaxis as well as treatment. If you know a patient is about to undergo treatment with a broad-spectrum antibiotic, you can consider one troche tid.

   f. There are dozens of other antifungals (I don't want to exaggerate and say hundreds, but there are probably thousands) available both by prescription and OTC. Find a treatment you like for thrush, for intertrigo, for fungal diaper dermatitis, and for vaginal yeast infections and then pull out that option when indicated.

   g. **Cumanda** is an herbal treatment used to treat fungal overgrowth and systemic fungal infections. Grapefruit seed extract may also be helpful.

h. **Mepron** (atovaquone) was originally developed as an antifungal.

i. The literature describes use of binding agents, such as cholestyramine, to bind mycotoxins. This therapy has been used in the sinuses when fungal infection has been intractable to systemic antifungals. This is more of a "detoxification" procedure and might be more appropriately discussed in Chapter 26: *Alternative Treatments*.

Common focus areas of Candida overgrowth:

1. If a fungal **diaper rash** appears, wash with mild soap and water. Pat or dab off the excess water. Don't rub. Then let the area air dry or use a cool to warm hair drier before applying creams. Keep the diaper off as long as you can tolerate even if it means a mess. (As with kids with diarrhea, this might be a good time to sit outside in the grass. Pick a sunny part of the yard so ticks are less likely.) Apply antifungal OTC creams or lotions. Your pharmacist can help you select. Treat a baby's butt like you would your own under the same circumstances. This rash can be excruciating. Prescription meds are available but usually unnecessary, since the active antifungal ingredients in OTCs are the same and much less costly. (The drug companies are playing with you. I know because I worked on these drugs. Even though the TV ads try to tell you that certain prescriptions are better, it is the *same* active drug in a different grade of petroleum jelly that you are overpaying for. Check the ingredient list.)

   If you see a RED, raised, thick, circumscribed patch in the diaper area it could be fungus. Sometimes there are a few small red satellite lesions associated with the fungus. Fungi LOVE warm, moist, dark places and no place is better than under a diaper for them to set up their household. Make the living conditions as unpleasant for them as possible. Avoid waterproof diapers and plastic pants during acute infection because they trap moisture.

   Do NOT use steroid antifungal cream. They work like a miracle, but are systemically absorbed by the thin, macerated skin and can cause significant side effects, especially in TBI patients.

   After the area is clean and DRY, a barrier antifungal cream or ointment can be used. Urine and stool can be irritating to already inflamed skin.

PEARL: Washing skin infected with fungus with an antibacterial soap can make the rash worse. Why? You have already wiped out the normal skin bacteria with a gorillacillin, allowing the fungus to overgrow. Washing with antibacterial soap will just keep the natural flora suppressed and allow more fungus to run wild.

2. Overgrowth of fungi in the mouth is called **thrush** (or candidiasis or monilia). Usually a caregiver will notice an isolated thick white bump that looks like a bit of cottage cheese on a baby's tongue, inside cheeks, or gums. The fungus can spread throughout the mouth to the tonsils and esophagus. Sometimes the area will bleed a little if the white bump is brushed off the mucous membrane. The lesions can be a little sore but usually are not painful. A breast-feeding baby and her mother can spread the fungus back and forth. Thrush is common in babies but less so in older kids and usually occurs after antibiotics are started or the child's immune system is being stressed in other ways. Thrush is treated by applying an antifungal, usually nystatin (Mycostatin), to the affected area. Nystatin is usually applied 3 or 4 times a day with half the dose dropped on each side of the mouth and sort of squished around to hit the affected areas. Brush all around the mouth, teeth, and tongue. For infants, you can wipe the inside of the mouth with a little gauze or infant mouth cleaner. Some drugstores have special cleaners for this purpose. Older kids can use formulations they can swish and spit. Since nystatin is poorly absorbed, the patient should not be harmed by swallowing this medicine. Treatment should continue for 7 to 10 days or until 3 days after all lesions are gone, whichever is longer. Sometimes miconazole is used in infants less than a month old.

3. Candida can also overgrow in the **vagina** and often when I give an adult female a broad antibiotic, I give her a prescription for an antifungal in case she needs it. Vaginal fungal infections usually involve thick, white, discharge and ITCH. There are many effective OTC preparations. If these do not seem to help, oral Diflucan (fluconazole) often works. In the case of a patient enduring a Herx, I might stay away from oral preparations since the topical can work just as well and will not compete for metabolism space in the liver. In a pediatric population, intravaginal creams and suppositories may be less appropriate than oral remedies.

4. Fungal **intertrigo** is an infection of the skin that occurs in skin folds such as under the breasts, in the gluteal cleft, under the arms, or in the groin. These spots are a fungal delight because they are warm, moist, and dark. Candida can overgrow in these areas even without the use of antibiotics, but with antibiotics the likelihood is greater. Treatment is essentially the same as for fungal diaper rash.

5. Overgrowth of **yeast in the GI tract** can cause gas, bloating, heartburn, dyspepsia, and post-meal fatigue. Once the yeast is in the alimentary canal, the next step could be systemic involvement as described below. Just like the rest of us, yeast love processed sugars and flour and all the high-glycemic delights such as potatoes and white rice. Even some fruits are quick to spike blood sugars. Avoid these high-glycemic foods if yeast is a potential risk. Probiotics may help. Blood sugars remain most stable if small frequent meals are consumed. Anti-yeast diets that avoid sugar, breads, hard cheese, and vinegar could improve the situation. Activated yogurt (without added sugar) and kefir may improve the natural balance of intestinal flora. If sxs continue, consider Diflucan.

6. In some cases Candida or other fungi get into the blood stream and the infection is said to be **systemic.** Since Candida is a normal flora, sometimes it's hard to tell when the line has been crossed. Chapter 18: *Ordering Appropriate Tests* discusses Ig testing for Candida. The fungus can penetrate the mucosa, especially in the GI tract and cause symptoms. That's why you can't just scrape off the fungus of athlete's foot and say you have a cure. The fungus can penetrate deep into the tissue. The problem here is that the symptoms of systemic yeast are similar to those of many infections, especially Lyme, and include: allergy-like symptoms, brain fog, anxiety, hyperactivity, inflammation, GI complaints, lethargy, eye problems, fatigue, rashes, urinary symptoms, localized yeast infections, dandruff, lactose intolerance, OCD, ADD, muscle and bone pain, weakness, dermatitis, itching, swelling, and white tongue. Probiotics can help restore balance in the GI tract. Treatment is that listed above in the general *Fungi* section. However, while local treatments will be useful for the local manifestations, a systemic antifungal will likely be needed to address the systemic infection. Diflucan is probably the most common choice in these cases.

PEARL: Not all patients on strong or long-term antibiotics will have either diarrhea or fungal overgrowth. Many factors combine to determine who might be affected. Often, after an initial imbalance the body adjusts to the antibiotic use and symptoms subside. Just be prepared.

H. Mold allergies

In the previous section, we discussed the consequences of fungal overgrowth, primarily yeast. While we are still talking about fungi, we now shift to mold and the possibility of hypersensitivity and allergic reactions. In addition to the familiar hypersensitivity signs and symptoms, allergies to mold have been associated with fatigue, brain fog, and a fibromyalgia-like syndrome.

Molds are everywhere. If you go away for a week without cleaning out your fridge, when you get back you will find mold. Although it's nice to think that *your* mold spontaneously generated from nothing, we both know that was not the case. The mold was there all along. Every sandwich we eat and every apple and every peanut probably has a hyphae or spore hanging on for the ride. A large component of dust in homes is actually mold, along with human skin cells. Kennett Square, PA, is the mushroom capital of the world and there is a reason for that. Kennett has many warm, dark, moist places, with lots of compost and leaves and the right blend of temperature and humidity to make a mushroom happy. Spores are everywhere and allergies to molds abound. Mushrooms have a distinctive smell and realtors often forget to tell prospective buyers that it's better to buy upwind of the mushroom houses.

Mold in homes is primarily found in poorly-ventilated, damp, dark, or moist places like bathrooms or basements, and are a particular problem after floods. That musty smell is mold. Bread can be covered in a few days. Car air filters and air conditioners are often filled with mold.

Some people get sick after floods or other exposure to static water. These individuals might experience symptoms 36 to 48 hours after water intrusion into walls, insulation, carpet, or other fabrics. The EPA says about 30% of US buildings have mold that can cause disease. The risk persists for a long time. One legend contends that when the tomb of Casimir IV, the last king of Poland, was opened in modern times about a dozen observers present died secondary to toxic mold exposure. He died in 1370.

In addition to direct complications of exposure, mold can cause hypersensitivity reactions and allergy symptoms. Most mold allergies are Type I hypersensitivity reactions. (I told you that *Gentle Immunology* chapter would come in handy.) These IgE-modulated responses can range from itchy eyes to life-threatening anaphylaxis. The type of signs and symptoms depends on where the allergen (antigen, spore) enters the body:

Eye contact:	Itchy, watery, irritated, or red eyes
Skin contact:	Itch, swelling, redness, hives, rashes
Nasal contact:	Itch, runny nose, sneezing, stuffy, sinus problems, sore throat
Inhalation:	Sneezing, swelling in airway, trouble breathing, SOB, wheeze
Ingestion:	GI complaints, nausea, vomiting

Treatments: In general, consider the antifungal treatments listed in the previous section. Here treatments for mold allergies are outlined.

1. Avoidance: As always, the first recommendation when dealing with allergies is to avoid the allergen. With mold everywhere, this is easier said than done. In general, keep the windows and doors shut when spore levels are high (unless the level in the house is higher than those outside the house. We have to consider that here in mushroom land. We do have a local Mushroom Museum.) Change furnace and ventilation filters frequently. Use a dehumidifier.

2. Remediation: Some buildings are so filled with mold that an entire industry has grown around identifying and eliminating mold from homes and businesses. Mold has been suggested by the WHO as one of the causes of Sick Building Syndrome and a number of buildings have been razed because the mold could not be adequately removed.

   You can test your home yourself for mold or have professionals do it. Since my husband is a PhD physical chemist, we figured we could handle this on our own. We tried to do so but when we checked the plates, we couldn't read them because they were all moldy. We assumed that was a positive test.

   Many remediation projects for mold have been undertaken after floods and storms where much fabric and wood has been soaked and cannot adequately dry. All moldy material must be removed. Dehumidifiers and desiccators can be tried and walls and hard surfaces scrubbed with borax. Even then the smell can be quite off-putting. Ozone fog machines have been used to remove the smell of mold and mildew (a pet name for a subclass of mold).

   If a TBI patient is not getting well and excessive mold is suspected in that patient's environment, consider having the area of potential exposure tested. If symptoms or amount of mold is significant, think about remediation by professionals.

PEARL: There are many resources in the phone book and on the Internet about how to address mold. That does not make assessment and remediation easy or clear. Be careful of unscrupulous vendors. In your zeal to get help you are an easy mark for people making unsubstantiated claims.

PEARL: While assessing the environment, the patient can also be tested for immune response to molds. Consider testing for serum Abs (IgE, IgG, and IgA) to stachybotrys and aspergillus.

3. Medicinal treatments: If you put the term "allergy treatments" into your search engine you will get 32,800,000 hits of which 4 are legitimate. The rest are people trying to sell you sheep bladders.

   a. Antihistamines: There are dozens of OTC and prescription antihistamines for kids and adults. The gold standard is Benadryl. I am so used to just saying Benadryl that I forget it has a generic name: diphenhydramine. There are so many store brands of this product in a variety of formulations that I cannot give dosing advice. Here is a good time to read the package directions. Usually little kids get about 6.25 mg and bigger kids 12.5 to 25 mg and the biggest kids 25 to 50 mg/dose. Dosing can be every 4 to 6 hours. Benadryl makes most kids drowsy. In contrast, there is a small but significant minority who actually become excited and hyper with a dose of Benadryl.

   b. Epinephrine is used in severe allergic and life-threatening anaphylactic reactions.

   c. Bronchodilators are used when allergies present with wheezing and respiratory tightness.

   d. Steroids: In general, steroids are not recommended in Lyme patients. As a former ER doctor, if I had a kid in front of me in anaphylaxis, the epi, the nebulizer, and the steroids would be in that kid so fast you wouldn't have time to say, "In general, steroids are not recommended in Lyme patients."

4. In cases where the patient seems to be having either a hypersensitivity reaction to molds or presenting with other clinical syndromes related to yeast or fungus, a change in diet may be warranted. Chapter 27: *Supportive Measures* discusses these options in more detail.

I. Steroids

In my opinion, steroids are the best of drugs, while they are also the worst of drugs. There is no question or controversy: STEROIDS WORK. At the first sign of poison ivy, I am getting myself a script for a Medrol dose pack. If the symptoms are sudden and severe, I am whimpering for an injection at my local "Doc-in-a-Box." For patients with colitis or respiratory problems or a number of inflammatory conditions, steroids save lives and make life worth living. Unfortunately, they can also kill you. With their effective anti-inflammatory action they can mute the immune response to such a degree as to leave the patient vulnerable to either a more virulent presentation of the infection than they already have or to all manner of opportunistic infections. Steroids can raise blood sugars to dangerous levels, cause rapid and significant weight gain, alter hormonal pathways, cause severe bloating which taxes the heart, as well as many other untoward events.

PEARL: Some authors suggest that steroids should not be used in Lyme patients because they activate low level infection. I'm not sure what they mean by that or which mechanism they blame for this possible phenomenon. Just be aware. As we gather more information in the future, this might all become clear.

Some Lyme-focused physicians say NO STEROIDS. Ever. Not ever. Not once. Not in topical creams, not in inhalers for asthma, not in joint injections, not in eye drops, not in oral preps of any kind. In all these cases, local steroid can be systemically absorbed and a surprisingly high blood level can be attained. In TBI patients, this can be enough to hamper or eliminate the immune defense that is already struggling to overcome the infection. Take a reasonable approach, using steroids in life-threatening conditions or in cases where the patient's recovery would be hampered by not using steroids. Of course, try to use the lowest dose for the shortest time while still achieving the desired result. Concomitant antibiotics may be prudent.

PEARL: Early in the evolution of theories on the clinical course of Lyme, one sage proclaimed that all symptoms that occurred in Lyme patients after 10 days of treatment were due to immune dysfunction and NOT infection. This announcement was made despite the fact that other researchers were finding live spirochetes in patients sick for long periods. Many of the chronic Lyme patients he labeled immunodeficient, rather than infected, had actually been treated with steroids: some with a lot of steroids, some for a long time. What a shock to discover they were immunosuppressed. Some current patients who remain sickest today are those who were initially treated with steroids. In general, Lyme patients treated with a steroid blast get worse over time.

In TBI patients avoid steroids, but don't be a fanatical fool about it. In cases of emergency such as anaphylaxis, severe flares of ulcerative colitis, life-threatening pulmonary conditions, etcetera, consider steroids at least temporarily until the patient can be stabilized. In Lyme cases, try to have appropriate antibiotics on board *before* starting the steroids. Don't allow a patient to be dangerously compromised in order to prove your point. You can be right another day.

PEARL: A new set of powerful anti-inflammatories is under development called JAK inhibitors. Janus-associated kinases are enzymes that contain some of the most important receptors for cytokines. Inhibition of these enzymes is thought to decrease inflammation. Could these immunosuppressors have a role for TBI patients in cases where steroids are a problem? Time will tell.

J. Allergies

I repeat here exactly the treatment options listed above for mold allergies which may be used for Type I hypersensitivity reactions caused by any antigen.

1. Avoid the allergen as much as possible. If the allergen is a medicine, discontinue immediately and call the prescribing HCP to discuss next steps. If pollen, stay inside with windows closed and the air conditioner on. If cats, get a rescue dog. You get the idea.

PEARL: Food allergies present differently from standard hay fever or drug allergies, but can cause significant symptoms including anaphylaxis. Of course, if a food allergy is uncovered, avoid the offending food.

2. In cases where the patient seems to be having either a hypersensitivity reaction to molds or presenting with other clinical syndromes related to yeast or fungus, a change in diet may be warranted. Chapter 27: *Supportive Measures* discusses these options in more detail.

3. Medicinal treatments: If you put the term "allergy treatments" into your search engine you will get millions of hits of which very few are legitimate. The rest are people trying to sell you shark scales.[2]

    a. Antihistamines: There are dozens of OTC and prescription antihistamines for kids and adults. The gold standard is Benadryl (diphenhydramine). There are many store brands of this product, so read the package directions. Small children receive 6.25 mg per dose and bigger kids 12.5 to 25 mg and older kids 25 to 50 mg/dose. Dosing is every 4 to 6 hours. Benadryl makes most kids drowsy, but a few become excited and hyper with a dose of Benadryl.

PEARL: Some patients with chronic Lyme have red ear pinnae (Winter's ear) which may signify high histamine levels. In these cases, the histamine may be contributing to symptoms such as brain fog and malaise. Antihistamines might attenuate these symptoms. Some HCPs use Benadryl to help patients through a Herx reaction. Consider whatever might work to help the patient.

PEARL: Antihistamines and decongestants are not interchangeable. Antihistamines reverse the histamines that cause the symptoms of allergic reactions. Decongestants unstuff noses. If you want both effects, get a product that does both. If you only want one effect, order one or the other.

---

2 *Sharks don't have scales.*

b. Epinephrine is used in severe allergic and life-threatening anaphylactic reactions. Epi is administered as a SQ injection by an HCP or in an auto-injector such as an EpiPen.

c. Bronchodilators are used when allergies present with wheezing and respiratory tightness.

d. Steroids: In general, steroids are not recommended in Lyme patients. As a former ER doctor, if I had a kid in front of me in anaphylaxis, the epi, the nebulizer, and the steroids would be in that kid so fast you wouldn't have time to say, "In general, steroids are not recommended in Lyme patients."

K. Anxiety

Of all the myriad TBI symptoms, I have the most empathy for patients with anxiety. Anxiety associated with TBIs especially Lyme, bartonellosis, and M. *fermentans* is biochemical and is not simply a way to annoy unsympathetic HCPs. Anxiety actually tangles our DNA, as shown by the impact of stress on the tips of the nucleic acid chains or telomeres.

Anyone who feels sick, usually also feels some anxiety, otherwise they have other problems outside the scope of this book. With TBIs this might be compounded, since patients often face considerable resistance to the idea that they are "really sick." When you have 4-year-olds having to defend themselves to people who took an oath to help them, you might have a little anxiety in play.

The anxiety that accompanies some of the TBIs can appear like a biochemical tidal wave, where the patient feels incapable of controlling the feelings and no rational attempts to "talk them out of it" will turn the tide.

Anxiety due to TBIs can range from nervousness about getting a blood test to full-blown panic attacks. Unfortunately, the anxiety displayed on the one end of the spectrum is treated very differently from the anxiety on the other end. In fact, treating a patient with GAD, OCD, or panic attacks with the medicines used for mild anxiety can sometimes make the situation worse.

If the TBI patient is experiencing anxiety out of proportion to the situation, or beyond what was usual for that individual in the past, consider the co-infections that are known to cause these kinds of responses. Look again or treat again for Bartonella and M. *fermentans* and make sure the Bb are under control.

Research at Purdue (okay, and elsewhere, too) has shown repeatedly that emotions are contagious. If the patient is nervous, the caretaker is nervous, and the HCP is nervous. Any of the three parties can be the anxiety-instigator here. But once one gets nervous, the anxiety spreads, in a domino effect. Care must be taken to address this symptom in all parties.

PEARL: Positive emotions such as confidence, courage, optimism, and happiness are just as contagious. Even "faked" positive emotion can influence a person constructively. This has been measured quantitatively using HR and BP, as well as cortisol and oxytocin levels. Even false smiles demonstrably decrease anxiety. And they're free.

If you are not comfortable treating anxiety or depression, make sure you know appropriate HCPs to consult. These issues will come up again and again and they must be addressed. Try to find a consulting HCP who is knowledgeable and empathetic to TBI patients.

Treatments:

1. Both talk therapy and cognitive behavioral therapy have been shown to help anxiety at all levels. A variety of techniques have been helpful. If you believe the patient is anxious enough to need medication, she is anxious enough to consider counseling. Many studies have shown that the combination of these two modalities may be the best approach.

2. Medication options:

<u>Mild to moderate nervousness:</u>

Benzodiazepines including the "pam" drugs such as lorazepam (Ativan), diazepam (Valium), and oxazepam (Serax). These drugs can make the patient sleepy and can cause dependency.

PEARL: At one point, I was the benzodiazepine physician for Europe. When the company decided to discontinue the benzodiazepines in France because the French system did not allow sufficient profit, there were protests and a near-riot. I had never seen the French so angry. When the word got out, I think every person in Paris called me. The company changed its mind. I believe they still sell benzos there at a loss. If you want the French to go to war, threaten to take away their benzodiazepines.

Antihistamines such as Benedryl (diphenhydramine) and hydroxyzine (Atarax, Vistaril) can alleviate anxiety. In kids, the dose of Benadryl usually ranges from 6.25 mg to 50 mg/dose q 4 to 6 hours depending on the size of the kid. Antihistamines make most people drowsy. But there is a small but significant minority who actually become excited and hyper with a dose of Benadryl.

<u>Severe anxiety or anxiety associated with GAD, OCD, and panic attacks:</u>

Benzodiazepines sometimes make these conditions *worse*. Unless addressing an acute episode, think about alternatives. They might best be reserved for the immediate relief of a panic attack.

Consider **SSRIs** or other indicated antidepressants. SSRIs are considered first-line treatment for anxiety disorders. I was the development physician for several of these drugs a few years ago. (I must say I am disappointed that one company has chosen the low road by taking what they are already selling and focusing on an isomer, changing its brand name in order to present it as a new drug, and advertising it as such. DDMAC, where are you?) Then, as now, the SSRIs were said to cause increased suicidal thoughts and actions in teens and young adults. Those of us working on the development of these medications thought that some of these kids were SO depressed that the antidepressant might make some of them feel well enough to actually have suicidal thoughts and actions. Does that make sense? The medicines got them mobilized to act. Some kids when started on SSRIs are almost paralyzed with depression. How sad that they had to feel a little better before they could even contemplate suicide. Of, course, watch teens (and everyone else on antidepressants) for suicidal thoughts. If you are not comfortable prescribing antidepressants, you may need to consult with another HCP. You keep managing the TBI. Despite some studies saying that antidepressants are no more effective than placebos, that has not been my experience. I have found that the majority of patients with significant anxiety or depression show improvement on SSRIs, especially when used in combination with talk or behavioral therapy. Do not discontinue SSRIs abruptly. Patients should be weaned from these medications, when it's time to discontinue.

PEARL: Lexapro (escitalopram) is an SSRI that has been used with considerable success in TBI patients with anxiety and panic attacks. Officially indicated for depression and GAD, this drug can be used in anxious patients whether they have depression or not.

PEARL: Don't get Lexapro (escitalopram) and Luvox (fluvoxamine) mixed up. Both work through serotonin reuptake and both have similar indications like depression and anxiety. I've had patients that have experienced considerable success on both these drugs, but they are distinct entities.

Additional medication options for anxiety:

The β-blocker propranolol has been used for performance anxiety and in treating the anxiety associated with PTSD. Alpha-adrenergics like Minipress and Catapres have been used for anxiety. Trazadone has been used to treat nighttime anxiety, GAD, panic, and PTSD. Mirtazapine (Remeron) has been useful in patients with nighttime anxiety associated with insomnia. Remeron is one of my first choices but it will increase appetite and blood sugars. This drug is a great choice for little old folks who can't sleep, and won't eat, and are worried about it. BuSpar (buspirone) is usually indicated for ADD but has been tried for GAD in adults. Klonopin is considered a benzodiazepine but has been used for panic disorders. B6, zinc, and trace minerals have been included as part of the treatment regimen for anxiety.

IN ALL CASES, IF THE ANXIETY IS DUE TO AN UNDERLYING, ON-GOING INFECTIOUS PROCESS, THE SXS ARE UNLIKELY TO RESOLVE UNLESS THE INFECTION IS ADDRESSED.

3. There are many ancillary modalities that may help with anxiety and depression including exercise, meditation, breathing techniques, etcetera, which will be discussed more thoroughly in Chapter 27: *Supportive Measures*.

L. Depression

Depression is a common manifestation in TBIs. In addition, the incidence and prevalence of depression are higher in all patients with chronic disease and chronic pain. Currently, there are a number of helpful antidepressants. Although very effective, the "older" agents like the MAO inhibitors are rarely used today, especially in the pediatric population, because of side effects and drug interactions. The most commonly used today are the SSRIs and their derivatives that work by trying to rebalance the brain chemistry, usually through serotonin or norepinephrine.

Treatments:

1. Counseling has been shown to be effective alone and in combination with medications. HCPs should work in collaboration with a TBI-aware therapist. If the depression is secondary to a TBI, neither condition will likely get better unless the underlying TBI is addressed.

2. There are many ancillary modalities that may help with anxiety and depression including exercise,

meditation, breathing techniques, etcetera, which will be discussed more thoroughly in Chapter 27: *Supportive Measures*.

3. One of the biggest impediments to recovering from depression is the on-going stigma associated with the condition. Many HCPs who should know better still have a "suck it up" attitude. If only treatment of depression were so simple, no one would be depressed. Even the strongest willpower cannot overcome biochemistry, and treatment options should be reviewed. There is no extra credit for suffering longer.

PEARL: Additional resources might be available through Depressioncheck, an iPhone application that helps assess depression risk – DBSAlliance.org that offers online support groups – HealthyMinds.org from the American Psychiatric Association – or @NIMHgov a Twitter handle for the National Institute for Mental Health.

4. Medications

   SSRIs and their offshoots are currently the most common medications used to treat depression in all age groups. Despite warnings about suicidal ideation and actions in teens and young adults, those of us who have frequently prescribed these medications have seen them be quite effective without excessive safety issues beyond those that would be expected in a depressed population. I have not experienced increased suicidal tendencies in kids that I have had on antidepressants. I sure have seen suicidal ideation and gestures in some kids who are not treated.

   Recent studies have touted the claim that SSRIs are not any more effective than placebo. This does not match my clinical experience. I have seen some truly depressed patients in my practice. Each person that I have started on antidepressants has improved. Of course, I counsel them and their caregivers about suicide risk and for some I have requested written no-suicide agreements. Here I had them sign a written promise to call before acting on any suicidal thoughts. Will this agreement stop a person determined to commit suicide? Probably not, but since we both have copies at least the patient has a list of people she can call if she is in trouble. If the risk of suicide is high, this is an individual that should not be alone and either in-patient or out-patient supervision should be considered.

   Do not prescribe or otherwise treat depression if you are not comfortable doing so. Refer quickly to a competent TBI-aware HCP. If you cannot bring yourself to ask, "Are you having any thoughts of hurting yourself or ideas about suicide?" then refer the depressed patient. Do not abandon the case. The TBI is still yours to manage.

   I tell all patients that antidepressant medicine will take about two weeks to work. These are not happy pills. They will not make a person jolly, but will hopefully smooth out the path and there will not be such low points. There can be side effects such as diarrhea, nausea, strange sensations, etcetera, but these tend to go away in short order. Just about the time they think they might be feeling better, they notice the side effects are gone. I have never had a patient stop an antidepressant due to a side effect. Generally, he was feeling so bad initially that a week of queasiness was thought to be worth the potential benefit.

   Follow up either by phone or a visit in two weeks or less. By then the patient should be feeling a little better. The more severe the depression, the shorter the interval before the follow-up.

   PEARL: TBI experts frequently choose Wellbutrin or Zoloft, and may incorporate Abilify if that addition might be clinically beneficial. Abilify is one of several atypical antipsychotics used in the treatment of schizophrenia, bipolar disorder, and depression. This medicine is commonly considered for treating irritability in kids with autism. If standard antidepressants are not working, Abilify can be used as an adjunct to other agents in treating depression.

   Do **NOT** stop these medicines abruptly. Remember the point is to rebalance the neurotransmitters in the brain. Shutting off the equilibrator can cause a rebound in symptoms and in some cases signs of withdrawal. To be discontinued these medicines need to be weaned. That does not mean skip one dose this Thursday and then come off entirely on Sunday. I like a long, slow, gradual **wean**. Why not? Slowly cut the dose and then gradually skip a day, etc. One approach is to alternate a half a tablet with a whole tablet for several weeks, then move to a half tablet daily, then every other day, then every second day, etc. Weaning should take weeks or longer. What's your hurry?

5. Treat the TBI.

M. Sleep Problems

Sleep problems can manifest in a number of ways. Remember that essentially every hormone and chemical in the brain can impact the sleep cycle. With any shift in the normal physiology, there is the potential for sleep disturbance. We know that Bb, Bartonella, and M. *fermentans* alter brain chemistry. All might be expected to have an effect on sleep.

Some TBI patients do almost nothing but sleep 18, 20, 22 hours a day. This excess sleep is not necessarily due to weakness or fatigue. This is **hypersomnia**. In TBIs this condition is likely due to the underlying pathology. While there are anti-narcoleptic drugs like Provigil (modafinil) on the market, in these cases digging harder for the underlying cause and aggressively handling that problem is likely to be more productive in the long-run. Of course, amphetamines are used all the time as stimulants, but we would be hard pressed to find an indication for their use in TBI patients. Caffeine is a commonly used stimulant but the results here are more likely jitteriness than revival. Caffeine can also be habit-forming, actually causing withdrawal symptoms in heavy users. Look for the reason why they are sleeping so much and focus on that.

In contrast to the hypersomniacs, there are those patients who cannot sleep and this manifests in two ways: those who have trouble falling asleep and those who have trouble staying asleep. These patients are said to suffer from **insomnia**.

Also, some TBI patients have disturbed sleep with restlessness, vivid dreams, posturing, spasms, abnormal movements, etc. TBIs do not seem to predispose to apnea unless the patient has other risk factors for this condition.

PEARL: Lyme and other TBIs can be associated with bizarre sleep patterns that go beyond just sleeping too much or too little. These manifestations might include: strange dreams, abnormal postures, immobility, terrors, etc. These syndromes should be assessed by a sleep expert, not just by the tech at the local sleep center where they are looking only for sleep apnea. If a TBI is the underlying cause, the symptoms are not likely to respond to conventional treatment unless the underlying TBI is also appropriately managed.

We are just beginning to understand the sleep cycle in children. Teens especially seem to have a clock that keeps them up late and wanting to sleep later in the morning. That is why having high-schoolers report to class at 7:15 a.m. is unnatural. Schools are trying to save money so the bus comes at 6:55; at least it does here in Unionville School District.

If a patient is having sleep problems and cannot function in the morning, the condition may be initiated or exacerbated by TBIs. This may require the HCP talking to the school and getting an adjusted schedule. Schools are not always sympathetic. Even with the best habits, sometimes sleep is elusive. Then treatment may be useful. Remember, if a sleep problem is due to a TBI, it is not likely to completely respond to conventional treatment unless the underlying TBI is appropriately addressed.

Treatments:

1. First, do all the good sleep hygiene things that the National Sleep Foundation recommends: warm baths, darkness, routine, cool room, limits on stimulation from caffeine, exercise, or electronics right before sleep, and warm tryptophan in milk, turkey, or tuna, etc. Make the sleep area a safe sanctuary. I am not a believer in letting a child cry it out, but that is just one of my controversial opinions.

2. If a person is suffering with sleep problems and not responding to conventional therapies, consider that an underlying, on-going infection may be contributing to the problem. Treat the infection.

3. Melatonin supplements are recommended by some but found not to be effective by others. Lavender is said to be relaxing. As long as the treatment is not harmful, try reasonable things that might help.

4. Progressive Muscle Relaxation or PMR is a technique that involves deep breathing while successively tensing and relaxing muscle groups. Theoretically, PMR slows the SNS and allows the patient to focus on something beside the fact that he can't sleep.

5. Medication:

   a. OTC sleep aids usually contain antihistamines like Benadryl and may be effective in many cases. As mentioned earlier, Benadryl has a paradoxical effect in some people making them hyper.

   b. There are a number of prescription medications that are quite effective. Some of the older generation sleep meds are benzodiazepines such as Dalmane and Halcion. While effective in helping patients sleep, they often cause considerable "hangover" the next day. They are not as commonly used today in most practices.

   c. Zolpidem (Ambien) is not recommended in patients under 18. Ambien is indicated for short-term treatment of insomnia and comes in 5 or 10 mg tablets. When starting a patient on this medicine, consider half a tablet to monitor effect. Ambien usually works in about 10 minutes but can cause vivid dreams (that some find unpleasant), poor judgment, impulsivity, memory impairment, sleep walking and talking, and abnormal eating, driving, and sexual behaviors. (Tiger Woods is not the only celebrity who has blamed bad behavior on Ambien.) Zolpidem seems to cause much less hangover in the morning, if the person sleeps a full course after dosing, compared to the older generation sleep aids. The young and the elderly may experience more side effects, while middle-aged folks just love the stuff. Use with caution with antifungals and rifamycin. Ambien keeps people asleep for about 8 hours and should not be taken by anyone who does not have a full 8 hours to sleep.

d. For those without a whole night to sleep or those who wake up in the middle of the night and have trouble falling back to sleep, consider Sonata (zaleplon) which is effective for about 4 hours.

e. Additional agents that have been used to promote sleep include: pregabalin, trazadone, quetiapine (Seroquel), and tiagabine.

f. Modafinil is an agent that has been used to promote **wakefulness** or to combat excessive sleepiness.

g. Some HCPs try an activating agent in the morning and a sleep promoter in the evening. BUT…

IN ALL CASES, IF THE SLEEP DISTURBANCE IS DUE TO AN UNDERLYING, ON-GOING INFECTIOUS PROCESS, THE SXS ARE UNLIKELY TO RESOLVE UNLESS THE INFECTION IS ADDRESSED.

N. Constipation

When I was in the Army, they had MREs (meals-ready-to-eat) for us to consume while in the field. A combat force (we were the supportive medical corps) must have food that is light, compact, and high energy. MREs were often dehydrated so that the heavy water did not have to be carried, low fiber so they would not take up too much space, and very high in calories to keep an army in fighting form. They were often quite tasty and we were ravenous and so we gobbled them up. For about two days. That's when we all became so constipated that we would sob if we had to go to the bathroom and sob if we didn't. Our entire focus was on the toilette and we all talked about our bowel movements as though we were old married couples who had known one another for 60 years instead of army docs who had only met the previous week. Needless to say, it is most difficult to focus on the mission when all your concentration is on one square inch of mucus membrane. We would cheer when any one of our comrades had any success in the latrine.

As a family practice doc going to visit patients in four Wilmington hospitals, my patients often were in the ICU with a half dozen specialists. They liked me best and do you know why? I was the only one who bothered to help make their bowels move. They would tell the cardiologist about their constipation and he would say that wasn't his job; and they would tell the pulmonologist and he would say that wasn't his job; and they would tell the nephrologist and she would say that wasn't her job. The neurologist in the bow tie would nearly faint. And then, here I would come with my small armamentarium of stool softeners, fiber, and mild laxatives.

By definition, constipation is infrequent bowel movements of less than 3 per week, often accompanied by straining, discomfort, and the eventual passage of hard stool. Severe constipation means less than one bowel movement per week. You definitely know constipation when it grips you or your child. The goal of treatment is one BM every 2 or 3 days without strain or discomfort.

There are many GI complaints with TBDs, constipation among them. Although diarrhea is the more common side effect of antibiotic use, constipation can be associated with other drugs, like opioids, used in TBI cases. A number of TBIs significantly impact the nervous system. We know that the GI tract is inseparably intertwined with the nervous system. Could Lyme or other co-infections be affecting the GI tract?

Treatments:

1. Find the underlying cause:

   a. TBI contribution?

   b. Some commercial weight-loss programs (often liquids and powders) cause significant constipation.

   c. Many drugs including opioids, some antidepressants, iron supplements, and certain anti-convulsants can be constipating. Sometimes the pain of a TBI is treated with opioids and the patients and caretakers are stunned by the severity of constipation. Don't let constipation come as a surprise. Review the medicine list.

   d. Underlying conditions such as diabetes and hypothyroidism

2. Diet: The best anti-constipation diet is one high in fiber and very low in processed foods. This means plenty of fruits and vegetables and whole grains. Not only are prunes high in fiber they have a slight stimulant effect.

PEARL: The food label must say whole grain not just whole wheat or whole rice. Just because something is 100% wheat doesn't mean they haven't processed all the fiber out of it. Whole grain usually means they left the fiber.

Dietary fiber does not work overnight and may take a week to 10 days to impact the regularity of bowel movements. At first, the higher the fiber the gassier the patient – think high fiber beans. This effect usually dissipates with time. Since constipation is easier to prevent than to treat, high fiber diets might be considered as a long-term life style choice.

3. Commercial fiber:

   a. Psyllium products (Metamucil) tend to be thick and gloppy. In my considerable time spent visiting rehab facilities over the last few years, I must say I have never witnessed so much lying, cheating, bribing, and just plain subterfuge as I saw when it came to consuming this stuff. Even my own compulsively honest mother would say it was "all gone" when the nurse checked to make sure. Nope, she pitched it. No treatment helps if it is never taken. I know psyllium is likely the most economical approach but sometimes you get what you pay for. I could never get a kid to take it.

   b. Synthetic cellulose (Citrucel) can also be unpleasant to get down.

   c. Benefiber (dextrin) is the fiber product with which I have had the most success. Tasteless, clear, and easy to mix, this product can be combined with most drinks and food. Patients will not notice.

PEARL: Do not get Benefiber mixed up with Beneful, which is a dog food.

   d. All these fibers, plus the dozens of others, alone and in combination, can cause gas, bloating, and rumbling. You may want to start with a low dose and work your way up. None work instantly.

4. Water: Fiber is a great remedy for constipation because it pulls water into the intestine, softening the stool and allowing it to move forward, No water, no progress. In fact, commercial fibers without water can compound the problem. Drink lotsa fluids, especially plain water. Caffeine and alcohol are thought to be dehydrating.

5. Lubricants: Oils, like mineral oil, make the fecal matter slippery and easier to pass. The oil stays in the intestinal tract and keeps water from being readily absorbed into the circulation. Theoretically, more water then stays with the stool. These oils are unpleasant to drink even when flavored, but mineral oil can be given in a suppository. Usually mineral oil is not absorbed from the GI tract. Rarely, a problem with the intestinal lining will allow mineral oil to be taken into the system causing inflammation. Mineral oil should not be used long-term because indigestible oils can impede the absorption of fat-soluble vitamins and some drugs.

6. Stool softeners such as Colace are wetting agents that improve the ability of water within the colon to penetrate and mix with the stool. More water means a softer stool. Colace can be used long-term but may take a week to work. Colace can be a blessing especially to those who have been straining or have developed hemorrhoids.

7. Saline laxatives act within a few hours and are often given at night for "relief in the morning." There are a number of these commercially available but the mildest and most commonly used is milk of magnesia (MOM). Now there is a vanilla-cherry formulation. MOM should not be used regularly but can help when the patient is struggling after trying other remedies.

PEARL: The salts in saline laxatives are thought to work using osmotic pressure to pull water into areas of higher salt concentration.

8. Stimulant laxatives: BE CAREFUL. These laxatives cause the muscles in the intestine to contract, propelling the contents forward. Examples include senna derivatives like Ex-Lax and Senokot.

PEARL: When the British chemical company ICI split in two, the employees were told to wait for the big announcement about the name of the new pharmaceutical division. Millions of dollars were spent on consultants to ensure that the selected name was not offensive in any language. The word came first by phone broadcast messages and word-of-mouth. For days we thought we had been renamed Senokot when it was really Zeneca. This is not a PEARL at all and will not be counted as one of the thousand.

Although some stimulant laxatives come in children's formulations, care must be taken with their use in any age group. They can cause severe diarrhea and explosive bowel movements which can result in dehydration and electrolyte imbalances, especially low K. Use of stimulants can cause cramping and chronic use can damage the colon. Dependence on these stimulant laxatives can worsen constipation. Be aware that these types of laxatives are commonly used by people with eating disorders. Bisacodyl stimulants (Dulcolax, Correctol) stimulate the nerves of the intestine and thereby stimulate intestinal activity. These can cause very powerful results and must be used with extreme caution in the pediatric and elderly populations.

9. Herbal remedies are occasionally recommended in the literature. Since these preparations are not regulated by the FDA, the ingredients as well as their quantity and purity are not clear. Most promotional claims are unsubstantiated. Phrases like "clinical proof" mean nothing. Since some of the herbal formulations do contain stimulant laxatives, be very careful before considering their use.

10. Mechanical treatments:

    a. Enemas should be used only as a last resort since they can be traumatic at any age. They are best saved for when stool seems to be impacted in the rectum. Care must be taken when giving an enema since too much fluid can be introduced and the mucosa can be injured or punctured by the enema apparatus. Warm tap water enemas are the most common but lubricants like mineral oil and saline laxatives like MOM are also used. Colace enema preps can soften the stool. The purpose is multifold: add water to the mix, provide lubrication to reduce the pain of evacuation, and to crowd the rectum with water. Sometimes the mechanical stimulation alone produces movement. Many preps used for enemas can be irritating. Proceed with caution.

    b. Suppositories can be irritating so know what you are inserting into the rectum. Glycerin is often used in suppositories but this can irritate the soft tissues. Again, the mechanical action alone of inserting a suppository into the rectum may be enough to spur evacuation.

    c. Manual disimpaction: Occasionally stool becomes so hard and packed inside the rectum that the feces must be manually removed.

11. Biofeedback: The GI tract is so connected to the nervous system that there has been some success in using biofeedback to try to influence the voluntary control of bowel movements.

12. Good bowel habits include: Avoid rushing. Go when you have to go. (Sometimes there is no bathroom available, but follow this advice as much as practical.) Don't hold it in. Don't strain if you can help it. Don't force yourself to go when you don't have to. Never try to force a little kid to go. Encouragement is one thing, yelling is another. Some people get comfortably into a routine, and others never do. Respect a routine, but don't be a slave to certain times or places. You can read, just not *War and Peace.* Read only while actively involved in toileting. When you're done, stop reading. There will be other opportunities to finish that chapter.

13. Exercise: If you remember, in James Michener's book, *Hawaii,* the missionaries walked and walked and walked, round and round and round the deck of the ship in desperate attempts to encourage bowel movements. Now, some sources say that exercise does not help constipation. Well, I can't imagine that it would hurt. I would walk the deck.

O. Miscellaneous ancillary treatments

1. **Gamma globulin** (GG, IVIG, IV IgG) may have potential as an ancillary treatment in selected TBI cases. For many years, intramuscular injections of γ-globulin has been used as a temporary protection against hepatitis. Igs from plasma have been used since the 50s to treat immune deficiency. In recent years, IV IgG has been studied as a treatment for a number of autoimmune conditions. If the Igs in the patient are deficient or malfunctioning, the IV IgG covers for them, impacting the immune system as it would if these were the patient's own healthy antibodies. Remember the *Gentle Immunology* chapter? These Igs step into the cascade in all the places that normal, healthy Igs would step in, picking up the slack for ineffective or misdirected Igs and perhaps encouraging the removal of defective antibodies. The literature around treatment with gamma globulin contains a broad range of outcomes.

   In TBI patients, innovative work is being done exploring a possible treatment role for IgG in patients with antineuronal antibodies. These antibodies are just beginning to be understood in association with an autoimmune response and are thought to contribute to a number of neuropsychiatric syndromes sometimes collectively called PAND (pediatric autoimmune neuropsychiatric disorders). Manifestations include tics, bipolar patterns, OCD, anxiety, ODD, manic depression, schizophrenia, psychoses, involuntary movement disorders, myoclonus, new-onset vocal and motor abnormalities, and unresponsiveness to psychotropics. Initially PANDs were thought to only be associated with Strep infections. Current thinking is that these autoimmune neuropsychiatric problems may also be associated with some TBI pathogens such as Lyme. Bartonella and M. *fermentans* could also be involved, but their role is theoretical at this point. PAND associated with TBIs have been treated with IV IgG, appropriate antibiotics, and then plasmapheresis to clean up debris. Antibiotics appear to be an important component of treatment in the TBI-associated PANDs.

2. **Probenecid** (Benemid) is sometimes given with Amoxicillin or other PCNs to increase efficacy. Probenecid competes with penicillins in line for renal

excretion and so there is a higher PCN blood level than would be achieved if PCN was used by itself. The anion transporter in the kidney usually prefers the probenecid to the amoxicillin, leaving the amoxicillin behind to do its work. During WWII, probenecid was used to extend the limited supplies of PCN. Probenecid is not used as much today to improve efficacy since many PCNs now have enhancers already added in combination products. Still probenecid is mentioned in the literature and used in developing countries. Probenecid should be taken with water. Adult dose is 500 mg q 8 hours. Adverse events include: headache, allergies, rash, nausea, vomiting, and abnormal LFTs.

3. Binding agents

Occasionally, TBI patients will need binding agents to capture bile salts before they can form gallstones in response to Rocephin treatment. Some HCPs use binding agents to trap heavy metals in cases of toxicity or to bind mold toxins (mycotoxins). The literature also mentions use of binders to capture Lyme toxins. Options include:

a. Cholestyramine (Questran) is a resin that sequesters bile salts in the GI tract to prevent their reabsorption. These bile salts are then removed from the body by forming insoluble complexes that are excreted in the feces. Questran comes in packets and usually 4 to 8 grams are given once or twice a day in adults with a maximum of 24 grams per day. AEs include constipation and problems with teeth after exposure to the suspension. Questran may alter the absorption of other drugs and should not be taken near other medications. Use 1 hour before or 4 hours after other drugs. There may also be interference with absorption of fat-soluble vitamins.

Cholestyramine is sometimes used to try to bind the toxins from fungus and has been considered for use in binding toxins made by TBI pathogens. These results are not conclusive. Since cholestyramine sequesters bile acids, and Actigall is a bile acid, these two should not be used together.

b. Ursodiol (Actigall) is a naturally occurring bile acid that is often co-administered with Rocephin to prevent or dissolve gallstones. Ursodiol changes the bile of patients with gallstones from cholesterol-precipitating to cholesterol-solubilizing. This can either prevent stone formation or dissolve stones that are already present.

Actigall comes in 300 mg capsules and is very bitter if the capsule dissolves in the mouth. Usually 1 to 3 capsules are given daily. In kids consider 8 to 10 mg/kg/day in 2 or 3 divided doses up to 600 mg/day.

GB stone dissolution may require months and complete resolution does not occur in all cases. Composition of bile acid returns to pretreatment levels about a week after Actigall is stopped. This drug will not help with calcified stones and stones can recur.

Do not use cholestyramine and Actigall concomitantly. AEs include abdominal pain, constipation, diarrhea, dyspepsia, nausea, vomiting, headache, and dizziness. US of the GB should be done at baseline and at regular intervals usually at least once a month if on Rocephin. Consider monitoring for 3 months after the Rocephin is discontinued.

4. Glutathione may help with brain fog. Additional information about glutathione can be found in Chapter 27: *Supportive Measures*.

5. Vaccines: Why would a topic as important as vaccination be tucked at the bottom of a miscellaneous treatment list after binding agents and supplements for brain fog? Simply because there are currently no human vaccines against the most familiar TBIs. Just as with so many other aspects of the history of TBI, the story of the Lyme vaccine is filled with incompetent development mixed with too many personal agendas. Add a big dose of hubris and greed and you end up with no vaccine. The fallout of this vaccine fiasco is that we are still stuck with diagnostic recommendations that were put in place to protect the vaccine developers and that should have no place in clinical decisions. But, I digress. Pam Weintraub outlines the history of the Lyme vaccine in humans very well in *Cure Unknown*. Because Bb seem to have the ability to frequently change protein coats, and for a number of other reasons, it will be hard to target one antigen to use in the development of the vaccine. The idea would be to select an appropriate antigen, and then purify, manufacture, and finally introduce this antigen in a non-virulent form into the organism you want to protect. The antigen would then inspire the manufacture of antibodies against that microbe. When the host is later exposed to the pathogen presenting that same antigen, antibodies are already present to offset the infection. The result is no disease in spite of exposure. I am not aware of any of the big vaccine producers working on a Lyme vaccine.

PEARL: I am not 100% sure but I believe my dog had a severe adverse reaction to a Lyme vaccine. I do not know what type or brand of vaccine since that vet retired. About 10 days after the dose our dog had incapacitating, migratory joint pain where he would pant and scream as well as what can only be described as a canine panic attack: extreme anxiety, hysteria, frantic circling, racing, gnawing, and panting. His joint pain seemed to move and he was very sensitive to touch. There were several repeat episodes.

II. COMMON ADJUNCTIVE TREATMENTS

In most cases the foundation of TBI treatment is antimicrobials. While always keeping that core concept in mind, many experts advocate adjunctive therapies. An adjunct therapy supplements the basic treatment regimen. Where clinically appropriate, make good use of the following modalities.

A. **Counseling:** Referral to psychiatric counseling including therapy provided by psychologists, psychiatrists, and social workers has benefited many patients. However, the person you choose as your consultant should be aware of the potential impact of the TBI pathogen on neuropsychiatric health. Counseling would be one part of the overall treatment strategy. A good therapist can help both the patient and caregiver understand that TBI-associated problems are not the result of lack of willpower or motivation. There is real underlying pathophysiology and repeatedly admonishing a patient to "suck it up" is probably not going to help. The counselor can provide insight as to why certain symptoms are present and then provide tools to manage the often intense manifestations of a TBI at work in the nervous system. Therapists can be valuable in helping teachers understand what is happening with a TBI patient and in encouraging schools and workplaces to make appropriate accommodations. Make sure the patient and counselor fit. A bad match here can be damaging. Just as in any profession, there are therapists who are mean, incompetent, and lack empathy. There are also those who change lives.

PEARL: Nearly 50% of anorexics maintained a healthy weight after family therapy compared to 23% for those who tried to go it alone.

B. **Neuropsychiatric testing**: A number of TBI clinicians advocate neuropsychiatric testing in appropriate cases. These assessments can provide useful information, especially in those patients presenting with significant cognitive or behavioral problems. There are, of course, many different types of NP tests. Depending on the patient's condition, the testing can be targeted to focus on memory, ability to learn new information, judgment, impulsivity, problem solving, attention span, concentration, distractibility, logic, abstract reasoning, use of language, organizing, planning, synthesizing, analyzing, spatial relationships, or visual-motor coordination. Many of these tests are used to assess patients for ADD, ADHD, HD, or PANDAS.

Consider NP testing in TBI patients who seem to have a disproportionate amount of cognitive or behavioral problems associated with their TBI. This type of presentation is not uncommon in Lyme, bartonellosis, or M. *fermentans* infection. NP testing may be indicated if a TBI patient is not achieving developmental milestones, or in those cases where the child was progressing normally but then seems to fall off the charts. Also consider NP tests in those TBI cases with significant CHANGES in cognition or behavior that is unusual for the individual such as noticeable decline in school performance, personality changes, difficulty adjusting socially, problems with making decisions, or suddenly using poor judgment.

The testing may take many hours and is usually conducted by an experienced examiner in a one-on-one setting. NP tests can be expensive, but often they are covered by insurance. Usually the individual's score is compared to scores from a matched population. The results can be used to see where one child stands compared to his peers and to define the current peak performance level. Further, a patient's individual results can then be evaluated over time to determine if the condition is improving or deteriorating. The results of these assessments may help the teacher understand a struggling child.

C. **Structural manipulation**: Both osteopathic physicians and chiropractors, as well as many physical therapists, use structural manipulation to enhance the body's innate ability to heal. Since structure dictates function, problems in the body's structure can impede normal processes and delay healing. Osteopathic and chiropractic manipulation focuses on the proper alignment of the spine and joints and maintenance of normal soft tissue. Many techniques are used to realign, balance, and equilibrate the body. These procedures encourage good drainage and allow for toxins to more readily leave the body. In TBIs, some patients experienced relief with cranial/sacral adjustments which theoretically allow better flow of spinal fluids from the base of the skull down the course of the spine. Some TBI patients who have had cranial manipulation felt a loosening of the fluids cushioning the brain. I'm not sure what that means, but many patients feel considerable relief.

Bb appear to have an affinity for collagen which is one of the foundation molecules of the body structure. If the structure is compromised, the function will also likely be impacted, especially around joints. This effect can impact motion, fluid flow, nerve conduction, and inhibit the patient's ability to heal. Structural manipulation serves to directly counter this pathology. Manipulation may help with joint motion, ROM, function, and fluid flow including circulation and lymphatic drainage. These techniques can help relieve pain and spasm and restore function so that the patient can participate in full AODL.

When something hurts, the body may subconsciously try to shield that part by splinting. Protective over-compensation can lead to imbalances, strains, spasms, and misalignment. When the structure is impeded, normal flow of fluids and normal nerve conduction can be impacted. Energy can be greatly diminished. All these pathologies can impede recovery.

One osteopath reported that Lyme seemed to change the character of the fascia, making it feel stickier and more adhesive. Fascia are the layers of fibrous connective tissue that surround muscles, blood vessels, and nerves, permitting these structures to slide and glide past one another. While stabilizing, fascia also facilitates motion. What makes up fascia? Collagen bundles. Bb have a particular penchant for collagen. Theoretically, with Bb present, the fascia is less able to allow free-flowing motion. This causes tension in the tissue, decreases the nerve conduction and tissue elasticity, and thereby, impacts ROM and coordination. In Lyme cases, the fascia feels restricted. Osteopathic techniques like fascial release have been reported to offer considerable relief in some patients.

Both chiropractors and osteopathic physicians should be well-versed in these manipulative methodologies. Physical therapists can also perform some structural modalities that may help with joint alignment, fluid flow, nerve conduction, flexibility, optimal ROM, and healthy posture. Anecdotally Lyme patients have reported relief with cranial manipulation, release of trigger points, lymphatic drainage, re-alignment of the spine, and myofascial release. When the underlying structure is intact, the patient may have the best chance for recovery.

PEARL: No matter how skilled the practitioner, any structural problems caused by an underlying TBI is not likely to respond optimally unless the TBI is also addressed.

D. **Physical and occupational therapy**: Depending on the individual case, PT and OT can offer many positive results. If the patient is physically limited, PT encourages movement, flexibility, balance, agility, and stamina. With TBIs, damage to joints and muscles can cause acute or chronic impairment. Sometimes either the disease or the prolonged bed rest can cause so much weakness and stiffness that the patient needs to rebuild almost from scratch. OT can suggest alternative ways to accomplish activities-of-daily-living and help the patient live with impairments. In some cases, physical trainers can offer fitness advice as well. Visits to the therapist can range from 1 to 5 times a week but usually 3 is reasonable depending on the patient and condition. Some insurance companies will not pay if the diagnosis is Lyme arthritis but will pay for arthritis. Therapy should continue as long as the

patient is benefiting and there are signs of progress. In some cases, PT/OT practitioners will come to the house.

Therapy can help the person in many ways including pain reduction and the return to more normal function. The goal of OT/PT is for the patient to become functional enough to advance in AODL and get the stamina to live on in better health. Therapy can be especially helpful as the patient transitions through different phases of recovery.

The therapist can teach the patient how to stretch, breathe, increase mobility, improve muscle tone, enhance strength, develop coordination, and re-establish balance. Further, the therapist should be able to advise on ways to protect any painful or limited joints with gradual improvement on ROM and avoidance of hyperextension. The therapist should encourage the individual to always have control of the movement unless she is working on passive ROM techniques. Going too far beyond capacity can cause injury in these patients. Often repetitions are more important than weight. Good form will be essential to avoid injury. An experienced therapist should be able to coach a patient on when she is doing enough and when to push herself sensibly.

With some patients this may be the first time they have exercised, or at least done so correctly. Novices may need constant supervision and considerable education. Previously athletic patients may be more difficult to treat since they may resent their weakness and infirmity. They may not be used to significant physical limitations. Many do not understand how incapacitating inadequately treated Lyme can be. Here the therapist may need to reel them back to prevent injury or exhaustion.

The most common PT approaches for TBI patients include both passive and active ROM, massage, heat, pressure, and ultrasound. Some of the literature counsels Lyme patients to avoid ice and TENS units.

OT provides alternative approaches for performing AODL. TBI patients may be shocked to experience the level of fatigue, pain, and disability associated with their condition. Unfortunately, Lyme that has not been properly managed or that has been allowed to progress to a chronic state, may leave residual impairments. This can result in frustration, anxiety, and depression. For long-term disabilities the occupational therapist will need to help the patient adjust both physically and emotionally to her new circumstances. This may require a creative collaboration between the patient, the caretaker, and the therapist in order to come up with solutions to everyday problems.

PEARL: PT/OT can be quite expensive. Make sure that something is happening in therapy that could not be done at home for free. Be wary of PT sessions with one therapist and a dozen or more patients at once. The other patients are not splitting the cost with you and you should get considerable individual attention. The cost of $400 an hour is a bit steep for 30 minutes of ice at the beginning, 2 minutes of stretching, and then 28 minutes of a heating pad at the end. Good PT/OT will be focused on the patient for the majority of the session.

E. **Cognitive rehabilitation**: Trauma is not the only way to damage a brain. Many pathogens, including those that cause TBIs, cross the BBB and cause harm:

1. Directly by burrowing or encapsulating

2. Through stimulation of potent immune chemicals that result in fogginess, lassitude, or confusion

3. By the manufacture of autoantibodies, such as the antineuronal antibodies likely associated with PANDAS

4. By releasing toxins that poison the tissue

5. Through a combination of factors or by way of modalities not yet identified

In TBIs, the purpose of cognitive rehabilitation is to return the conscious brain function to where it was before the injury. Many methods can be used here including computers tied into EEGs and biofeedback programs targeting different parts of the brain. Cognitive rehabilitation can help by facilitating the by-pass of the damaged parts of the CNS and encouraging the healthy parts to take over. This type of rehabilitation should be available at a children's hospital or an up-scale rehabilitation facility. Never underestimate the damage made possible by certain TBI pathogens. Some of these injuries will be permanent. However, we are learning that the brain is more resilient and reconstituting than previously thought. Cognitive rehabilitation might allow for the restoration of functions that were thought to be lost. While some of these techniques can be quite expensive, other approaches may be as simple and practical as specialized tutoring.

Chapter 26 ALTERNATIVE TREATMENTS – Detailed chapter contents

Chapter 26

ALTERNATIVE TREATMENTS

"They couldn't hit an elephant at this dista___."
Last words of General Jon Sedgwick just as he was shot and killed

There is a real website called Dubious Diagnostic Tests. It's actually pretty good and it lists dozens of medical tests of questionable value. Some of the listed tests are quite bizarre and you have to wonder how they would actually be performed. A number of these tests are so strange that I worry that some people, including HCPs, would actually think they are valid. I wish there were a similar website to evaluate some of the alternative treatments proposed for treatment of TBIs.

I would never presume to disparage any treatment that might have the potential to help someone who has been suffering. In fact, as a clinical researcher, I know that many of the therapies called alternative and non-traditional have as much solid supportive evidence as some of the treatments we spend thousands of dollars on in the US. For example, much traditional Chinese medicine has strong effects. Clearly, TCM often works. We just don't know how it works, the purity of the product, the side effects, or the best doses to use. I always found the role of TCM confounding when I was setting up clinical trials in Asia. How should these traditional therapies be managed? I soon learned that these agents were definitely going to be used by the study population. Just because we are not accustomed to some therapies, does not invalidate them.

Remember that many of the treatments that are so common today as to be boring (such as injections of botulinum toxin, the rasping of fat from our flesh, cutting out, banding, and stapling parts of our digestive tracts, chewing nicotine to help us withdraw from nicotine, and implanting various synthetic globules to make parts of our anatomy artificially large) might be considered outlandish in a different venue. However, these are all currently quite "acceptable" and many are covered by insurance. These modalities might be considered bizarre by other cultures or to those reading about them in the future. Just as we shudder when we read about George Washington being bled to death by leeches and the toxic treatments used to heal in the past, someday our kids might be shuddering about those things we found to be solid therapies.

With all that being said, use common-sense. I once observed a patient who was on over 100 supplements. The HCP was thrilled because the supplements on the office shelves were selling. This patient had a minute by minute daily chart that told her when to take 5 drops of this and 12 drops of that. Some days she increased the amount by 27 drops (like when she was feeling sluggish) and then later took another supplement to counteract the overdosage that made her feel jittery. I found that scenario bizarre, (not to mention a touch unethical on the part of the HCP). When asked when she ate, the patient said she had a hard time eating because she was usually full from those thousands of drops all day. She couldn't take most of her supplements with food anyway.

Many times, if you are not the first practitioner this person has seen for TBIs, you will inherit some treatments that you might not have initiated on your own. In these cases, keep treatments that seem to be helping and wean or discontinue any that seem to be hurting or not adding anything but confusion.

Do not overwhelm the patient. As a physician with a PhD analytical chemist husband, we were often overwhelmed with all the documentation and schedules and dosing for our son. If we didn't understand, who would? No treatment does any good if the regimen can't be followed or understood.

Teenagers especially burn out. "How much longer do I have to do this?" the usually quite sensible Chris Spreen asked at about month four. The HCP may need to prioritize therapies and emphasize the importance of each medicine or treatment. Be careful if the HCP is also a salesperson for alternative modalities. Most patients appreciate when the HCP makes supplements available in the office setting, since quality products can be hard to find in pharmacies, health food stores, and on the Internet. But there is a difference between making products conveniently accessible and insisting that the patient buy your merchandise.

In many cases, exploration of concurrent conditions can be prudent but do not get carried away with fads. Do you know how many times I have heard patients tell me they finally found the answer to all their medical problems by discovering molds or food allergies or heavy metals or radon or toxins, etc? Funny, they never seem to have the same passion for basic diet and exercise programs to solve their problems. When yet another trendy program eventually fails to fix everything, they are disappointed and desperate to move on to the next best thing.

When you tell your next HCP how you just failed the self-administered yeast spit test or the home armpit test for defective thyroid function or that your radioactivity monitor buzzed all night, she might wish you had gone to another doctor. I AM NOT SAYING that people do not have real problems with gluten allergies, radon, or toxins. I know these things hurt people. But if you start looking at some of these alternative therapies as the Holy Grail that will solve all your problems, you might come off as unbalanced or naïve.

One practitioner told me that a bizarre treatment worked because SHE HAD READ THE DATA. Knowing her, she had no more capacity to read the data scientifically than I would have in reading the structural outline for the B52 bomber. Just because someone is an HCP that does not make her a scientist. Let me remind you that hundreds of hours are spent at companies writing up this "data" in a way that makes sure you can find no flaws in the science. While this is not exactly lying, it is advertising, promotions, sales, and marketing. That is the reason that there is an FDA and other regulatory bodies around the world today. A long time ago, an enterprising entrepreneur discovered that people WANTED to believe that snake oil cured everything and the more ailments you said it fixed, the more they bought. By the time the consumer figured out that he was just drunk and not cured, the honest businessman was off duping the people in the next town. Be careful. Many people touting treatments do not care about you. They want to make money. They are not your friends. They do not care about your sick child. They want to make money.

Some of the treatments listed below may be useful for *some* patients at *some* points in their clinical course. Remember you are dealing with a very vulnerable population. Many of the caretakers have presented their sick children to dozens of doctors trying to find relief for these kids. I was one of them. We are willing to buy anything or try anything that might help. HCPs, please stay on the ethical high ground. The more big words and convoluted science in the promotional material, the more skeptical you should be. Take time to think before you agree to something that sounds too good to be true. I have been saddened and scared by TBI parents, patients, and HCPs who buy-in too readily.

I remember when one of my aunts taped a magnet to her forehead and my mother-in-law went through her papaya and progesterone gel phases. The best advice is: Don't believe everything you read. As I learned in working in drug development in China and the subcontinent, many traditional therapies work. Nonetheless, just as many do not work and may cause harm. We often do not know the purity of an herb and what other ingredients these formulations might contain. Since many of the sources are unregulated, we do not know if they have the same ingredients from one time to the next. I learned this concept the hard way, working for a company that thought it was great not to put active ingredient in medicines

distributed in Africa (much more profit that way). That makes it hard to know appropriate doses. But, no active drug in the formulation does make for few side effects. (If you have ever seen a drug made in a dark basement in India, you will know what I mean.)

Experienced TBI practitioners do not always suggest these alternatives, but if something is working and not doing harm they will tend to go with the program. Many are not especially enamored with patients taking multiple supplements. Some of these therapies are "way out there" and only included here because you might run into them. Use what's helpful and avoid what's harmful. If it seems kooky or too good to be true, it probably is. Just like the myriad weight-loss plans that say this is the last diet you will ever need. If it's so great, why is there even one chubby person left out there?

Many patients come into a TBI specialist already on one or more of these treatment modalities. If the therapies being employed are not compatible with a planned treatment, discuss it with the individual. Here the HCP and caretakers may need to prioritize treatments and understand the importance of each therapy.

Be willing to try any reasonable approach to help the patient feel better. Do no harm. Do not let the patient's core antibiotic regimen get crowded out by parsley, sage, rosemary, and thyme. Consider all options and select. A little sage might be good; too much is overwhelming.

I.   SORTING ALTERNATIVE THERAPIES

What should I do with this Pandora's box of possible remedies? No matter how I slice and dice, someone is going to be offended that I put their precious Neti pot in with potentially harmful treatments like intravenous peroxide. Just like Pandora, I am left only with hope. My goal in the next section is simply to introduce various options.

The following is a list of treatments that you may want to investigate. For each there are HCPs who swear by it and just as many others who believe it's quackery. In general, I added only those descriptions I felt might be useful and that I felt competent to present. For some I barely have a sentence. But for each of the following treatments I did find several mentions of use in TBI patients. I am sure there are many I missed. I have no idea what the risk/benefit ratio is of some of these purported remedies. If every one of these therapies worked as well as their advocates profess, there would be no one with any medical complaints. I list them here, in no particular order, to allow you to see what else might be available. I have limited my opinions unless I have direct experience or knowledge. This list is by no means all-inclusive. There are books written on each topic. If you find something that you believe might be useful, discuss with all parties the possibility that this treatment might help the patient in question. Go on an information search. I know how much you want to help this person, but don't let your eagerness cloud your judgment.

A. **Foods** that claim to cure: Advocates for certain foods assert that figs cure headaches, chard fixes osteoporosis, miso soup eliminates hot flashes, rice boosts brain function, tomatoes prevent cancer especially if cooked, turkey helps you sleep, celery cures HTN, bananas fix kidney stones, licorice is used for dyspepsia, ginger helps nausea and motion sickness, margarine blocks the absorption of cholesterol, and of course, everyone knows to drink cranberry juice if you have a urinary tract infection. EXCEPT, that for every article touting these claims there are matching published reports that refute these very same assertions. Do you know how much miso soup you'd have to consume to prevent one hot flash? I don't want to be the one trying to coax a kid to eat her chard. As always, use good sense. Do not imbalance a diet just to get in enough celery. Be cautious as you read claims. I know you want to believe so badly, because I wanted to believe as well. Think twice when you read about the proven Amish remedy that stops leg cramps in just one minute. Someday I will write a book telling you how to analyze data. Here you would want to ask: Who says? What kind of leg cramps? I live in Amish country and I don't see a lot of time-keepers running in and out of Amish farmhouses. How did they measure this? Who is benefiting by making this claim? If figs help relieve your child's headache, give her a fig. But be careful: Balance. Moderation. Practicality.

B. **Food supplements**: These compounds are not regulated by the FDA and so many claims are made, but few are delivered. Some supplements are important such as vitamins and minerals in those who are not likely to get their needs met through diet or moderate sun exposure. We have learned, with experience, however, that there can be too much of a good thing. Excess water-soluble vitamins are just peed out (if the kidney is healthy), but fat-soluble vitamins can build up with chronic overdosing. More is not necessarily better and untoward side effects can occur. Since many of these supplements compete with drugs for the liver's metabolic enzymes, HCPs must be cognizant that something might be backing up and reaching high systemic levels.

When I worked in drug development, we would see the same "great" idea pitched to us over and over. Everyone had a food supplement, since these are easier to get on the market with no FDA hoops to jump through. I hate to tell you how many times I listened to the capsaicin spiel (derivative of chili peppers), or how we could infuse Vitamin D into a foam base. There are a number of excellent, appropriate, and useful food supplements on the market that may be of benefit to TBI patients. There are just as

many shysters hawking ineffective supplements because presenting a remedy as a supplement, instead of a drug, eliminates most FDA approvals and GMP requirements. Please be careful and don't get your hopes up for cures from these supplements. Just as with diets, if they really worked, no one would be fat.

Too many supplements can be a problem. As I mentioned earlier, I witnessed a number of patients on a ridiculous number of supplements. There is no possible way these can all be taken as directed and there is no way that some of these supplements are not interacting and even at counter-purposes to one another. Be wary of an HCP who recommends a complicated protocol and then sells the supplements out of the office. (Good price, just for you! Limited time offer! Only two per customer!) I have seen spread sheets for keeping track of supplements that rival those used by Wall Street banks to defraud the government. Ask if this is really necessary and what exactly each supplement is supposed to do. When my son was sick, one HCP was pulling supplements off the display case like a frenzied snake oil salesman (Must have been thinking, "Here's a rich one. She is worried about her kid, so she'll buy anything.")

I am not a fan of direct-to-consumer advertising for medicines and food supplements on a good day. By far, my least favorite of these ads are those for canned nutritional supplements for the old and the young. Using scare tactics that suggest that your child is not getting proper nutrition, and to be a good mom you must buy their product, is in my mind unethical. The kids in the ads look healthy and more like they are training for the Olympics than in need of a fortified liquid dietary supplement. The kids who really need these supplements are in St. Jude's and I do not take this exploitative advertising lightly. Certainly, if a TBI patient is having a chronic problem with consuming enough balanced nutrients, consider commercial supplements, but in most cases, a little home cooking will do just fine.

PEARL: Would apricot kernels used as a treatment be considered a food, a food supplement, or an herbal?

C. **Herbals:** I am an advocate for select herbal treatments. Artemesia is one herbal recommended for all potential babesiosis cases. But there is a mindboggling array of other herbals that are purported to treat TBIs. Again, since these are not regulated by the FDA, we do not know the validity of claims, the purity of ingredients, or the safety profile. The information available for most of these products is provided by those who profit by selling them. Herbals run the gamut: everything from the African herb devil's claw for pain, to Chinese thunder god vine for arthritis, to the Native American use of butterbur, and thousands more. At least herbals are interesting. I am sure that some of these herbals do what their promoters allege. CAVEAT EMPTOR.

Reports suggest that TBI patients who are not progressing on traditional antimicrobial therapy might be more successful if certain herbals are added to the regimen. Aside from artemesia, the herbals most commonly used in TBI patients include:

Samento is a brand name of the herbal cat's claw obtained in the Amazon rain forest. This climbing vine has been used for over 2000 years to boost immune response and is currently used as an ancillary remedy in Lyme management. Samento is thought to create immune system balance and act as an anti-inflammatory and has been used to treat Bb and various co-infections. There are a number of dosing regimens in the literature. Start with one drop bid and work up slowly to 15 drops bid. Some patients can tolerate only a ¼ of a drop/dose and that amount is difficult to measure. A usual dose might be between 5 to 10 gtts two or three times a day. Each patient should work up to a tolerable dose over a period of weeks. The herb should be dropped into about 4 ounces of water and then the patient should wait about a minute before taking the dose. AEs include diarrhea which lessens after about a week of regular use. Some types of cat's claw contain tetracyclic oxindole alkaloids (TOAs) that diminish efficacy and may be toxic. Any cat's claw or Samento product should be labeled **TOA-free**.

Burbur is thought to enhance lymph drainage and to detoxify the system. Burbur may help ameliorate the Herx reaction.

Cumanda is considered to be an anti-Lyme, antifungal, and anti-inflammatory. Cumanda is thought to be effective against Bb and some of the co-infections and is sometimes used to treat the systemic effects of mold. Consider cumanda in patients who have been on antibiotics for a long time and are not progressing or those who relapse when antibiotics are discontinued. Herx reactions have been associated with cumanda when used to treat Lyme.

Astragalus is said to provide immune support.

Enula may be as effective as artemesia against protozoa such as Babesia. This herbal is discussed in more detail in Chapter 24: *Antimicrobials*.

Mora is used for microbial defense.

*PEARL: Work by Eva Sapi, PhD, suggests that **banderol** might help Lyme patients by impeding biofilm formation.*

Some patients Herx after these treatments, which suggests antimicrobial activity. Some HCPs use herbals after a course of antibiotics as a sort of transition off traditional therapy. Herbs, such as burbur, have also been used to ameliorate the symptoms of a severe Herx.

Dr. Lee Cowden has a protocol for the treatment of chronic Lyme with herbal therapies, which can be found at www.bionatus.com. Some patients swear by these treatments. I find some of the herbal regimens overwhelming, but I would be remiss if I did not introduce the option. There is a modified Cowden protocol for those who cannot manage the intricacies of the original program. The modified plan has been simplified and should be easier to follow.

In addition to treating the actual infection, there are thousands of herbals that might be considered for symptoms of TBIs, such as St. John's wort said to be effective against depression, and lavender, which is thought to enhance sleep. Each herbal remedy should be considered on a case-by-case basis with a risk/benefit analysis before each decision.

I am unaware of blinded, controlled studies that outline use of these herbs in the pediatric population. Just because a study is done in a "clinical" setting does not mean that it would withstand the rigors of review by the FDA or most European regulatory bodies.

If you inherit a patient already on herbals consider how these treatments will fit into your treatment plan. Keep what seems to be helping. Be aware of potential interactions with other agents. Simplify overly complex regimens to give the patient the best chance for compliance. Encourage discontinuation of any treatment that seems to be causing harm. Initiate herbals after careful consideration of how the treatment might benefit the individual. One size does not necessarily fit all and all herbals are not appropriate for all patients.

Practitioners who might be well-versed in herbal remedies include naturopaths, herbalists, or holistic providers.

D. **Traditional Chinese Medicine:** I may be more familiar with some aspects of TCM than many western physicians since I organized clinical trials in Asia for a number of years. One thing I know for sure is that much of TCM works. There is a reason that there are 1.4 billion Chinese alive today, most never having any access to western medicine. From energy balance to shark fin to marinated bird's nests to acupuncture, TCM offers many options. The focus of TCM is to remove blockages in energy flow and restore balance. Westerners are just beginning to understand the mechanism by which some of these approaches produce their positive effects. Of course, there are TCM modalities that do nothing and a number that are harmful, which sounds a lot like the medical milieu that we also find ourselves in every day. As always, make decisions in the best interest of the individual patient.

E. **Acupuncture:** Usually a component of TCM, acupuncture has been gaining more acceptance in western culture. Studies are underway to determine why these techniques work in many patients. Acupuncture involves the insertion and manipulation of needles into the body usually at specific locations depending on the condition being treated. The needle insertion is thought to redirect and balance energy, although detractors think any response is due to a placebo-effect. There are many variations and in the west, acupuncture is used primarily to treat pain and nausea and as an adjunct to anesthesia for the discomfort of childbirth. In Lyme patients, acupuncture is thought to fight the bacterial agent and to promote general health. As yet, few clinical studies have unequivocally supported the effectiveness of this modality, although there are many anecdotal reports. Detractors say that acupuncture is pseudoscience and nonsense needles and that the procedure is not without risk. Assess the risk/benefit ratio.

F. Treatments for **heavy metal** and other toxicities

While I believe that a number of people have suffered from exposure to heavy metals and other toxins, some HCPs have gone over-the-top in their obsession with these conditions, leaving the more reasonable practitioners to be painted with the same brush and potentially keeping real cases from getting diagnosed and treated.

There are dozens of books on this subject and hundreds of articles, many mixing etiologies and treatments, often making it seem as though the author couldn't tell if he was talking about heavy metal toxicity or celiac disease. I will focus here on the aspects of heavy metal toxicity that might impact TBI patients. While this section focuses primarily on heavy metals, recall that toxins can come from many sources. Pathogens can produce toxins including a number of tick-borne pathogens. Toxins can be found in molds and in the environment such as in pesticides, chemical exposures, industrial and landfill waste, and various pollutants.

Symptoms are often vague such as generalized aches and pains especially involving muscles, tendons, and soft tissues, malaise, fatigue, brain fog including confusion and forgetfulness, GI complaints, fungal overgrowth, allergies, dizziness, headache, vision problems, depression, and anxiety. These symptoms are similar to those found in many inflammatory responses including those found with Lyme and other TBIs. Heavy metals can cross the BBB and get into the CSF. Mercury can be especially neurotox-ic and signs might include numbness or electric, shooting, or burning sensations.

The differential diagnosis includes autism, celiac disease, MS, chronic fatigue, fibromyalgia, depression, food or mold allergies, Candida overgrowth, or infectious diseases such as Lyme. Consider heavy metal toxicity if you have a TBI patient who is not getting well despite appropriate treatment. Your patient history form might include questions that would provide insight into this area. For example, "How old is the home where you are currently living?" Although today you would not expect to find many patients with mercury fillings in their teeth, I learned long ago to expect the unexpected.

Heavy metals can be assessed by looking for the metals in hair, stool, and urine. Heavy metal toxicity is due to the buildup of certain metals in the body. While there are over 20 metals that can be considered "heavy" usually the term refers to lead (Pb), mercury (Hg), cadmium (Cd), or arsenic (Ar). Most people who are exposed to small amounts of these metals can excrete them normally in the feces or urine. However, when there is a large dose or chronic exposure over time, problems can occur. Also, in individuals with chronic medical conditions that impede excretion, or genetic predispositions that allow for an accumulation to toxic levels, poisoning can occur. As we know from many old murder mysteries, arsenic poisoning can be lethal. Many of these heavy metals can be found in varying concentrations in landfills and these types of environmental toxins are suspected as one cause of autoimmune disease.

What do heavy metals have to do with TBIs?

Toxic levels of heavy metals can confound the diagnosis of TBIs because of similar symptom patterns including poor concentration, decreased memory, tremors, and brain fog. Metals may impair the patient's ability to recover from a TBI because of their impact on the immune response. There are many theories around how heavy metal toxicity might impact Lyme disease:

1. Heavy metal toxicity might make Lyme worse by impeding the actions of the immune system.

2. They potentially cause autoimmune-like presentations with chronic fatigue, joint pain, and aches.

3. The Hg that is slowly released by chewing in patients with mercury fillings is hypothesized to stimulate the growth of Bb. I am not sure what evidence supports this claim, but I couldn't find anything to discredit it either. Still, the number of molecules released by chewing must be infinitesimal.

4. Anecdotally, metals such as aluminum and copper have been found in higher levels in some Lyme patients.

5. Toxins overtax the immune system leaving less resource to fight the TBI.

6. Heavy metals lower NK cells and increase autoimmune responses.

7. Metals can impact metabolism and take a toll on the liver, kidneys, adrenals, pancreas, and thyroid.

8. Some authors believe it is not the heavy metal toxin causing problems in Lyme patients but the toxins made by Bb itself. Is it Lyme or heavy metal causing the symptoms? Can it be both? Chelation therapy has been used in an attempt to bind those toxins. Some patients are speculated to have more difficulty removing the toxins from the body than others. Perhaps they need help. The jury is still out.

9. Consider that high heavy metal levels may be confounding the clinical picture especially where there are severe neurologic symptoms. Of course, this type of presentation could just be one of the big neuropsychiatric pathogens like Bb, Bartonella, or M. *fermentans* and have nothing to do with heavy metals at all.

10. Some think there are genetic reasons for toxins to accumulate more in some patients than in others. Certain authors believe it is prudent to detoxify a Lyme patient before starting antibiotics; yet others say treat the infections first and then do the detoxification. I say you will be lucky to think of both of these options at the same time.

11. Heavy metals and Bb like to congregate in the same body locations such as the CNS and joint spaces. This concept might explain why so many symptoms overlap.

12. Consider that heavy metals might be one reason why your TBI patient is not responding as well as you'd like. But unless there is a clear reason to suspect exposure, don't become obsessed.

Most of the dozen points listed above are speculation and I could find little supporting evidence for some of these assertions. Any, all, or none could be true. Nonetheless, it is prudent to keep in mind the possibility of heavy metals or other toxins complicating the clinical pictures in TBIs. Especially in kids who do not seem to be getting well despite what appears to be adequate and appropriate treatment, think of heavy metals. (I am frustrated because it took me so much time to write this section, when I wanted to move to other topics, For some reason, though, the topic of heavy metals comes up frequently in the TBI literature, so here I sit.)

The most common heavy metals that might be found in a TBI patient include:

Lead (Pb): Most lead exposure comes from lead-based paints in older houses built before 1978. While some of this old paint has been removed, much has been merely painted over. We used to see kids in the ERs in Philadelphia who had been nibbling on the old paint chips that flaked off the walls. Lead in pigments is still commonly found in ceramics and toys imported from other countries. The brightly painted puppets and souvenirs sold on Mexican beaches usually contain lead. Lead is often found in pipes in old plumbing. Lead affects calcium-mediated cell processes, reduces nerve conduction especially in the PNS and interferes with heme synthesis. Sxs include fatigue, encephalopathy with poor concentration, memory problems, sleep disturbances, depression, anxiety, irritability, and cognitive problems. Patients might also have kidney problems, anemia, abdominal cramping, and peripheral neuropathy.

Mercury (Hg): Most mercury exposure comes from:

a. Dental work using mercury amalgams: A few decades ago, mercury was often used in filling and repairing teeth. Many people still have mercury fillings in their mouths. If these fillings start to disintegrate the person can be getting a chronic low dose of mercury exposure. Some patients have felt better after careful removal of Hg fillings. The dentist must understand how to remove these old fillings or the patient could get another dose of Hg. Improper removal might be worse than leaving intact fillings stay in place.

PEARL: Alas, the debate over mercury fillings in teeth rages. Some authors believe that mercury fillings are an enormous health risk and must be removed from everyone immediately. Others think this is yet another tempest in a teapot fueled by overreaction. Of course, money would fuel this controversy since some dental plans will only cover mercury fillings, so the patient has little choice. Others will not cover the removal of these type of fillings. I don't know what is real but it seems prudent to avoid mercury if possible and to be careful about removal of old fillings. If the removal technique is poor, the person could end up with more mercury exposure than if the fillings were left alone.

b. Spills: Mercury spills occur in industrial settings or even in small amounts from broken mercury thermometers. Fortunately, there are alternative thermometers these days. But as recently as ten years ago, the "best" science teachers always had a vial of mercury in their desks for the kids to play with as a reward for good behavior. We would chase the mercury around the room as though it were alive.

c. Mercury emissions from coal-fueled power plants

d. Vaccine preservatives: The never-ending controversy around thimerosal, a mercury derivative found in many vaccines until recently, keeps this potential source of contamination in the news. Whether thimerosal did or did not contribute to autism, I don't know, but it was present in vaccines and millions were exposed. Most manufactures of vaccines today say that they no longer use thimerosal as a preservative.

e. Contaminated seafood: Both bottom-feeders, like oysters and lobsters, as well as certain deep sea species like tuna, mackerel, and swordfish, have been shown to have high mercury levels. Farm-raised salmon are thought to have higher levels than wild caught salmon.

f. Curing animal pelts: While this is no longer a common practice, making hats from pelts was standard into the 20th century. The phrase "mad as a hatter" came from the neuropsychiatric symptoms of those workers who made hats all day and breathed in the mercury fumes. Lewis Carroll, who created the character of the Mad Hatter in his *Alice in Wonderland* series, was raised in an English village where hat making was the primary trade. The mad hatters experienced numbness, vision problems, loss of hearing, slurred speech, hallucinations, irritability, depression, lack of coordination, and tremors. Since little was known about metal poisoning at that time, these workers were subject to considerable ridicule. Actually they were truly a sad lot who suffered and died in large numbers.

g. For a long time, mercury was the treatment of choice for syphilis.

Mercury penetrates nerves and interferes with receptors as well as the normal function of axons. This metal can affect the nerve fibers through a mechanism similar to the pathology found in MS. When Hg crosses the BBB, it can impede conduction of nerve impulses. Sxs include depression, fatigue, encephalopathy, joint pain, metallic taste, changes in hearing and vision, tremors, ataxia, cognitive problems, irritability, kidney and GI disturbances, and peripheral neuropathy.

Cadmium (Cd): Second hand smoke contains cadmium.

Treatment Options for heavy metal toxicity and other toxins:

Again, there are unscrupulous entrepreneurs trying to sell any manner of detoxification methods. Be careful.

a. Identify and remove the source of contamination. If one child was eating paint chips, better check the other kids in the house.

b. Diet: There are proponents of diets that may help detoxify the effects of the heavy metal poisons. Usually these diets seem to be healthy choices all of us might consider.

   i. Recommended foods are those high in antioxidants such as blueberries, cabbage, whole grains, all the orange foods that contain β-carotene, spinach, kale, red peppers, tomatoes, and watermelons. Glutathione is found in broccoli, spinach, and asparagus. Fiber may help with elimination.

   ii. Supplements that may be useful: Vitamins A, C, and E, Coenzyme Q 10, manganese, iodide, melatonin, lutein, and omega-3 fatty acids.

   iii. Some foods are discouraged such as refined carbohydrates, alcohol, caffeine, carbonated beverages, MSG, and yeasty foods.

c. Some suggest filtering all drinking water to decrease the chance of additional heavy metal consumption that might occur from lead pipes or from contaminated water supplies.

d. Exercise until you sweat.

e. Structural manipulation encourages good drainage and allows toxins to more readily leave the body.

f. Support for other body systems. The adrenals should be fully functioning in order to have effective detoxification. The pancreas and thyroid can be especially hard hit by heavy metal overdoses.

g. Detoxification: By definition, detoxification is the removal of a poison or toxin from the body or the process by which a toxin is rendered harmless. In current parlance, the word is also used to refer to getting all the drugs and alcohol out of an addicted person's system such as, "Before Lindsay went to rehab she went through detox." When I worked on the drug naltrexone for alcohol dependency, we had a heck of a time dealing with the dozens of "detox" facilities that seemingly popped up overnight. These detox centers made all manner of outrageous claims from 24 hour detox, to easy lemonade detox, to detox with Jesus. When the money ran out, the patients were literally left on the street. Some died. Be careful.

i.   If a patient does have heavy metal toxicity, do find a reputable institution to manage this condition. If you are the HCP, make sure you are referring to an experienced practitioner. Any "Two-for-the-Price-of-One" detox ads should make your run screaming for the door. (I do not make these things up.) Unfortunately, charlatans may keep patients with real problems from getting the help they need. Heavy metal poisoning in children can lead to life-long neurologic and cognitive problems and should not be taken lightly.

ii. As always, if the underlying problem is a TBI with a concurrent heavy metal problem, don't lose your TBI patient. You are still in charge of that part and you should oversee the management of the overall case. Real detoxification of heavy metals can take weeks or months and can have side effects. Of course, the patient could be coming to you with heavy metal toxicity as the primary complaint and the TBI could be the concurrent condition. Keep track of the big picture.

iii. Some HCPs consider various detox methods in treating chronic Lyme when other therapies have not been successful. IV GSH (glutathione) has been reported to be successful in a subset of resistant Lyme patients.

iv. Chelation is a detoxification method that uses various agents to draw out and bind the heavy metals and hopefully facilitate their excretion in the feces or urine. Chelating agents not only bind the toxin, they can also bind vitamins, minerals, and drugs, so proceed with caution. Make sure the liver and kidney are both in good form before initiating a detox regimen. Agents (it seems wrong to call them medicines) used for detoxification include:

• DSMA: Orally, DSMA is often used for lead, arsenic, and mercury poisoning. DSMA binds the metal and then moves with it as it is excreted in the urine. AEs include diarrhea, nausea, vomiting, and decreased appetite. DMSA is available in both oral and IV formulations.

• EDTA: Used primarily for chelation of lead but also for mercury and arsenic. IV EDTA is very powerful and should be managed carefully. EDTA is also available in suppositories.

• DMPS: The strongest and most specific chelator of mercury with a variety of formulations

• Glutathione: IV or suppositories. With IV glutathione make sure the person has sufficient B12.

• Questran has been used to bind toxins in the GI tract.

• Multiple other methods. Be careful with methods claiming to be a detox accelerator or enhancer.

PEARL: Some HCPs believe that a Herx reaction may be mollified by various detoxification methods as outlined above. Here the hypothesis is that the antibiotic treatment is eliminating a lot of pathogen at once. The antibiotic is causing apoptosis with a bunch of dead and broken cells in its wake. Both the toxins in the pathogen cells and the debris can initiate an inflammatory response with all the coincident signs and symptoms making the patient feel terrible (i.e., a Herx). The theory is that if detox therapy can remove the garbage, perhaps there will be less reactive inflammation and the patient won't feel so bad.

G. **Temperature** treatments: Some say that Bb hates the cold and that cold temperatures will make the pathogen burrow into the tissue, encyst, or go dormant. This can be good news in that the patient will feel better temporarily, since the spirochete is not currently active. At the same time, this is bad news since antibiotics have a hard time reaching the Bb when it is in hiding and also because as soon as the environment is more favorable the Bb will return, often with a vengeance. Others say that Bb hates the heat and that high temperatures are likely to damage or destroy the organism. This theory accounts for the many recommendations for heat therapy for Lyme including: saunas, infrared hot tubs, hot baths, warm drinks, heating pads, warm paraffin to joints, etc. Just as the body naturally raises the body temperature to fight pathogens, extraneous heat may serve the same purpose.

H. **Oxygen:** Hyperbaric oxygen treatment (HBOT) is a potentially useful treatment for Lyme. This therapy involves placing the patient in a chamber and providing oxygen at a higher than normal pressure. While some say that there is no proof of efficacy in Lyme patients, a number of patients have reported a positive response. HBOT is thought to increase cell healing by increasing the level of oxygen in the tissue, mobilizing stem cells in the bone marrow, and using a nitric oxide (NO) mechanism to help heal damaged tissue. The high O_2 concentration may be unfavorable to organisms such as Bb. While there are portable chambers for home use, most patients are treated in chambers used for treating decompression sickness and air embolism. HBOT is contraindicated in patients with suspected babesiosis since high pressure O_2 seems to make this condition worse. Bb and Babesia are common co-infections that are often unrecognized. Use caution in patients who cannot clear their ears and who have high fevers.

I. Miscellaneous Treatments

1. **Neti Pot:** This gadget looks like a cross between Aladdin's lamp and "I'm a little teapot." Saline solution is used to flush the nasal passages and is used to relieve nasal congestion, allergies, and sinusitis. Patients either love it or hate it. For older kids with chronic congestion, the Neti Pot can provide considerable relief and is available in most drug stores. Unfortunately, in early 2012 there were several substantiated reports of a rare pathogen spreading through use of Neti pots. Currently distilled, sterile, or previously boiled water is being recommended.

2. **Aroma:** The experts at the Monell Chemical Senses Center in Philadelphia report that smelling something pleasant is a rapid way to lift mood quickly. The olfactory system is a quick means to connect to the emotion centers of the brain. Citrus such as lemon oil appears to increase levels of norepinephrine, a mood regulator. While this may seem like a short-term solution, there seems to be no risk in trying.

3. **Biofeedback:** An increasingly accepted modality, biofeedback is used to treat pain and anxiety and a number of physiologic parameters. The patient is connected to an instrument that monitors things like heart rate, temperature, brain waves, muscle contraction, or respiration. By becoming aware of one parameter, the person can be trained to voluntarily control an associated parameter. For example, if the patient is learning to manage anxiety and the heart rate increases with the degree of anxiety, then the patient can learn to control the heart rate through feedback from the monitoring instrument. Theoretically, as the heart rate is lowered, so is the corresponding anxiety. Biofeedback has the potential to help with a number of TBI-associated issues including behavior and emotional problems. Although home units are available, biofeedback is best managed, at least initially, by a trained professional.

J. Heaven-only-knows-if-these-treatments work

What follows is a list of potential treatments for Lyme and possibly other TBIs. For a treatment to make the list below I had to find it referenced more than twice in relation to Lyme. Some were only a name on someone's list. Sometimes I could find more information and sometimes not. With the repeat mentions, I assume that someone somewhere was in some way helped by the listed therapy. Because a modality made the list does not mean I endorse it as a Lyme treatment. I just want you to be aware of the options. Heaven-only-knows…

1. Rife machines are said to kill bacteria by bathing them with electromagnetic waves, thereby decreasing the pathogen load. The MOA is unknown although negatively charged ions might be involved that adversely impact some microbes. The Rife machine might also be effective against some biofilms. There is considerable controversy around this treatment modality. Some patients swear by its positive effects, while others warn to avoid this therapy. At one point the American Cancer Society warned that Rife machines were being sold in a pyramid-like marketing scheme. At best, Rife machines appear to be supportive, not curative.

2. IV γ-globulin has been used to treat Lyme if the patient is found to be deficient, although what defines a deficiency is vague. The γ-globulin is speculated to help neuropathy in Lyme and may address the autoimmune component. IDSA does not approve of its use. This IV IgG use is a different regimen than the proposed use of γ-globulins beginning to be explored for the treatment of PANDAS.

3. Prolotherapy or proliferation therapy or regenerative injection therapy involves injecting an irritant into the body usually near painful ligaments and tendons to incite inflammatory action in the area. This stimulation causes new fibers to form and regenerate so fewer pain signals are sent. The ultimate goal is to strengthen the connective tissue.

4. LDN (Low dose naltrexone): A long time ago in a galaxy far, far away, I was the doctor working on the approval of a branded form of naltrexone for treating alcoholism. Naltrexone is an opioid antagonist that blocks certain receptors that are involved in addiction. You will see naltrexone mentioned in the media with some frequency since it is used in the treatment of celebrities with various compulsive behaviors like shoplifting. I was amazed to see it listed as an alternative treatment for Lyme disease because of its ability to balance the immune system, decrease inflammation, and diminish pain. This was all news to me. One patient referred to the LDN treatment as the best thing to come along in half a century. Mighty fine praise for a drug that a major pharmaceutical company didn't find worthy to promote. I do not know what they mean by

low dose and I do not know any studies done to corroborate these findings. Doses are variable but seem to hover between 1.5 mg and 3.0 mg per day. AEs are vivid dreams, increased urination, and sleep problems. I included LDN because I was stunned by the possibility of my old friend being used in Lyme and, in case you run across an HCP who recommends this approach, you will not be as shocked as I was. Unfortunately, the potential of LDN was somewhat muted in my mind when a case report touting the efficacy of this treatment proclaimed that a patient's LFTs were said to go from over a million to less than 50,000 on LDN. Since this claim is medically implausible, I have to wonder what other bogus claims are being made. Of course, if you have a Lyme patient who has the energy to shoplift, LDN might be a consideration.

5. Naturopathic medicine believes in vital energy and the body's ability to heal itself. Naturopaths prefer not to use surgery, antibiotics, or vaccinations. Since in this text, one of the foundation treatments for TBIs is appropriate antibiotic therapy, naturopathic medicine is not especially compatible with this philosophy. Naturopaths do use what they call natural products to aid in healing. There are references in the literature describing use of these compounds to break down fibrin and clots and possibly dissolve biofilms in chronic infections. There may also be a role in ameliorating Herx reactions. I could find no solid data to support many of these claims.

6. Homeopathy is a philosophy of medicine based upon the idea that substances that cause illness in healthy individuals at high doses can be used to cure or weaken similar symptoms when given in small doses. Samuel Hahnemann, the namesake of the Hahnemann Medical School in Philadelphia, did not like the way medicine was practiced in the 1790s. He felt that conventional medicine blocked the body's natural ability to heal itself. In fact, the AMA was originally formed to wipe out homeopathy. Since the 1800s, homeopathy has evolved and become more compatible with conventional practices. Today, certain principles of homeopathy make sense with regard to TBI patients, especially around use of steroids and management of Herx reactions. For example, if a patient has a rash, traditional medicine might try to obliterate the rash with steroids or antihistamines. Homeopathy prefers that the symptoms be expressed and the inflammation not be suppressed. Practitioners believe that suppression of symptoms causes more problems in the long-run creating worse chronic conditions. They prefer to stimulate the body to heal. Homeopaths tend to use one medicine at a time, at the lowest possible dose. They consider mental, emotional, and physical components of the overall condition and attempt to individualize treatment. Homeopathy believes that very small amounts of a substance that can cause a disease can help resolve it and their doctors formulate their medicines in very dilute concentrations. A nosode is a homeopathic remedy created from some part of the disease process itself such as secretions, mucus, pus, diseased tissue, or a sample of the pathogen. Treatment is customized. Homeopathy believes you should remove obstacles to wellness. Homeopaths would view a Herx reaction as evidence that the body is mobilizing its arsenal to get well.

7. Ozone therapy uses an oxidizer to create O_3. Ozone is often created during lightening storms and has a unique, but not unpleasant, odor. Ozone generators are often used to remove the smell of smoke and mold in buildings after fires and floods. O_3 is hypothesized to work in Lyme through electron transfer, thereby neutralizing toxins and decreasing free radicals that cause damage in chronic infection. Inside the patient, ozone is thought to work as a kind of detoxification. After my son's apartment building burned, ozone generators quickly and effectively removed the smoke odor.

8. Clofazimine is an old drug for tuberculosis and leprosy now being studied in autoimmune disease and implicated for the potential treatment of some aspects of TBIs. Clofazimine enters immune cells turning on the complex signaling system. Hypothetically, the MOA involves blocking the Ca influx into the immune cells and thereby shutting down the autoimmune cycle.

9. Transfer factors are molecules speculated to cause antigen-specific, cell-mediated immunity. They are purported to treat cancer, infertility, and a number of infectious diseases. These factors are thought to be messengers produced by T lymphocytes that relay or *transfer* information about how to recognize known pathogens to previously naïve white cells. One T cell tells another what to look for so that a better defense can be mounted. These molecules remember information about pathogens for which immunity has already been established. TFs are speculated to be one mechanism by which the mother transfers immune information to the infant through the colostrum. TFs are classified as food supplements and are often mentioned in the literature in conjunction with immune support as well as treating myriad other conditions. There has been no solid evidence of efficacy but some Lyme patients report relief with their use. While the underlying physiologic premise makes sense, TFs appear to be at that stage of development where entrepreneurs are more interested in their promotion than are the scientists. In one article an advocate wrote that transfer

factor increased the immune response by 437% (not 436% or 438%, but 437%). Do you realize that these kinds of wild claims weaken your case? When the FDA reads a "fact" like this, the few staff members they have left in the dietary supplement department roll their eyes in unison. They wave red flags until their little arms ache. When you read such a claim ask: Which of the million parts of the immune system were measured? Just one cell type or one kind of humoral molecule or the entire immune response? Were these results compiled from tests of one patient or many? Who did the measuring? Why did they assume that such an increase was a good thing rather than a sign of a hyper-response or a manifestation of autoimmunity? Who is making the claim? Who might benefit by making such a claim?

10. Reiki is a Japanese technique for stress reduction and relaxation that attempts to promote healing and involves gentle touch. I could find no evidence that this modality caused any harm, but I only explored the surface.

11. Reflexology or zone therapy involves the application of pressure to the feet, hands, or ears within specific zones or reflex regions.

12. Biophotons are mentioned as used in Europe.

13. Ozonides are also referenced in Europe.

14. Hydrotherapy

15. Large doses of Vitamin C

16. NMT: NeuroModulation Technique

17. EFT: Emotion Freedom Technique

18. TAT: Tapas Acupressure Technique

19. Footbaths

20. Core Energetics

21. Light therapy is purported to decrease pathogen load.

22. Plant stem cell extracts are said to boost the immune system.

23. Color therapy

24. Photon therapy uses electromagnetic fields to treat Lyme.

25. There are hundreds of additional treatments that have been proposed for Lyme and other TBIs. The ones listed appeared in my searches at least twice.

K. Sounds scary to me treatments:

The following modalities either have shown no benefit or have been documented to do harm. I have no experience with these methods so I cannot comment either way, except to say, "BE VERY CAREFUL." Always do a risk/benefit assessment before deciding on any course of treatment. Consider how each modality you add fits into the overall scheme. If it sounds too good to be true, it just might not be true. If a treatment cures everything, it just might cure nothing. If a therapy has no side effects, it might have no effects. Some treatments are harmful.

CAUTION:

IV peroxide

IV colloidal silver

MMS: Miracle Mineral Solution professes to cure everything, but sounds more like a cult than medical treatment.

Intracellular heat

Daily skin brushing until blood flows

High, harsh colonics

There were a number of treatments that were so bizarre, I didn't even know how to list them.

II. Summary:

I am not completely convinced that putting expensive sticky pads on my feet will draw out toxins and I don't plan to sign up for a coffee enema anytime soon. Nonetheless, when my kid was sick I would have purchased eye of newt if I thought it would help him. (Or even eye of Newt in an election year!) That is the problem with many of these unconventional treatments. In the world of TBIs, we are so desperate, we want to believe.

Any one of these alternative treatments may turn out, at some point, to be a great treatment for Lyme or other TBIs. Right now, there is not enough information to draw conclusions either way for most of these methods. I include this list (which is by no means all-inclusive) for completeness. You can find a "specialist" to help you with any of the alternatives listed. Gather as much information as you can but read with a critical eye. If the information is only coming from the company promoting the product, there may be a little bias. I tried to provide as much relevant information as I could find or comprehend. At least you will have an idea of the range of possibilities that are out there. Since appropriate antimicrobials are usually the foundation of treatment in many of these patients, I would advise use of these alternative treatments *only* as adjuncts to the core treatment regimen.

Use good sense. Don't be either the first or last to try a new treatment. You may need to prioritize therapies and emphasize the importance of each medicine or treatment. Don't overwhelm either the patient or the caregivers with too much treatment. Try not to select modalities that might be at cross-purposes.

I am not discounting any therapy unless I see it doing harm, but that doesn't mean that the experts would specifically recommend some of these therapies. I must say the most harm I have witnessed and experienced comes from not treating patients who could benefit from treatment. What is "alternative" today may be mainstream tomorrow. My philosophy after researching for weeks is: "When appropriate, use whatever helps and does no harm" and the soon-to-be-famous Spreen Corollary: "Be careful what you criticize, because tomorrow you might be begging for that treatment for your child."

Chapter 27   SUPPORTIVE MEASURES – Detailed chapter contents

Chapter 27

SUPPORTIVE MEASURES

Writing is easy. All you do is stare at a blank sheet of paper
until drops of blood form on your forehead.

Gene Fowler

Our bodies heal most efficiently when we give them the best chance to recover. We can use the right antibiotics, in the correct doses, for the ideal amount of time, yet the patient might still not get well if he is otherwise a physical or emotional wreck. Especially for patients with chronic disease, we must support their recovery efforts in every way possible. One or more of these modalities should be considered in managing TBIs.

I. NUTRITION/DIET

If I only knew the right answers to the questions: "What does it mean to eat right?" and "How do you lose weight and keep it off?" The fact that the majority of advertising today involves diet, weight loss, and reality shows about diet and weight loss, simply confirms that something is amiss with the way we eat. Most of us know how to eat properly, we just don't do it. Studies have repeatedly shown that kids left to their own devices will make remarkably sound choices. They will pick the cucumber slice over the cookie. As time goes on, children learn poor eating habits and society reinforces these lessons over and over.

In his 2009 book, *The End of Overeating,* Dr. David Kessler makes the strong case that processed sugars and wheat flour cause cravings that are nearly impossible to resist. The chronic overeating that results is one factor contributing to the current obesity epidemic that is spreading worldwide. Of course, fast food restaurants and the manufacturers of processed foods want to keep us craving. They do everything imaginable to pack as much sugar, salt, and fat into each portion. Sugar is thought to increase dopamine, a biochemical that is associated with pleasure and addiction. Most experts now accept that fat, sugar, and salt can be addictive and alter brain chemistry.

In this section, I will not be focused on how to remain svelte, but rather on how to fortify and nourish the body of a TBI patient. The individual must be able to mount the best defense against TBIs as possible. Of course, the wise food choices suggested for these patients tend to be good for most people in general.

BASICS: On June 2, 2011, the USDA introduced a revised food pyramid which is not a pyramid anymore, but a plate. While they still don't completely "get" the importance of avoiding processed foods, this iteration is an improvement over the old version, where the bad stuff had reached the top of the pyramid making it look like the good stuff.

While there will probably always be controversy over what is a good fat versus a bad fat and a good carb versus a bad carb, here are a few general principles to help steer food choices:

BASICS

A. PROTEIN

All cells contain proteins which are essential for both normal structure and function. Protein is required for all metabolic processes since enzymes are needed to catalyze chemical reactions including those involved with digestion, energy formation, and the ability to process medicines. Proteins are the foundation of immune response. Inadequate protein means inadequate immune defense. Antigen is just another word for protein.

Protein is necessary for the repair of old cells and the manufacture of new ones. This nutrient is especially critical in children, teens, and pregnant women, since protein is needed for growth and development. Protein is made of strings of amino acids, some of which we must obtain through diet. These are called essential amino acids.

If a dietary protein contains all the essential amino acids it is called a complete protein and these include meat, fish, poultry, eggs, and dairy. Soybeans are the only common plant source of complete protein. Other good, though incomplete, sources of proteins include beans, peas, nuts, seeds, peanut butter, and grains. Vegetarians must be careful to mix and match their plant sources of protein so that they get all the amino acids they need to stay healthy.

An appropriate portion size of a complete protein is the size of a deck of cards for an adult and even smaller for children. Consider that we might have been expecting kids to eat much larger portions than they actually required.

PEARL: Regular protein consumption is a good way to decrease cravings by keeping the blood sugar levels steady. One recommendation is that protein comprise at least 15% of the diet. Quinoa is a great grain. High in protein, fiber, and magnesium with a low glycemic index, quinoa covers many healthy bases.

Too much protein, such as that found in protein supplements used by athletes to "bulk-up," can severely tax the kidney. If the proportion of protein in the diet is high, the amount of water consumed should also be high.

The best sources of protein are probably the leanest and the lowest in fat. Low fat or skim milk and low fat cuts of meat are preferred. Lean meats and other good sources of protein also contain a number of other nutrients like vitamins and minerals. Meats and dairy have little fiber, but other sources of protein, such as beans and nuts can have both protein and fiber. Make sure that fish used as a protein source have low levels of mercury. Be cognizant that some meat sources have been fed hormones and antibiotics.

B.   CARBOHYDRATES

Structurally a mixture of carbon and water, carbohydrates are the primary source for quick energy in the body. Carbohydrates can also be stored for later use in the form of glycogen (similar to plant starch). While they do have a structural role in cell walls, carbohydrates are not essential in the diet. Other nutrients will eventually break down to glucose providing any sugar that is needed for energy or other functions. The brain can only use glucose (blood sugar) as an energy source.

Carbohydrates in the diet are divided into simple and complex. Simple carbs transform readily into glucose while complex carbohydrates take longer to digest. Fiber is a carbohydrate.

Unfortunately, simple carbohydrates are one of the primary reasons for the poor nutrition and obesity many of us struggle with today. Although Dr. Kessler explains this phenomenon clearly in his book, *The End of Overeating,* I will summarize briefly.

Simple carbohydrates in the diet rapidly turn into blood sugar. Once consumed, these simple sugars quickly raise the blood glucose level, insulin is pumped into the system to allow the sugar to enter the cells, and the cells gobble up the sugar as though they had never seen food before. As the sugar is consumed, the level in the blood plummets

and the cells start to wonder where all the sugar has gone. They get hungry again fast. They soon feel starved for more sugar. The person starts to focus on the next sugar fix. This is a craving and these cravings can be very powerful. In the meantime, the blood sugar levels peak and crash and peak and crash.

Over time, this kind of pattern leads to insulin resistance, metabolic syndrome, and obesity. Unless you are a diabetic whose sugar is now 32 and you are about to pass out, there is NEVER a NEED for more simple sugar in your diet. Some sources believe that simple sugars can be addictive with all the hallmarks of addiction including cravings, tolerance, and withdrawals. My own experience does not allow me to argue with that assertion.

PEARL: Just to add yet another twist – not only do we crave sugar because our blood levels are on a roller coaster, but also, sugar impacts the same neuro pathways as those used by narcotics. They stimulate the same pleasure centers. Just as heroin addicts crave more heroin, sugar addicts crave more sugar. Obviously the urge is compelling in both cases.

The speed at which carbohydrates begin to circulate in the blood as glucose can be measured using the **glycemic index** (GI). The GI describes how a carbohydrate acts as it enters the circulatory system. Simple carbs often enter the blood almost immediately and raise the blood sugar levels quickly. Complex carbohydrates are slower to digest and have lower values on the GI scale. Fiber might have very low values. Sucrose (table sugar made of glucose and fructose) has a GI of 100. Processed white flour like in yummy, soft, white bread often has a GI over 100. Fructose is fruit sugar and the GI of various fruits depends on fiber content and other factors. Grapes and oranges rank high on the GI. Jams, jellies, and many fruit juices are also quite high on the list. Lactose is milk sugar and many individuals of African and Asian descent lose the ability to digest this sugar after weaning. Maltose is actually a disaccharide made of two glucose molecules and is the sugar that results when barley is brewed or fermented. Maltose is also the delectable sugar that results when buns are caramelized at fast food restaurants that keep us coming back for more and more.

PEARL: Be careful with "No Sugar Added" products. This does not mean they are not high in simple carbohydrates. This label simply means that no one stood over the vat in the processing plant with a sugar bowl ADDING sugar to what may have already contained plenty of simple sugars. I have been fooled many times by this marketing gimmick. A good guideline is how badly you crave more after consuming something that says no sugar was added. If the label has ingredients ending in –ose you're likely eating simple sugars. Nothing with –ose should be listed in the first 6 ingredients on the food label if you are trying to avoid simple sugars. You should probably also be avoiding processed foods with more than 6 ingredients anyhow.

Since GI values can be surprising, a book of GI listings can be useful. The GI for essentially every food is also available on the Internet. Trust me when I say the food industry will not be rushing to add these numbers to their packaging. Often you can find a small 3 X 5 pamphlet in the checkout line at the supermarket right beside the candy.

Adjusting carbs in the diet can be one of the most difficult challenges in managing any patient. My mother, who was blind and had chronic pain, infection, and kidney failure from her diabetes, could never grasp the concept of the GI. She was quite intelligent and I suspect it was more fun not to understand. Twice I found her little blind self standing at the kitchen sink eating Betty Crocker cake frosting directly out of the can with a spoon. When her caregiver told her not to order the bun with her grilled fish at a local restaurant, she said she would just have spaghetti instead. Addiction is powerful, whether glucose or crack.

PEARL: I once heard a teenage Lyme patient complain to her physician that she was addicted to orange juice and drank gallons a day. When she couldn't drink it for an hour or two she became faint and felt she had to have it or she would collapse. To my chagrin, her doctor said to drink as much as she wanted, it was fruit after all. The teen's mother was aghast at this advice since this was equivalent to telling a junkie to mainline heroin as often as he liked since poppies grow naturally. Ask your doctor if orange juice is right for you!

Foods that commonly contain simple sugars with a high GI include: processed white foods such as white bread, white sugar, white flours, white rice, white pasta, and peeled white potatoes. If you are craving it, you should probably be avoiding it. No one ever CRAVED cauliflower. No one ever CRAVED a radish. The words, "I just have to have asparagus or I'll die," have never been uttered. Give me cabbage or give me death. There is a reason we only crave certain foods.

Individuals can get addicted to the bad carbs early and TV ads help them stay that way. From toaster pastries to breakfast cereals we are talking white flour and sugar. What kid doesn't love raman noodles with its fix of white flour, salt, and fat? What a relief for the caregiver that any third grader can make these all by herself. They can be purchased in bulk. Corn products often have high GI rankings.

PEARL: High fructose corn syrup is ubiquitous in processed foods. This corn-based ingredient has a high glycemic index. A recent flurry of criticism over its use has caused the corn industry to fight back. They are focused on the "natural" source and now may change the name to a much less tainted moniker of corn sugar. Be aware.

In the midst of all that surging blood sugar are the complex carbohydrates. Slowly digested with low GIs, these are nutritious and almost always a good choice. Complex carbs include most of the colorful fruits and vegetables including cabbage, lettuce, radishes, broccoli, cauliflower, kale, spinach, onions, asparagus, peppers, eggplant, squash, etc. Despite the name "sweet" potato, these vegetables have a lower GI than white potatoes. Some fruits like orange juice and watermelons have a high GI, so check the values before you overindulge. Grapefruit, lemons, and limes have relatively low GI values. Whole grains are usually good carb choices but make sure the term whole GRAIN is used.

PEARL: Be careful. Whole grain is NOT necessarily the same as whole wheat or whole rice. A cereal or flour can be composed entirely of wheat and still have had all the fiber removed. You want the entire grain to be present. Manufactures are very much aware of the public's confusion over this issue. We have become accustomed to soft textured white breads and the soft pasta in mac and cheese. We have to struggle a little to swallow the breads that look like they're made of sawdust. Fortunately, there are many more appealing choices now than there were just a few years ago.

I believe it is unfortunate that simple and complex carbohydrates share the same surname. When speaking of high carb and low carb diets, all carbs tend to be painted with the same brush. While there is never a need for more simple sugars in the diet, complex carbohydrates are the key to a *sustainable* healthy eating plan. While you can *almost* live on protein alone, you really need complex carbs (and a few fats) to balance out the nutritional requirements. Besides without fiber, you will suffer from stupendous constipation.

Of course, there are many diet plans that allege that some foods should only be eaten at certain times and only before or after other foods. Some proclaim the benefits of all raw, all primitive, all hot, all cold, all white, all red, and vinegar mixed with maple syrup, etc. Some say that a cold peeled potato has a lower GI than a hot peeled potato. Who knows? We all have a good idea about what makes sense. Extremes are probably not healthy.

The question around artificial sweeteners is raging. Better than sugar, worse than sugar, the same as sugar? Since added sugar is unnecessary for health, how can something be compared to the unnecessary? The jury is out but little packets of chemicals, "all natural" though they may be, might give you reason to pause. There is some fairly compelling new evidence that suggests that artificial sweeteners can spur cravings for additional sweet foods and that their use may actually impede weight loss.

Commitment from caregivers and from older patients themselves will be needed when trying to avoid simple sugars. This can be difficult especially when trying to find healthy choices in public places like schools, airports, and malls. Juices, sweetened chocolate milk, and soda can be at the top of the GI charts.

PEARL: The glycemic index is a useful tool to determine how fast a food converts to glucose in the blood. Processed white flour turns into blood sugar faster than eating a teaspoon of table sugar. The higher the glycemic index (table sugar is 100) the faster and higher the blood sugar peak and the lower the subsequent blood sugar crash that follows. The blood sugars plotted on a graph look like a roller coaster. The crash makes the cells cry out for more sugar since they perceive a deficit in the blood. They think they are starving. They MUST have more sugar.

Why care so much about simple sugars in relation to TBI patients?

- Simple carbs, especially white sugar and flour, are thought to increase inflammation.

- Some of the pathogens that cause TBIs (in addition to yeasts) are thought to thrive on processed sugars and wheat.

- One teaspoon of sugar is speculated to depress the immune system for 16 hours.

- A low glycemic diet is thought to help with the many skin problems associated with TBIs.

- Excess simple carbohydrates over time leads to insulin resistance which leads to metabolic syndrome (Syndrome X), which affects cholesterol, BP, DM, dementia, etcetera, which are all conditions associated with increased and chronic inflammation.

- People with TBIs can crave sugars due to a faulty carbohydrate metabolism. We know that Lyme affects both the GI tract and the endocrine system. While sugar consumption makes the patient feel better temporarily, it makes things worse over the long-run. We know that people with abnormal sugar metabolism (diabetes) heal much more slowly than the general population. TBI patients can experience

hypoglycemic fatigue where the blood sugar level crashes about every 2 hours and the graphed blood glucose levels look like the skyline of the Alps.

Make wise food choices to garner the best chance for recovery.

C. FIBER

Fiber is an important part of the diet and works to: keep the bowels regular, bind certain molecules like cholesterol and some toxins, and slow the absorption of sugars, thereby leveling blood glucose levels. Fiber also makes you feel full faster and may help you keep from filling up on empty calories. Although I do not understand the mechanism, mice that were fed diets high in soluble fiber like that found in oats and apples, showed less signs of disease when their bodies were later led to believe they were infected. There is debate about whether fiber helps decrease the risk of some cancers.

Dietary fiber has been divided into soluble and insoluble forms:

Soluble fiber: Legumes (peas, soybeans, beans), oats, barley, fruits such as prunes and some berries, sweet potatoes, onions, nuts, apples, and psyllium seed. This type of fiber ferments in the gut causing gas formation, but this gas subsides if these fibers are eaten regularly.

Insoluble: Whole grains, brans, potato skin, flax, and some fruit and vegetable skins. This fiber absorbs water as it passes through the GI tract and bulks up the stool.

*REPEATED PEARL: The food label must say whole **grain** not just whole wheat or whole rice. Just because something is 100% wheat doesn't mean they haven't processed all the fiber out of it. Whole grain usually means they left the fiber. Also, watch for cereal brands that advertise that they have more whole grain than any other ingredient. The second ingredient is probably sugar or processed grain.*

All manner of plants are the usual dietary source of fiber. Milk, eggs, and meat contain essentially no fiber. While the USDA is now talking new classifications of functional fibers, we have enough to worry about without splitting more hairs. Too much fiber can cause gas and bloating and too little can cause constipation. Actually, too much fiber without enough water can cause constipation as well.

The American Dietetic Association recommends that adults consume between 20 and 35 grams of fiber a day. The average actual consumption is about half that at 12 to 18 grams per day with teens consuming only about 20%

of what is recommended. Kids should take in fiber equivalent to their age in years plus 5 grams per day, so a 5 y/o should consume about 10 grams per day. Of course, the recommended amounts of fiber differ with various government agencies and professional groups.

The best way to get fiber into the GI tract is by eating sufficient amounts in the diet. Dietary fiber does not work overnight and may take a week to 10 days to impact the regularity of bowel movements. At first, the higher the fiber the gassier the patient. Think high fiber beans. This effect usually dissipates with time. Since constipation is easier to prevent than to treat, high fiber diets might be considered as a long-term lifestyle choice. Fiber pulls water into the intestine, softening the stool and allowing it to move forward. If not enough fiber is being consumed in the food, then fiber supplements may be needed. The *Constipation* section of Chapter 25: *Ancillary Treatments* lists fiber options. All the many fiber sources can cause gas, bloating, and rumbling. With commercial fibers you may want to start with a small amount and work your way up. None work instantly.

D. FATS

Those of us concerned with TBIs have two ways of looking at fat: either as a component of a healthy diet or as a condition where the body is storing too much adipose tissue. Since this chapter focuses on good nutritional choices, we will not dwell on obesity here except to say that immune function is markedly depressed in the obese, toxins often store in adipose tissue, and many co-morbidities are associated with excess weight. All these combine to impede recovery in TBI patients.

We need fat in our diet to:

1. Provide the essential fatty acids that we cannot synthesize ourselves. There are two EFAs required in the human diet:

    a. Alpha-linolenic acid, an omega-3 FA

    b. Linoleic acid, an omega-6 FA (You'd think they could have spelled these two fatty acids a little differently. It's not like we're running out of letters.)

2. Keep skin supple and healthy. Fats are part of cell membranes.

3. Participate in metabolic processes

4. Make food palatable. Fats do not usually taste great, (take a slug of Crisco and you'll see what I mean) but they sure do alter the texture of foods making them much more palatable and less "dry." Notice that when we decide that it is too unhealthy to fry chicken anymore, we replace the fat with sugar, white flour, and salt and call it Shake 'n Bake.

5. Allow for absorption of fat soluble vitamins. Note that when a low fat diet is combined with a product like orlistat (Alli, Xenical) to prevent further absorption of any remaining dietary fat, care must be taken that these consumers get enough fat soluble vitamins. Fortunately, when the users of these products start leaking smelly fecal oil, they stop taking the product and their fat soluble vitamins are safe again.

6. To use as fuel. While stored fat can be used as fuel, we don't NEED to put some away for a rainy day. Any nutrient will eventually convert to a fuel source and we really don't need to store fat in case the wooly mammoth herd is sparse this year.

7. In terms of TBIs and other infectious processes, EFAs are involved in 1) modulation of the immune response 2) regulation of mood and behavior, 3) DNA activity, and 4) formation of the lipid rafts that allow communication between cells. EFAs may also be needed for brain function operating at the level of the synapses. Adequate amounts may decrease depression. Omega-3 FAs are needed for repair of the myelin sheaths that cover the nerves. Further, EFAs may help with fatigue, aches, weakness, vertigo, dizziness, memory deficits, and concentration problems that are often part of the clinical presentation of TBIs. Along with Vitamins B and C, EFAs are necessary for normal adrenal function. Omega-3 FAs found in fatty fish are associated with relief from joint pain and arthritis. The mechanism of this anti-inflammatory action could have something to do with COX-2 inhibition.

PEARL: In addition to fatty fish, nuts, olive oil, and some teas, there are many fruits and vegetables as well as dark chocolate that are thought to decrease inflammation through COX-2 inhibition.

Fats have more calories per gram than either proteins or carbohydrates (9 grams verses 4 for the others). While we used to blame fats for obesity we are learning that fats are just one part of the bigger picture. Fat consumption may allow us to stop eating sooner because we feel more satisfied than when we can't stop ourselves from eating a whole loaf of white bread. While not politically correct to refer to a food as good or bad, we will make an exception for fats:

Good Fats: Polyunsaturated fats are found in vegetable oils (especially canola, peanut, flaxseed, and olive), fatty fish like salmon, trout, catfish, and shellfish, avocadoes, leafy vegetables, seeds such as pumpkin, sunflower, and flax, and nuts, especially walnuts. Fatty fish are the best source of omega-3 FAs. Olive oil can be a good source of the antioxidant Vitamin E. Good fats can reduce bad cholesterol and triglyceride levels and so decrease the risk of heart disease, which can start in childhood.

Bad fats: Can you say lard? How about bacon grease? Saturated fats are found in red meats, poultry skin, and full-fat dairy. Egg yolks have gotten a bad rap and do not raise cholesterol levels nearly as much as was believed. Coconut and palm oils also contain saturated fats. So, not all oils with a plant source are "good."

PEARL: *Processed low fat or no fat foods often mean higher sugar content.*

E. VITAMINS

By definition, vitamins are nutrients that we need that we cannot make for ourselves. For humans, ascorbic acid is a vitamin because we cannot make it ourselves (endogenously). We need to take it in from exogenous sources like citrus or supplements. In contrast, rats make their own Vitamin C. Sailors at sea, after eating the ship-board rats to keep from starving, found their scurvy cured. Various agencies have published minimum daily requirements for most vitamins and the commercial preparations usually list the percentage of this daily minimum that is contained in a dose of the product. The best way to get all the vitamins you need is by eating a variety of foods that contain these nutrients.

Fat soluble: Fat soluble vitamins can be retained in the system after absorption. Overdoses can cause buildup to the point of clinical symptoms.

A (retinol): Vitamin A is needed for vision in dim light, mucosal epithelial integrity, tooth development, and endocrine function. In the diet, Vitamin A is found in fish liver oils, liver, eggs, dairy, and green, yellow, and orange vegetables.

Deficiency due to prolonged diet scarcity can result in night blindness, trouble adapting to the dark, and growth retardation.

Vitamin A levels are usually increased by more orange foods in the diet, adding a variety of other food sources, or by oral supplements.

Too much Vitamin A can cause toxicity with vomiting, increased ICP, and yellow discoloration of the skin especially the palms and soles. Sclera usually do not discolor.

PEARL: *On June 16, 2011, an independent study from ConsumerLab.com noted that 1 in 3 multivitamins don't have the ingredients claimed in the label. The biggest problem was too much Vitamin A. There was no relationship between cost and quality with some of the cheapest having the best test results.*

D (calciferol): Vitamin D is actually a hormone which the body can make in sufficient amounts if exposed to enough sunlight (UV radiation). Vitamin D is currently THE vitamin these days since studies are showing many people are quite deficient. Since we have been slathering on the sunscreen over the last decade, many people including children in the US are lacking D. In addition, increases in air pollution have kept sun energy from reaching the skin in the first place.

Vitamin D is essential for immune function, the regulation of Ca and P metabolism, bone growth, bone maintenance, and normal kidney, bone, and parathyroid function. In clinical studies, kids given 1200 IU of Vitamin D daily were 60% less likely to come down with the flu during the study period than kids who took placebo. Low Vitamin D has been associated with higher cancer rates, body aches and cramps, hormone abnormalities, and balance problems. With significant deficiencies, bone can become weak and deformed, manifesting as rickets in children and osteomalacia in adults.

To increase Vitamin D levels additional sun exposure is suggested. This does not mean staying in the sun until you sizzle. Usually 10 or 15 minutes is sufficient for the chemical reactions necessary for the precursors in the skin to convert to the active molecule. Then slather on the sunscreen. You must be cautious if the patient is taking a TCN antibiotic since 10 minutes is enough for them to burn. In those cases, oral supplements and dietary changes might be preferred. Adults usually take 2000 to 4000 units a day if deficient, followed by a lower maintenance dose.

Vitamin D is found in fish liver oils, egg yolks, and fortified milk and dairy products. I remember as a little kid some vet deciding our chihuahua was Vitamin D deficient and we had to give him cod liver oil once a week, as though he wasn't crabby enough already. Some breastfed infants will need supplements.

Vitamin D is almost always low in those with chronic disease. Adequate amounts are needed to combat infection, regulate inflammation, and facilitate hormonal communication and the synthesis of a number of other hormones. All these functions might be important for TBI patients.

Excess Vitamin D can lead to toxicity with anorexia, kidney stones, vomiting, polyuria, weakness, nervous system problems, and renal impairment.

E (tocopherol): Poor Vitamin E! Once the king of the vitamins and now almost an after-thought. E is a powerful antioxidant needed for the proper formation of red blood cells, regulation of metabolism in tissues, and the efficient function of muscle and liver. Deficiency is uncommon. Some sources say that the healing power of Vitamin E has been somewhat overblown.

K: A group of molecules that serve as cofactors in blood clotting, the K comes from the German word koagulation. Vitamin K is found in green leafy vegetables like spinach and kale. Vitamin K is closely associated with the intestinal flora and so any disturbance of flora, such as a wipeout by strong antibiotics, can affect the Vitamin K levels. K should not be taken if the patient is on certain anticoagulants, since that would defeat the purpose.

Water soluble

C (ascorbic acid): Vitamin C is an antioxidant that protects the body from oxidative stress. This acid is used in collagen synthesis, numerous metabolic pathways, healing, scar formation, blood cell development, adrenal function, and bone and tissue growth. Scurvy has been recognized for centuries and was a common problem for sailors who were at sea for extended periods. In the late 1700s, the British navy started to give its sailors limes which not only stopped the symptoms but also resulted in the nickname "limey." Eventually, a lack of Vitamin C was recognized as the underlying problem.

Scurvy renders collagen non-functional and that affects all collagen-containing structures such as tendons, ligaments, cartilage, bone, blood vessels, valves, and spinal discs. Collagen is also found in connective tissue and in the gut. Collagen is only found in animals and is the most abundant protein in the body. (Albumin is the most common *circulating* protein.) Symptoms of scurvy include brown spots on the skin, blood oozing from capillaries and mucous membranes, spongy gums, and loss of teeth. Victims can be pale, depressed, and immobile. Scurvy can be fatal.

There is a high concentration of ascorbic acid in immune cells and the vitamin is rapidly consumed during infection. Since Vitamin C is involved with fatty acid transport into the mitochondria to make energy, without sufficient amounts the person will be lethargic. This vitamin also appears to act as a natural antihistamine.

Vitamin C will forever be associated with Nobel Prize winner Linus Pauling, who promoted its benefits with great resolve. Years of investigation have failed to demonstrate a role for Vitamin C in altering the onset, severity, or duration of the common cold. Although when I feel a cold coming on I always pop a few Vitamin Cs. Don't you?

Vitamin C is found in citrus fruits, green peppers, watermelon, strawberries, broccoli, and tomatoes. Of course, there are many oral supplements available.

Too much Vitamin C is usually just peed out, but high doses can cause GI complaints, flushing, and rashes.

PEARL: Strawberries are also thought to decrease levels of C-reactive protein, which is a measure of inflammation in the body.

B vitamins include:

B1: Thiamine is a necessary coenzyme for carbohydrate metabolism. Thiamine may also boost the immune system, improve mood and cognition, increase energy, decrease anxiety, and improve memory. B1 has been used in Alzheimer's patients in attempts to decrease symptoms. More than half of alcoholics are thiamine deficient and treatment is critical before withdrawal to prevent encephalitis. Thiamine is found in yeasts, grains, beans, nuts, and meat. Supplements can be administered orally or by IV.

B2: Riboflavin is a coenzyme in oxidation reactions and is needed for metabolism of fats, carbohydrates, and proteins, as well as energy production. B2 is found in milk, cheese, leafy vegetables, liver, yeast, legumes, and almonds. Riboflavin is the compound that makes the urine hyper-yellow after taking a multivitamin. This vitamin is destroyed by exposure to light. When neonates are treated with light therapy for jaundice, the light breaks down not only the bilirubin, but also the riboflavin. These kids will need supplements, or they can experience growth delays, failure to thrive, and epithelial lesions. Otherwise, deficiency is rare. Any excess is eliminated in the urine.

B3: Niacin is a coenzyme in carbohydrate and fat metabolism and is involved in numerous biochemical processes within the cell including DNA repair and production of steroid hormones in the adrenals. Niacin is found in a variety of foods including liver, chicken, beef, fish, cereal, peanuts, legumes, milk, eggs, yeast, mushrooms, and many fruits and vegetables. Deficiency is rare in the US, but when it occurs there are skin lesions and inflammation of the mouth and tongue. Since some forms of niacin may increase the good lipids in the blood, there has been an onslaught of direct-to-consumer advertising.

(I recall a frumpy-sibling series of ads.) Use of niacins as an adjunct for lipid management is not without side effects.

B4: Adenine is included for completeness but there is no clear association with TBI patients.

B5: Panothenic acid is included for completeness but there is no clear association with TBI patients.

B6: Pyridoxine is used to release energy from foods, develop RBCs, and is essential for the efficient function of the nervous system. Since B6 is a cofactor in the production of neurotransmitters and therefore necessary for proper brain function, adequate levels may be especially important in TBI patients. Pyridoxine is found in whole grains, fish, vegetables, beans, and organ meats. If neuropsychiatric symptoms are significant, consider B6 supplementation.

B7: Biotin is included for completeness but there is no clear association with TBI patients.

B8: Inositol is included for completeness but there is no clear association with TBI patients.

B9: Folic acid is a cofactor in nucleic acid metabolism and in the formation of heme and its incorporation into hemoglobin. Folic acid is especially important in pregnancy because of its role in cell division and growth. Deficiency in pregnancy can cause neural tube defects in the developing fetus. B9 is involved in the synthesis and repair of DNA. Deficiency can also be associated with macrocytic anemia. Some drugs can impact folic acid levels, so keep that in mind when monitoring blood work during treatment. The body does store small amounts so there may be a delay in the manifestations of a deficiency. When folic acid levels are low, the patient may experience nerve damage with weakness and numbness, mental confusion, forgetfulness, cognitive deficits, depression, sore tongue, irritability, and behavior problems. Folic acid is found in leafy greens, beans, and eggs. Many processed foods are now fortified with folic acid. This vitamin is often deficient in alcoholics.

B10: May be a derivative of para-aminobenzoic acid (PABA), which used to be called R factor. Lack of PABA may cause poor feather development in chicks. While I had trouble finding out what B10 really is and what it actually does in humans, there were plenty of people on the Internet who were willing to sell me some. PABA may be found in wheat germ, yogurt, and bran but there is no known deficiency. (Is this really a vitamin? If nothing bad happens if you don't have it and it isn't needed for anything in particular and you can kind of pick it up anywhere, why is it on this list? If they can cavalierly demote Pluto from a planet to a chunk of stuff in space, can't they ditch PABA as a vitamin? Is there anyone out there that powerful?)

B11: Carnitine is required for the transport of fatty acids into mitochondria for breakdown into energy. Originally identified as an essential growth factor for mealworms, carnitine is now touted as a supplement for weight loss. Naturally found in red meat and dairy, there are a number of oral supplements available. (See tirade accompanying B10.)

B12: Cyanocobalamin or cobalamin is needed by all cells but especially in the manufacture of RBCs and for proper function of the GI tract and nervous system. B12 is important for both RNA and DNA synthesis. This vitamin contains cobalt which is rare in biological systems.

Pernicious anemia can occur when there is an autoimmune destruction of the parietal cells of the stomach. These cells can no longer make an intrinsic factor necessary for absorption of B12. Without B12, there is not adequate RBC formation and anemia results. Patients with a severe gastritis may have a temporary reduction in intrinsic factor.

B12 is only found in animal products, so extreme vegetarians and vegans have to be careful. Excessive alcohol also impedes B12 absorption. Many drugs such as chloramphenicol, OCPs, and K supplements can interfere with B12. High doses of folic acid supplements can mask B12 deficiency.

Because B12 is so intimately related to brain and nervous system function and so many TBIs manifest CNS symptoms, adequate B12 levels should allow for optimum recovery in these patients. B12 is thought to enable normal function of the PNS thereby supporting effective immune function, fostering better sleep by contributing toward optimum day-night cycles, and regulating normal energy production. Adequate B12 seems to be needed for neurologic stability and is currently being assessed in Alzheimer's patients to try to enhance nervous tissue function, improve cognition, memory, and mood, and increase strength and energy.

Foods high in B12 include animal-derived foods such as fish, meat, and dairy. Many cereals and other foods are fortified with this and other vitamins. Vegans probably need supplements.

B12 is not absorbed well orally. Supplements can be injected IM or SQ and may be given intranasally. B12 may discolor the urine. Injections are sometimes given weekly or daily if the deficit is large. B12 shots are a lucrative business in some practices, whether the patient is deficient or not.

PEARL: After all that information, a broad-based multivitamin with minerals, along with a varied diet, will likely provide all the nutrition needed by the average TBI patient. A sick patient may be metabolizing nutrients at a faster rate than a healthy individual at steady state. When choosing a vitamin supplement, the most expensive are not necessarily the best. Even those at the specialty vitamin shops have been found to contain different amounts than the quantity stated on the label. Find a brand you think is reliable. Read the label. Make sure you are buying what the patient needs. Excess water soluble vitamins are just excreted by the kidney. In contrast, fat soluble vitamins can build up and cause symptoms of toxicity. If you are taking more than one product, make sure that you are not getting a double dose. This is especially true if you are taking a targeted product such as one labeled for "eye health" along with a routine multivitamin. You could end up with high levels of Vitamin A.

F. MINERALS

There are at least two dozen minerals necessary for healthy metabolism. Various agencies have set recommendations for daily consumption. Here I will discuss only those most likely to help TBI patients.

Calcium (Ca): Calcium is essential for normal bone growth and metabolism and proper development of teeth. Ca is involved with the parathyroid gland and Ca-P balance. Ca is active in many enzyme reactions, acid-base balance, lactation, nerve and muscle activity, and membrane permeability. Usually Ca levels in the blood remain fairly constant because if levels get low, more calcium will be pulled from bone to compensate. Of course, this only goes so far and if blood levels are consistently low and calcium is constantly pulled from bone, soon the bones will weaken. Calcium needs an activator like Vitamin D to be functional.

Deficits cause brittle bones and teeth, dental loss, tetany (muscle spasms due to nerve dysfunction), twitching, excessive bleeding, and irritability. If there is no calcium, there is no clotting. More calcium is needed in pregnant and lactating females. Calcium deficiencies may be more common in kids who cannot eat dairy due to lactose intolerance.

Good sources of calcium include dairy, salmon, sardines, anchovies (that slight crunch is itty, bitty bones that have a lot of calcium), broccoli, almonds, and figs. Milk fortified with Vitamin D is a good source of both nutrients.

Supplements are not always well absorbed and there is disagreement over which formulations work best. Some preparations combine Ca and Vitamin D. Too much calcium can result in nausea, constipation, or weakness.

Iodine (I): – Iodine is an essential component of the thyroid hormones, which influence much of the overall metabolism. Low iodine levels can result in hypothyroidism. Often the thyroid gland will enlarge to compensate for the deficit (goiter). In 1924, iodine was added to table salt in order to stem an epidemic of goiters. In children, on-going hypothyroidism can lead to mental, sexual, and physical developmental delays. Growing kids, teens, the chronically ill, pregnant women, and the severely stressed may need more iodine. We know that Lyme patients often have thyroid problems. Ensure that insufficient iodine is not a contributing factor.

We still get most of our dietary iodine from fortified table salt. Since table salt is out of favor these days, less iodine is in the diet. Food sources for iodine include seaweed, cod, some yogurts, and dairy. You can see that getting sufficient iodine might be a problem.

Iron (Fe): Iron is an essential component of the hemoglobin molecule and allows the heme to carry oxygen. Iron is also part of the myoglobin molecule in muscle.

Signs of deficiency include anemia, lack of energy, pale gums and conjunctiva, delayed development, and low hemoglobin.

Good sources of iron include red meats, organ meats, almonds, beans, oatmeal, and whole grain wheat. When possible iron should be obtained through food.

Babies may need iron supplements although this is, of course, controversial. In the first few months of life babies use up most of their iron stores. If breast fed they might not get enough iron in the mother's milk and may need supplements. If bottle fed, the formula may not have enough iron to meet the child's needs. The formula may need to be changed or supplements added. Food sources rich in iron can be added to the child's diet by about 6 months.

Not every patient needs added iron. Menstruating females often need more iron, and girls are menstruating earlier than in past decades. But if the patient is a 9 y/o boy who eats a couple of burgers a week, iron is probably not your biggest worry. Besides, Hb is one parameter that is easy to check.

The constipation associated with oral iron supplements you shouldn't wish on your worst enemy. (Wish it on my worst enemy instead.) Before starting a person on oral iron supplements, read the *Constipation* section in Chapter 25: *Ancillary Treatments.*

PEARL: Be careful of too much of a good thing. Too much copper, iron, and some of the fat soluble vitamins can cause problems.

Potassium (K): Potassium is essential to overall homeostasis including acid-base balance and osmotic pressure and is needed for control of muscle contraction, nerve impulses, and efficient kidney and heart function. Many foods contain K including cereals, peas, beans, and bananas. Rarely is there a deficit in kids except in cases of severe diarrhea and vomiting. Water pills (diuretics) can lower potassium, with symptoms of weakness, dizziness, thirst, confusion, and EKG changes. Excess potassium is seen in cases of renal failure and in severe burns.

Magnesium (Mg): Of the minerals listed here, Mg may be the most pertinent to the Lyme patient. Magnesium is part of the enzymes used to make energy through ATP. This element is needed for muscle contraction and protein synthesis. Magnesium may be useful to combat fatigue, since it is necessary to make the ATP essential to convert food to energy. Lyme patients with neurologic sxs might benefit from supplemental Mg.

Widely distributed in foods, magnesium deficiency is rare, EXCEPT in Lyme patients. Many HCPs have found low levels of Mg in these cases. Symptoms of deficiency include neuromuscular irritability, increased reflexes, tremors, twitches, cramps, muscle soreness, depression, irritability, anxiety, and heart skips. Patients with depleted Mg levels can experience weakness with low energy levels and impaired cognition. Magnesium also seems to be low when the person is under stress. In theory, Mg may allow the immune system to better target pathogens and may spur Bb to come out of hiding.

PEARL: Low magnesium is correlated with jumpiness and irritability and chronic inflammatory stress which is associated with sleep problems.

Even in patients with Mg levels WNL, supplements may help with weakness, anxiety, and especially the muscle twitching and cramping. In Chapter 19, I warn about the false security that can come when lab tests fall WNL, when, in fact, the listed value might not be normal for that individual patient at all.

Magnesium can be found in whole grains and many other foods. Even dietary Mg can be difficult to absorb and diarrhea can further impede absorption. Supplements seem to have a range of absorption potential. There is

considerable debate over which brand is absorbed better with proponents of one or another getting quite heated. If levels are low, consider parenteral formulations.

High doses may cause diarrhea. With Lyme patients, you may need to start with a low dose and build up as needed. Mg supplements shouldn't be taken at the same time as antibiotics.

PEARL: Low magnesium levels in Lyme patients seem to lead to many of the symptoms traditionally associated with Mg deficiency. Perhaps some of these symptoms that we have associated with Lyme are really a reflection of low levels of this mineral. Hypothetically, the Lyme could diminish the Mg levels through some unknown mechanism and then the deficit, in tandem with the underlying Bb, can contribute to the symptoms that have been listed as part of this combined pathology: neuromuscular irritability, twitching, cramping, increased reflexes, joint pain, agitation, anxiety, and depression. Another theory is that adequate magnesium allows better immune response with better aim at the pathogens and more Bb coming out of hiding. Whatever the underlying mechanism, Mg seems to affect Lyme and Lyme affects Mg.

Mg supplements can be administered orally, IM, or IV. If levels are low try a parenteral route until stable. Attempt to find an oral supplement that is better absorbed, but this may be easier said than done. Doses of 100 to 200 mg per day in adults is standard. Be careful with IV administration if there is kidney dysfunction.

PEARL: There is controversy about which salt of magnesium is better absorbed. Most say that citrate capsules are better, but there are the malate proponents.

Selenium (Se): Selenium supplements have been used in TBIs to decrease anxiety and depression and to provide support for thyroid function.

Zinc (Zn): Zinc is involved in most metabolic pathways as part of protein metabolism and as a cofactor in enzymatic reactions. Deficits cause loss of appetite, growth retardation, skin changes, poor wound healing, and impaired taste. If levels are low during pregnancy, developmental disorders can result. Dietary sources include meat, liver, eggs, and seafood. In TBI patients, zinc has been used to mitigate anxiety, stimulate immune response, and support the thyroid.

Manganese (Mn): This mineral, not to be confused with Mg, may help maintain joint cartilage, rebuild connective tissue, improve flexibility, and relieve joint pain, which in diseases like Lyme, might be useful. Nuts, beef, and spinach are all good sources.

G. ADDITIONAL SUPPLEMENTS

Hundreds of supplements are available and have been used in attempts to help TBI patients. I only discuss a few here that seem to have potential to help in TBIs and are mentioned most frequently in the literature.

Antioxidants: Oxidation reactions are a part of normal metabolism. These reactions can produce compounds called free radicals that can become involved in chain reactions. When these reactions occur inside a cell, damage or death can result. Antioxidants inhibit these oxidative reactions and thereby limit the damage done to the organism. The antioxidants remove the free radicals and stop the chain reactions by becoming oxidized themselves. They sacrifice themselves for the cause. Examples of antioxidants include Vitamins C and E and glutathione. Excess oxidation seems to be a component of many disease states, so antioxidants in supplements are used to try to counter the damage. Too much antioxidant can be harmful and the science supporting the benefits is equivocal.

In Lyme patients, free radicals are hypothesized to increase with the amount of infection and may account for some of the neurologic problems associated with the disease. Antioxidants may help protect the brain and other tissues from the damage caused by these free radicals. They act as scavengers, taking a hit for the team and sparing the host cell. Excessive production of free radicals can overwhelm the naturally available enzyme pathways. Theoretically, supplemental antioxidants can come to the rescue like the cavalry coming over the hill.

Two common antioxidants used in TBIs are:

Coenzyme Q 10 or ubiquinone is a part of the electron transport chain and makes energy in the form of ATP through aerobic cellular respiration. Organs with the highest energy requirements have the highest concentrations of CoQ 10 like the brain, heart, liver, and kidney. Ubiquinone can be synthesized by the body or ingested in the diet in sources like meats, fish, oils, nuts, and some fruits and vegetables. Chronic disease increases the demand for CoQ 10, presumably because the body needs additional energy to recover. CoQ 10 is commonly recommended for Lyme patients. Even Dr. Oz in an *O Magazine* article on Lyme disease offered CoQ 10 as a treatment option. So it must be really good stuff. Mepron may deplete CoQ 10.

Glutathione is a peptide that acts as an antioxidant to protect cells from free radicals. Produced naturally in cells, glutathione neutralizes free radicals and keeps other antioxidants like Vitamins C and E active. This molecule can detoxify a number of foreign molecules and appears to

be essential for full immune function. Glutathione helps to regulate immune response and is involved with both the cell-mediated and humoral responses and appears to help regulate apoptosis. The peptide is involved in the synthesis of DNA, proteins, and prostaglandins as well as amino acid transport and enzyme activation. Glutathione affects all body systems, especially the immune response, nervous system, GI tract, and lung. The molecule can be hard to absorb orally but concentrations can be increased by oral co-administration of S-adenosylmethionine (SAM-e) taken in the morning so as not to disturb sleep. Glutathione has been used in Alzheimer's, Lyme, the pain of arthritis, and depression. Some TBI patients have found glutathione helps with brain fog.

Essential Fatty Acids (EFAs): EFAs in humans include α-linolenic acid, an omega-3 FA, and linoleic acid, an omega-6 FA. These EFAs might help CoQ 10 enter mitochondria and so may mitigate fatigue and help lower insulin resistance. Fish oil seems to be one of the best sources of the omega-3 FAs and may help fatigue, dizziness, memory, concentration, depression, as well as decrease inflammation and provide support for the adrenals.

H. HERBS as dietary supplements

There are a thousand herbs used as dietary supplements. In Lyme, a few stood out and they were licorice and ginseng for adrenal support and cinnamon for insulin resistance and stabilization of blood sugars.

SPECIAL DIETARY CASES

- **Yeast and mold overgrowth** has been discussed extensively in Chapter 25: *Ancillary Treatments*. Nevertheless, I would like to reiterate a few principles of healthy eating that might make your body less inviting to fungus.

  At least during the time of active fungal infection, try to minimize the amount of processed sugars and white flours consumed. There are low glycemic and anti-yeast diets available that may help serve this purpose. Even high sugar fruits and juices can make a fungus feel like it is in fungal heaven, since these foods tend to cause a spike in blood sugar. The strict anti-yeast, anti-mold diets usually recommend no fermented products like wine, beer, vinegar, mushrooms, hard cheeses, or yeast breads. Yeast, unlike most of us, have no problem with cannibalism. Yeast, like the rest of us, LOVE sugars and white flours including rice and potatoes. Target the low end of the glycemic index scale. Not only do sugars feed the fungus, they probably feed the Lyme as well.

Symptoms of too much yeast in the digestive tract include gas, bloating, heartburn, dyspepsia, post-meal fatigue, and brain fog. Of course, the entire system might be overrun with systemic yeast in patients experiencing a more general presentation of symptoms.

While no one agrees on the best antifungal diet, foods that may help include activated plain yogurt with no sugar added, kefir, acidophilus supplements, and grapefruit seed extract.

• There are a number of problems with food and digestion that add complications to an already complex world. In this arena, there are almost as many contrasting and conflicting viewpoints as there are with TBIs. We are not talking just one condition here but a symptom-set that crosses a broad range. Some of these syndromes may have little to do with the others. Since I have no inclination to write a book on this subject, I will provide only a few terms and dietary considerations.

Celiac disease: For the majority of people, gluten is a protein found in grains like wheat, rye, and barley that makes bread fluffier and not so much like eating a wooden plank. In patients with celiac disease even a very small amount of gluten can cause a severe autoimmune reaction. Celiac disease seems to affect the small intestine and is probably genetic. This condition can lead to chronic diarrhea, failure to thrive, and fatigue. All the usual inflammatory signs may be present. Symptoms can be mild to severe. Celiac disease can interfere with the normal absorptions of nutrients and cause short-term discomfort as well as long-term problems. Escalation of symptoms may be due to more aggressive autoimmunity. About 1% of the population has celiac disease. Currently, "gluten-free" foods are very popular. This too will pass except for those who truly need to avoid gluten.

Gluten sensitivity: Gluten sensitivity is an allergic reaction to gluten with the usual signs and symptoms of a Type I hypersensitivity reaction: swelling, rashes, hives, and wheezing. This allergy can progress to difficulty breathing and anaphylaxis.

Food allergy: This scenario is underscored when you see the worried parents of kids with peanut allergies picketing schools and airlines for exposing their kids to allergens. Any number of foods including gluten, casein, shellfish, and nuts can cause hypersensitivity reactions. These allergies can cause mild symptoms, but they can also cause anaphylaxis and death. Some people say they are allergic to foods that they simply don't like. Once diagnosed with a true food allergy, consider an EpiPen.

Lactose intolerance: This condition is not a sensitivity at all, but an inability to digest milk sugar due to the absence of the lactase enzyme. The majority of people of African and Asian descent stop making lactase soon after weaning. If they consume milk sugar, they experience gas and loose stools.

What do food allergies have to do with TBIs? I'm not sure, although the topic comes up a lot in TBI literature. Unlike simple sugars, gluten does not seem to be a favorite food of either fungus or Lyme spirochetes. Some authors contend that gluten is pro-inflammatory but in patients without celiac disease or hypersensitivity to this protein, I could not find evidence that it is any more pro-inflammatory in Lyme patients than anything else. Certainly food sensitivities can occur concurrently with TBIs. Since they manifest with many of the same symptoms as TBIs, food sensitivities should be part of the differential diagnosis. Instead of occurring along with Lyme, a food allergy could be the reason for the symptoms instead of Lyme. Disease does occur outside the world of Lyme.

Always remember that with TBIs, more than one condition can be manifesting at a time. Be aware and try to recognize when a patient might benefit from addressing some of these concurrent conditions.

There are ways of testing for sensitivity reactions by looking for antibodies to specific antigens. The Celiac Disease Center does not seem to find tests for celiac disease especially reliable and, as you might have heard somewhere before, diagnosis of this condition is based on clinical judgment with lab results playing a supportive role.

Treatment for any of these conditions is primarily avoidance of the trigger allergen. In celiac disease this can mean avoidance of gluten in wheat or other gluten-containing grains. Some say no wheat whatsoever, but to achieve total avoidance you must be educated about what contains gluten or wheat or other gluten-containing flours. You will be surprised at what might include gluten, or peanuts, or ground chitin from shellfish, or lactose, or whatever it is you need to avoid. Read labels but don't necessarily trust them.

PEARL: Gluten-free is not the same as low carb or low calorie. This label has become the latest buzz word for marketers and now there are shelves of gluten-free cookie mix and beer. Gwyneth Paltrow will help you avoid gluten with tips on her website. Even communion wafers have gone gluten-free. Vendors have taught us that somehow gluten-free is healthier, organic, or "something" that makes us believe that paying more is a good idea. Most people who buy these products do not have celiac disease or sensitivity to gluten. Some things that never had any gluten in them in the first place are now labeled "free." Soon they will be packaging gluten-free radishes and pork roast. The manufacturers act as though they expended a big effort to extract gluten from these products. So far there are no government regulations saying what actually constitutes gluten-free. Nonetheless, when one enthusiastic entrepreneur labeled regular bread as gluten-free, and many people who really had a problem with gluten got sick, he was handed an 11-year prison term. Unfortunately, most mislabelers don't get caught. Gluten-free is not calorie-free as it has sometimes been touted. A gram still has 4 calories. Many gluten substitutes are high in sugars and fats.

- **Promotion of good intestinal flora**: The use of probiotics is discussed in detail in Chapter 25: *Ancillary Treatments*. Probably the best foods to maintain balanced intestinal flora include active yogurts, miso, and kefir. Kefir is a yogurt-like drink that may help inspire the beneficial flora. Kefir is fermented milk with active cultures that is easy to digest. I have never had kefir. I have never given my child kefir (the true test of whether I have bought into a concept). But to read the TBI literature, you would think this stuff was the fountain of youth being served in the Holy Grail. So far I have found no evidence that kefir is harmful in any way. Try it and let me know what you think.

  If buying yogurt at the supermarket, try the no-sugar-added types or you may defeat the purpose by providing yeast a banquet from which they can continue to overgrow.

  Probiotic supplements appear to be an effective way to re-establish normal intestinal flora. In addition, actual acidophilus is sold in health food stores either frozen or refrigerated. The usual dose is two with each meal. Different brands may help mix up the flora. (Somehow this sounds unappealing to me.)

PEARL: Recent work on intestinal flora suggests that each person has their own unique population of many diverse species. These organisms can be genetically distinct even from those in the same household. The microbes are sufficiently distinguishing to serve almost as a fingerprint. People in close proximity do show patterns more similar to one another than to outsiders and there have been

successful flora transplants between household members with remarkable success.

PEARL: This is interesting. Artificial sweeteners (as well as "natural" sugars) can alter the normal gut flora, thereby affecting satiety and inspiring additional eating. They might also increase inflammation in the gut through mechanisms not yet well-defined.

- **Diets recommended for the chronically ill**: In addition to all the dietary advice presented in this section, there are a few more points that were reinforced in the literature for the chronically ill:

  You can't adequately fight infection without a good supply of protein. Protein is the basis of immune response.

  Foods that may lower inflammation: oatmeal, brown rice, beans, olive oil, fatty fish, nuts, some teas, dark chocolate, foods high in Vitamin D, strawberries.

  Foods that may increase inflammation: dairy, corn, eggs, animal fats, margarine, corn oil, red meat.

  Vitamin D is almost always low in those with chronic disease. This nutrient is essential for building hormones and combating infection and inflammation.

  Sick people have increased nutritional needs such as B12 and magnesium.

  Nutrients such as fish oil and Vitamin C are thought to improve immune response.

  The modern, western diet of high calorie, low fiber, high glycemic, nutrient-depleted, processed foods is probably the least healthy diet in human history. These foods are most likely to trigger inflammation, even before assault, making it harder to heal and to mount an effective natural defense.

  Optimal function of the immune system requires adequate nutrition. Malnutrition clearly leads to immunocompromise.

  Obesity and diabetes are known to impede immune efficiency. Immune response seems to work best when the patient is in the normal weight range.

  Biotoxins bind preferentially to adipose tissue (i.e., fat cells). The more fat, the more toxins might be stored for indefinite periods. Biotoxins bound to cell receptors increase cytokines, which cause inflammation.

- **Diets targeted for Lyme patients**: A good deal of dietary advice is targeted specifically for the Lyme patient:

Lyme patients are thought to do better in an alkaline state, especially when Herxing. Warm lemon juice may help. I know that lemon juice is acidic and I just said alkaline is best but Chapter 28: *Understanding the Herxheimer Reaction* explains this paradox.

Some believe that many of the pathogens that cause TBIs (in addition to yeasts) thrive on processed sugars and wheat. Certainly, we don't want to make life easier for Bb.

Many people with Lyme have a magnesium deficit. Strive to find an oral supplement that is well absorbed.

Dairy may increase inflammation in some patients.

Some of the late symptoms of Lyme may be due to cellular damage and deficits in specific essential nutrients.

PEARL: Dr. Ken Singleton has developed a diet for Lyme patients. This eating plan involves elimination of certain foods that are thought to be inflammatory. Once the individual determines which foods might be triggering inflammatory reactions in her case, those that are not responsible might be re-introduced. A number of patients have reported improvement with this approach. Dr. Singleton's book, The Lyme Disease Solution*, details his theory. He also provides the foundation for the anti-inflammatory diet in the Foreword of* Recipes for Repair: A Lyme Disease Cookbook.

- **Vegetarian/Vegan** practitioners need to be especially vigilant in making sure they get enough protein and B12.

GENERAL DIETARY ADVICE:

1. The closer to the farm and the farther from the factory, the better.

2. A low glycemic, high fiber diet is probably best for everyone.

3. Well-balanced is good, but do not become obsessive. A child might only eat blueberries and cucumbers today but will balance that with an egg and milk tomorrow.

4. Forcing people to eat something they hate is cruel and ultimately doesn't work over time. There is always an alternative nutrient source.

5. Forcing kids to clean their plates teaches them to eat beyond when they are full, which is not a good lesson to learn.

6. Portions in restaurants are gigantic. Know reasonable portion sizes.

7. Eating smaller amounts at shorter intervals is probably healthier than three huge meals per day. This tends to keep blood sugar levels more even.

8. Really changing eating habits takes commitment from both the patient and the family. I was at an ice cream shop the other day and a child about 5-years-old came in with her mom and grandmother. The child pointed to a picture of an ice cream sundae and said, "Can I have that?" The mother was appalled, "You know you can't have dairy! You can have a lemonade." The mom and grandmother both got ice cream and the child got a lemonade. I happen to think that scenario was abusive. Why would you take a child to an ice cream shop if that child cannot eat ice cream? Even in our small community there are plenty of other places they could have gone for a treat. Everyone in the household does not need to eat the exact same things but if one person has restrictions, it is mean to flaunt that forbidden food in front of them.

9. Be cognizant of pesticides on fruits and vegetables as well as antibiotics and hormones in meat. Some authorities say that the antibiotics given to animals is a far greater risk for the development of bacterial resistance than treating a Lyme patient for an extended course. Organic foods are said to be "cleaner" in this regard, but again, some foods advertised as pesticide or hormone-free may not be.

10. The best source of nutrients is food, followed by supplements, if appropriate.

II. PETS

I am an advocate of pet ownership. Of all the science I have read on all sides of these controversial issues, there is one set of studies that consistently reach the same conclusions and seems to be controversy-free. Pets help people with chronic illnesses feel better and get better. Study after study has confirmed these findings. HOWEVER, if you are not a pet person, don't force yourself because I never want someone to have a pet only for it to be abused or neglected. Some people don't want a pet because they feel they will be hurt more than they are already hurting if they lose that pet. As with anything else, assess the pros and cons.

I believe pets can be therapeutic. Last year I suffered a very bad fall complete with a concussion that incapacitated me for

3 months and a face that looked like it was removed by an asphalt road, which it was. While my family was helpful and supportive, my dog was there 24/7. He cried when I cried. Who else would sit with you faithfully for 3 months without even a book or TV? He gave me a reason to get out of the chair.

Actually, I had to stop researching the health benefits of pet ownership because I found so much material. I could have kept listing for weeks. The bond between humans and pets is evidenced by the finding in Israel of a 12,000-year-old human skeleton with his hand on the skeleton of a wolf puppy. Here is a list of potential benefits of pet ownership based on articles I found in the general medical literature. I am not weighing scientific method here, just making points.

1. Pets ward off depression.

2. Pets increase immunity as measured by both immune cells and humoral markers.

3. Pets decrease blood pressure.

4. Several studies demonstrated how pets decrease overall health care costs by decreasing the number of office visits, length of hospital stays, and duration of illness.

5. Pets increase social interactions by serving as conversation starters and taking owners out where they are likely to run into other people.

6. Kids with pets feel sorry for people who do not have a pet.

7. Pets decrease stress.

8. Pets give a reason for getting up in the morning.

9. Pets decrease cholesterol.

10. Pet owners are better able to manage their weight, probably by being more active.

11. Pet owners exercise more, walking farther and faster.

12. Pets provide companionship, affection, and company.

13. When they snore, it's cute. (Okay, I didn't find this point in the literature and I know that snoring in snubnosed breeds can be a sign of apnea, which is *not* cute.)

14. Pets take the focus off the illness, at least temporarily, so life isn't all Lyme all, the time.

15. Pet owners are calmer.

16. Pet owners have more mobility and flexibility.

17. Psychologists assert that pets are very comforting to children, helping them learn empathy.

18. Pets are especially helpful in socializing autistic kids.

19. Pets decrease triglyceride levels.

20. Pets decrease loneliness and feelings of isolation.

21. Pets resulted in better survival rates after heart attacks.

22. Pets are funny. Really funny. And they know it.

23. Contrary to what we've been led to believe, kids with pets may have fewer allergies than those without pets. Furry pets resulted in lower incidence rates of allergies and asthma.

24. Caregivers feel less burdened, since the pet will sit with the patient for a while giving the caregiver a bit of a break.

25. Pets instill feelings of friendship, responsibility, and patience.

26. When asked who they talked to when they were upset, a large number of people named a pet.

27. Pets are sources of comfort and empathy.

28. A 1980 study showed that patients with heart attacks or angina had significantly better survival rates if they had a pet compared to those without - even if the pet was a snake. A 1995 study corroborated those findings but suggested that the best outcomes occurred when the pet was a dog.

29. Oxytocin spikes were documented after interactions with dogs, increasing feelings of trust and attachment.

30. Patients asked to count backwards by 3s performed better and felt less stressed when their dog was present.

31. Dogs make excellent social bridges. A 2008 study demonstrated that men made better connections with women when dogs were present to facilitate conversation.

32. Finnish researchers found that children who lived with a dog were 21% more likely to be healthy than those

who didn't and 44% less likely to have had an ear infection.

33. Pets stimulate the immune system of children so that the kids can do a better job of fighting infection.

34. Studies have shown that watching fish calms and relaxes essentially all people. One researcher claimed that observing fish made people nicer. I don't know if the science is valid but an aquarium probably wouldn't hurt.

35. Babies exposed to pets and dust are less likely to develop allergies and asthma.

36. Specially trained therapy animals have improved mood and decreased anxiety and provided pleasure in long-term care facilities.

37. Pets provide a sense of normalcy and routine, especially in a crisis.

38. Kids love the idea of saving a pet from the pound.

39. Most pet owners believe pets are a member of their family.

40. Animals don't need to be small and housebroken to afford health benefits. A group called Saddle Up provides equine therapy for kids with any number of health problems from autism to epilepsy. They have achieved amazing results. Both the kids and the providers benefit and the horses don't seem to mind.

41. Yes, pets carry ticks and are smelly, but so are we.

42. When the pros and cons are weighed, unconditional love always tips the scales.

III. HYDRATION

Drink water. Only in very rare cases such as diabetes insipidus or congestive heart failure, should a person be told to drink less water. Water removes toxins, flushes the kidneys, helps regulate body temperature, softens the stool, liquefies mucus, aids in the dissolution of medications, and improves the appearance of the skin. People with fevers and sweating should replenish the lost water. Is there anything a cool glass of water can't do?

It's hard to drink too much water. With little kids you may want to have them drink earlier rather than later in relation to their bedtime. Sometimes sugar-free ice pops can get water inside that would have otherwise stayed outside. Sipping and counting games may help a child take in a little more than they would ordinarily. Excessive thirst will be observed when a patient has high blood sugars, with steroid use, after sweating for any reason, and with fevers.

Patients with TBIs should be encouraged to drink. I have paid a penny a sip (with my mom, not my child. He was impervious to bribery, she was not.) Encourage drinking BEFORE thirst. If the patient is thirsty, she is already getting dry.

Drink water, not caffeinated beverages or alcoholic beverages, which can be dehydrating. Water. If the patient just has to have some flavoring, try lemon or lime juice, or mild herbal teas. Avoid sweet, carbonated drinks, first because of the sugar bolus, and second because the carbonation is theorized to leech calcium out of bone. Sports drinks are usually overkill unless there has been excessive vomiting, diarrhea, or drenching sweats. Water, water with ice, water in a squirt bottle, water with a straw. Water.

IV. EXERCISE

It's hard to overstate the benefits of exercise. Still, this is the world of Lyme, where everything is controversial. I did find sources that were quite opposed to any activity in Lyme patients. Remember, we're not training for the Olympics here. Exercise can mean ROM exercises encouraged by a therapist at the bedside. We're talking movement not World Wrestling Federation or Extreme Sports. Of course, for the acutely ill with 104° fevers, these patients just aren't going to feel well enough to do much of anything. For those who are stabilizing, however, consider the pros and cons of an exercise program.

Potentially bad things about exercise for Lyme patients:

1. Some authors say Lyme patients need to save all their energy for fighting the disease. Any energy spent exercising is energy that would be better used building the immune response.

2. T cell function and other immune processes may depress temporarily with exercise.

3. Too much exercise can exhaust a Lyme patient and require prolonged recovery.

4. Overdoing can lead to sore muscles and joints, which are already compromised in Lyme.

5. Too much exercise can deplete the adrenals and therefore decrease T cells.

6. Patients with an active babesiosis co-infection may not have the O_2-carrying capacity.

7. Once the patient starts to feel better she may overdo and may overestimate stamina and endurance.

8. The main problems with exercise for Lyme patients are exacerbation of pain and fatigue, which may make these individuals less likely to move at all.

9. Bb don't like too much oxygen. Some exercises cause a temporary depletion of oxygen in the adjacent tissue making the Bb happy.

Potentially good things about exercise for Lyme patients:

1. Weight can be controlled with the help of exercise. The immune system functions best when the individual is not at either extreme on the scale.

2. Activity often breeds more activity.

3. Exercise is associated with stress reduction.

4. Activity strengthens the heart.

5. Movement mobilizes waste.

6. Exercise builds endurance. Endurance is the measure of the ability to do cardiorespiratory work or how long a person can perform an activity. You don't need a lot of muscle strength to run a marathon but you need incredible endurance.

7. Activity builds stamina. Stamina is endurance plus strength. To cross-country ski you need to be strong and have plenty of endurance.

8. Bb don't like too much oxygen. In contrast to exercises that deplete oxygen levels in the tissue, other exercises raise the oxygen levels making the Bb unhappy. Some exercises increase tissue perfusion as well, again making the Bb unhappy.

9. Too much rest leads to deconditioning. Those of us who have taken care of in-patients know that 3 days of bed rest will have the patient so weak they can hardly sit up. Inactivity can lead to an unhealthy cycle. The more you lay there, the more you lay there.

10. Body temperature increases with exercise and Bb appear to be heat sensitive.

11. Exercise mobilizes lymph and decreases swelling.

12. Movement decreases the risk of clots.

13. Activity improves circulation.

14. Exercise lowers CRP, an inflammatory marker linked to heart disease, by about 10% after one year.

15. Cardiac workouts boost immune responses. Researchers at McMaster University in Canada examined the impact of exercise on the efficacy of the immune response. They found that regular aerobic activity boosts the immune system and helps reduce chronic inflammation.

16. T cell function and other immune processes may temporarily depress with exercise but then come back stronger (i.e., rebound).

17. A study released in July of 2012 says that inactivity is as deadly as smoking.

PEARL: Too much heavy aerobics can cause immune suppression. Gentle, non-aerobic exercise can be done daily, but strenuous workouts should be followed by a break. Very strenuous aerobic activity may be best avoided in the Lyme patient. If the patient decides to pursue aerobic activity, the more reasonable plan is to exercise several days a week with a day of rest in between. As stamina improves, the patient can increase duration and intensity.

18. Most patients feel better with exercise.

19. Strong muscles stabilize joints.

20. Weight stabilization and better glucose control result from activity.

21. Exercisers tend to have better flexibility.

22. There is an exercise to fit everyone no matter how physically limited.

23. Activity may rebalance hormones.

24. Movement usually results in a better mood.

25. Exercisers may respond better to vaccines.

26. The active seem to produce more antibodies.

27. Exercise promotes circulation.

28. Movement increases nutrient delivery to cells.

29. Exercise distracts the thinking away from the illness temporarily.

30. Activity provides a sense of accomplishment that counters the feelings of helplessness that can accompany chronic disease.

31. Exercise stimulates neurotransmitters that reduce stress.

32. Keeping fit is one of the few documented ways to stimulate neuronal growth.

33. Movement helps modulate excess emotion like anger.

34. Working out clears the head.

35. Oxygen supply to the cells is critical to good immune function.

36. Chinese medicine says exercise activates energy flow.

37. Slow and controlled exercise lowers inflammation.

38. Body heat itself may thwart Bb.

39. The more you do, the more you can do (i.e., stamina).

40. Fitness allows for more energy to be available for healing and mounting effective immune defense.

41. Satisfaction comes from accomplishment. Patients feel good when they make progress.

Components of a comprehensive exercise program:

1. **Strength:** The power to resist and exert force. To increase strength, use resistance to build muscle. How "strong" a sick person is will be measured by her capacity for exertion (endurance) and her overall ability to mount a defense. Strength can be increased usually through weight training or resistance bands. Heavy weights are not usually recommended until after puberty because of the potential impact on the growth plates of bone. In Lyme disease, patients may gradually be able to move to light free weights and other strengthening modalities as tolerated. Here about 3 or 4 sessions a week may be appropriate with a day of rest between each session. In strength training always use correct form and technique.

2. **Balance:** The ability to control position either when the body is static or in motion. Balance can be significantly affected in Lyme and other TBIs. Check balance during each exam. Is the patient tripping or tipping? Exercise can improve balance with practice.

3. **Flexibility:** The ability to achieve a full range of motion. This capability can vary in the same individual for different joints. Much flexibility is genetic but practice can improve flexibility within the patient's innate range. An individual who is "tight" may be more prone to injury when performing other activities.

4. **Coordination:** The interaction between muscles and nerves and can be impacted in TBIs. Coordination can include eye-hand coordination or the balance of actions between muscle groups. Coordination is the integration of various components of the nerve and structural systems. Exercise can improve coordination.

5. **Agility:** Ability to perform a series of movements in succession in different planes or directions. Usually the faster these tasks can be performed without error, the more agile the person. Practice can enhance agility.

6. **Cardiovascular fitness:** The heart's capacity to deliver blood to working muscles, and their ability to use it, is called cardiovascular fitness. To improve this parameter the patient must exercise at an intensity that increases HR and respiration. Fitness progresses with slow and steady advancement over time.

7. **Endurance:** The ability to do cardiorespiratory work or the capacity to perform a task over and over. How long can a person perform a certain activity?

8. **Toning:** Focus on shaping a muscle and appearance. While being toned is nice, that's the least of our worries.

9. **Conditioning:** Conditioning is any regimen used to train the heart to pump more efficiently, bringing more O_2 to muscles. Training helps improve a skill set over time. For example, a conditioned heart beats SLOWER and more efficiently than a non-conditioned one, which will beat faster, trying to pump enough blood to perform the same task. Intervals, where exercise intensity is varied from moderate to intense and back again in cycles, are often used to improve overall conditioning. Lyme can level some patients and they will need slow but steady conditioning.

10. **Fitness:** Ability to perform physical demands without exhaustion. In sick patients, fitness can be important both in terms of cardiovascular preparedness as well as overall strength. Functional fitness can be especially important in patients with chronic diseases so that the patient has sufficient energy to perform tasks important to daily life such as taking a shower or feeding herself. Usually, the more fit the person is at the onset of illness, the more rapid the recovery.

Possible exercises for Lyme patients:

1. **Breathing exercises:** Proper breathing is an essential component of all exercise. Cheap and easy, breathing can be done by anyone, anywhere, anytime. Yoga is mostly a series of postures that simply allows the

participant to breathe. I heard one fitness trainer say that aerobic exercise and strength training were both a waste of time if the person isn't breathing properly. Many meditation practices are focused on breathing. Deep breathing decreases stress and increases oxygen to tissues during exercise. Since Bb do not like too much O_2 in their environment, deep breathing can have mixed effects, either impeding the Bb life processes or causing the organisms to go into hiding. Deep breathing, also called diaphragmatic breathing, expands the chest and lungs in such a way that the diaphragm moves downward, making more room for the lungs and oxygen exchange. When performing any exercise, attention should be paid to proper breathing. While there are many proposed breathing techniques, here are two variations:

- The 4-7-8 breath: Breathe in for a count of 4, hold for a count of 7, and then breathe out for a count of 8. Depending on the source, these numbers vary such as the 6-7-8 breath or the 4-8-8 breath.

- During inhalation the chest should inflate and abdomen move in slightly as the diaphragm flattens. During exhalation, the belly button should move toward the spine.

2. **Range of motion exercises**: Even bedridden patients can do ROM exercises. These exercises involve moving the joints through their full array of flexion, extension, rotation, abduction, and adduction. Joints are limited by their natural range and should not be moved beyond that point. For example, a knee should not be forced to extend cephalad beyond 180 degrees of the normal line between the femur and tibia. ROM exercises increase circulation, move fluid, drain lymph, decrease swelling, prevent clotting, decrease stiffness, increase flexibility, avert contracture, and prevent muscles from weakening. These exercises can be passive, where a therapist or caretaker moves the joints, or active where the patient positions the area. Joints should not be forced, but if the movement is consistent with its natural ROM, the joint can be encouraged to move a little farther each session. These exercises can be performed several times a day. In-patients should almost always be doing some kind of ROM exercises and bedridden patients at home should be encouraged to do the same. A therapist can come to the house to teach the family or patient the proper ROM of each joint. ROM exercises can continue and expand into flexibility work as the patient gets stronger and has more tolerance. Just because other exercises become possible does not mean that the ROM exercises must stop.

3. **Warm-up exercises**: Many consider "warming-up" essential to any workout. Even the most fit should not go from 0 to 60 instantly. A warm-up prepares the muscles and joints for more intense activity and thereby helps prevent injury, promotes circulation, increases body temperature, and slightly raises the heart and respiratory rates, but not to the level experienced in the actual workout. Warming-up makes the muscles more flexible and receptive to activity and is recommended even before stretching.

4. **Stretching:** When stretching, a specific muscle or group of muscles is elongated to improve elasticity and to increase control. Stretching improves flexibility and is an important adjunct to ROM exercises. Stretching feels good, otherwise cats wouldn't do it. We know that stretching a muscle in spasm can relieve the cramp. (Boy, does that hurt!)

Recently, there has been debate around whether stretching before more strenuous exercise actually prevents injury. A few sources insist that stretching is damaging. With all the controversy, one would think that stretching was a cross between voodoo and pornography. Some say that stretching may make the individual more prone to injury and that this activity should be the reward after exercising is complete. They say that too much stretching might alter calcium metabolism in the muscle fibers leading to quicker fatigue. Nonetheless, many athletes stretch before rigorous exercise.

Of course, as with any activity, if done improperly, there can be problems. Don't stretch statically to the point of pain; only extend to the point of awareness of the stretch. Don't hold a stretch until it hurts or burns or stings. *Only to the point of awareness.* Don't bounce like a 1960's cheerleader. Static stretches can actually decrease performance by weakening the motor neurons and making them less reactive when you need them to respond.

Instead, dynamic stretching starts small and gradually increases the ROM. Move only as far as comfortable. Then take the muscles through the ROM you plan to use during your real workout. Five minutes or so of movement, gradually increasing the intensity, should improve flexibility, enhance performance, and decrease the risk of injury by getting more and more muscle fibers involved in the activity. Muscles and tendons that are warm and stretched are more pliable.

Many athletes feel too stiff to play unless they stretch first. Some football teams do ballet stretches to get ready for games. They believe that stretching enhances performance. Yoga uses stretching to elongate the various parts of the body and enable focused breathing. Here stretching is believed to strengthen muscle over time. In fact, stretching alone has been shown to be as effective as yoga in decreasing back pain.

Despite the controversy, most runners stretch before a run, and many stretch afterwards as well, to decrease the chance of injury. Individuals who are too flexible may stretch to the point of joint instability and this laxity may cause problems. I could find no real disadvantages to dynamic stretching in the TBI population, especially if they purr when they do it.

5. **Walking:** Walking is an excellent exercise and appropriate for any age group. By adjusting the pace, adding intervals, swinging arms, or interspersing stretches, a walk can be either a gentle or intense workout. Some sources say that a good assessment of overall fitness is how fast a person can walk a mile. A pedometer can be an excellent way to measure progress. Especially in the chronically ill, a few extra steps each day can provide a sense of accomplishment. While the length of a person's stride is fairly set by genetics, pace can be altered easily as endurance increases.

Advantages of walking

- Can be done alone or with others

- Everyone over the age of two has mastered the basic technique.

- Can be done indoors or outside: the treadmill allows for reading or watching TV and outdoors provides the benefits of being in nature. Treadmills or indoor tracks allow for walking in any kind of weather.

- Relatively easy on joints compared to running, tennis, basketball, etc.

- Can adapt intensity to underlying health. (The acutely ill may want to delay until feeling better.)

- Need only supportive walking shoes as equipment

- Easy to assess progress

- Easy to notch up or down

- Can alter distance or speed

- Low risk of injury

- Easy to stick with and can make part of everyday life

- Can alter route, add music, etcetera, to diminish boredom

- Enhances hippocampal function, which might help memory problems in Lyme

- Associated with many health benefits: increases calcium in bones, stabilizes blood sugars, decreases risk of stroke, increases good cholesterol, decreases body fat, helps in losing weight, enables maintenance of normal weight, decreases swelling in legs, relieves pain in joints, increases longevity, daily walking may add 1.3 healthy years, maintains lean muscle mass, decreases blood pressure, minimizes stress, benefits the heart, increases circulation, helps breathing, combats depression, boosts the immune system, and helps prevent osteoporosis.

Problems with walking

- Adding weights could increase stress on knees or ankles.

- Walking can get boring. Add music, intersperse intervals, or change routes

- Acutely "hot" joints, as in Lyme, may not be amenable to any but the shortest distances.

- Walking outside at night requires safety precautions.

- If the walk is too long or too intense, the activity can result in injury such as shin splints.

- Shoes can be expensive and must fit properly. Constant microtrauma of the toenail against the shoe can cause bruising and detachment of the nail. Blisters are painful and can get infected. Sweaty feet are fungal nirvana.

- Pedometers can be "off" and thus distracting.

Fundamentals of walking

- Non-aerobic walking can be done daily for maximum effect.

- The closer walking comes to jogging and running, the more breaks need to be taken away from daily workouts.

- Heel strike first then roll through the step to the toe.

- Walking is low intensity and low impact.

- Using walking poles and swinging arms can increase intensity of the workout.

- The more intense the activity, the closer the walking comes to speed walking and then to jogging and running. The faster the pace, usually the higher the heart rate.

- Usually walking burns carbohydrates first and then fats.

- With regularly paced walking, it's best to walk every day.

- Start slowly and build up whether through a faster pace or longer duration.

- If weight loss is the goal, there are a number of exercises that might be faster in helping to reach those goals.

PEARL: Walking poles can enhance the overall workout and can stabilize those who may have wobbly gait, balance problems, or a lack of coordination associated with TBIs.

6. **Jogging:** A jog is a slow to moderately-paced exercise that is faster than walking and slower than running. Speed walking and jogging are close in terms of overall benefits. Jogging burns 25% more calories than walking, but there is correspondingly more stress on joints. Jogging flushes toxins in sweat and often improves skin appearance. Jogging allows the individual to see results faster than walking, depending on the fitness goals. Jogging takes less time to achieve the same effect. Jogging and running can be addictive in that they cause the release of endorphins, making the person feel good after a run. As always, there is a risk/benefit relationship and jogging causes more stress on knees, ankles, and feet than walking. Walking may be the better choice in those who are chronically ill, have joint damage, or underlying heart problems. Jogging is a slow run at a steady pace and is often defined as less than 6 mph or 10 minute miles. Jogging is sometimes used as a warm-up for runners or other athletes. Jogging may cause too much impact on the knees, especially in Lyme patients with significant joint involvement.

7. **Running:** Once the pace becomes faster than 6 mph or you are moving faster than a mile in ten minutes, you are running. I wouldn't know since I don't think I have ever reached this speed.

Advantages of running:

- The faster the pace, the greater the increase in HR and blood circulation

- Running provides one of the fastest ways to achieve fitness goals (depending on the goals, of course) and is one of the best exercises for overall conditioning.

- Long distance runs can result in a "high" which is a state of euphoria or a clear and calm condition after an extended run. Also refers to the time when the runner hits the perfect stride during a run. This feeling is due to a rush of endorphins.

- Running is associated with many positive results:

    Rapid conditioning

    Enhanced toning

    Feelings of happiness and creativity

    More energy

    As a weight bearing exercise there is an increase in bone density and a decreased risk of osteoporosis

    Increase in overall and resting metabolic rate

    Enhanced circulation that increases brain function

    Stimulation of memory and learning centers

    Less muscle loss with age

    Increased longevity

- Running is an efficient way to burn calories, using about 100 calories/mile, depending on weight.

- Can be done alone, with a partner, or as part of a group

- Others can motivate the runner through support or competition.

- Decreases stress and clears the mind

- Improves speed and endurance

- Mood is enhanced through hormones called endorphins.

- Running improves mental focus, concentration, memory, and cognition, perhaps through new cells forming in the hippocampus and more protection of other cells in the CNS.

- Improves posture and coordination through fluid motion

- Stimulates immune response unless overdone

- Relieves depression and allows for better management of stress and anxiety

- Increases blood circulation and increases O_2 levels

- With committed running, there is possibly decreased risk of URIs and cancer.

- Because of augmented O_2 uptake there is an increase in cardiac function and a decrease in BP and fewer overall cardiac problems.

- Running allows for better insulin sensitivity.

Problems with running:

- Frankly, running may be too intense for chronic Lyme patients. Nevertheless, there are a number of athletes with Lyme, who when they are well enough, pester their doctors to resume training. Often that includes running.

- Intense running can be associated with bruising under the nail and subsequent loss of the toenail, shin splints, stress fractures, muscle cramps or Charley horses, dehydration, joint damage especially in those with pre-existing problems, and dampening of the immune response.

PEARL: Some muscle cramps respond to magnesium.

- Consistent running may cause irreversible breast sag, which can be limited by using a sports bra but cannot be reversed without invasive procedures.

- Running in the sun can result in burning and an increased risk of skin cancer.

- Skin on the inner thighs can chaff from the friction of rubbing against cloth or skin. A protective ointment like Aquaphor might help.

- Especially important for Lyme patients, running can be hard on even the healthiest knees.

Running advice:

- Unlike walking, you don't need to run daily for maximum benefit. The more intense the run, the more break days you need in between.

- Running may not be the best choice for Lyme patients, but since we all know how well patients follow instructions, make sure any patient who decides to run is at least aware of the risks and how to mitigate those risks.

- Take all safety precautions such as sunscreen, drinking water, reflectors at night, well-fitted supportive shoes, toe protection, antifungals, and sports bras. Don't run alone in risky areas.

- You can't start with sprints and marathons. Participants should start with walking, progress to fast walking, then jogging, and finally running if tolerated.

- Use a nice fluid motion with upright posture. Heel strike first then roll through to the toe.

- Overdoing leads to injury. Those who overdo are much more likely to quit.

- Large dogs like to run but don't let them overdo it either.

- Deciding that running is not right for you is fine. Select an exercise that is a better fit.

- Keep well hydrated. Water is the best choice unless distances are long or sweating profuse.

8. **Biking:** Exercise on a bike can be less hard on joints than running. Biking can also strengthen the muscles that help support joints which can be beneficial to Lyme patients. Unlike walking that is essentially free, prudent bike riding requires equipment such as a safe, well-maintained bicycle and a helmet. Yes, a helmet. No matter how tough you think you are, a concussion is tougher. TBI patients do not need any more damage to their neurons. While biking appears to focus on leg strength and stamina, the entire body gets a workout including the upper body, core, and the cardiovascular system. Biking increases overall strength and tone, builds endurance and stamina, and promotes balance and coordination. Again, balance and coordination can be impacted by Lyme and other TBIs. Riding a bike

may be a way to regain these skills. By significantly increasing the HR, biking can be a real calorie burner.

Biking can be done inside on tracks, a stationary bike, or in a spin class. Outdoor biking, however, can offer the benefits of nature such as decreasing stress, modulating anxiety, and improving mood. Indoor biking can be painfully tedious. Of course, biking in frenetic traffic can be unnerving. There are bike safety courses through many organizations such as the Boy Scouts, schools, and bike shops that should be considered before you start peddling up I-95. As with all exercise, start slowly and gradually increase either speed or distance. Bicycling can be deceptive in that many novices think they can do more to start than is reasonable.

Make sure traffic can see you and watch uneven surfaces. Follow the rules of the road and look out for traffic. Consider wearing long sleeves and long pants since skidding along a road top during a fall can cause severe abrasions that can become secondarily infected and leave scars. Do not wear baggy pants that can get tangled in the gears. Use sunscreen in exposed areas, especially on the skin on top of the knee where no one ever thinks they will get sunburned. This 4 X 4 plot of epidermis is uniquely exposed during biking. Never wear flip-flops to bike since they tangle in the pedals.

PEARL: We all sit on our ischia bones. No matter how plump you are and no matter how many jokes are made about "natural padding," when you sit it's pretty much skin and bone in direct contact with the seat. Biking shorts have built-in pads and seats can be cushioned and tilted to help minimize this problem.

Even young kids can bike and they often take pride in their biking skills. This exercise can be done as a family and many parks have biking trails where the biker does not need to worry about getting hit by a car. Here, though, you need to be cognizant of other bikers.

Stay hydrated. Bike riding can be a good choice for Lyme and other TBI patients offering a number of benefits. Biking is especially kind to the knee joints and strengthens the muscles and tendons that support the knee.

PEARL: Bicycle riding requires balance. Lyme can affect balance. My balance and proprioception were significantly altered by Lyme. I had to learn to ride all over again. The process was long and humbling. (Thanks to Dr. Kliman for suggesting the wider tires.)

9. **Strength training**: Strengthening exercises involve working the muscles in a way that will allow them to build the capacity to do more work. To increase strength, resistance must be used against muscle to build more muscle. A person's strength is usually measured by his capacity to work, which is defined as force over distance. Something has to be moved, whether it is a muscle fiber or a kettlebell, in order to meet the definition of work. Strength can be increased through weight training or resistance bands.

Strength training has been associated with positive health benefits including: weight loss using multiple repetitions with light weights, building of muscle mass with heavy weights and few repetitions, toning, improved cardiac function, better posture, enhanced support of joints, overall boost in BMR, increase in lean body mass, improved bone mineral density, stabilization of the entire body, and a decrease in the proportion of body fat. Muscle burns more calories at rest than fat cells, so the more proportional muscle, the greater the basal metabolic rate.

Resistance or weight training can involve using one's own weight as the resistance force or free weights, attached weights, weight machines, or resistance bands. When you do a push up, your own upper body is the weight being moved through distance to qualify as work. With resistance training, specific muscle groups can be targeted. When you increase weight you will be building more muscle. When you increase repetitions you will be burning more calories and conditioning.

- **Light resistance** usually involves hand-held free weights, attached ankle or wrist weights, weight vests, or easy to moderate resistance bands. Here the goal is to perform 8 to 12 repetitions using good form. In comparison to heavy weights, light resistance takes more time to achieve goals but allows for longer performance.

  Workouts with light weights might be appropriate for Lyme patients, since there is a decent strengthening component without taxing the system or risking joint damage. Resistance bands might be a good way to start.

PEARL: Be careful when adding wrist or ankle weights on patients who already have compromised hips, knees, or ankles.

- **Heavy resistance** more often involves machines and bars onto which additional weight can be added. Usually the weights are so heavy that only 3 to 6 repetitions can be done using good form. Once you are too fatigued to perform with good form, STOP. This is an anaerobic exercise with high intensity for short bursts.

The body is not burning oxygen at the time of the exercise and metabolic by-products build up until they can be removed. Lactic acid accumulation in muscle is the reason that the muscles feel so sore after heavy weight lifting. Muscles build during rest, not during exercise. To build more muscle, the foundation muscle must be stressed to the point where there is some muscle cell breakdown. Recovery prompts more protein synthesis causing muscle to grow thicker and bigger fibers. The healing process starts about 2 hours after a training session and can continue for 24 hours or more depending on how exhausted the muscles were after the session. If another workout follows too closely then there is not enough time to rebuild.

Use of very heavy weights requires spotters to prevent injury if the individual cannot hold the weight. Overdoing can lead to injury. Before attempting any exercise with heavy weights, the form should be perfected using light weights first.

Consider that workouts with heavy weights might not be the best choice for Lyme patients for several reasons. Their protein might be better used in making immune molecules and repairing tissue damaged by pathogens. Lifting heavy weights can put enormous strain on joints and Lyme patients may not have that functional capacity to spare. While lifting heavy weights can accomplish more strengthening in less time, is that really the highest priority for this individual?

PEARL: Be careful with teenage weightlifters. Desire to progress can lead to temptation with steroids, growth hormones, and protein supplements. If you see a five-year-old body builder, be very concerned about the caretakers and what supplements that child may be taking to look that way. Heavy weights are not usually recommended until after puberty because of the potential impact on the growth plates of bone.

10. **Cross training:** This term refers to participation in various activities to garner the benefit of each in an effort to improve overall fitness and performance. While cross training principles can be applied in many ways, I list it here in order to introduce the benefits of the elliptical machine, also called the cross trainer. This stationery exerciser is preferred by many Lyme patients because it was designed to minimize stress on the joints. Since the feet never leave the pedals, there is no impact on the joints in the lower extremities. The legs still bear weight so the bones gain the benefit of weight bearing exercises. Cardiovascular intensity can be adjusted.

General advice regarding resistance training to build strength:

- Lifting weights must be done in a slow controlled way.

- Good form is essential to garner maximum benefit and to prevent injury.

- Use enough weight so that you can exercise, using good form, until you cannot do another repetition. Sacrifice one more rep to form every time.

- While lifting the weight is important, lowering the weight is just as critical and must be done in a slow, deliberate, and controlled way. The lowering of a weight should never be termed a collapse.

- If you cannot manage the weight, reduce it for the next session.

- Progress is still progress, even if it is slow.

- Proper form should be mastered using light weights before attempting heavy weights.

- You must overcome inertia with each repetition. Each rep must be complete: fully raised and fully lowered. Do not let momentum do the work. In PT, my mother was the champ by swinging her half-pound weight up and down like a whirling dervish. In 20 reps she was lucky to reap the benefits of 2.

- Bad form results in injury.

- Try to balance out and work all muscle groups so you don't look like Arnold Schwarzenegger on top and Mark Zuckerberg on the bottom.

- Change the routine every 4 to 6 weeks.

11. **Swimming and aquatic exercises:** Swimming can be excellent for those who have painful joints, since the buoyancy of the water cushions the impact. Swimming is usually cheap requiring nothing but access to a pool and a Speedo. Swimming strengthens, conditions, and tones. Since water has 12 times the resistance of air, swimming builds strength and stamina. While swimming is easy on the joints, it can be tough on skin and eyes. Many people like the whole body workout, although others find swimming laps boring. Swimming serves as an individual challenge

and it is easy to measure progress. Swimming can be an excellent choice for Lyme patients with joint problems and can be good as a part of cross training. Professional athletes frequently use water therapy as part of their rehabilitation after injury. Laps are not the only thing to be done in the water and there are many alternate forms of aquatic exercises including aerobics and pedal boats. While swimming does increase the strength of the cardiac muscle, it is not the best exercise for weight loss. Nonetheless, with its overall workout, the ability to stretch, enhance flexibility, and perform ROM exercises, as well as its low potential for joint injury, swimming should be considered high on the list of exercise options for Lyme patients. Aquatics, or movement in water, provide the Lyme patient with a safe, supportive environment for relieving arthritis pain and stiffness. If done in warm water, aquatics allow arthritis patients to exercise without putting excess strain on joints.

12. **Dancing for exercise**: Dancing can also be a good choice for exercise in TBI patients. Dance has several advantages: the pace can be tailored to the individual and dances can be selected that spare the joints. Dance can be aerobic, burning calories as it strengthens muscles, builds endurance, and tones. Dancing is fun and many people will continue a dance program long after they quit other regimens due to difficulty or boredom. There are certified dance therapists who can set goals and measure progress. There are just about as many forms of dance as there are individuals and dance can be very socializing. Of course, with modern interactive technology, dance can be done alone with a number of programs available on systems like Wii. Dance has been demonstrated to improve symptoms of PTSD, decrease anxiety and depression, enhance self-image, promote healing, augment self-esteem, build confidence, increase lung function, improve endurance and stamina, build strong bones through weight bearing, increase circulation, develop coordination and balance, increase mental acuity, stimulate immune response, promote flexibility, increase endorphins for better mood and feelings of well-being and creativity, expand memory, enable weight loss, stabilize blood sugars, augment good cholesterol, and further agility, endurance, and stamina. Many references noted how dance lubricates joints. I am not sure what that means, or the mechanism by which it is achieved, but it sounds like a good thing. A good dance workout makes many people happy and all ages have shown interest in lessons.

While strenuous dancing can result in injuries such as muscle cramping, stress fractures, and sprained joints, this is rare in those who are just exercising for fitness and not competition.

You can even dance with your dog, as we learned when my uncle got a basenji-mix from the pound. This little wild man will dance on his two back legs as long as you dance with him. He actually dances better than my husband. With the many potential benefits and few downsides, dance can be considered a healthy choice in TBI patients.

13. **Yoga:** This may be one of the best overall fitness choices for Lyme patients. Yoga can be as gentle or as intense as the practitioner wants it to be. No equipment is needed, although a non-slip mat is nice. People of any age can appreciate yoga and many schools are converting old classrooms to yoga areas. Yoga is a practice and doing it once or even once a month probably isn't going to get you to your goals.

Yoga is a series of poses designed to allow the practitioner to breathe. These exercises combine stretching and conscious breathing with balance poses to shore up weak muscles and release muscle tension. Many studies have been done to measure the effects of yoga and the findings include a positive impact on flexibility, posture, balance, control, coordination, breathing, muscle strength, awareness, immune function, and lubrication of joints. (Again, I don't know what this means but it seems good.) Yoga appears to stimulate the PNS as opposed to the activation of the SNS which occurs with most other exercise programs. Yoga stretches the muscles and massages the organs and soft tissue. The novice begins by following more experienced instructors and correctly doing as much as they can. Then comes the practice.

Measurements of effect have shown that with yoga, patients have better efficacy from vaccines, better circulation with increased perfusion of tissue, lowered BP, lower RR with more lung efficiency, enhanced endurance, a more stable GI tract, better pain tolerance, additional appetite control, a more balanced metabolism, improved sleep cycles, additional energy, diminished stress, accelerated healing, increased lymphatic drainage, more good cholesterol, stabilization of hormone levels, more even blood glucose levels, less back and joint pain, and increased insulin production. Practitioners have better ROM, eye-hand coordination, dexterity, reaction time, concentration, endurance, and depth perception. Studies have documented positive increases in GABA levels, lower Alzheimer's risk, decreased triglycerides, additional RBCs, and more detoxification capacity. The weight-bearing in yoga strengthens bones and keeps more Ca in the bone.

Yoga improves mood, curtails depression, reduces anxiety, and enhances attitude, concentration, attention span, and level of calmness. Yoga has been found to be an excellent exercise program for patients with back pain, headaches, joint problems, constipation, and arthritis. In OCD patients, yoga decreases symptoms and there is less need for medication. Symptoms in carpal tunnel syndrome and asthma diminish. The slow deliberate movements and gentle pressure on joints relieve pain in arthritis. The origins of the Neti Pot to open sinuses and nasal passages is part of ancient yoga traditions. Back pain is eased by decreasing spinal compression and improving body alignment.

Yoga allows for whole-body conditioning and personal challenge. Usually the student is so focused on following the teacher and remembering to breathe, that there is no attention left for comparison with others. Yoga is non-competitive, unless you count the sage-tinted spandex worn by some of the class members and the jostling for the best mat position on the floor. You never hear about the next yoga tournament.

There is a meditative feel to a yoga practice which may help relax the Lyme patient. Since yoga relieves joint discomfort, relaxes muscles, helps with back pain, and diminishes headaches, yoga might be a good choice for fitness in TBIs. Yoga provides a balanced workout for all muscles including the jaw, tongue, face, and toes that many other regimens ignore completely. Yoga focuses on soft tissue, internal organ massage, lymphatic drainage, and stamina. A full ROM is employed and balance, eye-hand coordination, dexterity, and endurance all improve with practice. These positive results are just what might be needed by a Lyme patient. There are variations of the standard yoga practice with some including high room temperatures. While these hot yoga classes may provide additional benefit from the heat, usually these classes would be too intense and demanding for the average Lyme patient.

There is a very low risk of injury with yoga, since the person does only what she is comfortable doing. This makes yoga a valid option for Lyme patients. The patient can participate to the degree they feel up to or just rest on the mat. However, yoga just might be too slow moving for younger kids who will get ants in their pants as they wait for something to happen.

You feel so guilty saying anything bad about yoga since you think the Dalai Lama will somehow know and be disappointed in you. While most yoga sessions leave the individual with a sense of positive well-being and serenity, there are times when all that audible breathing is downright creepy. There are instances in yoga class when you want to be done so badly that you could scream and other times when you want to smack the practiced serenity right out of the instructor. (I am truly non-violent. I have never smacked anyone, ever.)

Yoga offers a very complete benefits package for the TBI patient. Yoga is probably a good choice for many Lyme patients especially older teens, who often think the somewhat exotic feel of yoga is cool. In my gym in West Chester, in the child care room, the caretakers sometimes conduct a baby yoga class while the parents are in the actual instruction area. The little kids look forward to this and don't seem to get restless, so maybe I'm wrong about the age groups that would benefit. Nonetheless, yoga may not be the best option for some 12-year-old boys.

Namaste.

14. **Tai chi:** Tai chi is a gentle exercise that combines meditation and martial arts. With SLOW, deliberate movements, tai chi has much to offer Lyme patients. Traditionally a part of both Chinese medicine and personal defense, the government in China encourages its practice in all age groups. On any given morning, you can witness hundreds of people outside practicing. Much scientific study has been done on tai chi to determine if it lives up to its billing. The practice is catching on in the west for its health benefits.

Tai chi is a meditative exercise where the mind clears through movement. This practice has been demonstrated to be immune-enhancing and practitioners get better response to vaccines through augmented CMI. Tai chi has been found to be especially beneficial in chronic conditions, improving the rate of healing and recovery. In fibromyalgia, tai chi decreased pain, fatigue, sleep disturbances, and depression and has been shown to improve balance, control, and flexibility. Fewer falls were documented in specific populations. Tai chi was also shown to be beneficial in stabilizing DM, modulating symptoms in ADHD, and in reducing pain in arthritis of the knee. On-going practice decreased LDL. Tai chi can be ideal for arthritis patients because it includes agile moves that do not require bending or squatting. Patients experience improved mobility, breathing, and relaxation.

A meta-analysis conducted by the US government found increased well-being, better mood, and decreased stress, anxiety, and depression with tai chi practice. These findings may be due to altered levels of norepinephrine and cortisol. The goal of tai chi is to decrease stress on mind and body and to balance the person and maintain homeostasis. Homeostasis is the preservation of a stable equilibrium between elements in the body, whereby the physiology adjusts as needed to keep metabolic processes on an even keel. If one aspect is disturbed, other components of the system compensate to re-establish balance. Tai chi promotes this homeostasis, which is critical to both physical and mental health.

While tai chi places almost no strain on joints, it does improve fitness. Even though tai chi is low impact, this exercise can burn more calories than surfing and almost as much as downhill skiing and has been shown to improve cardiovascular fitness. Tai chi has been associated with increased longevity and serenity.

Tai chi can be a good choice to promote fitness in Lyme patients, offering a number of the physical and mental health benefits they might need. Easy on the joints and flexible in intensity, tai chi may provide a good exercise option. Since tai chi can be sold as a martial art, the 12 y/o boys who I speculated might not be a good fit in yoga, might be sold on tai chi.

Personally, I found tai chi interminable, but the tai chi masters were ready for the likes of me. I read that the ancient practitioners said that anyone who could not embrace tai chi had difficulty because they were an unhealthy or uncomfortable person who could not comprehend the meditative aspect of tai chi and appreciate its effect on calm. They were right. Mediation makes me nervous, too. Nonetheless, I believe that for the right TBI patient, tai chi could be enormously beneficial.

15. **Conditioning exercises**: I include this as a separate category so that I can introduce any number of fashionable, trendy exercise regimens designed to enhance cardiovascular fitness in conjunction with other components of a comprehensive exercise program. From Zumba to Pilates to martial arts to Jazzercise, there are innumerable opportunities to improve on individual fitness. Pilates has been shown to be especially useful for patients with back pain by strengthening the core muscles that support the spine and improving flexibility. Note that **METs** or the metabolic equivalent of tasks can be used to assess the metabolic rate during a specific activity in relation to a reference rate at rest. Using METs allows for comparison between a number of conditioning programs. Of course, METs are not the only way to evaluate the right program for an individual, but it's one tool to use.

Selecting the best exercise program for a TBI patient will depend on the individual's personality and status of disease. The choice may change over time as the patient's condition changes and whenever the person might want to try something new. Any of these options

may fit into the fitness plan at different times in different stages. These choices are best discussed among the patient, caregivers, and HCPs. Steer the patient toward the program that will likely provide the most benefit and that does not damage the patient in light of the unique nature of his disease. Tennis and basketball may not be the best choice when a kid has a hot Lyme knee but may be considered later in the recovery process. Risk/benefit analysis works here.

16. **Aerobic exercises**: Aerobic exercises involve low to moderate effort over a long duration. Over time, all the body's available carbohydrate is used for energy to fuel the exercise and when it's depleted the body starts burning fat. For this reason, aerobics may be better for weight loss than anaerobic exercise. Aerobic means with oxygen and in these exercises oxygen is used to burn carbohydrate and then fat to power the activity, the same way oxygen is used to burn a fuel in a furnace. Lactic acid does not build up in the muscle. Aerobic exercise improves mental health, decreases BP, stabilizes DM, and increases the amount of RBCs. Although the HR increases during the exercise, usually the resting HR slows as the heart is trained to beat more efficiently and the heart muscle becomes stronger. There are all kinds of calculations for optimal HR and maximal HR and other parameters that can be considered when performing aerobic exercise. Running relatively long distances or dancing for an hour might both be considered aerobic exercises. In contrast, minute sprints and lifting heavy weights would be anaerobic. Intense aerobics are not usually recommended for acutely ill TBI patients. Aerobics may be possible later in recovery.

17. **Anaerobic exercises**: These activities involve high intensity for short bursts and are better for building muscle. As the name implies, anaerobic activity does not use O_2 to burn fuel to make energy *at the time of exercise*. Sugars are used but not combusted using O_2. The by-products of these anaerobic reactions, including lactic acid, build up in the muscle and it takes hours or days for these molecules to be metabolized away. The lactic acid accumulation is thought to be one reason for sore muscles after lifting heavy weights. While anaerobic activity is not great for weight loss, these exercises build muscle and muscle has a higher basal metabolic rate than fat cells. Therefore, over time, anaerobic activity can help maintain a healthy weight. Sprints and heavy weight lifting can both be anaerobic since they involve short bursts of intense effort. Extreme anaerobic exercise is not the best choice for acutely ill Lyme patients. Careful consideration should go into whether some forms of anaerobics would be appropriate later in recovery.

18. Interactive programs: Today there are interactive fitness programs such as Wii. This technology might be suitable for Lyme patients since just about everything a TBI patient might need to work on can be found. Software is available that focuses on coordination, balance, warm-ups, control, stability, strength training, flexibility, aerobics, conditioning, toning, dance, yoga, and most any kind of sport including archery, skiing, bowling, boxing, soccer, etc. Workouts can be done alone or with partners and can be competitive with your own past scores or the scores of others. Intensity ranges from beginner to advanced. Risk of injury is miniscule and activities can be selected that minimize impact on joints. I am not referring to interactive video games here but actual fitness programs that build physical, mental, and functional fitness. These programs can be expensive but more "used" units are becoming available. Many segments are fun and addictive in a good way. Most systems have ways to assess progress.

Advice applicable to any exercise program:

1. Do what you can tolerate.

2. A physical therapist or trainer can help you get started by assessing current status and helping to develop a fitness plan.

3. Usually frequent, short exercise sessions are better than occasional marathons.

4. Stay hydrated.

5. Try to select an activity that works on the various components of a fitness program, not just cardio or strength. All are important.

6. Overdoing is never a good idea.

7. Do what you enjoy so that you keep doing it.

8. Even gentle moderate exercise can lead to a positive habit. Some say it takes 30 days to form a habit, others say 90. Exercise can become a good habit. In contrast, three days may be all it takes to break a habit that you don't want to break.

9. The hardest part is getting started.

10. Capacity to exercise will depend on the person and stage of healing.

11. Don't compare yourself to anyone else.

12. Measure your progress by assessing how you do over time.

13. Some days you just won't feel like it. That's okay. Take a break.

14. A break is a day without exercise. Two days, be careful. You could be heading toward a long lapse.

15. Some days you do have to push yourself a little, unless you are acutely ill. Then you have my permission to take a rest.

16. Some recommend a gym or classes. Other people hate gyms and classes. There is no one right way to exercise.

17. Progress, no matter how minimal, is worth celebrating.

18. Don't get frustrated if progress is slow.

19. If you HATE to exercise, try all the different options until you find something you can tolerate or even enjoy.

20. Some people do better with a partner. Others can't stand the inane chatter. (Guess which side I fall on.)

21. Persistence will lead to results.

22. Never exercise to the point of exhaustion. That defeats the purpose. Challenge yourself to do a little more each time and save some energy for living.

23. If you have questions, ask a pro: trainers, instructors, PTs, OTs. (Many coaches know very little about safe, effective fitness programs. They have a different agenda.)

24. If you don't feel like it, try anyway. I have often heard people say "I wish I had worked out today." I have never heard anyone say, "I am so glad I didn't exercise today." Once you get started, you may get in the mood. If you just can't, you just can't.

25. Aim for an hour of activity a day. Try to complete the hour even if the intensity is limited when first starting. Adjust the activity in order to complete the hour, even if that means laying on a yoga mat watching the clock. At least you got on the mat. The next day's hour might mean a therapist moving your joints through ROM exercises. The hour can be broken into pieces but be careful here, since our minds have many ways of talking us out of the last 50 minutes.

26. Lyme can flatten some people and they will need to revert to a slow but steady conditioning program, even

if they were ready for the Olympics prior to their infection.

27. Gradually move to light free weights and other modalities as tolerated.

28. Some exercises like ROM and walking are best done daily in your hour of activity. More rigorous exercises can be scheduled about 3 or 4 days a week. Do not exercise muscles still sore from exercise on consecutive days. Rest these areas at least a day between sessions.

29. Stress correct form and technique.

30. Assess the effects of prior sessions before the next workout.

31. Too much rest leads to deconditioning. Those of us who have taken care of in-patients know that just 3 days of bed rest will have the patients so weak they can hardly sit up. Inactivity can lead to an unhealthy cycle.

32. Smile when you exercise even if you want to grimace. Studies at Purdue have shown that you can fool yourself into thinking you are happier than you actually are. The 12 Step programs have a saying "Fake it until you make it." No one wants to spend an hour hearing their own voice tell them how miserable they are. If a fake smile makes the exercise session a little easier, why not? Smiling sure doesn't hurt anything.

33. Consider changing the routine in some fashion every 4 to 6 weeks, so you don't get bored and the muscles don't get so accustomed to the same activity that they don't get as much benefit. With change, different muscle groups are used and there is more balance.

34. Don't do anything painful. I am not talking the soreness that might come from stretching a tired muscle or the discomfort that comes from that extra push. You know the difference between damaging pain and a motivating effort. If it is painful STOP, no matter what the coach says. Therapists in rehab will push you through non-harmful discomfort. That's okay. Don't let anyone make you damage yourself.

The Arthritis Foundation recommends the following paraphrased ways to protect your joints:

1. Move. Exercise protects joints by strengthening surrounding muscles.

2. Try to keep a reasonable weight. The heavier you are, the more stress on your joints.

3. Good posture protects joints.

4. Use the big joints to do big work. Use thighs to lift.

5. Good pacing with alternate periods of rest and activity is better than repetitive stress.

6. Pain tells you something. Listen. The kind of pain Jane Fonda referred to with "No pain, no gain" was the discomfort that comes from using new muscle, or pushing to achieve more stamina. That is not the pain referred to here. Don't overdo and don't exercise when you are in agony.

7. Change positions often to decrease stiffness.

8. Don't overdo after a period of inactivity. The weekend athlete can get hurt. Build up your stamina and endurance. Don't take on activities for which you are unprepared. Slow and steady.

9. Protect joints as needed with pads and other appropriate safety equipment. (Remember helmets. TBI patients do not need any more damage to brain cells.)

PEARL: The Arthritis Foundation, the National Sleep Foundation, the Association for the Blind, and the Lyme Disease Association are superlative advocacy groups. I have worked with all four over the years and my experience has been interaction with a group of dedicated, knowledgeable people with compassion and commonsense. Their missions to educate both the public and the professionals have helped millions.

PEARL: Watch out for sports like basketball and tennis that can be quite hard on the joints in the leg.

V. SLEEP

A long time ago, in a pub in Dublin, while a colleague crooned *Danny Boy,* I pledged my son's hand in marriage to the daughter of a renown sleep expert. We were working on a large, global clinical trial comparing treatments for insomnia. The expert was Tom Roth from Henry Ford Hospital in Detroit and our kids were about two at the time. Since they both had red hair, the engagement just seemed like a good idea. I learned a lot about sleep from Tom and I also learned over the years that after their weight, their depression, and their bowels, there is nothing patients like to complain about more than their inability to sleep. (Of course, in these days of erectile dysfunction, the priorities may have changed.)

Chapter 25: *Ancillary Treatments* discusses what to do if a person is having sleep problems. Here I want to focus on the role of sleep in TBI patients and the fostering of good sleep habits (or sleep hygiene as it might be called in a pub in Dublin).

The National Sleep Foundation has considerable information on its website on ways to foster a good night's sleep. But in Lyme patients it seems as though every imaginable factor is conspiring to disturb the normal sleep pattern. Sleep is critical to healing since all systems, especially the immune system, regenerate during sleep. Only one night of missed sleep can cause insulin resistance, which can increase inflammation and result in all the subsequent inflammatory signs and symptoms. This affects immune response to infection. High nighttime cortisol and inflammatory biochemicals can disturb sleep in Lyme patients. Most healing occurs during sleep including tissue repair, muscle growth, and protein synthesis.

The immune system is greatly impacted by sleep and rest. Immune function is greatly reduced by sleep deprivation. Complex feedback loops involving cytokines such as interleukin-1, produced in response to infection, appear to also play a role in sleep. Therefore the immune response may result in changes in sleep patterns and account for some of the symptoms associated with many infections and other diseases. Likewise, poor sleep can impact the ability of the immune system to mount a full response. Sleep is essential to recovery. If they aren't sleeping, they probably aren't healing.

Sleep problems in TBIs come in several forms: TOO MUCH, TOO LITTLE, and BIZARRE.

Some Lyme patients want to sleep essentially all day, waking only when forced. Note that sleepiness is not the same as weakness or fatigue, which can also be present. Sleepiness is the desire to sleep and the ability to sleep whether or not the situation is appropriate for sleeping. In Lyme this desire to sleep can be present even when the individual apparently slept long enough the previous night. We presume that the extended sleep hours have something to do with the recovery process, but we don't know that for sure. The excessive sleep may be due to an imbalance of biochemicals that are the result of the pathogen or the body's response to the pathogen.

Other TBI patients have trouble falling asleep or staying asleep. Little kids will fight sleep because they are afraid to be alone or they're anxious that they will miss something exciting. If only they knew how truly boring life is after dark for most adults.

We also know that kids, especially teenagers, are chronically sleep deprived. The sleep cycle in teens is skewed in one direction while society forces them in the other direction. Their melatonin often kicks in after midnight, so getting up at 6:30 am to catch the bus results in much dozing off in class. These kids aren't lazy or unmotivated, just sleep deprived. With after-school activities keeping them up and their sleep cycle

not conducive to falling asleep before midnight, we have a major disconnect.

Lyme and other TBIs can be associated with bizarre sleep patterns that go beyond just sleeping too much or too little. These manifestations might include: strange dreams, abnormal postures, immobility, terrors, etc. These conditions should be assessed by a sleep expert, not just by the tech at the local sleep center where they are only looking for sleep apnea. If a TBI is the primary cause, the symptoms are not likely to respond to conventional treatment unless the underlying TBI is also appropriately managed.

Add Lyme to this picture, and the problem becomes even more complicated. Many Lyme patients often have an afternoon energy crash, with severe fatigue and a desire to sleep. Naps and avoidance of processed sugars for lunch may help.

In our frenetic US society, naps have been frowned upon. The Puritan work ethic clearly stated that anyone caught napping was a lazy sluggard and so we all must keep busy at all times. Finally, we are recognizing that a short 15 to 20 minute nap may actually increase productivity. Companies that used to fire an employee on the spot if caught napping, now are installing napping areas.

The NSF says that 85% of mammalian species nap. Einstein, Edison, Napoleon, Churchill, and Kennedy were all nappers. While naps don't make up for inadequate nighttime sleep, a short nap improves mood, alertness, and performance. A nap longer than 20 to 30 minutes will allow the napper to fall into other stages of sleep and could interfere with nighttime sleep. Upon awakening from a prolonged nap, the person might feel groggy, disoriented, sluggish, and confused. Keep naps short to better serve their purpose.

Pleasant rituals like warm, tryptophan-laden milk, warm baths, herbal teas, lavender, gentle backrubs, white noise, and soothing reading, may all promote sleep. The NSF recommends turning off all electronics well in advance of the desired sleep time. Do not exercise or consume caffeine immediately before bedtime. Exercise during the day is helpful in falling asleep and staying asleep at night. Routine is conducive to good sleep hygiene. Going to bed at the same time and getting up at the same time each day is better for overall good sleep habits. While it is nice to dream about, you can't really put sleep into a bank to save for a rainy day. Pretty much, if you missed it, it's gone, except for a minor ability to replace.

PEARL: People sleep better when cool. Researchers at the University of Pittsburgh (which expert Tom Roth says is a good place for assessing complicated sleep issues) have tested a cooling cap that apparently helps sustain sleep. Otherwise, keep the room cool. Better to snuggle under a blanket than to have too high of an ambient temperature. A warm bath will relax the muscles and then the body will rapidly cool off and that will enhance deep sleep. I'm nodding off here.

Chapter 25: *Ancillary Treatments* reviews treatment options for the various sleep problems. With kids whose sleep patterns are greatly impacted by Lyme, consider talking to the school nurse to see if accommodations might be made. You just might get lucky.

PEARL: I am NOT a believer in letting babies cry it out. If I was so scared or confused that I had to scream for hours before I could collapse into an exhausted sleep, I would hold a grudge against those who didn't feel my pain. Many disagree with me. While the NSF recommends sleeping in complete darkness, many little kids and middle sized kids and me, prefer some dim light.

VI. STRESS MANAGEMENT AND EMOTIONAL SUPPORT

Life with Lyme can be a rough road filled with frustration, anxiety, and stress. Martin Seligman, a PhD from the University of Pennsylvania, has clearly established a link between emotion and healing. Attitude affects immunity and the rate of recovery. A patient's level of optimism can significantly influence overall health and well-being. Negative feelings increase cortisol, called the stress hormone, which suppresses the immune system. Therefore emotional support can be critical to the recuperation of TBI patients.

Unfortunately, many TBI patients are beset with neuropsychological manifestations of their disease, especially if they are infected with Bb, Bartonella, or M. *fermentans.* They can feel isolated and asking themselves questions like, "What is the matter with me? Am I crazy? Am I really sick? Does anyone else feel like this? Why did I get so sick when a lot of people get better right away? Why do I have to take so many medicines? Is there any hope? Did I do something wrong?" TBIs can be challenging enough for adults, let alone children trying to cope with feeling bad, while picking up the anxiety of their parents, and getting dismissed by HCPs.

Each patient had a baseline emotional state before she got sick and this baseline will be impacted depending on the severity and duration of the illness. The usual emotional condition prior to illness and the overall effect of the disease will determine what it means to get back to "normal." Well-established science has shown time and again that stress impacts the immune response. Stress can even alter DNA and affect immune function for years. Relaxation and pleasure can ease stress and help reverse any negative effects. The importance of stress management and emotional support cannot be overstated.

Several TBIs cause syndromes that include considerable anxiety, anger, depression, and behavioral changes. There are many modalities for emotional support in the literature that may be used to help Lyme patients and their families.

A. **Psychotherapy** is the treatment of mental and emotional disorders through talk therapy with a trained therapist such as a psychiatrist, psychologist, or social worker. A psychiatrist is a physician who can add medication to the psychotherapy. The goal of the treatment is to identify problems and view these problems realistically, gain insight into thoughts and actions, and change behaviors in a way that allows for better functioning in society including work and school. There are many types of psychotherapy and the best fit will depend on the patient situation and diagnosis.

1. Cognitive Behavioral Therapy - CBT is a type of talk therapy where the treatment is focused on solving problems in the here and now. CBT is underscored by the premise that thoughts can be redirected and behaviors changed. Using a systematic approach, with goal setting, CBT has been found to be especially effective in mood disorders, anxiety, personality problems, dysfunctional relationships, eating disorders, substance abuse, OCD, panic attacks, PTSD, bulimia, depression, insomnia, and phobias. CBT introduces new ways to think about old situations and provides a reality check. The therapist helps the patient to be in control of the situation and focus on the positive. Tools and techniques are introduced to help the patient cope with everyday situations, such as exposure therapy used to help with phobias and the thought recognition and acceptance modalities used in OCD. Usually a combination of tactics is used to get the patient fully functional.

In contrast to psychoanalysis that probes the underlying causes of thoughts and behaviors buried deep in the past, CBT focuses on getting rid of unwanted thoughts and actions to improve QOL and the ability to function in real world situations. Where psychoanalysis asks "Why?" CBT asks, "Who cares about why? How do I cope or change?" CBT worries less about understanding and more about adjusting.

Emotional problems due to TBIs are biochemical and so cannot be talked away. Nonetheless, CBT can provide tools that allows for more normal functioning until the underlying pathophysiology can be corrected. For many Lyme patients, CBT has been life-changing. Symptoms caused by TBIs can be managed with CBT, but treatment of the underlying pathogen will be the best way to eradicate the problem completely.

Patients are taught that they can choose thoughts and behaviors. CBT is often short-term therapy and the patient actively participates both inside and outside formal sessions. Homework might be assigned with skills to practice and material to read. The goal is to solve day-to-day problems step-by-step. CBT is very effective in motivated patients and can be used as an adjunct to a number of other treatment modalities.

2. Person Centered Therapy is talk therapy where the therapist is a facilitator creating a comfortable, non-judgmental environment of empathy and unconditional positive reinforcement. This approach is non-directive and the patient finds his own solutions to psychological and behavioral issues. The counselor does not diagnose or treat. This form of psychotherapy is effective and popular but may not be directive enough for children.

3. Many other approaches such as psychoanalysis are available. Considered the creation of Freud and his contemporaries, this form of therapy is less common than it once was. Analysis investigates the underlying causes of psychological discomfort using patient history, interpretation of dreams, and examination of the conscious and unconscious in order to bring up repressed feelings and unresolved conflicts. In contrast to CBT, analysis struggles to find the underlying causes of thoughts and behaviors and may take years of therapy. The therapist must be specially trained. This is not the type of counseling usually recommended for patients with TBI-induced emotional and behavioral problems, since in those cases we believe the underlying cause of the discomfort is the TBI infection. Psychoanalysis is included here since it is the form of therapy that might be the most familiar to readers and as a basis of comparison for other techniques. In current psychiatric practice, many therapists use tools from different approaches to help patients.

B. **Meditation:** A term used to describe a myriad of techniques used to clear the mind and bring on a peaceful inner milieu. Most approaches use a focus on the breath or a selected word or mantra to help settle the thoughts. Meditation takes practice and some folks never master the techniques, usually because they are trying too hard. When outside thoughts intrude in the practice, and they do with everyone, they are to be recognized and released. This is easier said than done and rumor has it that even the Dalai Lama ruminates on his shopping list from time to time.

Since the Beatles helped popularize meditation in Western culture in the 1960s, many scientific studies have confirmed that meditators do enter an altered state of consciousness that apparently has many measurable effects.

Considerable science supports the multiple health benefits. PET scans, recordings of brain waves, and measurements of immune molecules and other biochemicals have consistently demonstrated the positive results. Meditation is associated with mental tranquility and the reduction of anxiety and depression. Regular practice has been linked to lower blood pressure, heart rate, and respiratory rate, better concentration and focus, and more rapid and complete resolution of many medical conditions from infections to heart disease to cancer. With practice, the brain is said to be more active while cognition, memory, and attention all may improve. Meditation appears to take one's baseline attitude and kick it up a positive notch.

PEARL: Just two minutes of meditation lowers cortisol levels.

Transcendental Meditation, or TM, is one of the more familiar meditative practices. In the 70s TM was a big business as college kids flocked to classes to learn how to "do it." The student was to sit quietly for 20 minutes twice a day and using a unique mantra, practice clearing the mind. We never knew if our mantra was actually unique since we swore not to tell anyone.

Mantras can be meaningless sounds such as la, or traditionally sacred words such as om, selected so as not to distract the meditator. Mantras can also be a word such as peace, serenity, or hope, selected to steer the practitioner into a positive mind set. The author of *Eat, Pray, Love* took months to find a workable mantra. When she shared this mantra (something like ham-sha) which she felt represented the sound of her breath going in and out, I could not stop thinking about ham sandwiches, which didn't help my practice in the least.

The breathing in meditation tends to be different from the deep breathing of the exercises described earlier. While the breath is often the focus in meditation, breathing often becomes shallow and in some experienced practitioners, barely perceptible.

Meditation is an integral part of most religions, using the quiet mind to allow in God's message. For many years, a number of Christian traditions felt that meditation was a subversive practice and church members were warned away. The restrictions have been loosened especially since repetitive prayers like the Rosary were found to induce a meditative state. Most religions now recognize the quieting of the mind as a means of spiritual communication and nothing to fear.

Meditation can be a part of yoga practice and now is often incorporated into other exercises like walking meditation. Tea ceremonies are often adjuncts to meditation. We are now learning that the previously-prescribed, rigid 20 minutes twice a day is not necessary to garner benefit and 5 minutes once a day or 3 minutes twice a day and all manner of other variations are also beneficial. The most benefit does seem to come from doing something meditative each day. There is no need to berate yourself for never "transcending" the mundane conscious world. No longer is the lotus position *de rigueur* or the pre-practice food restrictions. Patients can benefit from meditation in all kinds of ways.

Kids tend to like to learn to meditate but for young kids a regular practice may be unrealistic. For some patients with OCD, meditation can be nerve-wracking since the more they struggle to clear the mind, the more the thoughts intrude. They can feel frustrated and inept. For these people a short session of focused breathing might be preferable. There is so little downside to meditation that consideration of even a trial-run might prove helpful.

C. **Hypnosis:** An induced mental state where the person is feeling calm and relaxed. In reality, she is in a heightened state of awareness where she is more susceptible to instruction and suggestion. The subject can concentrate intensely on one thought while blocking out distractions. The hypnotic state or trance can be induced by a hypnotherapist or self-generated. During hypnosis the subject is fully awake and focuses on one idea with decreased awareness of surroundings.

There is considerable scientific documentation regarding the effect of hypnosis. Hypnosis has contributed to the improvement of IBS, pain, anxiety disorders, and skin disease. Changes in brain activity have been documented. Throughout the process, the subject always has free will and doesn't lose control of her own behavior.

Hypnosis decreases anxiety and has been successful in changing habits such as smoking and overeating because the subject is more receptive to positive suggestions. Smokers have a 20% to 30% chance of stopping with hypnosis, which is similar to other stop-smoking programs. When hypnosis is used in conjunction with other quitting plans, the odds of success are greater than for either modality alone.

Hypnosis is often used as an adjunct to CBT, making the patient more receptive to the suggestions made by the therapist. Likewise, CBT can make people who are hypnotized more receptive to suggestions made by the hypnotist. Used together, these two supportive techniques can be very powerful.

There are many misconceptions about hypnosis. The subject is always in control of behavior and morals do not become loose and personality does not change while in a trance. One controversial aspect of hypnosis involves the concept of retrieved memories. Subjects have remembered things that they were not aware of when in their normal conscious states, such as sexual molestation and abuse. In at least a few cases, these retrieved memories may not represent actual events. A number of individuals were accused of crimes they did not commit. Others used the unreliability of retrieved memories as a defense, when they may have been guilty. Some authorities think that the therapists may have been too strong in making suggestions and false memories were planted in the subjects.

In TBI patients we aren't trying to retrieve memories, but rather bolster the ability to cope with their disease. Hypnosis should improve focus and concentration and allow the patient to be more receptive to modifying thoughts and behaviors. Hypnosis can increase positive expectations and motivation to either adopt healthy habits or at least reduce the number of bad choices. A healthier lifestyle should improve the chance of healing and recovery.

D. **Visualization:** Also called imagery, visualization is a means to imagine oneself well or symptom-free or in any number of alternate scenarios. This technique can be incorporated into meditation, deep breathing, yoga, or other practices. The images can be those of the patient in a better state of health or of pleasant scenes like a forest, waterfall, or ocean to induce tranquility. With kids, I have suggested imagining puppies with round tummies or pink bubbles floating through clouds. Visualization has been known to decrease pain, improve acne, increase healing, diminish arthritis, and provide relief for headaches, heart disease, ulcers, and UTIs. Important for TBI patients, visualization can decrease stress and anxiety and improve mood. Cancer patients and those with chronic infections have been told to imagine white cells roaming though the circulation, gobbling up disease. This type of imagery seems to have positive results. Free and easy, the only caution around visualization is to not focus on negative images. Patients with TBIs can be guided to imagine themselves healed.

E. **Yoga:** Yoga has been described at length in the previous *Exercise* section. Yoga is known worldwide and has been practiced for millennia because of the many ways it improves mood, sleep, and sense of well-being. For stress management and emotional support of TBI patients, yoga should always be high on the list.

F. **Anger management:** TBI patients with Bartonella, Borrelia, or M. *fermentans* infections can suffer with anger and hostility. If you see rage, think Bartonella. Some of these patients become violent. In these cases, the rage is due to infection that alters the normal physiology. Only treatment of the underlying cause will eradicate the problem. In the meantime, these people need to live in society and while we are figuring out what is really going on, they need ways to manage the anger. They require tools to be able to handle relationships at home, in school, and at work. While we have all been counseled that it isn't healthy to hold anger in, these individuals can behave uncontrollably with irrational raving, and more than a few have ended up in jail. Anger management should be considered early in the treatment process before someone gets hurt. This type of support is often a part of CBT, but there are also HCPs who specialize in the control of anger, oppositional behavior, and hostility. Please address any underlying infectious process, if appropriate.

G. **Socializing:** Having a positive social life can be very affirming. A recent study of men's health showed that one of the best predictors of longevity was strong friendships. Unfortunately, many Lyme patients don't feel well enough to go out and be social. Instead, consider inviting friends over where you can control the time and level of activity. Here is a good place for family to come in and interact with the patient. By now, the caregivers could probably use a little social interaction themselves. Spend time with others outside the Lyme setting. While other Lyme patients can provide tremendous support, do not allow your life to become all Lyme all the time. Make a conscious effort NOT to talk about Lyme with friends who do not have the disease. They will tire of that topic quickly. There is a whole world out there that does not revolve around Lyme. Explore this world with other people. Social media is not the same as interactions with real people. Recent studies have shown that too much social media may lead to isolation, inability to converse on the most basic levels, and difficulty making decisions because of information overload. Many times when you REALLY don't feel like going out, once you get out there, you're glad you went.

H. **Music therapy:** The use of music for healing can be said to have started around 900 CE when the Persian-Turk, Alpharabius, wrote about the therapeutic effect of music on the soul. Since the 1600s, healers have recognized that music and dance help alleviate mental illness, especially depression. Today, there are certified music therapists who use all aspects of music from creation, to active participation, to passive listening, in order to improve physical, emotional, mental, social, and spiritual health. Physiologic changes are measurable when a person listens to music.

Music therapy increases mental functioning including cognition, motivation, emotional development, behavior, and social skills. All this combines to improve the patient's QOL. Music is especially useful for rehabilitation after brain damage. In these cases, music appears to retrain the injured brain. We know that a number of TBIs damage the brain.

From the perspective of development, music enhances communication skills including the ability to express emotions and connect with others. Music has been able to reach some who were previously thought to be impenetrable. Music may be able to be of value in TBI patients in areas such as anxiety, mood, and depression. Music can increase motivation and stabilize emotions. Some people say that music enables them to express themselves and vent in a healthy way. Research has shown that the more impaired a brain damaged person is to begin with, the more benefit from music therapy. Further, the earlier the music therapy is started after the brain injury, the more help it brings, especially in areas of motor impairment, improved gait, and coordination. Music decreases anxiety, hostility, and fatigue. Music also provides the opportunity for social interaction. Playing music with others fosters cooperation, teamwork, a sense of accomplishment, and confidence. Remember that music can also reinforce sad emotions, as anyone who has ever listened to a true country-western song can attest.

I. **Gardening:** Horticultural therapy is an official clinical process with measurable objectives and outcomes. Trained therapists address behavioral problems. Universities have degree programs educating therapists to use gardening to induce the relaxation response and to decrease stress, anxiety, and violence. Even the color green is thought to be the most relaxing of colors. Usually this approach is done outdoors but sessions can be conducted in greenhouses as well, or even on a windowsill. Horticultural therapy has been used effectively in weight management, rehabilitation after brain injury, developmental delay, and to improve agility and coordination. Gardening can be done solo or as part of a group. Hoeing and weeding are good ways to release frustrations and vent emotions. Even very young children can appreciate a seed sprouting and growing into a sturdy plant. Progress is easy to see. Chronically ill kids have been shown to benefit from having a plant to care for. They can relate to how the plant needs water, light, and food to stay healthy. I found only a few references to gardening as therapy for Lyme patients, but this approach seems to be a simple, easy way to get positive results with very little downside. (Watch for ticks!)

J. **Art therapy:** This form of psychotherapy helps the patient to communicate, recognize feelings, and vent in a constructive way. People who have been sick for a long time often have considerable frustration and appreciate a means to express their feelings. Art therapy helps patients cope with symptoms, identify family dynamics, decrease stress, increase cognition, and allows the pure pleasure afforded by the creative process. Art can help improve relationships, resolve conflict, improve social and interpersonal skills, and manage behavior. Chronic TBI patients or those with significant neuropsychiatric symptoms may benefit from such an outlet.

K. Journaling: Keeping a dairy or journal of thoughts and feelings about life events can help some patients. The journal would not be just a log or chronology, but a record of perceptions and emotions. Journals have been especially useful in chronic illnesses as a way to vent frustrations, disappointments, boredom, and anger. The journal is best kept in confidence so the writer can feel free to express any emotion, even those that would not be politically correct if they were voiced aloud. Journals help patients identify feelings and gain self-knowledge. They help with problem-solving by the construction of pro and con lists. Decision-making can be clearer through brainstorming of options and identification of solutions. Writing can help process trauma, as I learned in working with torture survivors in my other life. Some of the literature recommends writing a letter to a person who has hurt you and then never mailing the letter. The emotions are released with no more damage done. Journaling uses both sides of the brain and over time improves cognition and concentration. Studies have shown that journaling decreases the symptoms of asthma and arthritis, increases immune response, and decreases stress. Journaling seems to be associated with healing and has been shown to increase T cells and decrease pathogen load. Journaling helps clear a cluttered mind. Recent examinations of the benefits of keeping a gratitude list have shown similar positive benefits.

Journaling can be especially helpful to those who are bedridden. There can be downsides to journaling if the entries are all negative or if the person is being forced to keep a diary "for their own good." Perfectionists can be more worried about who will read their writings after they're gone and how they will be perceived than in actually expressing their true feelings. Journaling is something you either love or hate. While some kids may see journaling as a record of their dramatic life, others would view journaling as a punishment, a heinous chore worse than homework. As with all these supportive measures, select those that may be helpful and let the rest sit. Maybe they will be useful some other time.

L. Affirmations: Statements declared to be true now or are hoped will be true in the future. Declarations such as, " I am well" or "I am fit," can be repeated over and over, either silently, aloud, or written, until they engram into the psyche. These positive reinforcing statements can be used alone or as adjuncts to other therapies such as hypnosis or meditation. "Every day, I'm getting better." "Today, I can take 100 more steps." "I believe." Affirmations can also be used as mantras during meditation, if they don't inspire deep thinking.

PEARL: One curmudgeon author derides affirmations as personal propaganda, lies we tell ourselves, that are especially harmful to those with low self-esteem. I say if it helps and doesn't hurt, try it. If affirmations aren't right for a particular person, put them aside. Positive affirmations can be used as mantras in meditation.

M. Breathing: Focused or conscious breathing can mitigate anxiety and stress as well as improve mood and enhance healing. Whether deep, as in diaphragmatic breathing, or shallow and aware as in meditation, conscious breathing alone, or as an adjunct to just about any other modality, is beneficial. Even a few minutes once or twice a day of focused breathing has been shown to be beneficial.

N. Biofeedback: An increasingly accepted modality, biofeedback is used to treat pain and anxiety and a number of physiologic parameters. The patient is connected to an instrument that monitors things such as heart rate, temperature, brain waves, muscle contraction, or respiration. By becoming aware of one parameter, the person can be trained to voluntarily control an associated factor. For example, if the patient is learning to manage anxiety, and the heart rate increases with the degree of anxiety, the patient can then learn to control the heart rate through feedback from the monitoring instrument. As the heart rate is lowered, so is the corresponding anxiety. Biofeedback has the potential to help with a number of TBI-associated issues including behavior and emotional problems. Although home units are available, biofeedback is best managed, at least initially, by a trained professional.

O. Acupuncture: Usually a component of TCM, acupuncture has been gaining more acceptance in western culture and studies are underway to determine why these techniques work in many patients. Acupuncture involves the insertion and manipulation of needles into the body, usually at specific locations, depending on the condition being treated. The needle insertion is thought to redirect and balance energy, although detractors think any response is due to a placebo-effect. Additional information on acupuncture is provided in Chapter 26: *Alternative Treatments.*

P. Massage: The manipulation of superficial and deep layers of muscle and connective tissue to enhance function and healing and to promote relaxation and well-being. Massage is performed by a number of types of HCPs, PTs, trainers, and certified massage therapists. There are more than 80 variations, from the massage of newborns to hot rock massage. The pressure varies and the lymph system and internal organs can also be affected. Usually massage feels good, but care must be taken to be gentle with Lyme patients who might have very tender muscles and joints.

Deep tissue massage has been found to lower levels of the stress hormone cortisol and increase WBC counts. Even a light massage has been shown to boost oxytocin, the neurotransmitter associated with contentment.

Massage can be beneficial for pain relief, relaxation of muscle tension, stress reduction, and the lowering of BP and HR, after just one session. Multiple sessions reduce pain, anxiety, and depression. EEGs and scans show increased perfusion and mental alertness and a decrease in stress hormones. Immune function is stimulated by increasing the number of lymphocytes.

Q. **Time management:** Chaos in life causes stress. Organizational skills, keeping an accurate calendar, and removal of clutter all lessen anxiety. Now, we don't expect a 3 y/o to be worrying about time management. Caretakers will need to be doing that for him. Older kids can start to manage their time in a way that reduces stress. Routines help decrease the stress of decision-making. Furthermore, lowering the stress baseline in the caregiver will lower the anxiety in the patient. Lower stress means a more normal body biochemistry and a better chance to heal.

One time management technique that even young kids can use and that I used with this book, when I didn't think I could sit at the computer one more minute, was the **Pomodoro method**. Developed by Francesco Cirillo and named after the red Italian pomodoro tomato, this method just makes sense. With my interpretation of the Pomodoro method, the participant commits to focusing on a task for a selected amount of time: 5, 10, 20, 30 minutes. Then there is a scheduled break. So no matter how miserable you are, you only have to do the task for another 20 minutes and then you have 5 minutes all to yourself to do whatever you want. I mostly went to the bathroom but that was good enough for me. Then you go back to work for another 20 minutes before break time.

During the time you are on task that is all you do. You do not look on the web for timber-framing courses, or at Facebook to see if that goof from elementary school is now a Rhodes scholar, you just do the task. Anything else that comes to mind you just put aside until the next break time. Then if you choose to look up the goof from grade school feel free, but I bet you'd rather go to the bathroom. Again, during the work time, you work. Nothing but the task until the break. Of course, if the house

is on fire, you have my permission to do something else, but otherwise stick with it.

At least to start, set a small enough time so that you can make it to the break without too much angst. The amount of time spent at work and on break will depend on age and severity of illness in the TBI population. Soon you will be able to spend more time working, confident that your break will really come.

I find when I use this approach, I am not wondering after 12 hours of work why I got so little done. Pomodoro helps you to keep the time from frittering away and helps prevent you from finding every reason under the sun to get distracted. The break is coming. This approach might help those TBI patients who have difficulty concentrating. You might have to start with two minutes on and one minute off, but you'd be surprised what can be done in two minutes by a kid who hasn't been able to accomplish anything for months.

R. **Humor:** I despise the movie *Patch Adams*, but then again so did the real Patch Adams. This movie tells the story of a physician who used humor to connect with patients. I agree with Adams' belief that HCPs must connect with patients and nurture the spirit, but I believe that you can do that without being so darn annoying. Patch also seemed to have all the time in the world to rehearse his comedy act. Actually, humor and laughter have proven to be extremely therapeutic. Laughter has been used to resolve both physical and emotional pain, relieve stress, help the chronically ill cope, accelerate healing, boost immune response with higher levels of B and T cells, decrease BP, lower stress hormones, and modulate interferons and endorphins. Laughter raises pain tolerance by submerging the brain in endorphins, those endogenous opioids that mute pain.

From *Groundhog Day* to *Shrek* to *Toy Story* and *Caddyshack*, there are a million funny movies. On TV, there are a number of comedies that are appropriate for kids of all ages including *I Love Lucy, Andy Griffith, The Cosby Show*, and *The Three Stooges* to name a few. (No, we didn't all grow up deranged from watching *The Three Stooges*.) Of course, there's always *Looney Tunes* and *Sponge Bob*. Kids love joke books and puns. The local library is full of these books and CDs.

S. **Reading:** Reading can provide solace to many patients. Good literature can help distract the patient as well as provide companionship and a sense of connection to others like you. While Mary Karr asks if "poetry is just a trick played on smart people," many find great pleasure and comfort in poetry. While self-help books can provide insight and useful pointers on how to navigate through life, they can also make the reader feel inadequate and frustrated. Some are too pessimistic and some are too simplistic. Those that are relentlessly cheerful are not only unrealistic, they're annoying. Read for pleasure and release, not for perpetual self-improvement. I have never seen a favorite book list that did not include *To Kill a Mockingbird*. Although somewhat dark, sick teens might find eventual consolation in *The Catcher in the Rye*.

T. **Nature:** We don't need scientific evidence to prove that spending time in nature is emotionally fortifying. We know it is. Unfortunately, spending time in nature is probably what got us in this mess in the first place. Review Chapter 32: *Prevention* and then go outside and run amok.

VII. GROUP THERAPY

Group therapy is a form of psychotherapy where a small group of patients meet to discuss common issues in strict confidence. Guided by an experienced counselor, the purpose is to gain insight into shared concerns, discuss options, and provide support. Lyme can be very isolating and being part of a group can help many patients. The role of the therapist is to keep one person from monopolizing the discussion, prevent misinformation from being presented as fact, steer the discourse so that the tone is not all negative, and to keep on topic. While the social connections may help some patients, others are uncomfortable in the group setting and do better with individual counseling.

VIII. FAMILY THERAPY

When one family member gets Lyme, the whole family can suffer. Especially when the patient is told it is all in her head or there is no such thing as chronic Lyme, the family can start to get frustrated, defensive, and paranoid. In a number of cases, one parent pits against another: one side saying the child is too sick to go to school or feed herself and the other saying, "She doesn't have anything that a good kick in the butt wouldn't cure." Sometimes siblings get less attention than "the sick one" and this can cause resentment. Life starts to revolve around Lyme and that isn't healthy. There is always some degree of anxiety and depression embedded with chronic illness and family therapy may be beneficial in redirecting the negative energy. If there ever was a time when a family needed to have one another's backs it is when they are going from doctor to doctor to doctor, desperate for help. Caregivers on duty 24/7 can have incredible stress and parents can feel guilty for allowing their child to get sick. Think family therapy sooner rather than later.

IX. SOCIAL MEDIA

Use of social media like blogs, chat rooms, and tweets are used by many people as a kind of group therapy without the therapist. BUT the lack of professional guidance can be a big problem. In researching this text, I have read thousands of pages of social media surrounding Lyme. While many people who post do so with the best of intentions, to share information or provide support, others are not so noble. More than a few posters get stuck in their own story, ruminating the same points over and over and over. The negativity can be contagious. While venting can be beneficial for Lyme patients, proceed with caution on these sites. A number of posts that seem sympathetic are covers for scams. Much information presented as fact is wrong, either intentionally or out of ignorance. Much of the discourse is obsessed with the past instead of addressing current issues. Once immersed in the negative, it can be hard to resurface. I reached a point where I could not read one more blog. I was surprised at some of the authors who identified themselves. A number were educated professionals who had bought into conspiracy theories about the government taking over the country through tick warfare or using Lyme to starve us all to death. Even though the ideas were irrational, many people had signed on hook, line, and sinker. The writing can be sexist, racist, and just plain bizarre. When you live all day in the asylum, the inmates start to appear normal. Communicating on Facebook is not the same as talking to a real human. Use a limited amount of social media for entertainment, comfort, encouragement, support, or emotional release only. These people are not real friends and they certainly are not your HCPs. Be very careful.

PEARL: The LDASEPA intern has a blog where she provides information to family and friends about her condition. She finds this an efficient way to communicate since it keeps her connected without having to repeat the answer to the question, "How are you?" over and over.

X. ADVOCACY GROUPS

Advocacy groups such as the LDA, Time for Lyme, CALDA (Lymedisease.org), and LDASEPA, are ready with information, referrals, and support. If you have reached a dead end, check the websites of these organizations to see if there is another option that you might not have considered. Contact your local organization to see how your involvement might be of mutual benefit. Patients may want to participate in supporting their local advocacy group.

XI. SPIRITUAL SUPPORT

If there is any topic more controversial than Lyme, then it must be religion. This section is included because many patients find solace in communication with God. Spirituality is a sense of peace or a positive feeling of connection to a higher being or to others. Although hard to measure, spirituality has been associated with higher CD4 levels and lower pathogen loads.

Spirituality may help with attitude and optimism. Numerous studies have demonstrated that a genuine feeling of gratitude can enhance the healing process. Spirituality can give a person an emotional foundation on which to build her opposition to her disease. Sometimes the feeling that God is in their corner can be empowering. People who believe they have a life purpose live longer. If spirituality results in inner peace, strength, serenity, positive attitude, and optimism, then more power to it.

In terms of patients, spiritual practice can be quite diverse:

A. **Individual prayer**: Communication with God can take a number of forms in which people pray to praise God, thank God, request forgiveness of sins, or ask for help or favors. When dealing with sick patients, many prayers take the form of requests for healing or relief from symptoms. Some say that praying is talking to God and mediation is God talking back. Meditation allows the brain to quiet down enough to listen. Unfortunately prayer can impede progress if the patients get too into "turning everything over to God" and then using that as an excuse to do nothing to help themselves. Which of us hasn't bargained with God? "God, if you will only make my child well, I will tithe 20% of my income forever." And we actually think God doesn't see right through these amateur negotiations.

B. **Group prayer**: Here we get more into organized religion than individual spirituality. A number of people find comfort in the social support they garner from being in a spiritual group. Essentially all religions call on God(s) to help the sick. Sometimes people look to clergy for counseling, which can be good if the clergy has been trained and is experienced in this area. With regard to Lyme disease, clergy might be able to help families cope in answering the question about why bad things happen to innocent people. Parents might benefit from discussions around forgiving themselves for things over which they had no control.

C. **Others praying for you**: This is an interesting area where the science is all over the place. Numerous recent studies have shown that praying for patients who are completely unaware of the prayers results in 1) a significant improvement in their condition, 2) a significant deterioration in their condition, or 3) absolutely nothing. The difficulty in finding matching populations for comparison and the size of the study group needed to make a valid assessment will keep this debate active for a long time. I was raised Catholic and Catholics spend a lot of time praying for the living and the dead. I confess to being a tad unnerved when I recently learned that the Catholic church was outsourcing some of its prayer requests to Hindus in India. The contract was won by the lowest bidder. This introduces a number of interesting questions. Is the God prayed to the God of the prayer or the prayee? Is there an extra charge for addressing both deities? Since Hindus have thousands of gods, is there a discount for multiple intercessions? Which plan has the best return on investment? Do you get your money back if the prayer doesn't work?

Spirituality may help TBI patients who are comfortable with this type of support. No one should be forced to participate in ways that make her nervous or pressured. You can take someone to a specific place of worship, but you cannot coerce belief.

XII. PASSIONS

Patients can be encouraged to develop a hobby or interest that gives them a reason to be committed and enthusiastic. Chronic illness can be disheartening and tedious: Day after day of pills and drops and cool compresses and tea and changing sweaty sheets. Whether the passion is Lady Gaga, or a hamster, or a hamster named Lady Gaga, encourage the person to pursue something she can get excited about. With kids this can change frequently, but that can be fun, too.

XIII. LITTLE THINGS

In support of TBI patients do all those things that might help them feel better. Within reason. A blanket when they're cold or mittens or warm packs. Ice chips when they're hot. Turn down the music and the lights. The sheet just might be too scratchy. Dark glasses might help. The texture of the food might be unappealing, not because she's a spoiled brat, but because her sensory integration is out of whack.

XIV. HEALTHY HABITS

In all my years of patient care, I only had one official complaint from a patient. Apparently, I had the audacity to suggest to a woman with severe pneumonia in the Fort Dix ER, that she might want to consider cutting back on her 2-pack-a-day smoking habit. She saw no connection between her COPD, her bilateral pneumonia, and her smoking. She saw no possibility that smoking might impede her recovery.

We all know what the healthy habits are. In the 1960s, cigarettes were advertised as a health aid that cleaned the lungs. For decades patients used the excuse that their doctors never told them that a certain habit was bad. If they weren't specifically told to stop, the behavior must be sanctioned by their doctor. My mom's former physician sat with her in his back office where they smoked and ate M&Ms. They had a great time together as she went blind and developed kidney failure, cancer, UC, chronic pain, and diabetes. The sugar and the smoking must be okay if the doctor was also addicted.

Today, excuses that anyone is ignorant of the consequences of drugs, alcohol, sniffing, snorting, processed foods, trans fats, no exercise, unprotected sex, are no longer valid. You can have the greatest treatment plan ever for your TBI patients and they just aren't going to do well if they are compromising themselves with poor health choices.

Simply put, if you are trying to recover from a TBI there should be little or no alcohol, no recreational drugs, no medicines not prescribed for you, no snorting and no sniffing. There must be at least minimal attempts for physical and mental stimulation.

Caffeine should be weaned. Look for caffeine in coffee, tea, and chocolate. Teens and college students are big on energy drinks and caffeine pills to stay awake. If they are drinking a lot of these they should wean, not just quit.

Make good food choices. Avoid toxins like BPA in plastics. Manage stress. Although a single bad habit is damaging, more than one will have cumulative effects and further diminish healing capacity. Pursue whatever help you need to work away from the bad habits. This may require anything from a 12-Step program to nicotine gum to a physical therapist. There are plenty of bad choices being made that can potentially be altered.

Encouraging the discontinuation of bad health choices is not a moral judgment by the HCP onto the patient. The goal should be to give each patient the best opportunity to heal. Avoid anything that wears you out or runs you down. Be vigilant for self-medicating patients. Making good choices will give the best chance for recovery.

Chapter 28

UNDERSTANDING THE
HERXHEIMER REACTION

I just felt like poisoning a monk.

Umberto Eco

Jarisch-Herxheimer Reaction, Herx, Die-off reaction,
Healing crisis, J-H, JHR,
Herxheimer Effect, Herxheimer Response

INTRODUCTION

When I first started seeing TBI cases in preceptorships, patients and parents were throwing around a term that I did not know. Four-year-olds were talking about "my Herx" and "his Herx." Apparently, a "Herx" always belonged to someone. I heard about "Joey's Herx" or "Emily's Herx" or the severity of a patient's last Herx. As is my nature, I was always empathetic and I nodded with concern. In truth, I had no idea what they were talking about. Nothing builds the ego like being out-maneuvered in medical terminology by a first grader. Of course, to eliminate the possibility of being identified as an impostor, I ran to look up the Herxheimer reaction.

The official name of this phenomenon is the Jarisch-Herxheimer Reaction, but it is more often referred to as the Herxheimer reaction or the Herx. Simply defined, some patients feel worse before they feel better after being started on treatment. Some feel much worse. Therapies that most often trigger a Herx reaction are those that actually kill some of the infectious organisms. For this reason, the Herx is sometimes referred to as a die-off response or a healing crisis.

The Herx reaction has been documented in other diseases such as syphilis. The causative agents for syphilis and borreliosis are both spirochetes. This treatment response was first described by an Austrian physician, Adolf Jarisch in 1895, who worked primarily with syphilitic skin lesions. He and Karl Herxheimer discovered that not only did treated patients experience renewed symptoms such as fever, chills, sweating, and nausea, but also the syphilitic skin lesions became bigger and more inflamed. These physicians noted that the more severe the reaction, the faster and more complete the eventual recovery.

I.   THEORIES ON PATHOPHYSIOLOGY

Over the years, theories have been formulated to explain the pathophysiology of the Herx reaction. Although a Herx response can feel terrible, the Herx is considered a normal response by the body when a large number of pathogens are being killed. These pathogens are thought to contain endotoxins. An endotoxin is a poison that is part of the structure (usually the cell wall) of a pathogenic organism. When that bacterium is killed, its cell lyses or breaks apart. Then the toxin is free to enter the circulation of the host.

The body recognizes foreign matter in the system and mobilizes to get rid of the broken cells and toxins. Even though the body tries to eliminate these poisons as fast as it can, it can't always keep up. In fact, as white cells gobble up the damaged bacteria, more toxin can be released as the cells are broken apart. Two things are happening here that can cause the increase in symptoms seen in a Herx.

First, the body's immune defense system is triggered. These natural protective mechanisms initiate a mind-boggling cascade of responses simultaneously. Many chemicals are released into the bloodstream that mobilize cells whose function is to clean up the dead bacteria and other debris. During a Herxheimer reaction, rapid increases in inflammatory cytokines, TNF-α, and various ILs have been measured.

PEARL: Both TNF-α and immune complexes have been implicated in the instigation and severity of the Herx reaction.

Broken cells that have released toxins are targeted as foreign and marked for phagocytosis (gobbling done by the body's clean-up crew). This kind of response causes the well-known signs and symptoms of inflammation. These are often the same signs and symptoms recognized as indicators of a Herx reaction and include fevers, pain, headache, and muscle and body aches.

Second, toxins from the broken pathogen are also roaming in the host's circulatory system. Poisons are usually detoxified in the liver and to a lesser extent in the kidney. Because detoxification is based on chemical reactions and there are only so many enzymes and reagents to catalyze these reactions, these assembly lines can get backed up. The toxins circulate and congregate as they wait their turn for annihilation. Remember these are the same endotoxins that contributed to the symptoms of the disease in the first place. Therefore, it is not surprising that some of the symptoms associated with a Herx reaction are the same as those of the actual disease process.

Once detoxified, these end-products are eliminated by the body's usual elimination processes. Depending on the chemical nature of these products, they may leave the body through urine, stool, respiration, or skin. That is why drinking plenty of fluids is often recommended during a Herx, since water will help with the internal flush needed to eliminate the endotoxins as quickly as possible.

There are at least two reasons for a patient to have symptoms during a Herx reaction: the usual symptoms that might be expected from an enhanced inflammatory process, and the symptoms associated with the toxins from the original specific infectious pathogen. This could explain why many Herx reactions have common symptoms of general inflammation along with symptoms aligned with the specific underlying disease process.

So there is good logic behind why some Herx signs and symptoms are common to all sufferers, while others are more individual. For example, both a Herx in a syphilitic patient and a Herx in a Lyme patient might have similar generalized fatigue, headache, apprehension, and low-grade fever, but then each could have symptoms more in line with their particular spirochete. For example, a patient with a Herx after treatment for syphilis might have worsening skin lesions, while a Lyme Herx might be expressed in more joint pain. Therefore, a combination of the body's immune reaction and the effect of the toxins are likely responsible for the increase in symptoms seen in a Herx reaction. Of course, all this is pathophysiologic speculation, but it does fit into the patterns observed with many Herx responses.

In general, the more killed and broken bacteria, the more toxin is set loose and the more inflammation is needed to respond and, therefore, the more intense the Herx. The Herx can be severe in patients who have a high bacterial load or if effective treatment is initiated when many of the Bb are in vulnerable life stages. A Herx is not always observed and a number of improving patients with effective therapy never experience a Herx. As with all these phenomena, individuality is the key to response. For patients who have previously experienced a Herx, the next Herx may be similar or totally different.

PEARL: The Herx reaction provides the best evidence in support of the active infection theory of chronic Lyme. How

could there be a kill-off reaction if there is nothing alive to kill off? Would the immune system suddenly burst into activity without any prompting? Why would Herx reactions only occur after antibiotics are started or adjusted? What would account for Herx sxs beyond those of general inflammation if not for the toxins released by the dying pathogens?

PEARL: A Herx reaction is the OPPOSITE of a flare although they can look alike. A Herx reaction is due to spirochetes dying. A flare is due to spirochetes living.

PEARL: Why do some patients Herx and others do not, all things being equal? Could the occurrence of a Herx be due to the life stage of the majority of the organisms at the time of the introduction of the antibiotic? We just don't know. This question troubles Doug Fearn from LDASEPA. Are the pathogens in all their various life forms concurrently? Does a Herx occur only when a certain level of Bb are in the spirochetal form? Is there some sort of threshold that has to be crossed? How do the encysted Bb know when the coast is clear? Is there a minimal number of the free-floating form needed to trigger a Herx? Would this explain the varying intensities of different Herx episodes? A Herx might present only when a minimum number of microbes are involved in the kill-off. Does this phenomenon involve biofilms and quorum sensing? Imagine, this all might be clear in a few years. As you might imagine, Doug is even less fun at a party than me.

II. CLINICAL COURSE

Herx reactions have been identified within hours of the start of treatment, but some may not manifest for weeks. The usual time before recognition of a Herx is 2 to 4 days. Some symptoms might occur sporadically throughout the Herx, while others can remain for the duration. For a number of patients on a longer course of antibiotics, the Herx may wax and wane. The symptoms may occur cyclically, say every 4 weeks. In Lyme, this pattern may be due to the spirochete burrowing within host tissue, corresponding to limits on how much access the antibiotic has to the pathogen. Or, the Herx cycles can occur in association with the particular life stage of the pathogen at the time the antibiotic was started.

An antibiotic challenge is hypothesized to cause pathogens like Borrelia to protect themselves by going into a cystic stage. These cysts have been known to remain dormant for extended periods. Cysts may not be vulnerable to certain antibiotics. They remain encysted until conditions are favorable for their reemergence in spirochete forms. This may account for a cyclic symptom pattern during a Herx. Hypothetically, in Lyme:

A. Borrelia are present in the host, possibly in a variety of life stages.

B. A threat, such as the presence of antibiotic, causes some pathogens to protect themselves inside cysts or hard-to-reach safe niches.

C. The free-floating spirochetal forms that are in the circulation are susceptible to antibiotics that hit cell wall pathogens.

D. When spirochetes are killed either by antibiotics or immune response, their cell walls are broken and endotoxin released.

E. Symptoms of Herx may occur.

F. Some spirochetes are again able to hide in cystic fashion.

G. When conditions are again favorable (like the discontinuation of antibiotics), spirochetes re-emerge, and the cycle starts over.

Therefore, one Herx may not be enough to define the end of the disease cycle. This type of life stage cycling could also explain the waxing and waning of symptoms in Lyme in general, independent of a Herx. For these reasons, the addition of a cyst-penetrating antibiotic like metronidazole (Flagyl) to the treatment regimen may be prudent. This inclusion could possibly lessen the chance of some pathogens hiding in cysts with each course of treatment.

Often, after each Herx, the patient is somewhat better. The *lack* of a Herx does not mean that the treatment is not working. If the child seems to be feeling better, maybe this kid's system is able to keep up with the internal processes needed to recover from the result of the pathogens dying off. Or the antibiotic dose could be just right for this specific individual in this particular course of treatment. There could be a hundred reasons why Herx responses vary. Observe and learn as much as you can from each one.

Herx symptoms most identified with Lyme treatment include apprehension, fatigue, headache, fever, sweats, chills, pain in joints or muscles, nausea, lower blood pressure, and elevated heart rate. Skin lesions are fairly common and this would make sense, since the body does like to use the skin to remove toxic substances. The skin signs may involve various rashes or hives. Sometimes the hives are mistaken for allergies. But a patient can be having a Herx *and* an allergic reaction, so don't miss anaphylaxis because you think the patient is only having a Herx. Some Herx manifestations are more classically Lyme, such as migratory joint pain, fasciculations, and EM rash. Anxiety, insomnia, depression, and feelings of panic have been associated with Herx reactions after treatment. Again, whether these are part of a Herx or part of the underlying disease is difficult to determine, and it does not matter unless the symptoms are so severe that they may cause

the patient to stop treatment. When describing her Herx, one teenager said, "I just wanted to die."

PEARL: IV regimens can prompt a severe and long-lasting Herx.

In general, a Herx will last about 3 to 5 days but this varies considerably from hours to weeks. The body needs time to adjust to the treatment and recovery process. The severity of the Herx reaction may depend on the pathogen load at the time treatment is initiated. In some cases, the sicker the patient is when antibiotics are started, the more intense the Herx. Other factors that might contribute to the severity of the Herx reaction are the general health of the patient and the efficacy of the treatment. If the antibiotic is a good "cidal" agent for the target organism and is at sufficient dose, a large number of pathogens will die in fairly short order. This will put in place all the elements needed for a Herx response. As the body mobilizes its defenses, the patient will begin to feel the effects of inflammation and then the results of an endotoxin bolus as the cells disintegrate. The patient will feel worse before she feels better. Symptoms subside as the body restabilizes.

Herx reactions have been noticeably severe in patients with tick-borne relapsing fever due to an infection with Borrelia *hermsii*. Usually tetracyclines have been the most effective antimicrobial for tick relapsing fever but these drugs may induce a significant Jarisch-Herxheimer reaction. Over 50% of the TBRF patients treated with TCNs have experienced a Herx. This reaction produces apprehension, diaphoresis, fever, tachycardia, and tachypnea. At least the miserable patient has the satisfaction of knowing the treatment is probably working.

III. MANAGEMENT OF A HERXHEIMER REACTION

Some authors consider a Herx response a natural detoxification process. While uncomfortable, the Herx is a signal that the body is in full gear trying to heal. For some HCPs, this suggests that you should not try to "cure the cure," and supportive treatments should be withheld to allow the inflammatory process to flourish. While stoicism may be admirable in boot camp, there is something to be said for doing what you can to help the Herx patient endure the reaction.

Do everything possible to support the immune system. Rest. There are worse ways to spend a Herx than sleeping through it. Compassionate nursing is great if you can get it. Drinking lots of water is the best therapy in all cases. The fluid allows the body to flush toxins more rapidly. Good nutrition helps. Try to avoid processed foods and drinks since these might contain chemicals that will just add to the workload of the already overloaded liver and kidneys. A multivitamin may help support the immune response, especially if the patient has a poor appetite or cannot eat because of nausea. Warm or hot baths may help with the aches or chills.

Do not overdo herbs or other supplements since they are also metabolized in the same organs that are trying to detoxify the excess toxins. Using nonsteroidals like ibuprofen (Motrin, Advil, etc.) or acetaminophen (Tylenol) can take the edge off the aches, pains, and fevers. You do not want the Herx to become so uncomfortable that the patient wants to stop treatment.

PEARL: Some HCPs use a variety of herbs to ameliorate the effects of a Herx including burbur, turmeric, or licorice. Since parsley has a detoxifying effect it may help facilitate the clean up after the die-off. Antimicrobial herbs such as cat's claw may trigger Herx reactions. I have no specific supportive data, so proceed with caution. Use common-sense in trying to help your patient endure.

Especially in patients who have had severe Herx reactions in the past, you may want to start at a lower dose of antibiotic to avoid a massive bacterial kill the first day. This gives the body's defenses a chance to mobilize while not getting backlogged right from the start. Of course, this approach might allow the surviving spirochetes to hide or encyst. If the Herx becomes intolerable, the dose of antibiotic can be lowered. Sometimes switching antibiotics is helpful. There may come a time when the patient and the HCP must decide if they want to have an intense Herx all at once or multiple milder Herxes over time…like pulling the Band-Aid off all at once or little by little. Of course, since these things are hard to predict, you may not get the exact path you think you have chosen.

If the Herx is severe, the regimen might need to be adjusted by lowering the dose or altering the frequency of administration. Be careful in stopping the medicine altogether since breaks in antibiotics can result in the need for longer or stronger treatment in the future. Although some authors recommend pulsing antibiotics in the case of a severe Herx reaction, others prefer to find ways to make the Herx tolerable. In fact, now might be a good time to add a cyst-buster to the regimen, so that when the Bb decide to encyst to save themselves, good ol' Flagyl will be waiting.

Some increases in symptoms may seem to be associated with a Herx but are not. For example, many strong antibiotics alter the flora in the digestive tract. (Remember, many broad spectrum antibiotics can't tell the difference between a good bug and a bad bug and so it wipes 'em all out.) This can cause cramps, gas, and diarrhea. The diarrhea can be severe and bloody. As the gut restabilizes, the symptoms usually resolve, but this can take days and result in dehydration. Probiotics can help salvage some of the digestive tract bacteria and more is said about these agents in Chapter 25: *Ancillary Treatments*. Some recommend eating active culture yogurt to help the GI tract rebalance.

Be vigilant for one more non-Herx related complication, and that is an allergic reaction. The nature of the allergic reaction is that a patient may not show signs of an allergy the first time he takes a specific antibiotic, but the second time, all Hades might break loose. Since skin lesions are a common manifestation of both Herx reactions AND the underlying TBIs, it might be hard to tell an allergic reaction from these other etiologies. Actual hives are not as common a skin problem in TBIs or Herx reactions as they are in allergies, so if you see hives, proceed with caution. I have been fooled by hives many times.

Benedryl can help with some of the histamine manifestations of the immune response whether the person has hives or not. However, be careful not to mask or mute a full-blown allergic reaction as you tell yourself that the hives are just part of the Herx. A patient with a Herx might also be a patient with impending anaphylaxis. (One of the major underlying themes of this book is that more than one thing can be happening at once.) If an individual has hives or other signs consistent with an allergic response, keep in close contact with the caregivers and assess before the next dose of antibiotic is given. Be especially vigilant if the person has other allergies to medicines, has asthma, or is decompensating in other ways.

If possible, the HCP and the caregivers should document the nature of the Herx. This helps if the patient will need to go through another Herx in the future, and it also helps the HCP to make on-going treatment decisions. Did the patient have a Herx in the past and then come out of it feeling better? Then maybe the antibiotic selected was a good choice. Maybe the dose was reasonable. If the reaction was severe, maybe a lower dose would be just as effective without being so uncomfortable next time. If the Herx seems never-ending, maybe you need to back off or hit harder. Again, all these decisions are judgment calls depending on the response of the individual patient. Learn from each Herx.

The best way to help a patient through a Herx is to tell him it might happen. Especially tell the caretakers. As both a TBI patient and a TBI parent, trust me when I say that the parents are suffering. Present the Herx as a positive phenomenon that is a *temporary* rough road on the way to getting better. Don't scare them to death, or you will have a reverse placebo-effect. Try something like this. "You may feel worse before you feel better. This is your body calling in all its defenses to fight against the disease. To do this, it has to heat up, swell up, and clean up from the inside out. This doesn't always feel great, but it is the way your body is helping you in the long-run. If it feels too bad, we will try to make you feel better through it." They should never feel that you are abandoning them when they are feeling their worst. Remind them that you will see them through to the other side of this reaction.

Pay attention to the patient and the caregivers to help them through the Herx. A severe Herx can affect compliance. Teenagers especially might be reluctant to take medicines that they believe are responsible for making them feel worse. Do what you can to encourage the patient to endure the Herx. Tell them that these symptoms are a sign that they are healing and that there is a light at the end of the Herx tunnel. But there is no extra credit for suffering to the point of torture. Don't punish the person in order to save him. No one likes surprises. Ask older patients, "Do you think you can make one more day?" If not, trust their decisions and adjust things to help them feel better. Here you must decide if the symptoms are due to a Herx, or if the treatment is ineffective and the disease is getting worse. This is a clinical judgment, but you should pay enough attention to make a valid determination. A few patients have reported suicidal thoughts when they Herx. Don't let them get that far. Make sure they know they can call you.

Consider one more perspective on the Herxheimer reaction. As I mentioned in the first paragraph of this chapter, I had no idea what a Herx was when I started to see TBI patients. If the HCP is not aware that a Herx might occur, he might feel frustrated when he gets a call 2 days after he started treatment and the child is sicker. The parent is mad at the HCP, and the HCP is mad at the patient for not getting better when she should. Many doctors feel a bit of trepidation when they first move into the controversial world of TBIs. Now they have a patient who is sicker than when they first saw her. Don't panic if the person feels worse before she feels better. Just keep an eye on her. The worst you can do is to mistake ineffective treatment for a Herx. Especially when you first enter the TBI world, keep a close eye and have the caregivers commit to calling you if there is a problem. After you have seen a few thousand TBI patients, you will be more confident.

Do not blame life-threatening symptoms on a Herx. Feeling miserable, yes. But breathing problems, heart problems, changes in consciousness, or anything else that scares the patient or the caregiver should be addressed.

Explain the Herx reaction to both patients and caretakers. People who have been through a Herx reaction in the past often seem to think that the end justifies the means. Most are not thrilled that it is upon them again, but I have been surprised at how much they want to get better. Many are more than willing to go through the Herx. If a patient cannot tolerate the severity or duration of a Herx, it is *not* a failure on anyone's part. Rethink, regroup, and consider alternatives.

Some antibiotics, as well as some pathogens are renowned for their association with Herx reactions. TCNs commonly cause reactions, as does Bicillin, maybe because they are working. If Bartonella is treated appropriately, expect a big Herx. In tick relapsing fever, a Herx occurs in over half the patients. Be aware and be prepared.

At least 10% of chronic Lyme patients don't Herx at all. Some fear the Herx, some avoid it, and some welcome it as the sign of increased inflammation because of all the work the immune system is doing. Experienced practitioners appreciate the Herx because it means the bugs are dying. Try to be empathetic in helping the patient and family move through the process.

Some think you can decrease the Herx by boosting the immune system so that it can better handle the symptoms that have been caused by work overload. Remember, there is a fine balance between too much immune response and not enough. We are not at that level of understanding just yet.

Since Bb toxins seem to be the biggest contributor to the Herx sxs, some HCPs try detoxification modalities to decrease the symptoms of the Herx. Chitosan, a derivative of shellfish, has been used as an absorbent. Many of the chelating agents have also been tried.

Supportive therapies have been suggested including warm lemon water, alkaline foods such as most fruits and vegetables, bananas, chocolate, orange juice, potatoes, spinach, watermelon, most vitamin and mineral supplements (Ca, K, Fe, Mg), and antacids. I have also seen eggs, wine, yogurt with active cultures, fermented foods, aged cheese, buttermilk, corn, meat, fish, fowl, coffee, and beans touted as helpful. I had to make sure I wasn't reading cures for a hangover. I thought it seemed strange to recommend lemon water and alkaline foods in the same sentence. Well, apparently lemon and other citrus fruits are acidic before they are consumed but leave alkaline residue after they are metabolized. Who knew? Probiotics are often recommended. As long as these suggestions don't seem to be causing any harm, try what helps.

IMPORTANT: Antibiotic therapy should be considered for 2 to 3 months after the last signs of the Herx have subsided. Enough of the Bb could have escaped to resurface at a later date when conditions again become favorable.

Chapter 29

EFFECTS OF TBIs ON INDIVIDUAL ORGAN SYSTEMS

"It does not do to leave a dragon out of your calculations, if you live near him."

J.R.R. Tolkien

This chapter would be much shorter if I discussed the body systems **NOT** affected by Lyme. Lyme impacts both the body structure through its invasion of connective tissue and collagen and, because of its damage to blood vessels and nerves, potentially compromises every tissue in the body. Either directly or indirectly, Bb have broad-based clinical significance. The longer a person is sick, the greater the potential for more organ systems to become involved. So the simple answer to the question "Could this symptom be Lyme?" is YES. Of course, nothing about Lyme is simple.

Initially, I kept lists of all signs and symptoms EVER associated with each of the TBIs. I alphabetized them, numbered them, and organized them by organ system. Eventually, I realized I was just transcribing the medical dictionary. Life was passing me by and I wasn't creating anything especially useful. Note that the listings below are NOT in order of severity or importance or frequency of occurrence – simply recognized findings associated with various conditions.

I decided to focus only on the manifestations in each body system that are especially suggestive of a TBI diagnosis. Each of the items listed below should make you think about a particular TBD. Some are subtle. The eye can't see what the brain doesn't know. So, be aware.

Out of curiosity, look at this list and see where the problems concentrate with Lyme. While the GI, endocrine, and joints are often impacted, the nervous system seems to take the biggest hit. This observation is not in any way a scientific or quantitative conclusion, but it's hard not to be impressed by the number of neurologic manifestations that seem to result from Bb infection. Also, the GI tract is highly innervated and the mechanism by which the GI sxs occur is probably at least partially mediated by borrelial impact on those nerves. Likewise, the endocrine manifestations are possibly due to biochemical and nervous system interaction. Do not allow limited or delayed treatment to change a temporary problem to a permanent condition.

Use the multifaceted nature of Lyme to your advantage. In managing TBIs, you will have dysfunction in many body systems, clouding the diagnostic process. Lyme with only one body system involved would be the exception not the rule. Be able to tell the forest from the trees. Do not let multiple end-organ manifestations take your focus off the underlying causal agent. The more diverse the sxs, the more you might want to get closer to the trunk of the tree instead of focusing on individual branches. You might find an explanation that covers all the manifestations you're seeing.

PEARL: TBIs affect many body systems in various ways. The key point of this chapter is that if a medical problem is Lyme-related, there is a much better chance for treatment success if you treat the Lyme as well as the end-organ symptoms. Without concomitant antimicrobials, Lyme-induced symptoms are less likely to respond to conventional therapies alone. This assertion has been demonstrated in cases of myriad neuropsychiatric conditions, seizures, sleep disorders, depression, joint pain, and cardiac problems. Yes, the signs and symptoms may be able to be mitigated without antibiotics, but a cure is harder to achieve without addressing the underlying infectious process. For example, a Lyme-induced conversion reaction will respond to antibiotics, but if the conversion reaction is developmental, it won't be affected by antibiotics. If your patient does not seem to be responding to conventional therapies in the way that you had anticipated, consider that Lyme or other TBIs may be influencing the outcome.

General:

Incapacitating fatigue	Lyme, babesiosis, CFS
Alterations in immune system	Lyme, babesiosis, M. *fermentans,* Bartonellosis
Headache	Ehrlichiosis, anaplasmosis, Lyme, Babesiosis, bartonellosis, TRF, RMSF
Herx reaction	Lyme, TRF, bartonellosis
Rigors/sweats	Babesiosis, tularemia
Abnormal LFTs	Q fever

Skin:

Pale skin, anemia	Babesiosis
Violaceous striae	Bartonellosis
Subcutaneous nodules	Bartonellosis, sarcoidosis, RA, RF
Primary (localized) EM rash	Deep red, oval lesion(s) near tick bite site/ Perhaps concentric circles, ONLY borreliosis (Lyme, STARI, TRF)
Secondary (disseminated) EM rash	Rare, transient, multiple. ONLY borreliosis
Progressive, red, pinpoint, petechial rash	RMSF
Ulcers	Tularemia

Scalp:

Perhaps tendency to lesions	Lyme

Eyes:

Various eye problems	Lyme, bartonellosis, tularemia, TRF, MS
Uveitis, iritis	Lyme, MS
Pale mucous membranes inside lids	Anemia, babesiosis
Dark circles	Lyme, babesiosis
Light sensitivity	Lyme, congenital Lyme
Coloboma, strabismus	Congenital Lyme
Lid twitching	Lyme
Punctated erythema on conjunctiva	Lyme eye
Astigmatism	Lyme
Blurred or "smeared vision"	Lyme
Floaters	Lyme
Flashing lights	Lyme

Ears:

Red pinnae	Lyme
Deformed or missing pinnae	Congenital Lyme
Tinnitus	Lyme
Underwater feel	Lyme
Hypersensitivity to sound	Lyme
Hearing impairment	Lyme

Mouth:

Pale mucous membranes	Anemia, babesiosis, Lyme

Throat:

Thrush	Fungal overgrowth, antimicrobial use
Bright red, injected tonsillar pillars	Lyme
Petechiae on palate	Lyme
Sensation of occlusion in throat	Lyme, HPV infection

GI:

GERD	Bartonellosis, Lyme
Reflux	Congenital Lyme
Vomiting	Congenital Lyme
Dysphagia	Lyme, mononucleosis, Strep, HPV
GI distress	Bartonellosis
Leaky gut syndrome	Lyme
Gallstones	Rocephin use
Omental trapping with abdominal pain	Lyme
Severe diarrhea/toxic megacolon	C. *difficile*
Pseudomembranous colitis	C. *difficile*
Gastritis	Bartonellosis, Lyme, some meds
Vague GI complaints	Lyme, bartonellosis, tularemia, other TBIs
Palsy of the gut vagus nerve	Lyme

GU:

Disproportionate interstitial cystitis	Lyme
Bladder irritability	Lyme
Incontinence	Lyme
Nonspecific urinary problems	Lyme
New onset enuresis w/o family history	Lyme
Chronic pelvic pain	Lyme
Kidney failure	Lyme

Cardiac:

Dysrhythmias, including atrial fibrillation	Lyme
Various heart blocks	Lyme
Valve problems	Lyme
Congenital anomalies	Congenital Lyme
Ventricular septal defect	Congenital Lyme
Carditis, endocarditis, myocarditis	Lyme, Q fever
Cause of death	Lyme

Respiratory:

Air hunger	Babesiosis
Pneumonia	Tularemia, M. *pneumoniae*, Q fever
Breathing difficulties	Babesiosis, tularemia, Q fever
Cough	Q fever, TRF, tularemia, RMSF
ARDS	TRF, late-stage Lyme

Blood/Circulation:

Dyscrasias	Most TBIs
Anemia	Babesiosis
Bleeding	Babesiosis, RMSF
Vascular damage	Lyme
Edema/swelling	Lyme
Cold extremities/Raynaud's	Lyme, bartonellosis
Lymphadenopathy	Lyme, mono, Strep, Bartonella, tularemia
DIC	Severe or end-stage disease
Hypercoagulability	Babesiosis, bartonellosis, Lyme
Hemangiomas	Congenital Lyme, bartonellosis

Endocrine:

Abnormal sugars, thyroid, cortisol	Lyme
Adrenocortical dysfunction	Lyme

Joints:

Pain in knees, shoulders	Lyme
Migrating joint involvement	Lyme
JIR-like presentation	Lyme
Small joint discomfort	Lyme
Popping joints/neck cracking	Lyme
Knees swollen	Bartonellosis, Lyme
Arthritis	M. *fermentans,* Lyme, RA, RF, Bartonella
Neck pain	Babesiosis, Lyme

Muscles:

Plantar fasciitis	Bartonellosis, Lyme, babesiosis
Migratory muscle pain	Lyme
Muscle pain	Ehrlichiosis, anaplasmosis, Babesiosis, fibromyalgia

Bones:

Severe shin pain	Bartonellosis

Immune:

Variable effects	May be significant in Lyme
General signs of inflammation	TBI co-infections, most infections
Possible antineuronal antibodies	Lyme, bartonellosis, Strep

Neurologic:

Hypersensitivity to any sense	Lyme
Multiple NP sxs	M. *fermentans*, bartonellosis, Lyme
Bell's palsy	Lyme, TRF
Fasciculations, tremors, twitches, tics	Lyme
Balance problems	Lyme
Cranial nerve dysfunction	Lyme
PDD including autism-like syndromes	Lyme
Asperger's-like syndromes	Lyme
Childhood Disintegrative Disorder	Lyme

Cranial nerve involvement	Lyme
Bell's palsy, CN7 defect	Lyme, TRF
Asymmetrical facial muscles	Lyme
Diminished coordination	Lyme
Confusion	Lyme
Cognitive impairment	Lyme, M. *fermentans,* bartonellosis
Brain fog	Lyme, heavy metal toxicity
Attention deficits/distractibility	Lyme, bartonellosis, ADD, ADHD
Problems with memory/judgment	Lyme
Encephalitis	Lyme, POW
Meningitis	Lyme
Neuropathies: mono and poly	Lyme, ehrlichiosis
Burning or crawling sensation/pins and needles	Lyme, Morgellon
Stammering	Lyme
Hypersensitivity to noise and touch	Congenital Lyme, Lyme
Seizures	Lyme, bartonellosis
OCD, ODD, panic, GAD	Lyme, bartonellosis
Emotional lability, aggression	Lyme, bartonellosis
Hypotonia	Prime sign of gestational Lyme in neonate
Hypersensitivity to pressure or temperature	Lyme
Pain	Lyme, bartonellosis, fibromyalgia
Delays in developmental milestones	Congenital Lyme, acquired Lyme
ANS damage	Lyme
Infection-induced encephalopathy	Lyme, bartonellosis
Neurotoxicity	Hg poisoning

Psych:

Rage	Bartonella
Irritability	Lyme
Conversion reaction	Lyme
Behavioral problems	Lyme, bartonellosis, M. *fermentans*
Broad psychiatric sxs	Lyme, bartonellosis, M. *fermentans*
Personality changes	Lyme, bartonellosis, M. *fermentans*

Chapter 30

SPECIAL POPULATIONS
(Pregnant, Nursing, and Gestational Lyme)

An diogann tu caratai credit: Gaelic for "Do you take credit cards?"

In drug development, special populations are those who need additional attention or instruction regarding use of a drug and most drug labels have a section titled *Special Populations*. These subpopulations most often include children, the elderly, those with liver or kidney problems, and pregnant or nursing women. Depending on the safety profile of the drug, sometimes distinctions are made based on gender, race, or ethnic group. Only the group distinctions applicable to Lyme or other TBIs will be vetted here. Since this book already discusses manifestations of TBIs in both the pediatric and adult populations, we will not expand on those groups in this chapter. Most experts do not recognize clinically meaningful differences in Lyme due to sex, race, or ethnicity, although these distinctions are theoretically possible. We know that a number of the TBIs do impact the liver and kidneys to varying degrees, as do several of the antimicrobials. All these contingencies are handled in other chapters. While the elderly could be considered a special population in this text, much of the material in the book is already applicable to them. Recognize that aging can alter liver and kidney function so pay special attention to these parameters as you manage TBIs in older patients. Their immune systems may quickly be overwhelmed by these pathogens and M&M might be higher.

The remainder of this chapter will focus on gestational transmission of TBIs, especially Lyme. Transmission through breast milk is also addressed, although in most cases very little is known about TBDs transferred through nursing. This material is presented as a series of *PEARLS*, because I was tired of the old format.

RANDOM TOPICAL *PEARLS*

PEARL: Gestational transmission of disease is infection of the fetus by active pathogens present in the mother during pregnancy.

PEARL: Congenital disease is disease present at birth.

PEARL: Statistics are sparse. One source says that about 10% of the patients in a TBI-only practice have disease due to gestational transmission. Who knows? The numbers don't matter as much as your ability to remember that gestational transmission of Lyme and other TBIs can occur, probably more often than we think.

PEARL: Bb are hypothesized to move across the placental barrier infecting the fetus. Syphilis, the much better known spirochete, has well-documented transmission from infected mother to child. Gestational LD closely parallels the diverse presentation of perinatal transmission of syphilis.

PEARL: Gustafson and Burgess demonstrated intrauterine transmission of Bb in dogs in 1993. In female dogs inoculated with Bb: 80% of the mothers became infected and 80% of those gave birth to infected pups as shown by DNA-positive tissues in PCRs and cultures. Most, but not all, of the pups were infected. Interesting...

PEARL: The most common sxs of gestational Lyme include: hypotonia (almost universal), irritability, cognitive problems such as learning disabilities and unclear thinking, mood swings, fatigue, lack of stamina, pain, low grade fevers, pallor, sickly appearance, dark circles under eyes, arthritis and painful joints with stiffness and decreased ROM, unspecified rashes, GERD, vomiting with coughing, frequent URIs and otitis, sensitivity to noise, light, and touch, developmental delay including language and speech problems, hemangiomas, night sweats, general muscle pains or spasms, and cardiac abnormalities such as palpitations, PVCs, murmurs, and MVP.

PEARL: Tone is the normal tension or responsiveness of a muscle or other tissue. In muscle, normal tone is a constant slight contraction that helps maintain posture and coordination.

PEARL: Hypotonia occurs in over 90% of children with gestational LD. Almost all kids with gestational LD have varying degrees of hypotonia. Many are limp like rag dolls. These children are described as floppy, deflated, wilted, or pillows full of pudding.

PEARL: The mechanism by which Bb causes this lack of muscle tone may be interference with sensory input from the muscles, or the muscles may not be able to respond to nerve activation, or there could be direct damage to the cerebellum. A combination of these factors might be involved. Or we may have no idea. All is speculation.

PEARL: Features of hypotonia include arms and legs hanging by the child's sides, decreased DTRs, little resistance to passive motion, decreased muscle tone, delay in the development of gross and fine motor skills, drooling, speech difficulties due to decreased muscle strength, rounded shoulders, and leaning. Hypotonic kids do not have normal muscle tension or responsiveness. They often present as excessively flexible.

PEARL: As a doctor who spent years in the world of pediatric GERD, I wonder if "hypotonia" of the sphincter leading into the stomach is causing the high incidence of GERD in these kids.

PEARL: As the child with gestational Lyme gets older, persistent irritability associated with impulsivity is seen in a high percentage of cases. This irritability is an on-going irritation that often accompanies impulsive acts. While irritability can improve with appropriate treatment, the impulsivity may never completely resolve. The irritation may result from the frustration associated with excessive impatience. Many of these kids:

- *Act without thinking*
- *Do not think things through*
- *Take unnecessary risks*
- *Have a short fuse*
- *Can't wait their turn*
- *Blurt*
- *Say the wrong things*
- *Interrupt*
- *Intrude*
- *Experience significant emotional lability*

PEARL: Neuropsychiatric sxs commonly associated with gestational Lyme include: irritability, headache, poor memory, developmental delay, vertigo, tics, involuntary movements, broad neuropsychiatric problems, anger or rage, mood swings, depression, ADD, ADHD, lack of concentration, hypersensitivity, motion sickness, cognitive problems, speech delays, articulation difficulty, reading/writing issues, word selection impairment, auditory or visual processing defects, dyslexia, anxiety, aggression or violence, emotional lability, suicidal thoughts, OCD, photophobia, and seizures.

PEARL: If the pregnant woman has Lyme, both the mother and fetus need to be protected. So now you have two patients. If the mom has LD, she needs to be treated in a way that gives the best chance of protecting the fetus from contracting the infection. If born with congenital Lyme, the neonate must be treated in a way that provides the most opportunity for eliminating the infection and reducing the potential for long-term damage. In both cases, antibiotics must be selected that will hit both the active and dormant states of the Bb and will not cause damage to the developing fetus or newborn.

PEARL: A registry tracking Lyme-infected mothers was maintained for a number of years. From this data, several conclusions were drawn. If a Lyme-infected mother was on adequate antibiotics during gestation: **NO** *babies were born with Lyme. In these cases, if two antibiotics were used that together would hit both the free spirochete as well as the intracellular form of Bb,* **NO** *Lyme babies resulted. In infected mothers treated with only one antibiotic, about 25% of the babies were born with Lyme. About half the babies born to untreated mothers had Lyme.*

PEARL: In treating the pregnant mother consider: Oral options: amoxicillin 1 g q 8, **OR** *cefuroxime (Ceftin) 100 mg q 12* **OR** *cefdinir (Omnicef) 300 to 600 mg bid* **PLUS** *azithromycin 500 mg bid. Parenteral options: Bicillin 1.2 million units IM 1 to 3 times per week,* **OR** *Rocephin (ceftriaxone) 2 g IV daily,* **OR** *Claforan (cefotaxime) 6 g daily either continuous infusion or as 2 g IV q 8* **PLUS** *azithromycin.*

PEARL: After birth, the maternal Lyme may no longer be mollified by the pregnancy hormones and sxs may return in full force. There may be profound fatigue and these women may need additional help post-pregnancy.

PEARL: Breast feeding should only proceed in actively infected Lyme patients IF the mom is on appropriate antibiotics. Live spirochetes have been isolated from breast milk.

PEARL: In evaluating the neonate, have a high index of suspicion. Although only subtle sxs may be present at birth, serious neurologic sequelae may result if not promptly diagnosed and treated. These problems can be severe and debilitating.

PEARL: Patients often have entrenched and chronic Bb-associated neurologic manifestations by the time the diagnosis is made. Kids tend to do well if treatment is aggressive and for sufficient duration

PEARL: Treatment options for kids: Combination of PCNs **OR** *CSs* **WITH** *macrolides. TCNs are not usually used in kids under 8.*

PEARL: If unsure whether to treat a mom or child consider Gardner's 1995 study of 161 cases of LD in the fetus or newborn. If mothers with active disease were treated with antibiotics then 85% of the neonates were normal and 15% were abnormal. If no antibiotics were used then only 33% of the neonates were normal (67% abnormal). Many serious events occurred in the abnormal outcomes such as miscarriage, stillbirth, perinatal death, congenital anomalies, sepsis, or chronic progressive infection.

PEARL: In 1989, Alan MacDonald documented the adverse outcomes in cases of LD during pregnancy. These AEs were found to occur irrespective of the trimester of initial infection and appear to be in excess of adverse outcomes compared to what is observed in matching uninfected populations. MacDonald found Borrelia spirochetes in stillborn infants. Since these children were in utero prior to examination, they could not have become infected with their Lyme through a tick bite. The transmission of pathogen had to be gestational.

PEARL: Untoward outcomes documented from Lyme infected moms include: prematurity, hydrocephalus, blindness, SIDs, toxemia, fetal death, CVS anomalies, growth retardation, respiratory distress, and hyperbilirubinemia. Children with gestational Lyme seem to have congenital anomalies in excess of those seen in kids without Bb infection. Anomalies that have been documented include syndactyly, congenital eye problems, prematurity, cardiac abnormalities, and congenital urologic anomalies.

PEARL: Confounders in recognizing congenital Lyme: 1) The child may be asymptomatic at birth, 2) First signs of LD may be delayed for varying periods causing the mom's Lyme during pregnancy to be forgotten, 3) When sxs are finally noted, they're commonly dismissed or attributed to something else, 4) Sxs may mimic other conditions leading to misdiagnosis, 5) Co-morbidities are common and may be masking Lyme, 6) Manifestations may affect multiple systems leading to pursuing wrong leads, 7) Sxs may wax, wane, and change with varying degrees of severity, 8) There is difficulty in gathering supportive lab data with many false negatives, 9) Many HCPs do not realize that negative lab results do not rule out disease, 10) The mom may have LD but if the disease is not currently active, may not know the child is at risk. In general, the longer the child goes without appropriate diagnosis and treatment, the more severe and complicated the clinical course.

PEARL: Recent work has demonstrated that protozoal parasites, certain viruses such as HIV, and some bacteria affect gene structure or expression in the host. Xiao demonstrated significant changes in rodent behavior due to alteration in gene expression after infection with the protozoal parasite Toxoplasma gondii. "T. gondii can play its infected rodent hosts like a piano, ..." HIV and other viruses, and bacteria such as Helicobacter pylori are known to alter gene structure and expression. Why not Bb? With Toxoplasma, different strains of the pathogen affected genes in different body systems, some preferring the nerve tissue and others the genetic material itself. This is especially interesting as we look at the effect Bb might have on babies infected in utero. We know that many viruses and bacteria impact the genetic material of the host either directly by changing the nucleotide sequences themselves, resulting in different molecular construction, or by altering the on-off switches involved with gene expression. Pathogens can also genetically affect the immune cells and therefore the response of the immune system to the infection.

PEARL: The other TBIs get short shrift in this section, so know that both Babesia and Bartonella can also be transmitted to the fetus. Neonates born with babesiosis are often critically ill with a high mortality rate. You must have a high index of suspicion here and be ready to act at the birth; otherwise you will not have time to respond as quickly as needed to save the child. Refer to Chapter 6 for additional guidance. Also, Mycoplasma easily cross the placenta. Be aware.

PEARL: Infected mothers will sometimes ask if they should get pregnant or not. If appropriately treated for long enough and with the right antibiotics there is little, if any, chance of gestational Lyme. In a case review, infected mothers who were treated with two targeted antibiotics delivered no babies with Lyme. Treatment with one antibiotic resulted in about 25% of the children with gestational transmission. Untreated mothers with active Lyme had about a 50-50 chance of transmitting Bb to their child.

PEARL: In the newborn with an infected mother take samples for Bartonella, Borrelia, and Babesia. Take these samples from the placenta, the cord, and foreskin if there is any suspicion. Even though yields are low for positive testing in all cases, the placenta and cord are your best bets. You will never have this opportunity again. Do not waste the chance to collect a decent sample.

PEARL: Tell the obstetrician prior to delivery that you would like specimens. You will need to specify exactly how to handle the samples and where to ship. Take the opportunity to collect these potentially useful samples. Unless the lab knows how to test for these pathogens, the samples will be wasted. Be prepared.

PEARL: If the mother is infected in the first 3 months of pregnancy while many of the major organs are forming, the child can have significant problems including cardiac anomalies, ventricular septal defect, and eye problems such as coloboma (a black, round hole or slit in or near the iris, sometimes called cat eyes) or strabismus (eyes do not line up).

PEARL: Meyer and others found that infections associated with strong immunological events early in gestation have a stronger neurodevelopmental impact that those that occur later in fetal life. This effect can cause abnormal cell differentiation and proliferation, problems with cell migration, and synapse development, all potentially resulting in multiple congenital abnormalities.

PEARL: Although neither scenario portends well for the infant, some TBI practitioners believe that children who are infected in utero do better than if they are infected in the first year of life. In both cases, a high index of suspicion on the part of the HCP is the child's best chance of getting appropriate treatment prior to permanent sequelae. In both cases, the child may be hypotonic with joint and body pain, irritability, and hypersensitivity. She may be born with a small windpipe, cardiac anomalies, and cataracts along with other eye problems. Soon after birth an excess number of URIs and pneumonias may be noted as well as GERD, and significant developmental delays. Cognitive deficits may be the most debilitating manifestation in these children.

PEARL: There are a number of interesting anecdotes. For example, an infected mother gave birth to fraternal twins, one with gestational Lyme and one without.

PEARL: The placenta does a good job in keeping most pathogens away from the fetus. Well-known exceptions include the microbes that cause rubella, syphilis, bartonellosis, and Lyme.

PEARL: Pathogens can harm the fetus several ways: Directly through invasion of the fetal cells or indirectly through the harm that can come from the harsh biochemicals delivered by the immune system's reaction to their presence.

PEARL: The fetal nervous system is very susceptible to pathogen interference. There may be inadequate cell migration, limited myelination, lack of differentiation, or poor synapse development. The presence of IL-6 might decrease the number of Purkinje cells. These findings have been confirmed from autopsy samples.

PEARL: In utero infections often result in eye problems including deformities in structure and diminished vision.

PEARL: The timing of the infection can be critical. Depending on when during gestation the infection occurs will determine what genes are affected and how this might influence the phenotype.

PEARL: Antimicrobials thought to be safe in pregnancy: PCNs, CSs, azithromycin, atovaquone. Caution in pregnancy: quinolones, clarithromycin, TCNs, metronidazole, and sulfa combinations. Options may be limited, so always do a risk/benefit analysis and discuss the alternatives with the patient.

PEARL: Teens and any population undergoing hormonal shifts may be especially affected by the hormonal impact of Bb. Lyme affects hormones and hormones affect Lyme. In pregnancy, there is considerable hormonal fluctuation.

PEARL: There is strong anecdotal evidence for Lyme being transmitted through breast milk. More than a dozen cases of breast-fed infants acquiring Bb through nursing have been documented. TBI experts usually recommend that infected mothers remain on antibiotics as long as they are nursing. One ID doctor told an infected mom that she was fine to stop antibiotics and continue nursing. Although all testing had been negative at birth and for months afterward, the child developed a classic EM rash and other symptoms consistent with Lyme and began to test positive. There was no possibility of tick bite since the mom was hypervigilant.

PEARL: Bb seem to be able to be transmitted transplacentally. Anecdotes describe contagion using IVF.

PEARL: There are anecdotes where an infected man is thought to have transmitted Bb to his partner who later delivered an infected child.

PEARL: Recognize that Lyme disease is becoming more prevalent and thereby opening up more opportunities for gestational transmission. Understand that Lyme can be a serious illness in children.

PEARL: Dr. Bransfield makes a good point. All these congenital manifestations of gestational Lyme could be PREVENTED if the mother is appropriately treated when pregnant.

PEARL: In Cure Unknown Pam Weintraub relates the case of a child born with Lyme. By 6 weeks the infant had eye tremors and frequent vomiting. By 6 months the child was blind and likely deaf. Please retain a high index of suspicion. You cannot manage a disease you don't consider. Never underestimate the damage that can be done by Lyme or other TBDs.

Chapter 31

A BALANCED LIFE
School, Relationships, and Stability

Newspaper correction: Sunday's Lifestyle story about Buddhism should have stated that Siddhartha Gautama (the Buddha) grew up in Northern India, not Indiana. Bloomington Herald Times

Chronic Lyme can take over your life. And your household. And depress your pets. And your spouse. I have been consumed with this book for four years. All day every day. Except when I serve as caretaker for people who have Lyme and other TBIs. Except when I am ill or injured or someone has died, Lyme has been my life. When I am not working on the book and I am otherwise well enough to be working, I feel guilty. I am convinced that guilt is a part of the disease. I know it is more common than a positive ELISA.

Of course, I took on this task without realizing just how complicated, controversial, and consuming Lyme can be. I have set personal deadline after deadline and watched them slip by as I made yet another 1500 mile round-trip to Purdue when the TBIs would flare in my son. It's been 4 years and I think the flares are not as severe and seem to be getting farther apart. Yet you never know when the other shoe will drop. Again. I am the least superstitious person on the planet, yet as I typed that last sentence I am looking for wood to knock, salt to toss, and a rabbit to assail.

Every time I think I am almost done, (Really. This time for sure.) Dr. Bransfield or Lorraine Johnson provide me with hundreds of additional references and I put on my snorkel and dive back in. Every time I think there could not be another book, article, or guideline that I haven't seen, something new turns up. Sometimes I daydream about what I will do when I am really, most sincerely, finished. Then I realize that if I don't get back to work I will never get done and Lyme prevails.

Often, Lyme has taken over my life and has impacted my health not just from spirochetes doing the backstroke in my right knee but in the mental effort it has taken to fight it as a patient, parent, and physician. This chapter will encourage the pursuit of reason and balance and the minimization of guilt, stress, and angst for the patient, caretaker, and family.

Two of the most stressful states in which humans find themselves are the experiences of chronic illness and the responsibility of being the caretaker for someone who is chronically ill. I know from both personal and professional experience. Balance. Ha! Most of us would be happy to take a bath.

In the US we tend to live frenetic, over-stimulated, competitive lives even when those lives are not complicated by severe illness. In the workplace many companies have introduced the concept of work-life balance. This idea would be great if it worked in practice as it does in theory. Only the Japanese are less likely to take all their allotted vacation days than Americans. Those employees who take advantage of the flexible Fridays and "work from home" often just leave more chores for those workers who don't have those options. If you have Lyme or your child has Lyme, you will often be trying to keep your head above water and you would consider yourself lucky to have time to worry about life balance.

Nonetheless, I encourage you to strive for balance and don't let your pursuit stress you even further. If you are already anxious, adding "relax" to your TO DO list probably isn't going to help. Even reading self-help books on how to achieve life balance can be stressful.

Keep in mind that if a caretaker is stressed, the patient will feel that tension. Under duress the adrenal cortex goes into overdrive, releasing the stress hormone cortisol, which causes a cascade of untoward effects. One of the most damaging consequences is cortisol's impact on healing. This problem can be cyclic. The sicker you are, the more anxious you become, and the more anxious you are, the slower your recovery. Of course, that makes you even more nervous.

Chapter 27: *Supportive Measures* reviews numerous suggestions for balancing life and reducing stress from yoga to journaling. The most proven components to life balance are probably positive socializing, pets, exercise, nature, solitude, and some kind of meditative or spiritual practice. There is something to be said for a walk in the woods, by yourself, as you clear your mind. For just a few minutes, a break from the constant input of the day can be revitalizing for both patient and caretaker. Breathe. Really. A few minutes of conscious, deliberate, deep breathing can reboot your psyche.

Remember that patients have both subtle and overt pressure on them to get well. This is stressful. Both the sick and their caretakers have guilt and appropriate situational sadness. Here gratitude and optimism, mixed with reality, can be useful. For goodness sake, try to stay away from the negative. I know when I watch the endless news cycles about the abuse at Penn State or the most recent political vitriol I become sad. Numerous studies have demonstrated that negativity is contagious as is happiness and many other emotions. Children especially should not be exposed to the perpetual pessimism of the 24/7 news.

Enough pontificating. This chapter needs to address several practical issues in the quest for life balance. Most of these tips apply to the caregiver, but the patient and HCP can also benefit. In some Lyme cases one person can be the patient, caregiver, and HCP. Use these balancing techniques to help yourself and the patient.

A. **GET ORGANIZED**: Easier said than done. The more clutter in your living space the more stress in your life. Likewise, the more clutter in your mind, the more stress in your psyche. Decrease the clutter and you will decrease the stress. Some people find that making lists decreases stress and enhances balance, while others are more stressed by lists. This book provides a number of ideas on how to organize drug regimens and other treatments using the medication tracking sheet. While this sample may work for you, it may not fit your style. You might have to devise an alternative. If more than two or three instructions need to be followed in the course of a day, adopt some kind of organizational strategy or you will miss something. That miss will increase stress and decrease your capacity for balance in your life and the life of the patient. Having to remember to give the medicine at 2:00 and then take the temperature at 4:00 and then eat so that the next drug can be taken with food is not humanly possible for more than a day or two, if that long. Adopt some organizational tools so that you can be free to better pursue that life balance. Use what works for you. Even a pill holder can help. Don't let the chaos of the day send your anxiety level off the charts. It takes about two weeks to get into a routine and about 3 months to form a positive habit. You might have to schedule the desired behaviors at first until they come naturally. You might have to shut off much of the extraneous input from electronic devices in order to organize your thoughts and regain your balance. Although getting organized may take some time initially, the effort might save time in the long-run and help keep your sanity.

PEARL: Some recommend goal setting as a positive way to get organized. Still, each day I set goals for weight loss, good food choices, exercise, and pages written. And each day I fail to achieve them. So use what works for you. One tip on goal setting is to remember that when you are deciding whether or not to do something in pursuit of your goal, a delay of 20 seconds can mean all the difference. Twenty seconds is enough time to talk yourself out of exercising or choosing the carrots over the corn chips. If you give yourself 20 seconds, you'll probably make the wrong choice. Set yourself up so that the walking shoes or the apples are so readily available you don't have 20 seconds to talk yourself into taking the wrong path.

PEARL: A recent theory on setting goals suggests that goals should be specific, measurable, achievable, realistic, and trackable (SMART).

PEARL: Superbetter.com is an on-line site that helps break down big health problems into manageable pieces with realistic goals. At least it was in October of 2012.

B. **GET HELP**: Accepting help is difficult for many people. Some do not like to admit weakness and others prefer that no one outside the house know their business. With the controversy around Lyme, some are even embarrassed by the diagnosis. Yet only in the last decade has the strain on caretakers been recognized. Clearly, we all need help when dealing with a long-term care situation. Aside from death, there is no life circumstance more emotionally taxing over time than taking care of a chronically ill person. There is no situation that has as many mixed emotions. Help can range from grandparents caring for the sick child for a few hours, to hiring someone to do the laundry, to getting counseling as an individual or family. An extra pair of hands can go a long way in helping achieve that elusive balance. Chapter 34: *Friendly Advice* provides additional information on finding resources that might provide assistance.

C. **BALANCE:** Work when you work and play when you play. Care when you're care-giving and then break when you break. Do not let your responsibility and your rest ooze into each other so that both are diluted and ultimately ineffective. I am opposed to ooze and believe that it interferes with life balance. Many of us never really relax because work is always intruding on play. Dalton Conley in *Elsewhere U.S.A.* invented the term *weisure* to describe the mix of work and leisure. For Lyme caretakers the responsibility can be around the clock 24/7/365. Conley advises energy management as opposed to time management. There is only so much of you to be spent. If you are not well, you will have nothing left to help others get well. Balance.

D. **RELIGION**: Spiritual endeavors can help provide life balance for many people. For older kids and caretakers, religious beliefs can provide strength, meaning, and serenity in some cases. Some find solace in rituals, while others benefit from the community. For children with debilitating fatigue, religious activities like youth group can provide time to socialize without being physically taxing. Services tend to be shorter than 6 to 8 hour school days. Both children and those who care for them might get spiritual and social support in their attempt to balance various aspects of their lives. Spirituality can provide a sense of peace or goodness and a connection to others. Besides, a strong sense of the spiritual has been suggested to increase CD4 levels and lower pathogen load. Be careful that the selected religious tradition enhances the healing process and does not contribute to pressure, guilt, or stress.

E. **WORK**: Because of the severity of illness in some chronic Lyme patients, a number will be unable to work. But many patients try to continue on the job and the majority of caretakers are employed outside the home. Nonetheless, more than a few have had to leave work, at least temporarily, to take care of a sick family member. Just as accommodations are often needed at school because of Lyme, the employer may have to try to adjust work responsibilities to allow for the disease. This is not always easy.

First, the patient or caregiver should check to see what family leave and flexible scheduling they might be entitled to. While many employers profess to be supportive, some are subtly or overtly miffed that a worker is asking to alter hours or change shifts, or whatever, to take care of herself or her ward. Co-workers could get irritated if they feel they have to take on more work because of prolonged absence. While many will be empathetic to start, their patience may wear thin as time goes on. If you are the requestor, be very careful not to be perceived as taking advantage of the illness to get out of work. Over time, you may have to give back more than you get in order to garner the flexibility you need.

I am board certified in occupational and preventive medicine and worked in this area for several years prior to moving into clinical research and drug development. In this role I spent a great deal of time struggling with the **Americans with Disabilities Act** (ADA). What a complicated jumble that can be! The ADA prohibits, in some circumstances, discrimination because of a disability. A **disability** is a physical or mental impairment that substantially limits a major life activity. Major life activities include walking, talking, reading, hearing, writing, etc. The decision around whether a particular condition is actually a disability is made on a case-by-case basis. Some conditions are excluded such as current substance abuse and visual impairment that can be corrected with lenses. The law was designed to be flexible to protect people with physical, mental, or cognitive deficits.

The ADA focuses on employment, access to public places, transportation, telecommunication, and education. In terms of employment, the ADA says you cannot discriminate against a "qualified" individual who must be able to perform the "essential functions of the job." The employer must make "reasonable" accommodations to enable the person to perform the work. Definitions of qualified and reasonable are often in the eyes of the beholder. For example, no amount of accommodation would turn me into an opera singer since I am not qualified for that job. While it may be reasonable to accommodate a blind medical student in her quest to become a psychiatrist, it may not be reasonable for that student to become a surgeon. These cases can become very complicated and contentious.

In terms of TBIs, the most difficult decisions likely involve the chronic nature of Lyme in some patients. Chronicity has been argued around diseases like CFS and fibromyalgia with regard to the ADA. The law says that episodic illnesses (those that wax and wane) are disabling even when the person is in remission *IF* they would be disabled when the disease is active, such as in the case of ulcerative colitis. With all the controversy around the chronic potential of Lyme, the arguments can get messy. Usually chronic is defined as a problem that lasts a year or more, limits what the person can do and requires ongoing care. Where does Lyme fit in? What happens to the patient who believes they are cured only to flare? Fatigue and pain may be especially disabling in this population. If attendance is considered an essential function of the job and a Lyme patient is too fatigued to show up for work, how much accommodation should be made before deciding that the worker cannot perform the fundamental job duties?

In making these determinations for individual cases in the workplace, usually the employee, her manager, the Human Resources person, and occupational medicine doctor meet and discuss what is reasonable. Input will be gathered from the employee's private HCP as well. The meeting should review the job description and recognize the challenges that the employee might be experiencing. The goal should be to develop strategies that might enable the employee to perform her duties. The needs of the worker should be balanced with the needs of the business. Management often starts out empathetic but can soon tire of the situation. Co-workers might feel awkward or resentful if they feel their workload has increased. Remember you can accomplish a lot with "free" accommodations like flexible hours, changes in shifts, or minor alterations in duties. Be creative. There are many parallels between work accommodations and the school accommodations required by Section 504 of the Rehabilitation Act within the ADA, which are described below.

F. **RELATIONSHIPS**: Patients with Lyme may feel isolated and alone. Caregivers of chronic Lyme patients can feel isolated and alone. The effort needed to keep relationships alive when overwhelmed by a chronic illness is considered worth the energy expended. A virus exposure study by Sheldon Cohen from Carnegie Mellon University found that those with the least social interactions got the sickest. The implication was that positive relationships impacted immune response in a constructive way so that the body could better defend against infection. Social interaction may relieve stress which might decrease cortisol levels which appear to exacerbate signs and symptoms of Lyme. Whether this hypothesis is valid in TBIs has not been demonstrated, but does it need to be? Some concepts just make sense.

G. **SIBLINGS/PETS**: One child with a chronic illness or disability can alter the family dynamics. Two sick kids can wreak havoc. Even if the siblings are "really good with him," there can be resentment and jealousy. Consider what siblings may be asked to sacrifice on the altar of the illness and be careful in assigning caretaker roles to kids. Open communication and counseling may be useful. Pretending that negative feelings do not exist can increase internal pressure and acting out. Here is where grandparents and other relatives might play an important supportive role. Even great grandpa can walk the dog or feed the cat or water the plant in an effort to regain family equilibrium. My friend's grandson was born one week before his 3-year-old brother was diagnosed with leukemia. I recently realized that I had never asked how the infant was, or is, or will be, although I ask constantly about the child with cancer. The infant is too young now to realize the disparity in attention, but that will change. Care must be taken that the disease does not completely define the family dynamic. Some marriages don't survive the chronic illness of a child. This isn't the time to turn on one another, but high stress levels can make us all lash out. Each family member has a role, both in the context of the disease and completely independent of it.

H. **ADVOCACY GROUPS**: I cannot say enough about the role that LDASEPA undertook in steering my son to appropriate medical care. They saved him. I also cannot repeat often enough the role that the national LDA and CALDA[1] played in the completion of this book. What do Lyme advocacy groups have to do with life balance? Dealing with chronic Lyme can be a lonely proposition. You see your family member getting sicker and no one seems to hear you when you beg for assistance. The Lyme groups help you realize that you aren't alone. Other people have been in your shoes and came out the other side. They educate, provide information, and help make connections. The role that Lyme associations play in life balance is a bridging function, linking patients and caregivers with sources of information. (I have found solid

corroboration for the information that I have seen and used provided by the local and national LDAs.) They have hot-lines and referral services to TBI-aware HCPs. They can suggest local support groups and legitimate on-line resources such as teen support sites. The work of advocacy groups has helped patients, caregivers, and HCPs. After they help you regain balance and your life stabilizes, you can give back by volunteering and donating to those who helped you.

I. **SCHOOL**: Since this book deals a lot with kids and since kids spend considerable time in school, this section will be large, long, and detailed. Lyme has been shown over and over to detrimentally impact learning unless properly managed by both the medical and education systems. School districts have provided some of the best advocates for Lyme kids and also some of their strongest detractors. Depending on the people you have to deal with, they can make your life heaven or hell. Learning to work within this system could be critical to establishing any type of balance within Lyme families.

1. In an academic setting the manifestations of Lyme most often encountered include:

   a. Debilitating fatigue that does not respond to sleep or rest

   b. Fuzzy thinking, brain fog, confusion

   c. Pain

   d. Exhaustion

   e. Anxiety, sometimes severe or incapacitating

   f. Visual and auditory problems that interfere with reading and communicating

   g. Difficulty processing information

   h. Problems concentrating, focusing, and sustaining interest

   i. Distractibility

   j. Cognitive deficits

   k. Memory loss: short-term, long-term, working recall

   l. Trouble organizing

   m. Attention deficit

   n. Behavior problems that can be debilitating

---

1 CALDA is now referred to as Lymedisease.org

o. Depressed mood and emotional lability

p. Various neuropsychiatric issues

q. Dyslexic-type manifestations

r. Patterns similar to those seen in the autism spectrum

s. Impairment of executive function including difficulties with planning, working memory, attention, problem solving, verbal reasoning, inhibition, mental flexibility, multitasking, initiation, and monitoring actions

2. Cognition and behavior problems are the most common complaints of both parents and teachers regarding Lyme disease in school children.

3. Pat Smith with David Dennis looked at 65 school kids with Lyme. They found more than 90% had neuropsychiatric manifestations including memory problems. About the same number complained of headache and fatigue.

4. Tager, Fallon, et al from Columbia University, looked at the long-term cognitive dysfunction in kids with Lyme. Twenty kids with new onset cognitive problems were compared with 20 matched controls. Each child was assessed using measures of cognition and psychopathology. The children with LD had significantly more cognitive and psychiatric disturbances than those not infected. Cognitive defects were still found after controlling for anxiety, depression, and fatigue. The authors concluded that LD may be accompanied by long-term psychosocial and academic impairments especially in areas of attention and memory. These researchers felt that including LD as part of the DD of kids with new-onset neurocognitive disorders in endemic areas was reasonable.

5. In some students, these problems are new-onset after infection with a TBI. In other cases, the child had gestational transmission. There are other kids who start out with some of these signs and symptoms for unrelated reasons and then get a TBI, which then exacerbates the problem.

6. In most cases where symptoms are associated with Lyme, antibiotic treatment improves the situation.

7. Lyme-induced sleep disturbances may make it hard for students to fall asleep and stay asleep and then get up early for school. Others feel the need to sleep continuously.

8. Problems with impaired executive function manifest in forgetting books and homework and in difficulties with scheduling and organizing.

9. One of the biggest problems that schools have with Lyme is the variable nature of the disease. Because Lyme can wax and wane and flare and remit, school officials can think that the child having one good day will never experience another bad day. Lyme can be an ever-shifting condition. With the picture changing week-to-week or even day-to-day and hour-to-hour, school officials might think they have been duped into accommodating a kid who is clearly faking an illness. Fluctuations in the clinical presentation can cause misunderstandings. Kids who look fine for a while and then crash are the ones most likely to be suspected of faking. The sxs in Lyme can come and go and the child will not look sick 100% of the time.

10. When school personnel see a child they have just excused from attending class out riding her bike or at the market, they feel as if someone has pulled a fast one over on the school. School administrators, I know you have heard it all in terms of excuses. (Remember I was an ER doc for many years who had to deal with virgin births and any number of wild explanations. I had the wool pulled over my eyes many times and when I discovered the ruse, I wasn't happy.) So, please remember that Lyme is rarely, if ever, the condition of choice in kids trying to get out of school. The condition is too complicated and variable. Lies (fake data) are usually simple and consistent. ("It's my story and I'm sticking to it.") Consider that the student with chronic Lyme might truly be suffering and that his parents are just as baffled by what is going on as you are. If a child were going to fake a condition, why would anyone choose Lyme? It's even harder to fake things like babesiosis or bartonellosis, or M. *fermentans*. With these TBIs, the HCPs have barely heard of the conditions let alone the 12-year-old who just feels miserable and doesn't know why she feels so nervous and tired and crazy.

11. In some cases, the educators think that the child is exaggerating the symptoms more than the disease. They believe that even very young children can profess to be "too tired" or "too sick" or have "too bad a headache" to go to school. I would say to these people that if a child is so miserable that she is faking sxs to stay out of school, there is a problem whether it is a TBI or not. Bother yourself to find out what is going on. The experts I consulted say they have found very few cases where the sxs described by the child were not real, although sometimes the sxs are hard for kids to explain.

PEARL: I have several friends who are school nurses. Their consensus is that they have far more problems with administrators and parents than they ever do with the kids.

12. Many of the behavior problems associated with Lyme can be mistaken for sloppiness, disrespect, opposition, and laziness. Especially when a previously good performer takes on a new academic persona, consider that there could be an underlying medical cause and it could be Lyme.

13. With all the associated cognitive difficulties, chronic Lyme patients may or may not be intellectually impaired. A study out of Columbia showed a drop of 22 IQ points in LD kids that later *corrected* with antibiotic treatment. There is great satisfaction in cases where children were labeled retarded and placed in special education classes, only to regain or surpass their baseline IQ levels and excel academically. With appropriate long-term treatment, a seemingly hopeless situation can be reversed. School officials might help recognize problems and identify those who might need further assessment. If just one child is found and helped, the effort would be justified.

14. Some ADD, ADHD, OCD, GAD, ODD, PDD students, as well as kids with new onset behavioral problems, developmental delays, or symptoms found on the autism spectrum, might appropriately be assessed for Lyme and other TBIs, ESPECIALLY if the condition is not responding to conventional therapy. What a shame if the child has a treatable problem that is not explored.

15. Some chronic Lyme cases are discovered too late and there are already permanent sequelae. These manifestations will likely need accommodation from the school.

16. In a study reported with Pat Smith, David Dennis was surprised at the "devastation" Lyme could cause in school children, especially the social costs. Student life is disrupted with dramatic declines in GPA, decreased extracurricular activities, and decreased time spent with peers. School performance of nearly all children with chronic Lyme fell, sometimes drastically, and in several instances was said to interfere with selection by colleges and universities.

17. Whatever the clinical presentation, the pupil will need validation of the condition from their treating HCP. The more knowledge the HCP has regarding TBIs, the more productive the communication with the school can be. If the HCP thinks the symptoms are "all in his head," the discussion about appropriate accommodations is likely to be stymied. If the attending physician is not an advocate for your child, consider finding another HCP.

18. Students could potentially be harmed by misdiagnosis and under-diagnosis due to the inadequate diagnostic criteria laid out in one guideline. Consider finding another HCP if the one you have denies the child is sick, says the symptoms are psychosomatic, or will not help pursue accommodation by the school, irrespective of diagnosis.

19. Especially in endemic areas, Lyme may be causing more learning problems within the schools than it is given credit for. Lyme case reports have increased by 40% in the last decade but as few as 10% of the real cases are captured. Therefore, there may be more kids with Lyme sitting in classrooms than we recognize. The presence of these kids is impacting education from all angles. Patricia Smith reports on a study where the CDC found that the median duration of chronic Lyme in the 64 students studied was 363 days, the mean number of school days missed due to illness was 103, median duration of home instruction 98 days, and more than a third of the families of affected kids had 3 or more members diagnosed with Lyme at some time including 40% of moms. Nearly 80% of the parents stated that their children experienced a fall in grades during the time of illness and 79% noted a decrease in friends.

20. The role of the **school nurse** can be especially important for the Lyme-infected students and their families. The National Association of School Nurses is committed to curtailing the prevalence of tick-borne disease and acknowledging the importance of prevention. There are a number of ways the nursing staff can be involved:

   a. If a child is inattentive and chronically tired, think Lyme.

   b. If there is a new onset of behavior problems or an escalation of known problems, think Lyme (or other TBI).

   c. With significant neuropsychiatric problems, especially those that are not responding to conventional treatment, think TBIs such as Lyme, bartonellosis, and infection with M. *fermentans*.

   d. Suggesting that a child have further medical evaluation may be the biggest favor anyone has ever done for an infected student.

e. You may be part of the team assessing the student's disability and designing IEPs and adequate accommodations. Your input can be the most valuable at the table since it can be the most objective. You can balance both the needs of the student as well as the perspective of the school. Yes, the child needs flexible school hours, but, no, the child does not need a school-supplied, personal yoga room.

f. Kids who already had conditions such as ADD, ADHD, OCD, ODD, or PDD when infected with Lyme may present with a much more complicated clinical picture. Lyme-induced symptoms, or those that are exacerbated by Lyme, will not likely improve unless the underlying Bb infection is treated along with treating the individual signs.

g. Know that depression and suicide are possible with any chronic illness and a higher incidence is hypothesized with Lyme. We do not know the stats, but we don't need to since the potential should be sufficient for us to be more vigilant. Pat Smith relays anecdotes of a NJ student who committed suicide when she felt no one understood her Lyme, as well as the case of a young male who stopped taking his medicine after a doctor told him he didn't have Lyme and all his symptoms were in his head. He killed himself when he could no longer bear the pain.

h. A prime role of the school nurse is to educate herself, her students, her patients, the staff, and the administration. She is likely the only information source available for many of these individuals. Kids will need to know that they cannot "catch" Lyme from another student no matter how sick that child is. PICC lines and IVs may need to be explained as well as why some students are "allowed" to skip school when others are not. The nurse might be able to explain that the sick child doesn't want to be away so much. While being away from school for a day or two can be fun, more time away than that is boring and lonely.

i. The nurse might also be expected to discuss tick bite prevention. There are a number of resources available from LDA and its local affiliates to aid in this endeavor. This book might also be used as a reference.

j. As the nurse, retain your compassion. Encourage the LD students to push themselves somewhat, but not beyond what they can do physically because of the disease.

k. The nurse can serve as advocate, cheerleader, and empathetic ear. A number of LD kids said that it was

helpful to know they could go to the nurse's office when they needed to rest.

l. The nurse can function as an advocate for the patient, conduit to the administration, and an overall knowledge source. Sometimes a nurse is the only support a Lyme disease student has at the school.

m. Communication between the parents and the nurse can be important and both parties should be interested in establishing an on-going dialog, leading to collaboration toward a common goal. Whether she wants to or not, the nurse may become the communication center: talking to the outside HCPs, discussing the situation with the teacher and administration, coordinating efforts with the parents, and helping the patient/student. The nurse can facilitate a cooperative environment in the best interest of the child.

n. A Lyme-infected child may be jumping around one minute and flat the next minute. She may have little spurts of activity but little stamina.

o. Smith and Dennis found that children with persistent Lyme in the school system often recovered on appropriate treatment but a number of them had to be treated for 2 to 4 years. The school nurse would likely be involved with this treatment, administering medications and monitoring for adverse reactions and other problems.

p. Unfortunately, chronically ill kids are seen as different and can be the target of bullies. Victims are often stressed to the point that they can be afraid to return to school especially after an extended absence. Some are ostracized when they return. There are cases of school phobia that have developed from intimidation at school. Recent reports of staff and teachers contributing to teasing and bullying have hit the media. The school nurse should be aware of the possibility of bullying and be prepared to help the victim.

q. With all that being said, most school nurses are BUSY. They have dozens of students vying for their attention on a daily basis. And, like the rest of the medical profession, they are inundated with paperwork, changing rules, and bureaucracy. Despite the best of intentions, there just might not be enough hours in the day to do all they would like to do.

21. **Teachers** are likely to have the most face time with the chronic Lyme students. Kids with behavioral problems from any cause can be hard to like. Recognizing that the manifestations of Lyme are potentially irritating and frustrating can be quite liberating. It's okay to

feel irritated and frustrated sometimes. In most cases, the child is not trying to annoy. The disease is doing that for him.

a. Clearly, a sick child who is in and out of the classroom can increase the workload of an already overworked teacher. Constantly having to set alternative test dates and put together separate homework packages can be exasperating. You are not an evil person or a bad teacher because you experience negative feelings in these situations. Still, you are the professional and it's best to direct the negativity at the disease and not the child, who is probably just as bewildered and frustrated as you.

b. The teacher must guard against the Lyme student disrupting the class and consuming a disproportionate amount of teacher time and energy. If this becomes the case, then the teacher needs to pursue additional resource and accommodation in the classroom.

c. Parents can be a colossal pain. Please remember that if their child has a chronic illness, especially one as potentially debilitating as Lyme, the parents have been through hell. They have probably had to wrestle with the medical establishment and are happy that their child is alive. Their home life has been turned upside down. They are confused and petrified that the changes they see in their child's health may be permanent and disabling.

d. On the other hand, there are parents and students who will milk a medical condition for both academic and personal advantages. They must realize that you have other students in need of your attention and you are not a private tutor for one student. They should expect you to be compassionate and fair. You should expect them to respect your role as teacher, value your time, and consider your professional opinion.

e. With Lyme, all sides might have to give the other the benefit of the doubt.

f. Lyme can go after nerve tissue and the many neuropsychiatric signs of Lyme can be mistaken for a lack of intelligence. In fact, appropriate treatment for Lyme has been shown to reverse even large dips in IQ scores due to infection. Many of these students have not only persevered, they have excelled.

g. Never give up on a student with Lyme. They may need treatment to overcome their learning and behavioral difficulties.

h. If you see a child with persistent fatigue or a new onset of behavioral problems or an exacerbation of a previous condition, talk to the nurse or the parents to see if there is an underlying medical condition to blame.

i. As the classroom teacher, you may be part of the panel assessing the child's ability to learn and developing IEPs and accommodations. Consider that if the child's problems are due to underlying infection, that the condition may change with appropriate treatment. Don't let a child be put into a box that she can never escape.

j. You know that any signs of weakness or being different can expose a child to a chance of being bullied. Be aware of the risk and know how you will handle a bully before you find yourself confronting the situation.

22. The **administration,** including the school board, is responsible for the local policies and procedures and for the execution of state and federal law. This ranges from implementation of laws around accommodation and individual education programs to the maintenance of the physical plant where ticks can wait to feed. Some areas of administrative involvement with Lyme are listed.

a. The administration can work to decrease the opportunity for tick bites on school property. Chapter 32: *Prevention* contains much information applicable to schools and students with regard to preventing bites. Ticks do not like well-manicured lawns but thrive in the border areas with the longer grass and foliage, often found at the perimeter of schoolyards. Leaf piles and the edge of woods are also prime habitats for waiting ticks. Play areas should be in dry, sunny spots since ticks prefer moist places and are not inclined to migrate to areas where they could desiccate.

b. While the actual education around tick-borne illness is likely performed by the nurse or outside speakers, the administration is responsible for providing the tools, time, and staff to educate students and school personnel.

c. The administration needs to provide adequate resource. Investment in prevention and management of current cases will be more cost-effective than letting ticks and disease run rampant. Once Lyme disease becomes chronic, accommodations can be costly. An ounce of prevention may be the most fiscally responsible approach. So instead of the press box and climbing wall we now have at the local school, could this money have been better spent in the nurse's office?

d. Schools, especially those in endemic areas, need to be aware of their responsibility to protect students from tick bites on field trips. There is at least one legal case where the child is alleged to have acquired Lyme disease on a school trip and the parents had not been informed of the risk. The www.lymedisease.org website contains a "Field Trip Tick Alert" that talks about risks and protection.

e. Recognize that because of Lyme, the family may be under considerable stress financially, medically, and emotionally.

f. Schools in TBI-prone areas might have a real drain on money and resources due to Lyme and the need to accommodate many kids at once. Better to plan ahead than waste energy by fighting every step of the way. These kids exist.

g. As administrators, do not view Lyme patients as adversaries or malingerers or consumers of a disproportionate amount of your budget. Negative feelings will not make these kids go away. Rather think of creative ways to integrate these children into your school system, using the resources you already have available. Flexibility on your part might be quite cost-effective. While a small minority might want more than they are entitled to by law, most parents will be willing to meet more than halfway to work out a plan that is fair and effective. You might be surprised at how far you can go with "free" accommodations such as adjusting school hours, pushing back the morning start times, or student note sharing services.

23. Just because someone works at a school, do not assume she knows the school's legal responsibilities to a sick child or a child with special needs. All states have their own education and accommodation laws. Note that state and local laws are superseded by federal laws unless the local law is more protective of the child. There are two national programs that are in place for any school system receiving government funding. This applies from pre-school through college.

a. A **504 plan** refers to Section 504 of the Rehabilitation Act within the Americans with Disabilities Act. This section says that no one with a disability can be excluded from participating in federally funded schooling. This law outlines the modifications and accommodations that will be needed for the students to have the opportunity to perform at the same level

as their peers. These adjustments have spanned everything from monitoring of medicine doses, home instruction, and flexible schedules.

• Possible accommodations to consider: part-time classes, homeschooling, tutors at school or at home, classroom aides, resource room, special education classes, speech or language therapy, IEP, cognitive remediation, cognitive testing, sensorimotor therapy, physical accommodations such as ramps, elevators, or wheelchairs, late start times, longer times for testing, flexible hours, lighter course loads, focus on core subjects only, classes over the summer and during breaks to make up for fewer classes during the school year, peer tutors, and creative approaches targeted to the individual case.

• The variable nature of the clinical course of Lyme can make accommodating these students more challenging. For a week they may be so debilitated they need to be able to rest in the nurse's office two hours a day and then the next week they might have much more energy. Accommodations may need to be flexible, allowing the child to do more when she can and less when necessary. Lyme is not the same as a structural deformity that might stay the same over time and the accommodations would be relatively static.

• Lyme cases can be unique in a way that Pat Smith describes as "transitory learning disabilities." Cognitive deficits and other Lyme-associated symptoms can vary over both short and long time periods. Flexibility might be built into the accommodations and individualized education plans, since conditions change so regularly. For example, one child might be home schooled for a time, then use at-home tutors, then try a part-time return to school, and gradually progress as tolerated. If the child relapses, then the educational plan may need to take a step or two back until the child can regain the lost progress. In all cases, try to take advantage of times when the child is more capable of learning. Just a visit to his old class may help dispel the isolation. Since one purpose of school is socialization, Lyme can result in big social deficits for kids who are stuck at home for weeks or months.

• With the 504 plan, anyone who has a physical or mental impairment that substantially limits one or more major life activities, such as working or learning, is entitled to be placed in the regular educational environment with the use of aids and services unless education in the regular environment with aid can't be achieved.

- Pat Smith quotes a CDC report: "Perhaps the greatest cost incurred by the study children were the social costs of the illness and its treatment. Schooling and extracurricular learning activities were seriously interrupted for most children. Often, children spent large blocks of time as semi-invalids, isolated from social groups and missing out on cultural, sports and social activities." Some schools have a policy where if a child is absent from school she is not allowed to participate in extracurricular activities. This can be a sad, unproductive rule for Lyme patients, since many are often desperate for social interaction. Extracurricular activities are different from a structured school day. Here the student can observe or participate as she is able and, if the activity becomes too demanding, the student can rest or leave. Social events like birthday parties or friends going to the movies might be tailor-made for Lyme patients who tend to have little stamina and may need to restrict participation to short or non-taxing events. Accommodations and IEPs should not be punitive and should enable sick kids to benefit from the social interactions that school can provide. Of course, the student should be expected to give her best effort in attempting the academic aspects of school and not just the social.

b. Individualized Education Programs or **IEPs** are mandated by the Individuals with Disabilities Education Act (IDEA) and are designed to meet the unique educational needs of the individual child who has a defined disability. The IEP must be tailored to the individual needs as determined by the IEP evaluation process. The IEP should help teachers and paraprofessionals understand the disability and how it might affect that child's ability to learn. The child should be assessed to determine learning strengths and weaknesses that will help determine the best education process for this particular student. The learning environment should be the least restrictive possible in accommodating the child's needs.

- Children with chronic Lyme might fit into the IDEA classifications in several ways.

- Here, disability refers to a physical or mental impairment which substantially limits one or more major life activities and specifically includes chronic conditions.

- Guardians are intended to be full participants in setting up the IEP for their child.

- An IEP is not intended to just deposit students in special education classes but to appropriately place them in an environment where they can learn.

- Services under IDEA depend on the severity of the illness and how the condition impacts learning.

- IEP programs that move beyond special education classes may be expensive and IEP committee members may be reluctant to spend money on accommodations they feel are excessive for just one child. These programs should focus first on what might be accomplished within the already existing framework and press for additional accommodations only as truly needed.

- Pat Smith, the current LDA president and long time school board member, makes a practical point. Although children with Lyme can be eligible for an IEP or 504 plan, sufficient accommodations might be negotiated between all parties so that a workable plan can be implemented without an "official" IEP or 504 program.

24. **Parents** are integral to the school/home balance.

a. Don't just go with what the school deems appropriate for your child. By law, parents have a right to input into IEP discussions and plans. You are the expert on your child. And remember, you catch more flies with honey than with vinegar.

b. If a staff member is doing his best to help you, show gratitude.

c. You should investigate what accommodations and additional services your child might be entitled to use.

d. Make sure you have an HCP who is knowledgeable enough with the provisions of the 504 plan, as well as the nature of TBDs, to help you work with the school.

e. Establish a strong working relationship with the school nurse and your child's teacher(s). If one or both of these individuals are impossible to work with, try everything possible to repair the relationship. If collaboration just isn't going to be possible, take your concerns up the chain.

f. Be reasonable. Enable your child to do what is possible within the already existing framework and press for those additional accommodations only as truly required.

g. Don't take advantage. One of my son's classmates, who aspired to be an astronaut, said he needed extra time on tests to perform at his best since he was a "slow thinker." Since most of the testing in aeronautical engineering is insanely time-sensitive, this was a distinct advantage to this student who showed no evidence of slow thinking when he was driving or performing other tasks, like doing homework. I do not know the diagnosis he used to justify his slow thinking but it makes you wonder how fast he might respond if this aspiring astronaut had to say, "Houston, we had a problem."

h. Don't take advantage. A mother in one practice wanted a note saying her child was too tired to attend school in any capacity so she would then be free to go on a year-long plush trip around the world. The plan was to go hiking and bungee jumping and scuba diving and indulge in multiple physically taxing adventures. This mom also wanted a free office visit since she needed to save money for the trip.

i. Try not to mimic the little boy who cried wolf. I know I was often frenetic when my child was sick. When you see things going downhill, your first impulse may be to panic or get aggressive. Try to pick your battles, so you don't waste your "pester" credits on a small matter when you might need something more important later.

j. Don't forget to make use of speech and/or language therapy offered through the school, if your child could benefit. Lyme can significantly impact a child's ability to communicate and process information. If such therapy is not offered, you might ask.

k. Because of the controversy around the diagnosis of Lyme, your child may have difficulty being recognized as a child with special needs. Your HCP will be essential in confirming the medical condition and helping to work out a program that is of practical benefit to your child. Some school administrators are skeptical that Lyme could genuinely affect energy and focus to such a degree. Others have accused Lyme kids of being lazy and unmotivated. Here is where your HCP advocate can again become involved. If your HCP is not up to the task, you may need to find another. Your local LDA affiliate may be able to refer you to HCPs in your area.

l. You may be your child's only advocate. You may have to be persistent. The squeaky wheel gets the oil. You don't want to be obnoxious, but you do want your child to get what she is entitled to under the law and to be treated with respect. When you read the writings of Pat Smith and Pam Weintraub, and you listen to the stories told by parents in the clinician's office, you will realize that you may have to become quite insistent to get what your child needs. You may have to make it easier for them to grant your request than to listen to your gripe one more time. If you get no satisfaction, take your request up the chain.

m. If your child has been out of school for an extended period, work with the staff to help ease the transition back into the classroom.

n. Remember that modifications may make more work for your child's teacher. Do whatever you can to help the teacher accommodate your child. Meet them more than halfway.

In working to balance school and chronic disease, always keep in mind that children with persistent Lyme, who are appropriately managed, have gone on to college and excelled. My son is a graduate student in rocket science in one of the top programs in the world. But his TBIs presented many challenges and obstacles. He had to exert superhuman effort to overcome a lack of concentration, distractibility, and problems with focus and persistence. These problems did not occur until after he was infected with TBIs. Re-treatment was necessary to resolve these issues. Willpower was not enough and he has the doggedness of a pit bull. Antibiotics were necessary. For a long time. Three times. So far.

If the school is dismissive, disrespectful, or punitive regarding their handling of the chronic illness, take your complaints up the chain. The law protects your child's right to an education. Make them live up to their responsibility. Fight like a tiger. With that being said, some situations are hopeless, and for whatever reason, if the administration is obstinate, inflexible, and unmovable, consider cutting your losses. If your child is miserable, think of your options. What would it take to rectify this situation? Is the juice worth the squeeze?

Despite the misery of the disease, the school should be trying to provide a positive learning environment that challenges the child without overwhelming him physically or emotionally. He should be expected to perform within the limits of his disease, pushing a little but not taxing the system as it heals. The student should be slightly challenged, but not overwhelmed. Recovery takes a lot of energy and that supersedes all else.

The HCP may need to interact with school personnel trying to arrive at the best learning environment for the patient. Be careful, some private schools can be reluctant to take on Lyme kids because they worry that their test scores could be compromised. Find ways to reassure them that with proper treatment, cognitive difficulties can resolve. Use examples provided in Chapter 17-N. "And with your exceptional program at (enter name of snooty school here), I'm sure little Albert will excel." Realize that schools who do not accept government funding do not have to follow the rules for accommodations and IEPs.

The various LDAs have information on websites and in the form of pamphlets available for students, parents, and educators. The national LDA has a pamphlet called "The ABC's of Lyme Disease." You may want to have such a pamphlet with you when you discuss your child's needs with the school staff. Or this book... or both...

FINAL THOUGHTS ON LIFE BALANCE AND LYME

Pam Weintraub laments the lost childhood of many kids with persistent Lyme. Please do not wait for total healing before you allow some peace and pleasure into your lives. There is life during and after Lyme.

Sheldon Cohen, PhD, from Carnegie Mellon University has done considerable work on levels of positive emotion (happiness, calmness, and liveliness) and the capacity for sickness and health. The lower the positive emotions, the more likely the subjects were to get sick. A positive mind set and an optimistic attitude mattered. Several studies say you feel better if you smile even if you're faking it. Friends mattered, because they tended to reduce high stress levels.

There is a strong connection between thoughts, beliefs, and healing. When a patient expects a treatment to work, the brain chemistry shifts to allow healing to happen by releasing endorphins and other chemicals that help improve immune function. Our minds and bodies know how to get well, we just need to help them. There is a strong mind-body connection where it is hard for one aspect of the self to be sick without impacting the other.

Relax, seek pleasure, stimulate the mind, and try art, music, or gardening. Do not become "all Lyme all the time." In the midst of a nasty Lyme flare, it can be hard to believe that there is anything else in life aside from Lyme. Do things you enjoy. But don't become so focused on the idea that your life SHOULD be more balanced that you become even more stressed.

Believe in SOMETHING. Have something to get excited about. People who believe they have a life purpose live longer. For many of us, who have had a child sick from Lyme and have struggled with the medical establishment, our passion becomes our advocacy for Lyme patients.

As an HCP, expect to do some counseling about emotional balance issues during each contact. Of course, if you are not comfortable in this arena, refer as appropriate. If you see a family becoming unstable and unbalanced because of the disruption caused by Lyme, address the issue. Do not wait to be asked. Do not ignore the situation, hoping it will go away. The more balanced the lives of the patients and caretakers, the greater the chance for a positive outcome.

Chapter 32

PREVENTION

Society is always taken by surprise at any new example of common-sense.
Ralph Waldo Emerson

Let me confess, I have come across a hundred ways to remove a tick. Every crusader on the planet has the ultimate, supreme, utmost, superlative, never-need-another method. From smearing the tick with fingernail polish, Vaseline, peanut butter, gasoline, lipstick, Vicks VapoRub, acetone, mayonnaise, liquid soap, olive oil, or Karo syrup, to burning it out with a lit match, I've heard them all. People who know I am working on this book continue to send me the "latest" even-better technique. This chapter will clearly define the least risky method of tick removal as well as outline a number of other prudent prevention modalities.

Prevention is paramount. Unfortunately, if you are assessing a patient for TBIs, it's too late to prevent *that* particular bite. Remember, though, that exposure to a number of these tick-borne pathogens does not seem to provide long-lasting immunity. For some patients, another bite that could transmit more of the same pathogens or a whole different crop, can be very bad news. In all cases, the most prudent course is to avoid a *second* bite.

While we are familiar with measures we can take to prevent the bite that causes the initial disease, we should also be mindful of the ways we can prevent **acute** disease from turning into a **chronic** condition. Much of the following has been contributed by Doug Fearn and Ron Hamlen, PhD, both from LDASEPA. I could write 10 books and still not know as much about ticks and TBI demographics as these two. Dr. Hamlen earned his PhD in plant pathology and nematology and did postdoctoral training in insect pathology and microbial insect control.

A number of practical tips can help avoid both acute and chronic TBDs.

I. WHO IS AT RISK?

While I would like to be able to define a specific population that is at the greatest risk, there is always the first case of a TBI in a new area. In any locale, HCPs may have been missing the diagnosis for quite some time before that first case is recognized. You don't want your child to be that case. Everyone in North America needs to be aware of the potential dangers of

a tick bite, especially people in areas where disease-bearing ticks have been identified.

I cannot emphasize prevention enough. When my son was in Boy Scouts, one leader begged the kids to watch for ticks. The kids thought she was hysterical and were very cavalier about tick bites, toying with many of the bad behaviors I am about to warn you against. Now, many of these same kids are dealing with the long-term consequences of repeated infections. If only they had listened.

A. **Predisposing activities**: After saying that everyone should be attentive, there are certain subpopulations at greater risk. Gardeners, hikers, hunters, fishers, golfers who wander into high vegetation, outdoor workers, campers, picnickers, city dwellers moving through planted areas or weeds, and park visitors. Kids are at special risk because they tend to take off into the tall grass without a second thought. Children on school-sponsored trips have also been found to be at additional risk.

B. **Age**: According to the CDC, children and teens account for more than 60% of yearly cases of Lyme. The ages most likely to have deer ticks removed are between 8 and 14. Of course, tick bites have been documented in all age groups from the youngest infants to centenarians. The younger the child, the thinner and softer the skin and the more vascular. Easy and rapid transmission is possible.

C. **Location:** TBIs, especially Lyme, have been reported in all 50 states. On my recent trip to Alaska, the locals said they had no TBIs. Yet they said there were plenty of ticks and each person we spoke to did know someone who had a cousin or a dog that "might have had Lyme disease." Many were still having problems or, in the case of the two dogs mentioned, had died. Who knows? Wherever you are, keep the possibility of TBI in mind.

There are parts of North America where tick-borne diseases are endemic. That means the implicated tick species are located in these particular areas in high concentrations. Individuals living or traveling in these regions should be on high alert.

PEARL: The term endemic refers to entities, in this case TBIs, that are found in a particular area or are affecting a particular population. Diseases that are caused by vectors native to a district are said to be endemic in that locale. Endemic means indigenous or native to a place.

Consider the following map compiled from data provided on Lyme disease incidence by the CDC-P.

Reported Cases of Lyme Disease—United States, 2010

One dot is placed randomly within the county of residence for each confirmed case. Though Lyme disease cases have been reported in nearly every state, cases are reported based on the county of residence, not necessarily the county of infection.

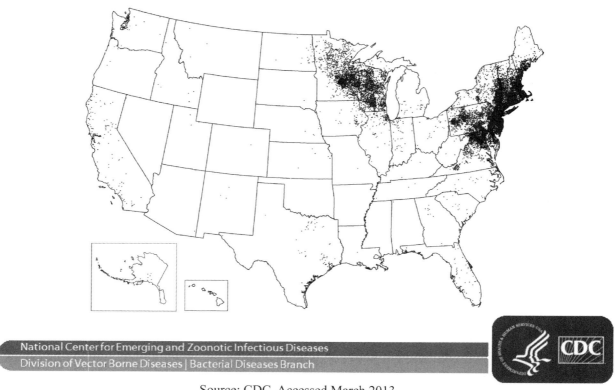

National Center for Emerging and Zoonotic Infectious Diseases
Division of Vector Borne Diseases | Bacterial Diseases Branch

Source: CDC. Accessed March 2013

While this map is frightening for those of us who live in the dark endemic areas, consider how frightened you should be when you recognize that this map is based only on those cases that meet the CDC surveillance criteria. Conservative estimates are that only about 1 out of 10 cases are identified using these CDC criteria. Imagine this map with 10 times the shading. The areas from southern Maine to Maryland, as well as the upper midwest and parts of California, are considered hyper-endemic. If you get bitten from a tick in these geographic locales you will want that creature OFF you as soon as humanly possible to minimize risk of disease transmission. Also, consider the use of prophylactic treatment.

PEARL: Robert Lane is a tick researcher in northern California. In his geographic area, 70% of human LD cases are due to the bites of tick nymphs. The adult males are not usually hazardous because they do not feed. There, fewer adult ticks are infected compared to nymphs because when the adult female feeds on a western fence lizard, the Bb do not survive. This destruction is due to proteins that are only expressed when the Bb are in the lizard. In California, a prime involved species is the squirrel. The point of this PEARL is never trust a tick. Any life stage, any gender, any reservoir, any location poses potential risk. Of course, some scenarios are riskier than others. Stay suspicious.

D. Habitat: Deer ticks like moist environments, not too hot or dry. They prefer moderate to cool temperatures but not freezing since freezing temperatures tend to make them enter diapause. The most favorable niches include: leaf litter, tall grass and weeds at the edge of yards, stone walls, stacked logs, adjacent wooded areas, and the sides of roads and trails. Unfortunately, suburban backyards often provide many of these compatible surroundings.

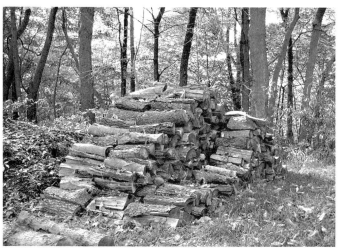

Stacked logs are a common place to find ticks.
Photograph by Doug Fearn, LDASEPA

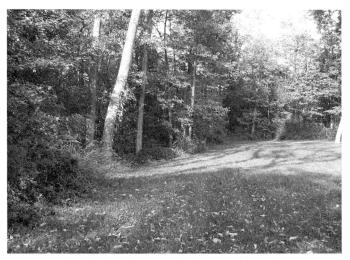

The border between the lawn and woods,
the suburban ideal, is a tick paradise.
Photograph by Doug Fearn, LDASEPA

E. Active times: Spring and summer tend to have the most tick activity since fall can be too hot and dry in some areas. Nonetheless, ticks can be active anytime the temperature is warm enough for them to move. Ticks have been known to mobilize even when the temperatures are below freezing. So, just when you thought it was safe to let your guard down, don't.

II. PREVENTION of TICK BITES

A. Be vigilant: There will be more active ticks in spring and summer and into the fall than in winter. There will be more ticks in leaf litter and wood stacks. There will be more ticks on trails near the woods. There will be more ticks when camping especially in old, rustic, wood cabins. There will be more ticks in suburbs where woods have been cleared to make way for houses and where deer and mice have free reign. Ticks can be found in the most unlikely and unexpected places. A commercial airline flight was recently delayed because a tick was found on board. Anyone who is immunocompromised (splenectomy, AIDS, chronically ill, the very young or very old) should be especially mindful of the risk of a tick bite. This caveat includes those who have been severely ill with a TBI in the past.

B. Protect Property: When in a tick-infested habitat like a wooded boundary area, don't sit directly on the ground, walls, fallen logs, stumps, or wood piles. Consider an impervious ground cover, like a piece of Gore-Tex fabric. Walk in the center of trails and try not to brush into the plants along the sides. Remember ticks can fall on you as well as attach onto you from low-growth foliage. For those in the suburbs, remove all standing leaf piles and stacked wood. Some sources recommend a gravel moat if the yard borders an overgrown area. Since ticks will not likely cross the hot, dry gravel, this barricade should keep them off the property. Since ticks require high humidity to survive, pruning trees to allow sunlight to reach the ground will lower the humidity in this low-lying area. Try not to disturb the foliage on the property border when mowing. Details on vector control, as well as pesticide spraying options, are provided below.

C. Clothing: Wear light colored clothes for easy tick discovery. Tuck pants into socks and shirt into pants so that ticks have a harder time crawling close to skin. Wear both long pants and high sox. A long-sleeved shirt is also recommended. Wear a hat and gloves if there is a chance for hand or head exposure. No bare feet, flip-flops, or sandals.

Use the insecticide permethrin on clothes. Spray until visibly damp or wet and let dry before wearing into infested areas. Some authorities also recommend that the clothes be sprayed again and allowed to dry before washing. Then wash in hot water and dry for at least 30 minutes in a hot dryer. One study showed that more than half of the ticks survived a hot water wash, but did not survive a hot drier. The dry heat desiccates the tick. Recommended drying times range from 30 to 60 minutes. This regimen is also good for sleeping bags. There are effective, but expensive, clothes, such as Insect Shield with built-in repellent, but spraying with permethrin seems to work well.

Rynoskin protective underwear is made of breathable material that ticks have trouble penetrating. This product is available in long sleeved tops and long bottoms, socks, hoods, and gloves.

D. Monitor: When engaged in outdoor activity, check every 2 or 3 hours for ticks on clothing or skin. If possible, brush off any ticks on clothing before skin attachment occurs. A thorough check of body surfaces for attached ticks should be done at the end of the outing. Remember new thinking is that even very short tick attachments can transmit pathogens. Of course, the longer the tick is attached and the more its saliva can mingle with the host's blood, the more likely is infection. Do not revel in the false sense of security that comes from thinking transmission can't happen in a short period of time. Wishing doesn't make it so. Especially with some of the co-infections, transmission can be quite rapid. Get in the habit of doing "tick checks." Check the dog and cat. Check clothes as well as skin. Do a full body review after bathing. Have someone else check the parts you cannot see yourself—it's that important. Holding up a mirror to your backside usually doesn't do the trick unless you are a contortionist. Check all hairlines, hair growth areas, scalp, and ears – all the nooks and crannies, especially where clothes were tight fitting like waistbands. Check bedding for several days after possible exposure. Check pets and their bedding regularly.

Also, monitor health closely after a tick bite. If any symptoms of infection appear such as headache, flu-like syndrome, fever, or rash, consult an HCP. Be especially vigilant for signs and symptoms in the first month, but the susceptible period may be longer. ILADS recommends the use of prophylactic antibiotics after a tick bite and these regimens are outlined in a later section. I am a strong proponent of prophylaxis.

E. Bug spray: Repellents on exposed skin can be effective in reducing bites, but their use is not without risk, especially if repellents are applied excessively or improperly. Repellents commonly available to consumers include many commercial brands of the following:

- DEET (N,N-diethyl-m-toluamide) – DEET products have been widely used for many years. DEET can be applied directly to the *skin*, but the eyes should be avoided. Use on all exposed skin areas. Commercial formulations generally contain 20% to 50% DEET, but 30% to 35% is the recommended strength. The American Academy of Pediatrics says up to 30% DEET can be used on kids over 2 months of age, but use only what you need since DEET can be absorbed.

DEET can be applied to the skin but only lasts a few hours before it needs to be reapplied. The higher the percentage of DEET in the formulation, the more hours of protection there are. DEET evaporates fast and must be reapplied often. Generally, 5% to 10% lasts about 90 minutes; 35% is effective for about 4 hours. If the person is sweating or swimming, reapply again when the skin is dry. If using a lower percentage formulation, reapply more often.

PEARL: Several sources noted that DEET might be more readily absorbed into the system if applied in lotions containing SPF.

Use caution in kids because DEET can cause adverse effects. Skin reactions (especially at DEET concentrations of 50% and above) and eye irritation are the most frequently reported health problems. DEET has also been associated with headaches.

A controlled release DEET formulation, Ultrathon is available as a cream, aerosol, or spray and is a highly effective repellent. This preparation provides longer residual and is believed to last 12 hours with one application.

- Picaridin (20%) is an effective non-DEET tick repellent.

- Permethrin – A formulation of 0.5% permethrin should be applied outdoors to minimize inhalation. Spray onto *fabric* and never directly onto the skin. Permethrin can cause eye irritation. Rather than acting as a repellent, permethrin kills ticks and insects that come in contact with the treated material. Use permethrin on clothes, footwear, gloves, hats, sleeping bags, bedding, and tents. Spray clothing until moist and let dry before going into infested areas. An application will last several days or even weeks. Some authorities recommend that potentially contaminated clothes be sprayed again and allowed to dry before washing. There are a number of brands, so follow the label directions. Note that permethrin is usually not found in drug stores but often must be purchased in outdoor supply shops or on-line. Pretreated clothing like Insect Shield are available from these same sources.

PEARL: Use the insecticide permethrin on clothes. Spray until damp or wet and dry before use. Subsequently, the clothing should be sprayed again and allowed to dry before washing. Then wash in hot water and dry for a minimum of 30 minutes in a hot dryer. While half the ticks will survive hot water they will not survive a hot drier. The dry heat desiccates the tick. Recommended drying times range from 30 to 60 minutes, which should also be good for sleeping bags.

- Of course, the literature is full of any number of other types of repellents. Botanical oils such as oil of geranium, cedar, lemongrass, soy, or citronella are available. Oil of lemon eucalyptus may offer protection against mosquitoes, but data are limited regarding its ability to repel ticks. Everything from Avon's Skin So Soft to smoke has been recommended to ward off insects. Usually, there is limited information on their effectiveness and safety when used as a repellent. Rosmarie Kelly, PhD, MPH, entomologist with the Georgia Division of Public Health, says that products with DEET are usually the best for fending off mosquitoes and ticks. If you want to go with something plant-based, oil of lemon eucalyptus (sometimes called PMD) may be as effective as repellents with 10% to 15% DEET. She does not recommend this oil in kids under 3. Just because something is "natural" doesn't mean it's safer. She would skip sprays made with citronella, geranium, basil, garlic, and peppermint since they generally don't work that well. Dr. Kelly also avoids repellent/sunscreen combos. Sunscreen usually needs to be applied at different intervals than repellents so some protection could get shortchanged. Since tick avoidance is so important, choose the most effective methods available to you.

If you decide to use a repellent, use only what and how much you need for your situation. In addition:

i.   Be sure to follow label directions.

ii. Use repellents only in necessary amounts, avoiding excessive repeat applications.

iii. Kids may be at greater risk for reactions to repellents, in part because their exposure may be greater. Some sources advocate applying the repellent to your own hands and then putting it on the child to minimize inhalation and ingestion. Do not apply to the hands of babies or children.

iv. Do not apply near eyes, nose, or mouth and use sparingly around ears.

v.   After returning indoors, wash treated skin with soap and water.

ADVICE THAT SHOULDN'T NEED TO BE GIVEN: Do not use a pet's flea and tick collar on yourself or your children.

F. **Vector and reservoir control:** In Chapter 2: *The Tick*, I referred to controlling the Lyme epidemic by managing the vector, the host, and the reservoir. Management of all three will likely be needed to get the situation back under human control.

Focus on the tick vector: Both scientists and government agencies have tried to control tick populations by applying pesticides and eliminating tick habitats such as leaf piles and brush. There has been some success on a small scale. Right now, the ticks are still winning and they are moving into areas that weren't prime targets in the past such as golf courses and urban centers. Since deer bring ticks into your yard, reducing the number of deer has been associated with a reduced number of ticks. Create an environment that is as unfriendly to ticks as possible. Consider the following options.

1. Increase sunlight into your yard to dry the ground, since ticks like moisture.

2. Use bark chips or gravel as edging instead of ground covering plants.

3. Move any play equipment into the sun.

4. Make a 3 foot or wider wood chip or gravel barrier between the yard and the forest.

5. Move gardens and play areas within this barrier.

6. Keep lawns and activity areas mowed and open.

7. Outdoor pesticide applications can be done by commercial companies or by the home resident with a hose applicator spraying toward the ground and on leaf piles and low bushes or foliage. (Remember you were supposed to remove those leaf piles.) There is evidence that pesticide sprays can diminish tick populations in the treated areas. Various pyrethroid formulations like permethrin as well as carbaryl insecticides like Sevin are most commonly used. These can be found in lawn and garden shops and some general department stores.

Focus on the mice and other rodents: Mice often have many deer ticks. *Damminix* tick tubes contain permethrin infused cotton balls. When placed near mice habitats, the mice use the cotton to build nests and the permethrin kills the ticks on the mice. We don't know if this method works with other small rodents that harbor deer ticks like chipmunks, voles, and shrews. In some areas, local governments are trying to curtail the rodent population. Patients and their advocates will need to continue to pressure the regional administrators if action is needed.

Focus on the deer: More control of deer and rodent populations is being attempted but a glance out my window suggests that this isn't working just yet. "Our" deer have scoffed at attempts to encourage them to try a different yard. (Yes, we have tried Ivory soap, blood, human hair, nail clippings, chicken drippings, dog hair, urine, ultrasound devices, flashing lights, noise makers, fences, netting, and extremely expensive, vile-smelling deer repellent, which has run off the neighbors but not the deer.)

Some authors believe that control of the deer population is the key to controlling the tick population. There are several studies that document the relationship between the number of deer, the number of ticks, and the diagnosis of Lyme. Apparently, the number of reported cases decline as the deer population declines. In looking at incidence and prevalence data for TBIs, always remember that rigid and contrived diagnostic criteria may have artificially decreased the number of cases. Nonetheless, the conclusion seems intuitive that if you have fewer deer, you would have fewer deer ticks, and thereby fewer TBDs. But not so fast. Unfortunately, another source notes that when the deer population decreases, the ticks just move to mice, and the number of infected mice increases in the area. We also know now that other tick species may be involved in disease transmission, not just those associated with deer.

The 4-poster deer treatment bait station was developed by researchers at the USDA and has been shown to be effective in reducing both Ixodes and Amblyomma ticks that use white-tailed deer as primary reproductive hosts. Ticks attached to the ears of the deer are treated with insecticide as the deer eat. Tick counts in tested areas showed that this device was effective in helping control the tick populations. Currently, several government agencies are using this approach.

Culling of the deer population continues to be used but is limited by human proximity to deer herds, especially in the suburbs.

Just in case you are worried that I missed something regarding tick avoidance: Do not hang deer carcasses near homes. Place a tub under a dead deer to catch any ticks that fall off, which they will start to do as the carcass cools. They will drop for days. Just because the deer is dead doesn't mean the ticks are. A hungry tick falling off a dead deer would be happy to latch onto a human.

Future possibilities: Some regions are trying new methods like using tick parasites such as fungi, nematodes, or tick predatory wasps to control the tick populations. Certain wasps may have potential to control the tick population by laying eggs in the tick. The emerging hatchling kills the host. In one study, guinea fowl were observed eating mass quantities of ticks. But a separate study showed no effect. Reportedly, a pair might clear as much as two acres a year. So far, Chester County, Pennsylvania remains guinea fowl-free (and quite tick-infested.)

An April 21, 2011, headline announced, "Scientists tweak mosquito genes to fight malaria." Ticks do not seem as easy to control as mosquitoes, where humans can try to dry any standing water to eliminate breeding grounds. And mosquitoes are difficult enough. Perhaps genetic manipulation of ticks will lead to eventual control of TBIs as well.

G. **Pets:** Definitely use flea and tick protection on your dogs and cats. There are many commercial brands and your veterinarian can recommend effective products. While flea and tick protection keeps the pet from tick bites it does not prevent the tick from being transported on the animal's fur and falling inside the home. That hungry tick can then latch onto a human. An unattached tick can survive for weeks indoors. Dr. Hamlen is a believer that pets should be either inside or outside but recognizes that this is not a popular stance with pet owners. In many households, pets have access to both human living areas and the outdoors. For this reason, pet caretakers must be vigilant in using tick repellent and checking pets regularly. Dr. Hamlen warns to not sleep with your outdoor pet.

H. **Disposal of live ticks:** While I am a fanatical animal lover, I am not opposed to disposing of a live tick to prevent future bites. You may discover a tick on you or in your living area and the tick you find may still be alive. There are almost as many folk tales about tick disposal as there are for tick removal. Just as you should run from the nail polish and Vaseline, most of the "great ideas" around tick demise are just as risky. Some sources recommend chopping the tick into pieces to ensure it is dead. This is NOT a good idea because in your zeal you could get contaminated fluids in you and get just as infected. Others recommend smashing the tick with your shoe. (I guess other blunt objects would work as well.) Again, viable pathogen may be discharged. To circumvent that complication, some propose putting the tick in a baggy before squashing it. Yet another suggestion includes flushing the tick down the toilet. Since ticks are known to survive this termination method, that approach seems to defeat the purpose. While smash-inside-a-baggy could be adequate, the safest method is probably drowning the tick in a sealable container of alcohol. This will 1) kill the tick, 2) prevent escape, 3) allow for easy transport if you want to show your HCP, and 4) reduce the chance of contamination.

PEARL: The Dr. Kliman fool-proof method: Fully encapsulate the tick in Scotch tape and dispose of in the trash. He has never witnessed an escape. This method does not squish the tick and it can be saved for later identification.

III. BITES HAPPEN

Despite the best intentions and all due diligence, tick bites occur. After potential exposure, do a meticulous tick check. Have someone else look you over as well. Since deer ticks are small and hard to see they can easily be missed or mistaken for specks of dirt. Take this exam seriously! The sooner an attached tick is removed, the less likely there will be transmission of potential pathogens. Look carefully at the waistband and hairline. Take a shower using your hands to run over all skin surfaces and scalp so you can feel the tiny firm speck that could be the deer tick. A soaped washcloth can be used to remove any unattached ticks.

IV. TICK REMOVAL

- Wear thin impermeable gloves, if available.

- Use fine point tweezers.

- Grasp the mouthparts with tweezers as close as possible to the attachment (skin) site. Don't grab just at the head/body juncture or you will pull the body off its head. Try to get down low enough (maybe by applying a little pressure to the skin with the curved part of the tweezers) to get the mouth parts.

- Be careful not to squeeze, crush, or puncture the body of the tick, which may contain infectious fluids. Do not apply any home remedies hoping to irritate the tick causing it to back away.

- Do not twist, jerk, or turn. Simply *pull back with a slow steady force.*

- If the mouth parts of the tick break off into the skin, use the tweezers to gently get them out, causing as little damage to the surrounding tissue as possible. I say this as a physician used to removing tick parts. The average layperson may do more damage than good in trying to dig out mouthparts. Do not macerate the flesh in trying to get the last bit.

- Wash the bite site with soap and plenty of water.

- Apply alcohol or other disinfectant.

- Wash your hands.

- Save the tick in a plastic bag, jar, or cellophane tape.

- Make sure the tick you just removed is the last tick on the person. Some people get so discombobulated over one tick that they miss others.

All the instructions say to just pull back gently, as though the head breaking off is rare. I have removed many ticks as an ER doctor and I have left mouth parts behind more often than I like to recall. What should you do if the mouthparts are still inside the wound? Some authors say not to worry about residual tick parts since damage done in the removal process can spread infection more than leaving things alone. Since it is the contaminated saliva we are trying to avoid, you will want to take the approach that causes the least exposure to that saliva. The attachment devices on the mouth of the tick are shaped like barbs, so they go in easily but come out only with difficulty. If you can do the removal without damaging the surrounding tissues, use a fine point tweezer and slowly and carefully remove. Do not damage the tissue. Wash and flush the area with soap and water. Flush but don't power wash. You want the germs flowing out, not forced in. Apply antiseptic.

PEARL: Use thin gloves if available. Infected fluids could get on bare hands and get transferred to the mouth or eyes. Err on the side of the conservative.

There are many tick removal devices on the market. For just $19.95 you can get, not one, but two. Call now for this limited time offer. Personally, I haven't found anything better than a slightly curved fine point tweezer and a steady hand. However, you may prefer the device and there are several reasonable alternatives.

If possible, wear gloves to remove the tick. After you remove the tick wash YOUR hands with soap and water since exposure to tick parts and fluid is known to transmit some co-infections.

Folklore removal techniques such as petroleum jelly may cause more harm than good. People say these methods will make the tick back out of the skin docilely on its own. For one thing, it can annoy the tick (imagine someone burning your butt with a match), causing it to reposition, regurgitate, and thereby release more contaminated saliva into the host. Essentially, the irritated tick will vomit, and any pathogens it is harboring in its saliva or GI tract will then go into the host, defeating the purpose.

PEARL: Do not be deceived into thinking you have plenty of time to remove the tick. Old thinking was that the tick had to be attached for 24, 36, or even 72 hours and be engorged for enough pathogens to be transmitted to cause disease. There are reports of patients who had full-blown, severe, Lyme with an attachment of only an hour or two. If you are engaging in a high risk activity in an endemic area, you might want to carry with you the implements you need to remove the tick and clean the bite site. Seemingly, in some cases, the second or third round of Lyme can be a more severe illness with greater potential for sequelae and more risk of chronicity.

V. SAVE THE TICK

"They" used to recommend that you save the tick for identification in case you become ill in the next weeks. Now "they" just ignore the tick (and you). One recommendation is to save the tick in a ziplock baggy in the freezer labeled with the date. Others want you to put the tick in alcohol in a jar. Today, showing the tick to the staff in the ER or office usually merits a stare or a roll of the eyes. Most don't know ticks from toenails. Especially now that we know that many kinds of ticks can transmit TBIs, identification of the tick is not as useful. In 2013, we can no longer safely say, "Oh, that's a dog tick, so you can't have Lyme."

With that being said, some doctors will not prescribe antibiotics, even with an EM rash, if you can't produce a tick. Since the majority of patients with Lyme and other TBIs never recall a tick bite, this attitude is irrational but still this is how some HCPs think.

Some state health or agriculture departments will identify ticks for you. They will tell you the species and the degree of engorgement as a way to tell how long the tick may have been present. Today, we know that absence of engorgement does not guarantee no transmission. In New Jersey (if lack of funding has not changed things), the state may test a tick for you. Inquire at 1-877-Tick-Test.

Better not to handle the detached tick with bare hands, since the fluids from a tick that was just pulled from its attachment site can contain pathogens. These infectious agents could enter the handler through breaks in the skin or mucous membranes, or through inhalation or ingestion. Why take chances? Some people seem to follow this advice when handling ticks they take off themselves or their kids, but ignore it when it comes to taking ticks off Muffin or Rascal.

VI. TICK TESTING

Despite how often we have been told to save the tick and show it to the HCP, no one really seems to care when you do. Occasionally a veteran TBI doctor will have the tick tested to see what pathogens may be lurking. This is done as much to see what infectious strains may be present in a specific geographic location as to diagnose the patient.

Nonetheless, a layperson can commission his own analysis of the tick if so inclined, no doctor's order needed. Clongen will do this testing if you use their special form. They will test for Lyme (Bb), Babesia *microti,* and Bartonella *henselea.* This test can be ordered by a layperson, *and,* if the specimen is not a tick, you will not be charged (Of course, they don't send your bug back, either.)

Mailing instructions from one lab: "A dead tick can be sent in a single ziplock bag. If alive, place the tick in two ziplock bags to prevent escape. A container with a tight seal can also be used. Label the bag/container with your name and send the tick with this form via standard US mail. Please do NOT use tape to attach the tick to paper. Payment is required to process your sample."

Other labs have other shipping requirements. One lab says put the tick in a jar with a moist cotton ball and no alcohol. Keep alive if possible. Another lab wants the tick shipped in alcohol. Still another tick identification service wants you to place the tick into a container with some foliage. Is the foliage to create a pleasant ambience? In all cases, they suggest closing the lid of the container to prevent escape.

Clearly, you should contact the specific lab or service and see how they want to receive the sample. Not following the directions could lead to inability to test the specimen.

Most Agricultural Extension services will just tell you what type of tick you have and will not test for pathogens. Since we now know that many different tick species are responsible for disease transmission, knowing if "your" tick *is* or is *not* a deer tick is less relevant than it was thought to be in the past.

Whatever the result, you might be able to use the information to convince an HCP that a patient actually has a TBI. Or, at least inspire him to look for a TBI in the person bitten by said tick. Or, as is often the case, the HCP might ignore you.

VII. PREVENTION OF ACUTE & CHRONIC LYME

We need to think about both the prevention of **acute** illness *and* **chronic** disease.

PREVENTION OF ACUTE DISEASE:

After a tick bite:

- If in an endemic area assume the tick is infected. If in a non-endemic area, remember anything is possible.

- ILADS recommends considering prophylactic antibiotics, especially in patients deemed high risk such as the immunocompromised, those with significant co-morbidities, a history of TBI in the past, or anticipating entry into a high exposure area. When my son was rebitten last summer, we had him on prophylactic antibiotics immediately.

- A reasonable prophylactic regimen in older kids and adults might include oral treatment for 28 days with a macrolide like azithromycin and a tetracycline like Doryx. Kids under 8 might be better served with amoxicillin in combination with azithromycin. Pregnant patients might use Amoxicillin 1000 mg q 6 hours for the duration of the pregnancy. Consider combining the amoxicillin with azithromycin for optimum results, otherwise Bb might hide intracellularly or encyst.

- You might have different prophylactic needs depending on whether the patient is going into a high risk situation versus those who have already had a tick bite. In the latter case you might want to select prophylactic agents that could hit co-infections known to be endemic in the hometown of the suspected tick. For example, if Bartonella or Ehrlichia are endemic, cefuroxime might be a prophylactic consideration.

PEARL: Even IDSA allows for prophylactic treatment for Lyme after a tick bite but the obstacles that must be overcome to get this papal dispensation are daunting.

1. *The tick must be a deer tick. (Most people never see the infecting tick and several kinds of ticks carry Bb. Further, the rare tick that gets seen may not even be the culprit.)*

2. *The tick must be attached for 36 hours. (How would you know? The sane response to an attached tick is to take it off as soon as it is discovered. Who would leave the tick in place for 36 minutes after discovering it? Where did they get that 36 hour number? Has no one in their experience ever been infected in 35 hours? Who held the stop watch?)*

3. *The prophylaxis is started within 72 hours after tick removal. (Who is the time keeper? No soup for you if you hit 73 hours. While I agree that prophylaxis should be started as soon as possible after recognizing that the regimen is indicated, sometimes the individual cannot reach the HCP within 72 hours. For example, many Boy Scout outings involve both ticks and remote locations for extended periods. Of course, if the kids are entering an endemic area, prophylaxis might be prudent anyway but, again, that would not fit into the rigid guidelines. So if a kid hikes out of Philmont after a week of tick bites, he would be denied prophylaxis because he had passed the 72 hour cut-off? What studies show that prophylaxis is not useful after 72 hours?)*

4. *The rate of Bb infestation of the local ticks is greater than 10%. (How would you ever find that out? Does Lilith[1] keep the latest stats in her pinafore? Who would you call? What if the person was bitten by a tick that was introduced from outside the local area? What if the patient had travelled to an endemic area? When was the last local tick count sample collected? Are those*

numbers still valid? Were they valid to start with? Who did the counting? Do these people even know Dr. Sapi?[2] I am immersed in all-things-Lyme and I don't know these numbers for my area. Would my son be treated based on the incidence in Pennsylvania where he sometimes lives, Maryland where he was most recently bitten, or Indiana where he went after the bite? We can't even get the local health department to answer the phone.

In my opinion, the above criteria are next to impossible to meet and place the patient at unnecessary risk. Not one of the four criteria makes medical sense for real people.

PREVENTION OF CHRONIC DISEASE:

If the patient has an acute TBI, take all appropriate steps to mitigate the risk of development of a chronic condition. These steps include:

- Aggressively treating the patient as early as possible in the course of the disease

- Treating with antimicrobials that will hit the suspected pathogen in its various life forms

- Treating for long enough to prevent sequelae and persistence

A pamphlet from ILADS titled *Top Ten Tips to Prevent Chronic Lyme Disease* includes the following paraphrased advice: A "wait and see" approach can be risky. Lyme is often misdiagnosed and so there can be a long delay in getting adequate treatment under the best circumstances. Lyme can present with no rash at all or many other kinds of rashes aside from a bull's eye. Lab tests are unreliable in making the diagnosis. Consider treatment options. Rule out similar conditions. If you aren't satisfied with the response of your HCP or you still feel sick, get another opinion. Look for an HCP who will work with you until you feel better.

If acute Lyme disease is not adequately treated, the problem can become a progressive condition that can leave permanent damage and impairment. People die from Lyme. Why take the chance when there are options that might mitigate the risk?

VIII. CONCLUSION

Education is the best prevention. *Preach prevention!* Remember the Boy Scout leader I mentioned who was always warning the boys to watch out for ticks. We scoffed and thought she was a flake. We owe you an apology, Jeanne. Know whether you live in a Lyme endemic area or a region where other TBIs have been reported. Just because TBIs are not well established

---

1 *See Glossary or Introduction for name origin*

2 *Eva Sapi is the researcher at the University of New Haven who actually knows how to do tick counts.*

in your area, does not mean a person was not exposed through travel or other unexpected flukes. A false sense of security is worse than insecurity since it delays diagnosis and treatment. Unfortunately, the patient you are looking at could be the first case in the neighborhood. Ben Franklin, who lived in an endemic area, must have been talking Lyme when he said, "An ounce of prevention is worth a pound of cure."

Chapter 33

FINANCIAL BURDEN OF TBIs

The longest journey begins with a single check.

Margaret Roach

To ask me about finances is like trying to explain economics to a little neck clam. Hapless. Hopeless. I have absolutely no interest, inclination, or expertise in that area. Nonetheless, the financial burden surrounding the diagnosis and treatment of TBIs is real, and in some cases, incapacitating. The cost issue needs to be addressed.

Insurance

Often a diagnostic code is required for insurance to accept the charge. With all the hoops that one must jump through to get an "official" TBI diagnosis, much testing and treatment is not covered. We all learned after-the-fact that some of the HCPs who helped contrive the diagnostic criteria for Lyme disease were in the pocket of the insurance companies, the pharmaceutical industry, or both. Now we're stuck with the repercussions of their bad decisions.

Insurance companies count on you not to contest a rejected claim. With each rejection, more clients give up the fight, and the insurance companies bank on that. By the third rejection, only a small percentage of patients are still fighting for coverage. This has nothing to do with the validity of the claim or if the person is really sick. Apparently, one company has the policy that *every* claim is initially rejected. In contrast, almost *all* claims are approved by the 4th or 5th attempt. Volumes have been written to educate the insurance claims adjuster. When it becomes more costly for them to keep denying your claim than to accept it, you will likely get approval. Don't be surprised if rejection letters are nearly incomprehensible so that you have no idea what is being said. They design them so they are within the law, yet leaving the consumer with no idea what the next step should be. They count on you giving up.

Work has been started by Lyme advocacy groups to demonstrate the lower cost of paying for early, appropriate treatment of TBIs compared to funding the long-term care for serious sequelae like PICC lines, cardiac valve replacements, pacemakers, and in my case, a new knee. But the person reviewing an individual claim only wants to get through the day without her supervisor berating her for approving too many requests. She is not in charge of long-term cost saving. She is more interested in keeping her job.

HMOs may limit referrals to specialists and restrict drugs on their formularies. When selecting insurance coverage, few expect that they will have a controversial, expensive, potentially chronic condition. It's easy to look back and wish you had picked different coverage, but none of us has a crystal ball.

Read your policy and make sure you know EXACTLY what you are entitled to. You deserve to get the care that is promised. An experienced manager in your HCP's office may know the coding system better than anyone else, identifying those codes that were accepted in the past and those that are more likely to be rejected on the same patient with the same condition.

Out-of-Pocket Expense

Some HCPs will make you pay before being seen, and then you are responsible for submitting your claim to insurance. So, in many cases money will need to change hands before the patient can even be examined.

Under the circumstances, some people view these large out-of-pocket expenses as the rainy day they have been saving for all along. Unfortunately, as they desperately try to get appropriate care, they sometimes have to go from doctor to doctor to doctor, and the bills pile up. Some can get their hands on the money, and others cannot. While we hope the crisis does not result in selling the house or pawning the wedding ring, the situation may come down to credit cards and loans. Ask if you can pay the bill over time. Many HCPs will allow a payment plan, but others adamantly refuse. Since there are so few practitioners who understand TBIs, choices might be limited.

Often the person is so sick you would do anything, travel anywhere, buy any medicine, and agree to any tests, if you think it will help. Find an HCP that you trust. I learned after the fact that a number of my son's lab tests were ordered more to appease the HCP's ego than to shed light on his case. The tests fed intellectual curiosity and the hubris of confirming brilliance. Ask what the test will do for you.

PEARL: Smith and Dennis looked at 65 school kids with Lyme. They found that the average duration of the disease

*was 363 days and 80% of these children had been hospital-
ized with a cost of $30,000. Further, 90% had been treated
with IV therapy with the cost around $63,000 per case. The
average overall cost was nearly $100,000 per patient. More
than a quarter recovered while on treatment, while the rest
had to be treated for 2 to 4 years. These numbers represent
real money irrespective of your tax bracket.*

Drug Costs

The gorilla-cillins used to treat many TBIs can be shockingly
expensive, especially if the patient needs a combination of
drugs. Mepron gets close to $1000 per prescription. The best
advice here is to shop around. Great differences in cost are out
there. We found a $200 disparity in the cost of Mepron within a
2-mile radius. The first probiotics that my son's doctor recommended were $36.00 at the organic food store. The next one we
bought was $4.99 at the chain drug store.

Some drugs are generic. I am no longer a big fan of generics
after working for a generic pharmaceutical company. Nonetheless, generics are often the only option, especially if you want
the insurance company to pay for the medicine. Use caution
if the active drug ingredient comes from a country where you
would not drink the water. Sometimes little, if any, active medicine gets into the pill. Unfortunately, a number of unscrupulous
companies know how to package in the US so that the medicine LOOKS like the drug came from Jacksonville, when it actually came from a place where you wouldn't drink the water.

Impact on the Family

Some of the financial burden of Lyme is apparent, while other
costs are more subtle. With Lyme and other TBIs, the gross
under-diagnosis and frequent misdiagnoses make quantification of overall expenses difficult to assess. Remember that both
time and money are spent. While we do not have a solid handle
on the cost of TBIs to an afflicted family, some interesting and
related work provides insight.

An ILADS survey tabulated some of the costs associated with
LD. More than 90% of the survey respondents saw multiple
doctors. Almost all (97%) felt that their disease was advanced,
severe, or chronic prior to finally getting diagnosed. The average patient visited 7 to 10 HCPs prior to diagnosis with a
wide range of specialties consulted. I can tell you that trying to
find an HCP who has both the technical expertise and patience
to make the diagnosis can tax your time, money, and endurance. Searching for adequate medical care can be consuming
in many ways.

Of the survey respondents, 95% experienced severe or debilitating pain, and a high percentage lost their jobs or quit due
to the physical symptoms of Lyme. Essentially all respondents
felt they experienced mental impairment. Consider the overall

impact both financially and otherwise that these statistics might
have on a family.

On March 19, 2012, the *Huffington Post* reported on a study
published in *Pediatrics* on the cost of treating autism. While
autism and Lyme are not interchangeable both can be chronic
conditions that impact not just the patient but the entire family
dynamic as well. The information gathered on autism can help
TBI families better understand what might be happening with
them and perhaps they won't feel that they are the only families
being impacted by disease.

The researchers attempted to quantify the financial toll of autism. The 2002-2008 Medical Expenditure Panel Survey data
was used because it tracks the cost and utilization of health
services in the US. Data was analyzed comparing families with
ASD children to those with other health problems and those
without significant medical issues.

David Mandell, a researcher for the study at the Center for
Mental Health Policy and Services Research at the University
of Pennsylvania, focused on the burden that can accompany
changes in the parent's employment. Families of kids with autism earn 28% less than families whose children have no health
problems. Women with kids with autism make 56% less than
those with kids with no health problems and 35% less than
those whose kids have other health issues. The mothers tend to
leave the work force altogether, or take lower paying jobs and
work fewer hours.

Mothers of kids with autism were 6% less likely to be employed than mothers of kids with no health problems and they
worked an average of 7 fewer hours per week. The authors
speculated that the mothers may have taken lower paying jobs
that allowed them more time with their sick kids, or did not
pursue additional education because of time needed at home.
The mom was the one that often had to cut back significantly
or even completely to care for the sick child. The research
did not find any differences in the father's income, only the
mom's, and the overall family financial state. The conclusion
of the study was if autism costs this much to treat, what would
the price be not to treat? Prospectively, the outlay would be
much greater both in dollars and emotional tolls.

*PEARL: I remember when my son was hospitalized as an
infant after febrile seizures. Back then, there was no family
leave or personal days, and I worked for one of the largest chemical companies in the country, where all men wore
white short-sleeved shirts and skinny black ties. I was the
only female physician out of 120 docs working for the company and just about the only one under 70-years-old. My
boss told me that I needed to prove I was as good as the
men by not missing work while my son was in the hospital.
I took all my vacation time to be with my child, and then,
my husband took all his allotted time so our son would not*

be alone in the hospital. (I believe everyone in the hospital needs a 24/7 advocate. You will be amazed at the number of errors you catch.) We were able to stretch our time so that all the in-patient days were covered and, of course, we stayed overnight in the world's most uncomfortable chair. By the time our son was released, my parents were there to watch him while we were at work. Because his grandparents were not comfortable with handling his medical condition, we hired an RN 10 hours a day to cover our work and commuting times. We were lucky. We had the money to cover these expenses. With my son's recent flares of TBIs, I have dropped everything to drive the 12 hours to Purdue to take care of him. He has been so incapacitated at times that there was no way he could manage on his own. One reason this book is a year past the original publication date is the cost in time and money that came with caretaking in a family of TBI patients.

As with autism, in a Lyme family affected children may have frequent doctors' visits and need to attend therapy or tutoring sessions. Consider the gas and time away from work and school. This all adds up to considerable time and money and it can become a full-time job taking care of these children. A number of caretakers need to quit work, miss work, or take leave. In addition, the family may need to pay for at-home help, as well as tutors and other ancillary support.

Recall that often more than one family member is affected, sometimes concurrently. There are times when a sick person is in both the role of patient and caretaker. Families can be so hard hit that they have to prioritize how to spend their resources.

With all that being said, be honest about financial limits. Don't cry poverty unless that is really the case. I saw one mother plead for financial indulgence as she was asking for a school note for the family's 12-month world cruise. If your child is in private elementary school, waiting to be accepted to Harvard, I am less sympathetic. If you are deciding between having your Mercedes detailed and buying Mepron, don't look to me for help.

One caretaker described financial chaos when all the therapy and counseling and testing and tutoring were in play. Don't panic. You know that these things do somehow work out.

Societal costs

In 2006, the Harvard School of Public Health estimated that it may cost more than $3 million to care for an autistic person over his lifetime. We don't know the comparable number for chronic Lyme, but we can theorize that the costs might be similar for similar conditions.

Insurers complain of the cost of treating chronic Lyme, but the cost of not treating is likely much greater. Many authors

have documented that the later treatment begins in Lyme, the more potential for long-term sequelae, which in some cases can be permanent. Neuropsychiatric conditions resulting from TBIs can be costly for the life of the individual. In these cases, preventing the early Lyme from becoming intractable is the most cost-effective solution. Insurers often take the penny-wise, pound-foolish approach. The insurance adjuster might be focused on how much he can save the company today and therefore make the best short-term decisions for the corporate bottom line.

PEARL: According to the National Academy of Science, every $1 spent on prevention of mental illness in kids will be paid back as much as 28 times over the course of a lifetime (savings in disability benefits, psychiatric care not needed, crime not committed, etcetera, although public policy experts rarely recognize this type of long-term practicality.

Furthermore, as far as I could find, no one has taken into account the financial burden of the Lyme-inspired pacemakers, sleep studies, cognitive testing, and myriad other interventions that are not recognized as being associated with Lyme. My knee replacement cost over $35,000, NOT counting the cumulative $12,000 bill resulting from the Bb eating away at my joint so that my leg length discrepancy contributed to a fall that resulted in multiple skin grafts and 3 months of an incapacitating concussion. (Orthopedics, podiatry, dermatology, plastic surgery, emergency medicine, neurology, and family practice all had a hand in putting me back together again.) Management of persistent sequelae, that have yet to be measured, can far outpace the cost of adequate treatment early in the clinical course. Potential disability and decreased productivity can cost society a great deal in terms of school accommodations and limited employment options. Think how much the prevention of chronic disease might save.

Returning to the autism analogy, since that is all we have, Bransfield postulates that if around 20% of the half million recognized cases of autism in the US could be either prevented or more effectively treated, society could potentially save billions per year. What if some of that autism is TBI-induced? His recommendation is to consider screening pregnant women, neonates, and autism patients when there is clinical suspicion that there could be a Lyme association. This would allow earlier and possibly more effective treatment and decrease the long-term problems that are so costly. Adequate treatment of pregnant women with active TBI could save money, morbidity, and suffering.

If even a fraction of the recognized autism is TBI-related, early intervention could lead to proper treatment, and perhaps spare some kids and families the overwhelming emotional and financial toll they currently endure. Wouldn't the overall savings greatly counterbalance the initial costs of treatment? I know that the APA has admitted to trying to decrease the I&P numbers of ASD diagnosis to save money, just as the CDC may be trying to decrease the I&P of Lyme by making diagnostic hoops almost impossible to surmount. These tricks will not save money in the long-run. Instead of paying for the antibiotic treatment for a kid with Lyme, they will instead be paying for his pacemaker. Of course, some insurers will be happy to save the money short-term and push as much of the cost as possible onto the already strapped families.

Remember we aren't just talking autism here. TBIs have many long-term sequelae such as heart problems, GI and GU conditions, and various neuropsychiatric problems such as depression, OCD, panic, GAD, ADHD, and sleep difficulties. Funny how insurers will pay for a dozen courses of Bactrim that doesn't work in interstitial cystitis and yet deny coverage of the same antibiotic in those TBIs where it might work. What if early intervention helped prevent even a small percentage of these problems? Think of the cost savings in terms of school and work over a lifetime.

> *PEARL: The APA is complaining about the epidemic of autism. The CDC is complaining about the increasing I&P of Lyme. The Red Cross is complaining about the contamination of the blood supply with Babesia. Every journal I read talks about the sky-rocketing increase in cases of OCD, panic, GAD, depression, cutting, ADHD, and sleep problems. I find it interesting that all these conditions are soaring at the same time. Is it just better recognition and detection? Or could there be an underlying infectious etiology to some of these diagnoses? Where is the next Willy Burgdorfer who can put this all together and make the connection?*

This chapter is about money but there is an even greater human cost to TBIs in terms of suffering and loss of potential. If you knew your child could be spared a lifetime of health problems through early intervention, would you not push for treatment? If you could return your child to achieving in school instead of struggling to process information, would you not want all treatment options presented and considered? Would you not hound the insurers? Would you not sacrifice anything to save your child? Would the human cost not trump the financial cost? Never give up.

Chapter 34

FRIENDLY ADVICE

You have enemies? Good. That means you stood for something.
Winston Churchill

Dear TBI HCP:

Please read this entire jumble of advice, but don't believe everything you read. Don't be afraid to march to your own drummer. Treat the patient not the test result. Never shout: "YOU DO NOT HAVE LYME!" She probably does and you will look deranged screaming at a four-year-old. Just because a proclamation comes from on-high doesn't mean it is right, correct, or ethical. Listen to the patient, even if they are only three-years-old. Listen to the caretakers. Believe them. Never give up, never.

Consider and present various options. If the patient is still sick, you're still on-duty. You may be right when you say, "It's all in your head," because antineuronal antibodies may be damaging the brain cells as you speak. Apologize to those you have doubted. Someday you might be appalled when someone doubts you. Forgive yourself. Admit when you don't know. Be willing to reassess, rethink, regroup. Admit when you are wrong. Have a plan B, and C, and D.

Care. This could be your child. No harm comes from not knowing, only from not caring. You can damage a patient by pretending to know things you don't know. Confidence should come from competence. And experience. The authorities aren't always right. Anesthesia in childbirth was vehemently opposed by the church for hundreds of years. In 1591 a mother in Edinburgh was burned alive for asking for pain relief during labor. The authorities aren't always wise or moral.

Don't act as if you're "not allowed" to make a diagnosis in the face of a negative lab test. Professional organizations are NOT your mother. Set aside enough time to address this extremely complicated and often obscure set of syndromes. Don't give patients the run-around. A good doctor-patient relationship results in better outcomes. Don't dump a patient on other doctors because the going gets tough and you are (bored, irritated, jaded, disinterested, frustrated, busy, annoyed, exasperated, humbled, overwhelmed) by the case.

Don't promise what you can't possibly deliver. Be optimistic. If you don't believe these patients can get better, you need to change fields. A negative test result proves nothing. Guidelines are just guidelines, not the Ten Commandments. (Interesting how many HCPs rigidly follow unscientific guidelines, who then ignore basic rules of civility.) Never scoff, roll your eyes, or dismiss a patient's genuine concern. Do not throw around terms and test results and medication instructions as though the 12 y/o and his frazzled parents know what you are talking about.

Don't feel smug and superior because deep down you know you just blew them away with your genius. Lions don't need to roar. Give them a blanket when they are cold. Don't interrupt; someone is trying to tell you something. Don't take it personally when a patient doesn't improve as fast as you would like. Never get so busy that you no longer have compassion. If it's not documented, you might not remember what you did or why you did it and it's terrifically hard to explain that in court. If it's not documented, it didn't happen. Provide directions to your office.

No two cases are alike. Don't be too eager to embrace each new medical fad. When the craze passes, you could look foolish. Science is often manipulated for secondary gain. Hubris is common in your field. Hubris killed most of the Greek heroes. If you are 100% certain about anything in medicine, you are delusional. Reading Chapter 17 is humbling.

Act in good faith with no other agendas but to help your patient. If you are in over your head, seek out the counsel of those who might know more than you, don't just give up. Work with other HCPs. Be aware of what they have ordered so you don't work at cross purposes. There is never any need to be mean to a sick person. Show respect. Know when and how to get help in managing a patient. Know what you don't know.

Build relationships with other HCPs such as specialists in cardiology, neurology, and psychiatry. Sometimes it's just nice to bounce ideas off someone else. If things aren't going well, you may have the wrong diagnosis or treatment plan. Could it be a co-infection that is ruining your day? If you inherit a patient from another HCP, you will be considered either the omniscient savior or a know-nothing galoot. You are neither.

If the previous plan hasn't worked, don't repeat the same plan you already know has failed. Remember, the caretakers are suffering, too. Take patient preferences into consideration. Understand the science before you proclaim malarkey from the rooftops. Don't be a sheep in following the opinion leaders. If it doesn't make sense to you, it probably doesn't make sense.

Be courageous in advocating for your patients in a system that discounts their every word. More than one thing can be going on at a time. Neither you nor your medicine is perfect and that's okay; you're giving it your best shot. Recognize that the people you are helping are very grateful. You really can save a life by caring for TBI patients. This is the real reason you went into medicine. Remember?

Sincerely,

KS

Dear Members of Advocacy Groups,

You people save lives. Never forget that your work saves lives. Countable, real lives. LDASEPA, you saved my son. LDA and Time for Lyme and CALDA (Lymedisease.org) you made this book possible. Also a special mention for Tin Cup (aka Lucy Barnes). And no one has done more for the Lyme community than Pat Smith. No matter how much your opponents rile against you, you are doing the right thing. You have helped more people than all your critics with their personal agendas and their pockets lined with special interest money. When you count your many achievements you will never have to be embarrassed about what you had to do to garner your success. Will your detractors be able to say the same thing?

I have never met so many people who were simply trying to help others. Imagine people without personal gain as their highest priority! So many individuals ready to sacrifice for the cause and continue to withstand so much pressure for the team. A number of you are so sick from TBIs that you can barely function. Still, you move ahead. No fighting over who was going to get credit or who would get the biggest share of the rewards. Everyone just rolling up their sleeves and pitching in. All doing more than their share.

Unfortunately, many of you were inspired to this work because of your own illness or that of a loved one. I know how hard watching your child suffer in an uncaring and oblivious system can be. Never stop. TBI patients still desperately need you. I look forward to the day when you can all take a rest. But that day is not here and won't be for a while. Eventually, step by step, you will triumph.

With gratitude, Dr. Spreen

Dear Authors of TBI Literature,

I just proofread my son's graduate level science project in which he compared different theories proposing mechanisms by which ejecta can flow after an impact by a meteor on the surface of Mars. This was rocket science and the four theories he compared were extremely robust, solid, and supported by considerable mathematical modeling and physical simulations. Yet the various authors disagreed, substantially.

The difference between these peer-reviewed scientific articles and the material I read by many purported TBI experts was mind-boggling. First, the authors disagreed with one another with respect. Second, they provided balanced reasoning on all sides of the issue. Their cited references could actually be found. They used spell check. They did not publish without proofreading. They valued the other person's opinion. Even though I did not understand the math and much of the physics, I could understand their prose. Their arguments were logical. They used a systematic approach to analyze work done at other institutions. (We're talking MIT, Purdue, JPL, UIC, and Stanford here.) They understood the scientific method and the concept of hypothesis testing. They understood statistics. Imagine! Respect. Civility. Science. Logic. Balance. Flexibility. If a number of PhD aeronautical engineers, who supposedly have no personalities, can get their acts together for their profession, don't we owe our professions, ourselves, and our patients as much?

Because of the shoddy work I was finding, I had to give up on citing all the references I used. First, the sources cited in the body of the work often didn't match the reference list. I found this time and time again. Many opinions were stated as fact with no supporting evidence. I found words misspelled in the titles of articles. Much of the science was confusing and contradictory (in the same article, sometimes in the same paragraph). I am not talking blogs here. I am talking published literature.

I found the same laxity on both sides of the controversial issues. I have analyzed data for nearly 20 years. I can pick out bias as easily as I can pick out a tick from a blond puppy's ear. I can see where statistics have been skewed to meet a political or personal agenda. I can see where an opinion once stated must be forever defended even if the logic was lost long ago. This does not make you look smart. The only reason you have gotten away with this sloppiness so long is because so few people understand this field and there is no one out there to call you on it. Please find a cousin who can proofread before you submit. That does not mean that this text is perfect and has no inconsistencies or typos. But the editors and I have read and reread and reworded the prose over and over. At least make it look like you tried.

I know some of you are motivated by your passion for helping TBI patients. But lack of discipline in your published work paints us all with the same brush. Advocates for TBI patients then look like radicals who do not understand the medicine. Know what you don't know. Being a physician doesn't make you a scientist, nor does being a scientist make you a physician.

With all that being said, some of the work out there, whether done by professionals or laypersons, is excellent. In general, the Lyme and TBI advocacy groups do a consistently superb job of getting their facts straight. Of course, they understand better than anyone how careless work can hurt their mission to help patients.

Please proceed with caution. Do your homework before you put pen to paper. The better we all look, the more we strengthen our argument.

Kathy

Dear Book Critics:

Because I have taken such clear positions on some of the controversial issues around Lyme, I suspect there may be some interest in my opinions from those with opposing views. Several quotations to soothe you as you rush to judgment:

> John Galbraith said, "Faced with a choice between changing one's mind and proving that there is no need to do so, almost everyone gets busy on the proof."

> Diane Ravitch said, "An opinion once stated is by necessity an opinion forever defended."

> Albert Einstein said, "Great spirits have always encountered violent opposition from mediocre minds."

> Abraham Lincoln said, "In times like the present, men should utter nothing for which they would not willingly be responsible through time and eternity."

> In the words of Nellie L. McClun "Never retract, never explain, never apologize; get things done and let them howl."

> And my favorite from Malachy McCourt, "Resentment is like taking poison and waiting for the other guy to die."

> Remember that Ursula LeGuin warns that to oppose something is to maintain it.

Kathy Spreen

> One evening an old Cherokee told his grandson about a battle that goes on inside people. He said, "My son, the battle is between two wolves inside us all. One is EVIL – it is anger, envy, jealousy, sorrow, regret, greed, arrogance, self-pity, guilt, resentment, inferiority, lies, false pride, superiority, and ego. The other is GOOD – it is joy, peace, love, hope, serenity, humility, kindness, benevolence, empathy, generosity, truth, compassion, and faith." The grandson thought about this for a while and then asked his grandfather, "Which wolf wins?" The old Cherokee replied, "The one you feed."

> Unknown source

Dear Members of Task Forces Assigned to Devise Diagnostic Criteria,

Accept that every patient presents in her own way. This is not a contest to see which patient can jump through the most hoops. Nor is it an opportunity for you to show how much more you know than the rest of us. There are real people impacted by your decisions and some of them are very sick kids.

I was not inspired to this tirade from any of the TBI literature, although I could have been. Rather, I became motivated to write this letter after reading the criteria for a PTSD diagnosis. As both a former army physician and a lecturer on medical care for torture survivors, I know a thing or two about PTSD. The criteria that I read did not allow any of the PTSD patients that I know an "official" diagnosis of the condition.

I am starting to believe that perhaps no medical opinion is valid unless it comes from a person who actually had the condition in question. If that is too restrictive, then the opinion should come from an HCP who has actually MANAGED more than one case of the disease under discussion. One of my big gripes about the FDA is that many physicians making decisions about future treatments never had the condition and have never seen a patient with the disease. Some of the government physicians I worked with had never seen a patient anywhere for anything. There is a difference between going to med school and being a physician. When you actually have the RESPONSIBILITY for the patient you see things in a different light.

Please stop splitting hairs and making diagnostic criteria harder to pass than entry into a Westchester pre-school. Think how your criteria will affect real people and consider allowing compassion to mix with ideology.

K. Spreen, DO MS MPH

Dear Caretakers,

Thank you for all you do. Studies have shown that no matter how much you love your ward, you still have the hardest job in the world. Whether you take care of a sick person a few hours a day or 24/7/365, there are times when your nerves are shredded and your patience is non-existent. You lose your temper. You snap at everyone. You feel guilty because you think somehow it's your fault the person got sick. You feel even guiltier because they stay sick. The reason for the illness must be your genes, your parenting, the time you let the kids have popsicles for dinner, the one time you forgot the medicine, or when you gave in and let them play in the yard. We have all been there. Think of me as a physician making decisions and then forever wondering if those choices hurt my son. We all know guilt. The only purpose guilt serves in TBI families is to be recognized and dismissed. Maya Angelou said, "You did then what you knew how to do, and when you knew better, you did better."

If you are the average TBI caretaker, you have been through hell. Dozens of doctors, hours in waiting rooms, witnessing medical testing as your child screams, and best of all the HCPs, like Lilith, who scoff and roll their eyes as though the patient's sole purpose in life was to annoy them. Your ward may have been called mentally ill, a brat, or a liar. You may have been called worse. If anyone understands what you've been through, it's me.

Advice to sustain you in the rough spots and a few practical pointers:

1. You can't turn back time no matter how much money or influence or religion you have. Just move forward.

2. Spend your energy only on the positive pursuit of your loved one's wellness.

3. Once they make you mad, they own you.

4. Don't ruminate on things you might have done better. I wasted years doing that and it doesn't change a thing.

5. You can't think clearly if you're furious.

6. Do take a break once in a while, even if you have to pay someone to step in.

7. If you have someone to share caretaking duties, split the time so "when you're on, you're on," but "when you're off, you're off."

8. When maneuvering through the health care system, don't lose your cool, don't raise your voice and don't let them intimidate you. Hold your ground.

9. Put the guilt behind you. I know you wish you had gotten more aggressive treatment for your child sooner. I know you wish you hadn't listened to the HCP who told you that your 2 y/o was not walking or talking just to annoy you. I remember the many women I've seen during preceptorships crying because they didn't insist on more aggressive Lyme treatment when they were pregnant. If the doctors didn't know, how were they to know? Forgive yourself.

10. You have the right to ask questions like "How will that test help Rusty? What will that tell us? Is there another way to get the information? What is our next step? Can we be more aggressive here in trying to get her feeling better?"

11. Be a part of the health care TEAM. You have the right to be involved in the decisions being made since you are the decision-maker on your child's behalf. Involve the patient if age-appropriate, as well.

12. You're not alone. More than 65 million Americans are caring for a sick or disabled family member.

13. You have the right to refuse any test, study, procedure, or referral that doesn't make sense to you. Just make sure you are refusing for the right reasons and not because you're trying to show them who's boss.

14. If you don't understand, ask. Ask again until you understand. Make them write it down. All those people in the waiting room are not your problem. You have the right to have your questions answered.

15. As long as you are making the best decisions you can in the best interest of the patient, with the information you have, you are not making a wrong decision.

16. Even if you keep all the records on your computer, get a BIG three ring notebook and put everything in there in chronological order. I even taped the Florastor label on a page. I didn't know what the stuff was when I bought it, so how would I remember it a month later?

17. Document everything. These cases get complicated beyond belief and no mere mortal can remember it all. You may have to update your records every day.

18. Rapidly changing medicine lists do best on the computer. Date them. Do not delete old ones. I promise you will need to go back and look something up. Use the computer to help you cut and paste multiple changes, so you don't have to handwrite "azithromycin" over and over and over again. Do not procrastinate. As soon as a medicine changes, change your list. Always have an updated version ready in case of a surprise ER visit. My son was so sick for so long that I kept one in my purse and one in the car. My mother's friend was recently admitted to the hospital with severe weakness and shortness of breath. When she was released $40,000 later she was given a medicine they said would really help her. The drug was the exact medicine she had already been on when she came into the ER. She had forgotten to tell them about that one.

19. Take a copy of the chronological record with you to each new HCP. NEVER give up your original. They can make a copy for their files.

20. Accept that everything you need to do within the medical system will take at least a half dozen phone calls and twice as many reviews of menu options. "Listen carefully because the options may have changed." When you finally pick an option you will either 1) hear recorded directions to the office, 2) be told that if you have an emergency go to the ER, 3) get a voice mailbox for someone who is smart enough to no longer work there, 4) be privileged to listen to blaring rap music for 17 minutes as they answer the calls in the order they were received, 5) get a voice mailbox like the one at the local hospital lab that says it is too full to accept any more messages and they don't intend to do anything about that situation for decades, 6) get the voice mail of a person who gets the message but has no intention of ever calling back, 7) get Lilith who was forced to cover the phones because the hospital was shorthanded. Don't worry; Lilith will handle your needs with all the compassion and insight that she bestows on her ER patients. My point here is if you EXPECT delays and obstacles you might not be so disappointed when they occur. Anything better than expected is then a gift.

21. Anyone who actually helps you on the phone should be thanked profusely. You don't need to weep, but I have.

22. If they say they will call you back and they do not, give them a little cushion. Then call them. No matter how "funny" you feel about being a pest.

23. Never stop being the patient's advocate.

24. Look for and accept support. Try: Family Caregiver Alliance (caregiver.org), National Alliance for Caregiving (caregiving.org), or strengthforcaring.com. Caring Bridge is a blog site that helps people stay in touch during a "health event." This on-line space enables patients or caretakers to connect with others and share and receive health updates. Friends and family can learn how the patient is progressing and leave supportive messages. Some users report feeling soothed by the site when overwhelmed by a health crisis. Some locales have a 211 phone service that provides information and referrals to community resources. Never be shy or embarrassed about asking for and accepting help.

25. Be careful with websites that end in .com. Look instead for .edu or .org or .gov. While there is no guarantee that these sites are legit, the suffix .com means it is admittedly a commercial site.

26. Do not settle. Know that the patient can improve with diligent case management. There is more than one way to reach the goal. Even if the TBI leaves residual damage, there are a hundred ways to work around it.

27. Don't let them break you. Don't let them get you down. The difficulty with being a Lyme caretaker is that you are not only fighting the disease, you are often fighting the medical system. I took part-time care of my blind, brittle diabetic,

cancer-ridden mom and I took care of my severely ill TBI-infected son. At least with my mother, no one spent energy trying to convince me that she was not blind, diabetic, and cancer-ridden.

28. Be careful of cons and scams. When you watch your child suffer, you become especially vulnerable. There are so many shysters out there who just want to sell you a little Chinese herb here and a little Malaysian muskrat there. There will be a special rate just for you because you seem so nice. Every time I would see some goofy gadget sold on one of those infomercials on TV, I would ask, "Who would be dumb enough to buy that?" I would then visit my mom and she would have purchased two, one for her and one for me. Please be cautious.

29. Be careful of blogs and chat rooms. While I know you need a lot of support when dealing with Lyme disease, blogs can be full of misinformation and chat rooms can be negative and depressing. Find the positive ones and stick with them. Some of these sites are just fronts for people trying to sell you something. Your new friend from the chat room, who found so much relief with the vacuum shoes that remove toxins, just might be the same guy selling vacuum shoes.

30. Be careful if the patient has more than one HCP. They could be prescribing treatments that are at cross-purposes. An HCP not familiar with the child's TBI condition might happily (and reasonably) order steroids for a case of poison ivy, not knowing that this may cause the child more problems in the long-run.

31. Remember there are HCPs out there who genuinely care. They are just well hidden.

32. If you have been a TBI caregiver for any length of time, you have probably educated yourself in this field far beyond the average HCP, especially those who have put up defensive walls. Denying Lyme makes their lives easier. Avoid the hostile doctors and when you find a kind and compassionate HCP, lead them without being smug. The goal should be a productive collaboration.

33. Don't let your other family members or pets become Lyme orphans. In some families the disease has become everyone's whole life. This is hard since TBIs can seem all-consuming.

34. You don't have to like an HCP to get good medicine out of him. That doesn't mean you and your ward have to submit to disrespect, ridicule, scorn, or abuse. You have the right to be treated with civility. If the guy is a pompous jerk but otherwise seems to know what he's doing and is helping the patient, tolerate his abrasiveness. If he is a pompous jerk whose primary goal is to sell you supplements off the display in the waiting room, consider finding a new doc. My mother's sole criterion for selecting a physician was whether or not the doctor was nice. As a result, she picked some inept nincompoops who accelerated her demise. There should be a balance.

35. Lyme and other TBIs can be challenging. Don't give up too soon. Sometimes progress is made in very small increments.

36. Don't agonize about seeking another opinion. If the HCP is not working out, that's okay. Happens every day. You worry that you will hurt someone's feelings or she will get mad. Truth is, she won't even know you're gone. She will never have to face the repercussions of her inadequacies.

37. You may have to travel a little to find good health care, but if you're reading this book, you already knew that.

38. If the HCP doesn't know what to do, show her this book or give her the number for the local Lyme advocacy group. Maybe she can get some ideas.

39. There is nothing more important than the effort you are currently putting toward your ward's health.

40. Never give up.

AND...the best piece of advice:

Contact your local Lyme disease advocacy group. These people are devoted to helping Lyme patients and their families. They know of support groups in the area and local physicians. They understand what you have been through. They have no other mission but to help you. Since HCPs knowledgeable about TBIs may be scarce as hen's teeth, they will help you find someone who matches the patient's needs. Better yet, become a member or send a donation. These folks are volunteers just trying to help people because they know how hard it was when they were in your shoes.

In an essay called "The Coping Conundrum" from the October 25, 2010, issue of *Time*, Nancy Gibbs describes the role of the caretaker this way: "There is guilt and mystery and anger and fear embedded in a process driven by love."

Caregiver, you are driven by love and will not regret what you did for your family member. You may be surprised at how grateful that person will be someday.

You are the salt of the earth.

Kathy Spreen

Dear Readers,

During the four years I spent writing this book, I felt connected to you. To me this was a conversation, sharing what I have learned so that you could benefit from my mistakes and not have to repeat them. I hope my style makes you feel like I am talking directly to you, because that is how I felt when I was writing. I genuinely want to spare you the angst suffered by me and my family due to TBIs.

Whether you are an HCP, a patient, or a caregiver, (and I have been in all those roles, sometimes concurrently), I am speaking to you. I have made some colossal mistakes and my son suffered for it. I don't want another child to suffer while his parents learn from scratch. Hopefully, your child will not need to endure what my child did because of ignorance.

I want to provide you with the benefit of my experiences, both good and bad. I really could have used this book when I was first encountering TBIs. Please use this text for all it's worth. My mantra is, "Take what helps you and leave the rest."

As part of the research for this book, I read and read and read. Even though mentally exhausting, typing and turning pages does not consume much energy. But if stress burned calories, I'd be a size 5. Nevertheless, I learned a great deal and in the process came across two works that I would like to recommend to you.

First, in *Flesh and Blood* by Gracie Dinkins, she warns about HCPs losing their ability to respond the way they used to. She says, "I think that is something a doctor should be vigilant about, because building up a residue of defensiveness and callousness isn't helpful. You miss clues that way. I also think you miss opportunities to grow and be blessed by patients. If you lose the ability to be affected, that's the equivalent to losing a little bit of living." I believe many HCPs today have lost their ability to "be affected" and that's a shame. Lilith has lost that ability, as has her physician counterpart in the local ER. If you are so burned out in your work that you no longer have any compassion and cannot even hear what people are saying to you, move along before you hurt anyone else. We had one doctor "correct" our son's history saying that what happened could not have happened that way, because it didn't fit into the conclusion already embraced.

Midway through my writing process I came across the book *How Doctors Think* by Jerome Groopman from Harvard. Read this book whether you are a patient, parent, caretaker, and especially if you are the HCP. You will see yourself there. In case you are pressed for time, here are my interpretations of some of Dr. Groopman's main points. I apologize if I misconstrued any of his concepts.

- Practice guidelines may be more about cost savings than patient care.

- You have to know a lot to know what you don't know.

- Evidence-based medicine is fine as long as it doesn't box you into patient care that requires no thought and forces patients into algorithms where they don't belong.

- Medical school teaches when you hear hoofbeats, think of horses not zebras. In real life, there are plenty of zebras. We pretend they are horses because we are more comfortable with horses. Actually, some docs are afraid of zebras.

- Once a doctor decides on a diagnosis, he will defend that diagnosis despite evidence to the contrary.

- Many feel that if a piece doesn't fit in the puzzle, either force it in or throw it out.

- Sometimes a good doctor is not sure. Many doctors have trouble with uncertainty and to remain in control will make pronouncements that may have no relationship to what is actually happening with the patient.

- The culture of conformity begins in medical school, where everyone is taught to think the same way. Should you think differently, you are ridiculed.

- The more specialized the doctor, the more likely he is to be certain of his own decisions and skeptical of those of others.

- Different people respond to treatment in different ways. Patients should be allowed to have their disease their way instead of having to conform to an artificial checklist.

- Listen without interrupting.

- You have to know that a diagnosis exists before you can diagnose it.

- Doctors tend to "do something" rather than admit they don't know what to do.

- In a study of radiologists looking at a set of X-rays (some duplicates) the readings were often wrong. More than 60% didn't see a missing clavicle. They disagreed with one another about 20% of the time and they disagreed with themselves 5% to 10% of the time. The worst docs tended to be the most confident.

- Where you stand depends on where you sit. Your specialty can affect your position. Once a doc adopts a position, he is loathe to give it up.

- Different specialty areas often take opposing sides on controversial issues. They tend to favor the tools of their trade. Surgeons want to cut, neurologists like EMGs, pain specialists like meds.

- Once a doctor catches the big diagnosis, she tends to ignore the other obvious problems.

- Both doctors and patients want a simple answer to a complex problem.

- Help patients understand their options.

- Docs dislike failure and patients who don't get well fall into that category. Physicians don't like patients who have little chance of improving or who could get sicker.

- Target the treatment to the individual case.

- Many docs refuse to put themselves on the line.

- Some doctors use magical thinking as though just saying something makes it so.

- There may be more than one answer to a problem and, unlike Ockham's razor, the best answer is not always the simplest.

- Accept when a treatment plan isn't working and try alternatives.

- Complicated things may take time to figure out.

Well, Lyme and TBIs are certainly complicated. As an HCP, consider these concepts as you see patients. As a patient or caregiver use these ideas to realize what you should expect from a good HCP.

Sincerely,

Kathy Spreen

FINAL THOUGHTS

If you take nothing else from this book, please remember:

- Lyme is a clinical diagnosis.

- Engage the patient.

- Guidelines are just opinions, not the law.

- Treat the patient, not the lab result.

- A tick need only be attached a short time to cause disease.

- Chronic Lyme exists.

- On-going infection contributes to persistent disease in many cases.

- Use combination antibiotics when treating Lyme, or an agent that hits the various Bb life forms.

- More than one thing can be going on at a time.

- Target the particular manifestations of disease in this unique patient.

- Making one diagnosis does not cure another.

- Treat infected pregnant women.

- Take patient preferences into account.

- Consider and present various options.

- The earlier treatment is started, the better the outcome.

- Stop treatment when the patient is better, plus a cushion.

- If sxs do not respond to conventional therapy, a hidden TBI might be the reason.

- For best treatment results, address the underlying infection as well as the more obvious signs.

- A negative diagnostic test proves nothing.

- Never rule out Lyme disease on the basis of a negative lab result.

- Not detected does NOT mean uninfected.

- Not detected does NOT mean cured.

- EM rashes are not as common as we have been led to believe.

- Don't wait for the rash to make the diagnosis.

- Neuropsychiatric complaints can be the most common, severe, and intractable.

- The importance of prevention cannot be overstated.

- Listen to the patient.

- Consider compassion.

- Never give up.

Appendix A

BIBLIOGRAPHY

Man is unique among animals in his practiced ability to know things that are not so.
Philip Slater

This textbook was designed to present a large amount of information, some of it conflicting, in an effort to construct a usable, practical, working reference. In many cases, I found similar ideas (including the opposite views) in multiple sources, all of which are listed in this bibliography. In other cases, I refer to the body of work of authors whose lectures, personal appearances, conversations, articles, books, guidelines, chapters, and electronic communications contributed substantially to the ideas presented in this text. In addition, discussions of causality assessment, drug safety, and understanding medicines have been informed by my years in the pharmaceutical industry and in occupational and preventive medicine. This knowledge has evolved over many years of interactions with government agencies and mentors, many of whom provided examples of what not to do. While it is not unusual for authors on any topic to disagree with one another, note that some authors on this subject actually disagree with themselves, often more than once. Regardless, I tend to rely on the guidance of the experts I consulted and those whose careful procedures, thought processes, and observations have led to consistent and intelligent conclusions. I tried to keep the focus on helping patients and caregivers and on increasing our understanding of tick-borne illnesses.

Books

ABC's of Lyme Disease. Jackson, NJ: Lyme Disease Association, Inc. 2009.

American Medical Association Council on Ethical and Judicial Affairs. Code of Medical Ethics. Current Opinions with Annotations 2002-2003. Chicago, IL: American Medical Association; 2002.

Bakerman S. ABCs of Interpretive Laboratory Data. 4th ed. Scottsdale, AZ: Interpretive Laboratory Data, Inc; 2002.

Bates B. A Guide to Physical Examination. Philadelphia, PA: J. B. Lippincott; 1979.

Burrascano J. Diagnostic hints and treatment guidelines for Lyme and other tick borne illnesses. In: Advanced Topics in Lyme Disease. 15th and 16th eds. Bethesda, MD: International Lyme and Associated Diseases Society; 2005; 2008.

Burrascano J. Lyme Disease. In: Rakel R, ed. Conn's Current Therapy. Philadelphia, PA: W.B. Saunders Co;1997:140-143.

California Jury Instruction Civil Committee. Duty of Physicians. In: California Jury Instructions, Civil: Book of Approved Jury Instructions. St. Paul, MN: West Publishing Co; 2002.

Conley D. Elsewhere, U.S.A. New York, NY: Pantheon Books; 2010.

Denby D. Snark. New York, NY: Simon & Schuster; 2009.

Drymon MM. Disguised as the Devil: How Lyme Disease Created Witches and Changed History. Brooklyn, NY: Wythe Avenue Press; 2008.

Edlow JA. Bull's-Eye: Unraveling the Medical Mystery of Lyme Disease. New Haven, CT: Yale University Press; 2003.

Fearn D. Lyme Disease and Associated Tick-Borne Diseases: The Basics. 5th ed. The Lyme Disease Association of Southeastern Pennsylvania, Inc. 2007.

Felder L. Fitting in is Overrated. New York: Sterling Publishing Co, Inc; 2008.

Field M, Lohr K, eds. Guidelines for Clinical Practice: From Development to Use. Institute of Medicine. Washington, DC: National Academy Press; 1992.

Gardner T. Lyme disease. In: Remington JS, Klein JO, eds. Infectious Diseases of the Fetus and Newborn Infant. Philadelphia, PA: WB Saunders; 1995:447-528.

Groopman J. How Doctors Think. New York: Houghton Mifflin; 2007.

Gutierrez Y. Blood apicomplexa: Plasmodium, Babesia and entopolypoides. Ch 9. In: Diagnostic Pathology of Parasitic Infections With Clinical Correlations. Philadelphia, PA: Lea Febiger; 1990.

Hamlen RA, Kliman DS. Lyme disease and tick-borne infections: Causes and physical and neuropsychological effects in children. In: Macabe PC, Shaw SR, eds. Pediatric Disorders: Current Topics and Interventions for Educators. Thousand Oaks, CA: Corwin SAGE India Pvt. Ltd; 2010:91-100.

Institute of Medicine. Committee on Conflict of Interest in Medical Research, Education, and Practice. Conflict of Interest in Medical Research, Education, and Practice. Washington, DC: National Academies Press; 2009.

Jacobs RA. Syphilis. In: Tierney LM, McPhee SJ, Papadakis MA, eds. Current Medical Diagnosis and Treatment, 42nd ed. New York: McGraw Hill; 2003.

Katzel J. Is there a consensus in treatment of Lyme borreliosis? In: Mermin L, ed. Lyme Disease 1991 Patient/Physician Perspectives from the US and Canada. Lyme Disease Education Project. PO Box 55412, Madison, WI: 1991.

Kessler D. The End of Overeating. Emmaus, PA: Rodale Press, Inc; 2009.

Langhoff PJ. The Baker's Dozen & the Lunatic Fringe: Has Junk Science Shifted the Lyme Disease Paradigm? Hustisford, WI: Allegory Press, LLC; 2008.

Louv R. Last Child in the Woods: Saving Our Children from Nature-deficit Disorder. Chapel Hill, NC: Algonquin Books; 2008.

Malaria. In: Beers MH, Berkow R, eds. Merck Manual of Diagnosis and Therapy, 17th ed. Hoboken, NJ: John Wiley & Sons; 1999.

Marquardt WC, Demaree RS, Grieve RB. Piroplasmea and piroplasmosis. In: Parasitology and Vector Biology, 2nd ed. San Diego, CA: Academic Press; 2000:221-224.

Muir Gray J. Evidence-Based Healthcare. How to Make Health Policy and Management Decisions. London: Churchill Livingstone;1997.

Office of Technology Assessment. United States Congress. Defensive medicine: Definition and causes. In: Defensive Medicine and Medical Malpractice. Washington, DC: US Government Printing Office;1994.

Ostfeld RS. Lyme Disease: The Ecology of a Complex System. Oxford University Press; 2010.

Piazza G, Piazza L. Recipes for Repair: A Lyme Disease Cookbook. Forward by Ken Singleton MD MPH. Peconic Publishing, LLC; 2010.

Rapini RP, Bolognia JL, Jorizzo JL. Dermatology. St. Louis, MO: Mosby; 2007.

Ravitch D. The Death and Life of the Great American School System. New York: Basic Books; 2010.

Ryan KJ, Ray CG, eds. Sherris Medical Microbiology, 4th ed. New York: McGraw Hill; 2004: 434-437.

Samuels DS, Radolf JD, eds. Borrelia. Molecular Biology, Host Interaction and Pathogenesis. Portland, OR: Caister Academic Press; 2010.

Scammell H. The Road Back. New York:M. Evans & Company, Inc; 1988.

Schaller, James. Treatment and Diagnosis of Human Babesiosis. Tampa, FL: Hope Academic Press; 2006.

Shah S. The Fever. New York, NY: Farrar, Straus and Giroux; 2010.

Singleton, KB. The Lyme Disease Solution. BookSurge Publishing; 2008.

Sonenshine DE. The biology of tick vectors of human disease. In: Goodman JL, Dennis DT, Sonenshine DE, eds. Tick-borne Diseases of Humans. Washington, DC: AMS Press; 2005:22-23.

Steere AC. Lyme Borreliosis. In: Fauci AS, Braunwald E, Kasper DL, et al, eds. Harrison's Principles of Internal Medicine, 17th ed. New York: McGraw-Hill Medical Publishing; 2008.

Tedlow RS. Denial: Why Business Leaders Fail to Look Facts in the Face – and What to Do About It. New York: Penguin Group; 2010.

Telford SR 3rd, Gorenflot A, Spielman A, et al. Babesial infections in humans and wildlife. In: Kreier JP, ed. Parasitic Protozoa, 2nd ed, Vol. 5. San Diego, CA: Academic Press; 1993:1-47.

Waisbren BA, Sr. Treatment of Chronic Lyme Disease: Fifty-One Case Reports and Essays in Their Regard. Bloomington, IN: iUniverse, Inc; 2011.

Weintraub P. Cure Unknown: Inside the Lyme Epidemic. New York: St. Martin's Press; 2009.

Published Journal Articles

Abbott A. Lyme disease: Uphill struggle. Nature. 2006;439(7076):524-525.

Adelson MA, et al. Prevalence of Borrelia burgdorferi, Bartonella spp., Babesia microti, and Anaplasma phagocytophila in Ixodes scapularis Ticks Collected in Northern New Jersey. J of Clinical Microbiology. 2004;42(6):2799.

Afzelius A. Verhandlungen der dermatologischen gesellschaft zu Stockholm (in German). Arch Dermatol Syphilis. 1910;101:100-102.

Aguero-Rosenfeld ME, Nowakowski J, Bittkner S, et al. Evolution of the serologic response to Borrelia burgdorferi in treated patients with culture-confirmed erythema migrans. J Clin Microbiol. 1996;34(1):1-9.

Aguero-Rosenfeld ME, Nowakowski J, McKenna DF, et al. Serodiagnosis in early Lyme disease. J Clin Microbiol. 1993;31(12):3090-3095.

Aguero-Rosenfeld ME, Wang G, Schwartz I, et al. Diagnosis of Lyme borreliosis. Clin Microbiol Rev. 2005;18 (3):484-509.

Amanda R, Marcia A, Richard WD, et al. What is a good decision? Editorial. Eff Clin Pract. 1999;July/August.

American Academy of Pediatrics, Steering Committee on Quality Improvement and Management. Classifying recommendations for clinical practice guidelines. Pediatrics. 2004;114:874-877.

Amore G, Tomassone L, Grego E, et al. Borrelia lusitaniae in immature Ixodes ricinus (Acari: Ixodidae) feeding on common wall lizards in Tuscany, central Italy. J Med Entomol. 2007;44(2):303-307.

Andres S, Schmidt H-M, Mitchell H, et al. Helicobacter pylori defines immune response through interaction with dendritic cells. 2011;61(2):168-178.

Arlen J, MacLeod W. Malpractice liability for physicians and managed care organizations. NY Univ Law Rev. 2003;78:1929-2003.

Armstrong PM, Datgavolos P, Caporale DA, et al. Diversity of Babesia infecting deer ticks (Ixodes dammini). Am J Trop Med Hyg. 1998:58:739-742.

Auwaerter PG, Aucott J, Dumler JS. Lyme borreliosis (Lyme disease): Molecular and cellular pathobiology and prospects for prevention, diagnosis and treatment. Expert Rev Mol Med. 2004;6(2):1-22.

Baker PJ. Perspectives on chronic Lyme disease. Am J Med. 2008;121(7):562-564.

Baldauf S. South Africa's wine country fights alcoholism scourge. The Christian Science Monitor. April 12, 2007. http://www.csmonitor.com. Accessed February 2009.

Ballantyne C. The chronic debate over Lyme disease. Nat Med. 2008;14(11): 1135-1139.

Battafarano DF, Combs JA, Enzenauer RJ, et al. Chronic septic arthritis caused by Borrelia burgdorferi. Clin Orthop. 1993;27:238-241.

Bayer ME, Zhang L, Bayer MH. Borrelia burgdorferi DNA in the urine of treated patients with chronic Lyme disease symptoms. A PCR study of 97 cases. Infection. 1996;24(5):347-353.

Belongia EA. Epidemiology and impact of co-infections acquired from Ixodes ticks. Vector Borne Zoonotic Dis. 2002;2(4):265-273.

Bernardino AL, Kaushal D, Philipp MT. The antibiotics doxycycline and minocycline inhibit the inflammatory responses to the Lyme disease spirochete Borrelia burgdorferi. J Infect Dis. 2009;199(9):1379-1388.

Bharadwaj A, Stafford KC III. Evaluation of Metarhizium anisopliae strain F52 (Hypocreales: Clavicipitaceae) for control of Ixodes scapularis (Acari: Ixodidae). J Med Entomol. 2010;47(5):862-867.

Bianchi GE. Penicillin therapy of lymphocytoma. Dermatologica. 1950;100(4-6):270-273.

Billeter SA, et al. Detection of two Bartonella tamiae-like sequences in Amblyomma americanum. J Med Entomol. 2008;45(1):176-179.

Bissinger BW, Zhu J, Apperson CS, et al. Comparative efficacy of BioUD to other commercially available arthropod repellents against the ticks Amblyomma americanum and Dermacentor variabilis on cotton cloth. Am J Trop Med Hyg. 2009;81(4):685–690.

Blevins SM, Greenfield RA, Bronze MS. Blood smear analysis in babesiosis, ehrlichiosis, relapsing fever, malaria, and Chagas disease. Cleveland Clin J Med. 2008;75:521-530.

Blum D, Chtarto A, Tenenbaum L, et al. Clinical potential of minocycline for neurodegenerative disorders. Neurobiol Dis. 2004;17(3):359–366.

Bolz DD, Weis JJ. Molecular mimicry to Borrelia burgdorferi: Pathway to autoimmunity? Autoimmunity. 2004;37(5):387-392.

Bouattour A, Ghorbel A, Chabchoub A, et al. Lyme borreliosis situation in North Africa (in French). Arch l'Institut Pasteur de Tunis. 2004 ;81(1-4):13-20.

Bransfield RC. Lyme disease, comorbid tick-borne diseases, and neuropsychiatric disorders. Psychiatric Times. 2007;24(14).

Bratton RL, Whiteside JW, Hovan MJ, et al. Diagnosis and treatment of Lyme disease. Mayo Clin Proc. 2008;83(5):566-571.

Breier F, Khanakah G, Stanek G, et al. Isolation and polymerase chain reaction typing of Borrelia afzelii from a skin lesion in a seronegative patient with generalized ulcerating bullous lichen sclerosus et atrophicus. Br J Dermatol. 2001;144(20):387-392.

Breitschwerdt EB, et al. Bartonella DNA in Dog Saliva. Emerg Infect Dis. 2007;13:938-41.

Breitschwerdt EB, Kordick DL. Bartonella Infection in Animals: Carriership, reservoir potential, pathogenicity, and zoonotic potential for human infection. Clin Microbiology Rev. 2000;13(30):428-438.

Brorson O, Brorson SH. A rapid method for generating cystic forms of Borrelia burgdorferi, and their reversal to mobile spirochetes. Apmis. 1998;106(12):1131-1141.

Brouqui P, Badiaga S, Raoult D. Eucaryotic cells protect Borrelia burgdorferi from the action of penicillin and ceftriaxone but not from the action of doxycycline and erythromycin. Antimicrob Agents Chemother. 1996;40(6):1552-1554.

Brown SL, Hansen SL, Langone JJ. Role of serology in the diagnosis of Lyme disease. JAMA. 1999;282(1):62-66.

Bunikis J, Garpmo U, Tsao J, et al. Sequence typing reveals extensive strain diversity of the Lyme borreliosis agents Borrelia burgdorferi in North America and Borrelia afzelii in Europe. Microbiology. 2004;150(Pt 6):1741-1755.

Burckhardt JL. Zur Frage der Follikel- und Keimzentrenbildung in der Haut (in German). Frankfurter Zeitschrift Pathol. 1911;6:352-359.

Burdash N, Fernandes J. Lyme borreliosis: Detecting the great imitator. J Am Osteopath Asso. 1991;91(6):573-574, 577-578.

Burgdorfer W, Barbour AG, Hayes SF, et al. Lyme disease - a tick-borne spirochetosis? Science. 1982;216(4552):1317-1319.

Burgdorfer W. Discovery of the Lyme disease spirochete and its relation to tick vectors. Yale J Biol Med. 1984;57:515-520.

Cabello FC, Godfrey HP, Newman SA. Hidden in plain sight: Borrelia burgdorferi and the extracellular matrix. Trends Microbiol. 2007;15(8):350-354.

Cadavid D. The mammalian host response to Borrelia infection. Wien Klin Wochenschr. 2006;118(21–22):653-658.

Cairns V, Godwin J. Post-Lyme borreliosis syndrome: A meta-analysis of reported symptoms. Int J Epidemiol. 2005;34(6):1340-1345.

Calcagni E, Elenkov I. Stress system activity, innate and T helper cytokines, and susceptibility to immune-related diseases. Ann NY Acad Sci. 2006;1069:62-76.

Calvo De Mora A, Garcia Castellano JM, Herrera C, et al. Babesiosis humana: aportacion de un caso de evolucion fatal. Medicina Clinica. 1985;85:515-516.

Cameron D, Gallo A, Harris N, et al. Evidence-based guidelines for the management of Lyme disease. Expert Rev Anti-infect Ther. 2004;2:S1-13.

Cameron DJ. Generalizability in two clinical trials of Lyme disease. Epidemiol Perspect Innovations. 2006;3:12-19.

Cameron DJ. Insufficient evidence to deny antibiotic treatment to chronic Lyme disease patients. Med Hypotheses. 2009;72:688-691.

Carroll JF, Benante JP, Kramer M, et al. Formulations of Deet, Picaridin, and IR3535 applied to skin repel nymphs of the Lone Star Tick (Acari: Ixodidae) for 12 hours. J Med Entomol. 2010;47(4):699-704.

Cary NR, Fox B, Wright DJ, et al. Fatal Lyme carditis and endodermal heterotopia of the atrioventricular node. Postgrad Med J. 1990;66(772):134-136.

Centers for Disease Control and Prevention (CDC) Summary of Notifiable Diseases - United States. MMWR. 2011b;58(53):1-100.

Centers for Disease Control and Prevention (CDC). Case definition for infectious conditions under public health surveillance. (Lyme disease surveillance case definition). MMWR. 1997;46(RR 10, 1-3):15-16.

Centers for Disease Control and Prevention (CDC). Notifiable diseases and mortality tables. MMWR. 2011a;60(36):1254-1267.

Chabria SB, Lawrason J. Altered mental status, an unusual manifestation of early disseminated Lyme disease: A case report. J Med Case Rep. 2007;1:62.

Change CC, et al. Coyotes (Canis latrans) as the reservoir for a human pathogenic Bartonella sp. J Clin Microbiol. 2000;38(11):4193-4200.

Chomel B. Tick-borne infections in dogs - an emerging infectious threat. Vet Parasitol. 2011;179:294-301.

Choudhry N, Stelfox H, Detsky A. Relationships between authors of clinical practice guidelines and the pharmaceutical industry. J Amer Med Assoc. 2002;287:612-617.

Cimmino MA, Accardo S. Long-term treatment of chronic Lyme arthritis with benzathine penicillin. Ann Rheum Dis. 1992;51(8):1007-1008.

Cimmino MA, Moggiana GL, Parisi M, et al. Treatment of Lyme arthritis. Infection. 1996;24(1):91-93.

Clark K. Borrelia species in host-seeking ticks and small mammals in northern Florida. Clin Microbiol. 2004;42(11):5076–5086.

Cohen S, Alper CM, Doyle WJ, et al. Positive emotional style predicts resistance to illness after experimental exposure to rhinovirus or influenza a virus. Psychosom Med. 2006;68(6):809-815.

Coleman JL, Gebbia JA, Piesman J, et al. Plasminogen is required for efficient dissemination of B. burgdorferi in ticks and for enhancement of spirochetemia in mice. Cell. 1997;89(7):1111-1119.

Connally NP, Durante AJ, Yousey-Hindes KM, et al. Peridomestic Lyme disease prevention - results of a population-based case-control study. Am J Prev Med. 2009;37(3):201-206.

Conrad PA, Kjemtrup A, Carreno RA, et al. Description of Babesia duncani n.sp. (Apicomplexa: Babesiidae) from humans and its differentiation from other piroplasms. Int J Parasitol. 2006;36(7):779-789.

Cook J, Fincham WJ, Lack CH. Chronic arthritis produced by streptococcal L-forms. J Pathol. 1969;99(4):283-297.

Cooper JD, Feder HM. Inaccurate information about Lyme disease on the internet. Pediatr Infect Dis J. 2004;23(12):1105-1108.

Coulter Peggy, et al. Two-Year Evaluation of Borrelia burgdorferi Culture and Supplemental Tests for Definitive Diagnosis of Lyme Disease. J of Clinical Microbiology. 2005;43(10): 5080-5084.

Coyle PK, Schutzer SE, Deng Z, et al. Detection of Borrelia burgdorferi-specific antigen in antibody-negative cerebrospinal fluid in neurologic Lyme disease. Neurology. 1995;45(11):2010-2015.

Coyle PK. Borrelia burgdorferi infection: Clinical diagnostic techniques. Immunol Invest. 1997;26 (1-2):117-128.

Coyle PK. Neurologic complications of Lyme disease. Rheum Dis Clin North Am. 1993;19(4):993-1009.

Dandache P, Nadelman RB. Erythema migrans. Infect Dis Clin North Am. 2008;22 (2):235-260.

Dattwyler RJ, Volkman DJ, Conaty SM, et al. Amoxicillin plus probenecid versus doxycycline for treatment of erythema migrans borreliosis. Lancet. 1990;336(8728):1404-1406.

de Mik EL, van Pelt W, van Leeuwen BD, et al. The geographical distribution of tick bites and erythema migrans in general practice in The Netherlands. Int J Epidemiol. 1997;26 (2):451-457.

Derdáková M, Lencáková D. Association of genetic variability within the Borrelia burgdorferi sensu lato with the ecology. Epidemiology of Lyme borreliosis in Europe. Ann Agric Environ Med. 2005;12(2):165-172.

Dolan MC, Jordan RA, Schulze TL, et al. Ability of two natural products, nootkatone and carvacrol, to suppress Ixodes scapularis and Amblyomma americanum (Acari: Ixodidae) in a Lyme disease endemic area of New Jersey. J Econ Entomol. 2009;102(6):2316-2324.

Donta ST. Late and chronic Lyme disease. Med Clin North Am. 2002;86(2):341-349.

Donta ST. Tetracycline therapy for chronic Lyme disease. Clin Infect Dis. 1997;25(Suppl. 1): S52-S56.

Donta ST. The existence of chronic Lyme disease. Curr Treat Op Infect Dis. 2001;3:261-262.

Dorward DW, Fisher ER, Brooks DM. Invasion and cytopathic killing of human lymphocytes by spirochetes causing Lyme disease. Clin Infect Dis. 1997;25(Suppl.1):52-58.

Dryden M, Hodgkins E. Parasites 100-vector-borne diseases in pets: The stealth health threat. Compend Contin Educ Vet. 2010;32(6):E1-4.

Dsouli N, Younsi-Kabachii H, Postic D, et al. Reservoir role of lizard Psammodromus algirus in transmission cycle of Borrelia burgdorferi sensu lato (Spirochaetaceae) in Tunisia. J Med Entomol. 2006;43(4):737-742.

Duffy DC, Downer R, Brinkley C. The effectiveness of Helmeted Guinea fowl in the control of the deer tick, the vector of Lyme disease. Wilson Bull. 1992;104(2):342-345. http://www.guineafowl. com/fritsfarm/guineas/ticks/tickstudy.pdf. Accessed March 2011.

Dvorakova HM, Dvorackova M. Babesiosis, a little known zoonosis. Epidemiol Mikrobiol Imunol. 2007;56(4):176-180.

Earnhart CG, Marconi RT. An octavalent Lyme disease vaccine induces antibodies that recognize all incorporated OspC type-specific sequences. Hum Vaccine. 2007;3(6):281-289.

Eisen L, Eisen RJ, Lane RS. The roles of birds, lizards, and rodents as hosts for the western black-legged tick Ixodes pacificus. J Vector Ecol. 2004;29(2):295-308.

Eisendle K, Grabner T, Zelger B. Focus floating microscopy: Gold standard for cutaneous borreliosis? Am J Clin Pathol. 2007;127(2):213-222.

Elenkov IJ, Iezzoni DG, Daly A, et al. Cytokine dysregulation, inflammation and well-being. Neuroimmunomodulation. 2005;12(5):255-269.

Elewa HF, Hilali H, Hess DC, et al. Minocycline for short-term neuroprotection. Pharmacotherapy. 2006;26(4):515-521.

Embers ME, Ramamoorthy R, Philipp MT. Survival strategies of Borrelia burgdorferi, the etiologic agent of Lyme disease. J Microbes Infection. 2004;6:312-318.

Engstrom SM, Shoop E, Johnson RC. Immunoblot interpretation criteria for serodiagnosis of early Lyme disease. J Clin Microbiol. 1995;33(2):419-427.

Ercolini AM, Miller SD. The role of infections in autoimmune disease. Clin Exp Immunol. 2009;155(1):1-15.

Ernst E, Canter PH. Investigator bias and false positive findings in medical research. Trends Pharmacol Sci. 2003;24(5):219-221.

Eskow E, Rao RV, Mordechai E. Concurrent infection of the central nervous system by Borrelia burgdorferi and Bartonella henslea: Evidence for a novel tick-borne disease complex. Arch Neurol. 2001;58(9):1357-1363.

Fahrer H, Sauvain MJ, Zhioua E, et al. Long-term survey (7 years) in a population at risk for Lyme borreliosis: What happens to the seropositive individuals? Eur J Epidemiol. 1998;14(2): 117-123.

Fallon BA, Keilp J, Prohovnik I, et al. Regional cerebral blood flow and cognitive deficits in chronic Lyme disease. J Neuropsychiatry Clin Neurosci. 2003;15(3):326-332.

Fallon BA, Keilp JG, Corbera KM, et al. A randomized, placebo-controlled trial of repeated IV antibiotic therapy for Lyme encephalopathy. Neurology. 2008;70(13):992-1003.

Fallon BA, Kochevar JM, Gaito A, et al. The underdiagnosis of neuropsychiatric Lyme disease in children and adults. Psychiatric Clin North Am. 1998;21:693-703.

Fallon BA, Nields JA. Lyme disease: A neuropsychiatric illness. Am J Psychiatry. 1994;151(11): 1571-1583.

Fallon BA, Schwartzberg M, Bransfield R, et al. Late-stage neuropsychiatric Lyme borreliosis. Differential diagnosis and treatment. Psychosomatics. 1995;36(3):295-300.

Fallon BA. Repeated antibiotic treatment in chronic Lyme disease. J Spirochet Tick Borne Dis. 1999;6:94-101.

Feder HM Jr, Johnson BJ, O'Connell S, et al. A critical appraisal of "chronic Lyme disease." N Engl J Med. 2007;357:1422-1430.

Feder HM Jr. Differences are voiced by two Lyme camps at a Connecticut public hearing on insurance coverage of Lyme disease. Pediatrics. 2000;105(4 Pt 1):855-857.

Ferris Tortajada J, Lopez Andreau JA, Salcede Vivo J, et al. Lyme Borreliosis (Letter). Lancet. 1995;345(8962):1436-1437.

Fikrig E, Narasimhan S. Borrelia burgdorferi - traveling incognito? Microbes Infect. 2006;8(5): 1390-1399.

Fivaz BH, Petney TN. Lyme disease - a new disease in southern Africa? J South African Vet Assoc. 1989;60(3):155-158.

Fletcher S, Fletcher R. Development of clinical guidelines. Lancet. 1998;352(9144):1876.

Food and Drug Administration. Lyme disease test kits: Potential for misdiagnosis. FDA Med Bull. 1999.

Freedman RM. The two Lyme camps. Pediatrics. 2001;107(6):1495.

Fried MD, Adelson ME, Mordechai E. Simultaneous Gastrointestinal Infections in Children and Adolescents. Practical Gastroenterology. 2004;November:78-80.

Furr PM, Taylor-Robinson D, Webster ADB. Mycoplasmas and ureaplasmas in patients with hypogammaglobulinemia and their roll in arthritis: Microbiological observation over twenty years. Ann Rheumatol Dis. 1994;53:183-187.

Gasse T, Murr C, Meyersbach P, et al. Neopterin production and tryptophan degradation in acute Lyme neuroborreliosis versus late Lyme encephalopathy. Eur J Clin Chem Clin Biochem. 1994;32(9):685-689.

Georgilis K, Peacock M, Klempner MS. Fibroblasts protect the Lyme disease spirochete, Borrelia burgdorferi, from ceftriaxone in vitro. J Infect Dis. 1992;166(2):440-444.

Gershon A: Unproven therapies don't belong in Lyme disease guidelines. South Med J. 2009;102:1088-1089.

Giery ST, Ostfeld RS. The role of lizards in the ecology of Lyme disease in two endemic zones of the northeastern United States. J Parasitol. 2007;93(3):511-517.

Goldenberg RL, Thompson C. The infectious origin of stillbirth. Am J Obstet Gynecol. 2003;189:861-873.

Goossens HA, Nohlmans MK, van den Bogaard AE. Epstein-Barr virus and cytomegalovirus infections cause false-positive results in IgM two-test protocol for early Lyme borreliosis. Infection. 1999;27(3):231.

Gorenflot A, Moubri K, Precigout E, et al. Human babesiosis. Ann Trop Med Paristol. 1998;92(4):489-501.

Grilli R, Magrini N, Penna A, et al. Practice guidelines developed by specialty societies: The need for critical appraisal. Lancet. 2000;355:103-106.

Grubhoffer L, Golovchenko M, Vancová M, et al. Lyme borreliosis: insights into tick-/host-borrelia relations. Folia Parasitol. 2005;52(4):279-294.

Guner ES. Complement evasion by the Lyme disease spirochete Borrelia burgdorferi grown in host-derived tissue cocultures: Role of fibronectin in complement-resistance. Experimentia. 1996;52(40):364-372.

Gustafson JM, Burgess EC, et al. Intrauterine transmission of Borrelia burgdorferi in dogs. Am J Vet Res. 1993;54(6):882-890.

Hajek T, Libiger J, Janovska D, et al. Clinical and demographic characteristics of psychiatric patients seropositive for Borrelia burgdorferi. Eur Psychiatry. 2006;21(2):118-121.

Hajek T, Paskova B, Janovska D, et al. Higher prevalence of antibodies to Borrelia burgdorferi in psychiatric patients than in healthy subjects. Am J Psychiatry. 2002;159(2):297-301.

Halperin JJ, Heyes MP. Neuroactive kynurenines in Lyme borreliosis. Neurology. 1992;42(1):43-50.

Halperin JJ, Shapiro ED, Logigian E, et al. Practice parameter: Treatment of nervous system Lyme disease (an evidence based review): Report of the Quality Standards Subcommittee of the American Academy of Neurology. Neurology. 2007;69:91-102.

Halperin JJ. Nervous system Lyme disease. Infect Dis Clin North Am. 2008;22(2):261-274.

Halperin JJ. Neuroborreliosis: Central nervous system involvement. Semin Neurol. 1997;17(1):19-24.

Halperin, JJ. Prolonged Lyme disease treatment: Enough is enough. Neurology. 2008;70(13):986-987.

Hamilton KS, Standaert SM, Kinney MC. Characteristic peripheral blood findings in human ehrlichiosis. Mod Pathol. 2004;17(5):512-517.

Hamlen RA, Kliman DS. Pediatric Lyme disease - a school issue: Tips for school nurses. NASN School Nurse. 2009;24:114-118.

Hannier S, Liversidge J, Sternber JM, et al. Ixodes ricinis tick salivary gland extract inhibits IL-10 secretion and CD69 expression by mitogen-stimulated murine splenocytes and induces hyporesponsiveness in B-lymphocytes. Parasite Immunol. 2003;25(1):27-37.

Hassler D, Riedel K, Zorn J, et al. Pulsed high-dose cefotaxime therapy in refractory Lyme borreliosis. Lancet. 1991;338(8760):193.

Haupl T, Hahn G, Rittig M, et al. Persistence of Borrelia burgdorferi in ligamentous tissue from a patient with chronic Lyme borreliosis. Arthritis Rheum. 1993;36(11):1621-1626.

Haycox A, Bagust A, Walley T. Clinical guidelines – the hidden costs. Br Med J. 1999;318:391-393.

Hayward RS, Wilson MC, Tunis SR, et al. Users' guides to the medical literature. How to use clinical practice guidelines. Are the recommendations valid? The Evidence-Based Medicine Working Group. J Am Med Assoc. 1995;274(7):570-574.

Healy TL. The impact of Lyme disease on school children. J Sch Nursing. 2000;16:12-18.

Hellerström S. Erythema chronicum migrans Afzelii (in German). Arch Dermato Venereol. (Stockholm). 1930;11:315-321.

Helmy N. Seasonal abundance of Ornithodoros (O.) savignyi and prevalence of infection with Borrelia spirochetes in Egypt. J Egypt Soc Parasitol. 2000;30(2)607-619.

Herwaldt B, Persing DH, Précigout EA, et al. A fatal case of babesiosis in Missouri: identification of another piroplasm that infects humans. Ann Intern Med. 1996;124(7):643-650.

Herwaldt BL, Cacciò S, Gherlinzoni F, et al. Molecular characterization of a non-Babesia divergens organism causing zoonotic babesiosis in Europe. Emerg Infect Dis. 2003;9(8):942-948.

Herwaldt BL, Kjemtrup AM, Conrad PA, et al. Transfusion-transmitted babesiosis in Washington State: First reported case caused by WA1-type parasite. J Infect Dis. 1997;175:1259-1262.

Hess A, Buchmann J, Zettl UK, et al. Borrelia burgdorferi central nervous system infection presenting as an organic schizophrenia-like disorder. Biol. Psychiatry. 1999;45(6):795.

Higgins R. Emerging or re-emerging bacterial zoonotic diseases: Bartonellosis, leptospirosis, Lyme borreliosis, plague. Rev Off Int Epizoot. 2004;23(2):569-581.

Hildenbrand P, Craven DE, Jones R, et al. Lyme neuroborreliosis: Manifestations of a rapidly emerging zoonosis. Am J Neuroradiol. 2009;30(6):1079-1087.

Hodzic E, Feng S, Holden K, et al. Persistence of Borrelia burgdorferi following antibiotic treatment in mice. Antimicrob Agents Chemother. 2008;52:1728-1736.

Hofmann H. Lyme borreliosis - problems of serological diagnosis. Infection. 1996;24(6):470-472.

Hojgaard A. Transmission Dynamics of Borrelia burgdorferi s.s. During the Key Third Day of Feeding by Nymphal Ixodes scapularis (Acari: Ixodidae). J Med Entomol. 2008;45(4):732-736.

Hunfeld KP, Brade V. Zoonotic Babesia: Possibly emerging pathogens to be considered for tick-infested humans in central Europe. Int J Med Microbiol. 2004;S37:93-103.

Hunfeld KP, Hildebrandt A, Gray JS. Babesiosis: Recent insights into an ancient disease. Int J Parasitol. 2008;38(11):1219-1237.

Hurwitz B. Clinical guidelines and the law. Br Med J. 1995;311:1517-1518.

Jackson LE, Hilborn ED, Thomas JC. Towards landscape design guidelines for reducing Lyme disease risk. Int J Epidemiol. 2006;35:315-322.

Jackson LE. The relationship of urban design to human health and condition. Landscape and Urban Planning. 2003;64:191-200.

Jacoby I. Consensus development at NIH: What went wrong? Risk - Issues in Health and Safety. 1993;4(2):133-142.

Jaenson TJT, Garboui S, Pålsson K. Repellency of oils of lemon, eucalyptus, geranium, and lavender and the mosquito repellent MyggA Natural to Ixodes ricinus (Acari: Ixodidae) in the laboratory and field. J Med Entomol. 2006;43(4):731-736.

Johnson L, Stricker RB. The Infectious Diseases Society of America Lyme guidelines: A cautionary tale about the development of clinical practice guidelines. Philos Ethics Humanit Med. 2010;5:9. http://www.peh-med.com/content/5/1/9. Accessed November 2011.

Johnson L, Stricker RB. Treatment of Lyme disease: A medicolegal assessment. Expert Rev Anti-infect Ther. 2004;2(4):533-557.

Johnson L, Stricker RB: Attorney General forces Infectious Diseases Society of America to redo Lyme Guidelines due to flawed development process. J Med Ethics. 2009;301:831-841.

Jowi JO, Gathua SN. Lyme disease: Report of two cases. East Afr Med J. 2005;82(5): 267-269.

Kaiser R. False-negative serology in patients with neuroborreliosis and the value of employing of different borrelial strains in serological assays. J Med Microbiol. 2000;49(10):911-915.

Kaplan RF, Trevino RP, Johnson GM, et al. Cognitive function in post-treatment Lyme disease: Do additional antibiotics help? Neurology. 2003;60(12):1916-1922.

Kersten A, Poitschek C, Rauch S, et al. Effects of penicillin, ceftriaxone, and doxycycline on morphology of Borrelia burgdorferi. Antimicrob Agents Chemother. 1995;39(5):1127-1133.

Khasnis AA, Nettleman MD. Global warming and infectious disease. Arch Med Res. 2005;36(6):689-696.

Kirsch M, Ruben FL, Steere AC, et al. Fatal adult respiratory distress syndrome in a patient with Lyme disease. JAMA. 1988;259(18):2737-2739.

Kjemtrup AM, Lee B, Fritz CL, et al. Investigation of transfusion transmission of WA1-type babesial parasite to a premature infant in California. Transfusion. 2002;42:1482-1487.

Klein JD, Eppes SC, Hunt P. Environmental and life-style risk factors for Lyme disease in children. Clin Pediatr. 1996;35:359-363.

Klein JO. Danger ahead: Politics intrude in Infectious Diseases Society of America guideline for Lyme disease. Clin Infect Dis. 2008;47(9):1197-1199.

Klempner MS, Hu LT, Evans J, et al. Two controlled trials of antibiotic treatment in patients with persistent symptoms and a history of Lyme disease. N Engl J Med. 2001;345(2):85-92.

Kordick DL, Breitschwerdt, EB. Intraerythrocytic presence of Bartonella henselae. J Clin Microbiol. 1995;33(6):1655-6.

Kraemer JD, Gostin LO. Science, politics, and values: The politicization of professional practice guidelines. JAMA. 2009;301(6):665-667.

Krause PJ, Foley DT, Burke GS, et al. Reinfection and relapse in early Lyme disease. Am J Trop Med Hyg. 2006;75(6):1090-1094.

Krause PJ, Telford SR III, Spielman A, et al. Concurrent Lyme disease and Babesiosis evidence for increased severity and duration of illness. JAMA. 1996;275:1657-1660.

Krause PJ, Telford SR, Ryan R, et al. Diagnosis of babesiosis: Evaluation of serologic test for detection of Babesia microti antibody. J Infect Dis. 1994;169(4):923-926.

Krause PJ. Babesiosis diagnosis and treatment. Vector Borne Zoonotic Dis. 2003;3(1):45-51.

Krupp LB, Hyman LG, Grimson R, et al. Study and treatment of post Lyme disease (STOP-LD): A randomized double masked clinical trial. Neurology. 2003;60(12):1923-1930.

Krupp LB, Masur D, Schwartz J, et al. Cognitive functioning in late Lyme borreliosis. Arch Neurol. 1991;48(11):1125-1129.

Lakos A, Solymosi N. Maternal Lyme borreliosis and pregnancy outcome. Int J Infect Dis. 2010;14(6):e494-e498.

Lane R, Steinlein D, Mun J. Human behaviors elevating exposure to Ixodes pacificus (Acari: Ixodidae) nymphs and their associated bacterial zoonotic agents in a hardwood forest. J Med Entomol. 2004;41:239-248.

Lane RS, Moss RB, Has YP, et al. Anti-arthropod saliva antibodies among residents of a community at high risk for Lyme disease in California. Am J Trop Med Hyg. 1999;61(5):850-859.

Lane RS, Mun J, Eisen L, et al. Refractoriness of the western fence lizard (Sceloporus occidentalis) to the Lyme disease group spirochete Borrelia bissettii. J Parasitol. 2006;92(4):691–696.

Lawrence C, Lipton RB, Lowy FD, et al. Seronegative chronic relapsing neuroborreliosis. Eur Neurol. 1995;35(2):113-117.

Ledin KE, Zeidner NS, Ribeiro JM, et al. Borreliacidal activity of saliva of the tick Amblyomma americanum. Med Vet Entomol. 2005;19(1):90–95.

Leeflang P, Oomen JMV, Zwart D, et al. The prevalence of Babesia antibodies in Nigerians. Int J Parasitol. 1976;6:156-161.

Lenhoff C. Spirochetes in aetiologically obscure diseases. Acta Dermatol Venreol. 1948;28:295–324.

Li M, Masuzawa T, Takada N, et al. Lyme disease Borrelia species in northeastern China resemble those isolated from far eastern Russia and Japan. Appl Environ Microbiol. 1998;64(7):2705-2709.

Liang FT, Jacobs MB, Bowers LC, et al. An immune evasion mechanism for spirochetal persistence in Lyme borreliosis. J Exp Med. 2002;195(4):415-422.

Liegner KB, Kochevar J. Guidelines for the clinical diagnosis of Lyme disease. Ann Intern Med. 1998;129(5):422.

Liegner KB. Lyme disease controversy: Use and misuse of language. Ann Intern Med. 2002;137(9):775-777.

Liegner KB. Lyme disease: The sensible pursuit of answers. J Clin Microbiol. 1993;31(8):1961-1963.

Little SE, Heise SR, Blagburn BL, et al. Lyme borreliosis in dogs and humans in the USA. Trends Parasitol. 2010;26(4):213-217.

Livengood JA, Gilmore RD. Invasion of human neuronal and glial cells by an infectious strain of Borrelia burgdorferi. Microbe Infect. 2006;8(14-15): 2832-2840.

Liveris D, Wang G, Girao G, et al. Quantitative detection of Borrelia burgdorferi in 2-millimeter skin samples of erythema migrans lesions: Correlation of results with clinical and laboratory findings. J Clin Microbiol. 2002;40(4):1249-1253.

Lo Re V, Occi JL, MacGregor RR. Identifying the vector of Lyme disease. Am Fam Physician. 2004;69(8):1935-1937.

Logigian EL, Kaplan RF, Steere AC. Chronic neurologic manifestations of Lyme disease. NEJM. 1990;323(21):1438-1444.

LoGiudice K, Ostfeld R, Schmidt K, et al. The ecology of infectious disease: Effects of host diversity and community composition on Lyme disease risk. Proc Natl Acad Sci USA. 2003;100(2):567-571.

Lopez-Andreau JA, Ferris J, Canosa CA, Sala-Lizarraga JV. Treatment of late Lyme disease: A challenge to accept. J Clin Microbiol. 1994;32(5):1415-1416.

Lubke LL, Garon CF. The antimicrobial agent melittin exhibits powerful in vitro inhibitory effects on the Lyme disease spirochete. Clin Infect Dis. 1997;25(Suppl. 1):S48-51.

Luft BJ, Volkman DJ, Halperin JJ, et al. New chemotherapeutic approaches in the treatment of Lyme borreliosis. Ann NY Acad Sci. 1988;539:352-361.

Luger S. Lyme disease transmitted by a biting fly. N Engl J Med. 1990;322(24):1752.

Ma Y, Sturrock A, Weis JJ. Intracellular localization of Borrelia burgdorferi within human endothelial cells. Infect Immun. 1991;59:671-678.

MacDonald A. Borrelia in the brains of patients dying with dementia. JAMA. 1986;256(16): 2195-2196.

MacDonald AB. Gestational Lyme borreliosis. Implications for the fetus. Rheum Dis Clin North Am. 1989;15(4):657-677.

Mackowiak PA, Lagace-Wiens P. Neutrophilic inclusions in a hunter. Fig. 1. Clin Infect Dis. 2012;51(9):1102-1103. http://cid.oxfordjpournals.org./content/51/9/1102.full. Accessed May 9, 2012.

Magnarelli L, Anderson J. Ticks and biting insects infected with the etiologic agent of Lyme disease, Borrelia burgdorferi. J Clin Microbiol. 1988;26(8):1482-1486.

Mahmoud AA. The challenge of intracellular pathogens. N Engl J Med. 1992;326(11):761-762.

Majláthová V, Majláth I, Derdáková M, et al. Borrelia lusitaniae and green lizards (Lacerta viridis), Karst Region, Slovakia. Emerging Infect Dis. 2006;12(12):1895-1901.

Maloney EL. The need for clinical judgment in the diagnosis and treatment of Lyme disease. J Am Phys Surg. 2009;14(3): 82-89.

Mantovani E, Costa IP, Gauditano G, et al. Description of Lyme disease-like syndrome in Brazil. Is it a new tick borne disease or Lyme disease variation? Braz J Med Biol Res. 2007;40(4): 443-456.

Marcus LC, Steere AC, Duray PH, et al. Fatal pancarditis in a patient with coexistent Lyme disease and babesiosis. Demonstration of spirochetes in the myocardium. Ann Intern Med. 1985;103(3):374-376.

Marshall GS, Jacobs RF, Schutze GE, et al. Ehrlichia chaffeensis seroprevalence among children in the southeast and south-central regions of the United States. Arch Pediatr Adolesc Med. 2002;156:166-170.

Massarotti EM. Lyme arthritis. Med Clin North Am. 2002;86(2):297-309.

Mast WE, Burrows WM. Erythema chronicum migrans and Lyme arthritis. JAMA. 1976;236 (21):2392.

Masters E. Spirochetemia after continuous high-dose oral amoxicillin therapy. Infect Dis Clin Prac. 1994;3(3):207-208.

Masters EJ, Grigery CN, Masters RW. STARI, or Masters disease: Lone Star tick-vectored Lyme-like illness. Infect Dis Clin North Am. 2008;22(2):361-376.

Masuzawa T. Terrestrial distribution of the Lyme borreliosis agent Borrelia burgdorferi sensu lato in East Asia. Jpn J Infect Dis. 2004;57(6):229-235.

Mathis A, Hilpertshauser H, Deplazes P, et al. Piroplasms of ruminants in Switzerland and zoonotic significance of Babesia. Schweiz Arch Tierheilkd. 2006;148(3):151-159.

McAuliffe P, Brassard MR. Memory and executive functions in adolescents with posttreatment Lyme disease. Appl Neuropsychol. 2008;1:208-219.

Mello M. Of swords and shields: The use of clinical practice guidelines in medical malpractice litigation. Univ Penn Law Rev. 2000;149(3):645-710.

Mencke N. Acaricidal and repellent properties of permethrin, its role in reducing transmission of vector-borne pathogens. Parassitologia. 2006;48(1-2):139-140.

Meyer U, Yee BK, Feldon J. The neurodevelopmental impact of prenatal infections at different times of pregnancy: The earlier the worse? Neuroscientist. 2007;13(3):241-256.

Miller NJ, Rainone EE, Dyer MC, et al. Tick bite protection with permethrin-treated summer-weight clothing. J Med Entomol. 2011;48(2):327-333.

Molloy PJ, Persing DH, Berardi VP. False-positive results of PCR testing for Lyme disease. Clin Infect Dis. 2001;33(3):412-413.

Moninger J. Cutting: Why teens hurt themselves. On the Edge. Family Circle. July 2011.

Moro MH, Zegarra-Moro OL, Bjornsson J, et al. Increased arthritis severity in mice coinfected with Borrelia burgdorferi and Babesia microti. J Infec Dis. 2002;186(3):428-431. Epub 2002 Jul 5.

Morriem E. From the clinics to the courts: The role evidence should play in litigating medical care. J Health Polit Policy Law. 2001;26(2):409.

Morris GH. Dissing disclosure: Just what the doctor ordered. Ariz Law Rev. 2002;44:313.

Mullegger RR. Dermatological manifestations of Lyme borreliosis. Eur J Dermatol. 2004;14(5):296-309.

Mulrow C, Lohr K. Proof and policy from medical research evidence. J Health Polit Policy Law. 2001;26(2)249-266.

Mursic VP, Wanner G, Reinhardt S, et al. Formation and cultivation of Borrelia burgdorferi spheroplast-L-form variants. Infection. 1996;24(3):218-226.

Mygland A, Ljøstad U, Fingerle V, et al. and the European Federation of Neurological Societies. (2010) EFNS guidelines on the diagnosis and management of European Lyme neuroborreliosis. Eur J Neurol. 2010;17(1):8-16.

Nadelman RB, Nowakowski J, Fish D, et al. Prophylaxis with single-dose doxycycline for the prevention of Lyme disease after an *Ixodes scapularis* tick bite. N Engl J Med. 2001;345:79-84.

Nichol G, Dennis DT, Steere AC. Test-treatment strategies for patients suspected of having Lyme disease: A cost-effectiveness analysis. Ann Intern Med. 1998;128(1):37-48.

Nigrovic LE, Thompson KM. The Lyme vaccine: A cautionary tale. Epidemiol Infect. 2007;135(1):1-8.

Noah L. Informed consent and the elusive dichotomy between standard and experimental therapy. Am J Law Med. 2002;28(4);361-408.

Nocton JJ, Dressler F, Rutledge BJ, et al. Detection of Borrelia burgdorferi DNA by polymerase chain reaction in synovial fluid from patients with Lyme arthritis. N Engl J Med. 1994;330(4):229-234.

Norris SJ. Antigenic variation in Lyme disease. Cell. 1997;89:275-285.

Norris SJ. Antigenic variation with a twist – The Borrelia story. Mol Microbiol. 2006;60(6):1319-1322.

Noskoviak K, Broome E. Images in clinical medicine. Babesiosis. N Engl J Med. 2008;358:e19.

Ogden NH, Lindsay LR, Morshed M, et al. The emergence of Lyme disease in Canada. CMAJ. 2009;180(12):1221-1224.

Oksi J, Kalimo H, Marttila RJ, et al. Inflammatory brain changes in Lyme borreliosis. A report on three patients and review of literature. Brain. 1996;119(Pt 6):2143–2154.

Oksi J, Marjamaki M, Nikoskelainen J, et al. Borrelia burgdorferi detected by culture and PCR in clinical relapse of disseminated Lyme borreliosis. Ann Med. 1999;31(30):225-232.

Oksi J, Nikoskelainen J, Hiekkanen H, et al. Duration of antibiotic treatment in disseminated Lyme borreliosis: A double-blind, randomized, placebo-controlled, multicenter clinical study. Eur J Clin Microbiol Infect Dis. 2007;26(8):571–581.

Oksi J, Nikoskelainen J, Viljanen MK. Comparison of oral cefixime and intravenous ceftriaxone followed by oral amoxicillin in disseminated Lyme borreliosis. Eur J Clin Microbiol Infect Dis. 1998;17(10):715-719.

Oldstone MB. Molecular mimicry and immune-mediated diseases. FASEB J. 1998;21(13):1255-1265.

Osorno BM, Vega C, Ristic M, et al. Isolation of Babesia spp. from asymptomatic human beings. Vet Parasitol. 1976;2:111-120.

Owen DC. Is Lyme disease always poly microbial? – The jigsaw hypothesis. Med Hypotheses. 2006;67:860-864.

Pachner AR, Delany E, O'Neill T. Neuroborreliosis in the nonhuman primate: Borrelia burgdorferi persists in the central nervous system. Ann Neurol. 1995;38(4):667-669.

Pachner AR, Steiner I. Lyme neuroborreliosis: Infection, immunity, and inflammation. Lancet Neurol. 2007;6(6):544-552.

Pachner AR. Neurologic manifestations of Lyme disease, the new great imitator. Rev Infect Dis. 1989;11(Suppl. 6):S1482–1486.

Papanicolaou DA, Wilder RL, Manolagas SC, et al. The pathophysiologic roles of interleukin-6 in human disease. Ann Intern Med. 1998;128(2):127-137.

Parola P, Raoult D. Ticks and tickborne bacterial diseases in humans: An emerging infectious threat. Clin Infect Dis. 2001;32(6):897-928.

Paschoud JM. Lymphocytoma after tick bite (in German). Dermatologica. 1954;108(4-6):435-437.

Patel R, Grogg KL, Edwards WD, et al. Death from inappropriate therapy for Lyme disease. Clin Infect Dis. 2000;31(4):1107-1109.

Patz J, Daszak P, Tabor G, et al. Unhealthy landscapes: Policy recommendations on land use change and infectious disease emergence. Environ Health Perspect. 2004;112(10):1092-1098.

Pavia C. Current and novel therapies for Lyme disease. Expert Opin Investig Drugs. 2003;12(6):1003-1016.

Perkins SE, Cattadori IM, Tagliapietra V, et al. Localized deer absence leads to tick amplification. Ecology. 2006;87(8):1981-1986.

Persing DH, Herwaldt BL, Glaser C, et al. Infection with a Babesia-like organism in northern California. N Engl J Med. 1995;332:298-303.

Persing DH, Mathiesen D, Marshall WF, et al. Detection of Babesia microti by polymerase chain reaction. J Clin Microbiol. 1992;30(8):2097-2103.

Petrovic M, Vogelaers D, Van Renterghem L, et al. Lyme borreliosis – a review of the late stages and treatment of four cases Acta Clin Belg. 1998;53(3):178-183.

Pfister HW, Preac-Mursic V, Wilske B, et al. Randomized comparison of ceftriaxone and cefotaxime in Lyme neuroborreliosis. J Infect Dis. 1991;163(2):311-318.

Piesman J, Dolan MC. Protection against Lyme disease spirochete transmission provided by prompt removal of nymphal Ixodes scapularis (Acari: Ixodidae). J Med Entomol. 2002;39(3): 509-512.

Piesman J, Stone BF. Vector competence of the Australian paralysis tick, Ixodes holocyclus, for the Lyme disease spirochete Borrelia burgdorferi. Int J Parasitol. 1991;21(1):109-111.

Piesman, J, Schneider BS, Zeidner NS. Use of Quantitative PCR to Measure Density of Borrelia burgdorferi in the Midgut and Salivary Glands of Feeding Tick Vectors. Journal of Clinical Microbiology. 2001;39(11):4145-4148.

Poland GA, Jacobson RM. The prevention of Lyme disease with vaccine. Vaccine. 2001;19(17-19):2303-2308.

Porcella SF, Schwan TG. Borrelia burgdorferi and Treponema pallidum: A comparison of functional genomics, environmental adaptations, and pathogenic mechanisms. J Clin Invest. 2004;107(6):651-656.

Pound JM, Miller JA, George JE, et al. Area-wide tick control project: Summary and conclusions. Vector-Borne and Zoonotic Dis. 2009;9(4):439-448.

Pozsgay V, Kubler-Kielb J. Synthesis of an experimental glycolipoprotein vaccine against Lyme disease. Carbohydr Res. 2007;342(3-4):621-626.

Preac-Mursic V, Marget W, Busch U, et al. Kill kinetics of Borrelia burgdorferi and bacterial findings in relation to the treatment of Lyme borreliosis. Infection. 1996;24(1):9-16.

Preac-Mursic V, Pfister HW, Spiegel H, et al. First isolation of Borrelia burgdorferi from an iris biopsy. J Clin Neuroophthalmol. 1993;13(3):155-161.

Preac-Mursic V, Weber K, Pfister HW, et al. Survival of Borrelia burgdorferi in antibiotically treated patients with Lyme borreliosis. Infection. 1989;17(6):355-359.

Puius YA, Kalish RA. Lyme arthritis: pathogenesis, clinical presentation, and management. Infect Dis Clin North Am. 2008;22(2):289-300.

Quick RE, Herwaldt BL, Thomford JW, et al. Babesiosis in Washington State: A new species of Babesia? Ann Intern Med. 1993;119(4):284-290.

Quill TE, Brody H. Physician recommendations and patient autonomy: Finding a balance between physician power and patient choice. Ann Intern Med. 1996;125(9):763-769.

Ramesh G, Alvarez AL, Roberts ED, et al. Pathogenesis of Lyme neuroborreliosis: Borrelia burgdorferi lipoproteins induce both proliferation and apoptosis in rhesus monkey astrocytes. Eur J Immunol. 2003;33(9):2539-2550.

Rand PW, Lacombe EH, Dearborn R, et al. Passive surveillance in Maine, an area emergent for tick-borne diseases. J Med Entomol. 2007;44(6):1118-1129.

Rand PW, Lubelczyk C, Holman MS, et al. Abundance of Ixodes scapularis (Acari: Ixodidae) after the complete removal of deer from an isolated offshore island, endemic for Lyme disease. J Med Entomol. 2004;41(4):779-784.

Raoult D, Houpikian P, Tissot Dupont H, et al. Treatment of Q fever endocarditis: Comparison of two regimens containing doxycycline and ofloxacin or hydroxychloroquine. Arch Intern Med. 1999;159(2):167-173.

Rasley A, Anguita J, Marriott I. Borrelia burgdorferi induces inflammatory mediator production by murine microglia. J Neuroimmunol. 2002;130(1-2):22-31.

Ratliff A, Angell M, Dow RW, et al. What is a good decision? Effective Clin Prac. July/August (1999). http://www.acponline.org/clinical_information/journals_ publications/ecp/julaug99/ essays. htm. Accessed February 2011.

Raveche ES, Schutzer SE, Fernandes H, et al. Evidence of Borrelia autoimmunity-induced component of Lyme carditis and arthritis. J Clin Microbiol. 2005;43(2): 850-856.

Rawlings JA, Fournier PV, Teltow GJ. Isolation of Borrelia spirochetes from patients in Texas. J Clin Microbiol. 1987;25:1148-1150.

Rhen M, Erickson S, Clements M, et al. The basis of persistent bacterial infections. Trends Microbiol. 2003;11(2):80-86.

Ribeiro JM, Mather TN, Piesman J, et al. Dissemination and salivary delivery of Lyme disease spirochetes in vector ticks (Acari: Ixodidae). J Med Entomol. 1987;24(2):201-205.

Richter D, Matuschka FR. Perpetuation of the Lyme disease spirochete Borrelia lusitaniae by lizards. Appl Environ Microbiol. 2006;72(7):4627-4632.

Rizzoli A, Hauffe HC, Carpi G, et al. Lyme borreliosis in Europe. Eurosurveillance. 2011;16(27):pii=19906. http://www.eurosurveillance.org/ViewArticle.aspx?ArticleId=19906. Accessed February 2012.

Ronn S. Rethinking Lyme guidelines within the spirit of the law. South Med J. 2009;102:1090-1091.

Rosenbaum S, Kamoie B. Managed care and public health: Conflict and collaboration. J Law Med Ethics. 2002;30(2):191-200.

Rothman DJ, McDonald WJ, Berkowitz CD, et al. Professional medical associations and their relationships with industry: A proposal for controlling conflict of interest. JAMA. 2009;301:1367-1372.

Rudenko N, Golovchenko M, Mokrácek A, et al. Detection of Borrelia bissettii in cardiac valve tissue of a patient with endocarditis and aortic valve stenosis in the Czech Republic. J Clin Microbiol. 2008;46(10):3540-3543.

Rupprecht TA, Koedel U, Fingerle V, et al. The pathogenesis of Lyme neuroborreliosis: From infection to inflammation. Mol Med. 2008;14(3-4):205-212.

Sabnis S, Zupan J, Gliddon M. Topical formulations of metaflumizone plus amitraz to treat flea and tick infestations on dogs. Vet Parasitol. 2007;150(3):196-202.

Sapi E, Kaur N, Anyanwu S, et al. Evaluation of in-vitro antibiotic susceptibility of different morphological forms of Borrelia burgdorferi. Infect Drug Resist. 2011;4:97-113.

Schabereiter-Gurtner C, Lubitz W, Rolleke S. Application of broad-range 16S rRNA PCR amplification and DGGE fingerprinting for detection of tick-infecting bacteria. J Microbiol Methods. 2003;52(2):251-260.

Schardt FW. Clinical effects of fluconazole in patients with neuroborreliosis. Eur J Med Res. 2004;9(7):334-336.

Schmid GP. Epidemiology and clinical similarities of human spirochetal diseases. Rev Infect Dis. 1989;11(Suppl. 6):S1460-S1469.

Schmidt B, Aberer E, Stockenhuber C, et al. Detection of Borrelia burgdorferi DNA by polymerase chain reaction in the urine and breast milk of patients with Lyme borreliosis. Diagn Microbiol Infect Dis. 1995;21(3):121–128.

Schneider BS, Schriefer ME, Dietrich G, et al. Borrelia bissettii isolates induce pathology in a murine model of disease. Vector Borne Zoonotic Dis. 2008;8(5):623-633.

Schoeler GB, Wikel SK, Modulation of host immunity by hematophagous arthropods. Ann Trop Med Parasitol. 2001;95(8):755-771.

Schofield S, Tepper M, Gadawski R. Field evaluation against mosquitoes of regular and polymer-based deet formulations in Manitoba, Canada, with comment on methodological issues. J Med Entomol. 2007;44(3):457-462.

Schutze GE, Buckingham SC, Marshall GS, et al. Human monocytic ehrlichiosis in children. Pediatr Infect Dis J. 2007;26(6):475-479.

Schutzer SE, Coyle PK, Belman AL, et al. Sequestration of antibody to Borrelia burgdorferi in immune complexes in seronegative Lyme disease. Lancet. 1990;335(8685):312-315.

Schutzer SE, Coyle PK, Reid P, et al. Borrelia burgdorferi-specific immune complexes in acute Lyme disease. JAMA. 1999; 282(20):1942-1946.

Scrimenti RJ. Erythema chronicum migrans. Arch Dermatol. 1970;102(1):104-105.

Seiler KP, Weis JJ. Immunity to Lyme disease: Protection, pathology and persistence. Curr Opin Immunol. 1996;8(4):503-509.

Seltzer EG, Gerber MA, Cartter ML, et al. Long-term outcomes of persons with Lyme disease. JAMA. 2000;283(5):609-616.

Setty S, Kahlil Z, Schori P, et al. Babesiosis. Two atypical cases from Minnesota and a review. Am J Clin Pathol. 2003;120(4):554-559.

Shadick GP. Epidemiology and clinical similarities of human spirochetal disease. Rev Infect Dis. 1989;11(Suppl. 6):S1460-S1469.

Shadick NA, Phillips CB, Logigian EL, et al. The long-term clinical outcomes of Lyme disease. A population-based retrospective cohort study. Ann Intern Med. 1994;121(8):560-567.

Shadick NA, Phillips CB, Sangha O, et al. Musculoskeletal and neurologic outcomes in patients with previously treated Lyme disease. Ann Intern Med. 1999;131(12):919-926.

Shaneyfelt TM, Centor RM. Reassessment of clinical practice guidelines: Go gently into that good night. JAMA. 2009;301:868-869.

Sherr VT. Human babesiosis - an unrecorded reality: Absence of formal registry undermines its detection, diagnosis and treatment, suggesting need for immediate mandatory reporting. Medical Hypotheses. 2004;63:609-615.

Silver W. The inadequacy of state legislative responses to ERISA preemption of managed care liability. NY Univ Law Rev. 2003;78(2):845-873.

Simecka JW, Ross SE, Cassell GH, et al. Interactions of mycoplasmas with B cells: Antibody production and nonspecific effects. Clin Infect Dis. 1993;**17**(Suppl 1):S176–S182.

Singh SK, Girschick HJ. Lyme borreliosis: From infection to autoimmunity. Clin Microbiol Infect. 2004;10(7):598-614.

Singh SK, Girschick HJ. Molecular survival strategies of the Lyme disease spirochete Borrelia burgdorferi. Lancet Infect Dis. 2004;4(9):575-583.

Sivak SL, Aguero-Rosenfeld ME, Nowakowski J, et al. Accuracy of IgM immunoblotting to confirm the clinical diagnosis of early Lyme disease. Arch Intern Med. 1996;156(18):2105-2109.

Skrabalo z Deanovic Z. Piroplasmosis in man; report of a case. Doc Med Geogr Trop. 1957;9(1):11-16.

Small PM, Fujiwari PI. Management of tuberculosis in the USA. N Engl J Med. 2001;345(3):189-200.

Smith RP, Schoen RT, Rahn DW, et al. Clinical characteristics and treatment outcome of early Lyme disease in patients with microbiologically confirmed erythema migrans. Ann Intern Med. 2002;136(6):421-428.

Smith SE, Li J, Garbett K, et al. Maternal immune activation alters fetal brain development through interleukin-6. J Neurosci. 2007;27(40):10695-10702.

Sniderman AD, Furgberg CD. Why guideline-making requires reform. JAMA. 2009;301:429-431.

Stanek G, Strle F. Lyme disease: European perspective. Infect Dis Clin North Am. 2008;22(2):327-339.

Steere AC, Angelis SM (October 2006). Therapy for Lyme arthritis: Strategies for the treatment of antibiotic-refractory arthritis. Arthritis Rheum. 2006;54(10):3079-3086.

Steere AC, Coburn J, Glickstein L. The emergence of Lyme disease. J Clin Invest. 2004;113(8):1093-1101.

Steere AC, Dhar A, Hernandez J, et al. Systemic symptoms without erythema migrans as the presenting picture of early Lyme disease. Am J Med. 2003;114(1):58-62.

Steere AC, Dwyer E, Winchester R. Association of chronic Lyme arthritis with HLA-DR4 and HLA-DR2 alleles. N Engl J Med. 1990;323(4):219-223.

Steere AC, Hutchinson GJ, Rahn DW, et al. Treatment of the early manifestations of Lyme disease. Ann Intern Med. 1983;99(1):22-26.

Steere AC, Malawista SE, Snydman DR, et al. Lyme arthritis: An epidemic of oligoarticular arthritis in children and adults in three Connecticut communities. Arthritis Rheum. 1977;20(1):7-17.

Steere AC, McHugh G, Damle N, et al. Prospective study of serologic tests for lyme disease. Clin Infect Dis. 2008;47(2):188-195.

Steere AC, Sikand VK, Schoen RT, et al. Asymptomatic infection with Borrelia burgdorferi. Clin Infect Dis. 2003;37(4):528-532.

Steere AC. Lyme borreliosis in 2005, 30 years after initial observations in Lyme, Connecticut. Wien Klin Wochenschr. 2006;118(21-22):625–633.

Steere AC. Lyme disease. N Engl J Med. 2001;345(2):115-125.

Steinbrook R. Conflicts of interest at the NIH – resolving the problem. N Engl J Med. 2004;351:955-957.

Steinbrook R. Guidance for guidelines. N Engl J Med. 2007;356:331-333.

Steiner FE, Ringer RP, Vann CN, et al. Detection of Anaplasma phagocytophilum and Babesia odocoilei DNA in Ixodes scapularis (Acari: Ixodidae) collected in Indiana. J Med Entomol. 2006;43:437-442.

Steiner I. Treating post Lyme disease: Trying to solve one equation with too many unknowns. Neurology. 2003;60(12):1888-1889.

Sternbach G, Dibble C. Willy Burgdorfer: Lyme disease. J Emerg Med. 1996;14(5):631-634.

Stone TW, Mackay GM, Forrest CM. Tryptophan metabolites and brain disorders. Clin Chem Lab Med. 2003;41(7):852-859.

Strasfeld L, Romanzi L, Seder RH, et al. False-positive serological test results for Lyme disease in a patient with acute herpes simplex virus type 2 infection. Clin Infect Dis. 2005;41 (12):1826-1827.

Straubinger RK, PCR-based quantification of Borrelia burgdorferi organism in canine tissues over 500-day post-infection period. J Clin Microbiol. 2000;38(6):2191-2199.

Straubinger RK, Straubinger AF, Summers BA, et al. Status of Borrelia burgdorferi infection after antibiotic treatment and the effects of corticosteroids: An experimental study. J Infect Dis. 2000;181(3):1069-1081.

Straubinger RK. Summers BA, Chang YF, et al. Persistence of Borrelia burgdorferi in experimentally infected dogs after antibiotic treatment. J Clin Microbiol. 1997;35(1):111-116.

Stricker R, Moore D, Winger E. Clinical and immunologic evidence for the transmission of Lyme disease through intimate human contact. J Invest Med. 2004;52(1):S151.

Stricker RB, Burrascano J, Winger E. Long term decrease in the CD57 lymphocyte subset in a patient with chronic Lyme disease. Ann Agric Environ Med. 2002;9(1):111-113.

Stricker RB, Johnson L. IDSA Lyme Guidelines: Response to Dr. Gershon's letter. South Med J. 2009;102:1089-1090.

Stricker RB, Johnson L. The American Academy of Neurology Lyme Guidelines: Through the looking glass. South Med J. 2008;101:672.

Stricker RB, Johnson L. The Infectious Diseases Society of America Lyme Guidelines: Poster child for guidelines reform. South Med J. 2009;102:565-566.

Stricker RB, Lautin A, Burrascano JJ. Lyme disease: Point/counterpoint. Expert Rev Anti-infect Ther. 2005;3:155-165.

Stricker RB, Lautin A. The Lyme wars: Time to listen. Expert Opin Invest Drugs. 2003;12(10):1609-1614.

Stricker RB. Counterpoint: long-term antibiotic therapy improves persistent symptoms associated with Lyme disease. Clin Infect Dis. 2007;45(2):149-157.

Summerton N. Lyme disease in the eighteenth century. BMJ. 1995;311:1478.

Sun Y, Xu R. Ability of Ixodes persulcatus, Haemaphysalis concinna and Dermacentor silvarum ticks to acquire and transstadially transmit Borrelia garinii. Exp Appl Acarol. 2003;31(1-2):151-60.

Swanson KI, Norris DE. Detection of Borrelia burgdorferi DNA in lizards from Southern Maryland. Vector Borne Zoonotic Dis. 2007;7(1):42-49.

Swanson SJ, Neitzel D, Reed KD, et al. Coinfections acquired from Ixodes ticks. Clin Microbiol Rev. 2006;19:708-727.

Sykes JE, Lindsay LL, Maggi RG, et al. Human coinfection with Bartonella henselae and two hemotropic Mycoplasma variants resembling Mycoplasma ovis. J Clin Microbiol. 2010;48(10):3782–3785.

Tager FA, Fallon BA, Keilp J, et al. A controlled study of cognitive deficits in children with chronic Lyme disease. J Neuropsychiatry Clin Neurosci. 2001;13:500–507.

Taylor R, Simpson I. Review of treatment options for Lyme borreliosis. J Chemother. 2005;17 (Suppl. 2):3-16.

The International Lyme and Associated Diseases Society (ILADS). Evidence-based guidelines for the management of Lyme disease. Expert Rev Anti-infect Ther. 2004;2(Suppl.):S1-S13.

Thomford JW, Conrad PA, Telford SR 3rd, et al. Cultivation and phylogenetic characterization of a newly recognized human pathogenic protozoan. J Infect Dis. 1994;169:1050-1056.

Thyresson N. The penicillin treatment of acrodermatitis atrophicans chronica (Herxheimer). Acta Dermatol Venereol. 1949;29(6):572-621.

Tilly K, Rosa PA, Stewart PE. Biology of infection with Borrelia burgdorferi. Infect Dis Clin North Am. 2008;22(2):217-234.

Tonks A: Lyme wars. BMJ. 2007;335:910-912.

Valentine-Thon E, Ilsemann K, Sandkamp M. A novel lymphocyte transformation test (LTT-MELISA) for Lyme borreliosis. Diagn Microbiol Infect Dis. 2007;57(1):27-34.

Van de Weyden M. Clinical practice guidelines: Time to move the debate from the how to the who. Med J Aust. 2002;176(7):304-305.

Varde S, Beckley J, Schwartz I. Prevalence of tick-borne pathogens in Ixodes scapularis in a rural New Jersey County. Emerging Infect Dis. 1998;4(1):97-99.

Vaughn MF, Meshnick SR. Pilot study assessing the effectiveness of long-lasting permethrin-impregnated clothing for the prevention of tick bites. Vector-borne and Zoonotic Dis. 2011;11(7):869-875.

Wahlberg P, Granlund H, Nyman D, et al. Treatment of late Lyme borreliosis. J Infect. 1994;29(30):255-261.

Walder G, Lkhamsuren E, Shagdar A, et al. Serological evidence for tick-borne encephalitis, borreliosis, and human granulocytic anaplasmosis in Mongolia. Int J Med Microbiol. 2006;296(Suppl. 40):69-75.

Walsh CA, Mayer EW, Baxi LV. Lyme disease in pregnancy: Case report and review of the literature. Obstet Gynecol Surv. 2007;62(1):41-50.

Wang G, van Dam AP, Schwartz I, et al. Molecular typing of Borrelia burgdorferi sensu lato: Taxonomic, epidemiological, and clinical implications. Clin Microbiol Rev. 1999;12(4):633-653.

Wang M. Resurgent paternalism. Virtual Mentor-Ethics. JAMA. 1994;6(2).

Waniek C, Prohovnik I, Kaufman MA, et al. Rapidly progressive frontal-type dementia associated with Lyme disease. J Neuropsychiatry Clin Neurosci. 1995;7(3):345-347.

Webster G, Del Rosso JQ. Anti-inflammatory activity of tetracyclines. Dermatol Clin. 2007;25(2):133-135.

Weinstein A, Britchkov M. Lyme arthritis and post-Lyme disease syndrome. Curr Opin Rheumatol 2002;14(4):383-387.

Weiss LM. Babesiosis in humans: A treatment review. Expert Opin Pharmacother. 2002;3:1109-1115.

Weissenbacher S, Ring J, Hofmann H. Gabapentin for the symptomatic treatment of chronic neuropathic pain in patients with late-stage lyme borreliosis: A pilot study. Dermatology. (Basel). 2005;211(2):123-127.

Wennburg JE, Fisher EF, Skinner JS. Geography and the debate over Medicare reform. Health Affairs (Millwood) (Suppl. Web Exclusives). 2002;21(2):W96-W114. http://www.dartmouth.edu/~jskinner/documents/WennbergGeographyandtheDebate.pdf. Accessed March 2010.

Wennburg JE, Peters GP. Unwarranted variations in the quality of healthcare: Can the law help medicine provide a remedy/remedies? Wake Forest Law Rev. 2002;37(3):925-941.

When a vaccine is safe. Nature. 2006;439(7076):509.

Wilske B. Epidemiology and diagnosis of Lyme borreliosis. Ann Med. 2005;37(8):568-579.

Wolfe F. Fibromyalgia wars. J Rheumatol. 2009;36(4):679-683.

Wolfram R. Connecticut Attorney General Investigation and Settlement Highlights Possible Applicability if Antitrust Standard Setting Law to the Development of Clinical Practice Guidelines. Antitrust Health Care Chronicle. May 2008:8-17. http://lyme.kaiserpapers.org/ pdfs/lymeantitrust.pdf.

Woolf SH, Grol R, Hutchinson A, et al. Clinical guidelines: Potential benefits, limitations, and harms of clinical guidelines BMJ. 1999;318(7182):527-530.

Wormser G, Masters E, Nowakowski J, et al. Prospective clinical evaluation of patients from Missouri and New York with erythema migrans-like skin lesions. Clin Infect Dis. 2005;41 (7):958-965.

Wormser GP, Dattwyler RJ, Shapiro ED, et al. The clinical assessment, treatment, and prevention of Lyme disease, human granulocytic anaplasmosis, and babesiosis: Clinical practice guidelines by the Infectious Diseases Society of America. Clin Infect Dis. 43(9):2006;1089-1134.

Wormser GP, Liveris D, Hanincová K, et al. Effect of Borrelia burgdorferi genotype on the sensitivity of C6 and 2-tier testing in North American patients with culture-confirmed Lyme disease. Clin Infect Dis. 2008;47(7):910-914.

Wormser GP, Nadelman RB, Dattwyler RJ, et al. Practice guidelines for the treatment of Lyme disease. The Infectious Diseases Society of America. Clin Infect Dis. 2000;31(Suppl.1):1-14.

Wormser GP. Clinical practice. Early Lyme disease. N Engl J Med. 2006;354(26):2794-2801.

Wright CB, Sacco RL, Rundek TR, et al. Interleukin-6 is associated with cognitive function: The Northern Manhattan Study. J Stroke Cerebrovasc Dis. 2006;15(1):34-38.

Xu Q, Seemanapalli SV, Reif KE, et al. Increasing the recruitment of neutrophils to the site of infection dramatically attenuates Borrelia burgdorferi infectivity. J Immunol. 2007;178(8):5109-5115.

Yoshinari NH, Oyafuso LK, Monteiro FG, et al. Lyme disease. Report of a case observed in Brazil (in Portuguese). Rev Hosp Clín. 1993;48(4):170-174.

Young D, Hussell T, Dougan G. Chronic bacterial infections: Living with unwanted guests. Nature Immunol. 2002;3(11):1026-1032.

Young JD. Underreporting of Lyme disease. N Engl J Med. 1998;338:1629.

Zajkowska J, Grygorczuk S, Kondrusik M, et al. (2006). New aspects of pathogenesis of Lyme borreliosis (in Polish). Przegląd epidemiologiczny. 2006;60(Suppl 1):167–170.

Zeller JL, Burke AE, Glass RM. JAMA patient page. Lyme disease. JAMA. 2007;297(23):2664.

Ziska MH, Donta ST, Demerest FC. Physician preferences in the diagnosis and treatment of Lyme disease in the USA. Infection. 1996;24(2):182-186.

Websites

Amber. http://www.ambericawest.com/tick. Accessed February 2010.

American Lyme Disease Foundation (ALDF). Southern Tick-Associated Rash Illness (STARI). http://www.aldf.com/stari.shtml. Accessed June 2009.

American Medical Association. Code of Medical Ethics. Current Opinions with Annotations 2002-2003. http://www.ama-assn.org. Accessed February 2010.

American National Standards Institute: ANSI Essential Requirements: Due Process Requirements for American National Standards. New York: American National Standards Institute; January 2008. http://www.asse.org/publications/standards/docs/2008%20 ANSI%20Essential%20 Requirements%20031108.pdf. Accessed February 2010.

Arthritis and Joint Conditions. http://www.arthritis.about.com/od/ lyme/. Accessed April 27, 2012.

Babesia life cycle. http://commons.wikimedia.org/wiki/ File:Babesia_life_cycle_human_en.svg

Babesiosis. http://familydoctor.org. Accessed January 2011.

Bach G. Recovery of Lyme spirochetes by PCR in semen samples of previously diagnosed Lyme disease patients. 14th International Scientific Conference on Lyme Disease. 2001. http://www.anapsid. org/lyme/bach.html. Accessed February 2010.

Baldauf S. South Africa's wine country fights alcoholism scourge. The Christian Science Monitor. April 12, 2007. http://www.csmonitor.com. Accessed February 2009.

Barnes L. Bartonella Alert. http://www.lymeinfo.net/bartonella. html. Accessed February 2010.

Barthold S, Hodzic E, Tunev S, et al. Antibody-Mediated Disease Remission in the Mouse Model of Lyme Borreliosis. http://iai.aom. org. Accessed May 9, 2012.

BBC News. Tick disease plea to moor users. May 27, 2009. http:// news.bbc.co.uk/1/hi/england/ south_yorkshire/8070935.stm. Accessed July 2009.

Booth A. What proportion of healthcare is evidence based? Resource Guide. University of Sheffield, School of Health and Related Research. http://www.shef.ac.uk~scharr/ir/percent.html. Accessed February 2010.

Borrelia burgdorferi.http://upload.wikimedia.org/wikipedia/ commons/f/f3/Borrelia_burgdorferi_%28CDC-PHIL_-6631%29_ lores.jpg

Bransfield R. Lyme Disease and Cognitive Impairments. http:// www.canlyme.com/cog.html. Accessed July 26, 2011.

Bransfield R. The Neuropsychiatric Assessment of Lyme Disease. http://www.mentalhealthandillness. com/tnaold.html. Accessed March 2012.

Brown SL, Hansen SL, Burrascano JJ. Diagnostic hints and treatment guidelines for Lyme and other tick borne illnesses. 14th ed. 2002. http://www.ilads.org/burrascano_1102.htm. Accessed February 2010.

Brown SL, Langone JJ, et al. Lyme disease test kits: Potential for misdiagnosis. FDA Med Bull. Summer 1999. http://www.mnlyme. com/files/ Lyme_Disease_ Test_Kits_ Potential_For_ Misdiagnosis. pdf.

California Lyme Disease Association (CALDA). http://www.lyme-disease.org. Accessed February 2010.

California Lyme Disease Association (CALDA). Notification of Field Trip, TICK ALERT: Please dress your child appropriately! 2001. http://www.lymedisease.org/resources/ pdf/tick_removal.pdf. Accessed August 2011.

Canadian Lyme Disease Foundation. http://www.canlyme.org. Accessed February 2010.

Centers for Disease Control and Prevention (CDC). Average Annual Incidence of Reported Cases of Lyme Disease by Age Group and Sex, United States, 1992-2004. http://www.cdc.gov/lyme/stats/ chartstables/incidencebyagesex.html. Accessed August 2011.

Centers for Disease Control and Prevention (CDC). National Center for Health Statistics. http://www.cdc.gov/nchs. Accessed February 2010.

Centers for Disease Control and Prevention (CDC). Preventing tick bites. http://www.cdc.gov/lyme/prev/ index.html. Accessed August 2011.

Centers for Disease Control and Prevention (CDC). Reported Cases of Lyme Disease by Year, United States, 1991–2005. October 2, 2006. http://www.cdc.gov/ncidod/dvbid/ lyme/ld_ UpClimbLyme-Dis.htm. Accessed August 2007.

Centers for Disease Control and Prevention (CDC). Southern Tick-Associated Rash Illness (STARI). http://www.cdc.gov/ncidod/ dvbid/stari. Accessed June 2009.

Centre for Evidence-Based Medicine Toronto. What are the limitations of EBM? http://www.cebm.utoronto.ca/intro/limit.htm. Accessed February 2010.

Children's Treatment Issue. Lyme Times. No. 42. Summer 2005. http://www.lymedisease.org. Accessed March 2012.

Cirillo F. The Pomodoro Technique. http://www.pomodorotechnique.com. Accessed June 20. 2011.

Columbia University Medical Center. Why is Chronic Lyme Disease Chronic? http://columbia-lyme.org/patients/ld_chronic.html. Accessed February 2011.

Connecticut Department of Environmental Protection - Wildlife Division. June 2007, 2nd ed. Managing Urban Deer in Connecticut, Figure 2, p.4. http://www.ct.gov/dep/lib/dep/ wildlife/pdf_files/ game/urbandeer07.pdf. Accessed May 2008.

Connor S. Glaxo chief: Our drugs do not work on most patients. The Independent. December 8, 2003. http://www.independent. co.uk/news/science/glaxo-chief-our-drugs-do-not-work-on-most-patients-575942.html. Accessed August 2012.

Cooper C. Safety of long-term therapy with penicillin and penicillin derivatives. Center for Drug Evaluation and Research. http://www. fda.gv/cder/drugprepare/pelongsafet.htm. Accessed June 2009.

Coyle M. Antitrust scrutiny of Lyme guidelines. Disease treatment probe by state AG. Nat Law J. 2007. http://lymeblog.com/modules. php?name=News&file=print&sid=828. Accessed February 2012.

Cunha BA, et al. Babesiosis. http://www.emedicine.medscape.com. Accessed June 2009.

Disease. http://www.disease.com. Accessed January 2012.

Edlow J. Tick Borne Diseases:Lyme. eMedicine. http://www.emedicine.com/emerg/ topic588.htm. Accessed June 2009.

Edlow JA. Lyme Disease. eMedicine. http://www.emedicine.com/ derm/ topic536.htm. Accessed August 2009.

EM rash. http://en.wikipedia.org/wiki/File:Erythema_migrans_-_erythematous_rash_in_Lyme_disease_-_PHIL_9875.jpg.

EM rash, secondary. http://www.sciencedirect.com/science/article/ pii/S0891552007001298

Erlichiosis/Anaplasmosis. http://www.columbia-lyme.org. Accessed February 2010.

Erythema Migrans Rash. http://en.wikipedia.org/wiki/File:Erythema migrans erythematous rash in Lyme disease – PHIL 9875.jpg. Accessed Oct 2012.

Erythema Migrans Rash. http://www. erwinadr.blogspot. com/2011/08/lyme-disease.html. Accessed October 2012.

Erythema Migrans Rash. http://www.sciencedirect.com./science/ article/pii/S0891552007001298 Accessed October 2012.

Erythema Migrans Rash. http://www.webMD.com. Accessed April 27, 2012.

Food and Agriculture Organization of the United Nations. Epidemiology. http://www.fao.org. Accessed February 2010.

Fowler F. The role of patient preferences in medical care. http:// www.fimdm.org/downloads/ patient_ Preferences_Fowler.pdf. Accessed May 2010.

Georgia Lyme Disease Association (GALDA). Lyme disease. http:// www.georgialymedisease. org. Accessed February 2010.

Greenberg D: Conflict of Interest at the NIH: NIH Looks the Other Way. The Chronicle Review. 2008. http://chronicle.com/blogPost/ cconflict-of-Interest-NIH/5647/. Accessed March 2010.

Grier T. ELISA and western blot: Lies that can kill you? http:// www.centurytel.net/tjs11/ bug/blot1.htm. Accessed March 2010.

Hamlen RA. Lyme disease prevention tips. 2011. http://www. lymepa.org/2011-0315_Lyme_ Disease_Prevention_Tips.pdf. Accessed August 2011.

Health Protection and Readiness. 2010. Permethrin-impregnated clothing. http://www.fhpr.osd.mil/factsheetDetail.jsp?fact=27. Accessed September 2011.

Hu L. Clinical Manifestations of Lyme Disease in Adults. http:// www.uptodate.com. Accessed May 2012.

Hypostome. http://www. Remove-ticks.com/tickhead.htm. Accessed October 2012.

Hypostome. http://www.tescan-usa.com. Accessed October 2012.

ICD-10-CM Diagnosis Code B60.0: Babesiosis. http://www.icd-10data.com. Accessed May 2010.

ICD-9-CM Diagnosis Code 088.82: Babesiosis. http://www.icd-9data.com. Accessed May 2010.

Infectious Diseases Society of America. Frequently Asked Questions about Lyme Disease. October 2006. http://www.idsociety.org/ lymediseasefacts.htm. Accessed June 2008.

Infectious Diseases Society of America: Final Report of the Lyme Disease Review Panel of the Infectious Diseases Society of America. http://www.idsociety.org/uploadedFiles/IDSA/ Resources/ Lyme Disease/Final Report/IDSA-Lyme-Disease-Final-Report.pdf. Accessed May 2010.

International Lyme and Associated Diseases Society (ILADS). Evaluation of antibiotic treatment in patients with persistent symptoms of Lyme disease. http://www.ilads.org/position2.htm. Accessed May 2010.

International Lyme and Associated Diseases Society (ILADS). What You Should Know About Lyme Disease. http://www.ilads.org/ lyme_research/lyme_articles6.html. Accessed October 2010.

Introduction to Ehrlichia spp: New Taxonomy of the Family Anaplasmataceae. http://riki-1bl. vet.ohio-state.edu/background.php. Accessed February 2010.

Jemsek JG. Lyme Disease in the Carolinas (1998). http://www. jemsekclinic/lymedisease.php. Accessed February 2010.

John.Carroll@ars.usda.gov. Lone Star tick. Accessed June 30, 2012 and August 2012.

Johnson RC. Leptospira. In: Baron S, ed. Medical Microbiology. 4th ed. Galveston, TX: University of Texas Medical Branch at Galveston; 1996. http://www.ncbi.nlm.nih.gov/books/ bv.fcgi?&rid=mmed.section.1965. Accessed June 2012.

Josselyn J. Account of Two Voyages to New-England Made during the Years 1638, 1663. Boston: William Veazie; 1865. Online facsimile edition at www.americanjourneys.org/aj-107/. Accessed February 2010.

Keller D. Infectious Disease Treatment Guidelines Weakened by Paucity of Scientific Evidence. Medscape Medical News 2009. http://www.medscape.com/viewarticle/712341. Accessed January 2010.

Leamy E, Gaynor J, Ferran L. Lyme Rage: Can Lyme Disease Affect Your Personality? ABC News, July 30, 2009. http://abcnews. go.com. Accessed January 2012.

Lewis D. National Guideline Clearinghouse: Extensive Resource Underused in Managed Care. www.managedcaremag.com/archives/0106/0106.guidelines.htm. Accessed February 2010.

Lukewarm Response To New Lyme Vaccine. New York Times. June 13, 1999. http://query.nytimes.com/gst/fullpage.html?res=9C05E4D 71238F930A25755C0A96F958260. Accessed July 2008.

Lyme and Tick-Borne Diseases Research Center. Columbia University Research Center. http://www.columbia-lyme.org. Accessed February 2010.

Lyme case map. http://commons.wikimedia.org/wiki/File:Reported_Cases_of_Lyme_Disease_2010.png

Lyme Disease Association of Southeastern Pennsylvania (LDASP). http://www.lymepa.org. Accessed 2010-2011.

Lyme Disease Association, Inc. (LDA). http://www.lymediseasesociation.org. Accessed 2009-2011.

Lyme Disease Association, Inc. (LDA). Lyme Disease and Children: Critical Issues. 2010. http://www.lymediseaseassociation.org/index.php?option=com_content&view=article&id=525:lyme-disease-and-children-critical-issues&catid=12:lyme-in-the-schools-&Itemid=147. Accessed August 2011.

Lyme Disease Diagnosis. U.S. Centers for Disease Control. October 7, 2008. http://www.cdc.gov/ncidod/dvbid/lyme/ld_humandisease_diagnosis.htm. Accessed July 2009.

Lyme Disease Gallery. http://www.rash-pictures.com. Accessed January 2012.

Lyme Disease. http://en.wikipedia.org/wiki/Lyme_disease - cite_ref-108. Accessed February 2012.

Lyme_Disease_Risk_Map.gif. Accessed July 2012.

LymeLight Newsletter. The Lyme Disease Foundation. http://www.lyme.org/trtcontrov.html. Accessed June 2010.

Maltese Cross. http://wwwnc.cdc.gov/eid/article/10/4/03-0377-f2.htm

Marasco AA: Standards Development: Are You at Risk? American National Standards Institute, 2000. http//www.astm.org/SNEWS/JUNE_2000/June_marasco.html. Accessed February 2010.

March of Dimes. http://www.marchofdimes.com. Accessed February 2010.

Marques A, et al. A randomized, placebo-controlled trial of repeated IV antibiotic therapy for Lyme encephalitis. http://www.neurology.org. Neurology, 2008. Accessed March 2012.

Mental Health and Illness. http://www.mentalhealthandillness.com. Accessed February 2010.

Mervine P, Keith RD. Review: Risk of Infection From Tick Bite vs. Duration of Attachment of Ixodes Nymphs. 2004. http://www.lymedisease.org/calda/articles_posters.html. Accessed March 2012.

Miklossy J. Alzheimer's Disease – Emerging Role of Infection. http://www.miklossy.ch. Accessed May 9, 2012.

Morgan M. Independent Review of Managed Care Decisions. California Society for Healthcare Attorneys. http://www.csha.calhealth.org. Accessed February 2010.

Morulae. http://www.cdc.gov/ehrlichiosis/symptoms/

Mothers of kids with autism earn less, study shows. Medline Plus. http://www.nlm.hih.gov/medlineplus/ news/fullstory_123086.html. Accessed March 2012.

MS Cure. http://www.abc.net.au/catalyst/stories/3572695.htm. Accessed September 2012.

National Guideline Clearinghouse: Summary of ILADS Guidelines for Lyme Disease. http://www.ilads.org/guidelines_ilads.html. Accessed February 2010.

National Institute of Allergy and Infectious Diseases. National Institutes of Health. Diagnosis of Lyme Disease. http://www.niaid.nih.gov/dmid/lyme/diagnosis.htm. Accessed February 2010.

National Institute of Allergy and Infectious Diseases. National Institutes of Health. Chronic Lyme Disease Fact Sheet. April 17, 2009. http://www.niaid.nih.gov/topics/lymedisease/understanding/ pages/chronic.aspx. Accessed February 2010.

New York State, Department of Health. Babesiosis. http://www.health.state.ny.us/ diseases/communicable/babesiosis/fact_sheet.htm. Accessed February 2010.

Nicolson G. (2007). Systemic Intracellular Bacterial Infections (Mycoplasma, Chlamydia, Borrelia species) in Neurodegenerative (MS, ALS) and Behavioral Disorders (ASD). Infect Dis Newsletter. http://www.immed.org/infectious%20disease%20reports/reports/SIBI. Accessed September 2011.

Nicolson G. Gulf War Illnesses Research. http://www.immed.org. Accessed May 9, 2012.

Nicolson G. Mycoplasma – Often Overlooked in Chronic Lyme Disease. http://www.betterhealthguy. com. Accessed May 9, 2012.

Oklahoma State University. Center for Health Sciences. Morgellons Disease. http://www.healthsciences.okstate.edu/morgellons/index.cfm. Accessed June 2011.

Parasites and Health. Babesiosis. http://www.dpd.cdc.gov/dpdx/HTML/Babesiosis.htm. Accessed May 2010.

Parry W. Iceman mummy may hold earliest evidence of Lyme disease. http://www.livescience.com. February 28, 2012. Accessed Feb. 29, 2012.

Patoine B. Guideline-making Gets Tougher: Action by State Attorney General Over Lyme Disease Guidelines Stirs Debate. http://annalsofneurology.wordpress.com/ page/2/?s= patoine.+lyme. Accessed February 2010.

Phillips S. Lyme Disease Review Panel Hearing, July 30, 2006. Infectious Diseases Society of America. http://lymewebcast.idsociety.org/. Accessed December 2010.

PR Web. Connecticut Attorney General Charges IDSA with Violating Lyme Antitrust Settlement Agreement. http://www.earthtimes.org/articles/slide/show/connecticut-attorney-general-charges-idsa.1155030.shtml. Accessed February 2010.

Risk Map. http://commons.wikimedia.org/wiki/File:Lyme_Disease_Risk_Map.gif

RMSF rash. http://en.wikipedia.org/wiki/File:Rocky_mountian_spotted_fever.jpg

Rubel J. Lyme disease symptoms and characteristics: A compilation of peer-reviewed literature reports. September 2005. http://www.lymeinfo.net/medical/LDSymptoms.pdf. Accessed May 2010.

Ryan, K. http://www.dartmoorcam.co.uk/dartmoortickwatch. Accessed March 2013.

Santaniello G. Lyme disease divide: A schism over treatment philosophies puts a Connecticut pediatrician's license on the line. Hartford Courant. 2006. http://www.courant.com. Accessed May 2010.

SCHOOL IPM 2015: A Strategic Plan for Integrated Pest Management in Schools in the United States. 2009. Version 1.1:137-141. http://www.ipmcenters.org/pmsp/pdf/usschoolspmsp.pdf. Accessed September 2011.

SCHOOL IPM 2015: Reducing Pest Problems and Pesticides in Our Nation's Schools. 2011. http://www.ipminstitute.org/school_ipm_2015/index.htm. Accessed September 2011.

Sherr VT. The Human Side of Lyme. http://www.thehumansideof-lyme.net. Accessed February 2010.

Sherr, Virginia. Bell's Palsy of the Gut. Practical Gastroenterology. 2006.

Sole Lyme Vaccine Is Pulled Off Market. New York Times. February 28, 2002. http://query.nytimes.com/gst/fullpage.html?res=9C00E5D71531F93BA15751C0A9649C8B63. Accessed July 2008.

Spirochetes. http://www.textbookofbacteriology.net/Lyme.html. Accessed March 2012.

Stafford KC. Connecticut Agricultural Experiment Station and Connecticut Department of Public Health. 2004; p. 46. http://www.ct.gov/caes/lib/caes/ documents/ special_features/ TickHandbook.pdf. Accessed August 2007.

STARI-Southern Tick-Associated Rash Illness. http://www.cdc.gov/stari. Accessed 2011- 2012.

Steere AC. Lyme Disease: Questions and Answers. 2003. Massachusetts General Hospital/Harvard Medical School. Archived from the original on 3/7/2008. http://web.archive.org/web/20080307191326/ http://www.mgh.harvard.edu/medicine/rheu/Q&ALYME.pdf. Accessed April 2009.

The Guardian. UK Dismisses Mugabe's Claim that Zimbabwe Cholera Crisis is Over. December 11, 2008. http://www.guardian.co.uk. Accessed February 2009.

Tick. http://www.ent.iastate.edu/tick.html. Accessed February 2010.

Tick. http://www.health.state.mn.us/ticks.html. Accessed February 2010.

Todar K. Borrelia burgdorferi and Lyme Disease. Todar's Online Textbook of Bacteriology, 2008-2012. http://textbook of bacteriology.net/Lyme.html. Accessed February 2011.

Top Ten Tips to Prevent Chronic Lyme Disease. http://www.ilads.org/files/2008/ Preventing_CLD_Top_Ten_Tips.pdf. Accessed February 2010.

Tunev S, Hastey C, Hodzic E, et al. Lymphadenopathy during Lyme borreliosis is caused by spirochete migration-induced specific B cell activation. PLoS Pathogen. http://www.plospathogens.org/ article/ info:doi. Accessed March 19, 2012.

United States Department of Defense (USDoD). Insect Repellent System. 2007. USACHPPM. http://phc.amedd.army.mil/PHC%20Resource%20Library/DODInsectRepellentSystemJustheFacts-June2007.pdf. Accessed August 2011.

United States Environmental Protection Agency (EPA). 2007. Pesticides: Topical and Chemical Fact Sheet, The Insect Repellent DEET. http://www.epa.gov/opp00001/factsheets/ chemicals/ deet.htm. Accessed August 2011.

UpToDate. http://www.uptodate.com. Accessed May 2010.

US Army Public Health Command (USAPHC): Using repellents on children. 2010. http://phc.amedd.army.mil/PHC%20Resource%20Library/UsingInsectRepellentsonChildrenJan2010.pdf. Accessed August 2011.

Vojdani A. Scientific facts versus fiction about Mycoplasma. www.fmcfsme.com. Accessed May 9, 2012.

Western black-legged ticks. www.doh.wa.gov. Accessed April 18, 2013.

Weis, J. University of Utah. http://www.path.utah.edu/research/cbi/janis-weis. Accessed February 2010.

www.ilads.org/lyme_research/lyme_publications_2html. Accessed 2012.

Zaidman GW. Lyme Disease. eMedicine Ophthalmology. http://emedicine.medscape.com/article/ 1202521-overview. Accessed August 2009.

Abstracts

Burrascano J. Failure of aggressive antibiotic therapy to protect the placenta from invasion by B burgdorferi in a pregnant patient with Lyme borreliosis. 6th Annual International Science Conference on Lyme Disease and Other Tick-borne Disease;1993. Abstract.

Horowitz R, Rodner D. A prospective study of heavy metal exposure among Lyme disease patients with chronic persistent symptomatology: Implications for treatment. 16th Scientific Conference on Lyme Disease & Other Tick-Borne Disorders; May 2003; USA. Abstract.

Horowitz R. Chronic persistent Lyme borreliosis: PCR evidence of chronic infection despite extended antibiotic therapy – a retrospective review. 13th International Scientific Conference on Lyme Disease and Other Tick-Borne Disorders, Connecticut. March 24-26, 2000. Abstract.

Horowitz RI, Atkinson-Barr M. Metronidazole therapy in the treatment of chronic Lyme disease. 12th International Scientific Conference on Lyme Disease and Other Spirochetal Disorders; April 1999; New York. Abstract.

Horowitz RI, Losicco-Yunker L. Lyme disease and pregnancy: Implications of chronic infection, PCR testing, and prenatal treatment.

16th Scientific Conference on Lyme Disease & Other Tick-Borne Disorders; May 2003; USA. Abstract.

Horowitz RI, Rodner D, Losicco-Yunker L. Borrelia burgdorferi & Bartonella henselea: A study comparing tetracyclines in combination with quinolones in co-infected Lyme patients. 16th Scientific Conference on Lyme Disease & Other Tick-Borne Disorders; May 2003; USA. Abstract.

Horowitz RI, Rodner D. Bartonella henselae: Limitations of serologic testing: Evaluation of ELISA and PCR testing in a cohort of Lyme disease patients and implications for treatment. 16th International Scientific Conference on Lyme Disease & Other Tick-Borne Disorders; May 2003; USA. Abstract.

Horowitz RI, Rodner D. Effects of shifting the acid-base balance among Lyme patients during Jarisch-Herxheimer flares: A small prospective study. 16th International Scientific Conference on Lyme Disease & Other Tick-Borne Disorders; May 2003; USA. Abstract.

Horowitz RI, Rodner D. Mycoplasma infections in chronic Lyme disease: A retrospective analysis of co-infection and persistence demonstrated by PCR analysis despite long term antibiotic treatment. 16th Scientific Conference on Lyme Disease & Other Tick-Borne Disorders; May 2003; USA. Abstract.

Horowitz RI. Bicillin therapy and Lyme disease: A retrospective study of the safety and efficacy of high dose intramuscular bicillin in the treatment of chronic resistant Lyme disease. 12th International Scientific Conference on Lyme Disease and Other Spirochetal Disorders; April 1999; New York. Abstract.

Liegner KB. Culture confirmed treatment failure of cefotaxime and minocycline in a case of Lyme meningoencephalomyelitis. Program and Abstracts of the Fifth International Conference on Lyme Borreliosis. 1992; Arlington, VA. Abstract.

Miscellaneous

Associated Press. Struck by Lyme disease, Parker Posey withdraws from Off-B'way Production. Huffington Post. August 26, 2009. http://www.huffingtonpost.com/2009/08/26/struck-by-lyme- disease-pa_n_269912.html. Accessed January 2010.

Attached deer tick. WebMD. Accessed April 27, 2012.

Babesia_life_cycle_human_en.svg. Accessed 2010 – 2012.

Billeter SA, et al. Infection and replication of Bartonella species within a tick cell line. Experimental and Applied Acarology. Published online: 26 February 2009.

Bransfield R. The Neuropsychiatric Lyme Assessment. http://www.mentalhealthandillness.com.

Bransfield R. New York State Assembly Committee on Health, chaired by Richard Gottfried. Albany, NY. November 27, 2001.

Britton C. Remarks before the New York State Assembly Committee on Health, Public Hearing, Richard Gottfried, Chair. Chronic Lyme Disease and Long-Term Antibiotic Treatment. New York, November 27, 2001.

Brown D. Bush apparently had Lyme disease. The Washington Post. August 9, 2007. http://www.washingtonpost.com/wp-dyn/content/ article/2007/08/08/ AR2007080802268.html. Accessed February 2010.

Buchman S. The Qualitative and Quantitative Implications of an Inadequate Diagnostic Test for Lyme Disease Patients. Public Policy Analysis. Academic Thesis. Advised by: Professor Worthington Mathew Sazinsky. May 1, 2009.

Burrascano J. Gestational Lyme. 2005. Accessed through lymedisease.org 2012.

Burrascano J. Lyme Disease Complexities. Presented at Kennett Friends Meeting. Sponsored by the Lyme Disease Association of Southeastern Pennsylvania, Kennett Square, PA. May 3, 2003.

California Business and Professions, Section 2234.1. Assembly Bill 592, passed August 29, 2005. ftp://leginfo.public.ca.gov/pub/05-06/ bill/asm/ab_0551-0600/ab_592_bill_ 20050831_ enrolled. pdf.

Chaconas G. Insight into spirochetal dissemination in vivo. Lyme & Other Tick-Borne Diseases. Conference Friday, October 17, 2008. San Francisco, California. Sponsored by Columbia University and Lyme Disease Association, Inc.

Coats D. DVM. 2010-2012. Personal communication.

Commonwealth of Massachusetts, 187th General Court. Administration of long-term antibiotic therapy upon diagnosis of Lyme disease. Chapter 112, Section 12DD. 2011. http://www. malegislature. gov/ Laws/GeneralLaws/PartI/TitleXVI/Chapter112/Section12DD. Accessed November 2011.

Cunningham, Madeline, PhD, University of Oklahoma. Personal Communication, 2011.

Daryl Hall back on tour following illness. Associated Press. August 3, 2005. http://msnbc.msn.com/id/8813408/site/todayshow/ns/ today-entertainment.

Diagnostic and Statistical Manual of Mental Disorders DSM-IV-TR. Fourth Edition. American Psychiatric Association. 2000.

Erlichia. Ohio State University website. Acessed 2010.

Expanding HIV/AIDS Treatment. The Week. Feb 20, 2009. p8.

Fallon BA. Testimony at public hearing re Lyme disease, State of Connecticut, Department of Public Health, January 29, 2004.

Fearn DW and the Lyme Disease Association of Southeastern Pennsylvania. Lyme Disease Population Survey in a Small SE Pennsylvania Township. 2004 LDA/Columbia and ILADS Conference.

Film Focuses on Lyme Patients. Washington Post. June 17, 2008. http://www. washingtonpost. com. Accessed September 2008.

Gibbs N. The Coping Conundrum. Time. October 25, 2011.

Grann D. Stalking Dr. Steere Over Lyme Disease. New York Times Magazine. June 17, 2001. http://www.nytimes.com/2001/06/17/ magazine/17LYMEDISEASE.html. Accessed June 2008.

Hitt J. The year in ideas: A to Z evidence-based medicine. The New York Times. December 9, 2001.

Hall SS. Iceman Autopsy. National Geographic. November 2011. http://ngm.nationalgeographic.com/2011/11/iceman-autopsy/hall-text. Accessed October 2011.

Horowitz R. Classical and integrative medical approaches in chronic Lyme disease: New paradigms in diagnosis & treatment. Lyme & Other Tick-Borne Diseases. Conference Friday, October 17, 2008. San Francisco, California. Sponsored by Columbia University and Lyme Disease Association, Inc.

Horowitz R, Burrascano J. Workshop: Fundamentals. Lyme & Other Tick-Borne Diseases. Conference Friday, October 17, 2008. San Francisco, California. Sponsored by Columbia University and Lyme Disease Association, Inc.

IDEXX Map. IDEXX Laboratories, Inc., Westbrook, ME USA, Accessed 2012.

Infectious Diseases Society of America (IDSA). Special Review Panel Unanimously Upholds Lyme Disease Treatment Guidelines: Short-term Antibiotics Proven to be Best Treatment for Patients. http://www.idsociety.org/Content.aspc?id=16501. Accessed April 2010.

Informed consent sample form http://www.lymedisease.org/resources/consent.html.

In the Matter of Joseph Burrascano v. New York State Bd. for Professional Medical Conduct, Determination and Order (No. 01-265) of Hearing committee dated November 6 2003 AND Natole v. Michigan Board of Medicine, (File no. 96-015560 AA-2) (1998) (2001).

Jones, CR, Smith H, Gibb E, Johnson L. Gestational Lyme Disease Case Studies of 102 Live Births. 2005. Accessed through lymedisease.org 2012.

Kelly R. Are there any non-DEET bug repellents that work? Woman's Day. June 16, 2009.

Kids and Mental Health. Time. November 1, 2010;176(18).

Landers SJ. Lyme treatment accord ends antitrust probe. American Medical News. http://www.ama-assn.org/amednews/2008/06/09/hlsa0609.htm. Accessed June 2008.

Lane R. Diversity of Borrelia burgdorferi genospecies and genotypes in California. 2011 Lyme and Tick Borne Diseases National Conference. Columbia University and Lyme Disease Association. Philadelphia, PA. October 1-2, 2011.

Liegner KB. Remarks before the New York State Assembly Committee on Health, Public Hearing, Richard Gottfried, Chair. Chronic Lyme Disease and Long-Term Antibiotic Treatment. New York, November 27, 2001.

Likits A. A clue to what makes Lyme disease tick. The Wall Street Journal. July 12, 2011.

Luft B. Diagnostics. 2011 Lyme and Tick Borne Diseases National Conference. Columbia University and Lyme Disease Association. Philadelphia, PA. October 1-2, 2011.

Lyme treatment: Doctor, patient should have freedom to decide on best course of action. PennLive.com. August 20, 2010. http://blog.pennlive.com/editorials/print.html? entry=/2010/08/ lyme_treatment_doctor_patient.html. Accessed November 2010.

MacDonald A. Borrelia Attack Models. Presentation. New Haven Lyme Conference, 2007.

Maloney E. The treatment of Lyme disease. 2011 Lyme and Tick Borne Diseases National Conference. Columbia University and Lyme Disease Association. Philadelphia, PA. October 1 -2, 2011.

Martinez B. Care guidelines used by insurers face scrutiny. Wall Street Journal. September 14, 2000.

McCoy JJ. Amy Tan, ticked off about Lyme. Washington Post. August 5, 2003. Lyme Disease Foundation. http://www.canlyme.com/amy.html.

Mead P. Statement by Paul Mead MD, M.P.H., Medical Epidemiologist, Division of Vector-Borne Infectious Diseases, Center for Disease Control and Prevention, US Department of Health and Human Services on Hearing: CDCs Lyme Disease Prevention and Control Activities. Public hearing re Lyme disease, State of Connecticut, Department of Public Health, January 29, 2004. http://www.hhs.gov/asl/testify/r040129.html.

Metzger D. Lyme disease and chronic pelvic pain. Lyme & Other Tick-Borne Diseases. Conference Friday, October 17, 2008. San Francisco, California. Sponsored by Columbia University and Lyme Disease Association, Inc.

Moeller JR. Functional neuroimaging findings in chronic LYD: Research as a tool to solve medical controversies. Lyme and TBD Research Center. Columbia University. 2007.

New Hampshire General Court. An ACT relative to the use of long-term antibiotics for the treatment of Lyme disease. House Bill 295, approved June 9, 2011. http://www.gencourt. state.nh.us/legislation/2011/HB0295.html.

Johnson, Lorraine, JD, MBA, at California Lyme Disease Association (CALDA). Personal Communication. (http://www.lymedisease.org).

Osterweil N. Extra antibiotics provide only transient improvement in Lyme encephalopathy. MedPage Today. October 11, 2007. http://www.medpagetoday.com/tbprint.cfm?tbid=6946.

Potrikus A. Shumer calls for education, research to prevent Lyme Disease and other tick-borne illnesses. The Post-Standard. August 4, 2011. http://www.syracuse.com/news/ index.ssf/ 2011/ 08/schumer_calls_for_education_re.html. Accessed October 2011.

Rhode Island Department of Health. Lyme Disease and the Law. Archived from the original on May 2, 2005. http://web.archive.org/web/20050502203519/http://www.health.state.ri.us/ disease/ communicable/lyme/law.php. Accessed July 2009.

Roth, Thomas, PhD. Director, Sleep Disorders and Research Center, Henry Ford Health System, Detroit, Michigan. Personal Communication, June 27, 2011.

Ryan, Keith, PhD. Personal Communication, March 2013.

Schoessler S, Schantz S. The "Tick-ing" Clock: School Nurses Intervene to Reduce the Risk of Tick-borne Disease. Promoting Community IPM for Preventing Tick-Borne Diseases Conference. U.S. Environmental Protection Agency, Arlington, Virginia, March 30-31, 2011.

Sherr VT. Unreported epidemic: Failure to count cases of babesiosis. Bucks County Courier Times. July 6, 2000;6A:1.

Singer S. No changes to Lyme disease treatment. Associated Press. April 22, 2010. http://www.msnbc.msn.com/id/36721207/ns/health-infectious_diseases/deck/news.mobile.msn. com/ent.mobile.msn. com/en-us/mny.mobile.msn.com/en-us. Accessed October 2010.

Smith P. New Jersey School Boards Association. September/October 2004 School Leader.

Spancake M. DVM. Personal Communication, 2012.

State of Connecticut, Office of the Attorney General. Attorney General's Investigation Reveals Flawed Lyme Disease Guidelines Process, IDSA Agrees to Reassess Guidelines, Install Independent Arbiter. Press Release, May 1, 2008. http://www.ct.gov/AG/cwp/view.asp? a=2795&q =414284. Accessed July 2009.

State of Connecticut General Assembly. An Act Concerning the Use of Long-Term Antibiotics for the Treatment of Lyme Disease. June 18, 2009. http://www.cga.ct.gov/asp/cgabillstatus/ cgabillstatus.asp?selBillType=Bill&bill_num=6200&which_year=2009&SUBMIT1.x=0&SUBMIT1.y=0&SUBMIT1=Normal. Accessed July 2009.

Stolberg S. Study says clinical guides often hide ties of doctors. New York Times. February 6, 2003.

Svonavec V. DVM. Personal Communication, 2011-2012.

Syphilis. USA Today. May 6, 2010.

Thandani V. Epilepsy update. 2011 Lyme and Tick Borne Diseases National Conference. Columbia University and Lyme Disease Association. Philadelphia, PA. October 1-2, 2011.

UK Dismisses Mugabe's Claim that Zimbabwe Cholera Crisis is Over. Dec. 11, 2008. http://www.guardian.co.uk. Accessed February 2009.

U.S. researchers find new disease carried by deer ticks.www.reuters.com. Accessed January 17, 2013.

Walter A. Update on ehrlichiosis and hemophagocytic lymphohistiocytosis. 2011 Lyme and Tick Borne Diseases National Conference. Columbia University and Lyme Disease Association. Philadelphia, PA. October 1-2, 2011.

Whelan D. Lyme Inc. Forbes. March 12, 2007. http://www.forbes.com/forbes/ 2007/0312/ 096.html. Accessed June 2008.

Xiao J. How Different Strains of Parasite Infection Affect Behavior Differently. Infection and Immunity. March 2011. As quoted in Science Daily, March 22, 2011.

Zeuzem S. A comparison of standard treatment versus dynamically individualized treatment in patients with chronic hepatitis C. Presented at the 54th Annual Meeting of the American Association for the Study of Liver Diseases, Massachusetts. October 24-28, 2003.

Various Additional Articles, Interviews, Reports, and Lectures by:

Robert Bransfield

Willy Burgdorfer

Joseph Burrascano

Brian Fallon

Richard Horowitz

Lorraine Johnson

Charles Ray Jones

Peter J. Krause

Kenneth Liegner

Alan MacDonald

Ed Masters

Garth L. Nicholson

Nancy L. Nicholson

Keith Ryan

Eva Sapi

Virginia Sherr

Ken Singleton

Patricia Smith

Raphael Stricker

Janis Weis

A bag of plain bagels with one onion bagel is really a bag of onion bagels.

Unknown

Appendix B

GLOSSARY

The greatest sin might be not living up to your potential and not using the gifts God gave you.
Maybe the purpose of prayer is not to change things but to change how we respond to things. Sometimes God
calms the storm and sometimes he lets it rage and calms his child instead.

Connie Patterson

A

Abducens nerve: (CN 6) Controls lateral and conjugate movements of the eye

Abduction: Motion that pulls a body part AWAY from the midline. Spreading the fingers apart is abduction. Raising the arms out to the side is abduction.

Abilify: One of several atypical antipsychotics used in the treatment of schizophrenia, bipolar disorder, and depression. Also indicated for irritability in kids with autism

Abscess: Collection of pus formed due to inflammation and infection of the soft tissue

Absorption: Taking in of a substance. The passage of material through a body surface. Process by which a drug, nutrient, or other molecule gets into the circulation. Absorption occurs when the matter crosses any number of barriers such as the skin, the mucous membranes, the GI tract, or muscle capillaries. If a drug is given IV, the molecules go directly into the vein, by-passing absorption issues.

Abstract thinking: Abstract concepts are those that do not have an immediate, obvious meaning and require some interpretation. Abstract thinking is the ability to use concepts that are not apparent and to understand generalizations. The capacity for abstract thought can be a measure of cognitive ability.

Acarology: Study of mites and ticks. From the Acari taxon of arachnids. Acarology was the last word I placed in the *Glossary* in late 2012. After 4 years of 20 hour days on this topic, I had never seen or heard this word. Spell check included astrologist and carpologist but not acarologist. If you have read this far, you may now qualify as an acarologist.

Accommodation: Eyes adjust so that clear vision is maintained when the gaze is shifted from far to near. By changing the curve of the lens, the eye can correct for varying distances so that it can focus an image onto the retina.

Accommodations: Actions taken to make a situation more suitable or in-line with specific needs. To furnish with something necessary. For example, accommodations may need to be made to facilitate learning in sick school children. These actions may need to be flexible, allowing the child to do more when he can and less when necessary.

Ache: Persistent discomfort. The term ache is often used to describe the joint pain or overall muted pain accompanying infection or inflammation. To suffer a dull pain

Acne: Inflammatory disease of the sebaceous (oil-secreting) glands and hair follicles of the skin characterized by comedones (whiteheads and blackheads), papules, and pustules. Cysts, nodules, and scars may develop, with eruptions mostly on the face, neck, and shoulders.

Acoustic nerve: (CN 8) Hearing and balance. Lyme involvement with CN8 can result in otic effects such as tinnitus, hearing loss, balance problems, and vertigo.

Acquired Lyme: Borreliosis due to a tick bite as opposed to gestational Lyme

Acrodermatitis chronica atrophicans: Progressive skin condition that leads to widespread atrophy of the skin. Some cases of the European version of Lyme have presented with this type of lesion that is unfamiliar in North America. Often associated with problems in the PNS such as polyneuropathy. The skin becomes like tissue paper. Usually the lesions begin in the extremities with a blush-red inflammation and swelling. The clinical course might last for years.

Acting out: Behaving on impulse in antisocial ways including drinking, doing drugs, shoplifting, behaving promiscuously, and throwing tantrums. Acting out may be a way to get attention but the behaviors are damaging to the person, others, animals, or property. Acting out helps express feelings that might be better expressed in more constructive ways.

Actinobacteria: Formerly called Actinomycetes, the Actinobacteria are of the genus Streptomyces known to synthesize components of certain antibiotics of the macrolide class

Acuity: Clearness, sharpness. Usually refers to eyesight, but also can refer to hearing as in visual acuity or auditory acuity

Acupuncture: Medical practice where fine needles are inserted into the body at specific points to relieve pain or treat a variety of conditions such as arthritis or fatigue. Usually a component of TCM, the premise is to balance the energy found in the body (yin and yang). This insertion and manipulation of needles is thought to redirect and balance the life force. Placement sites depend on the condition being treated. Detractors think any response is due to a placebo-effect.

Acute: Of short duration, not chronic or on-going. Acute conditions usually have a relatively sudden onset, sharp increase in intensity, and a limited course. Acute LD is often considered to be that condition where sxs occur shortly after the tick bite, but since the timing of that event is often unclear, the line between acute and chronic LD is often blurred.

Acute abdomen: Sudden onset of severe abdominal pain, often with other symptoms such as fever, guarding, and rebound tenderness. This is an emergency that must be addressed immediately and may need surgical intervention.

Acute renal failure: (ARF) Loss of kidney function which can have many causes. If not treated ARF can lead to progressive loss of kidney function and end-stage disease. Early signs are oliguria and azotemia.

Adam's apple: Laryngeal protuberance

ADD: Attention deficit disorder

Addiction: Compulsive use of a substance or the performance of a behavior that ultimately causes harm to the addict. Addiction is often framed in terms of dependency, tolerance, and withdrawal.

Addison's disease: Adrenal insufficiency where the adrenal glands do not produce enough adrenocortical hormones. Symptoms can include increased pigmentation of skin or mucous membranes, weakness, fatigue, hypotension, nausea, vomiting, diarrhea, abdominal discomfort, anorexia, and weight loss. Some hypothesized etiologies include infections and autoimmunity.

Adduction: Motion that pulls a part TOWARD the midline of the body. Dropping the arms to the sides, bringing the knees to touch each other, and pulling the toes together are all adduction. Think of "adding" a part to the whole.

ADHD: Attention deficit hyperactivity disorder

Adhesion: Fibrotic scars, most often in the abdomen and pelvis, which can bind organs that are not normally attached and thereby cause viscera to become matted together. On palpation the abdomen can feel stiff, immobile, and unnatural. Adhesions can cause discomfort and, in some cases, obstruction and loss of function. Often occur after surgery when the tissues scar as part of wound healing. They are also common after infection, inflammation, or trauma.

Adjunct: Adjuvant. A treatment added to an on-going regimen. For example, some physicians use cranial manipulation as an adjunct to antibiotics in treating Lyme disease.

Administer: To mete out or dispense to the patient

Adrenal: Literally next to the kidney. Usually refers to the adrenal glands

Adrenal gland: Crescent-shaped gland located on the top of each kidney. Function is controlled by the SNS. The cortex secretes steroid hormones such as cortisol, which regulate carbohydrate and fat metabolism, energy transformation, and salt and water balance. Cortisol is called the stress hormone and it has been found at high levels in patients with anxiety or panic. Addison's disease is a **hypo**active adrenal cortex, while a **hyper**active cortex can result in adrenogenital syndrome. The medulla secretes biochemicals that mimic the effects of the SNS including increased carbohydrate use for energy. Medullary hormones include dopamine (dilates arteries, increases cardiac output, and enhances blood flow to the kidney), norepinephrine (constricts small vessels, increases resistance to blood flow, raises blood pressure, and decreases heart rate), and epinephrine (also called adrenaline, which constricts vessels in skin and viscera, dilates vessels in muscles, increases heart activity, increases glucose in the blood, decreases GI activity, and dilates the bronchi by relaxing the airways which explains why it's used

in treating acute asthma. Epinephrine inspires whatever makes sense to help the organism survive in "fight or flight" situations). A hyperactive medulla can lead to pheochromocytoma.

Adult Respiratory Distress Syndrome: (ARDS) Severe air hunger with pulmonary compromise that has a high mortality rate. ARDS has been reported in severe cases of babesiosis and in end-stage Lyme.

Adverse event: Any unfavorable and unintended occurrence that might include an abnormal lab finding, symptom, sign, or disease associated with a medical intervention. Many synonyms such as adverse reaction, side effect, untoward result, etc.

Aerobic exercises: Aerobic means with oxygen. In aerobic exercises oxygen is used to burn carbohydrate, and later fat, to make energy to power the activity. This is the same way that oxygen is used to burn fuel in a furnace. Aerobic exercises involve low to moderate effort over a long duration. Over time, all the body's available carbohydrate is used for energy to fuel the exercise and when it's gone the body starts burning fat. For this reason, aerobics may be better for weight loss than anaerobic exercise.

Affect: General demeanor, especially the facial expression, indicating mood. The emotional reaction associated with an experience. A blunted affect is one where there is a muted emotional response to every situation. A flat affect is the absence of emotional reaction, no matter what the circumstances.

Afferent: Carrying an impulse or fluid TOWARD the center

Affirmations: Statements declared to be true or are hoped will be true in the future. Declarations such as, "I am well" or "I am fit," can be repeated over and over, either silently, aloud, or written, until they engram into the psyche.

Agglutination: Clumping. A type of Ag/Ab reaction used in lab testing to determine the presence of one or the other entity

Aggression: Ready to attack or confront, often without provocation. A forceful action or reaction that can be physical or verbal

Agility: Ability to perform a series of movements in succession in different planes or directions. Usually the faster these tasks can be performed without error, the more agile the person. Practice can enhance agility.

Agranulocyte: WBC usually with a one-lobed nuclei and few or no granules in the cytoplasm. Includes lymphocytes (B and T cells), monocytes (macrophages in the tissues), and others

Air hunger: Sensation that one cannot get an effective breath. Breathing does not feel adequate or satisfactory. The patient may not be able to sigh sufficiently. Air hunger can range from mild discomfort to respiratory distress. Can occur with acute babesiosis

Akinesia: Loss of muscle movement

Alanine transaminase: (ALT) Alanine-glyoxylate aminotransferase (formerly SGPT) is an enzyme that, when elevated, suggests damage to the tissue where it originates, such as the liver. ALT can be used as a biomarker of hepatic injury and levels can be correlated with liver function. When the liver cell is damaged, ALT leaks into the blood where it can be measured. ALT is a more specific indicator of liver problems than is AST, since AST is found in more kinds of tissue than is ALT. Transaminases are a measure of cell integrity. When there is an elevated ALT, damage to liver cells should be suspected.

Albinism: Partial or total lack of pigment in skin, hair, and eyes. Often with astigmatism, photophobia, and nystagmus (because the choroid is not adequately protected from light). Genetic, non-pathologic

Albumin: Protein made specifically by the liver and the primary protein found in blood plasma. Acts as a carrier molecule and helps maintain blood volume and BP and contributes to osmotic pressure balance. Albumin is a measure of cell function and levels suggest how well the liver is working to make proteins. If something is inhibiting the manufacture of protein in the liver, albumin levels will be low.

Algorithm: Sequence of steps used to make a decision or to solve a problem. Method of well-defined instructions. In medicine algorithms are designed to help with decision-making, diagnosis, and treatment. They provide a step-by-step approach to problem solving. Often involve sets of questions with Yes or No answers to lead the user down a path to a conclusion. While algorithms can be useful, they can also be restrictive and misleading.

Alkaline phosphatase: (ALP or AP) Enzyme found in the cells of the biliary ducts of the liver. Functions in the mineralization of bone and is also present in teeth, plasma, kidney, and intestine. Blood levels increase in obstructive jaundice, bile duct obstruction, cholestasis, or infiltrative liver disease and diseases of the pancreas, lung, and bone, as well as in malignancies. High in neonates. Also found in the placenta. AP is higher in kids since they have growing bones. AP can be used as a marker of liver or bone disease. Normals vary with age and pregnancy.

Allele: Alternate form of a gene

Allergy: An acquired, abnormal immune response to a substance (allergen) that does not usually cause a reaction in most other people. Sensitization. An initial exposure to the allergen is required for an allergic response to manifest upon second exposure. Subsequent contact results in a range of inflammatory responses.

Allopathy: Philosophy of medicine that uses various methods to combat disease such as drugs and surgery. In recent years allopathy has started to become more focused on wellness and disease prevention rather than simply eliminating symptoms. Physicians are called allopaths and usually have an MD degree.

ALT: Alanine aminotransferase

Alzheimer's disease: Progressive loss of cognitive function including judgment, abstract thought, and memory. Plaques and tangles in the grey matter in the cortex of the brain seem to be the focus of the pathology. Alzheimer's patients can't do most AODL and can't learn new things. This disease is rarely part of a pediatric practice, but appears on the differential diagnosis of Lyme in adults. Alzheimer's may have an underlying autoimmune mechanism. Alzheimer's disease presents as a dementia with a long clinical course that can be fatal.

Amantadine: Drug used for prevention and treatment of influenza A as well as sxs of Parkinson-like syndromes. Sometimes used as an efficacy enhancer for clarithromycin and azithromycin. Recently, amantadine was thought to help speed recovery in traumatic brain injuries.

Amblyopia: Reduced vision

Ameba: (Amoeba) Minute, one-celled protozoa. Changes shape by sending out fingerlike projections called pseudopods through which it moves and obtains nourishment. Some species can cause disease in humans.

Amebiasis: Infection with amebas

American malaria: Babesiosis

Americans with Disabilities Act: (ADA) Law that prohibits, in some circumstances, discrimination because of a disability. The ADA focuses on employment, access to public places, transportation, telecommunication, and education.

Aminoglycosides: Class of antibiotics rarely indicated for treatment of TBIs although they are sometimes used to treat tularemia and M. *fermentans*. However, if given for other reasons in TBI patients they might increase the risk of kidney damage. They include gentamicin, tobramycin, amikacin, kanamycin, streptomycin, and neomycin.

Amnesia: Inability to recall past experiences. Can be recent, distant, or both

Amoeba: Ameba

Amoxicillin: (Amoxil) Broad spectrum –cidal PCN antibiotic that works by impairing the cell wall. DOC as foundation antibiotic for combination therapy in Lyme disease in children

Amygdala: Part of the limbic system of the brain. The amygdala is associated with mood, arousal, and emotions both positive and negative. When this small area in the temporal lobe is stimulated, aggression and rage result. When the amygdala is removed the same subject is indifferent. The amygdala is responsible for identifying danger and is probably the seat of the "fight or flight" response. TBIs such as bartonellosis, M. *fermentans*, and Lyme can incite rage and aggression.

Amylase: Pancreatic enzyme that hydrolyses starch. Levels can be used to assess the status of the pancreas. A high amylase confirms pancreatitis but levels can return to normal even though the patient is still sick.

Amyotrophic lateral sclerosis: ALS or Lou Gehrig's disease is a combined UMN and LMN disorder that causes muscle atrophy. Onset is usually later in life and the condition is often fatal within 3 to 10 years after onset. Sxs might include progressive weakness in the arms, legs, and trunk, difficulty talking, chewing, swallowing, and eventually breathing. Death is due to aspiration or respiratory failure. Genetics is involved in many cases and the pathophysiology is likely an autoimmune reaction. There have been associations with infectious agents. Lyme is part of the differential diagnosis of ALS, as ALS is on the differential list of Lyme in older teens and adults. There is a small population of kids diagnosed with Juvenile ALS.

Anaerobic exercises: Exercise where the energy needed is provided without the consumption of oxygen. These activities involve high intensity for short bursts and are better for building muscle. Anaerobic activity does not use O_2 to burn fuel to make energy at the time of exercise. Sugars are used but not combusted using O_2.

Anaphylaxis: A Type I allergic hypersensitivity reaction to an antigen. Mediated by biochemicals released by mast cells and IgE. This is an Ag/Ab reaction. Systemic effects can lead to respiratory and vascular changes that can result in shock or death.

Anaplasmosis: Disease caused by the genus Anaplasma, closely related to Ehrlichia. Anaplasma *phagocytophilum* is the agent for HGA, human granulocytic anaplasmosis. Common TBI co-infection

Anasarca: Severe, general edema. Widespread swelling due to the seepage of fluid into the space between cells

Anemia: A decrease in the number or quality of RBCs leaving the blood unable to meet the oxygen demands of the body. Anemia is a symptom of a disease, not actually a disease itself. Sxs can include pallor of skin, nail beds, and mucus membranes, along with weakness, vertigo, headache, fatigue, sore tongue, malaise, SOB, and tachycardia.

Aneurysm: Localized defect in a blood vessel, most commonly an artery. The defect can pooch out like a bubble in an inner tube. Can occur in any artery but the most common sites are the aorta and arteries in the brain. The defect can dissect, meaning the blood gets between the layers of the artery wall and spreads. A broad pulsing mass in the abdomen might represent an aortic aneurysm. A bruit located over a pulse point suggests a flow problem, which could be an aneurysm.

Anger: Basic emotion of extreme displeasure or dissatisfaction in response to a person, object, or situation. Anger can help the person to respond to adverse situations and may contribute to survival. Anger can become out-of-control especially in association with certain infections like bartonellosis.

Angioedema: Swelling of the skin, mucous membranes, or viscera that may be due to an allergic response mediated by IgE

Angioma: An abnormal growth due to the dilation, or new formation, of blood vessels like those seen in bartonellosis

Anisocoria: Inequality in the size of pupils. May be genetic or due to pathology

Ankylosis: Stiffening, immobility

Ankylosing spondylitis: Chronic, progressive, degenerative condition involving the joints of the spine, the costovertebral joints, and the sacroiliac joints. Sclerosis (fibrosis) of the SI joints is the hallmark sign. The changes here are similar to those seen in RA. Ankylosis (stiffening, immobility) may occur, giving rise to a stiff, straight, immobile back. Usually the condition starts in the SI joint and low back, reaching the neck only late in the clinical course. There is significantly decreased ROM with spastic tenderness of muscles. The patient may need to turn his whole body to look sideways with the neck thrust forward. Other manifestations include increased reflexes and fasciculations.

Anorexia: Loss of appetite which can manifest in a number of conditions

Anorexia nervosa: A severe mental illness that presents with a disturbed sense of body image, a morbid fear of obesity, and refusal to maintain a minimum body weight. Self-imposed starvation can have multiple physical and emotional consequences.

Antabuse: (Disulfiram) Drug that causes a bad reaction to alcohol including nausea, vomiting, headache, flushing, cramps, and confusion. Used as a deterrent to excessive drinking with limited success

Antecubital fossa: Soft front of elbow. Bend of the elbow

Antibody: Immunoglobulin. Complex protein produced by B lymphocytes in response to an antigen. Proteins used by the immune system to identify and neutralize foreign agents such as bacteria and viruses. Abs are produced by specialized WBCs called plasma cells. All Abs have similar structures except for their tips where there is much variation. Each different tip can recognize and bind to a specific antigen. This diversity allows the immune system to recognize millions of different kinds of foreign material and either dispatch it or call others to get rid of it. An Ab binds only with its specific antigen in a lock and key fashion. Abs are all immunoglobulins (Igs).

Antigen: Protein on a cell surface that stimulates the production of antibodies by B lymphocytes. This protein can be foreign if it comes from a pathogen, allergen, or toxin OR a *self*-protein if the immune system is cleaning up cellular debris or there is an autoimmune malfunction. An antigen is any substance that causes the immune system to produce antibodies against it.

Antigen/antibody complex: Entity formed by the binding of an antibody to an antigen (also called an immune complex) that can then initiate further immune response

Antigen binding sites: Different tips on antibodies that allow the immune system to identify a wide range of antigens. Usually the antigen binds like a lock and key, one antigen to one antibody.

Antigenic variation: Some disease agents avoid the host's defenses by changing their surface proteins (antigens) so that the host's antibodies no longer recognize them and so they cannot be tagged for destruction. This has been well documented in trypanosomes and hypothesized in Bb.

Antigenic variety: Refers to the numerous serological types i.e., different strains of an organism. To be recognized as a separate strain, the surface antigens must be stable enough within a population to be identified as members of the same strain. Among strains, each one has to have a stable Ag surface protein identifier to be recognized.

Antihistamines: Agents that block the action of histamines. When histamines are causing sxs of an allergic reaction, antihistamines are often prescribed to ameliorate the discomfort.

Antimicrobial tolerance: Ability of a pathogen to resist damage by antibiotics (and host humors) by entering a state of transient, dormant, non-dividing existence. By being in the inactive state, they survive whereas their genetically identical cousins are killed by the antimicrobial or by the host's defenses. The dormant state makes them insensitive or refractory (or tolerant) to antibiotics. When such persistent cells can't be eliminated by the immune system, they are effectively a reservoir from which recurrent infection can develop. As long as the dormant Bb cells have the potential to reactivate into the free spirochete form, they have the potential to cause the sxs of disease. Persisters through antimicrobial tolerance may be the primary cause of relapsing and chronic infections.

Antineuronal antibodies: An antibody that attacks the nerve cells of the individual. This *self*-destruction might account for some of the wide ranging and intense neuropsychiatric sxs associated with Lyme. The human genome is about 90% identical to that of bacteria. Because of this molecular mimicry, when the immune system is assaulted and is in combat mode, it is understandable that some of the less specific components may mistake bacterial antigens for *self*-antigens. For organisms that are predisposed to nerve tissue, an autoimmune reaction might occur where neurons in the nervous system are mistakenly targeted for elimination. This phenomenon has been well-described in some children with a Strep infection. In other patients, association with Bb or Bartonella seems to result in this type of autoimmune reaction.

Antinuclear antibody: (ANA) Group of antibodies that react against normal cell protein. Found in a number of immune disorders such as lupus and other connective tissue diseases, ANA is likely present in many autoimmune conditions. Different patterns of ANA on immunofluorescent testing suggest different diseases like SLE, mixed connective tissue disease, RA, CREST, Raynaud's phenomenon, and others. ANA is present in lupus. If there is no elevation in ANA, the diagnosis is probably not lupus. ANA tests are best used to determine if there is more going on than meets the eye such as multiple etiologies or an underlying immune problem.

Antioxidants: Agents that prevent or inhibit oxidation. Oxidation reactions are a part of normal metabolism. These reactions can produce compounds called free radicals which are highly reactive and can become involved in chain reactions. When these reactions occur inside a cell, damage or death can result. Antioxidants inhibit these oxidative reactions and thereby limit the damage done to the organism. The antioxidants remove the free radicals and stop the chain reactions by becoming oxidized themselves. Antioxidants thereby help protect cells from damage. Excess oxidation seems to be a component of many disease states, so antioxidants in supplements are used to try to counter the damage. Examples of antioxidants include Vitamins C and E and glutathione. Too much antioxidant can be harmful and the science supporting the benefits is equivocal.

Antiphospholipid antibodies: Phospholipids are needed for normal blood clotting. In certain patients, the body mistakes normal *self*-phospholipids for foreign proteins and makes antibodies against them. In some circumstances, these patients are diagnosed with antiphospholipid syndrome which can manifest with hypercoagulation and miscarriage as well as numerous other sxs which can be similar to the clinical presentation of Lyme. Consider an antiphospholipid panel in patients with sxs of Raynaud's or otherwise cold extremities. Also, if the patient seems to have an autoimmune presentation, disorders of coagulation such as clots, or pregnancy complications including miscarriage, the possibility of antiphospholipid syndrome should be considered. There may be a cross-reactivity with Lyme antibodies.

Antiphospholipid syndrome: (Hughes syndrome) Antibodies against *self*-phospholipids can result in a disorder of coagulation often with excess clots and pregnancy complications including miscarriage. This condition can share a number of clinical manifestations with Lyme such as NP sxs and rheumatologic problems. There may be a cross-reactivity with Lyme antibodies. Antiphospholipid syndrome can stand alone but is often seen in the presence of other autoimmune conditions such as SLE. Can be hard to tell whether the clinical presentation is chronic Lyme or antiphospholipid syndrome, or both

Antipyretic: Fever-reducing agent

Antisocial personality: Pattern of disregard for and violation of the rights of others. Psychopaths and sociopaths. Sxs may begin in childhood. Callous, exploitative, with no remorse

Antitoxin: An antibody that is produced in response to a toxin. Can then bind and neutralize the toxin

Antivenom: (Antivenin) Term for the antibody produced if a toxin is from venom

Anus: Outlet for the rectum. Controls the elimination of feces and contains a series of sphincter muscles

Anxiety: Excessive feeling of nervousness, apprehension, uncertainty, worry, or fear. The feeling can be mild or paralyzing. The duration can be acute, intermittent, or chronic. Anxiety is associated with chemical changes in the body, especially in levels of cortisol and epinephrine. A number of the immune modulating chemicals have also been linked with increased anxiety levels. GAD manifests as excessive, chronic, usually daily anxiety and is a condition that can last for months or years. Anxiety is a common symptom in TBIs as it is with most disease state

Aorta: Main artery of the body carries blood from the heart to all body areas by way of its many branches

Aortic aneurysm: An aneurysm is a widening or dilation of a blood vessel, usually an artery, due to a weakening of the vessel wall. An abdominal aortic aneurysm is a wide pulsating mass located about midline near the back of the abdomen.

APGAR: System for evaluating an infant's physical condition at birth. Includes heart rate, respiration, muscle tone, response to stimuli, and color. Rated at 1 minute and again at 5 minutes after birth. Each factor is scored 0, 1, or 2 with a maximum total score of 10. Interpretation: 7 to 10 good to excellent, 4 to 6 fair, and less than 4 poor

Aphasia: Impairment of communication including speech due to some nervous system disorder or damage. Inability to produce or comprehend language

Aphonia: Loss of speech sounds from the larynx often causing a whisper

Aphthous ulcer: Oral lesion that is usually viral or secondary to excess acid. Small white ulcers surrounded by erythema that appear on the buccal mucosa and can be painful

Apical: Toward the apex or top of a structure

Apicomplexa: Large, diverse group of organisms that are almost entirely parasitic (no free-living). Formerly Sporozoa. Contain a group of organelles at the apical end of the organism called the *apical complex* that plays a role in the parasite-host interaction and how the parasite ultimately invades the host

Aplastic anemia: Aplasia is failure to develop normally. Aplastic anemia is caused by a deficit in RBC production due to bone marrow disorders.

Apnea: A period with no breathing with a pause of greater than 10 seconds is called apnea. Temporary cessation of breathing

Apoptosis: Disintegration of cells into particles that are then phagocytized. Programmed cell death where a cell breaks down and is cleaned up by the body's immune system. Allows for new cells to come into play. Without apoptosis there can be an overgrowth of certain cells such as in tumor formation. Apoptosis allows for the appropriate elimination of old or unneeded cells. This recycling of parts keeps the organism in balance i.e., homeostasis.

Appendicitis: Inflammation of the appendix

Appendix: Appendage, most often referring to the small piece of tissue attached to the cecum at the juncture of the small and large intestines

Apoplexy: Outdated term for stroke or bleeding into any organ

Apposition: Ability to put two parts in contact. Opposable thumbs allow humans to place the thumb in touch with the fingers of the same hand.

Apraxia: An inability to execute purposeful, previously known acts despite physical ability and willingness. Neurologic disorder in which the patient is unable to move or perform a requested task even though the command is understood and she is agreeable. Speech apraxia is trouble saying words correctly and consistently. There can be a rearrangement of sounds so that potato becomes topato.

Arachnid: Animal with 8 legs as an adult and no wings or antennae. Simple rather than complex eyes. Two main body segments: abdomen and cephalothorax which combines head and thorax. Includes: spiders, harvestmen, scorpions, ticks, and mites. Many are disease vectors.

Artemesia: (Artemisia) Version of a Chinese herb used to treat malaria and babesiosis. Many other spellings possible

Artemisia: Active herb found in artemesia and Arteminisin

Arteminisin: Version of a Chinese herb used to treat malaria and babesiosis

Arteritis: Inflammation of an artery

Artery: Vessel that moves blood AWAY from the heart under pressure that often can be felt as a pulse

Arthralgia: Discomfort, pain, or tenderness in a joint

Arthritis: Inflammation of a joint usually involving discomfort and limited function

Ascites: Accumulation of free fluid in the abdomen usually from liver disease

Aseptic: Germ-free. Without life forms

Aspartate transaminase: (AST, formerly SGOT) A liver enzyme that increases when there is damage to liver cells. Transaminases are a measure of cell integrity and AST serves as a biomarker of liver injury. If the hepatic cell is injured, AST will increase in the blood as it spills out of the cell. Similar to ALT in that both are enzymes in the liver cells that can be spilled into the circulation if the cells are damaged. NOT as specific to the liver as is ALT, AST is sometimes used to measure red cell damage as well as injury to heart cells.

Asperger's syndrome: Part of the autism spectrum of disorders. Condition primarily characterized by impaired social interactions. In contrast to other types of autism, there are no significant delays in language, cognitive, or developmental skills. In fact, many Asperger's patients are exceedingly intelligent and able to focus intensely for long periods within their area of interest. Severity may vary.

Aspirate: To draw in or out by suction. A foreign body can be aspirated into the nose. Aspiration pneumonia can be due to breathing GI contents into the lung. Fluid or tissue can be drawn from a cavity or organ for diagnostic or therapeutic purposes.

Assault: Intentional physical attack

AST: Aspartate transaminase

Asthenia: Loss or lack of strength. Weakness or debility, often from muscular or cerebellar disease

Asthma: Increased responsiveness of the tracheobronchial tree to various stimuli which results in paroxysmal constriction of the airways. Can be associated with infection, allergies, and irritants. Asthma can present with wheeze, cough, or no obvious symptoms aside from shortness of breath. A susceptible airway is triggered by a stimulus to constrict in paroxysms usually causing wheezing, which can progress to significant dyspnea.

Astigmatism: Inability of the eye to focus incoming light on one focal point in the retina due to differences in the curvature of the lens or cornea

Astrocytes: (Astroglia) Star-shaped glial cells of the brain and spinal cord. They provide biochemical support for the endothelial cells that form the BBB. They also supply nutrients to nervous tissue, stabilize extracellular ion balance, repair brain tissue after injury, release neurotransmitters, facilitate calcium communication channels, and signal neurons. Bb may alter the number of astrocytes.

Asymmetry: Lack of equality or balance between parts. One side is not the same as the other.

Ataxia: Deficiency in muscle coordination especially when voluntary muscle movements are attempted. Speech ataxia is due to muscle incoordination, usually a cerebellar problem.

Atelectasis: Deflated or collapsed lung tissue. Incomplete expansion of the lung can cause an airless condition that can result in collapse. There is no oxygen to be had in the area of atelectasis since there is no air there. Can be due to obstruction or infection. Dull to percussion with decreased or absent breath sounds

Atopic dermatitis: Inflammatory, chronically relapsing, pruritic skin eruption that is considered a type of eczema. The skin reacts abnormally and easily to irritation.

Atopy: Predisposition to develop Type I hypersensitivity reactions. May be a genetic susceptibility. The term can be used to refer to any IgE-mediated reaction or only to those that are excessive.

Atovaquone: (Mepron) Antiprotozoal agent used to treat malaria and is also effective against Babesia. Does not cross the BBB. Must take with fatty foods, otherwise is poorly absorbed. The product label has a horrendous list of AEs but these are likely due to the initial studies being done on late-stage AIDS patients. Hits only B. *microti,* not B. *duncani*

Atresia: Absence, restriction, or closure of a normal body opening or tube. Atresia can be congenital, surgical, traumatic, or metabolic.

Atrophy: A wasting or decrease in size of an organ or tissue. The wasting away of the skin can be caused by many mechanisms including cell death, resorption, diminished replenishment of cells, ischemia, pressure, poor nutrition, or hormone changes. The skin will appear thin, shiny, and translucent with decreased furrows. Repeated local steroid use can cause atrophy.

Attention deficit disorder: (ADD) Condition characterized by inattention, distractability, disorganization, procrastination, and forgetfulness. There is little or no hyperactivity or impulsivity.

Attention deficit hyperactivity disorder: (ADHD) Neurobehavioral condition characterized by inattention, hyperactivity, and impulsiveness.

Attention span: The ability to focus and maintain concentration on the environment

Attenuate: Lessen, decrease, weaken

Atypical autism: Part of the ASD, also called pervasive developmental disorder (PDD not otherwise specified or PDD-NOS). Probably the most common of the PDD diagnoses. Presents with significant social and communication deficits. The child will act differently than other kids his age. These patients do not connect well with others and have trouble reading expressions and social cues. They don't know how to respond when others laugh or cry. Thinking is quite literal and concrete with no sarcasm, irony, or figurative language. They do not babble, have delayed or limited speech, often repeat words, and have trouble with pronouns. They have poor non-verbal communication and a very narrow set of interests.

Auditory acuity: Sharpness or clarity of hearing

Augmentin: Brand name of a combination antibiotic with a broad-spectrum -cidal PCN and a β-lactamase inhibitor (amoxicillin and clavulanic acid)

Aura: A subjective sensation that precedes a paroxysmal attack. For example, before a seizure or migraine the patient may have an aura such as sensory, visual, or olfactory hallucinations.

Auscultation: Process of listening for sounds within the body

Autism: Part of the autism spectrum. Symptoms often start in infancy and are usually apparent by age two and include withdrawal, unresponsiveness, and impaired communication. Some live chaotically with no routine, while others stick rigidly to repetitive behaviors. Some have a compulsion for uniformity in their environment with everything precisely ordered. Infants may fail to react to touch or affection with a total lack of responsiveness. Some repeated behaviors can be self-destructive with head banging, eye scratching, or hair pulling. Arm flapping is not uncommon. Autistic kids can "look right through you" as though others aren't there. Both verbal and non-verbal language is impaired and they may repeat a word or sound over and over like an echo. These patients range from functional to total incapacity as they get older.

Autism-like disorder: While the controversy persists over the relationship between autism and Lyme, children with Lyme often present with an autism-like syndrome. In these cases, when the Lyme is treated with appropriate antibiotics the autism symptoms can regress.

Autism spectrum of disorders (ASD or Autism spectrum disorder or PDD) Pervasive developmental delay in multiple basic functions such as socialization and interaction causing severe impairment in thinking, feeling, communication, eye contact, and ability to relate. Includes autism, atypical autism, Asperger's syndrome, Rett syndrome, and CDD. These last two are less common and sometimes included in the spectrum and sometimes not. Since it is a spectrum, not all kids show the same signs, symptoms, or clinical course. One child may not fit exactly into any one category since there is such a wide range of involvement and severity. In addition, a child may shift on the spectrum as she does better or worse over time.

Autoantigen: Antigens on the host's own cells that should be recognized as *self*

Autoimmune disease: (Autoimmunity) Conditions that result when the body cannot distinguish *self* from non-*self*. The body attacks itself and the overall inflammation can grow out-of-control. Everyone has some degree of autoimmunity but usually the body keeps the response under control. Some components are genetic. The degree of autoimmune response may depend on the condition of the immune system when it confronts yet another insult. Autoimmunity can damage joints, skin, blood vessels, lungs, kidneys, heart, and brain. The condition can be chronic with flares and remissions.

Autoimmunity: Body produces antibodies against its own tissues. Abs bind to *self*-antigens activating complement and other biochemicals causing damage to organs, blood vessels, and other tissues.

Automatisms: In infants, reflex-like behaviors performed without thought

Autonomic nervous system: The ANS regulates the involuntary functions of internal organs. Working below the level of consciousness, the ANS controls the operation of the viscera including HR, digestion, micturation, RR, salivation, perspiration, pupil size, and sexual arousal. A few of these operations can also be influenced to a degree by conscious control like the respiratory rate and urination. The ANS has been categorized many ways including motor versus sensory, efferent versus afferent, PSNS versus SNS, and inhibitory versus excitatory.

Autosplenectomy: Situation where the spleen is so damaged, usually by fibrotic scarring, that it shrinks and becomes impalpable with limited function

A vitamin: (Retinol) Fat-soluble vitamin needed for vision in dim light, mucosal epithelial integrity, tooth and bone development, normal growth and maturation, and healthy endocrine function. Found in fresh water fish, fish liver oils, liver, eggs, dairy, and green, yellow, and orange vegetables. Deficiency due to prolonged dietary scarcity can result in night blindness, trouble adapting to the dark, and growth retardation. Too much Vitamin A can also become a problem.

Axilla: Under arm. Armpit

Axon: Long, slender process of a neuron that conducts impulses AWAY from the cell

Azithromycin: (Zithromax) Intracellular macrolide antibiotic. Excellent choice against Bb when used in combination with a cell wall antimicrobial

Azoles: Cyst-busting antibiotics such as metronidazole (Flagyl) and tinidazole (Tindamax). Can be an important part of combination regimen against Bb. Also may be effective against protozoa like Babesia. May be difficult to tolerate. Both Tindamax and Flagyl may be better tolerated if pulsed. Comparing Flagyl and Tindamax: Flagyl hits only the cystic form of Bb, whereas Tindamax is believed to hit all three life forms of Borrelia including the spirochetal form with a cell wall, the cell wall deficient L-form, and the cystic form.

Azotemia: Presence of nitrogen compounds, like BUN, in the blood. Increasing azotemia suggests decreasing renal function.

B

Babesia: (Formerly called Piroplasma) Tick-borne protozoa that infects the red blood cells of mammals

Babesia *divergens*: Primary Babesia parasite causing disease in humans in Europe

Babesia *duncani*: In addition to Babesia *microti*, causes disease in humans in the US. Does not respond to the same treatments as B. *microti*

Babesia *microti*: Primary Babesia parasite causing disease in humans in the US. Some recent literature calls B. *microti* by a new name: Theileria *microti*.

Babesiosis: Disease caused by the blood parasite Babesia characterized by high fevers, rigorous chills, fatigue, aches including headache, and air hunger. Different strains of the pathogen might present somewhat differently, with one causing more respiratory problems and others resulting in more anemia. Common TBI co-infection

Babinski response: Abnormal reflex. If the great toe dorsiflexes upon stimulation of the plantar surface of the foot, then there is a potential upper motor neuron lesion in the area of L4, L5, S1, or S2. The Babinski sign is abnormal after age 2.

Bacterin vaccine: Killed pathogen developed as a vaccine

Bacteriocidal: Antimicrobial that kills the pathogen

Bacteriostatic: Antibiotic that inhibits or slows the growth or reproduction of bacteria without directly killing them. They work by interfering with protein production, by impeding DNA or RNA replication, or by impairing some other metabolic process. To be effective these antibiotics must work with the immune system in order to decrease the bacterial load. The number of bacteria lessens over time because they cannot grow or reproduce. Some -static drugs become -cidal at high doses.

Bactrim: (Septra) Brand name of the combination of sulfa and trimethoprim. Sulfa drug thought to be effective against malaria, babesiosis, and possibly bartonellosis. Often used for UTIs, traveler's diarrhea, and bronchitis. Watch for allergies.

Balance: State of stability or equilibrium. Ability to maintain the center of gravity over the base of support. Normal balance allows for a position to be maintained both when the body is static and when in motion. Balance can be significantly affected in Lyme and other TBIs.

Banderol: Herbal that might impede biofilm formation

Bartonella-like organism: The bartonellosis transmitted by ticks may be due to Bartonella-like organisms (BLOs) and not the traditionally implicated B. *henslea*.

Bartonellosis: Disease caused either by pathogens of the genus Bartonella or by Bartonella-like organisms. The resulting syndromes can affect multiple organ systems including the immune system, GI tract, skin and subcutaneous tissue, coagulation and circulation, musculoskeletal, and especially CNS. NP sxs can be severe and incapacitating. Diseases due to Bartonella species are found worldwide and symptoms include fever, chills, headache, gastritis, weight loss, neurologic problems, sore throat, lymphadenitis, and red, papular skin lesions. Distinctive features of bartonellosis include severe pain in the tibia and sole, disproportionate neuropsychiatric symptoms, violaceous striae, and subcutaneous nodules. In the northeastern US, Bartonella may be a more common pathogen than Bb.

Basal ganglia: Masses of grey matter deep in the cerebral hemispheres of the brain. Involved with the subconscious aspects of voluntary motion so that the individual does not need to think about performing all components of every movement. The BG enables the acquisition of motor routines and habits. The BG will select which of several motor options to perform. Lesions in this area can cause abnormal movements such as those found in rheumatic fever, Parkinson's, and Huntington's disease. The BG has some function in emotion and behavior control and is linked to certain features of Tourette's and OCD. Hypothetically, the BG may be involved with abnormal movements and behaviors seen with several of the TBIs.

Basophil: Granulocytic WBC involved with inflammation, histamine, and allergies. May be the circulating form of the mast cell

B cell: Type of agranulocytic lymphocytic WBC. Activated B cells differentiate into either Ab-producing plasma cells that secrete soluble immunoglobulins or memory cells that survive in the body for years and recall Ags. Memory cells allow for more rapid immune response upon future exposure to the same antigen. After a B cell comes into contact with an antigen, the cell begins to mature and is able to independently identify foreign antigens. All B cells are antigen-specific and respond to only one foreign protein.

Behcet's disease: An immune-mediated, multisystem, chronic, recurrent syndrome marked by ulcers in the mouth and genitals, iritis, uveitis, arthritis, and thrombophlebitis. Joint pain, along with CNS and heart problems, may occur later in the clinical course. Lyme has some common features.

Bell's palsy: Facial paralysis of sudden onset due to impairment of the facial nerve (7th cranial nerve). In the past most cases were said to be of unknown etiology, but today many cases are associated with LD. Bell's palsy often presents with one-sided paralysis of the facial muscles innervated by CN 7. The patient may not be able to control salivation or lacrimation and in severe cases cannot close the eye on the affected side. Recovery is variable and if the eye cannot close it may need to be patched with moisture ointment.

Bias: A prejudice or inclination in one direction that causes the holder of the bias to maintain a perspective at the expense of equally valid alternatives

Bicarbonate: (Form of HCO$_3$) pH buffer helping to maintain acid-base balance in the body

Bicillin: (Benzathine PCN) An IM PCN, cell wall antibiotic, commonly used to treat Lyme

Bile: Enzyme-filled fluid made in the liver and stored and released by the GB into the duodenum where it emulsifies fats and aids in digestion

Biliary: Pertaining to bile or the gall bladder

Bilirubin: (BR) Breakdown product of heme which is part of the hemoglobin in RBCs. Bilirubin is taken up into the liver cells (hepatocytes), conjugated (modified to make it water soluble), and then secreted into the bile. Bile is then excreted into the intestine where the bilirubin helps give stool its brown color. The pigments in bilirubin also give urine its yellow hue and are responsible for the yellow-brown shades of bruises. The liver clears the blood of bilirubin. An increase in total bilirubin can cause jaundice and dark urine. Conjugated bilirubin is also called direct bilirubin and comparing levels of conjugated and unconjugated bilirubin may help tell the source location of a liver problem. Many neonates have excessive bilirubin which can be entirely separate from any consideration with TBIs.

Binge eating disorder: Chronic, excessive eating without purging. A large quantity of food is consumed in a short period of time. Binge eaters are often obese. Bingeing may be associated with addiction to carbohydrates, compulsions, and stress relief. This makes sense since people tend to binge on "comfort foods" that have high amounts of processed carbs, fat, and salt. Binge eaters cannot seem to stop eating.

Bioavailability: The rate and extent to which a drug enters the circulation and therefore has access to the site of intended action. Measurement of the fraction of the dose that reaches the systemic circulation is used to quantify absorption. After the drug is in the circulation, it almost immediately begins to clear and the plasma concentration decreases steadily after it reaches its peak.

Biofeedback: Training program used to help control the involuntary ANS. Biofeedback has been used to treat anxiety, pain, and high blood pressure. The patient is connected to an instrument that monitors things such as heart rate, temperature, brain waves, muscle contraction, or respiration. By becoming aware of one parameter, the person can be trained to attempt to reproduce the desired physiologic condition.

Biofilm: A biofilm is an aggregate of microorganisms in which cells adhere to one another and sometimes to a host surface. Organisms attach forming a bladder-like structure that may be protective of pathogens and allow nutrients and communication signals to pass. This shields the organisms from antibiotics and host immune response. Environmental triggers such as microbial crowding, nutrient depletion, and the introduction of antibiotics might promote biofilm formation. Both Bb and Bartonella are thought to form biofilms and this might explain the difficulty in treating these infections in some patients.

Biopsy: Obtaining a sample for analysis that is hopefully representative of the entire tissue. Usually done to make a diagnosis. Samples can be obtained surgically or by aspiration with a needle.

Biot's breathing: Several short breaths followed by long, irregular periods of apnea. Biot's breathing is seen in cases of significant increases in intracranial pressure.

Bipolar disorder: (Manic depression) In contrast to unipolar depression where sadness is the primary or sole feeling, the emotions in bipolar disorder alternate between highs and lows. The mood swings from euphoria to despair with spontaneous recoveries in between. The episodes are cyclic, although in most patients one extreme will dominate.

Bladder: Sac. Often a receptacle for secretions or for the storage of material

Bleb: Fluid-filled blister or bladder-like structure

Blister: A collection of fluid under or in the epidermis. Blisters can be due to friction or inflammation.

BLO: Bartonella-like organism

Blood: Cell-containing fluid that circulates throughout the body, pumped by the heart and distributed throughout the body by way of vessels. Used to transport nutrients, electrolytes, water, medicines, cells, immune responders, oxygen, and wastes. Blood is about half plasma and half cells: red, white, and platelets with RBCs predominating. Blood also contains clotting factors including fibrinogen. Blood can transmit diseases such as Babesia which is known to be transmitted though transfusions and is currently a public health problem.

Blood brain barrier: The capillary walls in the brain have special characteristics that prevent most of the potentially harmful molecules from moving out of the blood into the brain or CSF. Of course, this barricade also prevents some antibiotics and certain immune cells from entering an infected brain and helping get rid of pathogens.

Blood smear: A thin layer of peripheral blood is smeared onto a slide, stained, and examined under a microscope. Technicians can look at the type, number, and shape of white or red cells as well as platelets for diagnostic purposes. Evidence of some parasites such as malaria can also be noted. The most diagnostic findings with TBIs are Maltese crosses in red cells, indicative of babesiosis, and morulae in various white cells seen with Ehrlichia and Anaplasma.

Body dysmorphic disorder: An obsession with appearance and the feeling that the body does not measure up to unrealistic standards. This condition is most common in teen girls who think they are fat irrespective of their actual weight. This disorder may interfere with normal interactions with others. Teen males may become obsessed with body building, leading to excessive weight lifting, steroids, and protein shakes that can damage the kidneys.

Boggy: Soft and spongy

Bolus: 1) A mass of food ready to be swallowed. 2) A quantity of a substance such as a dye or medicine that can be dispensed all-at-once as an injection (IV, IM) or pushed over time as an infusion

Borderline personality: A disturbed personality with long-standing patterns of unstable or turbulent emotions leading to difficult relationships with others. Tend to have all-or-nothing thinking, mood disturbances, and impulsivity. These patients have an unstable self-image and they believe they were deprived in childhood and often feel empty, angry, and entitled. They may be relentless seekers of care. This is a very common disorder and can begin evolving in childhood. Borderline personalities can be very hard to like.

Borrelia *burgdorferi*: Causative pathogen of one variation of borreliosis, i.e., Lyme disease

Borrelial lymphocytoma: Discrete, purple bump appearing on the skin of the ear, nipple, or scrotum. Described in some cases of LD in Europe

Borreliosis: Refers to several diseases caused by pathogens in the genus Borrelia. Examples include Lyme borreliosis due to the microbe Borrelia *burgdorferi,* tick relapsing fever caused by Borrelia *hermsii,* and STARI from B. *lonestari.* Distinctions are not always clear, either between the species or the clinical syndromes.

Bradycardia: Heart rate too slow for the individual and circumstances

Bradypnea: Slow respiratory rate. Seen in end-stage disease, increased intracranial pressure, diabetic coma, and drugs that depress respiration

Brain fog: Probably the most common of the NP manifestations associated with LD and may be due either to an encephalitis or to the release of cytokines and other humors in response to the infection. Difficult to define but may include cognitive dysfunction with slow, weak, and inaccurate thought processes. Associated with confusion, forgetfulness, disorientation, and difficulty concentrating. Brain fog is a complaint in a high percentage of Lyme patients and is also commonly found in babesiosis, bartonellosis, and M. *fermentans* infection. The patient with brain fog complains of mental confusion and lack of mental clarity. Usually the fog is constant and doesn't wax and wane. The fog can clear with treatment. Brain fog is totally subjective and there are no physical findings. The person usually realizes there is something wrong with how they are thinking, but may be apathetic.

Brainstem: Base of the brain that connects the cerebral hemispheres with the spinal cord and is responsible for many processes that are independent of conscious thought such as breathing and heart rate. Input from all parts of the body goes back to the brain via the brainstem. CNs 3 through 12 originate there. The brainstem is an integrator, coordinating the heart rate, respiration, sensation, alertness, awareness, sleep cycles, and consciousness. The brainstem also has a role in proprioception, pain, itching, and temperature.

Brand: Name of a product designed to set it apart from all the others in the class. For example Kleenex and Puffs are brands of tissue. Brand names are designed to be easily recognized and remembered. In contrast, when selecting generic drug names, the non-brand name is purposely devised to be unpronounceable and impossible to recall so that doctors have no choice but to write for the brand product.

Bronchiolitis: Inflammation of the bronchioles in the lower pulmonary tree, usually caused by viruses such as RSV. The child presents with what appears to be a URI but then quickly deteriorates to respiratory compromise with wheezes, crackles, tachypnea, expiratory obstruction, tachycardia, hacking cough, circumoral cyanosis, and retractions. Bronchiolitis usually is diagnosed in children less than 18 months. They usually have no fever, but can be quite lethargic.

Bronchitis: Acute inflammation of the tracheobronchial tree which can be due to infections or irritations like dusts or fumes. Bronchitis is usually preceded by the signs and symptoms of a URI such as coryza (inflammation of the nasal passages with profuse clear discharge), malaise, mild fever, chills, aches, and sore throat. The beginning of the cough is probably the onset of the bronchitis. The cough starts dry and non-productive but soon sputum might be raised.

Brudzinski's sign: In meningitis flexion of the neck causes involuntary flexion of the knees. Sign of meningeal irritation. A positive test results when forward motion of the neck is impeded by pain and resistance suggesting meningeal inflammation.

Bruise: Ecchymosis, contusion, or blood in the skin. Bruising can be due to trauma, a problem with tissue integrity, or coagulation deficits. Blood is released from the vessels and if close enough to the surface will be visible under the skin.

Bruit: An audible murmur or blowing sound that indicates a problem with blood flow due to narrowing, ballooning, or other pathology. A vascular noise that sounds like a murmur that suggests an aneurysm. Common sites for the auscultation of bruits are the neck (carotid artery) and the abdomen (aortic aneurysm).

BSK medium: Barbour-Stoenner-Kelly formulation used to culture Bb, which is an exceedingly fastidious organism

Bulimia: Eating disorder marked by recurrent binge eating and then purging either by induced vomiting or diarrhea. The bulimic eating pattern consists of recurrent episodes of bingeing followed by purging. Bulimics may go to great lengths to hide their behavior. Like binge eaters, they can't stop eating, but they follow their binges with purging. They are also prone to using laxatives and fat blockers.

Bulla: (Bullae is plural.) Large (greater than 0.5 cm) lesions filled with serous fluid. A good example is a 2nd degree burn.

BUN: Blood urea nitrogen measures the amount of nitrogen in the blood in the form of urea. Useful measure of kidney function, hydration, and nutritional status. Only BUN will suggest the patient's hydration level, and readings can change quickly in response to fluids.

As a baseline test, BUN might be used to help make sure the kidney is healthy enough to handle the proposed treatment regimen.

Bunion: Enlargement of the bone and tissue of the 1st MTP. Usually the head of the metatarsal forms a large bump and the big toe may angle laterally toward the 2nd toe.

Bursitis: Inflammation of a bursa. A bursa is a sac or cavity lined with a synovial membrane and filled with fluid, which has the consistency of raw egg whites. The bursae provide a cushion for the joint and decrease friction allowing for free movement. Bursae can become inflamed due to stress on the joint, irritants, or infection. The most common sites of bursitis are the shoulder, knee, and elbow.

B1 vitamin: (Thiamine) Necessary coenzyme for carbohydrate metabolism. Also may boost the immune system, improve mood and cognition, increase energy, decrease anxiety, and improve memory. B1 has been used in Alzheimer's patients in attempts to decrease symptoms. More than half of alcoholics are thiamine deficient and treatment is critical before withdrawal to prevent encephalitis. Thiamine is found in yeasts, grains, beans, nuts, and meat. Supplements can be administered orally or by IV.

B2 vitamin: (Riboflavin) Essential coenzyme in oxidation reactions. Needed for metabolism of fats, carbohydrates, and proteins, as well as energy production. Important for tissue repair. B2 is found in milk, cheese, leafy vegetables, liver, yeast, legumes, and almonds. This vitamin is destroyed by exposure to light. When neonates are treated with light therapy for jaundice, the light breaks down not only the bilirubin, but also the riboflavin. These kids will need supplements or they can experience growth delays, failure to thrive, and epithelial lesions. Otherwise, deficiency is rare. Any excess is eliminated in the urine.

B3 vitamin: (Niacin) Needed as a coenzyme in carbohydrate and fat metabolism and is involved in numerous biochemical processes within the cell including DNA repair and production of steroid hormones in the adrenals. Found in a variety of foods including liver, chicken, beef, fish, cereal, peanuts, legumes, milk, eggs, yeast, mushrooms, and many fruits and vegetables. Deficiency is rare in the US, but when it occurs there are skin lesions and inflammation of the mouth and tongue.

B9 vitamin: (Folic acid) Cofactor in nucleic acid metabolism and in the formation of heme and its incorporation into hemoglobin. Especially important in pregnancy because of its role in cell division and growth. Deficiency in pregnancy can cause neural tube defects in the developing fetus. B9 is involved in the synthesis and repair of DNA. Deficiency can also be associated with macrocytic anemia. When folic acid levels are low, the patient may experience nerve damage with weakness and numbness, mental confusion, forgetfulness, cognitive deficits, depression, sore tongue, irritability, and behavior problems. Folic acid is found in leafy greens, beans, and eggs. Often deficient in alcoholics

B12 vitamin: (Cyanocobalamin or cobalamin) Needed by all cells but especially critical in the manufacture of RBCs and for proper function of the GI tract and nervous system. Important for both RNA and DNA synthesis. Contains cobalt which is rare in biological systems. Found in animal products, so extreme vegetarians and vegans have to be careful. Because B12 is so intimately related to brain and nervous system function and because so many TBIs manifest CNS symptoms, adequate B12 levels should provide the best chance for recovery in these patients. B12 is thought to enable normal function of the PNS, help support effective immune function by inducing better day-night cycles of immune responses, foster better sleep, and regulate normal energy production. Adequate B12 seems to be needed for neurologic stability and is currently being assessed in Alzheimer's patients to try to enhance nervous tissue function, improve cognition, memory, and mood, and to increase strength and energy.

C

Cachexia: State of very poor health with wasting as seen in AIDS, cancer, COPD, etc.

Calcium (Ca): Mineral essential for normal bone growth and metabolism and proper development of teeth. Ca is involved with the parathyroid gland, Ca-P balance, many enzyme reactions, acid-base equilibrium, lactation, nerve and muscle activity, normal heart function, the work of hormones, clotting, and membrane permeability. Usually Ca levels in the blood remain fairly constant because if levels get low, more calcium will be pulled from bone to compensate. Calcium needs an activator like Vitamin D to be functional. Deficits cause brittle bones and teeth, dental loss, tetany (muscle spasms due to nerve dysfunction), twitching, excessive bleeding, and irritability. If there is no calcium, there is no clotting. More calcium is needed in pregnant and lactating females. Calcium deficiencies may be more common in kids who cannot eat dairy due to lactose intolerance.

Callus: Skin can thicken in areas of persistent pressure like the ball, heel, and sole of the foot. Usually this thick skin is painless.

Candidiasis: (Thrush, Monilia) Yeast overgrowth in the mouth, vagina, or elsewhere from the Candida genus of fungus. Usually grows on moist surfaces. Can get in the blood and cause systemic infection. Monilia was the genus name of the fungi now called Candida.

Canine Lyme: Syndrome in dogs caused by Bb infection resulting in shifting leg lameness, joint swelling, fever, large nodes, and may also include metabolic abnormalities, blood dyscrasias, edema, and less frequently, myocardial disease with dysrhythmia. High morbidity and mortality

Carbon dioxide: (CO_2) By-product of cellular respiration in animals. Derived from breakdown of organic material. CO_2 travels in the blood from the tissue to the lungs where it is exhaled. In the form of bicarbonate, acts as a buffer to maintain normal acid/base balance. The body pH can be affected by foods, medicines, and the function of both the kidneys and lungs. Significant changes in CO_2, might indicate either metabolic or respiratory acid or base imbalances.

Carcinoma: Tumor in epithelial tissue. Neoplasm that can infiltrate and metastasize

Cardiomyopathy: Direct damage to the heart muscle (myocardium) due to disease or other modes of injury. Cardiomyopathy can impede the normal, effective contraction of the heart. Damage to the muscle can lead to fibrosis which can restrict motion. The sequelae can include metabolic disequilibrium that impairs normal efficiency. The degree of damage will determine the effect on function. Lyme is theorized to cause direct harm to the heart muscle in some cases.

Cardiovascular fitness: The heart's capacity to deliver blood to working muscles and their ability to use it. To improve this parameter the patient must exercise at an intensity that increases HR and respiration. Fitness progresses with slow and steady advancement over time.

Carditis: Nonspecific term referring to inflammation of several layers of the heart and can include pericarditis, myocarditis, or endocarditis

Caretaker: Any person who aids or helps a TBI patient. Can include parents, guardians, family, or friends involved in providing for the health, welfare, maintenance, or protection of the patient. In this text, the caretaker is usually viewed separately from the HCPs.

Carpal tunnel syndrome: Compression of the median nerve in the wrist. Can be unilateral or bilateral presenting with paresthesias, pain, and weakness in the radial palmar aspects of the hand. Pain can be incapacitating and is often more severe at night.

Carrier: An individual who is infected with a disease agent and able to spread that agent to others but shows no sign of clinical illness himself

Cartilage: A dense form of connective tissue made largely of collagen. Firm, compact, and able to withstand considerable pressure. The tip of the nose, the external ear, nasal septum, articular covering of bone, the area between the ribs and sternum, and tubes like the larynx, trachea, and bronchi are all made largely of cartilage. Cartilage does not have its own nerve or blood supply. Most of the skeleton of an embryo is cartilage and it retains its structural support role in the skeleton of adults. In joints, cushions the ends of bones and allows for easier movement

Cascade: Process continuing through multiple steps with each step initiating the next

Case study: Anecdote

Catch 22: Illogical set of rules that perplex well-meaning folks at every turn. Absurd reasoning

Catecholamines: Bioactive molecules such as epinephrine and norepinephrine with strong effects on the NS, CVS, metabolic rate, temperature, and smooth muscle activity

CAT scan: Computed axial tomography forms a 3-D image from pictures taken around a single axis of rotation. Images are taken in slices and then reconstructed in multiple dimensions. Although more expensive and less available than plain X-rays, CAT scans can focus in on the area of interest and can distinguish different soft tissues, one from the other.

Caudad: Toward the tail

Caveat emptor: Latin for, "Let the buyer beware." Be careful of slick salespeople.

CD: Clusters of differentiation are groups of protein markers on the surface of white blood cells that serve to identify and classify the cell types. Each marker has a specific function within the system like passing along biochemical signals.

CD57: Marker used by some practitioners to determine when treatment of Lyme can be discontinued. CD57 identifies a subpopulation of NK (natural killer) T lymphocytes. These are thought to be suppressed ONLY in Lyme disease (and perhaps some cases of autism). Measurement of CD57 looks at this specific subpopulation of NK cells. Low counts are seen in active Lyme disease. So in theory, the lower the CD57 level, the more suppression of these Lyme-specific NK cells and the more active the Lyme disease. Overall, the lower the count, the sicker the patient. Some believe that treatment for Lyme is needed until CD57 is greater than 150. During treatment there may be only small changes observed until late in the course, when values might increase dramatically. Possibly, the lower the number when treatment is stopped, the more likely a relapse. CD57 should be correlated with the *clinical condition* of the patient. Children do not make NK cells in the same quantity as adults, therefore, CD57 may not be as useful in monitoring Borrelia activity in kids as it may be in adults.

Ceclor: Cefaclor

Cefaclor: (Ceclor) A cephalosporin, cell wall, -cidal antibiotic. Used in combination with intracellular agent against Lyme

Cefdinir: (Omnicef) A cephalosporin, cell wall, -cidal antibiotic. Good choice against Bb in combination with intracellular agent

Cefotaxime: (Claforan) A cephalosporin, cell wall, -cidal antibiotic. Use in combination with intracellular agent against Lyme. Penetrates BBB

Ceftriaxone: (Rocephin) A cephalosporin, cell wall, -cidal antibiotic. Commonly used IV in Lyme. Gallstone risk. Use in combination with intracellular agent against Bb

Cefuroxime: (Ceftin) A cephalosporin, cell wall, -cidal antibiotic. Use in combination with intracellular agent against Lyme. Indicated for use against Borrelia

Celiac disease: Autoimmune reaction to gluten, which is a protein found in grains like wheat and rye. Celiac disease seems to affect the small intestine and is probably genetic. This condition can lead to chronic diarrhea, failure to thrive, and fatigue. All the usual inflammatory signs may be present. Symptoms can be mild to severe. Celiac disease can interfere with the normal absorption of nutrients and cause short-term discomfort as well as long-term problems. Escalation of symptoms may be due to more aggressive autoimmunity. About 1% of the population has celiac disease.

Cellulitis: Inflammation of the connective tissue, which may be due to infection. This condition can be dangerous in diabetics who have slow wound healing, poor vasculature, muted sensation, and trouble with antibiotic penetration to distal areas. Cellulitis is usually red, hot, and swollen. If the lesion gets bigger, the infection is spreading.

Cell wall antibiotic: A number of diverse drugs that are effective because of their ability to interfere with the cell wall of the pathogen. The cell wall is essential to the viability of these organisms. With regard to TBIs, the cell wall antibiotics that are pertinent include: PCNs, CSs, and cell wall synthesis inhibitors such as vancomycin.

Central nervous system: Command center of the body in charge of coordinating overall physiologic processes. Includes the brain and spinal cord

Cephalad: Toward the head

Cephalosporins: Cell wall, -cidal, antibiotics similar to PCNs in structure but have a broader range of action. Third generation CSs get into CNS better than earlier formulations. Since similar to PCNs in structure, when an individual is allergic to PCNs she may also be allergic to CSs.

Cerebellum: Region of the brain below the cerebrum near the brainstem. Coordinates voluntary muscle movements but does not initiate movement. The frontal lobe tells all the muscles to move, but it's the cerebellum that actually synchronizes the activity. Controls the various characteristics of movement like speed, acceleration, and trajectory. The cerebellum also allows for the intricate fine muscular interactions that permit writing, dressing, eating, playing musical instruments, and the smooth tracking of the eye muscles. Also maintains posture, balance, coordination, and the timing of movements so that the body is able to subconsciously pull off the complicated synergy needed to walk or run. The cerebellum is also involved in attention span and the emotions of pleasure and displeasure in ways we do not yet clearly understand. If the patient's disease is causing a lack of coordination, a change in balance, or an inability to learn a new motor skill like a new dance step that would have been easily mastered before, consider involvement of the cerebellum.

Cerebral cortex: Grey matter of the brain

Cerebral edema: Accumulation of excess fluid in the intra and extracellular spaces around the brain. Can be due to masses, inflammation, toxins, or infections

Cerebral palsy: Group of non-progressive, but often changing, motor impairment syndromes secondary to problems in the brain during early stages of development. Symptom complex rather than one specific disease often accompanied by seizures, retardation, and various neurologic deficits

Cerebral spinal fluid: Watery cushion protecting the brain and spinal cord. Pressure of this fluid can change for many reasons including infection, bleeding, or trauma. A change in volume of intracranial contents is usually rapidly compensated by alteration in the amount of CSF. The fluid maintains pressure which can be measured and samples can be examined looking for signs of pathology such as infection. A spinal tap can be done to relieve elevated pressure but care must be taken that pressure is not lowered too rapidly since brain tissue can herniate. CSF does not clot.

Cerebrum: Largest part of the brain divided into two hemispheres separated by a deep fissure

Challenge: To determine if a medicine is effective or causing a side effect, the drug can be administered, withdrawn, and then re-administered to see what happens after each step. If the patient is getting better on the drug and relapses after the drug is stopped, that is valuable information. Likewise if the patient again feels better when the treatment is resumed, that adds even more insight. In terms of adverse events, if the problem goes away when the drug is stopped and returns when restarted, the problem could be the drug. Be careful rechallenging especially if the AE is an allergy or other potentially serious condition.

Charcot-Marie-Tooth: A pediatric, progressive, neural based atrophy of the muscles that are supplied by the peroneal nerves

Chelicerae: Apparatus inside the palps of the tick mouth that protect the internal hypostome, or central feeding tube

Chemokines: Cytokines that cause chemotaxis by attracting certain immune cells to assist in the defense response

Chemotaxis: Cells move toward higher concentrations of certain "alarm" chemicals

Cherry-pick: To pick only the best or most desirable ideas or those which support your views as you ignore the rest

Cheyne-Stokes respiration: Breathing in a cyclic pattern where bouts of deep breathing alternate with periods of apnea. Not uncommon in children. Apnea from 10 to 60 seconds is followed by increased depth and frequency of respiration in older kids and adults. May be due to brain damage

Chiari malformation: Parts of the cerebellum protrude through the cranium into the spinal canal causing hydrocephalus

Chickenpox: (Varicella) Highly contagious viral disease caused by HHV-3, also called varicella zoster virus. Spread by airborne particulates from sneezing or coughing or by direct contact with rash secretions. Manifests with itchy vesicular rash in various stages of healing. Other sxs include myalgia, fever, headache, and malaise.

Childhood disintegrative disorder: One of the autism spectrum disorders. While relatively rare in general practice, a number of children with this diagnosis suggest the possibility of an association with infectious processes. Unlike other syndromes in the autism spectrum, CDD presents with a late onset of symptoms in a previously normal child. First signs occur between 3 and 10-years-old. These kids were developing normally when they regress. Attained skills are lost. The reversion can be rapid over days or weeks, but can take longer. Older kids can even ask what is happening to them as they watch themselves deteriorate. After a period of normal development, the child loses both expressive and receptive language skills, social interactions decline, and the ability for self-care is gone. There is loss of control over bladder and bowels and diminished play and motor skills. They have increasing problems with social interactions as they become progressively more retarded. Retardation can then become severe and CDD is considered a low functioning form of autism. Hallucinations and seizures may be present along with repetitive behaviors.

Chlamydia: Genus of intracellular parasites known to cause various diseases such as pneumonia. May be a TBI-co-infection

Chloramphenicol: Broad spectrum bacteriostatic antibiotic. Considered first-line for RMSF in pregnant women, patients with impaired renal function, or the severely ill. Crosses BBB

Chloride: (Cl) Electrolyte needed to maintain a normal fluid balance

Cholecystitis: Inflammation of gallbladder causing colicky pain due to spasms in the tubes of the biliary system

Cholestatic hepatitis: Inflammation and congestion of the bile ducts and the liver

Chloroquine: Quinine derivative occasionally used against babesiosis

Chorea: (Choreiform movement) Involuntary muscle movements. Usually brief, purposeless, non-repetitive movements of the distal extremities or face

Chronic: On-going, persistent

Chronic bronchitis: On-going inflammation of the membranes of the bronchi which carry the air in and out of the lung. This type of COPD causes hypertrophy of mucus glands with damage to the cilia lining the respiratory tract. Almost always mucus in the airways corresponds with a severe ventilation/perfusion imbalance. There is a frequent productive cough and exertional dyspnea.

Chronic fatigue & immune dysfunction syndrome: (CFIDS) Most recent name and acronym for what was traditionally called chronic fatigue syndrome

Chronic fatigue syndrome: (CFS or CFIDS) Crushing, disabling fatigue with headache, sensitivity to light, and widespread pain. Fatigue often devastating and overwhelming. While the individual sxs can wax and wane, overall the syndrome can be incapacitating. Can be hard to distinguish from Bb and some clinicians believe that all CFS is Lyme, just unsubstantiated by lab testing. CFS has been attributed to a number of other pathogens such as EBV. Very recently yet another viral etiology was suggested but that theory has also gone by the wayside.

Chronic Lyme: Syndrome of Lyme sxs beyond a short acute period of about 30 days. Alternatively called Category 4 Lyme, Persistent Lyme, Intractable Lyme, Recalcitrant Lyme, On-going Lyme, Unresponsive Lyme, Major Lyme, Post-Lyme, Long-term Lyme, and many other labels. Most ILADS members believe chronic Lyme is due to persistent Borrelia infection which may be complicated by co-infections and altered in its presentation by damage to the immune system or inadequate immune response.

Chronic obstructive pulmonary disease: COPD is long-term airway obstruction that decreases the lung's ability for efficient gas exchange. Divided into two primary presentations: chronic bronchitis and emphysema, but most patients have aspects of both. Both types of COPD present with dyspnea on exertion (DOE), hypoxemia, and abnormal PFTs.

Cinchonism: Quinine toxicity. Cinchonism is a cluster of symptoms which can occur after repeated doses with quinine. Quinine has a complex and poorly understood MOA, but appears to affect many body systems. Even at therapeutic doses the patient can develop cinchonism: ringing in the ears, headache, nausea, disturbed vision, and nausea. With on-going or higher doses, cinchonism can progress and can be fatal.

Ciprofloxacin: (Cipro) Fluoroquinolone sometimes used for treating Bartonella, M. *fermentans*, and Coxiella

Circulation: Movement of fluids such as lymph and blood

Circumcision: Removal of the foreskin of the penis. The foreskin remnant is one of the best sources of a sample for diagnostic testing allowing for greater sensitivity in cultures and Ag/Ab identification

Circumference: The perimeter of a body. Measuring the head or chest circumference is a common assessment in infants.

Cirrhosis: Chronic disease of the liver marked by dense connective tissue, degenerative changes of the liver cells, structural changes, fatty infiltrates, and loss of function. Resistance to blood flow can lead to toxic sequelae.

Claforan: Cefotaxime

Clarithromycin: (Biaxin) Macrolide antibiotic with excellent intracellular action. Good choice for Bb in combination with a cell wall antibiotic

Clavicle: Collar bone

Clearance: The measurement of the RATE of elimination. Each molecule has a specific clearance or elimination rate, almost like an identifying fingerprint. Most often this rate refers to how fast plasma is moving through the kidney and is usually measured per minute. Usually drugs are cleared through the kidney as part of elimination. Clearance occurs at different rates for different drugs in different people. After a single dose, only a fraction of the drug remains in the body. To maintain a therapeutic level another dose is needed before the clearance rate overtakes the bioavailability rate. Clearance measures the efficiency of drug removal and may involve a number of "passes" through the liver and eventually the kidney before the drug and its metabolites are all gone.

Clicks: Short high pitched heart sounds that may be associated with abnormal valve motion. Often associated with mitral valve disease

Clindamycin: (Cleocin) Bacteriostatic lincosamide. While most often considered a strong antibiotic for anaerobic bacteria, clindamycin is also quite effective in combination against protozoal diseases like malaria and babesiosis. Clindamycin does NOT penetrate into the CNS and is NOT for the treatment of meningitis. The bacteria Clostridium *difficile* is completely resistant to clindamycin, which is known for C. *difficile* overgrowth.

Clinical: Observable as a disease state *or* demonstrated in a health care setting

Clinical course: How a pathogen affects a host from the time of exposure, to infection, to symptoms, to signs, to damage, to resolution, to sequelae, to demise

Clinical PEARL: See PEARL

Clinical pharmacology: Describes the interactions between a drug and a body. Pharmacology is greatly affected by genetics, age, weight, gender, the current degree of pathology, concurrent medical conditions, compliance, and environmental factors such as the patient's hydration and nutrition. Individuals vary greatly in their response to an identical drug regimen. Even the same patient can respond differently at different times.

Clinical study: (Clinical trial) A test of a new treatment to evaluate the effectiveness and safety of that therapy. Can be controlled with placebo or run against other treatments for the same condition so that the results allow for conclusions and comparisons

Cloaking: Pathogens have been shown to strip away part of the B cell membrane and then wear the B cell as a cloak. Thereafter the presenting proteins are recognized as *self* instead of what they really are: non-*self*. In antigenic "cloaking" the host protein is bound to the surface of the pathogen.

Clonic: Alternating contraction and relaxation of a muscle

Clonus: Spasm between antagonistic (opposing) muscle groups (the flexors versus the extensors, for example) caused by a hyperactive stretch reflex from an upper motor neuron lesion.

Clostridium *difficile:* In many patients, C. *difficile* is part of the normal flora of the gut. When the patient is started on certain antibiotics, C. *diff* is often not susceptible to the action of these drugs as are other types of intestinal flora. While its neighbors are wiped out, C. *diff* has more room and resource to reproduce. The microbe now overgrows and becomes an opportunistic infection. The big problem comes when the C. *difficile* makes an endotoxin. The more C. *difficile*, the more toxin is made and released. This toxin can lead to severe colitis. This diarrhea is frequent, often explosive, watery, and may contain blood or mucus. Further diarrhea from C. *diff* can be accompanied by cramps, urgency, abdominal pain, and fever. A false or pseudo membrane can form over the intestinal lining. Symptoms can become severe and even fatal.

Clot: A sticky gel-like substance formed at the site of injury to a blood vessel that usually stops the blood flow

Clubbing: Enlargement of the distal finger phalanxes and the loss of the nail bed angle due to chronic pulmonary problems. Can be seen in infants with congenital disease and in other chronic respiratory conditions. The angle between the nail and base flattens and then the nail base becomes swollen with an increased angle. Clubbing is usually associated with long-term hypoxia but is also seen in IBD and endocarditis. Endocarditis is one possible cardiac manifestation of Lyme.

Clusters of differentiation: CDs are a group of protein markers on the surface of white blood cells. They are used to classify immune cell types and establish international nomenclature standards. Each marker identifies a cell with a specific function within the system, like passing along biochemical signals. CD levels are measured as a percent of total lymphocytes. T cells are mostly labeled CD1 through CD8, while B cells are categorized generally from CD19 to CD24.

Coagulation: Complex cascade of reactions that result in clot formation. Important part of hemostasis, which is the cessation of blood loss from a damaged vessel. The injured or leaking tissue is covered by a platelet and fibrin-containing clot to stop the bleeding and begin repair of the damaged area. Problems with coagulation include bleeding (hemorrhage) or obstruction (thrombus).

Coenzyme Q 10: (Ubiquinone) Part of the electron transport chain that makes energy in the form of ATP through aerobic cellular respiration. Organs with the highest energy requirements have the highest concentrations of CoQ 10 like the heart, liver, and kidney. Ubiquinone can be synthesized by the body or ingested in the diet in sources like meats, fish, oils, nuts, and some fruits and vegetables. Chronic disease increases the demand for CoQ 10, presumably because the body needs additional energy to recover.

Cogan's syndrome: Interstitial keratitis and inflammation of the cornea associated with tinnitus, vertigo, and deafness

Cognition: Ability to think. Awareness associated with reasoning, perception, judgment, intuition, and memory. Mental processes that allow for learning. Thoughts should be clear, realistic, and follow a logical flow. Cognition can be assessed using various methods. Cognitive deficits are very common in TBIs, especially Lyme.

Cognitive Behavioral Therapy: (CBT) Type of talk therapy where the treatment is focused on solving problems in the here and now. CBT is underscored by the premise that thoughts can be redirected and behaviors changed. Using a systematic approach along with goal setting, CBT has been found to be especially effective in mood disorders, anxiety, personality problems, dysfunctional relationships, eating disorders, substance abuse, OCD, panic attacks, PTSD, bulimia, depression, insomnia, and phobias. CBT introduces new ways to think about old situations and provides a reality check. The therapist helps the patient to be in control of the situation and focus on the positive. Tools and techniques are introduced to help the patient cope with everyday situations such as exposure therapy used to help with phobias and thought recognition and acceptance used in OCD. Usually a combination of tactics is used to get the patient fully functional. CBT focuses on getting rid of unwanted thoughts and actions to improve QOL and the ability to function in real world situations.

Cognitive deficits: Cognition is the ability to think. Bb and Bartonella impact clear thinking. In order to assess cognitive ability, look at basic knowledge, vocabulary, analytical ability, problem solving, logic flow, and the presence of a coherent line of reasoning. Cognition problems in kids can be the primary presenting sign in some TBIs and impaired cognitive function can make it hard to sustain attention, learn new things, and recall information.

Cognitive glitches can severely impact developmental milestones. Manifestations of cognitive difficulties in children with Lyme might include poor processing of incoming information, plodding thoughts, slow ability to catch on, illogical reasoning, trouble with reading or writing, word searching, limited recall, difficulty in learning new concepts, impaired concentration, confused ideas, and diminished ability to express thoughts.

Cognitive testing: Assessment of the capacity to think. Designed to measure various types of mental aptitude. Examples include an assortment of IQ tests, as well as evaluations of reasoning, memory, analytical ability, and multiple other parameters.

Colic: Spasm. A painful cramp in a hollow or tubular soft organ. Intestinal colic is a common condition in babies. Gall bladder colic is common in adults.

Collagen: A strong, fibrous, insoluble protein found in connective tissue, skin, tendons, ligaments, fascia, bone, teeth, non-enamel dental tissue, blood vessels, heart valves, and cartilage. Bb seem to have an affinity for collagen-rich areas such as joints.

Coloboma: A black, round hole or slit in or near the iris, sometimes called cat eyes. A gap in parts of the eye structure caused when the fetal eyes do not develop properly during pregnancy

Colorado tick fever: Viral TBI co-infection

Comedo: (Comedos, Comedones) Typical acne lesion. If closed: whitehead. If open: blackhead. If inflamed: pustule. Appear on face most commonly and also on back or chest

Co-morbid: Disease, condition, or disorder that occurs at the same time as another but is not necessarily related to it. Concurrent

Comparisons: Asking how two items are alike or different is one way to assess analytical ability

Compendium: A summary containing the essential information on a topic in a concise but comprehensive manner. A compilation that summarizes a much larger body of work. This *Compendium* condenses the material from thousands of articles and hundreds of books on TBIs and related topics.

Competent: Referring to a reservoir capable of passing an infection onto the feeding tick

Complement: Group of proteins that play an important role in immune response through a complex cascade of reactions. Antibodies can't do all the work themselves. They need their action to be *complemented* by this additional immune component. Complement is known to be consumed when antigen/antibody complexes are formed. These proteins then allow for lysis of foreign microbes. Complement impacts both innate and acquired immunity.

Complement fixation techniques: Blood assay used to determine if Ag/Ab reactions have occurred. After complement combines with antigen and antibody to form a complex, it is no longer available to lyse RBCs *in vitro*. The degree of complement fixation can then be determined by the number of RBCs destroyed, which indicates the amount of free complement not bound. Complement fixation can suggest the severity of an infection because it helps indicate the extent and effectiveness of the Ag/Ab reactions occurring in the system.

Complete blood count: (CBC) A laboratory test, often mechanized, that counts the amount of RBCs, WBCs, and platelets in a blood sample. The different types of WBCs are identified and counted. This test can provide clues regarding the etiology of symptoms including help in differentiating between bacterial, viral, parasitic, and allergic causes. Anemia with a low H&H may be a sign of Babesia infection. A high eosinophil count may indicate allergies rather than infection.

Complex partial seizure: Localized seizure. Often begins with an aura or sensation that the seizure is coming on. Include psychomotor and temporal lobe seizures. Complex partial seizures have been observed in patients with chronic acquired Lyme.

Concomitant: Treatments given at the same time. Usually refers to drug regimens. Compare to concurrent

Concurrent: Diseases occurring at the same time. Usually refers to medical conditions. Compare to concomitant

Concussion: Injury resulting from trauma to the brain. The mechanism of injury is the brain banging around inside the very hard and very confined space of the skull. The tissue is at least bruised and swollen. While no structural lesions are apparent, the patient may be dazed or confused immediately after the injury. There may be altered consciousness for seconds or minutes. The patient may be "knocked out." Pupils and other brainstem functions should all be intact. If they are not, consider that there might be a bleed or other reason for the problem. Loss of consciousness is no longer required for a diagnosis of concussion.

Conditioning: Regimen used to train the heart to pump more efficiently allowing more O_2 to muscles. Training helps improve a skill set over time. For example, a conditioned heart beats SLOWER and more efficiently than a non-conditioned one which will beat faster trying to pump enough blood to perform the same task. Intervals, where exercise intensity is varied from moderate to intense and back again in cycles, is often used to improve overall conditioning.

Conduction deafness: Problem with sound conduction through bone

Cone of light: Triangular area of reflected light on the eardrum

Conflict of interest: Situation where a person's official decisions might be influenced by personal agendas

Confounder/confounding: Factor that interferes. An extraneous variable that leads to confusion in drawing conclusions. These confounders can make relationships hard to discern. Confounding factors may go unrecognized. Does A cause B or is some inapparent 3rd factor influencing the observed effect?

Congenital: Present at birth

Conjunctiva: Visible membrane covering the sclera of the eye

Connective tissue: (Ct) Tissue that supports and joins one part of the body to another. Connects tissues. Connective tissue contains few cells and is primarily a collagen-protein matrix comprised mostly of intracellular substance. There are a number of kinds of connective tissue depending on location and function. Except for cartilage, connective tissue is highly vascular. Dense forms of connective tissue include cartilage, bone, and teeth (excluding enamel). Blood can be considered a Ct.

Connective tissue disease: Conditions where Ct is the prime target of pathology. Ct is made primarily of collagen and elastin, both of which can be impacted by inflammation or abnormal immune system activity such as autoimmunity. Ct disease can be inherited, autoimmune (such as SLE, RA, scleroderma, Sjogren's, or mixed Ct disease), as well as acquired as in the case of scurvy where a deficit in Vitamin C causes abnormal collagen. TBIs such as Lyme have much in common with some of these conditions.

Consistency: Level of performance that does not change greatly over time

Consolidation: Coalescence of fluid in the lung instead of air in the air sacs

Constipation: Infrequent bowel movements of less than 3 per week, often accompanied by straining, discomfort, and the eventual passage of hard stool. Severe constipation is less than one bowel movement per week.

Contraindications: All the reasons an individual should not use a specific drug. In other words, use of this medicine under certain listed conditions or circumstances may pose a particular risk. For example, a drug is contraindicated if the patient is allergic to any of the ingredients.

Controlled study: A clinical study that compares a group getting one treatment to a group not getting that treatment. The control group can receive a placebo, a different treatment, or no treatment at all.

Contusion: (Ecchymosis or bruise) Blood in skin that can imply trauma, coagulation problems, or leaky tissue

Convergence: Coordinated turning in of the eyes to focus on a close object. May be defective in Lyme

Conversion disorder: (Conversion reaction) A mental disorder that involves the involuntary loss of a body function without a reasonable explanation. This reaction can be sensory with loss of feeling, excessive sensitivity to strong stimuli, loss of the sense of pain, or tingling or crawling sensations. Conversion disorders can involve motor function as well, with involuntary movement of the arms, legs, and vocal cords or disorganized movements such as tics, tremors, twitches, even paralysis. Visceral conversion might include swallowing, burping, coughing, or vomiting. Anecdotally, infections have been implicated in conversion reactions. If the conversion reaction is due to an infection, the symptoms should diminish if treated with appropriate antibiotics. If the reaction is developmental and non-infectious, antibiotics will have no effect.

Coordination: The working together of various parts to produce a desired effect. For example, several muscles and nerves may need to act in tandem to produce a specific movement. Coordination can include such concepts as eye-hand coordination or the balance of actions between muscle groups. The cerebellum and a number of high level structures are probably involved in the timing and coordination of actions. Coordination can be significantly impacted by some of the TBIs.

Corn: A corn is a painful cone shaped thickening of skin over a pressure point. Corns most often develop on the thin skin on the foot over boney prominences like the 5th toe ball and sole.

Cornea: Curved, transparent front cover of the eye that serves as a refractive medium

Cortex: Outer layer of an organ

Cortisol: (Hydrocortisone) Steroid hormone produced in the adrenal gland. To be active, cortisone is converted to cortisol, which then helps regulate metabolism of fats, carbohydrates, Na, K, and many other bio-entities. Cortisol has been found to be associated with the normal function of many organ systems. Measurement of cortisol is done to assess function of the adrenal cortex. Levels vary with time of day! High cortisol levels are found in chronic inflammation, on-going anxiety, and obesity. Sometimes called the stress hormone, cortisol is well-known to suppress the immune system. Imbalance may result in a number of the symptoms associated with Lyme.

Coryza: Inflammation of nasal passages with profuse clear discharge

Costochondral: The rib and its cartilage

Costochondritis: Inflammation of joints between ribs and sternum

Costovertebral: Referring to the area or joint between a rib and a vertebra

Cough: A sudden explosive expiration designed to clear the airway

COX-2 inhibitors: COX is cyclooxygenase, an essential enzyme needed to synthesize the prostaglandins, which are associated with fever and dilation of blood vessels. Cox-2 inhibitors are drugs that function as anti-inflammatories.

Crackles: (Rales) High pitched, discontinuous lung sounds almost like the noise made by the crinkly plastic bubble wrap used by the post office

Cradle cap: Seborrheic dermatitis in infants. Scaly, crusty patches on scalp in first three months of life

Cramp: Spasm

Cranial manipulation: Treatment approach designed to enhance healing by balancing the motion, tissues, and fluid in the skull using structural manipulation techniques. Anecdotally, many Lyme patients report symptomatic relief after cranial manipulation.

Cranial Nerve: One of 12 pairs of nerves arising from the brain or brainstem

CN 1 Olfactory:	Smell
CN 2 Optic:	Vision
CN 3 Oculomotor:	Eye movement
CN 4 Trochlear:	Downward and inward movement of the eye
CN 5 Trigeminal:	Motor: Jaw clench with masseter and temporal muscles and lateral movement of the jaw. Sensory: Facial sensation
CN 6 Abducens:	Lateral and conjugate movements of eye
CN 7 Facial:	Motor: Muscles of the face. Sensory: Taste on the forward 2/3 of the tongue
CN 8 Acoustic:	Hearing and balance
CN 9 Glossopharyngeal:	Sensory input from the pharynx and middle ear. One muscle innervation

CN 10 Vagus: Motor: Movement of palate, pharynx, and larynx. Ability to swallow. Sensory: Pharynx and larynx

CN 11 Spinal Accessory: Motor: Sternomastoid and upper trapezius

CN 12 Hypoglossal: Motor: Tongue

C-reactive protein: (CRP) An abnormal protein detectable in blood only during active phases of certain illnesses. One hypothesis suggests that IL-6 and TNF-α produced through inflammatory processes induce CRP production. CRP is therefore associated with the presence of inflammation and used to help rule out autoimmune disorders. In TBI patients, CRP is considered a nonspecific marker of inflammation and is occasionally useful for discriminating among diagnoses and for monitoring clinical course.

Cream: Absorbs faster than an ointment but slower than a lotion. About half oil and half water, creams don't flow. They are appreciated for not being as greasy as an ointment, but are usually more protective than a lotion.

Creatine phosphokinase: (CPK or creatine kinase) An enzyme found in muscle (both skeletal and cardiac) and brain. Damage to these areas will cause the enzyme to leak into the blood, where it can be measured. By measuring the specific CPK isoenzymes, the site of injury might be determined. Muscle-derived CPK might be high in babesiosis, where this finding could be due to the intense muscle activity associated with rigors.

Creatinine: Breakdown product of muscle metabolism and, depending on muscle mass, is produced at a fairly constant rate by the body. Creatinine levels in the blood compared to the urine can be used to calculate creatinine clearance which reflects how fast the kidney is filtering and is one of the best measures of kidney function. Creatinine levels are a common gauge of the work of the kidney and a rise in creatinine suggests damage to kidney cells. Baseline levels can be compared to subsequent results to follow renal effects of the disease or to provide information regarding adverse drug reactions.

Crepitation: Crackling sound heard with some pneumonias, broken bones, or when joints move over rough or irregular articular surfaces. A crepitant neck is a common complaint in Lyme.

CREST syndrome: A form of scleroderma that manifests with C - calcinosis, R - Raynaud's, E - esophageal dysmobility, S - sclerodactyly, and T- telangiectasia. Probably autoimmune

Crohn's disease: Type of IBD. Inflammatory condition of the intestine. Crohn's and UC present similarly, the difference being the location and nature of the inflammatory changes in the gut. Crohn's can impact any part of the GI tract from mouth to anus in what are called skip lesions. UC affects the colon and rectum. Both can affect body systems outside the alimentary canal such as the liver, joints, skin, and eyes. Crohn's is thought to be autoimmune, while the consensus is still out on UC. Both may be associated with cytokine response and both present with diarrhea, abdominal discomfort, and cramps. Symptoms can be incapacitating and affect the ability to go to school and work.

Cross-reactivity: A reaction between an antibody and an antigen that is different from the original antigen that inspired the formation of the antibody (although it is probably very similar)

Croup: Viral respiratory inflammation characterized by stridor on inspiration and respiratory distress. The child may present with a barking cough often at night, seeming suffocation, retractions, long inspirations, and distress. The airway can spasm. Presenting mostly in kids 6-months to 3-years-old, fever is present in only about half the cases. Intense hydration and humidification can alleviate symptoms and the child may need to be hospitalized.

Crust: Dried blood, serum, or pus as can be found in a number of skin conditions such as impetigo infections caused by Staph or Strep

Cure: Restoration of health or wellness or the return of lost function and the ability to pursue AODL. In many conditions, cure is hard to define. One definition in Lyme is the absence of symptoms for a year or more following antibiotic treatment.

Current jelly stool: Combination of blood, mucus, and feces

Cushing's syndrome: Excess corticosteroid hormone from the adrenal cortex. May be due to a problem in the adrenal gland, over-stimulation of the adrenals by the pituitary, or prolonged use of steroid hormones. Sxs might include: protein loss, fatty infiltrates, fatigue, weakness, osteoporosis, amenorrhea, impotence, capillary fragility, hair overgrowth, abnormal blood sugars, skin discoloration, and striae.

C vitamin: (Ascorbic acid) Antioxidant that protects the body from oxidative stress. Essential for collagen synthesis, numerous metabolic pathways, healing, scar formation, blood cell development, adrenal function, and bone and tissue growth. Acts as an intercellular cement in many tissues especially capillary walls. Lack of Vitamin C results in scurvy which renders collagen non-functional and that affects all collagen-containing structures such as tendons, ligaments, cartilage, bone, blood vessels, valves, spinal discs, and connective tissue. Symptoms of scurvy include brown spots on the skin, blood oozing from capillaries and mucous membranes, spongy gums, and loss of teeth. Victims can be pale, depressed, and immobile. Scurvy can be fatal. There is a high concentration of ascorbic acid in immune cells and the vitamin is rapidly consumed during infection. Since Vitamin C is involved with fatty acid transport into the mitochondria to make energy, insufficient amounts may result in lethargy. This vitamin also appears to act as a natural antihistamine.

Cyanocobalamin: Vitamin B12

Cyanosis: Discoloration of the skin and mucous membranes indicating not enough oxygen in the blood. Fingers, toes, and lips are common sites of the blue color that suggests that the blood there is poorly oxygenated.

Cyst: 1)A closed sac or pouch with definite boundaries that contains fluid or other materials. An abnormal structure caused by infection or obstruction of ducts. Examples include the cysts of acne and pilonidal cysts. 2) Refers to a structure formed by certain pathogens where they are enclosed inside a capsule (cyst) and become inactive until environmental conditions are more favorable. In Bb infection, the spirochete will encyst in response to stressors like the presence of antibiotic. When the stress is gone, the cyst converts back to the spirochete.

Cyst-buster: Antimicrobial that is able to break through the cyst capsule of a dormant microbe and damage the pathogen. The best cyst-busters for Lyme are Flagyl and Tindamax.

Cystitis: Inflammation of the bladder most often due to infection but can be caused by irritants or trauma

Cytochrome P450: A cytochrome is an enzyme needed to catalyze many metabolic reactions. There are many varieties such as cytochrome P450, which represent a group of enzymes important in metabolism including the transformation of many substances and detoxification of medicines, toxins, or pollutants. If the system gets overloaded, the process can back up, increasing the blood levels of the molecules waiting their turn. Many medicines are processed through the P450 and related biochemical cascades. Some of these molecules are known to up-regulate or down-regulate the system resulting in high or low levels of other drugs, sometimes referred to as drug interactions. These deviations from the expected can result in lack of efficacy or toxicity.

Cross reactivity: A reaction between an antibody and an antigen that is different from the original antigen that inspired the formation of the antibody (although it is probably very similar)

Cytokines: Various distinct proteins produced primarily by WBCs. Each cytokine is secreted by a specific cell in response to a specific stimulus. Includes ILs, IFNs, TNFs, etc. Provide signals to regulate immune processes. Release of cytokines may be responsible for a number of symptoms associated with inflammation, so while they are helping the cause, they may be making the patient very uncomfortable.

Cytomegalovirus: (HHV-5) Type of herpes virus that can cause cytomegalic inclusion disease which has a wide range of presentations. Often unnoticed, CMV can remain asymptomatic indefinitely without sequelae. However, CMV can be a life-threatening condition in the immunocompromised. Latent infection can activate in pregnancy or when immune response is dampened. Can be transmitted to the fetus and congenital CMV can cause problems in the newborn, later manifesting with retardation and motor development delays. This infection can be especially problematic in babies also at risk for a congenital TBI, where it can confound diagnosis and recovery. Most problematic in those with an already compromised immune system. Once present, the virus stays for life.

Cytotoxic T cell: Type of lymphocytic WBC that destroys targets

D

Dandruff: Seborrheic dermatitis. Can be greasy, scaly patches on scalp with flaking, or dry, white scales. Many cases have a fungal component

Decision tree: Series of yes or no questions used to help HCPs make decisions about diagnosis and treatment. For example, the decision tree for TBIs might start with: Tick bite? Yes or No? Be careful, however. A "no" answer to this question does NOT preclude the existence of a TBI. Many people do not recall a tick bite or never noticed the bite. Decision trees can be very useful, but don't climb a tree you can't get down from.

Deep tendon reflexes: Involuntary responses to stimuli. DTRs are predictable and rely on intact neural pathways between the stimulus and the organ called reflex arcs. Deep reflexes can be assessed at insertions of the major tendons into bone. Normal response is a quick extension and contraction and reflexes should be symmetrical and compared side to side.

Defensins: Proteins that kill pathogens or inactivate poisons

Dehydration: Lack of water. Dry

Delayed hypersensitivity: Antibody-<u>in</u>dependent, cell-mediated, immune memory response

Delirium: An acute state of confusion common in kids with high fevers, often with disorientation to time and place. Possible illusions and hallucinations with decreased coherence and aimless thinking

Delusions: A false belief without supportive rationale. Thoughts inconsistent with actual knowledge or experience. Delusions may be associated with certain TBIs.

Dementia: Cognitive deficit that may incorporate memory problems, poor abstract reasoning, cloudy thinking, and impaired judgment

Demographics: Characteristics of a population such as age, sex, ethnic group, special populations, etc.

Dendrite: Short branching extension of a nerve cell that gathers information and transmits it to the neuron. Receives information and passes it centrally

Dendritic cell: Specialized phagocytic Ag-recognizing cell of the immune system with long outgrowths that help engulf microbes

Dependency: Addiction is often framed in terms of dependency, tolerance, and withdrawal. When a person first starts what will become an addiction, he uses a substance for pleasure and enjoyment. The first cigarettes and the first beers are used for fun or to feel relaxed. As the addiction develops, the individual has to use the substance just to feel normal. That is dependency, since the person "depends" on the substance to be normal. A person can be physically dependent, psychologically dependent, or both.

Depression: Movement in an inferior direction as when the shoulders unshrug

Depression: (Unipolar depression) Abnormal mood that may include feeling of sadness, apprehension, and gloom where the patient takes no pleasure in usually pleasant experiences such as food, friends, hobbies, or entertainment. The sad feelings occur just about every day and can also include changes in weight or appetite, altered sleep patterns, hopelessness, low energy or motivation, feelings of worthlessness or guilt, difficulty concentrating, and recurrent thoughts of death or a wish to end it all. Depression is the most common psychiatric disorder and is often coupled with anxiety. Common in children and associated with several TBIs

Detoxification: Removal of a poison or toxin from the body or the process by which a toxin is rendered harmless

Developmental milestones: Set of skills that can be used to assess where a child stands in terms of how she is developing compared to her peers. Usually aptitude in several areas are observed such as gross motor, fine motor, language, cognition, and social interaction. These skills can be quite variable but documenting milestones can be especially useful in TBI patients because the HCP can see how the child is doing now compared to past performance.

Diabetes: (DM) Disease of abnormal glucose metabolism usually marked by hyperglycemia and glycosuria secondary to the inadequate production or use of insulin. DM affects both the nervous system and circulation to all areas, which explains why diabetics get kidney dysfunction, neuropathy, and blindness from their disease.

For example, in the foot, the diabetic patient is less able to feel sensations of pain, heat, and cold. Poor glucose control is common in LD.

Diagnose: Use of a systematic approach to explain a set of signs and symptoms

Diagnosis: (Diagnoses) A disease or condition

Diagnostic and Statistical Manual of Mental Disorders: (DSM) Handbook that contains all currently accepted psychiatric diagnoses. The most recent edition is the DSM-IV.

DSM-5: Is scheduled for release early in 2013.

Diapause: Dormant state in tick life cycle where the tick awaits more favorable living conditions

Diaper rash: (Diaper dermatitis) Irritation in diaper area. Usually red and uncomfortable. If thickened and raised, likely fungal

Diaphragm: Dome-shaped muscle separating the abdomen from the thorax

Diarrhea: Loose stool defined by frequency not consistency. On physical exam, bowel sounds may be loud and rapid. Percussion may show considerable air and fluid. Palpation may result in generalized discomfort, but not specific localized pain. Frequent, loose stools are common in TBI patients, either as part of the disease process or as a side effect of antibiotic therapy. Look also for signs of dehydration. With diarrhea due to C. *difficile,* remain vigilant for complications like megacolon. Diarrhea can be a serious and even fatal condition in children and the elderly.

Diastasis recti: Separation of the two halves of the rectus abdominis muscles of the abdomen. Not a hernia, but an acquired partition of the two superficial abdominal muscles caused by pregnancy, obesity, or other strains

DIC: Disseminated intravascular coagulation or consumptive coagulopathy. Pathologic over-activation of the clotting cascade

Differential: Demonstrating a difference or showing a distinction. Within the context of this text, the differential count refers to blood cells and the differential diagnosis applies to parsing a set of signs and symptoms down to the most likely causal agent.

Differential cell count: The number and type of blood cells as determined by microscopic exam of a thin layer of blood smeared across a slide. For example, the number, size, and shape of the cells can be assessed. The different types of WBCs can be documented as well as a platelet count.

Differential diagnosis: (DD) Using the information gathered from the H&P and ROS, along with the process of elimination, a symptom set is reduced to the most likely causality. The probability of each candidate is reduced down to negligible levels.

Direct hernia: Because of weakness of the fascial floor of the inguinal canal, the direct hernia sac protrudes through the abdominal wall.

Disability: A physical or mental impairment that substantially limits a major life activity

Discomfort: Absence of comfort or ease. Disturbance of the equilibrium. This sensation is perceived to be less severe than pain and is more of an un-ease.

Discrimination: Ability to tell the difference between two sensory stimuli. Assessment of two-point tactile discrimination uses sharp objects like pins to stimulate two places at once. How close can the pins get and the patient still tell if it is two stimuli instead of one?

Dislocation: Displacement of any part. Usually refers to the temporary dislodging of a bone from its normal position in a joint

Disseminate: Spread

Disseminated intravascular coagulation: (DIC or consumptive coagulopathy) An overuse of clotting materials often observed in the end-stages of many diseases. DIC leads to the formation of small clots inside the blood vessels throughout the body. These multiple small clots use up the coagulation proteins and platelets and disrupt all aspects of normal coagulation. Abnormal bleeding occurs with seeping into the skin, GI tract, and pulmonary tree. Wounds won't stop oozing and small clots disrupt kidney function and normal blood flow to organs, which can quickly malfunction. While probably not the sole cause of M&M, DIC is often associated with death.

Disseminated Lyme: Bb that has spread from the local area into the circulation and tissues

Distal: Distal is further from a reference point, while proximal is closer

Distended: Stretched or inflated

Distractibility: Ability to be turned away from the original point of interest or focus. Able to be diverted. Attention wavers

Distribution: 1) The dispersion of a drug throughout the body usually traveling with fluids such as blood or lymph. Thereafter, the drug starts to find its way into the tissue cells and the space between cells. Depending on the chemical nature of the drug, some can cross the BBB and the placenta and others get into the CSF and breast milk. These distribution characteristics may be important in drug selection. 2) The location or arrangement of an entity on a map

Disulfiram: (Antabuse) Drug that causes a bad reaction to alcohol including nausea, vomiting, headache, flushing, cramps, and confusion. Used to discourage drinking in alcoholics, although it is minimally effective. A number of drugs used to treat TBIs such as metronidazole (Flagyl), some cephalosporins, and TCNs, especially doxycycline, can cause an Antabuse-like reaction.

Diverticulitis: Also called left-sided appendicitis. Diverticuli are little out-pouches of tissue in the colon, like bubbles on an old inner tube. They remain asymptomatic until they become inflamed. Acute cases are similar to the presentation found in appendicitis and care must be taken that a diverticuli does not rupture leading to peritonitis. Chronic problems with flares can lead to worsening constipation, mucus in the stool, and intermittent episodes of gripping abdominal pain. Since most people do not want to have a repeat episode they are advised to eat a diet high in fiber, consume non-irritating foods, and drink plenty of water.

Dizziness: Sensation of lightheadedness or fading consciousness. Patients will use this term interchangeably with weakness, sleepiness, malaise, vertigo, and many other labels making it difficult to tell what they are actually experiencing.

Doll's eye phenomenon: Normally when an infant's head is rotated quickly from one side to the other, the eyes will move TOGETHER to the opposite side. The doll's eye phenomenon will manifest if there is any problem with some of the EOMs. Here the child will not move his eyes when his head is turned and the eyes will remain in the starting position. This phenomenon may suggest brainstem or oculomotor damage.

Dormant: Period of time in an organism's life cycle when growth, development, and activity are temporarily stopped. Metabolism slows and energy consumption is significantly reduced. A dormant state is closely associated with environmental conditions. Dormancy is a time of metabolic slowdown. A survival strategy, dormancy allows an organism to move past a period of external stress.

Dorsiflexion: Movement of the entire foot toward the head as though you were going to scratch your eyebrow with your toe

Doryx: Enteric-coated doxycycline. Because the coating protects the drug allowing it to survive into the SI, more may be absorbed and there may be less GI side effects.

Dose: Quantity of medicine given at one time or at stated intervals. To administer a treatment. A loading dose is an initial higher dose given at the beginning of a treatment regimen before the amount is dropped to the usual maintenance dose. A loading dose allows for faster achievement of desired blood levels but may also increase side effects.

Dose-response curve: Graph that shows the effect of a drug or its blood level after a specific dose over time. The effect may plateau, after which more drug does not cause more effect. Americans tend to believe that more is better even if the data does not support this idea.

Double-blind: A study design where neither the investigator nor the subject know which treatment is being administered. Both are unaware of (or blind to) the actual treatment being given. Used to decrease the potential for bias

Doxycycline: (Vibramycin. Doryx is the enteric-coated formulation of doxycycline) Cidal antibiotic with a broad set of indications. DOC for the spirochetal form of Bb in adults and older kids in combination with intracellular agents. Also used for RMSF, ehrlichiosis/anaplasmosis, and may also be effective against malaria. Doxy should not be used as a solo agent against Bb infections, since the spirochete might then go intracellular or encyst. This would then allow for a reservoir of Bb which will resurface when conditions are more favorable.

Dressler's syndrome: Post-myocardial infarction syndrome

D vitamin: (Calciferol) Group of fat soluble vitamins needed to absorb Ca and P from the gut thereby allowing for the normal development of bones and teeth. An intrinsically-made hormone which the body can synthesize in sufficient amounts if exposed to enough sunlight (UV radiation). Vitamin D is essential for immune function, the regulation of Ca and P metabolism, bone growth and maintenance, as well as normal kidney, bone, and parathyroid function. Additional sources come from sun exposure and foods such as milk, butter, egg yolks, and cod liver oil. Most Americans, especially children, are lacking in Vitamin D. Deficiencies in this vitamin can lead to symptoms that may mimic Lyme symptoms including difficulty concentrating and balance problems. Low Vitamin D can cause rickets, while high levels can also cause problems.

Dysarthria: Slurred speech due to motor problems involving lips or tongue. Muscle weakness affecting speech, even while the mental function is intact

Dysautonomia: Disease impacting the ANS that can manifest as mental retardation, lack of motor coordination, vomiting, frequent infections, and seizures

Dysbiosis: Microbial imbalance. Most often recognized in the GI tract or skin but can present in any tissue with a mucosal surface such as the vagina, lungs, mouth, etc.

Dyscrasias: Term with a long and varied history but now used to refer to problems in the blood

Dysesthesia: Distortion of any sense, especially touch. Unpleasant sensation. Abnormal sensation after normal stimuli or unusual sensation without any stimuli

Dysgeusia: Distorted taste. Taste may be perverted to the degree that normal flavors are perceived as bad or totally different from the usual, accepted taste of a particular food

Dysmenorrhea: Painful or uncomfortable menstruation with cramping and mild lower abdominal discomfort

Dysphagia: Difficulty swallowing. Common finding in gestational Lyme

Dysphasia: Errors or uncertainty in word choice

Dysphonia: Raspy, hoarse voice. Difficulty speaking

Dysphoria: Intense feelings of depression, discontent, and apathy. Significant unhappiness. A symptom of disease, not a disease itself. With dysphoria, the depressive symptoms can begin subtly in childhood and may remain low-grade for many years. The clinical course may be punctuated with periods of major depression.

Dysplasia of hip: Dislocated or malpositioned femur

Dyspnea: Shortness of breath. Dyspnea is the unpleasant sensation of breathlessness where the person feels as though she is not getting enough oxygen. Dyspnea can be exhausting and as the body realizes it needs more oxygen it begins to compensate with use of accessory muscles, retractions, faster respiratory rate, increased heart rate, and nasal flaring. The patient will perceive that more oxygen is urgently needed and may experience a tight chest and feel the need to rest.

Dysrhythmias: Abnormal heart beat patterns. Usually the heart beats in a normal sinus rhythm, where the electrical stimulus is initiated in the sinus node and continues throughout the heart in the flow that nature intended. Many things can alter the electrical conductivity and cause the impulse to either originate elsewhere or impede the normal conduction. Causes include congenital problems, some medications, inflammation, infection, and multiple underlying disease states. Bb have been associated with various abnormal heart rhythms including atrial fibrillation, skipped beats, extra beats, premature beats, and flutters. Lyme patients frequently complain of palpitations. A palpitation is a perceptible fluttering of the heart. In contrast, many dysrhythmias occur without the individual ever being aware.

Dysthymia: A form of chronic depression thought to be less severe but lasting longer that major depressive disorder. Dysthymia may actually be more of a personality problem since the underlying temperament is gloomy and pessimistic, with no sense of humor or capacity for fun. The patient may be passive, lethargic, skeptical, hypercritical, complaining, self-denigrating, and preoccupied with failure and negativity.

Dysuria: Painful or difficult urination

E

Ecchymosis: (Contusion, bruise) Irregular hemorrhage area in the skin, mucous membrane, or other visible area. Implies trauma. Extravasation of blood into tissue

ECP: Eosinophil cationic protein

Ectopic: Tissue presenting in a location outside where it is normally found

Ectopic pregnancy: Implantation of a fertilized ovum outside the womb, most often in the fallopian tube. There may be considerable pain to palpation. A ruptured ectopic pregnancy can result in an acute abdomen and shock with all the associated clinical signs.

Eczema: Dry, scaly, red, itchy skin lesion. Found in all age groups, eczema is a cutaneous inflammation that can include redness, papules, vesicles, pustules, scales, crusts, or scabs. Eczema can be wet or dry in presentation and can itch and burn. Secondary infection can cause pus formation and oozing. The etiology has not been determined but eczema can be aggravated by irritants, allergens, infections, extreme temperatures, and stress. Persons with dry, thin skin are more susceptible. If long-term, the skin can become thick. What's the difference between eczema and psoriasis? Both are chronic skin conditions that cause red, scaly lesions and tend to involve some of the same body parts like the scalp. Psoriasis is often thicker than eczema and tends to be dry. Eczema tends to be more moist and oozing. Psoriasis tends to affect the back of the elbows and front of the knees (the extensor surfaces), while eczema hits the back of the knees and the front of the elbows (flexor surfaces).

Edema: Fluid, usually referring to too much tissue fluid. Excess fluid can be localized or general

Effect: Result or consequence. Something brought about by a causal agent

Effective: Successful in achieving the intended outcome. Adequate to accomplish a purpose

Efferent: Conduction AWAY from a central point. E.g., nerves that carry impulses away from the nerve are efferent. Opposite of afferent

Efficacy: Ability to produce the desired outcome. Term used most often to describe treatment results

Effusion: An escape of fluid into an area where it is not normally present in such amounts. E.g., a joint effusion is increased liquid in the joint space, which can be comprised of synovial fluid, inflammatory material, blood, serum, or pus. An effusion in a joint can be due to trauma, infection, or inflammation such as arthritis. A pleural effusion is fluid between the lung and the pleura.

Ehrlichia: Parasites that invade specific parts of the host's cells. Mostly settle in the cell vacuoles where nutrients are stored and waste released. Early on, the Ehrlichia were classified by the type of blood cell they most commonly infected. This turned out to be premature and misleading since the Ehrlichia species have been found in other cells beside their primary target cells. Further, more than one species may cause a certain disease. The blood cells used to sort the diseases include granulocytes, monocytes, platelets, and lymphocytes.

Ehrlichiosis: Diseases caused by certain parasitic genuses of Ehrlichia such as HME or HGE. Can be TBI co-infections

Ejection click: An abnormal sound a valve makes when fluid is expelled inefficiently

Electrolytes: Charged ions. Since they can conduct electricity in solution they are called *electro*lytes. Most body processes at the cellular level rely on electrolytes. Too much or too little can cause cellular and system malfunction. Ions help regulate the balance between salts and water and the acid/base equilibrium. Electrolytes are essential for normal heart rhythms, muscle contraction, nerve conduction, and kidney function.

Electrophoresis: A separation technique that uses an electrical field to move particles based on their size and charge. A complex mix of antigens is placed on an agar gel. Wherever there is an antigen/antibody reaction, a precipitate will form on that section of the gel. The more reaction, the more precipitation. Depending on the specifics of the technique the precipitate can be visualized using dyes, radioactivity, or fluorescence. This testing is used as a qualitative analysis when looking at a mixture of antigens.

> *PEARL: Do not confuse phoresis (the movement of particles in an electric field) with pheresis (extracorporeal treatment that removes and separates cells).*

Elevation: Movement in a superior direction as when the shoulders shrug

Elimination: Act of removal or getting rid of something no longer desired. The GI tract and kidneys eliminate wastes and the body metabolizes and eliminates drugs.

ELISA: (Enzyme-linked immunosorbent assay) Technique used to detect the presence of an antibody or antigen in a sample. Usually an unknown amount of antigen is fixed on a surface. Then a specific antibody is washed over that surface giving it the opportunity to bind with the antigen. A dye is added so that a visual demonstration of the formation of antigen/antibody complexes can be observed. Antigens usually bind only with their matching antibody and vice versa.

Emboli: A travelling clot with the potential to snag or occlude anywhere within the vasculature. Can result in tissue ischemia especially of the heart, lungs, or brain

Emesis: Vomiting

EMLA: Topical anesthetic

Emotional IQ: (EQ) Evolution of the ability to recognize and manage emotions in a way that allows for life satisfaction and stable relationships with others

Emphysema: Chronic pulmonary disease marked by increase in the size of the air spaces in the peripheral lung tissue with damage to the bronchial walls. Lungs are chronically inflamed, enzymes destroy tissue and scarring and fibrosis result. The lungs lose their elasticity and become overinflated and the patient has a hard time exhaling the old air out of his lungs so that fresh, O_2-rich air can replace it. DOE gets gradually worse. The patient will have a chronic cough and need to use accessory muscles to breathe. SOB is the primary symptom.

Empiric: Guided by experience and observation. Practical approach rather than theory

EM rash: Erythema migrans. Pathognomonic for borreliosis

Encephalitis: Inflammation of the brain, often caused by mosquito or tick-borne pathogens. Usually there is a sudden onset of fever. Additional sxs might include: headache, nausea, projectile vomiting, stiff neck and back, nuchal rigidity, malaise, restlessness, ataxia, opisthotonos, seizures, pupil irregularities, motor dysfunction, involuntary movements, changes in vital signs, ptosis, tremor, increased DTRs, paralysis, paresis (partial paralysis), abnormal sleep, and behavior changes. Encephalitis might also present with impaired cognitive abilities, personality changes, inability to concentrate, lethargy, changes in consciousness, and in some cases, nystagmus. There can be intense lymphocytic infiltration of brain tissues and the meninges, causing cerebral edema. Degeneration of ganglion cells and diffuse nerve cell destruction can occur. The infectious agent may directly damage the tissue. After an acute phase, the signs and symptoms may persist for days or weeks. Encephalitis can leave permanent damage and can be fatal. The overall syndrome that can accompany brain inflammation is called encephalopathy.

Encephalopathy: Deterioration of brain function through some acquired mechanism such as organ failure, metabolic disease, inflammation, or infection. Characterized by a change in mental status, encephalopathy can include loss of cognitive abilities, personality changes, inability to concentrate, lethargy, irritability, combative behavior, agitation, decreased consciousness, sleep problems, depression, restlessness, twitching, tremors, changes in muscle tone, nystagmus, neuropathy, and seizures. Encephalopathy is the symptom complex associated with encephalitis.

Endemic: Indigenous or native to a place. Entities found in a particular area or affecting a particular population. Present in a specific locality

Endocarditis: The endocardium is the endothelial membrane that lines the chambers of the heart, the valves, and is continuous with the lining of the arteries and veins. Endocarditis is inflammation of this membrane due to infection or immune processes. Infectious etiologies are usually bacterial but fungus is found in some cases and vegetative growths comprised of fibrin, pathogen, platelets, white cells, and other debris can accumulate on valves and vessels. Endocarditis can be fatal and there is a significant mortality even if aggressively treated. Severe and permanent valve damage leading to insufficiency and subsequent heart failure can ensue. Initial signs and symptoms can be nonspecific such as weakness, fatigue, weight loss, anorexia, arthralgia, and night sweats. More than 90% have intermittent fever. Symptoms can last for weeks. If they resolve, they can recur. Usually a loud regurgitant murmur is heard. Lyme has been associated with endocarditis.

Endocardium: Endothelial lining of the chambers of the heart, valves, and blood vessels

Endocrine: Referring to an internal secretion such as a hormone. A gland that secretes directly into the blood

Endogenous: Produced or originating from within a cell or body. Compared to exogenous which originates outside the system

Endometriosis: Presence of endometrial tissue outside the uterine lining. This ectopic tissue usually remains in the pelvis but can show up in various body locations. This is functional tissue and will go through all the tissue changes that the endometrium inside the uterus will undergo, so discomfort will be cyclic. Presents with constant pain in the lower abdomen that may increase with palpation. The pain is usually cyclic with the menstrual cycle.

Endothelial cell: Thin, flat cell layer that lines the surface of ALL the blood and lymph vessels. Bb gets into the endothelial cells. Endothelium is everywhere from the heart to the smallest terminal capillary. If you want to disseminate, get yourself into the endothelium. Inside the heart the endothelium is called the endocardium. From the endothelium, the Bb have access to EVERYTHING and this presence might help explain the multisystemic nature of LD.

Endotoxin: Toxin retained within the cell body and released when the cell is destroyed. Endotoxins released by damaged Bb pathogens may account for some of the sxs associated with the Herx reaction.

Endpoint study: Clinical study where the outcome is clearly predefined. When the subject reaches that endpoint the result is documented. The time to reach the endpoint is often one of the measured study parameters.

Endurance: Measure of the ability to do cardiorespiratory work. Length of time a person can perform an activity. Capacity to perform a task over and over

Engorgement: Swelling to the point of congestion. To feed ravenously. Some estimates suggest that the body of an adult female tick might swell 200 to 600 times its unfed size in order to accommodate the blood it draws from the host.

Enteritis: Inflammation of the intestines. Causes abdominal discomfort, increased BSs, and diarrhea. Common in all age groups. There is no point tenderness on palpation, just vague general discomfort. Add nausea and vomiting and you have gastroenteritis. Etiology is almost always viral.

Enula: Herbal remedy for protozoal infections such as the pathogens that cause malaria and babesiosis

Enuresis: Involuntary urination after the age where control is possible. Bedwetting is normal up to about 3 y/o and can be due to delayed neuromuscular maturation. Bedwetting associated with Lyme may be due to spirochetal damage to the bladder or other organs or pathogen impact on the ANS.

Eosinophil: WBC granulocyte focused on parasites and allergic reactions

Eosinophil cationic protein: (ECP) Biomolecule released during degranulation of eosinophils and is related to inflammation, asthma, and parasitic infections. ECP testing is sometimes used to assess level of inflammation, disease progression, and response to treatment. ECP is toxic to neurons so in patients with neuropsychiatric symptoms, elevated ECP may provide additional information.

Epidemic: Condition affecting an unusually large number of individuals within a defined population

Epidemiology: The science of disease patterns, looking for signals or trends, and analyzing this information in order to better predict and prevent disease

Epigastrium: (Epigastric) Area just below xiphoid in upper midsection of abdomen

Epilepsy: Recurrent, paroxysmal disorder of brain function with sudden, brief episodes of altered consciousness and abnormal motor or sensory activity (seizures). For seizures to be diagnosed as epilepsy there must be some recurring pattern. Seizures are the result of abnormal electrical discharges within a focal area of the brain.

Epiphysitis: An epiphysis is an ossification center of a bone. Epiphysitis is inflammation of this ossification center. Heel pain in kids can be epiphysitis of the calcaneus.

Epitope: One-of-a-kind region on an antibody that allows it to recognize its matching antigen

Epstein-Barr Virus: (EBV or HHV-4) Part of the Herpes family of viruses, EBV is thought to be one cause of infectious mononucleosis. Generally provides adaptive immunity. Presents with huge lymphadenopathy, severe sore throat, fever, and incapacitating fatigue.

Equivocal: Can go either way. Open to interpretation. Ambiguous. Opposite of unequivocal

Erosion: Loss of epidermis often seen after rupture of a superficial blister or chicken pock that do not bleed or scar

Erythema: Redness

Erythema chronica migrans: A historical or alternative name for EM rash

Erythema migrans: Skin manifestation often associated with LD. Pathognomonic for borreliosis. If an EM rash is observed you're likely dealing with Borrelia. Nonetheless, the EM rash is not as common as we have been led to believe. Incidences range from less than 10% to around 50%. Either way, the majority of patients do not experience an EM rash and the manifestation of such a rash may be due to the status of the immune system or to the infecting Bb strain. If you rely on the appearance of an EM rash before making the diagnosis of LD, you will be missing at least half the cases and maybe as many as 90%. Two types of EM rash are associated with Borrelia:

- Primary EM rash: Demonstrates localized Bb infection. The primary EM rash is most often a single, homogeneous, oval, red lesion. Often the bite site remains dark red and possibly slightly indurated. While the outer rim of the lesion remains reddish, the area in between can clear, causing the rash to look like a target or bull's eye. While there *might* be rings, there is usually no central clearing. EM rashes are called *expansive* lesions since they occasionally move outward to form concentric circles. Spirochetes enter the skin and begin replicating usually near the bite site since that's where they happen to be. As the population increases the microbes move out from the bite spot in all directions. This causes concentric circles, which are not always perfectly drawn since some pathogens may move faster and farther than others. Here the spirochete is present and active and moving and replicating. Bb have been isolated from biopsies taken at the edge of these lesions.

- Secondary EM rash: Quite rare, a secondary EM rash suggests disseminated Bb spirochetes. Now the pathogen is on the move. These are usually multiple lesions that appear as a result of Bb migrating through blood vessels and lymph channels. They can look like primary lesions but they come and go quite freely as the free-floating spirochetes traverse the circulatory system. These secondary rashes are *evanescent* in that one lesion, or multiple lesions, seem to pop up briefly, display, and recede. A secondary EM rash tends to be multifocal and can appear in any area where the Bb are migrating. The absence of a secondary EM rash doesn't mean that the Bb has not or will not spread.

Erythrocyte: Red blood cell

Erythrocyte sedimentation rate: (ESR) Nonspecific measure of the speed at which erythrocytes settle out of unclotted blood. Normally the rate is less than 10 mm/hr for males and slightly higher in females. The clumping of the cells depends on proteins released during inflammation. Therefore, the ESR can suggest the presence of inflammation and is used to monitor the onset and progress of inflammatory disorders. In TBI patients, ESR can be used to detect the presence of inflammation and to help rule out autoimmune disorders. ESR is more often normal in LD distinguishing it from conditions like RA and SLE which have higher levels of this inflammatory marker.

Erythromycin: Macrolide bacteriostatic antibiotic that stops the growth of a pathogen without killing it directly. Take doses at evenly spaced intervals because this antibiotic works best at a steady blood level.

Erythropoietin: Hormone that controls the manufacture of RBCs. Considered a cytokine

ESR: Erythrocyte sedimentation rate

Essential fatty acids: (EFAs) Fats needed for metabolic processes, not just as fuel, which the body requires but cannot synthesize. In humans include α-linolenic acid, an omega-3 FA, and linoleic acid, an omega-6 FA. Fish oil seems to be one of the best sources of the omega-3 FAs and may help fatigue, decrease inflammation, and provide support for the adrenals.

Etiology: Cause

Eukaryotes: Organisms with cell membranes and complex structures such as a membrane-enclosed nuclei. Eukaryotes include the parasite Babesia.

Evanescent: Soon passing out of site. Quickly fading. Likely to vanish

Evan's Syndrome: Autoimmune disease characterized by thrombocytopenia and hemolytic anemia

Eversion: Movement of the sole of the foot AWAY from the body midline. Turning outward

Evidence-based medicine: (EBM) Philosophy of medicine where all diagnostic and treatment decisions are based on strict interpretations of available data. These methods are helpful in steering HCPs in the right direction and are well suited to routine conditions. However, EBM also can result in inflexibility, especially with conditions where there is little data and prospective clinical trials would take too long to draw conclusions. This approach becomes less effective when a case is complicated or a patient has numerous concurrent conditions. Conservative adherents to this methodology believe no changes should be made in assessment or treatment options until data supports the change. This delay may take too long to help many individuals who need help now.

E vitamin: Fat soluble vitamin that stops the production of reactive oxygen species formed when fat undergoes oxidation. Previously a popular supplement, data has not supported its health benefits. Deficiency is rare since Vitamin E is found in many oils.

Exacerbation: Aggravation of symptoms or an increase in the severity of a disease

Excoriation: An abrasion or scratch. Sometimes patients with intense itching will excoriate their own skin.

Excretion: The elimination of wastes from the body such as the removal of material filtered out of the blood by the kidney

Executive function: Term used to describe cognitive functions such as self-control, planning, reasoning, and abstract thought, believed to be located in the frontal lobes of cerebral cortex

Exfoliation: Shedding or sloughing usually referring to skin or mucous membrane

Exhaustion: Extreme fatigue to the point of incapacity

Exocrine: Secretions to a surface or through a duct as opposed to those secretions that go directly into the blood. Sweat is an exocrine secretion.

Exogenous: Produced or originating outside a cell or body. Compared to endogenous which originates inside the system

Exostosis: Exaggerated bone growth at the place where bone typically grows

Exotoxin: Toxin released by a bacteria or other organism into its environment

Exposure: State of being introduced. Contact so that infection is a possibility. Proximity in a way that would allow for pathogens to enter a host

Extension: Movement that INCREASES the angle between two parts. When shaking hands, the fingers are fully extended. At 180°, as when standing, the knees are extended.

Exudate: Accumulated fluid in a space. Can also refer to material that penetrates though tissue or the oozing of serum or pus

F

Facial nerve: (CN 7) Motor: Muscles of the face. Sensory: Taste on the forward 2/3 of the tongue. In Lyme, Bell's palsy is paralysis of CN 7.

Factor H: A control protein involved in the alternative complement pathway, ensuring that the immune response targets the pathogen and not *self*-tissues

False negative: Poor specificity. A negative test result when the case is actually positive. The test says there is NO disease when there is. Common in Bb testing

False positive: Poor sensitivity. A positive test result when the case is actually negative. The test says there IS disease when there is not. Exceedingly rare in Bb testing

Fascia: Ct that holds things in place. Fibrous membrane that separates one tissue from another. Allows tissues to slide past each other. Fascia is largely composed of collagen and Bb's affinity for collagen may explain the fascial pain often associated with Lyme. Bb may change the character of fascia making it more adhesive.

Fasciculation: Muscle twitch that is a small, local, involuntary contraction visible under the skin. Most common in the eyelid. Sometimes called tremors, but tremors may be more often due to nerve dysfunction whereas fasciculations are more likely a muscle problem. Distinction can be difficult.

Fasciitis: Inflammation of fascia, which is a fibrous membrane-covering that supports and separates muscles. Plantar fasciitis is a common complaint in Bb and bartonellosis. Bb may be attracted to the collagen in the Ct comprising the fascia.

Fatigue: Feeling of tiredness or weariness. Sustained sense of exhaustion resulting in a decreased capacity for physical or mental activity

Fat soluble: Able to dissolve in fat, but not water. Fat soluble vitamins can be retained in the system after absorption. Overdoses can cause buildup to the point of clinical symptoms.

Fauna: Animal life. Bacteria have been classified as both flora and fauna, but most often end up with the flora.

Fear: A negative emotion caused by a real or perceived threat. Basic survival mechanism causing animals to move away from the source of the fear such as pain or risk. When experiencing fear, a human will usually resort to fight-or-flight, although in extreme cases the person might be paralyzed with fear. In contrast to anxiety, fear usually has an identifiable source, whereas anxiety can be general or vague.

Febrile seizures: Seizure activity often associated with a too abrupt CHANGE in body temperature rather than the actual number on the thermometer. Hypothetically, fever could lower the seizure threshold in certain individuals allowing for tonic/clonic seizures, or partial seizures with posturing.

Femoral: In the area of the groin. Near the femur

Fever: Body temperature above the normal range usually attributed to inflammation or infection. Elevated temperatures due to hyperthermia is usually not referred to as fever.

Fibroblast: Cell that makes collagen, connective tissue, elastin, reticular protein, and cartilage. Bb apparently gets inside the fibroblasts in joints and the NS.

Fibromyalgia: Despite "official" criteria for diagnosis, fibromyalgia remains a poorly defined and understood condition. This is a chronic, widespread pain syndrome that often presents with broad musculoskeletal aches, pains, stiffness, soreness, fatigue, and sleep problems. Common pain sites include neck, back, shoulders, hands, and pelvic girdle, but any part can be affected. Can be mild to severe and flare and regress, just like Bb infection. Often misdiagnosed. Should be on the TBI list of DD, especially when considering Lyme. Pain is almost always present in combination with tenderness at "tender points," widespread soft tissue discomfort or aching, persistent fatigue, generalized stiffness, and non-refreshing sleep.

Fibrosis: Abnormal formation of fibrous tissue. Excess fibrous tissue as a result of inflammation, irritation, infection, or healing after damage such as trauma. The result of repair work as seen in scarring

Filariasis: Nematode infection often affecting the lymphatic system

FISH: Fluorescent in-situ hybridization assay looks for RNA from the pathogens of interest.

Fissure: Crack, tear, or furrow in the lining of tissue. Often seen with fungus in the foot, in the mucous membranes near the anus, in chapped lips or hands, or as furrows in the tongue epithelium which seem to increase in the elderly

Fistula: Canal that forms in the tissue that allows pus or other fluids to drain. Abnormal tubes that form that allow communication between two areas, usually from one cavity inside to the outside surface, or into another cavity

Fitness: Ability to perform physical demands without exhaustion. In sick patients, fitness can be important both in terms of cardiovascular preparedness as well as overall strength. Functional fitness can be especially important in patients with chronic diseases where the patient has enough energy to perform tasks important to daily life such as taking a shower or feeding themselves. Usually the more fit the person at the onset of illness, the more rapid the recovery.

Flaccid: No tone, limp, weak, lax, soft. Paralyzed muscles are flaccid.

Flagyl: (Metronidazole) Antiprotozoal and antibacterial. Cyst-buster. Often used as part of combination therapy in TBIs

Flank: Part of the body between the ribs and the top of the hips. Sides of the torso

Flare: Resurge

Flaring: Dilation of the nostrils during inspiration. Infants (and all age groups) in respiratory distress will unconsciously flare their nostrils in an attempt to get more air into the lungs.

Flat feet: Abnormal flatness of the sole and arch of the foot. Usually inconsequential, but may interfere with normal function. A normal foot arch should have concavity. In the case of flat feet, also called fallen arches, the entire sole will be flat across the floor. This is most apparent when the patient stands, since there is no visible arch and the entire length of the sole touches the floor. Flat feet can be tender on long walks, and they keep you out of the army.

Flexibility: Ability to achieve a full range of motion. This capability can vary in the same individual for different joints. Much flexibility is genetic but practice can improve flexibility within the patient's innate range. An individual who is "tight" may be more prone to injury when performing other activities. Look at hypermobile kids since they may be predisposed to more joint involvement in TBI infections. Flexibility also refers to your ability to see things my way.

Flexion: Movement that DECREASES the angle between two parts such as bending the elbow or clenching the fingers into a fist. When sitting, the knees are flexed at 90 degrees.

Flora: Plant life. Bacteria have been classified as both flora and fauna, but most often are included with the flora.

Fluorescent in-situ hybridization: (FISH) Technique that looks for **RNA** from the pathogens of interest

Fluoroquinolones: Bacteriostatic antimicrobials that are very effective but have been associated with numerous and significant adverse effects including black box warnings on their labels

Foam: Air pushed through creams or lotions creates a foam that can be used to deliver medicines.

Folic acid: Vitamin B9

Food poisoning: Disease acquired by eating food contaminated with pathogens. The causative organisms often produce toxins. Examples include Salmonella in peanut butter and E. *coli* in undercooked hamburger.

Foreskin: Loose, retractable fold of skin that covers the head of the penis. Also called the prepuce, this is the skin that is removed during circumcision. This remnant is an excellent sample choice for diagnostic testing since tissue usually allows for more sensitive testing than blood.

Formication: Sensation of bugs crawling. Tactile hallucination

Formulation: Various combinations of ingredients or preparations used to deliver drugs. Goal is to get the medicine into a form that is stable and acceptable to the patient. E.g., tablets, capsules, suspensions, patches, creams, etcetera, can all be used to deliver the same active pharmaceutical ingredient.

Fossa: (Fossae is plural) A furrow or slight depression

Fovea: Pit in the center of the macula where the retina thins to a layer of tightly packed cones causing it to be the area of the most acute vision

Fractures: Breaks in bone, cartilage, and occasionally other organs that usually present with point tenderness

Freckles: Hyperpigmented areas, especially on skin, where the body sends out melanin to protect itself from UV rays

Free radical: A chemically unstable molecule that contains an unpaired electron, making it highly reactive. These molecules will try to steal an electron from a nearby stable molecule. When oxygen is involved this process is called oxidation. Inside the cell, DNA can be damaged by free radicals and if not curtailed, permanent damage may result. Antioxidants can stabilize free radicals before they have a chance to harm the cell. In Lyme patients, free radicals are hypothesized to increase with the amount of infection and may account for some of the neurologic problems associated with the disease. Antioxidants may help protect the brain and other tissues from the damage caused by these unstable molecules.

Fremitus: (Thrill) Vibrations palpable through the chest wall when the patient is speaking or coughing. If both hands are placed on either side of the chest the vibrations on one side can be compared to the other side. Alternatively, a stethoscope can be used to auscultate fremitus. Fremitus decreases in pleural effusions, emphysema, lung collapse, edema, or with large masses. Vibrations may be more noticeable when there is obstruction of one bronchus. Ask the patient to repeat the number "99" to evaluate fremitus.

Frenulum: Fibrous tissue that attaches the bottom of the tongue to the floor of the mouth

Frequency: The number of times an event repeats in a given time. Increased urinary frequency can suggest infection.

Friction rub: Crackling heard when two rough or dry surfaces chafe together. Sometimes rubs are described as squeaking, grating, or the sound of walking on crunchy snow. Rubs are heard in pericarditis, pneumonia, pleural effusions, and pleurisy. Here the pleura lining the lung is rubbing against the pleura of the chest cavity. Since the rubbing occurs each time the pleura moves, the rub is heard on both inspiration and expiration. Rubs occur when membranes are inflamed and lose their lubrication. A rub does not usually change after a cough.

Frontal lobes: Parts of the brain located in the front of the cerebral hemispheres. Control voluntary muscle movements including the motor area for speech. The frontal lobes contain the majority of the dopamine-sensitive neurons that are associated with reward, attention, short-term memory, planning, and motivation. The frontal cortex is where most of what we would consider "thinking" goes on. These lobes are the seat of personality, behavior, intellect, judgment, and problem solving. They are responsible for what is termed "executive function" which includes self-control, reasoning, and abstract thought. These capabilities might be considerably impacted by TBIs, especially Lyme, Bartonella, and M. *fermentans*.

Frozen shoulder: The shoulder joint can stiffen to the point of immobility and non-function, often secondary to splinting

Functional: Term used to suggest a finding is benign, innocent, or non-pathologic

Fundal exam: Examination of the back part of the eye as seen through an ophthalmoscope

FUO: Fever of unknown origin

G

Gait: Manner of walking

Gallbladder: Pear-shaped sac under the right lobe of the liver that serves to concentrate, store, and release bile into the duodenum

Gallops: Extra, or adventitious, heart beats that sound like a horse galloping. Usually a third sound constitutes a gallop, although sometimes an S3 and S4 combine. S3 is benign in kids, athletes, and some pregnancies, later this ventricular gallop can mean heart failure. Lyme has been associated with heart failure. Gallops can be due to volume overload.

Gallstones: Bile is concentrated in the gall bladder by removing water. Anytime the conditions are such that the cholesterol and salts can't remain in solution they can precipitate out forming gravel and stones.

Gamish: Big mess

Gamma globulin: A type of Ig or antibody. Given by injection to boost immune function in order to fight certain diseases like hepatitis or to help overcome immune deficiency

Gamma-glutamyl transpeptidase: (GGT) Reasonably liver-specific enzyme that will go very high for even minor subclinical liver problems. GGT can be helpful in identifying a one-time elevation in LFTs.

Ganglion: (Ganglia is plural) 1) Cystic, round, non-tender, swelling along tendon sheaths of joints, and 2) Clumps of nerves forming small centers of activity positioned on both sides of the spinal cord

Gangrene: Tissue necrosis or death, often due to poor blood supply or infection

Gastritis: Inflammation of the stomach

Gastroenteritis: Inflammation of the stomach and intestine

Gastroesophageal reflux disease: (GERD or heartburn) Backflow or reflux of the acidic stomach contents into the lower esophagus, which is not designed to handle that low pH. Can be due to increased intra-abdominal pressure or lax sphincters, both of which can be impacted by Lyme damage to the nerves in the area. Sxs include sub-

sternal pain and burning. Reflux is the most common GI feature of LD. GERD is very common in gestational Lyme.

Gastroparesis: Deceased ability of the stomach to empty its contents even though there is no blockage. Perhaps due to partial paralysis of the gut. Also called delayed emptying. Makes the person feel full and bloated. Has been associated with LD

Gel: A mixture of oil and alcohol. With a high viscosity, gels often melt at normal body temperatures. These vehicles tend to be *drying* because of the alcohol component and they can sting if they contact broken skin. Because of the alcohol and other additives, they may predispose to hypersensitivity reactions. Gels may be a good choice when you are treating fungus since they can be drying and fungi like it nice and moist.

General anxiety disorder: (GAD) These patients are always anxious about everything. Can't ever relax. Always in an unpleasant and uncomfortable state, worrying about both reasonable and unreasonable things. Although GAD can begin any time, initial sxs often begin early in childhood. GAD manifests as excessive, chronic, usually daily anxiety and is a condition that can last for months or years.

Generalized: Not restricted to one area

Generic: Non-proprietary drug or product. Not protected by a trademark. Not branded. Less regulated

Genital warts: Growths caused by HPV and most often seen in the genital/anal area

Genotype: Genetic code used to make the phenotype

Gentamicin: Aminoglycosides are a class of antibiotics rarely indicated for treatment of TBIs although they are sometimes used to treat tularemia and M. *fermentans*. However, if given for other reasons in TBI patients they might increase the risk of kidney damage. They include: gentamicin, tobramycin, amikacin, kanamycin, streptomycin, and neomycin.

Genus: Grouping of organisms below Family and above Species with common characteristics that distinguish it from other groups

GERD: Gastroesophageal reflux disease

Gestalt: Idea that something is more than the sum of its parts. Intuitive feel

Gestational: Acquired *in utero*

Gestational Lyme: Transmitted from mother to child *in utero* resulting in congenital disease

Giardiasis: Conditions caused by the Giardia genus of protozoa which sport flagella and attach to the mucosal walls and thereby cause disease

Gilbert's syndrome: Hereditary cause of increased bilirubin found in 5% to 10% of the population and only rarely causing jaundice. AST and ALT are normal but direct and indirect bilirubin are high. These patients have a decreased capacity to metabolize bilirubin which is thought to be a genetic variant and not pathologic.

Gingivitis: Inflammation of the gums usually manifesting with redness, swelling, and tendency to bleed. A distinctive odor suggests infection. Can cause a low grade inflammation that may interfere with the body's immune response to infection and impact recovery time

Glasgow Coma Scale: A tool for evaluating and quantifying the degree of coma by determining the best motor, verbal, and eye-opening responses to stimuli. Offers a quick standardized account of consciousness. A score of 15 is normal, 7 indicates coma, and brain death is 3 or lower. Comparison of results over time or after an intervention can be used to assess progress or deterioration.

Glial cells: The non-nerve or supporting tissue of the brain and spinal cord. Bb is believed to be able to get inside the glial cells within the CNS.

Glomerulonephritis: Inflammation of the glomeruli of the kidney, often due to infection. Glomeruli are the functional, filtering units of the kidney. Relatively familiar sequela to untreated Strep throat or skin infections. Abs formed to fight the Strep infection bind to segments of the glomeruli in the kidney. Can also be secondary to autoimmune conditions such as lupus

Glossopharyngeal nerve: (CN 9) Sensory input from the pharynx and middle ear. Also, one muscle innervation

Glutamate: A neurotransmitter that may be involved in the MOA of Rocephin and may contribute to the pathophysiology of ALS

Glutathione: Peptide that acts as an antioxidant to protect cells from free radicals. Produced naturally in cells, glutathione neutralizes free radicals and keeps other antioxidants like Vitamins C and E active. This molecule can detoxify a number of foreign molecules and appears to be essential for full immune function. This peptide is involved in the synthesis of DNA, proteins, and prostaglandins as well as amino acid transport and enzyme activation. Glutathione affects all body systems especially the immune response, nervous system, GI tract, and lung. Glutathione has been used for treating Alzheimer's, Lyme, the pain of arthritis, and depression. For TBI patients, some have found glutathione helps with brain fog.

Gluten: Protein found in wheat and some other grains. Some patients have an autoimmune reaction to gluten, called celiac disease, and others experience gluten sensitivity

Gluten sensitivity: Allergic reaction to the gluten protein

Glycemic index: Tool to determine how fast a food converts to glucose in the blood. The speed at which carbohydrates begin to circulate in the blood as glucose. Simple carbohydrates often enter the blood almost immediately and raise the blood sugar levels quickly. Complex carbohydrates are slower to digest and have lower values on the GI scale. Table sugar ranks at 100, but processed white flour as in some pastas and breads can rank even higher. Foods with high values cause blood sugar levels to roller coaster, resulting in cravings. Low GI foods keep blood glucose stable.

Goodpasture's syndrome: Uncommon autoimmune disease with antibodies depositing in lung and kidney tissue causing pulmonary hemorrhage and glomerulonephritis

Gout: Arthritis caused by deposits of uric acid crystals in the joint space causing inflammation. Usually one joint is involved initially, most often the MTP joint of the great toe. The toe presents red and swollen and the pain can be excruciating and crippling. Joints can lose function.

Gram stain: Method of staining bacteria in order to help in their identification. Organisms are said to be either Gram positive or Gram negative depending on the color they retain after being exposed to an iodine solution. Antimicrobials are often selected for use based on their ability to affect either Gram positive or Gram negative organisms. Staph is Gram positive and E. coli is Gram negative and Bb are Gram neutral.

Grand mal: Generalized seizure. Usually the patient loses consciousness and falls. The body stiffens and the tonic-clonic part of the seizure begins. Skeletal muscles spasm and relax rhythmically, most obviously in the extremities. A grand mal seizure may include incontinence and tongue biting. The seizure usually lasts 2 to 5 minutes. In the postictal state, the muscles can be sore and the patient complains of confusion, headache, or weakness. Grand mal seizures have been linked to congenital Lyme but causal association is unknown.

Granulocytes: WBCs that contain granules in their cytoplasm and have multilobed nuclei. They are sometimes called polymorphonuclear leukocytes or PMNs. Include neutrophils, eosinophils, and basophils

Granulomas: Small growths or nodules comprised of granulation tissue made from various immune cells. These tumors are thought to occur when macrophages can't destroy the foreign material and the phagocytes accumulate and become part of the abnormal growth.

Grave's disease: Probable autoimmune condition causing excess thyroid hormone resulting in nervousness, heat intolerance, palpitations, and weight loss

Gray baby syndrome: Associated with IV chloramphenicol. Some newborns, especially the premature, do not yet have the fully-functioning enzyme systems needed to metabolize and excrete chloramphenicol. As a result, the medicine can build up in the system. This toxicity can be fatal. The child may vomit and not suckle. Respirations can become irregular and rapid and cyanosis can result. The baby becomes flaccid and ashen gray.

Grey matter: Neurons

Grippe: Archaic term for influenza

Groin: Inguinal area

Group therapy: Form of psychotherapy where a small group of patients meet to discuss common issues in strict confidence. Guided by an experienced counselor, the purpose is to gain insight into shared concerns, discuss options, and provide support. Lyme can be very isolating and being part of a group can help many patients.

Growing pains: Nonspecific term used to refer to pain felt in the joints or limbs of growing children. There is no evidence that the pains have anything to do with growing. Of unknown etiology, growing pains are very common in the elementary school age group. I wonder if some of what we called growing pains over the years might have been associated with TBIs, especially the shin discomfort of bartonellosis. There is also a possible association with rheumatic fever.

Growth charts: Standard grid that allows for the recording of measures of height, weight, and head circumference. Can be used to compare one child to others of the same age and sex and to follow the individual child's progress over time. Usually expressed in terms of percentiles

Grunt: Quick, harsh sound of forced expiration against a closed glottis. A grunt temporarily halts expiration and is sometimes heard in pneumonia, pulmonary edema, and painful ribs. A newborn with atelectasis will grunt. Infants in respiratory distress may grunt as the body tries to keep air in the lung and keep up the O_2 level.

Guarding: Occurs when the patient voluntarily tries to protect the sore spot by tensing the muscles. Commonly found with acute abdominal pain and musculoskeletal problems

Guillain-Barré syndrome: (GBS) An inflammatory, autoimmune destruction of myelin in the nervous system often showing progressive, rapid loss of symmetrical motor function. GBS most often occurs after acute viral infection. Paresthesias often precede a loss of motor function that can lead to paralysis. The immune response targets parts of the nervous system causing numbness, weak limbs, and in severe cases paralysis.

Gynecomastia: Enlargement of breast tissue in males

H

Habitus: Set of learned dispositions, skills, and actions acquired through AODL. The person's sensibilities. Both the physical attributes and attitudes of a person

Half-life: ($t_{1/2}$) The time it takes for 50% of the drug to be eliminated. The time it takes for the drug concentration to fall to half its previous value. Knowing how long the drug remains in the body impacts many aspects of dose determination.

Hammer toe: Uncommon in small children, the 2nd toe presents with a hyperextended MTP and a flexed PIP. This kind of deformity can affect any toe and more than one toe at a time.

Haptoglobin: A protein that binds to Hb that has been released from lysed red cells. Haptoglobin binds *free* Hb that's released from RBCs and thereby decreases the oxidative capacity of the *bound* Hb. The haptoglobin-Hb complex is then removed, usually by the spleen. Measurement of haptoglobin can be used as a screen for hemolytic anemia. If the patient has sxs of anemia but haptoglobin is normal the anemia is not likely due to hemolysis. If haptoglobin is low, then hemolysis could be the underlying etiology. Can be measured serially in babesiosis to track anemia status. Increased in some inflammatory conditions and decreased in hemolytic disorders

Headache: Cephalgia. Head pain. Common manifestation of TBIs

Health care providers: (HCPs) physicians, psychologists, nurses, nurse practitioners, chiropractors, physician assistants, physical therapists, or any professional providing health care

Heart block: Refers to an impediment in the normal electrical conduction of the heart. Conductile tissue fails to convey impulses normally from the nodes in the atrium to the ventricles. Cardiac problems associated with Lyme often include conduction system problems. The most common site of blockage is thought to be at the AV node. Pacing may be needed in about a third of these patients and they may present with chest pain, palpitations, syncope, and dyspnea.

Heart failure: A temporary or on-going condition resulting from the inability of the heart to maintain adequate circulation of the blood. Pump failure

Heat rash: Prickly heat. Blockage of the pores that lead to sweat glands. Most common in infants since infants do not usually sweat.

Characterized by white or clear milia on face, chest or back. Will usually go away on its own when child in a cooler environment

Heavy metal damage: (Toxicity) Heavy metals can cross the BBB and get into the CSF. Hg can be especially neurotoxic and symptoms include burning, numbness, and electric shooting sensations. The term "mad as a hatter" refers to those exposed to high levels of mercury used in the manufacturing of felt hats in England in the 18th century. These workers would present with dementia, emotional lability, memory problems, excessive salivation, and insomnia. Other heavy metals such as lead and cadmium can also cause sxs that can be mistaken for manifestations of TBIs. Heavy metal exposure might also prolong or intensify Lyme sxs.

Heel spur: Sharp point that develops below the heel because of repeated insult to the area. Most often spurs are due to the pull of the plantar fascia on the heel. Spurs can also develop in people with unequal leg length, almost as a protective callous as the one heel repeatedly hits harder than the other. The pain of a heel spur can mimic plantar fasciitis and the sole pain associated with Bartonella.

Helicobacter *pylori*: Causative organism in many cases of GI ulcers

Helper T cell: Subpopulation of T cell lymphocytes unique in that they have no phagocytic or cytotoxic activity themselves. They activate and direct other cells and help facilitate multiple immune functions

Hemangioma: A benign tumor of dilated blood vessels, not uncommon in Lyme and Bartonella infections. May appear as small bright red, raised dots. Also called red nevi. Cavernous hemangiomas are dilated, thin-walled blood vessels also known as cherry angiomas.

Hematuria: Blood in the urine

Hemoglobin: Iron-containing pigment in the RBCs which carries oxygen from the lungs to the tissues

Hemoglobinuria: Presence of Hb in the urine free from RBCs

Hemolysis: Destruction of the membrane of the RBCs with the liberation of Hb

Hemoptysis: Blood in the cough product may be from the respiratory system, oral cavity, GI tract, or pulmonary tree.

Hemorrhoid: Varicose vein of the rectum or anus

Hepatic: Referring to the liver

Hepatitis: Inflammation of the liver, which is most commonly due to viral agents, is also caused by bacteria, parasites, and chemical irritation from drugs, alcohol, or other toxins. Clinical findings include an enlarged liver and jaundice. Usually a prodromal stage presents with malaise, fever, anorexia, nausea, vomiting, muscle aches, fatigue, headache, dark urine, and clay-colored stools. The condition then progresses to an icteric stage where jaundice worsens and other signs and symptoms progress. Pruritis can occur and the liver is large and tender. Lab tests including antigen and antibody screens and elevated liver enzyme levels support the diagnosis. Hepatitis is common and is often part of the differential diagnosis in TBI cases.

Hepatocytes: Liver cells

Hepatotoxin: Something that damages the liver

Hernia: Rupture or protrusion of an organ or part of an organ through the wall of the cavity that normally contains it. Common hernias include inguinal, abdominal, and umbilical. A hernia can become an emergency when the contents become incarcerated or strangulated.

Herniated disc: Protrusion of the cushion between the vertebra which may impinge the nerve

Herx: (Herxheimer reaction) Response to massive kill-off of pathogens resulting in excess toxin release and the sxs associated with the subsequent manifestations of an immune response clean-up. When effective antibiotics are started the patient may feel worse before he feels better.

Hesitancy: Delay in starting urination

HHV: Human herpes virus

HHV-1: (HSV-1) A human herpes virus thought to be the cause of cold sores

HHV-2: (HSV-2) A human herpes virus thought to be the cause of genital herpes

HHV-3: (HHV-3) Human herpes viruses thought to be the cause of chicken pox (Varicella) as well as shingles and herpetic neuralgia (Zoster)

HHV-4: (Epstein-Barr virus) A human herpes virus thought to be the cause of infectious mononucleosis that generally provides adaptive immunity with huge lymphadenopathy, severe sore throat, fever, and incapacitating fatigue

HHV-5: (Cytomegalovirus) A human herpes virus, CMV often goes unnoticed and remains an asymptomatic infection indefinitely. CMV can be a life-threatening condition in the immunocompromised. As with many of the HHVs, CMV can remain latent in the body for long periods. HHV-5 can be transmitted to the fetus and congenital CMV can cause problems in the newborn. About 1 in 150 neonates is born with CMV. This infection can be especially problematic in babies also at risk for a congenital TBI, where it can compromise diagnosis and recovery. Once present, the virus stays for life.

HHV-6: This herpetic virus can cause roseola, also called exanthum subitum

Hip dysplasia: Infant hip is either dislocated or out of position due to congenital, developmental, or traumatic causes. While not painful, hip dysplasia can lead to impaired walking and early arthritis. Relatively common. Females and breech deliveries have a higher incidence of dysplasia.

Hippocampus: Part of limbic system of the brain with a role in memory

Histamine: Biochemical involved with a number of immune reactions, especially allergies. Manifestations can include redness, swelling, and bronchial constriction.

Histiocyte: General term for any monocyte that has become a resident in tissue, i.e., a macrophage

Hive: (Wheal, urticaria) Often part of an allergic reaction with a sudden eruption of pale or reddish evanescent swollen lesions associated with intense itching. Can be singular, several, or general

HLA markers: Part of the MHC system, human leukocyte antigen markers are found primarily on white cells and serve to help distinguish *self* from non-*self*. HLAs are some of the thousands of protein markers on the surface of our cells that identify us as "us." HLAs are located on the surface of leukocytes and help determine what molecules our immune system will confront and to what degree. We have thousands of HLA identifiers (proteins/antigens) on our cells to prevent us from eating ourselves up.

HLA-DR2 and HLA-DR4: Specific HLA markers found in a sub-population of the general populace. These are just two of the millions of antigen markers present in humans. Their presence suggests which patients will tend to respond to Bb infection with an autoimmune presentation. About 15% of individuals in the general population have specific HLA markers that identify them as a singular group that will not react predictably to the B. *burgdorferi* infection. About 15% have HLA-DR2 markers, and about 15% have HLA-DR4. Some have both. This autoimmune presentation may be more severe and may include increased joint involvement and muscle pain, along with a more aggressive inflammatory response, since, in addition to attacking the foreign Bb, they are also assaulting the *self*.

Holistic: Approach to medicine looking at all the parts of a patient including physical, emotional, and spiritual

Homeostasis: Stable equilibrium between elements in the body whereby the physiology adjusts to keep metabolic processes level. If one aspect is disturbed other components of the system compensate to re-establish balance. Maintained by the constantly changing feedback and regulation in response to both external and internal fluctuations

Hormone: Compound, usually a peptide, produced by one tissue and transported via the circulation or across interstitial fluids to cells of another tissue, on which it has an effect

Host: Any animal that the tick feeds upon

Hughes Syndrome: (Antiphospholipid syndrome) Autoimmune, hypercoagulable condition secondary to antibodies attacking the phospholipids in the cell membrane

Human chorionic gonadotropin: (hCG) Hormone present in the urine of pregnant women

Humor: Biochemically active molecules such as hormones, ILs, etcetera, or the fluid carrying such molecules

Humoral immune response: Part of the immune system that does not involve cell-mediated response including the work of antibodies and the myriad other biochemicals involved with mounting a defense

Hydrocele: Collection of serous fluid in the scrotal sac

Hydrocephalus: Accumulation of CSF within the ventricles of the brain. Buildup of fluid in the brain either from too much being present or the inability of the fluid to drain. Hydrocephalus can cause a bulging fontanelle and papilledema and the pressure can cause damage to the motor neurons and other parts of the NS.

Hydroxychloroquine: (Plaquenil) Antimalarial and anti-inflammatory. May be good choice for Lyme patients who test positive for HLA-DR2 or HLA-DR4 or patients who clinically present with autoimmune-like sxs associated with Lyme. Consider for LD when arthritis is a predominant manifestation. Also used for babesiosis and M. *fermentans*. Consider as part of a combination regimen for Q fever endocarditis

Hyper-: Prefix meaning excess or more than normal. *Hyper-* before a motion such as hyperextension means the joint is moving beyond what is normal and this excessive motion may stress the joint.

Hyperacusis: Increased sensitivity to sound which might cause the patient to become phonophobic (avoid sound). Sensitivity to noise is common in newborns with Bb.

Hyperbaric oxygen: (HBO) Medical use of oxygen under conditions greater than atmospheric pressure. Administered in a pressure chamber. Most often used for decompression sickness, gas gangrene, and carbon monoxide poisoning. Recent use in cerebral palsy, MS, and Lyme with anecdotal reports of efficacy

Hypercalcemia: Excess amount of calcium in the blood. If blood calcium is too high, some will be stored in bone and the rest excreted into the urine and stool.

Hypercoagulation: Excessive clotting. Increased ability to form clots and sometimes the clotting cascade does not know when to stop. Sequelae of hypercoagulation can include thrombus (a stationary clot within the vascular system which can impede blood flow), or embolus (a travelling clot with the potential to snag or occlude anywhere in the vasculature).

Hyperkalemia: Excess potassium (K) in the blood. High potassium can be due to decreased kidney function, medicines such as steroids, muscle necrosis, IV or other K supplements, or acidosis. Hemolyzed blood samples or repeated fist clenching during a lab draw can artificially increase K.

Hypernatremia: High sodium (NA) in the blood. Kidney disease, low water intake, or loss of water due to diarrhea or vomiting can all increase Na levels.

Hyperpnea: Rapid, deep breathing found after exercise, anxiety, metabolic acidosis, or hypoxia. Deeper than normal breathing is expected after exercise. Hyperpnea is seen with pain, respiratory disease, fevers, cardiac problems, certain drugs, hysteria, and high altitude. Hyperpnea is a compensatory measure, trying to get things back to normal. The difference between hyperpnea and hyperventilation is that hyperpnea is an <u>appropriate</u> response to the patient's metabolic state while hyperventilation is an <u>inappropriate</u> response.

Hypersensation: (Hypersensitive, hypersensitivity) Excess perception or extreme awareness of a sense or feeling. Common and often severe problem in kids with Lyme and other TBIs. One of the most common complaints of TBI patients. Can include extreme sensitivity to touch, sound, light, taste, or smell. Hypersensitivity can also refer to certain kinds of allergic reactions or psychological overreaction to emotional stimuli.

Hypersomnia: Excessive sleep time in a 24 hour cycle after which the person does not feel refreshed. An increase in daytime sleepiness

Hyperthyroidism: Condition where on-going excess production of thyroid hormone causes sxs which can be subtle or obvious. One type is Grave's disease which can present with tachycardia, tremor, increased blood pressure, increased reflexes, eyelid lag, palpitations, nervousness, and weight loss.

Hyperventilation: Increased ventilation which results in blowing off CO_2 that may result in hypocapnia. Patients can hyperventilate in cases of asthma, acidosis, anxiety, pulmonary embolism, or pulmonary edema. Treatment involves slowing the rate of CO_2 loss. The difference between hyperpnea and hyperventilation is that hyperpnea is an <u>appropriate</u> response to the patient's metabolic state while hyperventilation is an <u>inappropriate</u> response.

Hypo-: Prefix meaning below, under, beneath, suboptimal, less than

Hypocalcemia: Low blood calcium. If blood calcium becomes too low, bones release more to bring the levels back to normal.

Hypochondriasis: Abnormal concern about one's health. Hypochondriacs are preoccupied with their bodily functions and health and they fear acquiring disease. These patients are suffering, it just isn't for the reason they think.

Hypoglossal nerve: (CN 12) Motor: tongue

Hypokalemia: Low blood potassium (K). Can be due to excess urinary excretion, GI loss, or redistribution of K from the extracellular space to inside the cells. The most common causes include medications such as diuretics and penicillins, kidney disease, excessive loss due to heavy sweating associated with high fevers or other causes, vomiting, diarrhea, eating disorders, abnormal aldosterone, increased Na, hypercalcemia, malabsorption, cancers, DKA, or severe B12 anemia.

Hyponatremia: Low sodium (Na) in blood. Often due to liver disease, kidney dysfunction, heart failure, burns, or excessive sweating

Hypospadias: Urethral meatus found on ventral surface of penis

Hypostome: Central feeding tube found inside the palps of the tick mouth protected by the chelicerae. Blood and saliva are exchanged through the hypostome.

Hypothalamic-pituitary adrenocortical axis: (HPA) Hormonal cascade involved with steering overall endocrine function and balance. One hormone affects the next and that hormone affects a third, etcetera, and disturbances anywhere along the line can have significant repercussions. TBIs, especially Lyme, can impact the HPA. LD is well-known to impact the normal endocrine balance in the body and this disturbance is likely modulated through the HPA. TNF-alpha influences the HPA and M. *fermentans* activates the system causing a number of limbic sxs. Because disturbance of the HPA can be so pervasive, diagnosis and treatment can be challenging.

Hypothalamus: Part of limbic system of the brain. Involved with the maintenance of homeostasis where all physiologic processes are kept in balance including water, salts, sugars, and fats along with the regulation of temperature and release of certain hormones. The hormone leptin influences appetite through the hypothalamus and may be associated with obesity. The hypothalamus integrates the SNS and PSNS and regulates hunger, thirst, and response to pain and pleasure. This part of the limbic system is concerned with sexual satisfaction, anger, and aggressiveness. The hypothalamus is involved with the EXPRESSION of emotion, not its generation. So this organ determines how a person reacts to fear or panic and may explain why some people itch for a fight. Neurosecretions are the modulators of the activity of the hypothalamus through the ANS and the pituitary.

Hypothyroidism: Deficit of thyroid hormone leading to a decrease in basal metabolism, obesity, dry skin and hair, lower blood pressure, slow pulse, sluggishness, less muscle activity, and intolerance of cold

Hypotonia: Lack of normal tissue or muscle tone. Cardinal sign of congenital Lyme. Child will appear floppy and limp.

Hypoxia: Low oxygen in blood

I

Iatrogenic: Adverse consequence due to the effects of treatment or actions of HCPs or the health care system

Icterus: Jaundice

Idiopathic: Unknown cause. Fancy way of saying, "I don't know." Be careful you don't stop looking for the underlying cause while hiding behind the idiopathic disclaimer. Medical term for, "Who knows?"

Ileus: Problem with the normal motility in the GI tract. A stoppage of intestinal movement or peristalsis. Material can no longer be propelled forward. Ileus can be due to inflammation or infection. Drugs like opioids cause severe ileus. Neurologic problems or injury can cause a paralytic ileus with atony.

Imagination: Ability of the mind to create something that did not exist before

Immune paralysis: When overwhelmed, the immune system can shut down until it has a chance to regroup. Possible causes include a massive bolus of pathogen such as seen with multiple co-infections or vaccine overload

Immune response: All the activities undertaken by a body in order to defend itself from external assault

Immune system: Various parts of an organism that work together to resist infection or protect the body from a disease, toxin, or other insult

Immunization: (Vaccination) Process of developing or creating immunity to a specific disease

Immunodeficiency: (Immunocompromised) Immune system lacks the normal capacity to respond effectively. Having an immune system unable to handle a given assault. May be due to genetics, steroids, or infectious agents that impair the immune response

Immunofluorescence assay: (IFA) Technique used to detect antibodies in a sample. IFA uses a single antibody that is chemically linked to a fluorescent molecule. The antibody recognizes the target antigen and binds to it causing the fluorescence.

Immunoglobulins: Antibodies

IgA – Antibody most often found in mucosal areas. Thought to prevent colonization of pathogens. IgA is found in the mucus of saliva, tears, and respiratory secretions. When the GI, GU, and pulmonary tracts are infected, IgA might be present in the discharge. Low IgA is a commonly recognized deficiency of antibodies but the significance of this finding in TBI patients is not clear.

IgD - IgD may help grow and develop B cells but its role is not yet clearly outlined. IgD might function as a receptor on cells that have not yet been exposed to antigens. The function of IgD is less defined than that of the other isotypes. When a B cell begins to express IgM as well as IgD, it is considered mature, so IgD may help develop its parent B cell.

IgE – Antibody elevated in allergies, asthma, and parasitic infections. IgE is found in mucus. Functions with mast cells in allergic and anaphylactic reactions. Binds to allergens and triggers histamine release. Involved in the body's defense against parasites including parasitic worms

IgG – Antibody that comes into play later in the immune reaction after IgM and remains after the infection is gone. Indicative of past, on-going, or chronic infections. Also present when there is an autoimmune component to the immune response. Most of the Ab-based immunity is due to IgG fighting against invading pathogens. Crosses placenta to give passive immunity to fetus. IgG is more likely to be detected when IgM starts to decrease.

IgM – Antibody high in early infectious states especially viral, parasitic, and autoimmune diseases. Found on the surface of B cells. Eliminates pathogens early on in B cell-mediated immunity. IgM does the job BEFORE there is enough IgG. IgM is thought to be the first antibody formed after exposure to a new antigen. IgG comes when IgM starts to decrease. New theories regarding the function of IgG and IgM suggest their roles may be somewhat reversed in Lyme patients, with IgM persisting far longer in the clinical course than previously expected. Some say IgG is the only antibody to cross the placenta, but others believe IgM can as well.

Impaction: Packed firmly. Pressed together. Fixed in place. A hard solid mass made of feces can compact in the rectum secondary to chronic constipation. A tooth can become impacted if there is not enough room for it to erupt from the gum.

Impetigo: Staph or Strep skin infection characterized by pustules which ooze and crust

Incarcerate: Tissue that is trapped, confined, or constricted. If blood flow is impeded, tissue may die.

Incidence: The number of individuals who develop a condition over a period of time

Incidence rate: Number of times a disease occurs over a period of time compared to the number of individuals in the population at risk at the midpoint of the time period

Incompetent: Referring to a reservoir species that is not capable of passing the infection on to a feeding tick, even though infected

Incontinence: Inability to retain urine or feces usually because of lack of tone or sphincter control

Indications: "Official" reasons to use a drug or treatment. Usually based on the results of clinical trials that are referenced in the product label. This does not mean that a drug is not effective for other conditions.

Indigenous: Native to a specific locale

Indirect hernia: Rupture or protrusion of an organ or part of an organ through the wall of the cavity that normally contains it. In the case of an indirect hernia, a weak internal ring allows tissue to descend through the inguinal canal into the scrotum or labia.

Individualized Education Programs: (IEPs) Mandated by the Individuals with Disabilities Education Act (IDEA) these plans are designed to meet the unique educational needs of the individual child who has a defined disability. Here, disability refers to a physical or mental impairment which substantially limits one or more major life categories. An IEP should be based on the individual's strengths and weaknesses and ability to learn.

Inducibility: Ability to be changed, activated, or expressed due to a stimulus

Induration: Firmness or hardness. An area of tissue that is firmer than normal

IEP: Individualized Education Program

Infant automatisms: Actions performed without thought in newborns and babies. These are sometimes called reflexes but there are slight differences.

Infection: Presence and growth of an organism inside a host that, in some cases, may eventually cause tissue damage or disease. The invasion of a host by an outside organism. If the organism is able to establish itself and multiply, disease may occur. If this reproduction then causes illness in the host, the organism is called a pathogen. Infected is not necessarily synonymous with diseased. Infections can be acute, chronic, persistent, on-going, localized, disseminated, systemic, recurrent, relapsing, subclinical, etc.

Infectious arthritis: Inflammatory reaction in the joint space that occurs in response to a pathogen, usually bacteria

Infertility: Inability to produce offspring

Inflammation: Nonspecific immune response that occurs in reaction to any type of bodily insult, from cuts, to foreign bodies, to poisons, to pathogens. Manifested by calor, dolor, tumor, and rubor

Inflammatory Bowel Disease: IBD is a group of inflammatory conditions of the intestine, the most common of which are **Crohn's disease** and **ulcerative colitis**. These two present similarly, the difference being the location and nature of the inflammatory changes in the gut. Crohn's can impact any part of the GI tract from mouth to anus in what are called **skip lesions.** UC affects the colon and rectum with a **continuous** area of inflammation including contiguous ulceration. Both can affect body systems outside the alimentary canal such as the liver, joints, skin, and eyes. Crohn's is thought to be autoimmune, while the consensus is still out on UC.

Infusion: Liquid introduced into the body usually through a vein for treatment purposes

Ingrown toenail: Common in older kids, the edge of the nail digs into the flesh causing inflammation and infection. The soft tissue around the nail becomes tender and red with the overhanging nail fold often oozing pus.

Inguinal: Groin

Inguinal hernia: Protrusion of a hernia sac containing intestine into the inguinal canal

Injection: The introduction of fluid into a vessel, cavity, or tissue usually IM, IV, or SQ. Can be bolus or infusion over time

Insect: Animal with 3 pair (6 actual) legs in contrast to Arachnids where the adults have 8 legs. Some insects are disease vectors.

Insomnia: Difficulty falling or staying asleep

Insulin: Hormone made in the pancreas which is essential for glucose metabolism

Institute of Medicine: (IOM) Independent non-governmental arm of the National Academy of Science, involved with providing guidance in medical decision-making

Intelligence: Ability to think and thereby understand relationships, solve problems, and adjust to new situations. Capacity to learn

Intelligence quotient: Measure of intellectual ability. IQ tests have individual strengths and weaknesses that may impact results and conclusions.

Intention tremors: These tremors occur during deliberate movements, such as when reaching or pointing, and are likely due to cerebellar lesions.

Interferons: Group of biologically active proteins involved with immune response

Interleukins: Cytokines (biomolecules) that help regulate the immune system, inflammation, and the formation of blood cells. Various IL families are made by different cells and have unique roles. ILs appear critical to normal function of the CNS in ways not clearly understood but seem to impact the hippocampus and its role in memory, learning, and nerve signal potentiation.

Intermittent: Coming and going. Not continuous. Intervals of activity

Interstitial: Many interpretations but here refers to the space between cells. Can also be a vague reference to the tissue comprising an organ

Interstitial cystitis: (IC) A chronically irritated and painful inflammation of the bladder. Poorly understood. Presents with frequency, nocturia, hesitancy, urgency, and suprapubic pain. This condition presents exactly like a bacterial UTI except no bacteria is recovered on routine cultures. Symptoms do not resolve with traditional antibiotic regimens. Remember that Bb has been recovered in some of these cases.

Intertrigo: Symptomatic fungus in the skin folds

Intervention: Action taken to improve on a bad situation or to modify an outcome

Intestine: Tubular portion of the alimentary canal from the pylorus of the stomach to the anus. Aids in the digestion, absorption, and elimination of food and fluid balance. GI tract inexorably associated with the nervous, immune, and endocrine systems

Intracellular: Within the cell

Intracranial pressure: Force exerted by fluid inside the cranium or skull. If high, infants may show signs of infection and be fretful and refuse to eat. Vomiting can lead to dehydration and this dryness may prevent bulging of the fontanelle which might otherwise occur. The swollen fontanelle is a sign of increased ICP, which can be found in meningitis.

Intractable: Incurable or resistant to therapy

Intraerythrocytic: Within the RBC

Intramuscular: (IM) Medicine is inserted into the skeletal muscle either through a needle attached to a syringe or through a pellet embedded in the muscle.

Intrathecal: Within the spinal canal

Intravenous: (IV) Medicine is administered directly into a vein either in a single dose **injection** (bolus) or more slowly in a dilute **infu-**

sion over time (that is, a syringe and needle or a hanging IV bag). IV dispensing goes right into the circulation and thereby circumvents any potential absorption problems. IV allows for the best plasma titrations and the most rapid onset of action.

Intrinsic factor: Glycoprotein secreted by the gastric mucosa that is essential for the absorption of Vitamin B12

Intussusception: The telescoping of a part of the bowel into a distal portion of the intestine is most common in boys under age two and may be the result of viral or other infections. This is an acute abdomen and needs to be addressed immediately. Otherwise, intussusception can be fatal within 24 hours.

In utero: Occurs in the uterus

Inversion: Movement of the sole of the foot TOWARD the body midline. Hyperinversion is usually what occurs when an ankle is sprained.

In vivo: In a living system

In vitro: In a non-living system

Iodine: (I) Essential mineral in thyroid hormones, which influence much of the overall metabolism. Low iodine levels can result in hypothyroidism, Often the thyroid gland will enlarge to compensate for the deficit (goiter). In 1924, iodine was added to table salt in order to stem an epidemic of goiters. In children on-going hypothyroidism can lead to mental, sexual, and physical developmental delays. Growing kids, teens, the chronically ill, pregnant women, and the severely stressed may need more iodine. We know that Lyme patients often have thyroid problems.

Iris: Colored portion of the eye. Inflammation can occur in Lyme. Iritis, also called anterior uveitis, is frequently associated with LD.

Iron: (Fe) Essential component of the hemoglobin molecule that allows the heme to carry oxygen. Iron is also part of the myoglobin molecule in muscle.

Irritability: Easily annoyed or irritated. Abnormally sensitive to stimuli. Very common complaint in LD

Irritable bowel syndrome: (IBS) Spastic colon. Symptoms include chronic abdominal pain, general GI discomfort, bloating, and alternating bowel habits. Possible miscommunication between the nervous system and the GI tract. Either diarrhea or constipation can be dominant in the clinical picture. IBS may start after an infection, stressful event, or the onset of puberty. An incomplete differential diagnosis includes malabsorption, lactose intolerance, celiac disease, parasites, and IBD. There may be associations with thyroid dysfunction and bacterial or fungal overgrowth. IBS patients have a higher incidence in connection with certain co-morbidities such as depression, CFS, fibromyalgia, headache, endometriosis, interstitial cystitis, and various chronic pain syndromes.

Ischemia: Local deficiency in blood supply often secondary to obstruction

Ixodes tick: (Ixodid) Genus of ticks that include important vectors of disease

J

Jacksonian seizure: Initially localized seizure with spasms or other signs confined to one body part or one group of muscles. This seizure begins locally and then spreads. There will be jerking and tingling in an extremity. For example, the thumb may begin the process and then the seizure activity spreads to the hand and arm.

JAK inhibitors: Janus-associated kinases are enzymes that contain some of the most important receptors for cytokines. Inhibition of these enzymes is thought to decrease inflammation.

Jarisch-Herxheimer reaction: "Official" name for the Herx reaction

Jaundice: (Icterus) Condition characterized by yellowing of the skin, whites of eyes, mucous membranes, and body fluids. Due to excess bilirubin in the blood depositing pigments in the tissues. In newborns, severe jaundice can damage cells in the brain that could lead to permanent sequelae.

JIR: Juvenile inflammatory arthritis, formerly called JRA

Jogging: Slow to moderate-paced exercise that is faster than walking and slower than running

Journaling: Keeping a dairy or journal of thoughts and feelings about life events can help some patients. A record of perceptions and emotions that may be a useful tool in allowing individuals with chronic illnesses to vent frustrations, disappointments, boredom, and anger

JRA: Juvenile rheumatoid arthritis, now referred to as JIA

Judgment: Ability to make considered decisions, come to reasonable conclusions, and to decide between options

Juvenile inflammatory arthritis (JIA) Formerly called JRA. Type of chronic arthritis in children usually presenting between 6 months and 16 years of age. Poorly understood autoimmune mechanism. Can involve few or many joints with pain and swelling. Typically positive for arthritis markers. LD and JRA present similarly and both should remain on the DD list until one can be safely ruled out.

K

Kawasaki's disease: (Lymph node syndrome, mucocutaneous disease, polyarteritis) Autoimmune disorder that causes inflammation of medium-sized blood vessels. Often associated with a pre-existing viral infection. Fever may present on the first day and last several weeks. Irritable, lethargic, bilateral conjunctival congestion, and deep red oral mucosa called "strawberry tongue." Lips can be dry and cracked and several days into the disease the palms and soles can get red with feet swollen and skin peeling. May be fatal long after the acute syndrome presents. Sometimes treated with IV IgG

Kefir: Fermented milk with active cultures that's easy to digest. Yogurt-like drink that may stimulate beneficial flora in the gut

Keloid: Hypertrophied scar

Kernicterus: Jaundice in infants usually in the first week of life. The NS can be flooded with bilirubin. If untreated, can have poor prognosis

Kernig's sign: In meningitis, pain limits the passive extension of the knee. A reflex contraction and pain in the hamstrings when attempting to extend the leg

Ketek: Telithromycin

Kidney: One of a pair of organs in the back of the abdomen outside the peritoneum that forms urine by filtering blood plasma. Important regulator of water, electrolyte, and acid-base content of the blood. Primary site of drug excretion

Kinete: Zygote in the life cycle of Babesia

Knee: Mid-leg joint at the articulation of the femur and tibia. Common site of Lyme joint pain

Kupffer cells: Macrophages in the liver

K vitamin: Fat soluble molecule that is needed for normal clotting. Both dietary sources as well as bacterial synthesis in the gut

Kynurenic acid: Neuroprotective biomolecule. Discovered by a German chemist in dog urine after which it was named

Kyphoscoliosis: Lateral curve of the spine that can be deforming with an A-P hump

L

Label: Package insert. Provides information on a drug based on manufacturer and regulatory agency agreement

Lactate dehydrogenase: (LDH) Enzyme found in many body tissues including the liver. When tissue containing LDH is damaged, the enzyme increases in the blood. In humans, LDH is found in several isoenzyme forms and recognizing which kind is circulating will point to the tissue that is damaged.

Lactose intolerance: Inability to digest milk sugar due to lack of the enzyme lactase causing GI sxs

Langerhans cells: Macrophages in the skin

Lanugo: Fine, downy-hair covering most newborns

Lariam: (Mefloquine)Treatment for babesiosis and malaria. Crosses the BBB but associated with significant CNS AEs

Lassitude: Weariness

Latent: Not active. Host is infected but pathogen does not replicate or grow for a period of time. Host is asymptomatic during this interval. Dormant refers to the pathogen and latent refers to the disease. Lurking

Lateral: Direction AWAY from the midline. Toward the side

Lateralization: Localizing a sensation or response to one side or the other. E.g., hearing can be tested to determine conductive versus neurosensory loss based on the lateralization of sound.

Leaky gut: Hypothesized condition causing increased permeability of the gut wall allowing substances through. Theorized to be due to infections, toxins, medications, or other potential etiologies. Might be due to, or might cause, an abnormal immune response

Legg-Calve-Perthes: (LCP disease) Necrosis of the hip joint occurs when blood flow is compromised causing cells to die. This condition can lead to permanent damage and arthritis.

Legumes: Plants in the Leguminosae Family including peas, soybeans, beans, and peanuts

Lesion: Area of pathology in tissue. Can be due to injury, irritation, wound, infection, or any other abnormal process

Leukocytes: WBCs including granulocytes (neutrophils, eosinophils, basophils) and agranulocytes (lymphocytes i.e., B and T cells, as well as monocytes, which are called macrophages in the tissue)

Leukoplakia: A thick white patch on the mucous membrane like dried paint, which can be pre-malignant

Levaquin: Fluoroquinolone antibiotic

Level of consciousness: (LOC) The degree of awareness of the patient is an important indicator of neurologic function. The LOC can range from alert and interactive to comatose. Failure to respond even to painful stimuli can suggest significant problems.

Levofloxacin: (Levaquin) Fluoroquinolone antibiotic. May hit Bartonella and M. fermentans. Use with caution

L-form bacteria: Bacteria that lack cell walls. There are at least two types of L-forms: those that are unstable and can revert back to their original form and those that are stable and remain as L-forms. L-forms are derived from bacteria that start out with cell walls. The morphology of L-forms can be quite different from that of the original bacteria and most are spheres. Although L-forms can come from either Gram positive or negative bacteria, all L-forms are Gram negative. Since the cell wall is important for cell division, which is usually accomplished by binary fission, replication is disorganized giving rise to a variety of cell sizes. Bb spirochetes are thought to make L-forms. This would be significant since the presence of L-forms may render cell wall antibiotics ineffective and provide another way for Bb to persist in the host. The Bb without the cell wall resist PCNs and CSs.

Lid lag: When the eye is looking from the upper to the lower field of vision, the normal lid slightly overlaps the iris throughout this movement. With lid lag, the upper lid lags behind the upper edge of the iris as the eye moves down. Lid lag and poor convergence can be seen in hyperthyroidism.

Ligament: Strong, fibrous band connecting bone to bone

Lilith*: Pseudonym for a real nurse at the local ER. To me, this person was the epitome of all that is hideous and evil about contemporary healthcare. Since I knew I would need to refer to this person often to tell my son's story, I needed an appropriate alias. I wanted to find the name of the most vile creature ever known. Since the real nurse's name began with an "L," I soon found the perfect pseudonym in Lilith. Biblical lore has Lilith as Adam's first wife in the Garden of Eden. She ran away from Adam (purportedly with a fallen angel). When other angels were sent to find her she responded, "Leave me alone. I was created only to cause sickness in infants." She refused to return to paradise after she hooked up with her wayward archangel. Her name means mean-spirit and she is now associated with demons, the occult, witchcraft, the spread of disease, and human sacrifice. Lilith was said to roam the streets like a stray dog, terrorizing the weak and stealing children. She is also associated with jackals, hyenas, and goats. The local Lilith was rude, arrogant, and technically inept. She acted bored and demonstrated no compassion. She rolled her eyes repeatedly and scoffed as she made numerous incorrect pronouncements. Lilith needs to pursue a new career path before she causes more harm. Just like her namesake the local Lilith is a storm demon; the bearer of disease, illness, and death. In Jewish lore Lilith appeared as a night hag and screech owl. Some folklore suggests that Lilith rapes Adam; others that she is the queen of demons and even better, that she is the serpent who tempts Eve. I selected this name as the alias for the local ER nurse because she was totally vile and abusive to all the patients within my hearing. She is not a composite. She was ONE nurse who harmed children.

Limbic system: A group of structures in the temporal lobe of the brain including hypothalamus, hippocampus, and amygdala with multiple connections and functions. Associated with emotions including aggression and repetitive behaviors. Some memory is also housed here. Involved with behavior and arousal and also impacts the endocrine and other systems. The significant NP sxs associated with LD, bartonellosis, and M. *fermentans* may be associated with impact on the limbic system.

Linea alba: White line of Ct in the middle of the abdomen from the sternum to the pubis

Lipase: Pancreatic enzyme that elevates when there is damage to the pancreas. Levels take longer to increase than amylase, but stay elevated longer

Liver: Largest organ in URQ of abdomen under the diaphragm with multiple metabolic functions. Primary site of drug metabolism

Liver functions tests: (LFTs) Laboratory tests that check for liver damage. When the liver cells are injured, contents such as enzymes can leak into the bloodstream. Patients with TBIs that are treated with medications that can cause liver damage should have regular LFTs. LFTs include: ALT, AST, GGT, and bilirubin.

LMN lesions: Skeletal muscle is innervated by a group of neurons called lower motor neurons which project out from the spinal cord to the muscle cells. A lesion to a LMN might affect the nerves traveling from the spinal cord to specific muscles. The signs and symptoms are OPPOSITE to those of an UMN lesion and include flaccid paralysis like that found in Bell's palsy, muscle loss, muscle atrophy, fasciculations, hypotonia, and hyporeflexia. There is no Babinski sign. Examples include polio, Guillain-Barré syndrome, muscular dystrophies, and peripheral neuropathies. A characteristic finding in children with gestational Lyme is hypotonia, although the pathophysiologic mechanism is not yet understood.

Loading dose: An initial higher dose of drug given at the onset of treatment before dropping down to a lower maintenance dose. Best used in those drugs that are slowly eliminated from the body and only need a low maintenance dose to maintain effective blood levels. These drugs are also presumed to take a long time to reach adequate blood levels and a loading dose may allow more rapid attainment of this level.

Localized: Restricted to one area

Logic: Ability to think using evidence, proof, and inference. Building one concept reasonably upon another. Assessment of a patient's ability to think logically is one way to check cognitive function.

Lotion: Mixtures of oil and water that can be used to deliver medications. Good at getting into crevices and folds such as those found on scalp and skin. Most medicated shampoos are lotions. Lotion has a light, flowing consistency and is less thick than a cream. With a low to medium viscosity (thickness), lotion can spread more thinly than other formulations. This allows more surface area to be covered with the topical medication.

Lower limit of normal: (LLN) Lab normals often fall into a range based on the compilation of data gathered from large populations.

The lower end of this range is called the LLN. If the value goes below that limit, the patient would be considered abnormal. Watch for patients who start out near the LLN and move to the ULN. While still "normal," this type of change could suggest a problem in this individual.

Lumbar puncture: (Spinal tap) Diagnostic (and sometimes therapeutic) procedure performed in order to collect cerebrospinal fluid (CSF) for analysis. Usually the test is done looking for confirmation of meningitis.

Lupus: (Systemic lupus erythematosus or SLE) Collagen vascular disease that can present with severe arthritis, rash, extreme photosensitivity, hair loss, kidney problems, lung fibrosis, and constant joint pain. SLE is an autoimmune, multisystem condition most common in young women. Many body parts are potentially affected including joints, skin, kidney, heart, lungs, blood vessels, and brain. Characteristic butterfly rash on face. On differential diagnosis of Lyme. MOA in lupus may be Ab against *self*-DNA that can then affect many tissues. Both lupus and Lyme involve collagen in their pathophysiology.

Lyme arthritis: Diagnostic term initially used to describe Bb infection before the pathology was well understood. In the past, if there was no arthritis there was thought to be no Lyme. Now the term is used to describe the joint inflammation that may be part of a larger infectious process.

Lyme disease: (LD) Borreliosis. Multisystem infectious disease caused by Borrelia *burgdorferi.* Lyme disease can be acute or chronic, localized or systemic, etc.

Lyme eye: Punctated erythema on the conjunctiva associated with LD

Lyme rage: Intense anger that accompanies borreliosis in some cases. Is it Lyme, or bartonellosis, or M. *fermentans*?

Lyme shrug: Noisy popping and cracking of the neck upon movement

Lymph: Plasma that diffuses from the blood in the general circulation and surrounds most tissues. Part of the interstitial fluid that is found around cells. Eventually the lymph returns to the lymph vessels, gradually moving through nodes and onto a reconnection with the blood circulation. Like blood, lymph has both a liquid and cellular component. Lymph is plasma PLUS the WBCs, but NO red cells. Lymph often carries pathogens or other foreign proteins to the nodes where they are phagocytized. Lymph carries WBCs (especially lymphocytes), bacteria and other microbes, and small proteins. Lymph differs in composition in various parts of the body. Near the intestine, the lymph (called chyle) contains more fat than lymph from other areas.

Lymphadenopathy: Enlarged lymph nodes suggest body is mounting a defense. The actual swelling is usually white cells and pathogen.

Lymphangitis: Inflammation of a lymph vessel usually manifesting as a red streak from the point of infection moving toward the central vasculature

Lymphocytes: Agranulocytic WBCs which include B and T cells

Lymphocytoma: Discrete, purple, skin bump associated with Bb infection that has been reported in Europe

Lysis: Destruction, dissolution, decomposition, usually by breaking the cell wall or membrane

Lysosome: A cell organelle involved in the digestion of nutrients, using enzymes capable of breaking down proteins and certain carbohydrates. Enzymes in lysosomes can be involved with phagocytosis.

M

Macrolide antibiotic: Any of several antibiotics containing a large (macro) lactone ring that are produced by Actinomycetes of the genus Streptomyces. Inhibit bacterial protein synthesis. Growth inhibitor with a bacteriostatic effect, but can be -cidal at high doses. Do well against intracellular pathogens such as when Bb enters the tissue cells. E.g., Zithromax (azithromycin) and Biaxin (clarithromycin)

Macrophage: General term for any monocyte that has become a resident in tissue, also called a histiocyte. Super-phagocyte. Can recognize and ingest foreign or damaged cells or materials. Named for their location within the body: Kupffer cells in the liver, Langerhans cells in the skin, microglia in the brain, etc. Monocytes (macrophages) may be the predominant cellular responders to Bb infections.

Macula: Yellow spot in the center of the retina close to the optic nerve

Macule: Non-palpable, small, flat lesion up to 1 cm (e.g., freckles, petechiae)

Magnesium: (Mg) Mineral with critical role in normal muscle, nerve, enzyme action, and protein synthesis. Involved in reactions involving energy use and part of the enzyme systems needed to make energy through ATP. Many symptoms associated with Lyme such as fatigue, twitches, weakness, and speech problems are also associated with low magnesium levels. Widely distributed in foods, magnesium deficiency is rare, EXCEPT in Lyme patients. Symptoms of deficiency include tremors, twitches, cramps, muscle soreness, depression, and heart skips. Patients with depleted Mg levels can experience weakness with low energy levels and impaired cognition.

Magnetic resonance imaging: (MRI) By using magnets and radio waves the nuclei of atoms can be realigned and the magnetic field that is produced can be detected by a scanner and recorded to produce an image. Because different nuclei resonate at different speeds, different tissues can be distinguished resulting in a clear image. MRI uses no ionizing radiation but still provides good soft tissue resolution making it especially useful in assessing the brain, heart, muscles, and connective tissue.

Maintenance dose: The usual dose of medicine selected to keep the blood levels optimal for that drug

Malabsorption: Inadequate absorption of nutrients or medication from the GI tract. Many causes and contributors. May lead to inadequate blood levels of drugs or nutrient deficits

Malaise: Disquiet, unease, or indisposition often secondary to infection. Patients will often use the word malaise interchangeably with weakness, fatigue, sleepiness, lassitude, and even dizziness.

Malaria: An acute and sometimes chronic infectious disease caused by the protozoal genus Plasmodium invading RBCs. Transmitted to humans by the bite of the mosquito. Initially presents as a minor fever with malaise, headache, fatigue, abdominal discomfort, and muscle aches followed by shaking chills and fevers around 104 with altered consciousness. Symptoms can cycle, i.e., wax and wane around every 48 hours. Malaria can cause anemia and an enlarged spleen. The tick-borne babesiosis is so similar that it is sometimes called North American malaria. Malaria is often fatal in underdeveloped areas and accounts for nearly 250 million cases each year with nearly a million annual deaths.

Malarone: Combination of atovaquone and proguanil. Antiprotozoal that has been used against Babesia

Maltese crosses: Formations of replicating protozoa in red cells infected with Babesia. If the time is right in the clinical course, Maltese crosses might be visible on a blood smear viewed under a microscope.

Manic depression: Bipolar disorder

Mantras: Sounds used to facilitate meditation that can be meaningless such as la, or traditionally sacred words such as om, selected to help the meditator focus. The mantra can also be a word such as peace, serenity, or hope, chosen to allow the practitioner to move into a positive mind set.

Massage: Manipulation of superficial and deep layers of muscle and connective tissue to enhance function and healing and to promote relaxation and well-being

Mast cell: Immune cell found primarily in tissue. The mast cell may be the tissue counterpart of the circulating basophil but appears to contain some bioactive chemicals that basophils do not. Involved with histamines, allergic reactions, and inflammation. Common around blood vessels of the skin and in the bone marrow

Mastitis: Inflammation of the breast usually due to bacterial infection. Responds to antibiotics

Mastoid process: Part of the temporal bone located just behind the ear

Maturation: Process of development where the individual reaches certain milestones and eventually becomes independent. Overall maturation is an integration of physical, mental, intellectual, emotional, and social components. Emotional IQ, or EQ, is the evolution of the ability to recognize and manage emotions in a way that allows for life satisfaction and stable relationships with others.

McBurney's point: Spot in RLQ where pain from appendicitis usually localizes

Meatus: Opening

Mechanism of action: (MOA) Description of how a drug works. Information on MOA may help when combining drugs to get better efficacy. There are hundreds of ways that drugs work, but the most common MOA is probably through some kind of receptor binding.

Meconium: First bowel movement of the newborn

Medial: Direction TOWARD the midline

Meditation: Term used to describe a myriad of techniques used to clear the mind and bring on a peaceful inner milieu. Most approaches use a focus on the breath or a selected word or mantra to help settle the thoughts. A number of positive physiologic effects have been documented.

Mefloquine: (Lariam) Antimalarial that crosses the BBB and may be effective against Bb and Babesia as well. May be associated with severe CNS problems in some patients

Megacolon: Extremely dilated colon

-megaly: Suffix meaning enlarged

Memory: Ability to retain and recall information. Normal memory can recollect material over both the short and long-terms.

Memory cell: Type of B lymphocyte that recalls previously identified antigens and allows for rapid response upon future exposure to that antigen

Meningitis: Inflammation of the meninges, the covering of the brain and spinal cord. Most commonly the inflammation is the result of an infection, although there can be other reasons. Signs of meningitis are initially those of infection: fever, chills, and malaise. As the disease progresses there will be signs of increased ICP such as headache, vomiting, change in consciousness, photophobia, irritability, drowsiness, confusion, and papilledema. Soon the signs of meningeal irritation develop including nuchal rigidity. Meningitis can be viral, bacterial, fungal, or aseptic.

Meniere's disease: Recurrent and often progressive symptom set that might include gradually worsening deafness, ear ringing, dizziness, ear pressure, and sensation of fullness. May have intermittent attacks and one or both ears might be involved

Meningoencephalitis: Inflammation of both the brain and the covering of the brain and spinal cord

Meniscus tear: Damage or rupture of the fibrocartilage cushion in the knee. Local tenderness or pain on adduction or abduction of the knee. An audible click also suggests a torn meniscus. Sxs may mimic Lyme.

Mental status: Functional state of mind as judged by behavior, appearance, responses to stimuli, speech, cognition, abstract thought, memory, and judgment

Mepron: Atovaquone

Mesenteric adenitis: Inflammation of lymph nodes in the membrane that attaches the intestines to the abdominal wall. These enlargements occur mostly in kids and teens and can present with abdominal discomfort and may be a sign of bartonellosis.

Metabolic syndrome: (Syndrome X) Combination of factors that when considered together increase the risk of CVD and DM. Might include chronic stress, excess weight, sedentary lifestyle, abnormal lipids, pre-existing heart conditions or diabetes, older age, insulin resistance, and a history of certain psychiatric and rheumatic conditions. May have some sxs in common with LD.

Metabolism: 1) The sum of all the physical and chemical actions within an organism. E.g., growth, digestion, maturation, and energy transfer can all fall under the term metabolism. 2) Transformation or alteration of a drug, usually in the liver, prior to excretion

Metronidazole: (Flagyl) Azole antibiotic. Important cyst-buster and common selection for combination therapy for Bb. Likely also effective against Babesia

METS: Metabolic equivalent of tasks. Calculation that can be used to assess the amount of energy expended during a specific activity in relation to a reference rate at rest

Microaerophilic: Organisms that require oxygen for survival but the levels needed are at a lower concentration than that found in the atmosphere

Microangioma: A small, sometimes microscopic, enlargement of tissue due to the dilation or formation of new blood vessels as seen in bartonellosis or Morgellons disease

Microglia: Macrophage in the brain

Micturition: Urination

Migrating pain: Pain that moves from site to site. With Lyme, pain may start in one joint and then move to another with or without resolution at the original pain site.

Milia: Characteristic lesion of heat rash. White, pinpoint-sized areas on the face caused by sebum plugging sebaceous glands. These may be present at birth or appear within the first weeks. They spontaneously resolve.

Minocin: Minocycline

Minocycline: (Minocin) TCN-type antibiotic. Often the preferred TCN in the pediatric population. May have less phototoxicity than some of the other TCNs. If the patient complains of dizziness, consider vestibular toxicity and determine how the symptom needs to be addressed. You may need to consider an alternative drug since lowering the dose is not usually the best option in TCNs.

Miscarriage: Loss of fetus

Mitochondrial disease: Loosely defined syndrome where food cannot be properly metabolized for energy

Modality: Way of performing an action or delivering a treatment

Moisture: Damp. Wet. Can refer to either how lubricated the skin is with oils or how much water is present

Mold: Molds and yeasts are types of fungus. Molds grow multicellular filaments called hyphae and they use spores to reproduce. The connected network of branching hyphae tubules are considered all one organism, which is called a colony. Fungi tend to grow in circles like ringworm, which causes a round skin lesion that is often mistaken for the EM rash of Lyme.

Mole: Nevus. Discolored spot-lesion elevated above the surface of the skin

Molecular mimicry: The human genome is about 90% identical to that of bacteria. Because of this similarity when the immune system is assaulted and is in combat mode, it is understandable that some of the less specific components may mistake *self*-antigens for bacterial antigens. This phenomenon is termed molecular mimicry. An autoimmune reaction may result where neurons are mistakenly targeted for elimination. This phenomenon has been well-described in some children with a Strep infection and is believed to occur in cases of borreliosis as well.

Monilia: Candidiasis, thrush, fungal overgrowth, often in the mouth. Monilia was the genus name of the fungi now called Candida.

Monocyte: Type of agranular WBC that circulates for about a day before moving into the tissue as mature macrophages. Bb may inspire a primarily monocytic immune defense.

Montauk knee: Lyme arthritis

Mood: Usual emotion sustained by a person over time that affects that individual's perception of the world

Mood disorder: Disturbance of feelings that falls outside what could be considered a normal range. While everyone has variations in mood over time, a mood disorder involves the abnormal mood becoming the predominant characteristic of the personality to the detriment of the patient.

Morbidity: 1) A diseased state 2) Number of sick people or cases in a population

Morgellons disease: Rare, multisystem condition with a likely infectious etiology where dermal hair-like extrusions are associated with sensations of movement. Pathophysiology is obscure, although excessive cytokines, immune dysfunction, and chronic inflammation are all probably involved. Physical sxs are followed by behavioral problems. Often pronounced Mg deficiency. When first discovered, considered psychosomatic because patients felt they were infected even though there was no proof of infection. Accused of having delusions of parasites. Currently, the dermal filaments are hypothesized to be a parasitic infestation. In 2009, 13,000 self-registrants from all US states and 15 countries were listed on the Morgellons website. Other sxs can include: skin lesions, problems with the hair and hair follicles, fatigue, decreased stamina, recurrent fever, skin filaments, sensation of movement, painful shallow skin ulcers, orthostatic hypotension, microangiomas, short-term memory problems, emotional lability, dysrhythmias, slight increase in pulse, increased insulin levels, and multiple NP associations such as bipolar manifestations, ADD, and OCD. Many sxs overlap with Lyme, especially the NP manifestations and the impact on the endocrine system including the thyroid, pancreas, parathyroid, and the overall adrenal-cortical cascade. Poorly understood and controversial. http://www.morgellons.com

Mortality: 1) Death 2) The likelihood of a disease causing death 3) The death rate associated with a condition

Morton's foot: (Morton's toe) A short, hypermobile 1st metatarsal with a long 2nd toe. May cause mobility problems and discomfort throughout the foot. Morton's toe is a relatively common finding in the TBI patient population. If the toe is symptomatic, a pad under the 1st metatarsal may help. With the 2nd toe longer, the patient may be prone to flat feet, genu valgum (knock knees), femoral anteversion, and have a tendency toward foot, shin, knee, hip, and tibialis anterior pain. This finding may be important when assessing patients who have LD or bartonellosis.

Morton's neuroma: A neuroma is a mass of nerve cells tangled in vascular tissue that may be uncomfortable. In the foot, these masses usually reside in the tissue between the digits, most commonly at the base of the 3rd toe. These spots can hurt especially when pressure is applied.

Morulae: (Morula is singular.) Form of Ehrlichia found in circulating white cells especially monocytes or granulocytes. May be visible under the microscope. Diagnostic of ehrlichiosis but can be hard to discern on blood smear.

Motor function: How the nerves are stimulating and working with the muscles

Motor neuron lesions: Group of neurologic conditions that selectively affect motor neurons which, in turn, control the muscle activity involved in speaking, walking, breathing, swallowing, and movement of the skeletal muscles. Skeletal muscle is innervated by a group of neurons called lower motor neurons which project out from the spinal cord to the muscle cells. The LMNs themselves are innervated by upper motor neurons (UMNs) that come from the motor area of the cortex of the brain. By careful physical examination, an HCP can determine whether the UMN or the LMN is the source of the problem. Lyme can present both kinds of lesions.

MRI: Magnetic resonance imaging

Multiple myeloma: Neoplastic disease with infiltration of the bone marrow and myeloma cells forming multiple tumors which eventually cause fractures

Multiple sclerosis: Progressive demyelination of the white matter of the brain and spinal cord. Sporadic patches of demyelination cause widely disseminated and diverse neurologic symptoms. MS is a chronic autoimmune inflammatory disease of the CNS. One cause is hypothesized to be an insidious infection triggering an autoimmune response, but toxins and allergies have also been implicated. MS is probably multifactorial with both genetic and environmental contributors. MS and Lyme should always be on both differential diagnosis lists. They have many factors in common including a nervous system target, a vague and confusing symptom set with waxing and waning symptoms, and minimal diagnostic support from testing. Signs and symptoms depend on the extent of demyelination and flares may be brief or last for hours or weeks. The pattern is unpredictable, with symptoms hard to describe. The first sign may be vision problems including double vision. Sensory impairment includes numbness (paresthesias) and tingling in one or more extremities, trunk, or face. Then comes muscle dysfunction including weakness and clumsiness. Emotional lability, apathy, and lack of judgment are common. An MS personality may present with a flat, artificial, chronic happiness. Often on physical exam, there is CN involvement, abnormal reflexes, optic neuritis, and impaired cutaneous sensation. The ANS can be affected as evidenced by urinary incontinence and other urinary symptoms. Many patients present with vision changes, muscle weakness, urinary problems, tremors, spasms, cognitive deficits, and mood disorders that can be very similar to the CNS manifestations of Lyme. While MS can progress steadily it can also wax, wane, flare and remit, just like Lyme.

Munchausen syndrome: Repeated fabrication of signs and symptoms of disease in order to get medical attention. While Munchausen's appears to be similar to hypochondriasis, this condition is more malevolent. While hypochondriacs worry about trivial matters, their concern is real and motivated by some valid perception. In contrast, Munchausen patients make things up, often in dramatic and convincing fashion to get attention. When one doctor tires of them, they will doctor shop and start over. They have been known to purposely harm themselves, change normal test results, and pry open healing wounds in order to continue the ruse. Their whole life revolves around keeping the charade going. Children rarely, if ever, present with Munchausen syndrome.

Munchhausen by proxy: A caregiver fabricates medical problems for another, usually a child or other vulnerable person, in order to get attention. These individuals have been known to falsify medical history, alter records, lie about previous test results, or cause injury in order to garner attention or some other benefit. Exceedingly rare

Murmurs: Abnormal heart sounds associated with turbulent blood flow usually originating at the site of one of the heart valves. Apparently there is enough disruption either through **stenosis** (constriction) or back flow (**regurgitation**) to make some noise. Often classified as **physiologic** (benign or part of the normal physiology) or **pathologic** (abnormal and potentially problematic)

Murphy's sign: A sharp increase in pain when the inflamed gallbladder is disturbed by an examining finger

Muscle: Tissue composed of contractile fibers that allow for movement

Muscular dystrophies: Group of hereditary diseases that cause progressive muscle weakness

Mute: Inability to speak

Myasthenia gravis: Autoimmune disease characterized by muscle fatigue due to defects in the synapses between the nerves and muscle fibers. May have trouble with eye movement as well as difficulty chewing and swallowing

Mycotoxins: Harmful chemicals made from fungi such as molds or yeast

Mydriasis: Abnormal dilation of the pupils

Myelin: Fatty layer covering the neuron

Myocarditis: Inflammation of the cardiac muscle. Can be acute or chronic and occur at any age. Early symptoms can be nonspecific with fatigue, dyspnea, palpitations, and fever. Often myocarditis comes from an infection that started elsewhere in the body and became systemic. The originating pathogen can be viral, bacterial, and occasionally fungal. Other etiologies include autoimmunity, RF, radiation, heat stroke, chemicals such as alcohol, and numerous parasites such as helminths. The patient may present with a heart beat that sounds weak at the apex, an irregular rapid pulse, dysrhythmias, and tenderness over the precordium.

Myocardium: Heart muscle

Mycoplasma: Genus of microbes that lack cell walls and are slow growing and not especially susceptible to traditional antibiotic regimens. At least a dozen Mycoplasma species infect humans and several are likely co-infections.

Mycoplasma *pneumoniae*: This pathogen is NOT the Mycoplasma *fermentans* listed with the potential TBI co-infections. M. *pneumoniae* is the causative agent for atypical pneumonia also called "walking pneumonia."

Mycotoxins: Chemicals produced by molds (a type of fungi) that can be pathologic to host organisms

Myopathy: Abnormal striated muscle. If muscles are weak proximally, then you likely have a myopathy. If weak distally, then neuropathy should be suspected.

Myositis: Inflammation of muscle tissue especially voluntary muscles

N

Namaste: Common saying at the end of yoga classes usually accompanied by a slight bow and hand gesture. Roughly translated to "I bow to you," or "The light in me recognizes the light in you."

Narcissistic personality: Abnormal perception of superiority. Exploit others because they believe they are entitled to do so. Impulsive and irresponsible, they do not handle frustration well and do not anticipate the consequences of bad choices.

Natural history: Takes into consideration the usual life cycle of an organism as it normally progresses. The natural history encompasses the creature's life including such things as development, metabolism, behavior, physiology, reproduction, interactions, demise, etc. In fact, the term life cycle is almost a synonym for natural history.

Natural killer T cells: Subset of T cells. Vicious creatures that bind and lyse and release cytokines that can cause sxs in an individual

Naturopathy: Drugless approach to therapy that prefers natural treatment modalities such as light, heat, water, air, massage, etc.

Nausea: Unpleasant sensation of impending emesis

Necrosis: Areas of tissue death

Neologisms: Made-up words as seen in schizophrenia

Nephritis: Inflammation of the kidney usually due to bacterial infection or bacterial toxins. Strep is a well-recognized etiology.

Nephrotic syndrome: End result of numerous diseases that harm the capillaries of the glomerulus. There might be protein spilled in the urine and low albumin in the blood.

Nephrotoxin: Something that damages the kidney

Neuralgia: Pain that follows the distribution of a nerve. The pain of shingles is herpetic neuralgia. Usually, neuralgia is severe sharp pain along the course of a nerve that is caused by pressure on nerve trunks, nerve damage, toxins, inflammation, or infection.

Neuritis: Inflammation of a nerve. Term is used often in association with Lyme. Neuritis can manifest in many ways.

Neuroborreliosis: Bb infection of the CNS

Neurogenic bladder: Any of the many problems that can come from interruption of normal innervations to the bladder including incontinence or retention. Neurologic problems can be spastic and hypertonic or flaccid and hypotonic. Signs and symptoms will depend on the underlying cause and the extent of ANS involvement.

Neurogenic pain syndrome: Experience of so much pain that the brain is set to respond abnormally even to the smallest amount of discomfort. The pain threshold is altered.

Neurologic exam: Includes evaluation of mental status, cerebral and cerebellar function, motor activity, muscle strength, balance, gait, reflexes, operation of cranial nerves, coordination, and sensory perception including pain

Neuron: Nerve cell

Neuropathic pain: Nerve-generated pain. Chronic pain can occur after an insult to any level of the NS and may be the result of aberrant communication between the sensory and motor systems.

Neuropathy: Problem with nerves due to damage or disease. If muscles are weak distally, then you likely have a neuropathy.

Neutrophil: WBC granulocyte often called a PMN. Elevated levels traditionally viewed as the harbinger of bacterial infection but Bb may stimulate more of a monocytic activation as opposed to a neutrophil response

Nevus: Mole. Discolored spot or lesion elevated above the surface of the skin

Niacin: Vitamin B3

Nidus: The focus of an infection. Origin-site of an infection

Nit: Egg of a louse

NK cells: Type of cytotoxic lymphocyte that kills by causing the targeted cell to die by apoptosis. Kills or destroys entities that aren't *self.* Activated by a signal such as a cytokine that tells the NK cell that something foreign is around

Nocturia: Excessive urination at night

Nodule: A bump, knot, knob, protuberance, swelling or cluster of cells. A small node usually ranging from 0.5 to 2 cm. Often deeper and firmer than papules. Subcutaneous nodules can be found along the legs and triceps in Bartonella infections. Nodules under the skin can also suggest RA or RF. Nodules under the tongue can be normal.

Non-*self:* Not possessing host protein markers (antigens). Foreign material present in the body

Normal pressure hydrocephalus: (NPH) Excess spinal fluid collects in small pockets in the brain and interferes with the electrical circuitry. More common in the elderly who might present with shuffling feet, incontinence, and memory loss

Normal muscle tone: Balanced between contraction and relaxation

Norovirus: Common cause of gastroenteritis

Nosode: Homeopathic remedy created from some part of the disease process such as secretions, mucus, pus, diseased tissue, or a sample of the pathogen

Nuchal: Nape or back of the neck. Bottom of the skull

Nuchal rigidity: Neck stiffness or the inability to flex the neck forward (actively or passively) due to increased muscle tone and stiffness. Found in 70% of those with meningitis

Nymph: Developmental stage in some Arthropods between the larval forms and adults. Larval ticks become infected while feeding on infected mammals and then become dormant and transform into the nymph form, which are primarily responsible for transmitting disease to mammals.

Nystagmus: Rhythmic, fine pulsing of the eye. They beat or oscillate. Involuntary, constant rhythmic movement which might be in any direction. A few beats are normal but beyond that is abnormal. Observed in a number of neurologic conditions

O

Obdurator sign: An inflamed appendix may be in contact with a portion of the obdurator muscle. Moving the muscle in a way that touches the appendix should cause discomfort if the appendix is inflamed.

Observational study: Clinical study where the patients are not randomized to a specific study group. Subjects are assigned to a group outside the control of the investigator and then the results are observed and documented. Observational studies are often used to draw conclusions about treatment effects.

Obstipation: Intractable constipation

Obstructed airway: Blocked air passage. Common reason for respiratory distress. Can be due to foreign bodies, masses, or allergies from medicines and other sensitizers. Allergies might cause the airway to swell, eventually occluding the passage and this presentation can be part of an anaphylactic reaction.

Obstruction: Blockage of a structure in a way that prevents normal function such as the blockage of a blood vessel, airway, or the intestine. Intestinal obstruction is the mechanical or functional blockage of the intestine that prevents normal movement of the products of digestion. Can be at any location within the intestine. Sxs depend on location and duration. In general, there is abdominal pain and distension, vomiting (sometimes of fecal material), diminished BSs, and constipation. X-rays can show distinct air-fluid levels. Vomiting can lead to dehydration and electrolyte imbalances. Distension of the abdomen can press up on the diaphragm and compromise respiration. The most serious complications include ischemia, perforation, and death. In partial obstruction there can be anorexia, vomiting, and tenderness to palpation.

SI obstruction: Presents with colicky pain with intermittent cramping. Spasm can last a few minutes with central and mid-abdominal pain. Vomiting usually occurs before constipation. Causes of SI obstruction include: adhesions, hernias, IBD, strictures, tumors, intussusception, volvulus, and foreign bodies including gallstones. In babies, atresia is a common cause of bowel obstruction. Neonates can have a meconium obstruction. "Never let the sun set on a small bowel obstruction."

LI obstruction: With large bowel obstruction, pain is present lower in the abdomen and spasms last longer than with SI obstruction. Constipation begins earlier and there is less vomiting, Causes of LI obstruction include: tumors, hernias, IBD, volvulus, adhesions, constipation, fecal impaction, atresia, strictures from diverticuli, and endometriosis.

Obstructive breathing: When there is a barrier in the airway there will be prolonged expirations because the chest gets overfull (air trapping)

Occipital lobe: Region of the brain that interprets visual stimuli

Occult: Not readily apparent or visible. Hidden

Occupational therapy: Methodology that teaches skills and provides alternatives in accomplishing AODL

OCD: Obsessive-compulsive disorder

Ockham's razor: The simplest answer is usually the correct one. Shave away the unnecessary assumptions to get to the most basic explanation. With TBIs, the explanation might not be the simplest but as more is understood the resulting elucidation usually does make sense.

Oculomotor nerve: (CN 3) Eye movement. EOMs

ODD: Oppositional defiant disorder

Off-label: "Officially" a drug is usually only approved for one or a few indications, based on the clinical studies conducted by the company that wants to sell the drug. That does not mean it cannot do other things very well. Any use other than that defined in the label including variations on dosing, regimens, or conditions being treated

Ofloxacin: (Floxin) Fluoroquinolone that might have efficacy in treating Bartonella and M. *fermentans*

Ointment: Formulation made of about 80% oil and 20% water. Stays on the skin longer than a cream or lotion. If there are active ingredients in the ointment, they often take longer to be absorbed. Ointments are viscous, semi-solids that are often referred to as greasy. They can be used by themselves as a treatment for dry skin since they effectively keep moisture in contact with skin or as an occlusive dressing. Used to deliver API, either as a treatment or as a prophylactic

Olecranon bursitis: Swelling and other signs of inflammation of the bursa around the elbow. This condition may result from trauma or from arthritis such as found in Lyme, gout, or RA.

Olfactory nerve: (CN 1) Smell

Oliguria: Too little urine

Omental trapping: Free flow of omentum can be impeded by adhesions and entrapment by hernias and can cause abdominal pain. Known to occur in some Lyme patients

Omentum: Double folds of peritoneum attached to the stomach and draping over a number of abdominal organs

Omnicef: (Cefdinir) A cephalosporin, cell wall, -cidal antibiotic. Good choice against Bb in combination with intracellular agent

Oncogene: Cancer inducer. A gene that has the ability to cause a cell to become malignant

Onycholysis: Separation of the nail from the nail bed

Opisthotonos: Spasm in which the back and extremities arch backwards so that the weight rests on the head and heels. Sometimes seen in meningitis

Opportunistic: Taking advantage of a situation to your benefit with no regard to how the outcome might impact others

Opportunistic infections: Situation where a pathogen takes advantage of a debilitated or immune-deficient host in order to survive and proliferate. Disease could result that might otherwise have never manifested. There are a number of opportunistic infections associated with HIV and Bb is hypothesized to be opportunistic in some cancer cases.

Opposable: Ability to move one part into contact with another. The human thumb is opposable with reference to the other fingers.

Oppositional defiant disorder: (ODD) An on-going pattern of disobedient, hostile, or defiant behavior, with a total disregard for authority. Stubborn with excessive and persistent anger manifesting with temper tantrums, outbursts, and the desire to annoy others on purpose. Blame others for their problems and are easily annoyed. They are rigid, resentful, and seeking revenge. Their behavior causes distress to others and interferes with academics and social relationships. Bartonella can manifest with persistent tantrums, arguing, and angry or disruptive behavior toward authority figures.

Opsonins: Substances in the serum that coat the membrane of foreign molecules and thereby increase the rate of phagocytosis by macrophages. Opsonization is the coating of a microorganism with antibody and/or complement making them easier to identify.

Optic ataxia: A spatial perception distortion. Here the patient has a hard time targeting movements in space. He will bump into doorways even when trying hard not to. Has been observed with LD

Optic disc: Head of the optic nerve. Lack of rods and cones here causes a break in the visual field called the blind spot

Optic nerve: (CN 2) Vision

Organomegaly: Enlargement of an organ

Organotropism: The attraction of certain chemicals or microbes to specific tissues or organs in the body. The special affinity of drugs, pathogens, or tumors for a particular tissue. Organotropism is important in understanding the pathophysiology of Bb and may help explain some of its sxs. E.g., Bb apparently love nerve cells and tissues containing collagen, which may provide reasons why so many of its manifestations involve the nervous system and any area that contains collagen such as joints, heart valves, and blood vessels in the GI tract.

Orientation: Sense of time, place, and person. Ability to understand and place oneself in the true circumstances

Osgood-Schlatter disease: (Osteochondrosis, OS, OSD) Painful inflammation of the epiphysis of the tibial tubercle. A common knee ailment in kids, this condition is probably due to cumulative trauma in bones before complete fusion of the epiphysis to the main bone. The most commonly involved area is the site of the insertion of the patellar tendon which serves as the anchor for all the thigh muscles. Severe disease can result in permanent tubercle enlargement. OS could be important during the differential diagnosis phase of TBI management, since the knee is a common target of Bb.

Osteoarthritis: (OA, degenerative joint disease, DJD) Arthritis due to wear and tear of joints and cartilage. is the most common arthritis affecting both large and small joints of the hands, feet, back, hip, vertebral column, and knee. OA begins in the cartilage and leads to the two opposing bones eroding into each other so the patient ends up with bone on bone. At first there is minor pain, but then the joint pain becomes continuous and may be problematic at night. The discomfort can be debilitating and often prevents normal activities. Important to consider in the DD of TBIs

Osteochondrosis: (Osgood-Schlatter disease) Painful inflammation of the epiphysis of the tibial tubercle

Osteomalacia: Vitamin D deficiency in adults

Osteomyelitis: Pyrogenic bone infection that can be acute or chronic. Can be hard for antibiotics to penetrate and may need aggressive and prolonged treatment

Osteopath: Fully licensed physician. Doctor of Osteopathy. Uses physical manipulation techniques in addition to allopathic methods to diagnose and treat patients. Believes that structure affects function

Osteopathic lesion: (Somatic lesion) Describes a structural restriction of motion often in the spine or other joints that can impede function

Osteopathy: Philosophy of medicine based on the idea that the body is a vital organism where structure and function are interdependent and both are equally important to health and recovery. Structural manipulation can be an important part of treatment in combination with medicines, surgery, and other modalities.

Osteophytes: Spurs on bone

Osteosclerosis: Thickening on bone

Otitis media: Middle ear infection. Earache manifested by pain, redness, and protuberance of the drum and loss of the cone of light

Ototoxicity: Any situation that causes an adverse effect on the 8th cranial nerve or the sense of hearing. Has been associated with use of vancomycin

Otzi: A 5300-year-old mummy discovered in the Alps about 20 years ago. Found to have DNA from Bb and is now considered to have had the first recognized case of Lyme disease

Outcome study: Type of clinical trial where the desired outcomes are prospectively described and when the patient reaches the designated endpoint, that box is checked. The group results can then be compared to an untreated population. Outcome research can be used to assess the effectiveness of treatments in the real world by pooling the results from large numbers of patients. Might be more practical than controlled trials because the efficacy of an intervention can be assessed in real-world settings. May eventually prove to be the best choice for studying persistent LD

Outer surface protein: (Osp) An antigen on the surface of Borrelia species. Includes OspA, OspB, and OspC, among others

Ovarian cyst: Usually benign sacs of fluid on the ovary. Often asymptomatic but torsion or rupture of an ovarian cyst can result in an acute abdomen

Overdosage: Intentional or unintentional over-consumption of a drug which can potentially cause untoward effects

Overwinter: Period of rest (inactivity) by which insects survive the winter

Oxidation: Biochemical reaction where a substance combines with oxygen

Oxytocin: Hormone secreted by the pituitary and probably certain specialized neurons. Long known to be essential for numerous roles around reproduction and childbirth, oxytocin is now recognized as the nurturing and social hormone. Important for bonding, empathy, and reducing anxiety, oxytocin is sometimes referred to as the love hormone. Research has found that compassion causes the frontal lobes of the brain to light up and increases oxytocin levels. In contrast, low levels of oxytocin have been correlated with sociopathy, psychopathy, narcissism, and manipulation.

P

Package insert: Drug label

Pain: Unpleasant sensory and emotional experience caused by actual or perceived tissue damage. Pain can range from mild discomfort to excruciating and incapacitating sensations. Pain is a complex awareness reflecting real or believed tissue damage and the affective response to this perception. Pain can be acute or chronic.

Acute: Pain associated with a recent event such as trauma or other tissue damage that remains for the short-term as the damaged sensory tissue heals. Usually defined as lasting less than a month. At the onset of pain the SNS may be stimulated causing tachycardia, increased respirations, elevated BP, sweating, and dilated pupils.

Chronic: Pain that persists beyond a month can be the result of on-going tissue damage, scarring, or abnormal pain loops within the nervous system. Long-term pain is probably multifactorial. Chronic pain can be difficult to manage and the patient may experience frustration, depression, lassitude, or sleep disturbances.

Pain amplification syndrome: Limbic involvement in the pain cycle causing enhanced perception of pain with no change in the underlying pathology. Pain has a productive role in communicating signals to the body that something should be done to eliminate the cause. Usually, once the acute damage is resolved, the pain alarm goes off, but sometimes the pain cycle continues. The limbic system gets involved and the more the pain cycle continues, the more the pain is perceived to be increasing. The perception of the pain is amplified.

Pallor: Lack of color. Paleness. Can suggest anemia, bleeding, shock, etc. On one episode of *Mad Men,* Betty is told she looks "wan." In this case, she was pale because she was pregnant.

Palp: Part of the mouth piece of a tick

Palpable: Able to be felt or discerned

Palpation: Use of touch to examine the body in order to gather information about the structures beneath the skin and procure evidence of disease

Palpitation: Perceptible fluttering of the heart

Pancarditis: Inflammation of all the structures of the heart and so would include myocarditis, pericarditis, and endocarditis

Pancreas: Both an exocrine gland behind the stomach that makes digestive enzymes and an endocrine organ making insulin and glucagon, which regulate carbohydrate metabolism

Pancreatitis: Inflammation of the pancreas. Can be acute or chronic

PAND: Pediatric autoimmune neuropsychiatric disorders

PANDAS: Pediatric autoimmune neuropsychiatric disorders associated with Streptococcal infections. Probably an autoimmune response involving antineuronal antibodies manifesting with significant neuropsychiatric symptoms. In these patients, during or after a known Strep infection of the throat or scarlet fever, there can be a sudden onset of neuropsychiatric symptoms such as OCD, tics, or Tourette's. The mechanism may be similar to rheumatic fever after Strep infection except instead of the autoimmune system attacking the heart, valves, and joints, the antibodies attack the brain cells. The basal ganglion seems to be the primary target and this is the site responsible for movement and behavior, explaining the abnormal involuntary movements and actions associated with PANDAS. In RF the antibodies attack the *self* cells of the heart, valves, joints, and apparently parts of the brain. This same mechanism could also be the case for PANDAS with the brain being the focus instead of the heart. PANDAS cause a dramatic, almost overnight onset of symptoms with motor or vocal tics, emotional lability, anxiety, OCD manifestations, enuresis, and deterioration in hand writing.

Pandemic: Occurrence of illness affecting a higher than expected number of individuals in an area

Panic attack: Time of intense fear or apprehension that may be accompanied by palpitations, sweating, trembling or shaking, a feeling of shortness of breath, smothering, or choking, chest discomfort, flushing, GI discomfort, dizziness, numbness or tingling, unsteadiness, detachment from the feeling, loss of control, and the fear of going crazy or dying. The patient may have a sense of imminent danger or doom and an overwhelming urge to escape. The attack is sudden with a peak in about 10 minutes.

PANS: Pediatric Acute-onset Neuropsychiatric Syndrome is one new name for PANDAS, incorporating the possibility of other infectious etiologies aside from Strep.

Papilledema: Edema and inflammation of the optic nerve at the point where it connects with the eye globe. Swelling in optic disc. Can be a sign of increased ICP but ICP has been known to increase in LD without the corresponding papilledema, especially in infants. Absence of papilledema does not rule out high ICP. Whenever there is papilledema there can be vision changes. High ICP is often affiliated with headache.

Papule: Palpable, raised lesion up to 0.5 cm such as a nevus or pimple

Paralysis: Temporary or permanent loss of function especially of voluntary muscles, but also can refer to nerves in the GI tract or to the perception of sensation

Paranoia: Persistent delusions of persecution, conspiracy, or jealousy

Paranoid schizophrenia: Condition of extreme delusions with scattered irrational thoughts of persecution and conspiracies. Patients hear voices telling them what to think and do and they believe that life is outside their control. Believe that others are running the show and they are just watching

Parasite: Organism that lives at the expense of its host. Depends on another for existence or support without helping or being useful to the host. Survives off another without contributing

Parasitemia: Parasites in the blood

Parathyroids: Glands behind the thyroid involved with Ca and P metabolism. Indirectly affects muscle activity. If parathyroid hormones are low, tetany might occur. If high, reabsorption of bone and renal stones could result.

Parenchyma: Cells performing the functional work of an organ and not just providing structure

Parenteral: Any method of drug administration EXCEPT for oral

Paresis: Incomplete paralysis

Paresthesias: Symptom most often described as numbness and tingling. Can also refer to sensation of prickling, increased sensitivity, decreased sensitivity to the point of numbness, itching, perverted sensation, tactile hallucinations, abnormal or bizarre sensations, pricking, "pins and needles," or formication (the feeling of bugs crawling on skin or inside the body). Caused by damage to nerves or interference with nerve conduction. One of the most common complaints in LD

Parietal lobes: Parts of the brain that help coordinate and interpret sensory information including skin senses

Parkinson's disease: Chronic neurologic condition often presenting with fine, slowly spreading "pill-rolling" tremors, rigidity, loss of muscle movement, flat affect, and a strange gait where the feet barely clear the floor. Specific areas of the brain seem to be involved as is the neurotransmitter dopamine. There have been Parkinson-like syndromes noted in conjunction with Bb infection, but any causal relationship is unknown.

Paronychia: Inflammation usually with infection (often accompanied with pus and redness) at the edge of a nail

Paroxysm: Sudden spasm or burst

Partial seizure: A local brain malfunction with symptoms specific to the area with the dysfunction. A partial seizure may start locally and then move to become generalized.

Passive-aggressive personality: Behavior in interpersonal relationships that is ultimately viewed as obstructionist or hostile but that is expressed in a passive or subtle manner. Pattern of denied negativity, passive resistance, "learned helplessness," procrastination, hostile humor, or deliberate repeated failure to accomplish any task for which they were explicitly accountable. These submissive charades are designed to control, manipulate, and avoid responsibility. Formerly considered a personality disorder, this syndrome is now in the *Appendix* of the DSM. That doesn't mean I know any less people with these annoying traits.

Passive immunity: Acquired immunity through the transfer of antibodies or activated T cells from an immune donor to the recipient, as when a mother transfers antibodies to her fetus. Usually short-term, lasting a few months

Paste: Combination of oil, water, and powder. Essentially an ointment with powder added. Used as a vehicle for drug delivery or skin protectant

Pasteur: Louis Pasteur was a French scientist who put forward the idea that germs cause disease. Heavily ridiculed by many physicians and scientists until he provided scientific evidence to support this theory in the mid-1860s

PAT: Paroxysmal atrial tachycardia

Patella: Knee cap. Sesamoid bone that sits in the tendon of the quadriceps muscle

Patellar-femoral syndrome: Condition characterized by pain originating in the contact area at the back of the kneecap where it meets with the femur. Common diagnosis in sports medicine. Presents with grinding or loosening of the structures in the area

Pathogen: Organism capable of causing disease in a host. Can be bacterial, viral, fungal, or other agent

Pathognomonic: A sign that only occurs in one condition. If you observe the sign, the condition is present. Distinctive feature of a particular condition which, when it appears, can only mean that condition is in operation. E.g., the EM lesion of borreliosis. "It can only be…"

Pathologic: Abnormal and potentially problematic

Pathology: Study of changes from normal or the deviations from the healthy state. Study of the nature and causes of disease due to changes in structure or function. Deviations from normal that can cause altered function that results in disease. Pathology can be studied in the macro state such as gross anatomical pathology or at the molecular level.

Pathophysiology: Abnormal processes resulting in dysfunction. When normal physiology is disrupted, the resulting damage to a cell, tissue, organ, or system can occur resulting in disease or injury. Ways normal physiologic processes are changed by disease

Patient Information Sheets: Designed to make the material contained in the package insert more comprehensible to the lay user

PCR: Polymerase chain reaction looks for DNA from the suspect pathogens

PEARL: A bit of wisdom bestowed upon a student by a mentor

Pelvic inflammatory disease: (PID) Infection of the internal reproductive organs and adjacent tissues can lead to acute abdomen, organ damage, septicemia, shock, and infertility if untreated. Usually bacterial

Pemphigus: Autoimmune disease characterized by successive crops of bullae that come and go leaving pigmented spots. Sad cases

Penicillins: (PCNs) Cidal, cell wall antibiotics that are effective against the spirochetal form of Bb since it has a cell wall. E.g., Amoxil, Augmentin, Bicillin

Percussion: Use of fingertips to tap the body to determine size, position, and consistency of underlying structures

Perforation: A hole in tissue

Pericardial effusion: Fluid inside the pericardium

Pericarditis: Inflammation of the protective membrane that covers the heart, which can be due to a number of causes including infection. Can be acute or chronic. The underlying pathophysiology can be fibrous or effusive with purulence or blood in the pericardial sac. Chronic forms are mostly due to constrictive fibrous formations like scarring that can thicken the pericardium. RF with cardiac manifestations can cause pericarditis with friction rub. The patient can present with pleuritic pain that increases with deep inspiration and decreases when position is changed. Pain can be of sudden onset and continue for days. Suspected in some cases of cardiac Lyme

Pericardium: Thin, protective, membranous sac that encloses the heart and the bases of major vessels

Perineum: The external region between the anus and scrotum in the male and the anus and vulva in the female

Periodic breathing: Normal respiratory variant in infants where the child will breathe rapidly for a few breaths and then have a short pause and before she resumes breathing

Peripheral: Located on the outside or AWAY from the center

Peripheral blood: Blood obtained from the systemic circulation remote from the heart

Peripheral nervous system: (PNS) Network of paired nerves that connects the CNS to remote body parts and that sends and receives messages from these locations. Peripheral means OUTSIDE the CNS. The PNS includes the 12 pairs of CNs and 31 pairs of spinal nerves.

Peristalsis: Intestinal movement. A progressive, involuntary, wave-like movement in the GI tract

Peritoneum: Serous membrane that lines the abdominal cavity and many of the abdominal organs

Peritonitis: Inflammation of the peritoneum which may be caused by irritation from exposure to pathogens or intestinal contents, infection, rupture in the female reproductive tract, surgical penetration, or sepsis. Peritonitis is an emergency requiring immediate attention. If any of the physical findings for an acute abdomen are observed, peritonitis could be present. Signs include involuntary rigidity, rebound, guarding, or spasm of abdominal muscles. These are all indications of peritoneal inflammation.

Periumbilical: Around the belly button

PERLA: Pupils equally reactive to light and accommodation

Persistent: Unrelenting. On-going, often despite what is thought to be appropriate treatment

Personality disorders: Traits and long-standing behaviors that contribute to distress or disability with regard to relationships with others. Patterns of interaction deviate from what is usually expected. People with personality disorders are inflexible, irritating, and annoying. They are outside the norm for the cultural standards and this causes distress in others who go out of their way to avoid them. These patients may not respond to emotional stimuli and cues in the same way as other people. There are many kinds of personality disorders.

Person-centered therapy: Talk therapy where the therapist is a facilitator creating a comfortable, non-judgmental environment of empathy and unconditional positive reinforcement. This approach is non-directive and the patient finds his own solutions to psychological and behavioral issues. The counselor does not diagnosis or treat. This form of psychotherapy is effective and popular but may not be directive enough for some patients.

Pervasive developmental disorder: (PDD) Delays in development of multiple basic functions such as socialization and communication. PDD is also called the autism spectrum of disorders or ASD. Spectrum of conditions that can range from barely perceptible to totally incapacitating, and even dangerous. Controversial. I&P increasing. LD can present with an autism-like syndrome and the association between LD and the various PDDs is unknown.

Petechiae: (Petechia is singular.) Small, deep red or purple hemorrhagic spots on the skin usually indicative of severe illness. Spots of blood outside the vessels. Lesions are usually small and purplish and do not blanch with pressure. Petechiae can be associated with severe fevers. They can be a significant finding in toxic shock syndrome and DIC and in these cases can be quickly fatal. Petechiae are seen in the typical rash of RMSF.

Petite mal: Type of generalized seizure. Absence seizures occur primarily in kids and present with a change in consciousness, blinking, an eye-roll, blank stare, and slight mouth movements. The patient retains her posture throughout the episode. A petit mal seizure only lasts a few seconds but can occur many times a day.

PET scan: (Positron emission tomography) Imaging technique that looks at function not just structure by measuring accumulation of radioactivity in areas of more intense metabolism. More active sites are often the place of dysfunction or disease and show up brighter on the scan. PETs show blood flow and chemical activity. These studies are especially useful for examining neurologic, cardiac, and cancer problems. Cancer cells show up brighter because they have a higher metabolism than surrounding tissue.

Phagocytes: Cells with the ability to ingest, lyse, or otherwise destroy unwanted material like pathogens and debris. Neutrophils and macrophages are the primary phagocytes of the immune system.

Phagocytosis: Ingestion and digestion of pathogens and debris by phagocytes

Phalanges: Digits. The bones of the fingers and toes

Pharmacodynamics: (PD) All the things the drug does *to the body*

Pharmacokinetics: (PK) All the stuff the body does *to the drug*

Pharmacovigilance: Process by which professionals gather safety data on medicines and then watch this data over time to see if there are identifiable patterns or trends. The idea is to gather clues that might identify potential safety issues before they happen.

Pharynx: Throat

Phenotype: Set of observable characteristics that are made using the genetic code, or genotype

Pheromone: Chemical released by an animal into its surroundings that affects the behavior or biochemistry of other animals. Deer, humans, and possibly other creatures seemingly release pheromones that attract certain tick species. Most likely the chemical developed in the potential hosts for other purposes and the tick evolved in a way that allowed them to detect this biochemical and thereby find preferred hosts. The amount of pheromone released can be quite individual.

Phlebitis: Inflammation of a vein with pain along the course of the affected vein. The area is usually red, firm, and swollen.

Phobias: Persistent, unrealistic, and intense fears that impact behavior. Usually the anxiety is focused on a specific object, event, or other stimulus. The most familiar phobias include: agoraphobia (the fear of open space or of leaving the house), claustrophobia (the fear of enclosed spaces like an MRI tube), fear of flying, fear of germs, or fear of public speaking. Children can be phobic of the dark, strangers, storms, or animals. Phobias can be affiliated with panic attacks, GAD, and OCD. These fears are real whether the threat is real or not. Reasoning and logic will not make a phobia go away. CBT can help.

Phonophobia: Fear or avoidance of sound or noise. May be associated with the hypersensitivity to sound observed in some TBI patients

Phoresis: The motion of particles in a field

Photopheresis: Technique where certain WBCs are separated from the rest of the blood for testing or treatment with light and then reintroduced back into the system. Patient is treated with a chemical that gets into the T cells but is only active after exposure to UV light. Cells are removed, separated, and then treated with UV light. T cells die within about two days. Photopheresis is extracorporeal treatment since it is performed outside the body.

Photosensitivity: Abnormal sensitivity to light. Some medicines are thought to cause chemical changes in the skin that makes the skin more susceptible to light. The person then might develop a rash or burn when exposed to the sun. TCNs are likely to cause photosensitivity.

Phototoxic reaction: Sun sensitivity. Excessive reaction to UV exposure such as that seen after dosing with certain drugs such as TCNs

Physical therapy: Various treatment modalities designed to help decrease pain and increase motion and function

Physiologic: Benign as part of the normal condition

Physiology: Study of normal function in an organism. Processes that allow for usual function in a life form such as digestion, movement, and reproduction. Physiology may be studied on a tissue, organ, or cellular level as well as from the perspective of an entire system such as the circulatory system or the endocrine system. When something disrupts a normal process then disease or injury can be present and then the term would be pathophysiology.

Pilonidal cysts: Cysts over the coccyx area in the gluteal cleft at the base of the sacrum or coccyx. Most common in older teenage males. These cysts can contain hairs and become infected producing abscesses and a draining sinus or fistula.

Pinna: (Pinnae) Auricle or external ear

Piroplasma: Former name of Babesia. A tick-borne protozoa that infects the red blood cells of mammals

Piroplasmosis: Former name of babesiosis. This term is still used for the disease in some animal species and in older literature.

Pitting: Depression in nails or in soft tissue after indention that does not immediately resolve. Can be seen in psoriasis in nails and is a sign of edema or fluid overload

Pituitary: Gland located under the hypothalamus of the brain. Some consider the pituitary the "master gland" of the body. Secretes a number of hormones that ultimately regulate many bodily functions including growth, reproduction, and metabolism. The posterior pituitary produces oxytocin, the comfort hormone, and antidiuretic hormone, which affects water absorption in the kidney. Problems with the posterior pituitary can cause diabetes insipidus. The anterior pituitary is involved with growth, sexual development, skin pigmentation, thyroid balance, and adrenocortical function. Lack of hormone from the anterior lobe can cause dwarfism and decrease the overall endocrine performance of the other glands. Hyperactivity results in acromegaly in adults and giantism in children. Lyme is hypothesized to impact the full hormonal cascade including the pituitary, which helps explain the multisystem nature of the disease.

Placebo: An inactive substance given to provide the perception of treatment either to help the patient believe they can improve or as a control in a clinical trial so that comparisons can be made between the placebo and the active treatment being tested

Placebo-controlled: One type of study design for clinical trials where variables are tested by comparing active treatment with a sham regimen. If blinded, the participants cannot tell which treatment they received. Placebo-control minimizes bias and allows for more powerful comparisons between groups.

Plan 504: Refers to Section 504 of the Rehabilitation Act within the Americans with Disabilities Act. No one with a disability can be excluded from participating in federally funded schooling. This law outlines the modifications and accommodations that might be needed for the student to have the opportunity to perform at the same level as his peers. With the 504 plan, anyone who has a physical or mental impairment that substantially limits one or more major life activities, such as working or learning, is entitled to be placed in the regular educational environment with the use of aids and services unless education in the regular environment with help can't be achieved.

Plantar fasciitis: Inflammation along the fascial plane on the bottom of the foot. Sole pain is a frequent complaint in bartonellosis, babesiosis, and occasionally Lyme. The mechanism by which these pathogens affect the fascia is unknown. Usually the cause of plantar fasciitis is mechanical, with repeated pressure and stress causing irritation. Fasciitis may present as a stress fracture.

Plantar flexion: Movement at the ankle that takes the foot AWAY from the head as though pushing on the gas pedal

Plantar warts: Warts on the bottom of the feet (the plantar surface) usually caused by HPV. Appear as a dark spot with stippling. As pressure is placed on the wart, a callus can appear. These can become tender as the callus presses into the softer underlying tissue. This viral infection can be dormant for months (or forever for all we know) before symptoms appear. HPV can present as one wart or several that form a cluster. Often these warts are self-limited.

Plaque: Palpable lesion larger than 0.5 cm, which can have both flat and raised regions such as a grouping of papules. A patch on the skin or mucous membrane

Plaquenil: Hydroxychloroquine

Plasma: Liquid part of both blood and lymph. Mostly water. Plasma does contain fibrinogen, a clotting factor, proteins (primarily albumin), glucose, ions, hormones, CO_2, and wastes. Plasma is an important transporter of wastes.

Plasma cell: (Plasmacyte) A type of specialized B white cell that makes antibodies (immunoglobulins)

Plasmapheresis: Blood purification procedure used most often to treat autoimmune disease. Involves removal, separation, intervention, and return of components of the blood plasma to and from the circulation

> *PEARL: Do not confuse phoresis (the movement of particles in an electric field) with pheresis (extracorporeal treatment that removes and separates cells).*

Plasmid: DNA molecules that are separate from the chromosomal DNA and can replicate independently. Plasmids may contribute to antibiotic resistance.

Plateau: State of little or no change after a time of progress. Can refer to recovery, healing, learning, training, etcetera, when progress is slow or flat compared to earlier phases

Platelets: Sticky cell fragments critical to the clotting process

Pleocytosis: An increased cell count. The term is used primarily to refer to a high white cell count in CSF.

Pleural effusion: An excess of fluid in the pleural space which may be due to either increased production or decreased removal. Normally, the pleural space has just enough fluid to keep the surfaces slippy. With effusion, there is a fluid imbalance and a pressure differential that allows fluid to be forced into the area between the lining of the lung and the lining of the chest wall. A significant effusion can crowd the lung and restrict full expansion decreasing the efficacy of respiration. The patient may complain of shortness of breath and chest pain.

Pleurisy: Inflammation of the membranes lining the chest cavity and the lungs. There can be sharp, stabbing pain that increases with respiration, which can significantly limit the movement of the chest on the affected side. Presentation can include significant SOB along with a pleural friction rub, which is a coarse, creaky sound heard during late inspiration and early expiration. Over the area of inflammation, coarse vibrations can be felt.

PMDD: Premenstrual dysphoric disorder

PMN: Polymorphonuclear neutrophils. WBC granulocyte

PMS: Premenstrual syndrome

Pneumonia: Inflammation of the lower respiratory tract due to infection or chemical irritation. Pneumonia can affect an entire lobe or just a section. The actual lung parenchyma is involved including the alveoli and interstitial tissue. With bacterial pneumonia, the patient may be more acutely ill but may respond more rapidly to treatment than with viral etiologies. Mycoplasma *pneumoniae* is the most common pathogen causing pneumonia in 5 to 35-year-olds. Recent tick drags have recovered M. *pneumoniae*. Pneumonia can occur in TBIs including Q fever and tularemia.

PNS: Peripheral nervous system

Pock: Scar left by a pox

Point tenderness: Localized discomfort. Sometimes an acute abdomen starts out with generalized aches, but then the pain settles in a more specific location demonstrated by point tenderness.

Polio: Viral inflammation of neurons that causes atrophy of muscles. Through vaccination, polio was nearly eradicated from the planet, except in places like pockets of India where local leaders feel vaccination is a government conspiracy. There polio thrives.

Polymerase Chain Reaction: (PCR) Technique that looks for DNA from the suspect pathogens

Polymorphonuclear neutrophils: (PMN) Granulocytic WBC. Contain granules in their cytoplasm and have multilobed nuclei. There are three types of granulocytes: neutrophils, eosinophils, and basophils. Overall granulocytes comprise 50% to 70% of all WBCs. Since neutrophils are by far the most prevalent type, sometimes the term PMN is used to refer to the neutrophil.

Polymyalgia rheumatica: Poorly defined condition most often found in older women. Pain and weakness in the shoulders and pelvis with an increased ESR and considerable stiffness in the morning and after prolonged inactivity

Polyuria: Too much urine

Pomodoro method: A time management technique that can be adapted for young children and those with difficulty focusing. The participant commits to concentrating on a task for a selected amount of time: 5, 10, 20, 30 minutes. Then there is a scheduled break. During work time, the entire focus is on the work. The break should be entirely work-free. In the TBI population, the amount of time spent at work and on break will depend on age and severity of illness.

Porphyria: Genetic enzyme disorder that causes sxs affecting skin or NS

Position: Location in space. Place occupied. Knowing where the body is in space is called proprioception or position sense

Position sense: Proprioception

Positive predictive value: Proportion of the subjects with positive test results that are correctly diagnosed. Important measure of the performance of a diagnostic test

Post-concussion syndrome: After head trauma, a patient can be affected for months with headache, dizziness, a dazed feeling, difficulty concentrating, varying degrees of amnesia, depression, apathy, and anxiety. All these symptoms may be due to neuronal damage.

Post-herpetic neuralgia: Pain, often intense, that occurs in conjunction with an HHV infection. In the case of HHV-3, post-herpetic neuralgia can be thought of as shingles without the skin lesions. The term "post" here is probably inappropriate, since there is nothing "post" about this active infection.

Post-Lyme syndrome: While there are certainly some patients who are left with residual sequelae after Lyme is cured, this term was coined specifically to discount the possibility of an active infection contributing to the signs and symptoms occurring in some patients with persistent Lyme. In these cases the term on-going, persistent, or chronic Lyme syndrome is preferred by most TBI specialists. Whenever you see the term post-Lyme syndrome, look carefully at the context.

Post-traumatic stress disorder: (PTSD) Because of an overwhelming traumatic event or series of events, a patient with PTSD mentally re-experiences the incident with intense fear, anxiety, helplessness, and horror. The person relives the experience through flashbacks or nightmares. She will go to great lengths to avoid a stimulus that will trigger these flashbacks. PTSD is common after abuse, rape, abandonment, assault, crime, torture, violence, and severe accidents. Persons with PTSD might numb themselves against emotion. They can startle easily, have short tempers, suffer problems sleeping, and feel angry as though they are always on guard. They may have a heightened sense of arousal and be hypervigilant. PTSD can impact normal life functions.

Postural tremors: During a prolonged posture, tremors can occur that may be exacerbated by anxiety and hyperthyroidism.

Potassium: (K) Electrolyte necessary for cell function, especially the regulation of heartbeat, nerve conduction, and muscle operation. Severely low potassium can be quickly fatal.

Powassan viral encephalitis: (POW) Flavivirus TBI co-infection

Powder: Vehicle that can be sprinkled on skin or hair or that can be inhaled (as with cocaine). Often used as a drying agent. Good choice for carrying antifungals since fungi do not like dry environments.

Prebiotics: Foods (usually fibers) that provide nourishment for the good flora in the intestine

Precautions/Cautions: This section of a drug label involves forewarnings regarding what you should know before you put a patient on the drug. Typical "cautions" include: the need for adequate liver and kidney function prior to drug use, no significant mental health issues present before starting therapy, a negative pregnancy test documented prior to initiating the first dose, or the need to avoid the sun after starting the medicine. Precautions are more of a recommendation regarding vigilance than a desire to keep the drug from being used.

Premenstrual dysphoric disorder: (PMDD) Can cause significant depression, irritability, and tension prior to menses. PMDD is considered more severe and potentially disabling that PMS.

Premenstrual syndrome: (PMS) Consists of a wide range of symptoms that occur a few days prior to menses and usually stop at the onset of bleeding. PMS may be due to changes in hormones and we know Lyme can affect hormone balance. PMS can include physical, behavioral, and emotional signs and symptoms, some of which can overlap with the endocrine or NP effects of LD.

Prepatellar bursitis: Inflammation of the bursa of the knee. Also called housemaid's knee or coal miner's knee. Superficial swelling sharply limited to the area in FRONT of the kneecap

Prevalence: The number of individuals who have a condition at a specific POINT in time

Prevalence rate: The number of people who have the disease at a point in time COMPARED to the number of individuals who are in the population at the same point in time

Probiotics: Potentially living organisms given to people (or animals) to enhance the growth of the helpful flora in the gut

Prodrome: Period of time before clear onset of disease symptoms. Indications of approaching disease

Prolapse: The dropping or falling of an organ into an area where it does not belong

Pronation: Motion or position that leaves a body part facing DOWN

Prone: Belly DOWN position. Facing or moving down

Proprioception: Knowing where the body is in space. Position sense. Awareness of posture, movement, and changes in equilibrium. Lyme has been known to cause significant problems with proprioception but often the connection is never made.

Prospective: Looking forward at data such as in a controlled clinical trial

Prostaglandins: Large group of bioactive molecules with diverse physiologic functions

Prostration: Collapse. Absolute exhaustion

Protein: Class of compounds comprised of amino acids and synthesized by all living organisms. E.g., antigens, nutrients

Protists: (Protozoa) Eukaryotic organisms that may cause diseases including babesiosis, malaria, and dysentery

Proton pump inhibitor: Drug used to decrease acid in the stomach. Often used to relieve sxs of GERD

Protozoa: (Protists) A vague classification of one-celled eukaryotes such as Amoebas (that cause dysentery), plasmodium (that cause malaria), and Babesia (that cause babesiosis). Many protozoa have both an active phase and a dormant cystic phase. These are single-celled parasites with flexible membranes and the ability to move.

Proverb: Short statement of truth or wisdom condensed into a few words that are easy to remember. Proverbs may need some thought to be understood by those who are unfamiliar with them. Their interpretation is one way to assess capacity for abstract thought.

Proximal: Proximal is closer to a reference point, while distal is farther

Pruritis: Itch

Pseudomembranous colitis: A false or pseudo membrane can form over the intestinal lining due to the C. *difficile* toxin. Characterized by severe diarrhea, dehydration, electrolyte imbalances, abdominal pain, fever, and mucus and blood in the stool. Toxic megacolon and death have been documented.

Pseudotumor cerebri: A reference to increased intracranial pressure. Usually this increased ICP is accompanied by papilledema but that is not always the case, especially in infants. The diagnosis of pseudotumor cerebri is only made after non-benign causes of increased ICP are ruled out.

Psoas sign: The psoas muscles are found internally in the loin. Because an inflamed appendix can rest near a part of the psoas muscle, movement of the muscle will cause pain in the inflamed area.

Psoriasis: Common chronic skin disease characterized by red papules that may coalesce to form plaques with distinct borders. If ongoing, silver-white scales can develop anywhere but the most common areas are scalp, knees, elbows, genitals, and umbilicus. New lesions can form at sites of irritation or trauma. Variable clinical course, but the underlying pathology appears to be a rapid turnover of epidermis. Some patients have associated arthritis. Etiology unknown but may have genetic component and infection, some medications, climate, and hormones could play a role. When distinguishing from eczema, psoriasis is often thicker and drier and tends to affect the back of the elbows and front of the knees (the extensor surfaces).

Psoriatic arthritis: In about 5% of psoriasis patients there is an accompanying arthritis. Usually skin lesions present first and later arthritis with joint pain, stiffness, and swelling. There are periods of remission and then recurrence. May be appropriate for the TBI DD list

Psychosis: A group of diseases where the patient withdraws into herself and fails to distinguish reality from fantasy. The disturbances can be of such severity that there is personality disintegration and loss of contact with reality. Symptoms can start as early as middle school, but the first episode can occur anytime throughout the teen years and into early adulthood. There is a significant personality change with unusual emotional responses. Psychoses are chronic conditions that handicap the patient in social interactions, in school, and at work. Thoughts are disorganized and the individual pursues extreme withdrawal into her own fantasy world. Behavior is often bizarre and inappropriate in ways that make sense only to that person. The first signs may be a strange pattern of fatigue, insomnia, and headache. In schizophrenia the person loses interest in real life. She is confused and agitated, with no capacity for abstract thought. Psychotics become very literal and very concrete. They may have distorted vision and auditory senses with a flat affect and low motivation. Hallucinations are common in some cases with the patient

seeing, hearing, or otherwise sensing things that aren't real. They may be plagued by delusions which are false beliefs that are not supported by fact. She might think the radio is talking to her or the government is trying to control her. Delusions seem to focus on sex, politics, and religion. Government and church conspiracies are common themes. Voices may tell the patient to make abrupt, life-changing decisions. There is a feeling that life has changed and no longer seems real. Sad cases

Psychotherapy: The treatment of mental and emotional disorders through talk therapy with a trained therapist such as a psychiatrist, psychologist, or social worker. A psychiatrist is a physician who can add medication to the psychotherapy. The goal of the treatment is to identify problems and view these problems realistically, gain insight into thoughts and actions, and change behaviors in a way that allows for better functioning in society including work and school. There are many types of psychotherapy and the best fit will depend on the patient, situation, and diagnosis.

Pterygium: Conjunctival thickening. Bunching of the conjunctiva that is visible over the sclera. Unattractive, but usually benign

Ptosis: Drooping eyelid

Pulmonary edema: Effusion of fluid into the alveoli and interstitial tissue of the lungs. May present with a cough productive of frothy, blood-tinged foam. While the problem appears to be in the lung parenchyma, the real trouble often lies with ineffective pumping by the heart. If the pump is broken, fluid will back up into the lung and swelling may occur elsewhere in the body. Children with weak hearts can develop pulmonary edema as can kids who have heart damage secondary to infections.

Pulmonary embolism: An embolus is an obstruction of a blood vessel by a clot or other substance. When the embolus is in a vessel supplying the lung, there can be a sudden loss of blood supply to the lung tissue. Most often a thrombus breaks off from a DVT in the leg. Signs and symptoms include: SOB, pain, tachycardia, cough, tachypnea, pleural friction rub, gallop, and rales. A pulmonary embolism can be hard to diagnose early on because the signs and symptoms can be nonspecific and vary in intensity. Symptoms can present within minutes although an infarct due to an embolus may take longer to manifest. A scan to compare the ventilation to the perfusion may be needed to make the diagnosis.

Pulse: 1)Palpable tap than can be heard or felt due to the expansion and relaxation of arteries as blood moves along under pressure. Rhythmic throbbing in time with the heartbeat. 2)Method of drug administration where the drug is given for a period of time and then withheld for an interval. Pulsing can be done for reasons of safety, efficacy, or tolerability. With some drugs, like artemesia, the metabolism of some formulations of this herbal dictates the need for pulsing.

Pupillary reflex: Light entering the retina causes pupil constriction of that eye (direct light reflex) and of the other eye (consensual light reflex)

Purging: Self-induced vomiting either by sticking a finger down the throat or using emetics

Purpura: Bleeding into the skin with various presentations and probably as many etiologies. The red/purple discoloration turns into yellow/green and then brown before resolution. The bleeding can be into skin, mucous membranes, internal organs, and other tissue. The discoloration usually disappears within to 2 to 3 weeks. There is no blanching on pressure. Purpura can be allergic, autoimmune, due to vascular inflammation, or idiopathic.

Pus: Mixture of white cells, pathogen, and debris at or near an infection site

Pustule: A blister filled with pus such as those seen in acne and impetigo

Pyelonephritis: Bacterial infection of the kidneys, most commonly due to E. *coli* but Staph, Strep, and Pseudomonas are also common etiologic pathogens. The microbes spread from the bladder, up the ureters, to the kidneys. Diabetics are more prone to infection as are those who cannot completely empty the bladder. Symptoms may develop rapidly over a few hours and include fever, chills, pain on urination, hematuria, flank pain, frequency, burning, urgency, and nocturia. Recurring infection can cause a chronic pyelonephritis with scarring (fibrosis) of the kidney and compromised function.

Pyuria: Pus (white cells, pathogen, and debris) in the urine

Q

Q fever: TBI co-infection caused by the Rickettsial pathogen, Coxiella burnetti

QT interval: The part of an EKG tracing that extends from the start of the Q wave to the end of the T wave. Some medications prolong this interval, and in some cases this lengthening results in problems for the patient. When using a medication known for QT lengthening or when treating a patient who might be particularly susceptible, watch to make sure that the QT is not getting progressively longer and longer to the point where there is no further electrical activity. Before I became obsessed with hyphens, I spent an inordinate amount of time talking to the FDA about QT intervals. I can't decide where I had more fun. One company tried to tell the FDA that their drug did not prolong the QT because some of the dogs in the animal studies had better cages than the others and that's why their QTs were longer.

QTc: QTc is the QT corrected for heart rate. QTc is the term that will appear more often in the literature.

Qualitative: Research methods that deal more with meaning than with measurement. Subjective. Considered a "softer" approach than quantitative testing. E.g., a yes or no answer on an Ag/Ab test would be qualitative, whereas measuring the amount of precipitate on the test would be quantitative.

Quantitative: Research methods that deal more with measurement and measurable parameters. Objective. Measures the numerical amount

Questing: Process used by ticks to find a host. The tick crawls up a stem and waits until clued by environmental signals like CO_2 concentration and warmth to leap aboard the new host.

Quinine: Original malaria drug. Considered the TOC for malaria for centuries. Still in use today but largely replaced by agents that are as effective but with fewer side effects. Only consider if there are no other options OR in cases of severe cerebral malaria. Can be hard to tolerate and has been associated with a number of AEs including visual problems, ototoxicity, and CNS complaints

Quinolinic acid: Neurotoxin involved with receptors associated with learning, memory, and synapse plasticity

Quinolones: Antibiotic class that blocks DNA synthesis by inhibiting one of the enzymes needed in the process

Quotes: Two quotes that I was itching to use but I just couldn't make them fit anywhere since they are a tad mean-spirited are: "'My country right or wrong' is like saying 'My mother, drunk or sober'." G.K Chesterton and "I wonder if anybody ever reached the age of 35 in New England without wanting to kill himself." Barrett Wendell

Quotessperescent: Word made up by Chris Spreen just for fun. Lieve Vandeplassche from Belgium caught this on editing.

R

Radial head subluxation: (Nursemaid's elbow) Dislocation of the elbow caused by a sudden pull on the extended arm. While not especially painful, the child will sit with the arm flexed and pronated. He will not be able to supinate. The radial head needs to be repositioned back into its proper place.

Radioimmunoassay: (RIA) Technique used to identify either antigen or antibody. With some pathogens, RIA is very sensitive and specific and can be used to measure the concentration of antigen by use of its corresponding antibody. Although there are a number of variations, a radioactive label is placed on a protein and then the amount of radioactivity is measured if the Ag/Ab reaction occurs.

Rales: Crackles that signify interstitial lung disease. Rales are discrete, non-continuous breath sounds most audible on inspiration. This crinkling noise can be heard in CHF, bronchitis, near-pneumonia, and fibrosis. Rales are higher pitched than rhonchi.

Range of motion: The full extent of motion through which a joint can progress

Range of motion exercises: These activities involve moving the joints through their full array of flexion, extension, rotation, abduction, and adduction. Joints are limited by their natural range and should not be moved beyond that point. These exercises can be passive, where a therapist or caretaker moves the joint, or active where the patient positions the area.

Rash: General term used to refer to a skin eruption

Rate: How fast something goes in time

Raynaud's: The term Raynaud's is used to describe at least two conditions, one fairly benign and one perhaps not. Raynaud's can be a spastic disorder of the arteries. The vessels can undergo episodic vasospasm of the smaller peripheral arteries, which seems to be precipitated by cold or stress. This condition is bilateral and affects primarily the hands but sometimes the feet, which might present with cold, pale, blue, cyanotic digits. Raynaud's is most often seen in females in puberty and young adulthood. But some Raynaud's appears to be associated with autoimmunity and connective tissue diseases like lupus and scleroderma. This type seems to be progressive. So, while some of the literature presents Raynaud's as a benign condition of nervous teenage girls, others see it almost as prodromal to more serious conditions. Raynaud's symptomatology is observed in a number of TBIs including Lyme and bartonellosis where it may be due to the presence of pathogen in the endothelial cells causing vasoconstriction.

Rebound tenderness: On abdominal examination, pain is increased with the sudden release of firm pressure suggesting peritoneal inflammation. When the pressure is suddenly removed, the muscle wall rebounds, causing discomfort.

Rechallenge: To determine if a medicine is effective or causing a side effect, the drug can be administered, withdrawn, and then re-administered to see what happens after each step. If the patient is getting better on the drug and relapses after the drug is stopped, that is valuable information. Likewise if the patient again feels better when the treatment is resumed, that adds even more insight. In terms of adverse events, if the problem goes away when the drug is stopped and returns when restarted, the problem could be the drug. Be careful performing a rechallenge especially if the AE is an allergy or other potentially serious condition.

Recrudescent: Return after abatement. To break out again after a period of quiescence, Recurrence despite standard treatment

Rectal prolapse: Part of the rectal mucosa can fall down or protrude through the anus

Rectum: Lower part of the large intestine. Contains the centers for the defecation reflex. Collects the final waste material which is then expelled through the anus

Recur: (Recurrent) Return of sxs after remission. Occurring again or repeatedly

Red herring: An item that serves to distract from the truth. Diversion to keep from seeing the real point

Red man syndrome: A mast cell reaction that releases histamine and causes flushing and a red rash on the face, neck, and upper torso when vancomycin is infused too rapidly. Hypotension, swelling, and shock may occur. This reaction usually occurs within a few minutes after the start of a too-rapid infusion. Slow infusion prevents this syndrome and antihistamines may help decrease the signs and symptoms.

Red reflex: When light shines into the pupil from a particular angle, this light should normally reflect back as a red glow. Absence of a red reflex can suggest eye disease such as an opaque lens from a cataract.

Reducible: When the contents of a hernia or prolapse can be manipulated back where it belongs without too much difficulty

Referred pain: Pain that seems to be in one place but is actually originating someplace else. This is common with dental pain, and in pain in the ear, jaw, gallbladder, heart, and appendix.

Reflexes: Involuntary responses to a stimulus. Reflexes are predictable and purposeful and adaptive. They rely on an intact neural pathway between the stimulus and the responding organ called the reflex arc. The end-organ can be a muscle or gland.

Reflex sympathetic dystrophy: A chronic pain condition secondary to dysfunction, irritation, or abnormal excitation of the nervous tissue

Refractory: Not responsive to treatment

Regulatory T cell: Type of lymphatic WBC that used to be called a suppressor T cell. Role is primarily to moderate (regulate or suppress) the immune response so there is not an overreaction

Regurgitation: Backflow or movement in the opposite direction from normal or desired. Can refer to a backflow of blood in the heart causing a murmur or the backflow of stomach contents causing vomiting. Going the wrong way

Reinfection: Refers to a new infection as opposed to one that has been dormant and recurs

Reiter's syndrome: Syndrome that usually begins with urethritis followed by arthritis and conjunctivitis. Most often caused by Chlamydia

Relapse: Return of sxs after a period of improvement or stability. Deterioration after progress. Reversal in clinical course

Reliability: Consistency of measurement. The degree to which the tool measures the same way each time under the same conditions. Repeatability

Remission: A lessening in intensity or an abatement of sxs

REMS (Risk Evaluation and Mitigation Strategy) Formerly called pharmacovigilance. Acronym referring to techniques used to identify, evaluate, understand, and prevent safety problems that could arise from the use of certain drugs. Taking what is known about a compound, a plan is written to try to anticipate and circumvent any problems that might appear in an individual patient.

Reservoir: A reservoir can be anything that harbors a pathogen allowing it to live and multiply. A species can be a competent reservoir, which can pass the infection on to a feeding tick, or an incompetent reservoir, which cannot. A reservoir is part of the pathogen's life cycle and is not incidental. Without the reservoir, the pathogen would die out, so the pathogen needs the reservoir to survive. A reservoir can be considered a storage place or depot. A species is considered a competent reservoir only if it is capable of infecting the next tick that bites it. Humans are not competent reservoirs, no matter how sick we are, because it is highly unlikely that we could infect a new tick that happens along and bites us. Deer are not reservoirs since they do not infect the ticks that feed on them. The only reservoir species known for the Lyme-carrying ticks are the white-footed mice, chipmunks, shrews, and maybe voles. Additional species may be uncovered as we learn more, but right now those are it. Reservoir animals do not get sick from the pathogen they harbor (that would be counterproductive to the pathogen), although there is speculation that the reservoir's behavior might be modified by certain microbes such as Bb in order to better serve its needs. For most other TBIs, the reservoir animals are not always well-defined.

Resistance: Any one of many mechanisms employed by microbes in order to survive. Most often, resistance refers to the ability of microbes to avoid damage from antibiotics or the host's immune system.

Respiratory failure: Gas exchange is impeded to the point of impending compromise and is seen at the end-stage of nearly every disease. The oxygen level drops markedly compared to what is normal for this individual and the carbon dioxide level might increase.

Respiratory rate: How often a breath occurs. The average RR is about 44 per minute in infants and 16 to 20 in adults. Anything over 60 in infants is considered rapid. The RR will increase for a number of non-pathologic reasons including crying, exercising, and overheating. Fevers can increase the breathing rate. The RR slows when sleeping.

Respiratory syncytial virus: (RSV) Lower respiratory tract infection that can be fatal in infants and young kids. By causing the formation of cell masses connected by a syncytium (multinucleated cell made from multiple cell fusions), RSV can result in pneumonia and bronchiolitis. Hard to diagnose early, this condition can confuse many differential diagnoses. Most cases occur in winter and early spring and present with dyspnea, cough, wheeze, and fever. Severe signs and symptoms may require hospitalization before the diagnosis is made.

Resting tremors: Tremors occur when extremities are at rest

Restless: Can't get comfortable

Retardation: Can refer to mental, physical, or maturation delays. Most often the term is used to refer to below average intellectual function. Retardation is sometimes recognized early and can include impaired learning, weak cognition, and problems with social adjustment and maturation. IQ measures are often inaccurate. Retardation can be genetic or from infections early in gestation. The cause is probably multifactorial and includes metabolic disorders, syphilis, birth anoxia, injuries, toxins, and environmental exposures. The term retardation has largely been replaced with more specifically-termed cognitive impairments.

Retina: Inner part of the eye that contains the rods and cones needed to see. Here the light waves come into focus. Normally red, but pale in anemia

Retraction: Drawing or pulling in. When struggling to breathe the accessory muscles of the chest are sucked in between the ribs and above and below the clavicle. Soft tissues in the neck and intercostal spaces will appear to hollow due to negative intrathoracic pressure. The abdominal muscles may also retract in acute respiratory distress in infants. Retractions during inspiration indicate some degree of respiratory distress and should not be ignored. Babies born with babesiosis can be struggling to breathe and be retracting.

Retrospective: Looking backward at data. Seeing what a group of patients who have already been diagnosed and treated have in common

Rett syndrome: Multiple developmental disorder more common in females and usually recognized between 6 and 18 months. Can present with hand wringing, breath holding, hyperventilation, seizures, impairment of hand skills, cognitive decline, slowing of head growth, and loss of communication skills. Hand dexterity is lost along with a decline in motor abilities. There is decreased social interaction and finally retardation. Rett's is uncommon and is sometimes included as part of the autism spectrum and sometimes not.

Reye's syndrome: Acute encephalopathy and fatty infiltrate of the liver and other organs. Usually in kids under 15-years-old after an acute viral infection. Severity of the CNS involvement is associated with the mortality rate. Recognition of the association with aspirin has decreased the incidence of this syndrome. I was in elementary school when my teenaged neighbor died of Reye's syndrome. I can remember the screams of the family echoing throughout the tiny coal-mining town as if it were yesterday. We had never heard of Reye's syndrome. We didn't know of anything aside from aspirin as a treatment for fever or pain in kids.

Rhabdomyolysis: Muscle wasting that can occur from debilitating diseases, long-term pressure on a muscle, or from taking certain drugs like statins or fluoroquinolones. This type of breakdown of muscle fiber, leading to a spill of myoglobin into the blood that can ultimately damage the kidneys, is known to occur in tularemia.

Rheumatic: Having to do with joints

Rheumatic fever: (RF) Systemic inflammatory disease of childhood that can be recurrent after a Strep infection. Early heart signs can occur with chronic valve problems developing later. Damage can be permanent. Systemically, the child may present with migratory joint pain, polyarthritis and swelling, redness, and effusion in the joints. There may be skin lesions and a small percentage may display red lesions with blanched centers called erythema marginatum. Subcutaneous nodules on or near joints and on the scalp and hands might be observed. Early neuropsychiatric symptoms include irritability, decline in legible writing, and inability to concentrate which can progress to chorea with purposeless, non-repetitive, involuntary muscle movements, along with problems with coordination and muscle weakness. Some type of carditis develops in about half of the RF patients. With pericarditis there may be an audible friction rub. A myocarditis can develop with Aschoff's bodies which are small nodules composed of pathogen and white cells found in the cardiac tissue. There can be cellular swelling and fragmentation of collagen leading to fibrosis and scarring of the valves. The valve leaflets can swell and erode. Debris and deposits can form bead-like vegetations in and on the valves. These can break off as emboli and affect other organs. Endocarditis from RF affects the mitral valve most in females and the aortic valve in males and the tricuspid can be affected in both genders resulting in a cacophony of loud murmurs. Long-term antibiotics are an accepted treatment for chronic cardiac manifestations of RF. Autoimmune dysfunction may be a reason why some kids get RF in conjunction with Strep and others don't.

Rheumatoid arthritis: Autoimmune group of diseases where the body attacks its own joints causing inflammation of the synovium and associated cartilage. While the joint problems in RA happen to be the most obvious component, many other body systems can also be affected. RA is a symmetrical arthritis that affects fingers, wrists, knees, and elbows and can lead to severe deformity. Usually RA affects people 20 years and older and may take weeks or months for full presentation of symptoms. The hands can provide many diagnostic clues, especially the PIP and MCP joints. There are clear signs of inflammation including swelling, fatigue, and low grade fever. Severe deformities may evolve including ulnar deviation of digits, spindle shaped joints, swan neck anomalies, and other debilitating defects of the hand that severely limit function. On X-ray, findings include narrowed joint space, bone erosion, and multiple malformations. Lab tests often show anemia and a positive ESR and RF. Extra-articular features are common including fatigue, malaise, anorexia, and lymphadenopathy. RA is often treated with steroids and other immunosuppressants.

Rheumatoid factor: (RF) An immunoglobulin (antibody) present in the serum of 50% to 95% of patients with rheumatoid arthritis. Without either great sensitivity or specificity, the IgM of RF is present in the serum of patients with a variety of infectious processes. The presence of RF might support the presence of an inflammatory process but will not give you a TBI diagnosis.

Rhonchi: Secretions in the moderate and large airways can cause loud, coarse, gurgling, almost snore-like sounds that are due to a partial blockage of the tube. Usually low-pitched and sonorous. Since they demonstrate only partial obstruction, they can be heard on both inspirations and expirations. Rhonchi can also be caused by swelling and masses. Rhonchi can change after a cough since the fluid can shift.

Rhythm: Regularity with which something occurs such as the beating of a drum or the pacing of a bass or the timing of a heart beat

RIA: (Radioimmunoassay) Technique used to identify either antigen or antibody. Very sensitive and specific and can be used to measure the concentration of antigen by use of its corresponding antibody

Riboflavin: Vitamin B2

Ribosome: Cell organelle made of RNA and protein. Assembly site for protein synthesis

Rickets: Vitamin D deficiency in children causing problems with bone and cartilage development. Bones can be soft with abnormal shape and structure. OJ Simpson had rickets as a child.

Rickettsia: Genus of bacteria. Widely distributed and a common agent of disease and a TBI co-infection

Rifamycin: (Rifampin, Rifadin, Rimactane, Mycobutin) -Cidal antibiotic that penetrates the BBB. Likely effective against Bartonella, Bb, and possibly Ehrlichia. Because of rapid bacterial resistance against rifamycin, do not use as a solo agent and try not to interrupt a course of this drug. Have a back-up in place to pick up the slack. Anecdotally, rifamycin is very effective against bartonellosis in combination regimens.

Rigidity: Involuntary contraction of the abdominal muscles where the abdominal wall can be board-like. Also, some conditions can be associated with rigid postures. Tenseness, immobility, stiffness

Rigors: Intense, severe, almost convulsive chills, where the entire body quakes as seen in malaria and babesiosis. Alternating severe paroxysms of fever and chills. Cold stage: sudden high temperature with feeling of chills. Hot stage: sense of heat and profuse drenching sweats

Rinne test: Compares bone and air conduction. Place a vibrating tuning fork on the mastoid process behind the ear until the patient can no longer hear it. Then quickly place the still vibrating fork NEAR the ear canal on the same side. Can the patient still hear it? Usually the patient can hear it longer through air than through bone.

Risk/benefit: Analysis to determine if the benefits outweigh the risks of a certain treatment. A pro and con list

Rocephin: Ceftriaxone

Rocky Mountain spotted fever: TBI co-infection caused by Rickettsia *rickettsii*. Widely distributed disease with characteristic pinpoint rash. If suspected treat. Doxy is DOC.

ROM: Range of motion

Romberg sign: Inability to maintain balance when the eyes are shut and the feet are close together. If the patient sways or falls when eyes are closed, she is Romberg positive.

Rotation: Motion that occurs when a part turns on its axis. The head rotates on the neck when a child shakes her head "no."

Rotator cuff: Group of muscles and tendons that serve to stabilize the shoulder and allow it to revolve on its axis.

Rub: A scratching, creaking high-pitched noise that results when two surfaces move against each other. There can be rubbing if there is not enough lubricant or if there is too much swelling or fluid in an area. Patients with pericarditis or pleural effusion may present with audible rubs. Rubs are dependent on body position and can change frequently and rapidly.

Rule out: (r/o) Use of scientific methods to exclude certain diagnoses from consideration in a process of elimination. Here, the HCP gathers all available information and creates a mental sign and symptom list. Then possible candidates that could account for those signs and symptoms are reviewed and subsequently removed from consideration as it becomes clear that they do not fit the clinical presentation. To eliminate or exclude from further consideration

Running: A rapid gait. Pace faster than 6 mph

S

Safety: Condition free from danger, risk, or injury. Drug safety is the monitoring of harmful drug effects with the goal of preventing harm in the future.

Safety profile: The entire scope of knowledge about a drug's side effects

Saprotrophic: Organism that feeds off dead matter

Sarcoidosis: (Sarcoid) Chronic multisystem disease characterized by infiltration of the affected organs by T cells and other phagocytes forming granulomas that change the tissue structures. An autoimmune condition characterized by granulomas in the blood vessels, connective tissue, skin, lungs, eyes, nodes, joints, and muscles. May have subcutaneous nodules that can be mistaken for those in bartonellosis

Scale: Exfoliated skin with thin flakes as seen with dandruff, psoriasis, or severe dry skin

Scar: Replacement of damaged tissue with fibrous material leaving a less flexible healed area. Initially a scar will be a red or purple mark that eventually becomes white. A keloid is a hypertrophied scar more common in dark-skinned races.

Schizogonic: Active phase of a Babesia organism from the invasion of RBC until cell rupture

Sciatica: Inflammation of the sciatic nerve that can cause extreme discomfort. This nerve passes from the pelvis down the back of the thigh and inflammation causes pain that runs down the back of the thigh and down the inside of the leg. The pain is sharp and shooting and movement makes it worse. There can be numbness and tingling. Sciatica might be due to compression, trauma, or inflammation. Infections such as Lyme have been associated with sciatica.

Sclera: Whites of the eyes

Scleroderma: Chronic, progressive systemic sclerosis in which the skin is taut, firm, and edematous, severely limiting motion. Autoimmune condition resulting in increased connective tissue in skin and blood vessels. Connective tissue can build up in organs like the kidneys, lungs, heart, and GI tract leading to organ failure.

Sclerosis: Fibrosis or scarring

Scoliosis: Lateral curve of the spine

Scotoma: Island-like blind spot in a visual field

Seborrhea: (Seborrheic dermatitis) Disease of sebaceous glands with increased sebum secretion. In kids less than 3 months manifests as cradle cap and in older people as dandruff. Greasy, scaly, crusty patches on scalp

Seizures: Paroxysmal event associated with abnormal electrical discharges of neurons. There is an electrical instability that triggers a seizure once the signal goes beyond the individual's seizure threshold. The presentation of the seizure depends on the size of the stimulus and the location of the abnormal event.

Selective mutism: Expectation to speak can cause a child to panic with temporary paralysis of the vocal cords. Child speaks only in certain situations such as when alone or to mom

Self: Protein markers or antigens identify cells as "belonging" as opposed to being foreign

Self-harm/cutting/self-aggression: Behaviors that result in physical or emotional injury perpetuated by the individual or that put the person in additional risk of harm. Many theories: 1) Need to break through the feeling of numbness, 2) Desire to punish oneself or self-hatred, 3) Longing to have one area of life that can be controlled. Incidence appears to be increasing but may just be more recognized

Sensation: A feeling or awareness of conditions within or outside the body due to stimulation of sensory receptors. Perception of the information picked up by the nerve dendrites and sent back to the brain for interpretation. Examples include the skin sensations: pain, temperature, light touch, position, vibration, and discrimination.

Sensitivity: The probability that a test will be positive if the disease is present. A measure of the proportion of those with the disease who are correctly identified by a diagnostic test. A positive when positive. How capable is the test in detecting the disease?

Sensory Deficit Disorder: (SDD) Many terms and acronyms that may or may not be describing the same condition: sensory integration defect, sensory integration disorder, sensory integration dysfunction, SID, multiple sensory disintegration, sensory processing disorder. How this phenomenon may or may not be associated with the hypersensitivity to sensory input observed in many TBI patients is not well understood. These conditions may be part of the same pathophysiology, share some of the underlying pathologic foundations, or be entirely separate sets of circumstances. Countless bits of information enter the NS each moment from the various senses and monitoring systems. The brain must sort and integrate all this data and then respond. If the circuits get overloaded, the person just can't effectively process or manage all the input. The response to this excess stimulation can range from numbness to hypersensitivity. The system either shuts down or tries to integrate all the input. Symptoms can include hyper-awareness of noise, light, or touch. Additional manifestations of what appear to be processing problems include a variety of abnormal behaviors and perceptions from hand flapping, to walking on tiptoe, to abnormal awareness of pain or temperature. In all cases, the inability to sort and integrate information will have a lot to do with how well the child is able to communicate and learn. If she can't efficiently process sensory input, she is going to be at a real disadvantage during social interactions and in traditional learning environments. Notice that autism, ADD, and Lyme share some of these manifestations. We do not know enough about the involved circuitry to know which sxs might belong to which syndrome. Many of the neuropsychiatric complaints associated with Lyme may be processing problems. At least consider the possibility of an underlying infection.

Sensory hypersensitivity: A number of Lyme patients complain of hyper-awareness to one or more senses including light, smell, sound, taste, or touch. Some need to be in a darkened room because even minimal light is too intense. Some want no sound and even soft music is overwhelming. Others cannot stand any clothing touching,

even the softest cloth. Kids with Lyme often experience excessive sensitivity to any of their senses. There are several hypothesizes attempting to explain why this might be so. Bb may cause direct harm to cranial nerves thereby impeding normal function. This phenomenon could also be due to problems processing sensory information, that is, a sensory integration problem. If the body cannot process all the sensory data that is gathered, then the patient can be subjected to either too much sensory response or too little response to the input. Thereby, the patient can suffer a range of sxs from numbness to intense perception of the involved sense. Hypersensitivity can manifest in all senses as well as with pain and temperature, but light, sound, and touch are the most common. Some patients respond with attempts to decrease the input by asking for dim lights, no clothes, or barely audible music. Others prefer additional input such as firmer and longer hugs in order help them process the clearer, more consistent input. While it is too early for us to put this all in perspective, be aware that some Lyme patients may be unable to process information normally. Hyperacusis or hypersensitivity to sound is common in newborns with Bb. Hypersensitivity is one of the most common complaints of TBI patients.

Sensu lato: Term referring collectively to the three primary disease-causing Borrelia

Sensu stricto: The one primary species of Bb causing LD in NA

Sentinel species: Animal species first to manifest a particular disease in an area. Can serve as a warning to humans

Sepsis: Systemic infection. The spread of infection from its initial site to the bloodstream initiating a systematic response

Septicemia: Presence of pathogens in the blood

Sequelae: Consequences of a previous action or event. Results of a prior condition. After-effect. Complication. Sequela is singular.

Serology: Study of the components of serum. The term serologic testing refers to the process of dilutions and titer measurements looking for Ag/Ab complexes. Any number of approaches might be used to obtain these results. Take the term serology as a general moniker for a wide variety of methodologies looking for evidence to support diagnosis, especially the identification of antibodies in the serum. E.g., serologic testing can be looking for antibodies against an infectious agent, foreign proteins in a mismatched blood transfusion, or one's own proteins in cases of autoimmune disease.

Serum: Fluid part of the blood AFTER clotting factors are removed. Fluid is called lymph when it is part of the interstitial material that is found between cells and tissues. In contrast, fluid is called serum when found within blood vessels carrying circulating blood. While lymph can have WBCs present, serum has: NO cells! NO clotting factors! No fibrinogen! But, YES, serum has all the proteins that are NOT involved in clotting. A sample of blood from a patient is often spun in a centrifuge to remove the cells, leaving a serum sample to be used in lab testing. Blood without cells

Sesamoid bone: Oval nodule of bone or cartilage in a tendon working over a boney surface

Shingles: HHV-3 or zoster virus causes both shingles and herpetic neuralgia. The virus can remain dormant in the dorsal root ganglion for many years after a bout of chicken pox. When conditions are favorable the virus can again manifest with a painful skin rash with blisters on only one side of the body following a specific nerve distribution or dermatome. Pain can be exquisite.

Shin splints: Pain in the tibia usually mid-anterior often following strenuous or repetitive exercise. Also associated with TBIs especially Bartonella and Lyme

Shock: Circulatory system collapse associated with inadequate perfusion, hypotension, and hypoxia. The peripheral blood flow may be inadequate to return enough blood to the heart to allow for normal function. Tissues do not get adequate oxygenated blood and become hypoxic

Shortness of breath: SOB or dyspnea

Sibilant: Sibilant sounds are hissing noises like a persistent "s" or "sh." Sibilant breath sounds are the whistling or hissing heard in conjunction with pulmonary rales

Sickle cell anemia: Abnormally shaped red cells can hook and sickle, snagging on the endothelium on the inside of blood vessels. Interference with capillary blood flow can impede oxygen exchange thereby suffocating the surrounding tissue. The obstructed flow can lead to ischemia causing severe pain in the abdomen and other organs. Acute presentation might involve fever and severe pain in joints and belly, which may look like an acute abdomen. Low ambient oxygen such as found in high altitudes and dehydration may precipitate a "crisis." In some sickle cell patients there can be sequestration of both red and white cells in the spleen and liver causing engorgement and enlargement. In other patients there can be an essential "autosplenectomy" where the spleen is so damaged by fibrotic scarring that it is shrunken and impalpable.

Side effect: Any action of a drug beyond what is expected. Usually considered unfavorable

Sigh: A deep inspiration followed by a slow audible expiration. Pathologic sighing as a sign of incomplete respiration is found in babesiosis.

Sign: What the HCP observes or measures. <u>Objective</u> evidence of disease

Significance: Importance

> <u>Clinical</u>: Possibly meaningful to the patient. Shown to have value in a patient-care setting. Clinical significance does not automatically correlate with statistical significance. Be very careful. Marketers inappropriately use the terms "clinically significant" and "clinically proven" all the time. In these scenarios, the terms are meaningless.

> <u>Statistical</u>: Possibly meaningful to the population. The likelihood that an event did not occur by chance based on the use of scientific method and hypothesis testing. A scientific study can have robust statistical significance and absolutely no relevance in the clinic for the patient.

Sjogren's Syndrome: (Sicca syndrome) Chronic, slowly progressing autoimmune condition that targets moisture producing glands causing dry eyes and mouth and fissured tongue. Recurrent enlargement of the salivary glands. May occur in conjunction with other syndromes such as RA, SLE, or scleroderma. Sjogren's syndrome involves chronic inflammation with decreased lacrimal and salivary production. Sjogren's can be part of the differential diagnosis of Lyme because it is also a multisystem disease involving joints, skin, thyroid, heart, bladder, brain, and other organs. Some Sjogren's patients describe brain fog.

S layer: Part of the covering of a cell made of glycoproteins. Offers protection, stabilization, and resistance to adverse environmental conditions like changes in pH

SLE: Systemic Lupus Erythematosus

Snaps: Cracking sound of abnormal valve movement

Social phobia: Intense anxiety in social situations. Can apply to a specific event or to social situations in general. This is more than shyness where the person feels vaguely uncomfortable until she warms up. Phobias can impede social interactions and limit relationships. A social phobic will avoid the scenarios that trigger her anxiety and may become isolated.

Sodium: (Na) Electrolyte important for salt and water balance and electrical conduction. Na is also critical for brain, nerve, and muscle function. Sodium allows electricity to flow and thereby enables communication between cells. Sodium "obligates" water, so wherever there is too much sodium, the ion will be pulling water toward it. If there is too much sodium *inside* a cell, water will flow in and expand (or explode) the cell. If there is too much sodium *outside* the cell, water will flow out, shriveling the cell.

Somatoform disorder: Disorder where the sxs can't be objectively explained. One scholar, who believes that children make up the sxs of chronic Lyme, says that these kids have a somatoform disorder with physical complaints that are just part of the routine anxieties of life. One 11-year-old Lyme patient was told she merely had female stress disorder. She had no idea what female stress disorder was and neither do I.

Sonorous breath sounds: Deep, resonant, snore-like noises heard when there is fluid in a bronchus such as the breath sounds heard in bronchitis. Rhonchi can be sonorous.

Spastic: Muscle tone in state of continual tension as though on the verge of spasm

Specific Developmental Disorder: (SDD) Developmental delays that are specific to one area such as motor coordination, speech, language skills, socialization, or learning

Specificity: The proportion of those who do NOT have the disease who are correctly called disease-free by the test. True negatives. Proportion of negatives correctly identified as such

SPECT scan: Single-photon emission computerized tomography shows the function of organs. A radioactive substance is used to create 3-D pictures illustrating how blood flows and what tissue areas are more or less active.

Speech: Verbal expression of thoughts

Sphincter: A circular muscle that constricts an orifice or opening. The sphincter contracts to close the orifice and relaxes to open the orifice.

Spinal accessory nerve: (CN 11) Motor: Sternomastoid and upper trapezius

Spinal tap: Lumbar puncture

Spirochete: Organism belonging to the phylum of double-membraned bacteria. Usually with long helically coiled, spiral-shaped cells. Most have flagella or axial filaments which enable a twisting motion. E.g., Borrelia which cause LD and relapsing fever and Treponema which cause syphilis and yaws

Spleen: Specialized, large organ in ULQ of the abdomen. Acts as a filter in immune response. Removes old RBCs and holds them as a blood reserve if needed. Recycles iron. Removes antibody-coated bacteria. Contains the majority of the body's monocytes (about half) that eventually turn into macrophages in the tissues. Functions as a giant lymph node. If removed then increased risk of infection and decreased response to some vaccines. May have a role in the dissemination of Bb

Spondylitis: Inflammation of a spine joint

Spondylosis: Degeneration of a spinal disc

Spore: Term sometimes used to refer to the resistant form of some bacteria that enable them to resist unfavorable conditions such as harsh temperatures. Many antibiotics cannot penetrate

Sporozoa: Class of strictly parasitic protozoans that have a complicated natural history and often need two or more dissimilar hosts to complete their life cycle. Usually intracellular and include the parasites that cause malaria and babesiosis

Sporozoite: Infective stage of the Babesia parasite

Sprain: A stretch or tear of a joint capsule or a ligament connecting bone to bone. A sprain threatens the stability of a joint. Often occurs after a joint is forced beyond its normal ROM such as a twisted ankle. Symptoms include pain, swelling, and difficulty moving.

Sputum: Slippy material in the pulmonary tree that is expelled by coughing or clearing the throat. Can contain many things: mucus, cellular debris, blood, pus, and pathogens. Cheesy or caseous material is found in infections like TB. If sputum is available, look at it and collect a sample for testing. If there are squamous cells present, the specimen came from high in the respiratory tract above the larynx. This will not yield reliable results. A "good" sputum sample has macrophages from deep in the alveolar sacs. The presence of eosinophils indicates allergies or parasites. Neutrophils suggest infection since they are the primary component of pus. Gram stain might help categorize the pathogen.

Stagnation: Cessation of metabolic activities

Stamina: Endurance plus strength

Stammer: Tripping over words. Common in Lyme

Standard of care: The level at which the average, prudent provider in a given community would practice medicine or how a similarly qualified HCP would manage a patient's care under similar circumstances

STARI: Southern Tick-Associated Rash Illness is a borreliosis that is not always distinguishable from Lyme

Stasis: Impediment of the normal flow of fluid

Status epilepticus: Continuous seizure episode that can occur with most types of seizures

Steady state: Stable blood level of a drug that does not fluctuate significantly over time. To achieve steady state, usually lower, more frequent dosing is used.

Stem cell: Fundamental cell of the immune system. Most blood cells begin as a stem cell before they differentiate into their more mature role. Must be able to renew itself through mitotic cell division (while remaining undifferentiated) *and* have the potency to evolve into many other distinct cell types. In adults, these cells act as a repair system, fixing many kinds of broken tissue. In the embryo, stem cells evolve into all manner of specialized cells capable of performing distinct functions *and* at the same time, they regenerate cells in organs such as blood, skin, and the GI tract. The more potent a stem line is, the more kinds of cells it can form.

Stenosis: Constriction. Narrowing, often referring to a tubular structure

Stereognosis: The ability to discern the identity of an object through touch alone

Steroid: 1) Sterol compounds manufactured by many animal species that are highly biologically active. 2) Group of drugs that are unparalleled in effectiveness in modulating the immune response but have significant side effects

Steroid withdrawal: If long-term steroid use is discontinued too rapidly without weaning, sxs of adrenal insufficiency can occur. During a prolonged steroid regimen, adrenal function is suppressed to such a degree that the adrenals no longer provide adequate response to infection or other insult. This ineffective response can extend for months after stopping the steroids and the patient might not feel well. Steroid use must be weaned and not stopped abruptly.

Stevens-Johnson syndrome: (SJS) Life threatening condition where the skin sloughs off the body due to an adverse reaction to medications or infections. Part of a continuum of adverse conditions probably beginning with erythema multiforme or even hives, progressing to SJS, and then more uncommonly and even more dangerous, to TENS. Poorly understood pathologic mechanism but allergic, immunologic, and genetic factors probably apply. SJS is a medical emergency.

Still's disease: JRA or JIR

Strabismus: The two eyes cannot focus on the same object at the same time

Strain: A stretch or tear of a tendon connecting muscle to bone occurs when the muscle is stretched and then suddenly contracts. This can occur when running or jumping. An acute strain causes pain, spasm, or tightness, diminished strength, and decreased ROM. Chronic strain can develop from overuse or repeat stress such as the tendonitis of tennis elbow.

Strangulate: To choke, cut-off, or suffocate. Constricted so that air or blood cannot pass

Strength: Capacity to do work which is defined as force over distance. The power to resist and exert force

Streptococcal-associated glomerulonephritis: Autoimmune reaction resulting in bilateral inflammation of the glomeruli of the kidney. Symptoms present in conjunction with a Strep infection of the throat or skin such as impetigo. Most common in boys 3 to 7 y/o, but can occur at any age. Most kids recover if appropriately treated. About 5% develop long-term renal problems. Glomerulonephritis can become chronic with inflammation, scarring, and progressive failure.

Streptomycin: An aminoglycoside antibiotic which is part of a class of antibiotics rarely indicated for treatment of TBIs, although it is sometimes used to treat tularemia.

Stress fracture: Fine hairline break in the bone that may be point tender but is hard to see on X-ray. These fractures are common in kids and are the result of repetitive microtrauma as seen with long-distance running. Non-supportive and uncushioned shoes on hard surfaces can exacerbate the problem. Point tenderness is the primary finding, although there may be swelling as well. The stress fracture can recur if not enough healing time is allowed.

Stretching: The lengthening of a muscle as part of an overall exercise program. May be static or dynamic

Stria: (Striae is plural) Lines that appear primarily on the abdomen or lower back. Striae may be slightly elevated or depressed and differ in color or texture from the surrounding tissue. Violaceous striae are an indication of bartonellosis.

Stricture: A narrowing or constriction of a tube, duct, or organ. Can be congenital or acquired due to infection, trauma, fibrosis, irritation, or pressure

Stridor: A somewhat musical sound audible without a stethoscope and most predominant during inspiration. Stridor means there is some obstruction of the upper airway.

Stroke: (CVA) Bleeding or blockage causes low oxygen supply to a particular brain area resulting in residual damage or death of brain cells. A cerebrovascular accident or brain attack presents with sudden, one-sided, impairment. The site where the injury occurs will dictate where the symptoms appear.

Stutter: Speech that includes hesitations, repetitions, and pauses which the speaker refers to as blocks. There can be prolongation of some sounds or the repetition of the first syllable of a word in a spasmodic fashion like C - C - C- Cat. Anxiety is not associated with the onset of stuttering, but can develop in social situations after the person is known as a stutterer.

St. Vitus dance: Sydenham's chorea

Subclinical: An infection or other phenomenon that is confirmed by various methods, such as diagnostic testing, but does not manifest sxs. The victim is unaware of a problem. Disease is present but under the body's radar.

Subcutaneous: (SC, sq, sub-Q) Under the skin. E.g., drug can be placed under the skin usually by a (hypodermic) needle where a small deposit of medicine is left for later dissolution.

Suicidal behaviors: Might include thoughts, actions, ideation, attempts, gestures, death-wish behaviors, or risky conduct focused on harming or killing oneself. While the majority of people with suicidal behaviors have pre-existing depression, a number do not. Never lightly dismiss any suicidal ideation or behavior.

Suicide: Intentional and voluntary ending of one's life

Sulfonamide antibiotics: Sulfa drugs including Bactrim that may be effective against malaria, babesiosis, and bartonellosis

Superficial: Located near the surface. Not deep

Superficial reflexes: A skin reflex caused by gentle stimulation of an area. Most often demonstrated in the abdominal, plantar, or gluteal regions

Superinfection: A new infection caused by an organism that likely mutated from the pathogen that caused the original disease

Supination: Motion of forearm that leaves palm facing up (like holding a bowl of soup)

Supine: Belly up position like a "s(o)up" bowl. In contrast to prone position with belly down. Also refers to palmar movement where the supine palm cups the bowl for the soup

Suppressor T cell: Former name of regulatory T cells

Symbiosis: Relationships involving the coexistence of multiple species usually in close proximity. The relationship can be beneficial (commensal) or harmful (parasitic).

Symmetry: Balanced shape, size or position on both sides of a body

Symptom: What the patient experiences. Awareness of a deviation from the normal state. Subjective perception of disease, but no less valid than an objective sign

Syndrome: A group of signs or symptoms, often found together, that loosely defines a condition. A diagnosis can be a sign and symptom "package" such as IBS which can occur for a number of reasons that might not be clear initially.

Synergy: Working together. Cooperation. The harmonious action of two or more entities such as muscles, organs, or drugs producing an effect that neither could have achieved alone

Synkinesis: An involuntary movement that accompanies a voluntary movement. E.g., blink synkinesis in Bell's palsy can be used to assess clinical status.

Synovium: Lining of the joints

Syphilis: An infectious, potentially chronic disease marked by lesions that can involve almost any tissue but primarily nerve, skin, lymph nodes, and mucous membranes. Can remit then relapse. May be latent for years. Caused by the pathogenic spirochete Treponema *pallidum*

Systemic: Throughout the body. Generalized as opposed to localized

Systemic lupus erythematosus: (SLE, lupus) Autoimmune, multisystem, inflammatory, collagen vascular disease most common in young women. Many body parts potentially affected including joints, skin, kidney, heart, lungs, blood vessels, and brain. Many features in common with Lyme and should always be part of the differential diagnosis. Marked by flares and remissions. Characterized by polyarthralgias, rashes, fever, malaise, vasculitis, nephritis, severe pain, extreme photosensitivity, hair loss, lung fibrosis, and cardiac involvement

T

Tabes dorsalis: Slowly progressing degeneration of the spinal cord that occurs in tertiary syphilis a decade or more after initial infection. Pathophysiology might include sclerosis of the posterior column of the spinal cord. Possible presentation: lightening-like pain, lack of coordination, ataxia (wobbliness), instability when eyes closed, staggering gait, dysfunction of optic nerve, pain, paresthesias, incontinency, loss of position sense, and degeneration of joints

Tachycardia: Heart rate that is too fast for the individual and circumstances

Tachypnea: Rapid, shallow breathing, with the definition of rapid depending on age

Tai chi: Gentle exercise that combines meditation and martial arts. With SLOW, deliberate movements, tai chi has much to offer Lyme patients. Tai chi is a meditative exercise where the mind clears through movement. This practice has been demonstrated to be immune enhancing and practitioners get better response to vaccines through augmented CMI. Tai chi has been found to be especially beneficial in chronic conditions improving the rate of healing and recovery. Easy on the joints and flexible in intensity

Tanner stages: Scale of physical maturation in children and teens. Uses primary and secondary sexual characteristics to determine where the individual is on the maturation timeline. Development of pubic hair, male genitalia, and female breasts are the staging criteria. Due to natural variation, individuals pass through Tanner stages at different rates that depend on genetics, nutrition, and general health status. Useful in determining where an individual stands when compared to others in the same age group in reaching the various stages. Tanner stages can be helpful in Lyme patients to see how the patient is progressing in areas governed by hormone levels, which can be significantly impacted by Bb.

Tardive dyskinesia: Slow, rhythmic, involuntary movement of the tongue or other muscles that can occur with the use of certain medicines. Predominant abnormal movements occur as a late complication of long-term use of certain psychotropic drugs. Most often the dyskinesia affects the tongue, lips, and face. There can be repetitive opening and closing of the mouth, grimacing, protrusion of the tongue, or deviation of the tongue and jaw.

Target level: Therapeutic concentration that provides a drug with the optimal chance to work

Taxonomy: Classification scheme for living organisms. The microbes that cause tick-borne illnesses are classified into Kingdom, Phylum, Class, Order, Family, Genus, and Species. Taxonomic classifications can change and an organism that was a certain genus or species one day can be reclassified another day.

T cells: Types of agranulocytic white cells that form one of the bases of CMI with many subpopulations and numerous functions. Includes helpers, killers, regulators, and cytotoxic cell types

Telithromycin: (Ketek) An erythromycin-like antibiotic used to treat borreliosis, babesiosis, bartonellosis, and M. *fermentans* infections. Black box warning regarding liver damage but this drug is likely the most effective drug in its class against Lyme. Use risk/benefit analysis

Temperature: 1) Measurement of the heat of a body. Body temperatures are measured to assess above normal readings indicating a fever. Fever patterns might provide information on infectious etiology. 2) Sensory nerves in the skin can distinguish a range of temperatures. The nerve damage in diabetics can cause them to lose this ability and they can unintentionally burn or freeze their skin.

Temporal lobes: Part of the brain that serves as a center for taste, hearing, smell, and interpretation of spoken language

Temporomandibular joints: Synovial joints that connect the jaw to the temporal bones of the skull. Can become inflamed. May be a target of the migratory joint pain found in Lyme

Tenderness: Sensitivity to pain upon palpation, touch, or movement

Tendon: Fibrous connective tissue that connects <u>muscle to bone</u>

Tendonitis: Inflammation of a tendon

Tenesmus: Anal spasm

Tennis elbow: Inflammation involving the tendon insertion at the lateral epicondyle of the humerus

Tenting: Slow return of pinched skin to normal level likely due to dehydration. Rapid return to normal indicates adequate hydration. Slow resolution or visible tenting of the skin suggests dryness.

Tetany: Muscle spasms due to nerve dysfunction. May lead to tonic spasms, usually of the extremities. Has been noted in gestational Lyme

Tetracyclines: (TCNs) Class of bacteriostatic antibiotics that inhibit protein synthesis. The TCN doxycycline is the DOC for LD in persons over 8 y/o. Should be used as part of a combination regimen, since solo usage can cause Bb to go intracellular, or encyst, and thereafter serve as a reservoir for pathogens, which will re-emerge when conditions are more favorable

Texture: Visual, tactile, or surface characteristics of the skin or other tissue

Theileria *microti:* Some recent literature calls B. *microti* by a new name, Theileria *microti,* apparently because RNA comparison found this microbe to be more like the Theileria genus than the Babesia. Perhaps that explains why the distinct Babesia species respond to different treatment regimens. This nomenclature shift has not yet been widely recognized.

Therapeutic window: Amount of medicine between the dose that gives an effective concentration and the amount that does more harm than good. Level of drug that is effective without causing unacceptable bad effects. This window can be broad or narrow.

Thiamine: Vitamin B1

Thickness: Viscosity

Thorax: Chest

Thought disorder: Disorganized and irrational thought processes

Thrill: Abnormal, palpable vibration accompanying a vascular or cardiac murmur. E.g., mitral valve disease often presents a thrill.

Thrombophlebitis: Inflammation of a vein in association with the formation of a thrombus usually in the leg. Need to treat to prevent the thrombus from becoming an embolus

Thrombus: Stationary clot within the vascular system which can impede blood flow. Can be superficial or deep. Once formed, pieces of the clot can break off causing thrombotic emboli to circulate in the blood. These clots can land in the lung, causing a pulmonary embolus, or in the brain causing a stroke.

Thrush: Fungus in the mouth Candidiasis (Monilia)

Thymus: Organ anterior to the heart, critical to the development of the immune response in the newborn

Thyroid gland: Endocrine gland in lower neck. Involved with how the body uses energy and metabolic rate. Indirectly influences growth and nutrition. Lyme can affect thyroid function.

Thyroiditis: Inflammation of the thyroid. Autoimmune condition of the thyroid gland where the organ is underactive causing fatigue, weakness, weight gain, cold intolerance, and muscle aches.

TIA: Transient ischemic attack

Tic: An involuntary spasmodic muscle contraction usually involving the brief, rapid movement of the face, eye muscles, mouth, head, neck, or shoulder. Tics can be simple or complex and are usually stereotypical and repetitive but NOT rhythmic. Simple tics include things like blinking or repeatedly clearing the throat. Tics often begin in childhood and mimic parts of normal behavior. Complex tics can include both motor movements and vocalizations and are disabling in some cases. Tics are associated with PANDAS and are common in TBIs.

Tic douloureux: (Trigeminal neuralgia) Irritation of the trigeminal nerve causing severe lightening-like stabs of pain. Location of pain will depend on which branch of the nerve is involved. Pain is momentary, lasting seconds or minutes along the sensory distribution of the trigeminal nerve. Something is impinging on the nerve or its pathway. Can occur repetitively for hours. The condition can subside for months and then return.

Tick-borne disease: (TBD) Interchangeable with tick-borne illness. Any of the various infectious conditions that can occur due to a tick bite

Tick-borne illness: (TBI) Interchangeable with tick-borne disease. Any of the various infectious conditions that can occur due to a tick bite

Tick drag: One method for collecting ticks in the wild. Usually involves pulling a piece of cloth on a pole through an area suspected of harboring ticks for the purpose of counting and identification

Tick paralysis: Condition caused by a neurotoxin found in the saliva of certain ticks. Fatigue is followed by flaccid paralysis.

Tick relapsing fever: Borreliosis secondary to B. *hermsii* characterized by remission and relapse. Hard to distinguish from Bb. Could this be Bb when there is no presenting rash?

Tigecycline: (Tygacil) Antibiotic closely related to the TCNs. Can be -cidal or -static depending on conditions. Unlike doxy can get into the cells where Bb may be hiding. Seems to kill Bb. May also be effective against Babesia. May be hard to tolerate

Tindamax: Tinidazole

Tinea pedis: (Athlete's foot) Foot fungus presenting with red, itchy, burning patches of dry, peeling cracked skin

Tinea versicolor: Yellow or buff colored patches on skin probably due to fungus

Tinel's sign: Pain or tingling after tapping on the lateral lower fibula in the path of the superficial peroneal nerve

Tinidazole: (Tindamax) Azole antibiotic cyst-buster. Excellent choice for the treatment of Bb since it can penetrate the cysts where Bb may be dormant. Tindamax hits all 3 Bb life forms: spirochetal,

intracellular, and encysted, i.e., those Borrelia with and without the cell wall. Better tolerated than Flagyl in some patients

Tinnitus: Sensation of ringing or buzzing in the ear. Common in Lyme

Titer: Concentration of a substance in solution. For example, the concentration of antibodies present in a sample can be calculated by determining the lowest concentration (highest dilution) where those antibodies are still able to combine with a known amount of antigen. If the concentration of antibody is too low (the dilution is too high), there will not be enough present to react with the antigen. Therefore, there will not be sufficient amounts of reaction product to measure. E.g., agglutination titer is the lowest concentration or highest dilution that allows for the clumping of the test substrates.

Titration: Estimation of the concentration of a solution by adding amounts of standard reagents until the detection of a chemical or physical change. Process by which a measured amount of one solution is added to a known quantity of another solution until a reaction between them is complete (as defined by some preset parameters). By measuring a quantity, such as a specific reaction product that forms between the known and unknown substances, the concentration of the unknown entity can be calculated. This is the premise on which many of the tests used to determine the presence of an antibody or antigen is based.

TNF: Tumor necrosis factor

TNF-α: Cytokine that is sometimes measured to assess the degree of chronic inflammation and on-going infection. This molecule is a growth factor for both immune cells and for osteoclasts.

TOA: Some types of cat's claw contain tetracyclic oxindole alkaloids that diminish efficacy and may be toxic. Any cat's claw or Samento product should be labeled TOA-free.

Tolerability: How well a patient can handle the totality of an administered drug

Tolerance: The capacity for enduring a large amount of a substance such as alcohol, food, drug, etc. Addiction is often framed in terms of dependency, tolerance, and withdrawal. Tolerance means that you have to use more and more of the addictive substance to get the same high. More is needed to get you to the same place.

Tone: Amount of tension, resistance, or responsiveness to movement in a muscle. In muscles, normal tone is a constant slight contraction that helps maintain posture and coordination.

Toning: Focus on shaping a muscle and appearance

Tophi: Crystal deposits in tissue near joints as seen in gout

Topical: Surface. Placing the medicine either on the site of desired action or on the skin or mucous membranes in the hopes of absorption

Torsades de pointes: Very rapid ventricular tachycardia characterized by a changing QRS complex on the EKG. Can be self-limiting or progress to ventricular fibrillation

Torsion: Twisted

Torticollis: Sternocleidomastoid muscle of the neck spasms, causing a painful shortening of the neck to one side, a bending of the head to the contracted side, while the chin goes in the opposite direction. Can be congenital or acquired. Muscles involved are often those innervated by the spinal accessory nerve.

Tourette's syndrome: An inherited multiple tic disorder that begins in childhood and can include both motor and vocal tics. A neurologic rather than psychiatric problem. Might present with lack of muscle coordination, involuntary purposeless movements, tics, grunts, barks, spontaneous obscenities (coprolalia), and social adjustment problems. Episodes may come and go. Simple tics may progress to complex and multiple tics including respiratory and involuntary vocalizations. The vocal tics can begin as grunting and evolve to compulsive inappropriate utterances. Severe cases can be physically and socially disabling. Similar tics are found in association with PANDAS.

Toxemia: Distribution throughout the body of poisonous material. Toxins can be produced by certain pathogens or acquired from other sources.

Toxic megacolon: Acute distension of the colon which can become very dilated, hence the term "mega" colon. Can be congenital but also an acquired complication of conditions like inflammatory bowel disease or the sequelae of C. *difficile* overgrowth and pseudomembranous colitis. Can present with fever, pain, and tenderness. A key finding is an accompanying tachycardia. Toxic megacolon can lead to sepsis, shock, and death. Perforation can lead to significant blood loss. This is an emergency.

Tracheomalacia: In neonates with gestational Lyme, cartilage in the trachea (windpipe) has not developed properly which might manifest as floppy, noisy, high-pitched breathing problems.

Transaminases: Enzymes that catalyze reactions in the liver. Damage to liver cells causes these enzymes to leak into the blood circulation where they can be measured. Higher than normal levels may mean there is a problem with full hepatic function. Normal levels vary with gender, race, and body fat.

Transcendental meditation: (TM) Meditation technique using a mantra to focus the breathing and clear the mind. Many documentable health benefits

Transient ischemic attack: (TIA) CVA that clears within a day or two. In contrast, a stroke leaves residual damage.

Transstadial: Passage of a parasite from one developmental stage of the host to another. Arthropods that undergo metamorphosis appear to have the capacity to pass a pathogen from one developmental stage to the next. One stage becomes infected and the next stage transmits the pathogen. If different stages feed on different hosts, transstadial transmission can provide the mechanism for interspecies transmission of disease agents.

Tremor: Fasciculation. Repetitive rhythmic movement caused by muscle contractions and relaxations that are described by: 1) pace of the rhythm slow to rapid, 2) amplitude, 3) distribution or location, and 4) whether at rest or when performing intentional movements. Parkinson's has a resting tremor while cerebellar disease has an intention tremor.

Triad of Neurologic Lyme: Meningitis, radiculopathy, and involvement of cranial nerves

Trigeminal nerve: (CN 5) Motor: Jaw clench with masseter and temporal muscles and lateral movement of the jaw. Sensory: Facial sensation

Trigeminal neuralgia: Tic douloureux

Troche: Vehicle to dispense medication. Usually a disc of medicine is implanted in a dissolvable lozenge

Trochlear nerve: (CN 4) Downward and inward movement of the eye

Trophic: Regarding a hormone or its effect. Stimulating the activity of another endocrine gland

Tropic: The turning or bending movement of a part, or an organism, to or away from a stimulus. Organotropism is important in understanding the pathophysiology of Bb and may help explain some of its sxs. E.g., Bb apparently love nerve cells and tissues containing collagen, which may provide reasons why so many of its manifestations involve the nervous system and any area that contains collagen such as joints, heart valves, and blood vessels in the GI tract.

Tularemia: Occasionally tick-borne bacterial disease caused by Francisella *tularensis* that can affect numerous organ systems

Tumefaction: Swollen area either from excess fluid or the formation of new tissues

Tumor: Growth, swelling, or enlargement which can be benign or malignant

Tumor necrosis factor: (TNF) A cytokine or protein mediator released primarily by macrophages and T lymphocytes that help regulate the immune response. Can cause cell death (apoptosis)

Tuning fork: Instrument used to assess vibratory sense and compare bone versus air conduction in hearing

Turgor: Indicator of pressure or tension inside a cell

Twitch: Muscle fasciculation. A small, local involuntary muscle contraction visible under the skin, most common in the eyelid

Two-tiered testing approach for Lyme: Scheme where ELISA must be used as a screen for Lyme disease. Only those with a positive ELISA result can move on to more definitive testing. This approach has been fully discredited by multiple professional groups and agencies. Many false negatives result.

Tympanic: Involving the middle ear or eardrum

U

Uit waaien: Dutch for walking in the wind for fun

Ulcer: Loss of skin surface that is likely to bleed and scar. An open lesion on skin or mucous membrane with sloughing of inflamed tissue

Ulcerative colitis: (UC) Type of IBD with inflammatory ulcers in the top layer of the lining of the lower large intestine causing abdominal pain, cramps, and diarrhea. Might be associated with cytokine response. Sxs can be incapacitating.

Ultrasound: (US) Imaging technique using high frequency (ultrasonic) sound waves to measure the energy as the sound moves through tissue. If anything impedes the flow of the sound, the energy will be reflected back in what is called an echo. The echo signal can be received and recorded and thereby tell the location, size, and other features of the entity that interrupted the path of the wave. Allows for good visualization of subcutaneous tissues such as tendons, muscles, joints, and internal organs.

Umbilicus: (Belly button) Scar that marks where the umbilical cord attached to the mother

UMN lesions: Skeletal muscle is innervated by a group of neurons called lower motor neurons which project out from the spinal cord to the muscle cells. The LMNs themselves are innervated by upper motor neurons (UMNs) that come from the motor area of the cortex of the brain. Lesions in the UMN will lead to increased muscle tone (hypertonia) in the extensors of the legs and/or the flexors of the arms. May present with a clasp knife response, clonus, spasticity, brisk reflexes, and pathologic reflexes like a positive Babinski. With UMNs there is NO muscle wasting. Examples of UMN disorders include MS, stroke, brainstem lesions, cerebral palsy, symptoms from injuries, and symptoms accompanying hydrocephalus.

Undescended testicle: A testis remaining in the abdominal cavity or inguinal canal. May be present at birth or develop later

Urinary Tract Infection: (UTI) Infection that can involve the upper part of the urinary tract (kidney and ureters) or the lower segments (the bladder and urethra). Lower UTIs are one of the most prevalent bacterial diseases in all ages. Manifestations might include: frequency, urgency, hematuria, pyuria, nocturia, and pain. Interstitial cystitis, very common in Lyme, might be a UTI where the pathogen has not yet been identified.

Unequivocal: Not open to interpretation. Conclusive. Clear

Upper limit of normal: (ULN) Lab normals often fall into a range based on the compilation of data gathered from large populations. If the value goes any higher, the patient would be considered abnormal. Watch for patients who start out near the LLN and move to the ULN. While still normal, this type of change could suggest a problem in this individual.

Upper motor neuron: (UMNs) Innervate LMNs. UMNs come from the motor area of the cortex of the brain. Lesions in the UMN will lead to increased muscle tone and hyperreflexia

Urethritis: Infection of the urethra can be a part of a UTI or an STD. The meatus in both sexes can be red and inflamed.

Urgency: Sudden and sometimes uncontrollable feeling of the need to void or evacuate

Urticaria: Wheals or hives spread usually over a large skin area. A vascular reaction of the skin characterized by a sudden general eruption of pale wheals or papules. Usually itchy

Uvea: Middle layer of the eye that provides blood to the retina. Inflammation is common in Lyme.

Uveitis: Autoimmune condition involving the structures of the inner eye including the iris and blood vessels. Associated with certain diseases such as ankylosing spondylitis and RA. An inflamed uvea has been found in a number of cases of Lyme disease.

V

Vaccination: (Immunization) Inoculation with an Ag from a pathogen or toxin in order to establish a defense upon re-exposure

Vagus nerve: (CN 10) Motor: Movement of palate, pharynx, and larynx. Ability to swallow. Sensory: Pharynx and larynx

Validity: Strength of conclusions. Best approximation of the truth. "Am I right?"

Valsalva maneuver: Method in attempt to equalize pressure behind ear drums (clear the ears). One way is to hold nose, shut mouth, and swallow.

Valve: Flap of tissue found in a hollow organ or passageway that is designed to keep fluids flowing in one direction. The GI tract and the circulatory systems have many valves so that flow should go only one way.

Vancomycin: (Vancocin) Glycopeptide antibiotic given orally for C. *difficile* overgrowth. Good for MRSA. Excellent IV drug for Bb but perceived toxicity limits use. Pulse to decrease adverse events

Varicella: (Chickenpox) Highly contagious disease caused by an HHV-3 virus. Characterized by successive crops of skin eruptions that go through stages: macules, papules, vesicles, crusts. "Dew drop on a pink petal."

Varices: Varicose veins

Varicocele: Varicose veins in the spermatic cord present like a "bag of worms."

Varicose veins: Distended, swollen, knotted, twisted, superficial vessels. Can occur in any part of the body but are most common in the lower legs and esophagus. A hemorrhoid is a varicose vein. There can be a genetic predisposition to develop these varicosities, but pressure and other strains can also increase the incidence.

Vascular endothelial growth factor: (VEGF) Elevated levels *might* mean that the person is infected with Bartonella since this pathogen might use this factor to enter into the cells making up the blood vessels.

Vasculitis: Inflammation of lymph or blood vessel. Can occur with Lyme

Vector: Carrier of disease. Transmits pathogen from infected to uninfected. A vector is a living organism (often an Arthropod or Insect) that transmits a pathogen from a reservoir to a host.

Vegetation: Deposits on heart valves or other tissue that are a combination of pathogen, fibrin, white cells, and debris that preclude the proper operation of the valve. Vegetations may be one mechanism by which Bb cause heart problems.

Vein: Vessel that moves blood toward the heart with the help of skeletal muscles and valves

Ventilation/Perfusion scan: (V/Q scan) Diagnostic modality that compares lung area with air to lung area with blood perfusion looking for evidence of obstruction by emboli

Vertigo: Sensation of moving in space or having the room or objects moving around the stationary subject. Sometimes term used as a synonym for dizziness or lightheadedness but they are not interchangeable. Dizziness is a fading while vertigo is a spinning. Vertigo is an equilibrium disturbance.

Vesicles: A small elevation of skin with free fluid in the layers such as those that occur with friction blisters or herpes simplex. Vesicles on the tongue or oral mucosa usually indicate viral infection.

Vestibular toxicity: Disturbance of the vestibular system controlling balance and equilibrium. Symptoms include dizziness, ataxia, nausea, and vomiting. Has been associated with minocycline use where sxs start soon after the initial dose and then resolve quickly after the drug is discontinued. This appears to be a dose-related reaction in susceptible individuals.

Vibration: Oscillating or moving back and forth around a point in a regular, periodic fashion. Quivering. 1) Vibration allows sound waves to be interpreted in hearing. 2) Vibratory sense is the ability to perceive vibrations by the senses.

Violaceous: Violet, purple

Violence: Inflicting physical injury

Viscera: Organs within a cavity, usually referring to the abdominal cavity

Viscosity: Thickness

Viscous: Thick. Resistant to flow. Dense. Less fluid

Visual acuity: Sharpness or clarity of vision. A measure of the resolving power of the eye

Visual fields: The area within which objects can be seen when the eye is fixed

Vitamins: Nutrients that need to be acquired because the organism cannot make them in sufficient amounts

Vitiligo: Autoimmune attack on the skin destroying pigment-making cells. White patches appear surrounded by normal-colored skin. May be associated with several systemic diseases or present alone

Vocabulary: Number of words a person is able to use or understand. One way to assess intellect is by the extent of vocabulary.

Volvulus: Twisting of the intestine which can result in compromise of blood flow. Usually abdominal distension along with severe pain. A mass may be palpable. Can be fatal

Vomit: Emesis

W

Wane: Fade

Warm-up exercises: Prepares the muscles and joints for more intense activity and thereby helps prevent injury, promotes circulation, increases body temperature, and slightly raises the heart and respiratory rates, but not to the level experienced in the actual workout. Warming-up makes the muscles more flexible. Many consider a warm-up essential to any workout.

Warnings: A black box warning, named after the black border that appears around the words, is the strongest message that the FDA sends in a drug label. The intention is to alert consumers that something very bad, even life threatening, can occur while taking this particular medicine.

Wart: Elevated skin eruption caused by hypertrophy of elements in the epidermis due to papilloma virus

Water soluble: Able to dissolve in water. Eg., B and C vitamins

Wax: Return. Flare. Recur

Weakness: Lack of physical or mental strength, energy, or vigor. NOT a synonym for sleepiness, dizziness, or malaise

Wean: Gradually reduce the intake

Weber test: Assessment of lateralization of hearing. Place a lightly vibrating tuning fork firmly on the patient's head or forehead and ask where he hears the sound. Does he hear the vibration on one or both sides? A normal test is heard equally on both sides or in the midline. If the patient has unilateral hearing deficit due to a <u>conductive</u> problem, the sound will be louder in the bad ear. If the deficit is <u>neurosensory</u> then the sound is louder in the good ear.

Wegener's granulomatosis: Autoimmune problem affecting small and medium-sized blood vessels throughout the body especially lungs and kidneys.

Western blot: (WB) Laboratory test used for detecting antigens

Wheal: (Hive): Irregular, often round, skin reaction that occurs in response to allergies and insect bites (even in those bites not associated with allergy). Swollen bump that can be red with a white area in the center. Can be isolated or can be disseminated over large skin areas and, in those cases, the reaction is called urticaria. Itchy. Generally wheals are transient, but some forms of urticaria last for years.

Wheeze: Continuous, high-pitched, sibilant, musical sound caused by narrowing of the respiratory tubes. Whistling produced by difficult breathing. Heard both on inspiration and expiration. To create a wheeze, air flow must be obstructed at some level which can be caused by constriction, swelling, secretions, or masses. Commonly associated with SOB. Asthma is the most usual cause of wheezing, although allergies and URIs are close behind. A monophonic wheeze over a single location indicates localized obstruction like a tumor or FB. Wheezes often start high pitched and treatment usually lowers the pitch to the point where the sounds are more like rhonchi than wheezes.

Wilson's syndrome: Hereditary syndrome characterized by the accumulation of copper in organs. Pigmented ring at the outer margin of the cornea is pathognomonic. Might manifest with abnormal function of the brain and liver. Muscles can exhibit movement problems with difficulty swallowing. Psychiatric manifestations are common.

Winter's ear: Red pinnae that may be associated with high histamine levels. Sometimes seen in chronic Lyme

Withdrawal: Addiction is often framed in terms of dependency, tolerance, and withdrawal. Withdrawal symptoms are the physical and psychological consequences of stopping the addictive substance. Alcohol withdrawal can be fatal.

WNL: Within normal limits

X

Xiphoid process: Base of the sternum

X-ray: Image produced on photographic film made by passing radiation through a body part. X-rays are best at distinguishing gas from liquid and liquid from solid, especially bone.

Y

Yawn: Normal involuntary action where a large slow breath is inspired usually in association with fatigue or sleepiness. Some speculate that yawning is an attempt to increase the oxygen levels in the individual. Yawns have been reported as a muscular tic in cases of neuropsychiatric manifestations of diseases. Inefficient and frequent yawns may be part of the air hunger seen with babesiosis.

Yeast: Budding, single-celled fungus

Yoga: Meditative exercise program that uses breathing and maintenance of poses to achieve focus and relaxation. May be one of the best overall fitness choices for Lyme patients. Yoga can be as gentle or as intense as the practitioner wants and is easy on the joints. Yoga is a practice. Many studies have reported the positive effects of yoga including enhanced flexibility, posture, balance, control, coordination, breathing, muscle strength, awareness, immune function, and lubrication of joints.

Z

Zoonosis/Zoonotic: Disease passed from animals to humans

Zoster: Type of HHV-3 that causes shingles and herpetic neuralgia

Zygote: Cell produced by the union of two gametes. Fertilized ovum. In Babesia called the kinete

SOLEMN VOW: Life is too short. I have wasted too much of mine reconciling and standardizing hyphens. As of Friday, January 18, 2013, at 5:04 a.m., I vow to NEVER use another hyphen. Never again. Never. Not one. I am thinking of getting a special keyboard made. Of course, I am also thinking of never using a keyboard again. My cousin Lindy thinks I won't be able to do it. Never again.

When I stand before God at the end of my life, I would hope that I would not have a single bit of talent left and could say to God, "I used everything you gave me."

Erma Bombeck

INDEX

A science career for women is now almost as acceptable as being a cheerleader.
Myra Barker

nodule, 91, 92, 322, 324
nursing, 22, 24, 36, 699–702
nutrition/diet, 647
nystagmus, 341
nystatin (Mycostatin), 616

O

obsessive-compulsive disorder (OCD), 146, 147, 150, 156, 164, 440
obstructed airway, 363
obstruction, 144, 320
occlusion, 144, 349
occupational therapy, 630
ofloxacin (Floxin), 565
omental trapping, 380
Omnicef. *See* cephalosporins
on-going Lyme. *See* Lyme disease
oppositional defiant disorder (ODD), 443
opsonins, 25, 36
oral (po), 176, 532
organotropism, 105, 117
orientation, 409
osteochondrosis, 403
outer surface protein (Osp), 15, 49, 120, 121, 122, 126
oxygen, 640
oxytocin, 124

P

P450, 527, 538
pain, 142, 148, 353, 415, 425, 607
 ache, 426
 acute, 426
 chronic, 426
 growing pains, 427
 migratory, 397, 426
 neuralgia, 426
 neurogenic pain syndrome, 426
 neuropathic pain, 426
 pain amplification syndrome, 426
 referred pain, 426
pancreatitis, 380
PANDAS, 43, 125, 156, 349, 435, 441, 448, 489
panic, 150, 156
panic attacks, 164, 441
PANS, 147, 156
paralysis, 345
parents, 710, 712
paresthesias, 142, 143, 144, 146, 147, 160, 189, 425
 burning sensation, 424
Parkinson's disease, 428
passions, 684
pathognomonic, 508, 511, 516
patient autonomy, 226
patient preferences, 178, 222
pattern, 453, 468, 506
PCR. *See* polymerase chain reaction (PCR)
Pediazole, 570, 571
pelvic discomfort, 155, 383, 390, 695
penicillins, 178, 558

amoxicillin (Amoxil), 168, 178, 559
amoxicillin plus clavulanate (Augmentin), 178, 560
benzathine penicillin (Bicillin), 168, 178, 560
Pepto-Bismol, 612
pericarditis, 158, 360, 370
peritonitis, 382
permethrin, 718
persistent, 102, 111, 112, 205
persisters, 115, 135
personality, 146, 151
personality disorders, 443
pervasive developmental disorder. *See* autism spectrum of disorders (ASD)
petechiae, 324, 344
pets, 660, 706, 720
PET scan, 456
phagocytosis, 22, 25, 26, 30, 33, 34
Phenergan (promethazine), 609
physical exam, 305–316
physical therapy, 630
placenta, 96, 126
plan 504, 711
plantar fasciitis, 91, 404
Plaquenil (hydroxychloroquine). *See* hydroxychloroquine (Plaquenil)
plasma cells, 27, 32
plateau, 137, 169
platelet count, 478
pleural effusion, 356, 360, 361
PMN, 127, 476
pneumonia, 320, 364
polymerase chain reaction (PCR), 72, 92, 98, 161, 460, 500
Pomodoro method, 682
popping joints, 151
post-traumatic stress disorder (PTSD), 446
potassium, 484
Powassan viral encephalitis (POW), 59, 230, 461, 517
precautions/cautions, 535
preference, 178
pregnancy categories, 529
pregnant, 168, 699–702
premenstrual dysphoric disorder (PMDD), 391, 439
premenstrual syndrome (PMS), 391, 439
prevention, 715–724, 722
 acute Lyme, 722
 bites, 721, 727
 chronic Lyme, 722, 723
 risk, 715
 tick control, 719
Primaxin, 562
probiotics, 167, 610, 659
problem solving, 410
processing, 146, 340, 431
processing difficulty, 431
prophylaxis, 169, 189, 722
proprioception, 413, 415
prostaglandin, 28

This Compendium provides a comprehensive overview of tick-borne diseases including descriptions, diagnostic approaches, treatment options, and an array of management plans. The text was designed to educate health care providers, patients, and caretakers about the risks posed by tick-borne illnesses. Previously, the contradictory, confusing, and inflammatory rhetoric available made proper diagnosis and treatment of these cases difficult, if not impossible. Because Dr. Spreen compiled, interpreted, and consolidated expert opinion, medical literature, and hands-on experience into one volume, the reader finally has an accessible resource that will aid in collaborative, practical, and compassionate decision-making.

Dr. Spreen focuses on creative strategies that allow the best chance for successful outcomes. She dispels harmful myths and provides a solid scientific foundation for the practical guidance incorporated into this text. You are no longer alone in your attempt to combat these complex and confusing conditions. This book will help you to never lose hope and to NEVER GIVE UP.

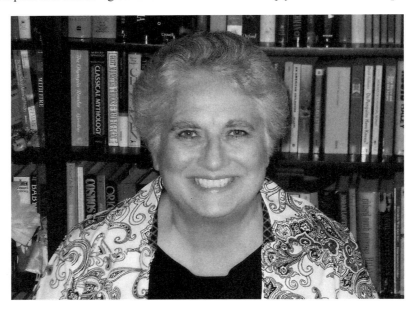

Kathy Spreen is a physician interested in educating professionals, patients, and caretakers about the potential risks posed by tick-borne illnesses. Her goal is to provide both information and support for all those impacted by these complex diseases. She is a doctor, Lyme patient, and caretaker. Dr. Spreen earned Master's degrees in biochemistry and public health and board certifications in preventive medicine and family medicine. She was a physician in the military working in emergency medicine as well as writing the procedures currently used to manage chemical and radiation casualties. During many years in the pharmaceutical industry, she substantially contributed to over a dozen successful new drug applications as she conducted clinical research trials around the world. She was closely involved with medical communication and managed large groups of scientific writers and editors as she garnered numerous performance and technical awards. Her diverse experience and common-sense approach make her uniquely qualified to gather, interpret, and condense this information into a usable and practical form. She lives with her husband and elderly dog in an area known by some as the tick and mushroom capital of the world.